THE ENDOMETRIUM

REPRODUCTIVE MEDICINE & ASSISTED REPRODUCTIVE TECHNIQUES SERIES

Series Editors

David K Gardner DPhil
Colorado Center for Reproductive Medicine, Englewood, CO, USA
Jan Gerris MD PhD
Professor of Gynecology, University Hospital Gheni, Ghent, Belgium
Zeev Shoham MD
Director, Infertility Unit, Kaplan Hospital, Rehovot, Israel

Published Titles

Gerris, Delvigne and Olivennes, *Ovarian Hyperstimulation Syndrome*
ISBN 9781842143285

Sutcliffe, *Health and Welfare of ART Children*
ISBN 9780415379304

Tan, Chian and Buckett, *In-vitro Maturation of Human Oocytes*
ISBN 9781842143322

Keck, Tempfer and Hugues, *Conservation Infertility Management*
ISBN 9780415384513

Pellicer and Simon, *Stem Cells in Human Reproduction*
ISBN 9780415397773

Elder and Cohen, *Human Preimplantation Embryo Solution*
ISBN 9780415399739

Tucker and Liebermann *Vitrification in Assisted Reproduction*
ISBN 9780415408820

Forthcoming Titles

Balen, *Infertility in Practice, 3rd Edition*
ISBN 9780415450676

Gardner, Howles, Weissman and Shoham, *Textbook of ART 3rd Edition*
ISBN: 9780415448949

THE ENDOMETRIUM

Molecular, Cellular, and Clinical Perspectives

Second Edition

Edited by

John D Aplin MA PhD
Maternal and Fetal Health Research Group
University of Manchester
Manchester
UK

Asgerally T Fazleabas PhD HCLD
Department of Obstetrics and Gynecology, Center for Women's
Health and Reproduction
University of Illinois at Chicago
Chicago, IL
USA

Stanley R Glasser PhD
Institute of Biosciences and Technology
Texas A&M University System Health Sciences Center
Houston, TX
USA

Linda C Giudice MD PhD MSc
Department of Obstetrics,
Gynecology,and Reproductive Sciences
University of California
San Francisco, CA
USA

informa
healthcare

First edition published in the United Kingdom in 2002

Second edition published in the United Kingdom in 2008 by Informa Healthcare, Telephone House, 69–77 Paul Street, London EC2A 4LQ. Informa Healthcare is a trading division of Informa UK Ltd. Registered Office: 37/41 Mortimer Street, London W1T 3JH. Registered in England and Wales number 1072954.

Tel: +44 (0)20 7017 5000
Fax: +44 (0)20 7017 6699
Website: www.informahealthcare.com

A CIP record for this book is available from the British Library.

Library of Congress Cataloging-in-Publication Data

Data available on application

ISBN 10: 0 415 38583 0
ISBN 13: 978 0 415 38583 1

Distributed in North and South America by
Taylor & Francis
6000 Broken Sound Parkway, NW, (Suite 300)
Boca Raton, FL 33487, USA
Within Continental USA
Tel: 1 (800) 272 7737; Fax: 1 (800) 374 3401
Outside Continental USA
Tel: (561) 994 0555; Fax: (561) 361 6018
Email: orders@crcpress.com

Distributed in the rest of the world by
Cengage Learning Services Limited
Cheriton House
North Way
Andover, Hampshire SP10 5BE, UK
Tel: +44 (0)1264 332424
Email: tps.tandfsalesorder@thomson.com

Composition by C&M Digitals (P) Ltd, Chennai, India
Printed and bound in India by Replika Press Pvt. Ltd

Contents

SECTION I: DEVELOPMENT

SECTION II: MATURE FEMALE REPRODUCTIVE TRACT

SECTION III: REGULATORY BIOLOGY

SECTION IV: ESTABLISHMENT OF PREGNANCY

SECTION V: THE ENDOMETRIAL STROMA

SECTION VI: PLACENTATION

SECTION VII: IMMUNOBIOLOGY

Contributors

Rupasri Ain PhD
Institute of Maternal–Fetal Biology
The University of Kansas Medical Center
Kansas City, KS
USA

John D Aplin MA PhD
Maternal and Fetal Health Research Group
University of Manchester
Manchester
UK

David F Archer MD
Department of Obstetrics and Gynecology
Eastern Virginia Medical School
Norfolk, VA
USA

Erkut Attar MD
Istanbul Medical School
Department of Obstetrics and Gynecology
Istanbul
Turkey

Mira Aubuchon
Department of Obstetrics and Gynecology
University of Cincinatti
Cincinatti, OH
USA

Indrani C Bagchi PhD
Department of Veterinary Bioscience
University of Illinois at Champaign-Urbana
Urbana, IL
USA

Milan K Bagchi PhD
Department of Molecular Integrative Physiology
University of Illinois at Champaign-Urbana
Urbana, IL
USA

David T Baird MD DSc
Division of Reproductive and Developmental Sciences
University of Edinburgh
Centre for Reproductive Biology
The Queen's Medical Research Institute
Edinburgh, Scotland
UK

Philip N Baker DM FRCOG
Maternal and Fetal Health Research Centre
St Mary's Hospital
Manchester
UK

Breton F Barrier MD
Department of Obstetrics, Gynecology
   and Women's Health
University of Missouri-Columbia
Columbia, MO
USA

Fuller W Bazer PhD
Department of Animal Science
Center for Animal Biotechnology
   and Genomics
Texas A&M University
College Station, TX
USA

Kathleen E Bethin MD PhD
Department of Pediatrics and Herman B Wells
   Center for Pediatric Research
Indiana University School of Medicine
Riley Hospital for Children
Indianapolis, IN
USA

Robert M Bigsby PhD
Indiana University School of Medicine
Indianapolis, IN
USA

Robert M Brenner PhD
Division of Reproductive Sciences
Oregon National Primate Research Center
Oregon Health & Sciences University
Beaverton, OR
USA

Jan J Brosens MD PhD
Institute of Reproductive and Developmental Biology
Imperial College London
Hammersmith Hospital
London
UK

John E Buster MD
Reproductive Endocrinology and Infertility
Baylor College of Medicine
Houston, TX
USA

Serdar E Bulun MD
Division of Reproductive Biology Research
Northwestern University Feinburg School of Medicine
Chicago, IL
USA

Art Caplan PhD
Center for Bioethics and Department of Medical Ethics
University of Pennsylvania
Philadelphia, PA
USA

Bo Chen
School of Life Sciences
Fudan University
People's Republic of China

Kristof Chwalisz MD PhD
Women's Health
TAP Pharmaceutical Products, Inc.
Lake Forest, IL
USA

Yvonne Collins MD
Division of Gynecologic Oncology
University of Illinois-Chicago
Chicago, IL
USA

Catherine MH Combelles
Biology Department
Middlebury College
Middlebury, VT
USA

Hilary OD Critchley MD FRCOG
Division of Reproductive and Developmental Sciences
University of Edinburgh
Centre for Reproductive Biology
The Queens Medical Research Institute
Edinburgh, Scotland
UK

James C Cross DVM PhD
Department of Comparative Biology
   and Experimental Medicine
Faculty of Veterinary Medicine
University of Calgary
Alberta
Canada

Gaurang S Daftary MD
Department of Obstetrics,
   Gynecology and Reproductive Sciences
Yale University School of Medicine
New Haven, CT
USA

Vibeke Dantzer PhD
Department of Basic Animal and Veterinary Science
Section of Animal and Cell Biology
The Royal Veterinary and Agricultural University
Gronnegaardvej
Frederiksberg
Denmark

Francesco J DeMayo PhD
Department of Molecular and Cellular Biology
Baylor College of Medicine
Houston, TX
USA

Joëlle Desmarais PhD
Center of Research in Animal Reproduction
College of Veterinary Medicine
University of Montreal
St-Hyacinthe, Quebec
Canada

Peter Dockery
National University of Ireland
Galway
Ireland

Francisco Domínguez PhD
Fundación IVI (FIVI)
Valencia University
Valencia
Spain

Allen C Enders PhD
Department of Cell Biology and Human Anatomy
University of California
Davis, CA
USA

David A Eschenbach MD PhD
University of Washington
Harborview Medical Center
Seattle, WA
USA

John V Fahey
Department of Physiology
Dartmouth Medical School
Lebanon, NH
USA

Asgerally T Fazleabas PhD HCLD
Department of Obstetrics and Gynecology
    Center for Women's Health and Reproduction
University of Illinois at Chicago
Chicago, IL
USA

Susan J Fisher PhD
Departments of Cell and Tissue Biology,
    Pharmaceutial Chemistry, Anatomy,
    and Obstetrics, Gynecology and
    Reproductive Sciences
University of California at San Francisco
San Francisco, CA
USA

Caroline E Gargett BApplSci MApplSci PhD
Centre for Women's Health Research
Monash Institute of Medical
    Research, and Monash University
Department of Obstetrics and Gynecology
Clayton, Victoria
Australia

Stacie E Geller PhD
Department of Obstetrics and Gynecology
University of Illinois at Chicago
Chicago, IL
USA

Birgit Gellersen PhD
Endokrinologikum Hamburg
Hamburg
Germany

Jane E Girling PhD
Centre for Women's Health Research
Monash Institute of Medical Research
    and Monash University
Department of Obstetrics and Gynaecology
Clayton, Victoria
Australia

Linda C Giudice MD PhD MSc
Department of Obstetrics, Gynecology, and
Reproductive Sciences
University of California
San Francisco, CA
USA

Stanley R Glasser PhD
Institute of Biosciences and Technology
Texas A&M University System Health Sciences
Center
Houston, TX
USA

Ruth Grümmer PhD
Institut für Anatomie
Universiättsklinikum Essen
Essen
Germany

Amy Hakim MD
Division of Gynecologic Oncology
Northwestern University Feinberg
    School of Medicine
Chicago, IL
USA

Amy Hamilton
Department of Obstetrics, Gynecology,
    and Reproductive Sciences
University of California
San Franscisco, CA
USA

Lynda K Harris PhD
Maternal and Fetal Health Research Centre
St Mary's Hospital
Manchester
UK

Alexander EP Heazel MBChB(Hons)
Maternal and Fetal Health Research Centre
St Mary's Hospital
Manchester
UK

Sylvia C Hewitt PhD
National Institute of Environmental
    Health Sciences
National Institutes of Health
Research Triangle Park, NC
USA

Joan S Hunt PhD DSc
Department of Anatomy and Cell Biology
University of Kansas Medical Center
Kansas City, KS
USA

Jean A Hurteau MD
Division of Gynecologic Oncology
Northwestern University Feinberg
    School of Medicine
Evanston, IL
USA

Mary Anne Jamieson MD
Division of Reproductive
    Endocrinology and Infertility
Queen's University
Kingston, Ontario
Canada

Gregory A Johnson PhD
Department of Veterinary
    Integrative Biosciences
Center for Animal Biotechnology and Genomics
Texas A & M University
College Station, TX
USA

Carolyn JP Jones PhD
Maternal and Fetal Health Research Center
St Mary's Hospital
Manchester
UK

Rebecca L Jones PhD
Maternal and Fetal Health Research Centre
St Mary's Hospital
Manchester
UK

Hey-Joo Kang MD
The Center for Reproductive
    Medicine and Infertility
Weill Cornell Medical College
New York, NY
USA

SM Alam Khorshed MD PhD
Institute of Maternal–Fetal Biology
The University of Kansas Medical Center
Kansas City, KS
USA

Susan J Kimber PhD
Faculty of Life Sciences
University of Manchester
Manchester
UK

Toshihiro Konno PhD
Institute of Maternal–Fetal Biology
The University of Kansas Medical Center
Kansas City, KS
USA

Kenneth S Korach PhD
Program Director
Environmental Disease Medicine Program
National Institute of Environmental
    Health Sciences
National Institutes of Health
Research Triangle Park, NC
USA

Graciela Krikun PhD
Department of Obstetrics,
    Gynecology and Reproductive Sciences
Yale University School of Medicine
New Haven, CT
USA

Takeshi Kurita PhD
Division of Reproductive Biology Research
Northwestern University Feinburg
    School of Medicine
Chicago, IL
USA

James V Lacey Jr PhD
Division of Cancer Epidemiology and Genetics
National Cancer Institute
Rockville, MD
USA

Kevin Lee PhD
Department of Molecular
    and Cellular Biology
Baylor College of Medicine
Houston, TX
USA

Rudolf Leiser DVM Dr Med VET Drhc
Department of Veterinary Anatomy,
    Histology and Embryology
Justus-Liebig University
Giessen
Germany

Bruce A Lessey MD PhD
Department of Obstetrics and Gynecology
University of South Carolina
Greenville, SC
USA

Laura A Lindsay PhD
Cell and Reproductive Biology Laboratory
School of Medical Sciences
University of Sydney
Sydney, NSW
Australia

Charles J Lockwood MD
Department of Obstetrics,
    Gynecology and Reproductive Sciences
Yale University School of Medicine
New Haven, CT
USA

Flavia L Lopes DVM PhD
Center of Research in Animal Reproduction
College of Veterinary Medicine
University of Montreal
St-Hyacinthe, Quebec
Canada

Julie Lukic MBBS FRANZCOG
Fellow in Reproductive Medicine and Endocrinology
McGill Reproductive Centre
Royal Victoria Hospital
Montreal, Quebec
Canada

Marcy Maguire MD
Department of Obstetrics and Gynecology
Tufts University
Boston, MA
USA

Larry Maxwell MD
Walter Reed Army Medical Center
Washington, DC
USA

Peter G McGovern MD
Division of Reproductive Endocrinology
    and Infertility
UMDNJ-New Jersey Medical School
Newark, NJ
USA

Bruce D Murphy PhD FCAHS
Center of Research in Animal Reproduction
College of Veterinary Medicine
University of Montreal
St-Hyacinthe, Quebec
Canada

Christopher R Murphy PhD
Cell and Reproductive Biology Laboratory
    School of Medical Sciences
University of Sydney
Sydney, NSW
Australia

Susan C Nagel PhD
Department of Obstetrics, Gynecology
    and Womens Health
University of Missouri-Columbia
Columbia, MO
USA

Hisae Nakamura
Department of Cancer Endocrinology
BC Cancer Agency
Vancouver, BC
Canada

Jose M Navarro MD PhD
Centro Clínico Al-Andulus and
Hospital Victoria Eugenia (de la Cruz Roja Española)
Unidad de Cirugía Endoscópica y Ginecología
Seville
Spain

Andrea Niklaus PhD
Department of Pathology
University of California
Los Angeles, CA
USA

Romana A Nowak PhD
Department of Animal Sciences
University of Illinois
Urbana, IL
USA

Justine Nugent MRCOG
Maternal and Fetal Health Research Centre
St Mary's Hospital
Manchester
UK

Troy L Ott PhD
Department of Dairy & Animal Sciences
The Pennsylvania State University
University Park, PA
USA

Haiyan Pan
Department of Microbiology
Columbia University
New York
USA

Margaret G Petroff PhD
Department of Anatomy and Cell Biology
University of Kansas Medical Center
Kansas City, KS
USA

Christiane Pfarrer
Department of Obstetrics and Gynecology
Justus-Liebig University
Giessen
Germany

Patricia A Pioli
Department of Physiology
Dartmouth Medical School
Lebanon, NH
USA

Jeffrey W Pollard PhD
Department of Developmental and
    Molecular Biology and Obstetrics and Gynecology
    and Women's Health
Albert Einstein College of Medicine
Bronx, NY
USA

Alex J Polotsky MD MSc
Division of Reproductive Endocrinology
Department of Obstetrics/Gynecology
    and Women's Health
Albert Einstein College of Medicine
Bronx, NY
USA

Catherine Racowsky PhD
Director, IVF Laboratory
Associate Professor of Obstetrics
    and Gynecology

Vardit Ravitsky PhD
Center for Bioethics and
    Department of Medical Ethics
University of Pennsylvania
Philadelphia, PA
USA

Kristy Red-Horse PhD
Genentech Inc.
San Francisco, CA
USA

BJ Rimel MD
Department of Obstetrics and Gynecology
Northwestern University Feinberg
    School of Medicine
Chicago, IL
USA

Sarah A Robertson PhD
Research Centre for Reproductive Health
Department of Obstetrics and Gynaecology
University of Adelaide
Adelaide, SA
Australia

Peter AW Rogers PhD
Centre for Women's Health Research
Monash Institute of Medical Research
Monash University Department of Obstetrics
    and Gynaecology
Clayton, Victoria
Australia

Zev Rosenwaks MD
Reproductive Endocrinology and Infertility
The Center of Reproductive Medicine and Infertility
Weill Medical College of Cornell University
New York
USA

Lois A Salamonsen PhD
Prince Henry's Institute of Medical Research
Melbourne, Victoria
Australia

Joseph S Sanfilippo MD MBA
Magee-Women's Hospital
Pittsburgh, PA
USA

Nanette Santoro MD
Division of Reproductive Endocrinology
Department of Obstetrics/Gynecology and
    Women's Health
Albert Einstein College of Medicine
New York
USA

Todd M Schaefer
Department of Physiology
Dartmouth Medical School
Lebanon, NH
USA

Glenn L Schattman MD
The Center for Reproductive
    Medicine and Infertility
Weill Cornell Medical College
New York, NY
USA

Frederick Schatz PhD
Department of Obstetrics, Gynecology
    and Reproductive Sciences
Yale University School of Medicine
New Haven, CT
USA

James H Segars MD
Reproductive Biology and
    Medicine Branch
National Institutes of Health
Bethesda, MD
USA

Charles L Sentman
Department of Microbiology
    and Immunology
Dartmouth Medical School
Lebanon, NH
USA

Aimee Seungdamrong
Department of Obstetrics/Gynecology
    and Women's Health
UMDNJ-New Jersey Medical School
Newark, NJ
USA

Andrew M Sharkey PhD
Department of Pathology
University of Cambridge
Cambridge
UK

Kathy L Sharpe-Timms PhD
Department of Obstetrics, Gynecology
    and Women's Health
University of Missouri-Columbia
Columbia, MO
USA

Li Shen
Department of Microbiology
    and Immunology
Dartmouth Medical School
Lebanon, NH
USA

Mark E Sherman MD
Division of Cancer Epidemiology and Genetics
National Cancer Institute
Rockville, MD
USA

J Robert A Sherwin MRCOG
Department of Obstetrics and Gynaecology
The Rosie Hospital
Cambridge
UK

Carlos Simón MD PhD
Fundación IVI (FIVI)
Valencia University
Valencia
Spain

Ov D Slayden PhD
Division of Reproductive Sciences
Oregon National Primate Research Center
Oregon Health & Sciences University
Beaverton, OR
USA

Michael J Soares PhD
Institute of Maternal–Fetal Biology
The University of Kansas Medical Center
Kansas City, KS
USA

Thomas E Spencer PhD
Department of Animal Science
Center for Animal Biotechnology and Genomics
Texas A&M University
College Station, TX
USA

Laura Studee MPH
Center for Research on Women and Gender
University of Illinois at Chicago
Chicago, IL
USA

Said Talbi PhD
Department of Cell and Tissue Biology,
    Pharmaceutical Chemistry, Anatomy, and
    Obstetrics, Gynecology and Reproductive Sciences
University of California at San Francisco
San Francisco, CA
USA

Seang Lin Tan MBBS FRCS MMed(O&G) FRCOG MBA
Department of Obstetrics and Gynecology
Royal Victoria Hospital
McGill University
Montreal, Quebec
Canada

Hugh S Taylor MD
Department of Obstetrics, Gynecology
    and Reproductive Sciences
Yale University School of Medicine
New Haven, CT
USA

Wei Tong PhD
Department of Pediatrics
University of Pennsylvania Medical School
Philadelphia, PA
USA

Jinrong Wang
Department of Molecular and Cellular Biology
Baylor College of Medicine
Houston, TX
USA

Alistair Williams
Department of Pathology
University of Edinburgh
Royal Infirmary at Edinburgh
Edinburgh, Scotland
UK

Virginia D Winn MD PhD
Department of Obstetrics and Gynecology
University of Colorado Health Science Center
Aurora, CO
USA

Elke Winterhager PhD
Institut für Anatomie
Universitütsklinikum Essen
Essen
Germany

Charles R Wira PhD
Department of Physiology
Dartmouth Medical School
Lebanon, NH
USA

FB Peter Wooding PhD
Physiology Department
Cambridge University
Cambridge
UK

Steven L Young MD PhD
Department of Obstetrics & Gynecology
Division of Reproductive
    Endocrinology and Infertility
University of North Carolina at Chapel Hill
Chapen Hill, NC
USA

Liyin Zhu
Department of Developmental and
    Molecular Biology and Obstetrics
    and Gynecology and Women's Health
Albert Einstein College of Medicine
Bronx, NY
USA

Preface to the first edition

The Endometrium is a research-oriented text devoted to a comprehensive multidisciplinary account of the uterine endometrium. This book is the first to focus on the endometrium in terms of defining the regulatory biological interrelationships between epithelial and stromal cell phenotypes, endothelial cells, extra-cellular matrix and immunobiological elements. The aim is to provide a parent language and the principles to translate our diverse understandings of reproductive cyclicity and embryo–endometrial interrelationships into a vocabulary common to all investigators and students. This base will also serve to establish the endometrium, intellectually and technically, as a singular, productive, fundamental biological model system for investigators from a broad spectrum of disciplines interested in the regulatory biology of cell–cell, cell substratum and reciprocal paracrine communication. This cardinal information will be complemented by emerging studies of oncology, aging and gene expression.

To accomplish these goals authoritative authors were enlisted. All are active in studies of the structure-function principles that govern endometrial biology. They were encouraged to go beyond cataloging basic information and build on emerging conceptual and technical motifs to critically reexamine the established database. This approach would support new directions and concepts and discourage insularity of ideas and practice thereby fostering an open forum that would promote a new interdisciplinary interrogation of benefit to all members of the diverse community of reproductive sciences. Avenues would then emerge for the exchange of ideas, materials and technology, which is central to integration of fundamentals and the basis for continued discussion.

Until late in the 19th century our knowledge of the female reproductive system was fragmentary, limited to observations of gross morphology and physiology. These relatively uncompounded methods of study persisted until the 1920s when microscopically discernable changes replaced other forms of observation. The discovery of sex steroid hormones served to motivate and expand the scope of study of reproductive biology beyond the directly observable. Steroid biochemistry was later augmented by the discovery of the trophic hormones of pituitary and placenta. Post World War II access to pure steroid and polypeptide hormones allowed the production of specific antibodies and the application of immunobiologic strategies. From studies, focused predominantly on hypothalamic regulation of the pituitary, evolved the concept of negative feedback and the clarification of the basic principles of homeostasis. Electron microscopy revealed fascinating new vistas of cellular structure.

The application of the intellectual and technical assets of molecular biology then created a new atmosphere in reproductive sciences. The beginnings of an understanding of gene expression emerged. Advances in gene targeting technology crystallized the linkage between hormone receptor complexes and the cell specific nuclear genetic apparatus. It is sobering, however, that of the more than 50 gene knockout models in which the implantation process in the mouse is compromised, none has yet yielded a satisfactory molecular mechanistic explanation of embryo–endometrial interaction. Thus we are learning that the challenge for today's science is to pass beyond reductionist biology and embrace a diversity of analytical procedures and tactics even greater than available to investigators in other times. The application of both *in vivo* and *in vitro* methods, across disciplines extending from molecular biology to systems physiology, is an opportunity not previously available. It is in this context that lessons learned from the elucidation of endocrine/paracrine signaling pathways in species of varying cellular complexity will enlarge the prospect of altering reproductive processes. We may, in the future, be able to modulate physiological responses in different living organisms through the understanding of a series of common mechanisms.

There is no organ other than the uterus that, in the exercise of its normal functions, displays so great a range of cyclic complexities in growth and adaptation. Mammals in general, their reproductive systems more generally, testify to the adaptations, the diversion of strategies that have evolved to serve a common goal, i.e. a successful outcome of the sum of the processes, species and adaptations, which regulate gestation. Historically the uterus has not occupied the centre of reproductive biology research. Rather, it has played a role secondary to the analysis of ovarian and testicular function and gametogenesis. Yet these studies contributed to the recognition of the unique cyclicity of the endometrium in different mammalian species, particularly as it applied to the stringently regulated transient period during which the embryo is permitted to attach and implant. The fundamentals of this unusual program of regulatory cell endocrinology were utilized effectively to develop the technologies that allowed embryo transfer into the uterus to yield live offspring. Yet in almost five decades of investigation we have cannot been able to resolve the most critical problems of infertility, pregnancy wastage and fetal growth restriction. Many of the contributions to this book relate the development and exercise of ideas and research programs that seek to enlarge our understanding of endometrial interactions with embryos and the outcome of pregnancy in a range of different mammalian species.

Two major issues, one cultural, the other technological have impeded our understanding of endometrial biology. Anthropocentricity has driven interest and funding to focus on efforts to develop experimental models from human systems. The bias favoring hemochorial placentation has deflected attention from non-primate systems that provided the intellectual driving force for many early studies of embryo–endometrial interactions. Using contemporary analytical and judgemental tools, past investigators identified the hierarchy of processes that includes embryo attachment, initiation of placentation and the maintenance of pregnancy.

These studies established a conceptual framework that proved valuable in human studies which are necessarily limited by ethical, financial and societal considerations, as well as the relative inaccessibility of the organ. This has led to the increasing use of cell culture systems. However much remains to be done, particularly improving our ability to culture specific primary cells. For example, despite the massive proliferative activity in the trophoblast that follows implantation and without which the conceptus is not viable, it still is not possible to produce sustainable proliferation in primary human trophoblast cultures. Nor have we the art and technology to develop cultures of primary endometrial cell phenotypes that respond faithfully to specific regulatory factors.

A few, too few, investigators continue to direct their attention to animal models for both comparative biology and species conservation purposes. Judging these data we are learning how to maximize the assets of comparative biology. The remarkable diversity of reproductive strategies to be found amongst mammalian species obligates every investigator to analyze *in vivo* and *in vitro* models, but to do so with caution. The programs that coordinate endometrial cell proliferation, growth and differentiation in different species afford the thoughtful investigator models in which both similarities and differences can prove instructive. It is to be hoped that studies of primates and other species will continue in the future with renewed vigor.

Even as this book was being organized it was apparent that our understanding of endometrial biology was in active transition. In the last decade genomics has evolved into a real scientific discipline. The sequencing of the genome has introduced astonishing technical advances and an unbelievable mass of data. With the first draft in hand, we are indeed entering the second genetic revolution. How will biology, reproductive science specifically, evolve from being a data-deplete to a data-replete science? How will the intellectual and technical level of effort and imaging advances in cell biology reshape our understanding of the endometrium and its interactions with the developing embryo?

Perhaps our next step in this second revolution, the focus of the next book devoted to the endometrium, will be the practices of functional genomics and proteomics. These emerging disciplines and their spin-offs will provide the information, interpretable on many different levels of biology, from which will materialize new perceptions of endometrial biology. Synthesis of data acquired using different tools (protein–protein interactions, mutational loss of function, computer derived ontogenesis) will require coordinated efforts to develop the algorithms and database correlates to integrate the data acquired by different tools and disciplines. The potential use of functional genomics will be the ability to utilize the data presented in this book and formulate protocols that will allow the simultaneous monitoring of many events, regardless of their level of expression, in an organism whose genome is entirely known.

Analysis of the genome will presage a new era of drug discovery in which therapy will be tailored to aberrations in the DNA sequence. Even if a free market economy will not support analytical and treatment practices based on specific single nucleotide polymorphisms (SNPs), a new molecular biology will emerge. Reproductive science has proved profitable for the pharmaceutical industry and will be a target field for the new pharmacogenomics. In time we will realize the promise that sequencing the eukaryotic genome will facilitate the solution of problems related to fertility, pregnancy wastage, endometriosis, cancer, reproductive aging and nuclear transfer technology and advance the design of novel contraceptives. New insights into the regulatory mechanisms integral to genetically controlled pathways will add a new dimension to the investigative abilities of the reproductive scientist. Promise approaches reality and as T.S. Eliot wrote, 'and the end of all our exploring will be to arrive where we started and know the place for the first time.'

Stanley R Glasser
John D Aplin
Linda C Giudice
Siamak Tabibzadeh

Preface to the second edition

The 5 years that have elapsed since the first edition of *The Endometrium* was published have seen the emergence of influential new technologies both in the laboratory and the clinic. Their impact on human reproduction is raising questions that reverberate in society at large. In the laboratory, genomics, transcriptomics, proteomics, and metabolomics are dramatically exposing the gene hierarchies responsible for endocrine and local regulation of reproductive systems; mouse genetics is being effectively used for reproductive studies, with often surprising results; the gradual maturation of our understanding of immune influences on normal reproductive function has led to a realization that cytokines and leukocytes have a profound influence on non-immune pathways; the importance of stem (or at least, progenitor) cells in adult reproductive tissues has been glimpsed; and the presence of both naturally occurring and man-made chemicals in our environment has had a marked impact on the endocrine and reproductive status both of human beings and other species with whom we share this planet.

Our intention in the second edition of *The Endometrium* continues to be to educate and stimulate. We stretch beyond the limitations of a review or paper and bridge the intellectual and cultural divide between basic science and clinical research communities. The second edition is updated in all its dimensions by former authors as well as additional experts, and is notably expanded with new chapters on endocrinology, puberty, progenitor cells, transgenics, transcriptomics, placental development, trophoblast biology, infection, and cancer.

We have aimed to provide a challenging, comprehensive, historically grounded, and factual account of endometrial physiology and pathology in development, during the years of mature reproductive function, and in later life. Our hope is that the book will help invest researchers, clinicians, basic scientists, and students with enthusiasm for the fascinating, complex, and crucial processes of reproduction. Ultimately we seek a readership sympathetic to the urgency of understanding the scientific foundations upon which emergent technologies operate, and examining critically the implications of the results.

John D Aplin
Asgerally T Fazleabas
Stanley R Glasser
Linda C Giudice

Color Plates

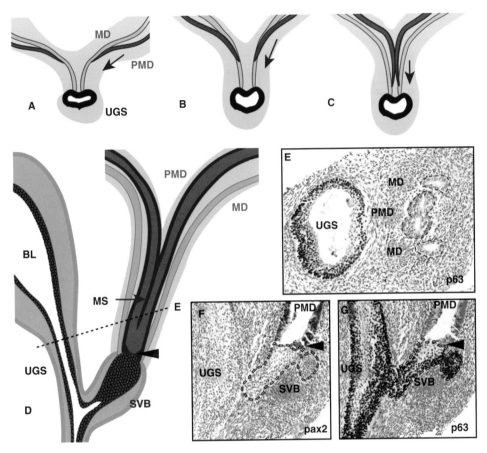

Figure 1.1 Initial development of the paramesonephric duct. CE, coelomic epithelium; MD, mesonephric duct; PMD, paramesonephric duct; UGM, urogenital mesenchyme. (**A**) Schematic drawing of PMD formation and growth. (**B, C**) Pax2 immunohistochemistry (IHC) on developing PMD of the E13.5 female mouse embryo. (**B**) The arrow indicates opening of PMD to coelom. (**C**) The numbers in this section correspond to the ones indicated in A. (**D, E**) H&E-stained sections of a human fetus (Carnegie stage 19). (**D**) A cross-section of developing MD and PMD at the cranial portion (corresponding to ① in A and E). PMD and MD are segregated by intervening mesenchymal cells. (**E**) A longitudinal section of developing human MD and PMD. PMD makes contact with MD at the caudal end. PMD arises as an invagination of coelomic epithelium at the cranial end of the urogenital ridge. The site of infolding remains open throughout development (arrows). PMD grows caudally through the UGM and the tip comes into contact with the MD within a common basement membrane. Later, the tip of growing PMD maintains close contact with MD while the cranial portion is dissociated from MD. Cross sections reveal three distinct special arrangements of PMD and MD: ① PMD and MD, each surrounded by basement membranes, are separated by intervening mesenchymal cells; ② both ducts are surrounded by individual basement membranes that are in contact on one side; and ③ direct contact between paramesonephric and mesonephric duct epithelial cells without an intervening basement membrane.

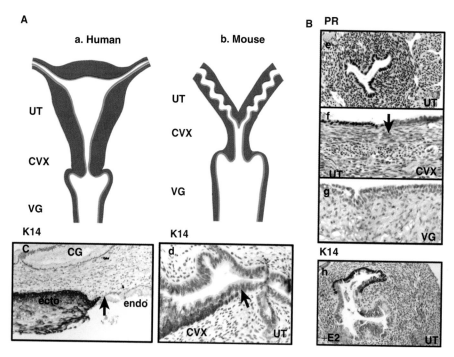

Figure 1.3 Adult uterus, cervix, and vagina. (**A**) Anatomy of human and mouse uterus. UT, uterus; CVX, cervix; VG, vagina. The location of the squamocolumnar junction is indicated by an arrow. (**a**) Simplex uterus of the human. The fused portion of the paramesonephric ducts forms a single uterus with one cervix and one vagina. The squamocolumnar junction is located between the endocervix and ectocervix. (**b**) Duplex uterus of mouse. The lateral fusion of the paramesonephric ducts does not occur at the uterine level, but does occur at the vagina and in the middle of the cervix. Two uterine canals open into two independent cervices, and the two cervices are connected into a single common cervical canal. The squamocolumnar junction is located between the uterus and cervix. (**c**) Keratin 14 expression in the human cervix. It is expressed in epithelial cells of the ectocervix (ecto) but not in those of the endocervix (endo). CG, cervical gland. (**d**) Keratin 14 expression in the mouse cervix. K14 is expressed in the epithelial cells of the cervix (CVX) but not in the uterus (UT). (**B**) Squamocolumnar junction in the postaxial hemimelia (px) mouse. (**e–g**) Immunohistochemistry (IHC) for progesterone receptor (PR); (**h**) IHC for K14. Female *px* (spontaneous *Wnt7a* mutant) mice were ovariectomized at postnatal day 35 and the expressions of PR and K14 were analyzed at postnatal day 60. In these mice, PR was constitutively expressed in the uterine epithelium (**e,f**), indicating normal uterine epithelial differentiation.[55] In contrast, PR was absent in the cervical and vaginal epithelia (**f,g**). The PR expression pattern was abruptly changed at the squamocolumnar junction (arrow in **f**). Cervical and vaginal epithelia were positive for K14, while such expression was absent in uterine epithelium in the ovariectomized *px* mice (not shown), indicating normal uterine and cervicovaginal epithelial differentiation. However, when the ovariectomized *px* mice were treated with 125 ng estradiol/day for 3 days, K14-positive stratified squamous epithelium appeared in a region of the uterus (**h**). These observations indicate that Wnt7a is required to maintain proper epithelial differentiation in the adult uterus, while it is dispensable for uterine and vaginal epithelial differentiation in the neonatal stage.

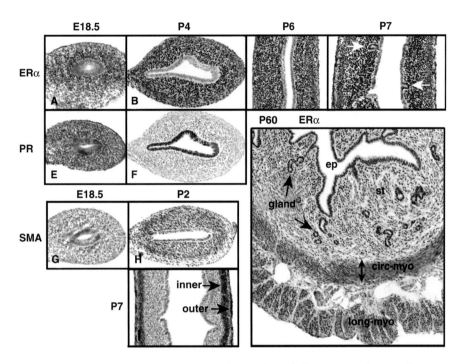

Figure 1.4 Morphogenesis of C57/B6 mouse uterus: ep, luminal epithelium; st, endometrial stroma; circ-myo, circular (inner) myometrium; long-myo, longitudinal (outer) myometrium. Immunohistochemistry (IHC) for estrogen receptor α (ERα) (A–D, J), progesterone receptor (PR) (E,F) α-smooth muscle actin (SMA) (G–I). Epithelial differentiation: at embryonic day 18.5 (E18.5), ERα (A) and PR (E) are not expressed in the uterine epithelial cells, while the mesenchymal cells show strong immunoreactivity for ERα (A). From a late embryonic stage to postnatal day 3 (P3), the uterine epithelium forms a simple tube with an oval-shaped lumen in a transverse view (H). At P4, the uterine epithelial tube shows a sign of morphogenesis as several epithelial evaginations protrude into the surrounding mesenchyme (B,F). At this stage, epithelial cells are mostly negative for ERα (B) but already strongly positive for PR (F). Although the epithelial evaginations can be observed as early as P4, uterine glands are totally absent at P6 (C) and cannot be observed until P7 (D, arrows). In the adult uterus (P60), the uterine epithelium forms an irregular, tubular shape with many folds that protrude into the stroma (J). Fully developed uterine glands are projected from the uterine canal deeply into the endometrial stroma (J). The entire epithelium is positive for ERα. Stromal differentiation: α-smooth muscle actin (SMA) was undetectable in the embryonic uterine mesenchyme (G). At P2, the expression of SMA is detected in the outer layer of the unorganized uterine mesenchyme (H). By P7, smooth muscle layers are organized into inner circular and outer longitudinal myometrial layers (I). Most inner layer surrounding the epithelium differentiates into endometrial stroma. In the adult uterus (P60), the myometrial layers form a thick circular inner myometrium (circ-myo) and a longitudinal outer myometrium (long-myo) with bundles of smooth muscle (J).

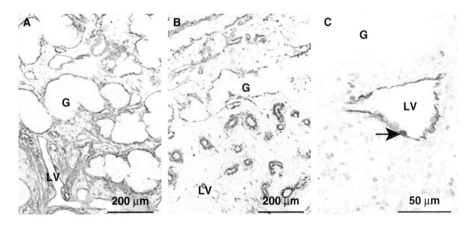

Figure 6.3 Photomicrographs illustrating lymphatic vessels immunostained with antibodies against D2-40 (stained blue) and α-smooth muscle actin (α-SMA, stained brown) in (A) functionalis and (B) basalis from human endometrium during the late secretory phase of the menstrual cycle. (C) Example of a proliferating lymphatic endothelial cell (arrow) immunostained brown using an antibody against PCNA.

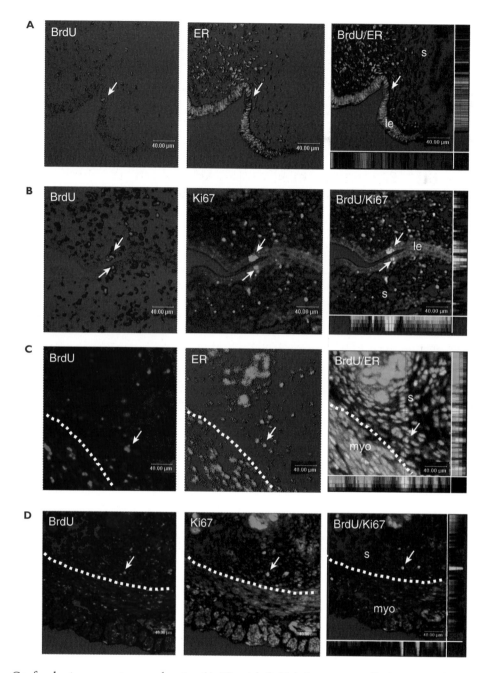

Figure 10.5 Confocal microscopy images showing (**A, B**) epithelial label-retaining cells (LRCs) and (**C, D**) stromal LRCs in mouse endometrium. Postnatal bromodeoxyuridine (BrdU)-labeled mouse endometrium double immunofluorescent stained for BrdU (red) and ERα (green), showing (**A**) lack of co-expression in a single epithelial LRC in the luminal epithelium at 8 weeks chase (blue arrows) but ERα expression in mature epithelial cells, and (**C**) co-localization of BrdU and ERα in some stromal LRCs near the endometrial–myometrial junction at 12-weeks chase (white arrows). Endometrium from postnatal BrdU-labeled, (**B**) 4- and (**D**) 8-weeks chased, ovariectomized mice double immunofluorescent stained for BrdU (red) and proliferation marker, Ki-67 (green) to visualize estrogen-stimulated proliferation of (**B**) epithelial LRC (blue arrows) and of (**D**) stromal LRCs (white arrows). The x/z and y/z planes are shown on the far right and underneath the merged pictures, demonstrating true co-localization of the two markers within individual whole nuclei. Dotted line indicates endometrial–myometrial junction; le, luminal epithelium; s, stroma; myo, myometrium (scale bars = 40 μm)

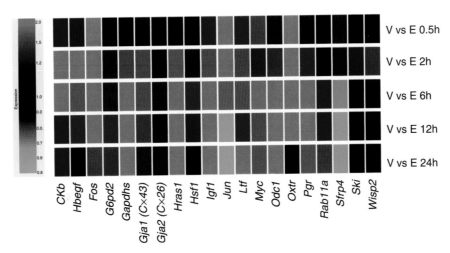

Figure 12.3 Heat map display of estrogen-regulated uterine genes from Table 12.1 showing values from microarray analysis. Ovariectomized animals were treated with E and sampled after 0.5, 2, 6, 12, and 24 hours. Each comparison is a pair of samples (vehicle compared to E_2 treatment at that time point) with red indicating higher transcript level in E_2 compared to vehicle and green indicating lower transcript level in E_2 treated compared to vehicle. *Ckb*, creatine kinase b; *Hbegf*, heparin-binding EGF-like growth factor; *Fos*, FBJ osteosarcoma oncogene; *G6pd2*, glucose-6-phosphate dehydrogenase 2; *Gapdhs*, glyceraldehyde-3-phosphate dehydrogenase, spermatogenic; *Gja1*, gap junction membrane channel protein alpha 1 (connexin 43); *Gjb2* gap junction membrane channel protein beta 2 (connexin 26); *Hras1*, Harvey rat sarcoma virus oncogene 1; *Hsf1*, heat shock transcription factor 1; *Igf1*, insulin-like growth factor 1; *Jun*, Jun oncogene; *Ltf*, lactotransferrin; *Myc*, myelocytomatosis oncogene; *Odc1*, ornithine decarboxylase, structural 1; *Oxtr*, oxytocin receptor; *Pgr*, progesterone receptor; *Rab11a*, RAB11a, member RAS oncogene family; *Sfrp4*, secreted frizzled-related sequence protein 4; *Ski*, Sloan-Kettering viral oncogene homolog; *Wisp2*, WNT1 inducible signaling pathway protein 2.

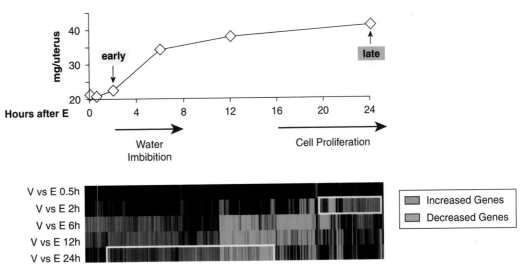

Figure 12.4 Analysis of uterine gene responses by microarray. The top panel is a schematic representation of the experimental design. It shows the trend in increasing uterine weight in an ovariectomized mouse following a single injection of estradiol (E). The initial weight increase is a result of water imbibition: cell proliferation begins and continues after 16–24 hours. Uteri were collected after 0.5, 2, 6, 12, or 24 hours, and the gene profiles relative to vehicle treated samples were obtained by microarray. The bottom panel is a heat map representation of the transcripts significantly different from corresponding vehicle control by at least two-fold at $p < 0.001$ showing the increases in red and the decreases in green. The yellow and gray boxes highlight transcripts that are characteristic of early and late time points, respectively. In subsequent studies the 2- and 24-hour time points were sampled as representative of early and late responses, as they appear to include most uterine responses and can provide a 'snapshot' from minimal sampling.

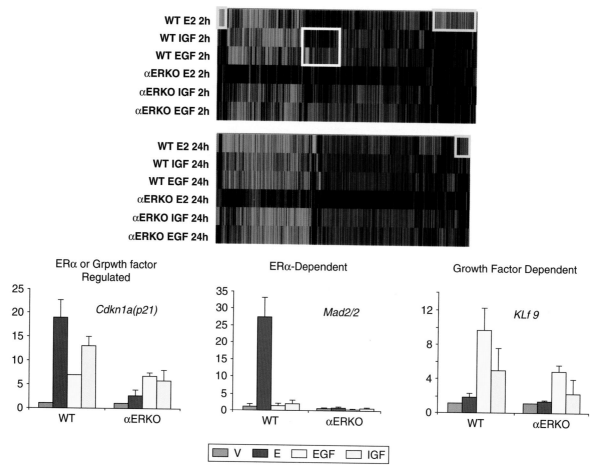

Figure 12.5   (A) Microarray comparison of WT and αERKO uterine gene responses to E_2 or growth factors epidermal growth factor (EGF) or insulin-like growth factor 1 (IGF) for 2 or 24 hours. Growth factor responses are ERα independent. Examples of ERα-dependent (yellow boxes) and growth factor-dependent (white box) clusters are highlighted. (B) Examples of regulatory modes observed by microarray. (1) ERα or growth factor regulated: RT-PCR analysis of *Cdkn1a* (p21) shows it is increased by either E_2 or growth factors; the E_2 induction requires ERα, as E_2-mediated increase is attenuated in the αERKO, whereas the growth factors increase them in both WT and αERKO, indicating the growth factor regulation is independent of ERα. (2) ERα dependent: RT-PCR analysis of *Mad2l1* (MAD2 [mitotic arrest deficient, homolog]-like 1 [yeast]) indicates it is increased by E, not by growth factors, and is dependent on ERα. (3) Growth factor-dependent: RT-PCR analysis of KLf9 (Kruppel-like factor 9) shows it is increased by growth factors and is not dependent on ERα.

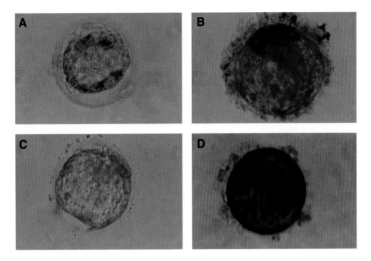

Figure 19.2 Inmunolocalization of chemokine receptors CCR2B and CCR5 in human blastocysts. (A) Negative control and (B) CCR2B. (C) Negative control and (D) CCR5. (Reproduced from Domínguez et al,[34] with permission.)

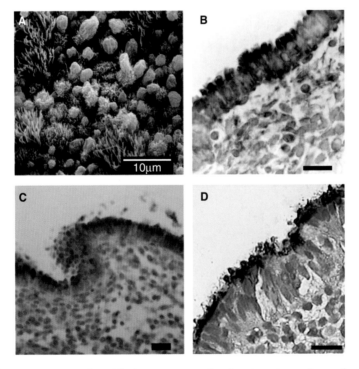

Figure 20.4 Scanning electron micrographs and photomicrographs showing pinopods on the mid-secretory endometrial surface. By scanning electron microscopy, classic pinopods can be seen (A). Using various specific antibodies to surface proteins, luminal pinopod-like structures can be visualized by high-powered microscopy for the $\alpha_v\beta_3$ integrin (B), osteopontin (C), and the ligand for L-selectin (D). Relative size is indicated by the bar, which is equal to 10 μm.

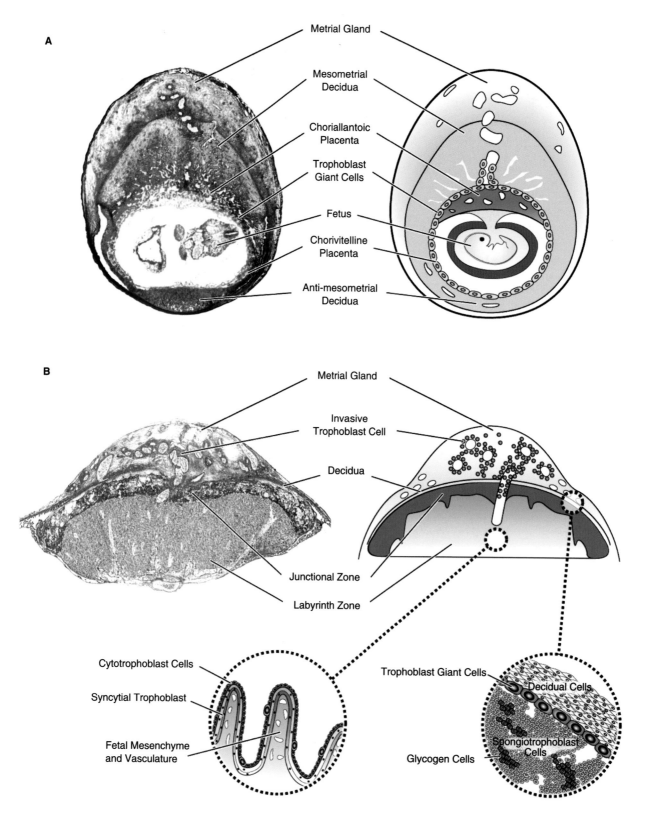

Figure 23.1   Mid and late gestation uteroplacental compartments. (A) Hematoxylin and eosin-stained tissue section of the mid gestation rat uteroplacental compartment (left, day 11 of gestation) and a corresponding schematic diagram (right). (B) Hematoxylin and eosin-stained tissue section of the late gestation rat uteroplacental compartment (left, day 18 of gestation) and a corresponding schematic diagram (right) with highlighted expanded views of the labyrinth and junctional zones (lower panels). (Reproduced in modified form from Ain et al,[103] with permission from Humana Press.)

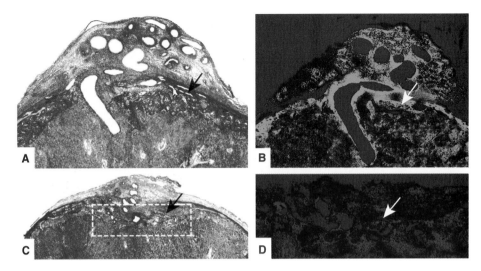

Figure 23.2   Identification of invasive trophoblast cells in the rat and mouse. Rat and mouse placentation sites were recovered at day 18 of gestation, and 10 μm sections prepared. Trophoblast cells were identified by cytokeratin immunostaining. (**A**) Hematoxylin and eosin staining of the rat placentation site. (**B**) Cytokeratin immunolocalization with the rat placentation site. (**C**) Hematoxylin and eosin staining of the mouse placentation site (the area shown in the box is present in **D**). (**D**) Cytokeratin immunolocalization within the mouse placentation site. All magnifications are at 100×. Arrows indicate the trophoblast giant cell boundary between the placenta and decidua. (Reproduced from Ain et al,[7] with permission from Academic Press.)

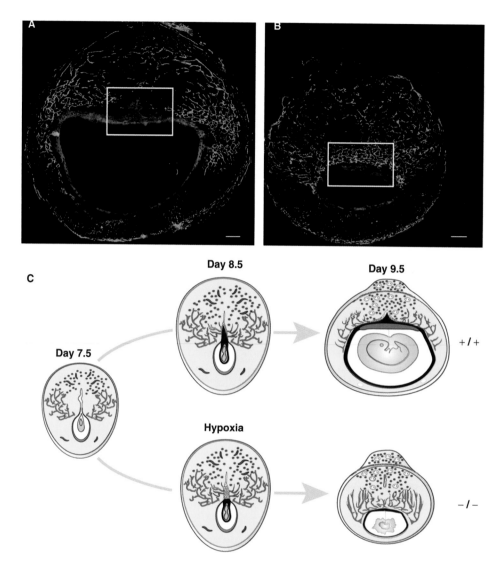

Figure 23.4   Defect in hemochorial placentation and trophoblast–vascular interactions in PLP-A null mutant mice exposed to hypoxia. Double immunohistochemical staining for trophoblast cells by using a cytokeratin-8-specific antibody (TROMA-1) and for endothelial cells by using an endoglin antibody within implantation sites of wild-type and PLP-A null mutant mice after 48 hours (**A** and **B**) of hypoxia starting on gestation day 7.5 (scale bars = 250 μm). (**C**) Cellular dynamics at implantation sites of wild-type and PLP-A null mutant mice exposed to hypoxia for 48 hours starting on gestation day 7.5. Note the lack of trophoblast expansion into the mesometrial chamber on days 8.5 and 9.5 of pregnancy in PLP-A null mutant mice after exposure to hypoxia. Also note the aberrant vasculature and underdeveloped placentas at the implantation sites on day 9.5 of pregnancy in PLP-A null mutant mice exposed to hypoxia. (Reproduced in modified form from Ain et al,[74] with permission from the National Academy of Sciences of the USA.)

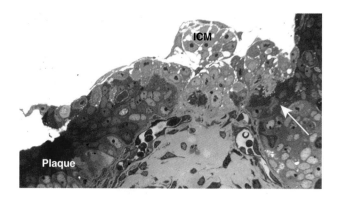

Figure 28b.1 Implantation site of a rhesus monkey 1 day after the onset of implantation (day 10). In this trophoblastic plate stage, trophoblast beneath the inner cell mass (ICM) has invaded into a gland. A cleft (arrow) has developed in the syncytial trophoblast that has invaded the gland on the right. The trophoblast has not penetrated the residual basal lamina of the uterine luminal epithelium or into the underlying capillaries. This is the first stage in which an epithelial plaque reaction is found. ×200.

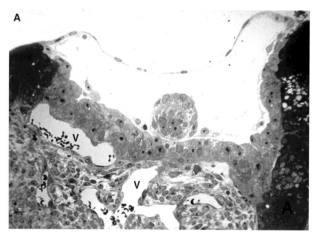

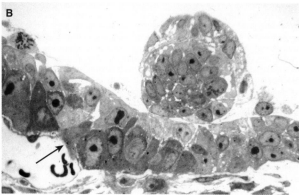

Figure 28b.2 Implantation site of a baboon, trophoblastic plate stage. (**A**) Note the dilated superficial vessels (v) underlying the trophoblastic plate. (**B**) Enlargement of an adjacent section, showing where syncytial trophoblast (arrow) has penetrated into the maternal vessel in one area. **A**, ×200; **B**, ×520.

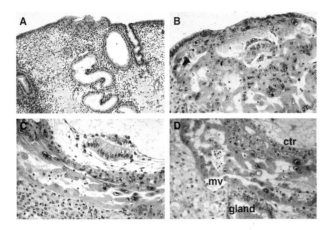

Figure 28b.3 Human implantation sites, photographed from slides in the Carnegie collection. (**A**) In stage 5a, the trophoblast of the trophoblastic plate consists of both cellular and syncytial trophoblast, and is largely above the level of the residual basal lamina of the luminal epithelium. (**B**) Early lacunar stage (stage 5b). At the bottom and right, lacunae with only partially expanded clefts can be seen (*). (**C**) A later lacunar stage (stage 5c). The lacunae are anastomotic, and the beginnings of decidualization can be seen in the underlying endometrial stroma. (**D**) Margin of a late lacunar stage (stage 5c), showing the continuity of the syncytial trophoblast lining the lacunae with the endothelium of a maternal vessel (mv). Note the continuous layer of cytotrophoblast (ctr) adjacent to the forming exocoelom, and the cluster of cytotrophoblast cells (*) initiating a primary villus. **A**, ×80; **B–D**, ×200.

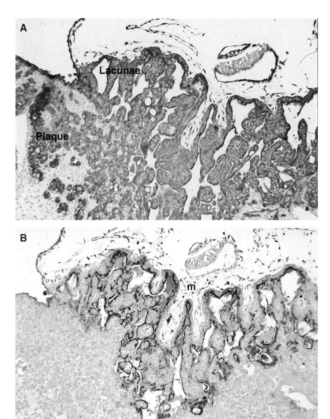

Figure 28b.4 Implantation sites of a cynomolgus macaque at the transition from the lacunar to the villus stage (day 13). (**A**) This section was immunostained to indicate localization of cytokeratins. Note that the embryo and the trophoblast of the villi stain, and also the uterine epithelium including the epithelial plaque cells. (**B**) Section adjacent to that in Figure 28b.4A, immunostained for pregnancy-specific β-1 glycoprotein (SP1). This antibody stains syncytial trophoblast but not cellular trophoblast or uterine epithelium. Note the extraembryonic mesenchyme (m) indenting the villi just beneath the embryo. ×80.

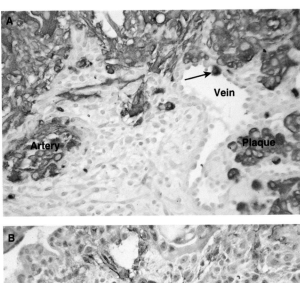

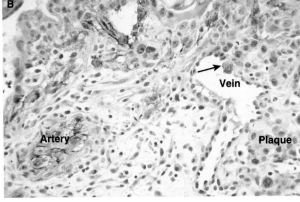

Figure 28b.5 Junctional zone of the implantation site shown in Figure 28b.4. (A) This section was immunostained for cytokeratin. Note the multiple cytokeratin-stained cytotrophoblast cells in the artery on the left, and the single cytokeratin-stained cytotrophoblast cell in the vein. (B) Section adjacent to that in Figure 28b.5A, immunostained for NCAM. Note that this cell adhesion molecule marks the surface of migratory cytotrophoblast cells. The lumen of the artery is filled with cytotrophoblast cells, whereas only a single cytotrophoblast cell forms part of the wall of the vein. ×200.

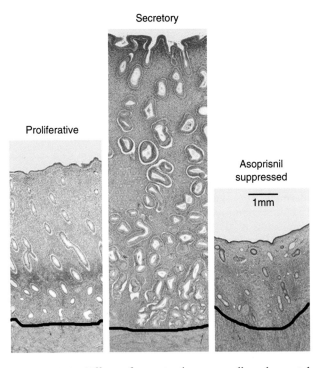

Figure 39.4 Effect of asoprisnil on overall endometrial histology of intact cynomolgus macaques. Photomicrographic comparison of endometrial histology of typical control animals (proliferative and secretory phases) vs asoprisnil-treated (90 mg/kg) animals. Original magnification ~ 4×. (Reproduced from Chwalisz et al[32] with permission.)

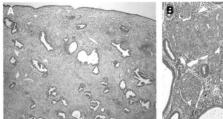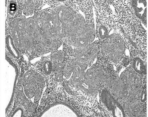

Figure 39.5 The 'SPRM endometrial effects' of asoprisnil after treatment for 3 months. (**A**) Representative full-thickness section of the endometrium from a hysterectomy specimen of a patient with symptomatic leiomyomata. Glands show a sinuous or serpentine profile, similar to the architecture of glands seen in the midsecretory phase of the menstrual cycle, with focal mild cystic dilatation. The stroma is compact, but non-decidualized. (**B**) Thick-walled muscularized vessel in endometrial stroma.

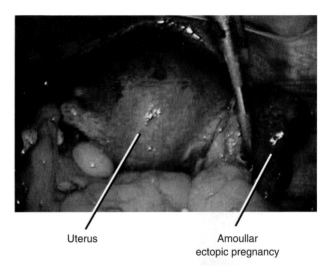

Uterus   Amoullar
                   ectopic pregnancy

Figure 49.2 Ampullary ectopic pregnancy. Many ampullary implantations abort spontaneously with few symptoms. (Courtesy of Dr David Zepeda.)

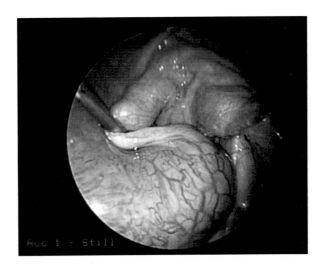

Figure 49.4 Cornual ectopic pregnancy. Cornual implantation may rupture catastrophically if diagnosis is delayed. (Courtesy of Dr David Zepeda.)

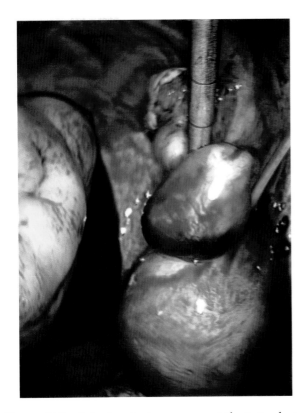

Figure 49.3 Isthmic ectopic pregnancy. Isthmic implantations have a higher likelihood of rupture than ampullary sites. A high percentage of isthmic implantations are associated with methotrexate failure. (Courtesy of Dr David Zepeda.)

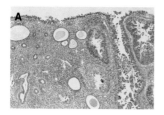
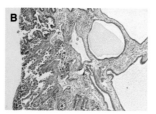
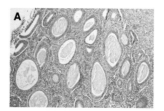
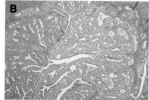

Figure 55.3 (A) Endometrial intraepithelial carcinoma (EIC) showing replacement of surface epithelium and superficial gland necks by malignant cells. Note: invasion through the basement membrane is not identified. (Adapted from Sherman et al.[8]) (B) Minimal uterine serous carcinoma (probably EIC) involving surface of endometrial polyp.

Figure 55.2 (A) Slightly crowded dilated glands compatible with non-atypical simple hyperplasia. (B) Substantially crowded glands with minimal intervening stroma (right) approaching glandular fusion (left) compatible with atypical complex hyperplasia with features of early endometrioid carcinoma, grade 1.

1 Embryology of the uterus

Takeshi Kurita and Hisae Nakamura

Synopsis

Background

- The two paramesonephric ducts of mesodermal origin, also called the Müllerian ducts, differentiate into oviducts, uterus, cervix (in all mammals), and the cranial portion of the vagina (in eutherian mammals), in a cranial to caudal order.
- Just before the paramesonephric duct tips reach the urogenital sinus, they join and fuse vertically with the sinovaginal bulb.
- The laterally fused portion of the paramesonephric ducts becomes the uterus, cervix, and/or vagina (Müllerian vagina), depending on the species.
- The complete fusion of the paramesonephric ducts in the uterine segment forms a simplex uterus in higher primates, including humans.

Basic science

- Epithelial cells taken from the paramesonephric duct, not from the sinovaginal bulb or the mesonephric duct, can be induced to become uterine epithelium when combined with uterine mesenchyme.
- The presence of the caudal two-fifths of the vagina in *Tfm* (testicular feminization mutation)-affected male mice provides evidence for vaginal development from these two discrete primordia.
- *Tfm* is a spontaneous mutation of androgen receptor causing insensitivity to testosterone. In the affected XY individual, the male reproductive tract does not develop due to the insensitivity to testosterone, and the paramesonephric duct also regresses due to the MIS/AMH produced by the testis.
- Therefore, the remaining short vagina in *Tfm* male mice is thought to be derived from the urogenital sinus.
- The Müllerian vaginal epithelium may displace the sinus vaginal epithelium during maturation.
- Alternatively, the entire vagina may be formed as a caudal growth of the paramesonephric duct with some involvement of themesonephric duct.
- Vitamin A deficiency in rats causes agenesis of the paramesonephric ducts.
- The morphogenetic effects of retinoids (vitamin A and metabolites) are mediated by two families of nuclear receptors: retinoic acid receptors (RARs) and retinoid X receptors (RXRs). Compound mutant mice lacking RARα + RARβ or γ, or RXRα + RARα, β or γ, show partial or complete agenesis of the paramesonephric duct.
- In mice lacking Wnt5a, the posterior growth of the paramesonephric duct is affected; thus, most of the cervix and the entire Müllerian vagina are absent.
- The location of the epithelial squamocolumnar junction is determined by the regional difference in the inductive activity of the uterine and cervical/vaginal mesenchyme.
- ERα, ERβ, and PR are dispensable for perinatal morphogenesis of the mouse uterus. However ERα is present throughout uterine development in mesenchymal cells.
- In both humans and mice, postnatal uterine stromal differentiation into endometrial and myometrial layers is dependent on the epithelium. Wnt7a is a candidate signaling molecule.
- p63, a homologue of the p53 tumor suppressor, is expressed in epithelial cells of the cervix and vagina, but not in the uterus. In its absence, the mouse cervical/vaginal epithelium differentiates into a uterine epithelium.
- p63 is induced in the paramesonephric duct epithelial cells by cervical/vaginal mesenchyme.
- Regulatory information encoded by *Hox* genes in the mesenchyme at different levels of the tract determines gene expression, which in turn directs organ-specific cytodifferentiation of associated epithelial cells.

Clinical

- Knowledge of uterine embryology is important in understanding the clinical complications of uterine abnormalities.
- The estimated prevalence of congenital uterine anomalies such as didelphic, bicornuate, or septate uterus varies significantly in different studies.
- Higher rates of abnormality are found in infertile women, implicating a causal association with adverse pregnancy outcome.
- The possibility that the vagina may have two developmental origins is consistent with features of the Mayer–Rokitansky–Küster–Hauser syndrome in which the caudal portion of the shallow vagina, presumably originating in the urogenital sinus, exists, but the most paramesonephric duct derivatives (from the uterus to the upper vagina) are rudimentary or completely missing.
- In humans, endometrial glands appear in the fetal period; however, they are initially shallow, and further growth occurs postnatally.
- DES (diethylstilbestrol), a synthetic non-steroidal estrogen, was prescribed during the 1940s–1960s for pregnant women at high risk of miscarriage.
- If DES was given to mothers before gestational week 8, more than a third of daughters developed adenosis of the cervix/vagina, a precursor to clear cell adenocarcinoma.
- Inhibition of p63 expression leads to the development of uterine epithelial cells in the cervix/vagina and these become cancerous.
- Thus, transient disruption of a developmental process by an exogenous signal can result in an irreversible developmental defect.

INTRODUCTION

Reproduction is the fundamental activity of organisms to ensure the continuation of a species from one generation to the next. Study of the reproductive system is central in understanding the basic biology as it touches every aspect of life. Particularly, the pivotal role that the uterus plays in reproduction is essential to acknowledge, for this is the very site where some of the mysteries of life begin to unfold.

Over the course of many centuries, numerous attempts have been made to learn about the function and structure of the uterus. However, it was only after the introduction of a new discipline, study of development, that the true biology of this organ was unraveled.[1,2] Therefore, to fully appreciate the morphological and functional knowledge of the uterus, it is of unquestionable value to explore its developmental process in depth. Furthermore, the knowledge of normal uterine development provides insights into how imperfection in such a process can lead to congenital anomalies that often affect pregnancy and healthy delivery of offspring. Thus, it is important to gain extensive knowledge of the embryology of this organ to comprehend the clinical complications of uterine abnormalities. In this chapter, the development of the uterus is discussed in detail from anatomical and molecular perspectives. Also, some of the recent findings from mouse-targeted mutagenesis studies, which have greatly enhanced our knowledge in this field during the last decade, are introduced.

Although the descriptions of developmental processes in this chapter are mostly based upon mouse and human studies, they are intended for all mammals.

DEVELOPMENT OF THE PARAMESONEPHRIC DUCT

In mammals, the uterus arises from a pair of paramesonephric ducts of mesodermal origin, which were first noted by a German physiologist, Johannes Müller, in 1825, and are also called the Müllerian ducts. These ducts differentiate into oviducts, uterus, cervix (in all mammals), and the cranial portion of vagina (in eutherian mammals), in a cranial to caudal order.

The timing of key events in paramesonephric duct development of humans and mice is summarized in Table 1.1.

Development of excretory systems

The reproductive system is closely related to the urinary system in origin and developmental processes.

Table 1.1   Comparative timetable for female reproductive tract development in humans and mice

	Human			Mouse
Event	Post-ovulation day	Gestational weeks	Carnegie stage[98]	Day
MD appears	24–26	—	11	E9.5
MD joins cloaca	28	—	12	E10.5
UGS distinguished	37–41	—	16–17	E11.5–12
Coelomic epithelial invagination	41–45	—	17–18	E11.5
PMD reaches MD	44	—	18	E12
Caudal PMD changes its position inside	52	—	21	E12.5–13
SVB appears	54	—	22	E14.5
PMD fuse together	56	8	22–23	E14–15
PMD tip reaches UGS	56	8	23	E13.5
MD starts regression	—	8	—	E15
Uterus distinguishable as an organ	—	9	—	~E16
PMD fuses with SVB	—	11	—	E15
MD disappears	—	14	—	E16
Vaginal plate appears	—	15	—	~ E17
Layers of uterus defined	—	17	—	P3–5
Smooth muscle differentiation	—	18	—	P2–3
Uterine glands appear	—	19	—	P7
Squamocolumnar junction noticeable	—	~26	—	~P5

The dates indicated are approximate estimates based upon multiple literatures.[7–9,17,21,30,31,34,35,46,48,56,99,100]
PMD, paramesonephric duct; UGS, urogenital sinus; MD, mesonephric duct; SVB, sinovaginal bulb; E, embryonic day; P, postnatal day.

Structures involved in both systems develop from a common mesodermal ridge (intermediate mesoderm), which lies between the paraxial (somites) and the lateral plate mesoderm along the posterior wall of the abdominal cavity.[3] Three developmentally overlapping excretory systems – the pronephros, mesonephros, and metanephros – are formed during embryogenesis in the amniotes (a group of vertebrates including reptiles, birds, and mammals). While the pronephros is functional as an embryonic kidney in lower vertebrates such as amphibia and fish, it is rudimental and nonfunctional in mammals.[4] Nevertheless, its formation is a prerequisite for subsequent urogenital development. In mammals, the pronephros is initially represented by clusters of cells in the cervical region, which regress before more caudal clusters are formed. The pronephric duct forms in the upper thoracic region and elongates caudally in the cleft between the somite and the lateral plate mesoderm.[4] The caudal part of the pronephric duct is incorporated into the mesonephros to form the mesonephric (Wolffian) ducts in both male and female embryos.

The second kidney, mesonephros, forms in the urogenital ridge caudal to the pronephros. As the mesonephric duct grows caudally, it induces transformation of urogenital ridge mesenchymal cells into an epithelial cell mass, which eventually develops into the mesonephros. The formation of the mesonephros proceeds in a craniocaudal direction.[5] The mesonephric ducts continue to grow caudally until they reach and fuse with the cloaca, which is of endodermal origin.

Metanephros is the permanent kidney in mammals. It develops from the ureteric bud, an outgrowth of the mesonephric duct close to its entrance to the cloaca. Metanephric mesenchyme induces the neighboring mesonephric duct to form the ureteric bud, which penetrates the metanephric mesenchyme and induces epithelialization of mesenchymal cells.[6] Complex molecular interactions between the ureteric bud and the metanephric mesenchyme to form the metanephric kidney is beyond the scope of this chapter and, thus, is not covered.

Role of the mesonephric duct in paramesonephric duct development

Shortly after the formation of the mesonephric ducts, the paramesonephric ducts arise as craniocaudal invaginations of thickened coelomic epithelium (Müllerian plaque) at the upper end of the urogenital ridge on the lateral aspect of the corresponding mesonephric duct (Figure 1.1A).[7,8] The site of the infolding remains open throughout the development of the paramesonephric ducts (Figure 1.1B) and becomes the abdominal ostium of the oviduct.[9] The paramesonephric ducts grow caudally through the urogenital mesenchyme (Figure 1.1A). During the caudal

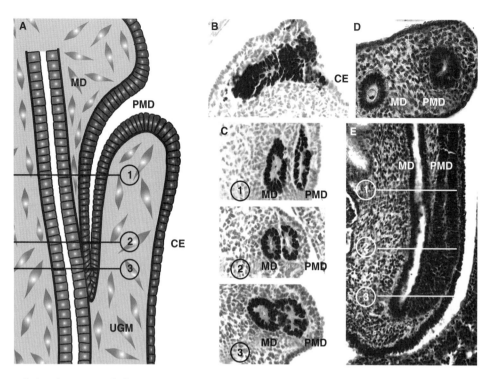

Figure 1.1   Initial development of the paramesonephric duct. CE, coelomic epithelium; MD, mesonephric duct; PMD, paramesonephric duct; UGM, urogenital mesenchyme. (**A**) Schematic drawing of PMD formation and growth. (**B, C**) Pax2 immunohistochemistry (IHC) on developing PMD of the E13.5 female mouse embryo. (**B**) The arrow indicates opening of PMD to coelom. (**C**) The numbers in this section correspond to the ones indicated in A. (**D, E**) H&E-stained sections of a human fetus (Carnegie stage 19). (**D**) A cross-section of developing MD and PMD at the cranial portion (corresponding to ① in A and E). PMD and MD are segregated by intervening mesenchymal cells. (**E**) A longitudinal section of developing human MD and PMD. PMD makes contact with MD at the caudal end. PMD arises as an invagination of coelomic epithelium at the cranial end of the urogenital ridge. The site of infolding remains open throughout development (arrows). PMD grows caudally through the UGM and the tip comes into contact with the MD within a common basement membrane. Later, the tip of growing PMD maintains close contact with MD while the cranial portion is dissociated from MD. Cross sections reveal three distinct special arrangements of PMD and MD: ① PMD and MD, each surrounded by basement membranes, are separated by intervening mesenchymal cells; ② both ducts are surrounded by individual basement membranes that are in contact on one side; and ③ direct contact between paramesonephric and mesonephric duct epithelial cells without an intervening basement membrane.

growth, the tip of the paramesonephric duct comes into intimate contact with the mesonephric duct within a common basement membrane[10] (Figure 1.1A,C3,E). The anatomical relationship between these two duct systems was well described by a classical study, which identified an essential role of the mesonephric duct in the development of the paramesonephric duct. In this study, a surgical disruption of the mesonephric duct caused discontinuation of the caudal elongation of the paramesonephric duct in a chick embryo.[10] This notion has also been confirmed in mice; conditional inactivation of the *Lim1* gene in the epithelium of the mesonephric duct induces regression of the already formed mesonephric duct by E11.5 (see Table 1.1), and the elongation of the paramesonephric duct is subsequently blocked at the breakpoint in the mesonephric duct.[11] It was further noted in this study that the initial formation of the paramesonephric duct appears to be independent of the presence of the mesonephric duct, unlike its elongation process. In this conditional knockout mouse, the invagination of the coelomic epithelium occurs even when the most cranial portion of the mesonephric duct, adjacent to the region of the paramesonephric duct formation, is absent.[11]

ORIGIN OF PARAMESONEPHRIC DUCT EPITHELIUM

The initial segment of the paramesonephric duct is formed as an invagination of coelomic epithelial cells into the urogenital ridge mesenchyme (see Figure 1.1). However, the cellular origin of the paramesonephric duct during its caudal growth is not fully established. One of the three theories currently proposed states that the paramesonephric duct forms solely by proliferation of the coelomic epithelium into the underlying mesenchyme, and the mesonephric duct simply acts as a guide for the paramesonephric duct growth.[9] In the second theory, the paramesonephric duct totally or partially splits off from the mesonephric duct after they make intimate contact with each other.[10] It has also been speculated in the third theory that the growing tip of the paramesonephric duct may induce transformation of the surrounding mesenchymal cells into paramesonephric duct epithelium. Such a phenomenon has been observed in the caudal growth of the mesonephric duct in *Xenopus*.[12]

The cellular origin of the paramesonephric duct epithelium, as proposed by these theories, may be revealed by performing transgenic mice experiments using cell-lineage labeling specific for the mesonephric duct epithelium (e.g. *Hoxb7-Cre* mice)[13] or paramesonephric duct mesenchyme (e.g. *Amhr2-Cre* mice).[14] For example, crossing the *Hoxb7-Cre* mouse strain with a reporter mouse for cre-recombinase activity (e.g. *ACTB-Bgeo/GFP* mouse)[15] would elucidate the mesonephric duct involvement in the formation of the paramesonephric duct.

Establishment of sexual dimorphism in urogenital organs

Both mesonephric and paramesonephric ducts form in male and female embryos; however, the mesonephric ducts in females and the paramesonephric ducts in males regress as embryos develop. Initially, embryos have bipotential gonads, which can develop into either testis or ovary. In males of the mammalian species, expression of the *Sry* gene (sex-determining region on the Y chromosome) activates a molecular signaling cascade, leading to the testicular differentiation of the bipotential gonad.[16] In the absence of *Sry* expression, the indifferent gonad differentiates into an ovary, and the embryo becomes a female as default. The developing testis in embryo with Y chromosome produces two key hormones for male urogenital development: (1) Müllerian inhibiting substance (MIS) or anti-Müllerian hormone (AMH) produced by Sertoli cells and (2) testosterone produced by Leydig cells.

MIS/AMH is a glycoprotein belonging to the transforming growth factor β (TGFβ) superfamily, and its action through receptors in mesenchymal cells induces apoptosis of the paramesonephric duct mesenchymal and epithelial cells, resulting in regression of the paramesonephric ducts in male embryos.[17] In females, the paramesonephric ducts remain due to the absence of MIS/AMH and eventually develop into the oviduct, uterus, cervix, and vagina.

Although the initial formation of the mesonephric duct occurs independent of testosterone, this male hormone is essential for survival and further development of this duct into epididymis, vas deferens, and seminal vesicle. In female embryos, the mesonephric duct degenerates due to the absence of testosterone.[18]

Lateral and vertical fusion of the paramesonephric ducts

Originally, the cranial portion of the paramesonephric duct lies laterally to the mesonephric duct within the mesenchyme of the urogenital ridge (Figure 1.2A). As the right and left paramesonephric ducts approach the urogenital sinus, they cross the mesonephric ducts ventrally to join (Figure 1.2B) and fuse with each other in the midline (Figuer 1.2C,D)[8] (see Table 1.1). A recent human embryological study has demonstrated that the caudal tips of the paramesonephric ducts remain separated to keep physical contact with the mesonephric ducts on both sides, while the midportions of the paramesonephric ducts remain fused together.[19] In this fusion process, the external walls of the paramesonephric ducts fuse, then the common wall (median septum) degenerates (Figure 1.2D) forming the 'genital canal' or so-called 'uterovaginal canal' in humans.[9]

Just before the paramesonephric duct tips reach the urogenital sinus, they finally become united and proceed with vertical fusion with the sinovaginal bulb[19] (see Table 1.1). The laterally fused portion of the paramesonephric ducts becomes the uterus, cervix, and/or vagina (Müllerian vagina), depending on the species (see 'Uterine types of mammals' section).

Origin of vaginal epithelium

Dual (urogenital sinus and paramesonephric duct) origin model

Despite the homogeneous differentiation process, the epithelium in the adult vagina is widely believed to have a dual origin.[20] In this view, the upper portion of the vagina develops from the caudal portion of the fused paramesonephric ducts (Müllerian vagina), and its lower portion develops from the urogenital

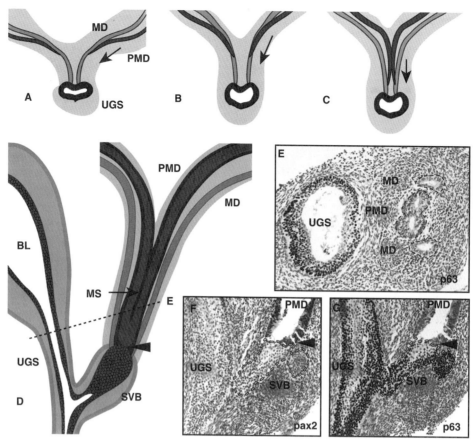

Figure 1.2 Caudal growth and fusion of the paramesonephric ducts. PMD, paramesonephric duct; MD, mesonephric duct; SVB, sinovaginal bulb; UGS, urogenital sinus; BL, bladder. (**A–D**) Schematic drawings of the developing paramesonephric ducts. PMDs remain in contact with MDs and use them as a guide during their caudal growth (**A**). As PMDs grow caudally, they cross over MDs (**B**) and meet in the midline to fuse with each other (**C**). The caudal tips of the paramesonephric ducts remain separated to keep contact with MDs (**C**).[19] Just before the PMD tips reach the urogenital sinus, they finally become united and proceed with the vertical fusion with SVB (**D**).[19] The boundary between PMD and SVB is indicated by a black arrowhead. The dotted line in **D** corresponds to the cross section **E**, at which level, canals of fused PMDs are still divided by the median septum (arrow, MS). (**E**) Immunohistochemisry (IHC) for p63 on a cross section of developing female urogenital ducts at E16.5. Epithelial cells in UGS are positive for p63. Remaining MD (circled by dotted blue lines) and two PMDs with the median septum dividing two canals (circled by a dotted red line) are observed. (**F, G**) Longitudinal sections of the E16.5 female mouse embryo at the PMD/SVB fusion. The origin of epithelial cells is highlighted by IHC. Pax2 staining indicates PMD origin in **F** and the p63 staining indicates UGS origin in **G**. The boundary between these two structures is indicated by a black arrowhead. (See also color plate section.)

sinus (sinus vagina). In female embryos, the paramesonephric ducts reach the urogenital sinus and the solid tip of the fused paramesonephric ducts fuses with the precursor of sinus vagina, the sinovaginal bulb, which is a projection of a solid epithelial cord growing out from a dorsal wall of the urogenital sinus (see Figure 1.2D,F,G).[20,21] The union of these two structures forms a solid epithelial cord without lumen (vaginal plate) connecting the paramesonephric duct and urogenital sinus.[8] In the dual-origin hypothesis, the vaginal plate consists of both paramesonephric duct and urogenital sinus epithelial cells. The growth of the vaginal plate is synchronized with canalization of the solid epithelial cord to form the caudal portion of the vagina.[20]

The dual-origin theory explains very well the developmental process of some human conditions such as the Mayer–Rokitansky–Küster–Hauser (MRKH) syndrome. In a patient with MRKH syndrome, the caudal portion of the shallow vagina, presumably urogenital sinus origin, exists, but most paramesonephric duct derivatives (from the uterus to the upper vagina) are rudimental or completely missing.[22] This observation raises the possibility that the vagina may have two developmental origins.

The presence of the caudal two-fifths of the vaginae in *Tfm* (testicular feminization mutation)-affected male mice also provides a strong support for the dual-origin model.[23] *Tfm* is a spontaneous mutation of androgen receptor causing insensitivity to testosterone.[24] In the affected XY individual, the male reproductive tract does not develop due to the insensitivity to testosterone, and the paramesonephric duct also regresses due to the MIS/AMH produced by the testis. Therefore, the remaining short vagina in *Tfm* male mice is thought to be derived from the urogenital sinus.

Another line of evidence to support the dual-origin theory comes from grafting experiments of mouse vaginal anlagen. In late embryonic and newborn mice, the vagina can be easily divided into sinus-derived (sinovaginal bulb) and paramesonephric duct-derived regions. When isolated vaginal anlagen are grafted separately under the kidney capsules of adult female hosts, both the sinovaginal bulb and the caudal portion of the paramesonephric duct will develop into a mature vagina.[25–27]

Tissue recombination experiments have clearly demonstrated that the epithelial cells in the paramesonephric duct and the sinovaginal bulb have different origins. For example, epithelial cells taken only from the paramesonephric duct, not from the sinovaginal bulb or the mesonephric duct, can be induced to become uterine epithelium when combined with uterine mesenchyme.[25,28] In contrast, epithelial cells only from the sinovaginal bulb can be induced to become prostatic epithelium by urogenital sinus mesenchyme.[25,28] These results suggest that the epithelial cord in the sinovaginal bulb is of endodermal origin, not of mesodermal paramesonephric or mesonephric duct origin.

It has been suggested that the dual origin of the vaginal epithelium may not be maintained in the adult mouse. Boutin and Cunha made vaginal tissue recombinants in which the Müllerian or sinus vaginal epithelia were combined with the Müllerian or sinus mesenchyme. They found that only the recombinants with the Müllerian epithelium exhibited normal differentiation in response to hormonal treatment, although both types of the recombinants containing the Müllerian and sinus epithelia formed morphologically normal vagina.[26] Based upon this result, they proposed that the vaginal epithelium is initially derived from both paramesonephric duct and urogenital sinus, but the Müllerian vaginal epithelium displaces the sinus vaginal epithelium during maturation. The replacement of the sinus vaginal epithelium by the Müllerian vaginal cells is thought to result from a higher proliferation rate observed in the latter tissue than the former.

Paramesonephric and mesonephric ducts'
origin model

In comparison with the theory stated above, some believe that the entire vagina is formed as a caudal growth of the paramesonephric duct with some involvement of the mesonephric duct.[7,29] A 3D reconstruction study performed by Drews et al demonstrated that the small caudal portions of the paramesonephric and mesonephric ducts remain attached to the urogenital sinus in *Tfm* mice, reflecting the possibility of the ductal remnants contributing to the formation of the sinovaginal bulb and the short vagina of *Tfm* mice. Therefore, the originally believed urogenital sinus origin of the vaginal pouch in *Tfm*-affected male mice is in doubt. In this alternative view, the normal vagina is thought to arise entirely by downward growth of the mesonephric and paramesonephric ducts. Furthermore, the presence of remaining mesonephric duct epithelial cells at the junction between the paramesonephric duct and sinovaginal bulb in female embryos has been well documented.[7,8,21,30] In addition, Forsberg suggested that the mesonephric duct contributes to the formation of the vaginal plate epithelium in humans because the cellular morphology and histochemical characteristics of the vaginal plate appear similar to those of the mesonephric duct epithelium.[21]

The contribution of the mesonephric duct to vaginal development may be delineated in mice using cell-lineage labeling specific for the mesonephric duct epithelium, as previously discussed in the 'Origin of paramesonephric duct epithelium' section.

Molecules involved in the development of the paramesonephric duct

The emergence of gene-targeted mutagenesis studies has unquestionably expanded our knowledge in the field of biology, and has provided a wealth of information on key molecules involved in embryogenesis for almost two decades. This section of the chapter presents some of the critical genes and their roles in the development of the paramesonephric duct.

Lim1 plays a primary role in the formation of the mesonephric and paramesonephric ducts, as such ductal systems have been shown to be lacking in *Lim1*-null mutant mice.[31] A study by Kobayashi et al has highlighted the essential role of Lim1 in the paramesonephric duct epithelial differentiation.[31] When *Lim1-/-/Rosa26* ES embryonic stem cells were injected into wild-type blastocysts, the resulting chimeric female mice developed the paramesonephric duct, uterus, and oviduct normally. However, *Lim1-/-* cells contributed only to the mesenchyme of these structures, not to the epithelial cells,[31] indicating that Lim1 expression is essential for differentiation of the paramesonephric duct epithelium.

Wnt4 is another molecule that is involved in the initial formation of the paramesonephric duct and is expressed in the coelomic epithelium and the mesenchyme surrounding the paramesonephric duct.[32] The distinctive phenotype of the *Wnt4*[-/-] mice is the lack of invagination of the coelomic epithelium. Interestingly, *Lim1* expression persists in these mutant mice in the coelomic epithelium at the anterior end of the mesonephros, where the invagination would be expected to occur in normal mice. These observations suggest that Wnt4 is required for the invagination of the coelomic epithelium but dispensable for differentiation of the paramesonephric duct precursor cells.[31]

A study of *Wnt9b*[-/-] mouse demonstrated that the paramesonephric duct fails to grow caudally to converge with the mesonephric duct despite the formation of the initial segment.[33] This phenotype in the paramesonephric duct disappears when loss of Wnt9b is compensated by targeted expression of Wnt1, which presumably can activate the same signaling cascade as Wnt9b, in the mesonephric duct epithelium. This indicates that the expression of Wnt9b in the mesonephric duct epithelium is essential for the elongation of the paramesonephric duct towards the mesonephric duct.[33] It can be speculated that paracrine interactions between these two duct systems may exist even before they make physical contact, and that Wnt9b may play a primary role in such interactions.

Pax2 is not required for the formation of the initial segment of the paramesonephric duct; however, it appears essential for the survival and caudal elongation of this duct.[31,34] Pax2 is normally expressed in the epithelial cells of the mesonephric and paramesonephric ducts. In the *Pax2*[-/-] mouse, the mesonephric duct initially forms by E9.5, but its caudal growth is arrested and starts to regress by E12.5. Similarly, only the cranial segment of the paramesonephric duct forms by E11.5 in the *Pax2*[-/-] mouse, and it degenerates by E16.5 in both sexes.[34]

Emx2 is expressed in the coelomic and paramesonephric duct as well as in the mesonephric duct epithelial cells. In *Emx2*[-/-] mice, the mesonephric duct forms normally, but its degeneration can be observed by E11.5 and the paramesonephric duct never forms.[35] Since Emx2 is normally expressed in the coelomic epithelium, it may be involved in the differentiation of the paramesonephric duct epithelial cells, which is thought to be the initial step of

paramesonephric duct development. Furthermore, Emx2 has been shown to play a role in maintaining Pax2 expression in the mesonephric duct epithelium,[35] whose presence is essential for par mesonephric duct survival.[34]

Retinoids (vitamin A and metabolites) act as morphogens during embryogenesis and also play an important role in the formation of the paramesonephric ducts. It has been previously shown that vitamin A deficiency in the rat causes agenesis of the paramesonephric ducts.[36] The morphogenetic effects of retinoids are mediated by two families of nuclear receptors – retinoic acid receptors (RARs) and retinoid X receptors (RXRs) – each consisting of three types (α, β, and γ) with several isoforms of each type. A null mutant mouse for a single type of RAR or RXR appears developmentally normal, probably due to the functional redundancy among RAR/RXR receptors. However, the compound mutants for RARα + RARβ or γ, or compound mutants for RXRα + RARα, β, or γ show a partial or complete agenesis of the paramesonephric duct.[37,38]

One of the mechanisms through which retinoids specify body axis during embryogenesis is by regulating *Hox* gene expression.[39] This may be the case in paramesonephric duct development. In the developing paramesonephric duct, *Abdominal B Hox* genes are expressed in a coordinated way,[40,41] and their gene products control specification of the paramesonephric duct-derived organs (see 'Genes regulating differentiation of the paramesonephric duct' section). Knockout studies showed that the caudal portion of the paramesonephric duct is missing in *Hoxa13*[-/-] embryos, and the fusion between the paramesonephric duct and urogenital sinus is incomplete or missing in *Hoxa13*[+/-]/*Hoxd-13*[+/-] mutant mice.[42]

The essential role of *Hox* genes in paramesonephric duct formation is also suggested by the phenotype of the *Pbx1*[-/-] mouse, which has the intact mesonephric duct but lacks the paramesonephric duct. Pbx1 is a cofactor for Hox transcription factors, and it is expressed in the mesenchymal and epithelial cells of the paramesonephric duct.[43] Impaired function of *Hox* genes in *Pbx1*[-/-] mice may, thus, cause the failure in paramesonephric duct development.

Wnt5a has been demonstrated to regulate the proximal–distal outgrowth of diverse structures (e.g. limb, external genitalia, and tail) during embryogenesis.[44] In the null mutant mouse for *Wnt5a*, the posterior growth of the paramesonephric duct is affected; thus most of the cervix and the entire Müllerian vagina are absent.[45]

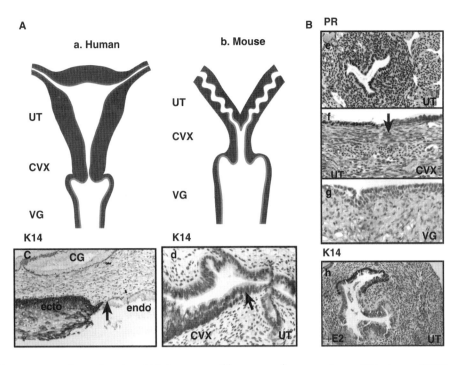

Figure 1.3 Adult uterus, cervix, and vagina. (**A**) Anatomy of human and mouse uterus. UT, uterus; CVX, cervix; VG, vagina. The location of the squamocolumnar junction is indicated by an arrow. (**a**) Simplex uterus of the human. The fused portion of the paramesonephric ducts forms a single uterus with one cervix and one vagina. The squamocolumnar junction is located between the endocervix and ectocervix. (**b**) Duplex uterus of mouse. The lateral fusion of the paramesonephric ducts does not occur at the uterine level, but does occur at the vagina and in the middle of the cervix. Two uterine canals open into two independent cervices, and the two cervices are connected into a single common cervical canal. The squamocolumnar junction is located between the uterus and cervix. (**c**) Keratin 14 expression in the human cervix. It is expressed in epithelial cells of the ectocervix (ecto) but not in those of the endocervix (endo). CG, cervical gland. (**d**) Keratin 14 expression in the mouse cervix. K14 is expressed in the epithelial cells of the cervix (CVX) but not in the uterus (UT). (**B**) Squamocolumnar junction in the postaxial hemimelia (px) mouse. (**e–g**) Immunohistochemistry (IHC) for progesterone receptor (PR); (**h**) IHC for K14. Female px (spontaneous *Wnt7a* mutant) mice were ovariectomized at postnatal day 35 and the expressions of PR and K14 were analyzed at postnatal day 60. In these mice, PR was constitutively expressed in the uterine epithelium (**e,f**), indicating normal uterine epithelial differentiation.[55] In contrast, PR was absent in the cervical and vaginal epithelia (**f,g**). The PR expression pattern was abruptly changed at the squamocolumnar junction (arrow in **f**). Cervical and vaginal epithelia were positive for K14, while such expression was absent in uterine epithelium in the ovariectomized px mice (not shown), indicating normal uterine and cervicovaginal epithelial differentiation. However, when the ovariectomized px mice were treated with 125 ng estradiol/day for 3 days, K14-positive stratified squamous epithelium appeared in a region of the uterus (**h**). These observations indicate that Wnt7a is required to maintain proper epithelial differentiation in the adult uterus, while it is dispensable for uterine and vaginal epithelial differentiation in the neonatal stage. (See also color plate section.)

ANATOMY OF THE UTERUS

The basic structure

Although morphology of the uterus is quite diverse among species, its basic structure is common among all mammals. The uterine corpus(es) (body), where the embryo (egg for monotmers) develops, tapers to a narrow neck (cervix), and the cervix opens into the vagina (Figure 1.3A). The body of the uterus consists of endometrium and myometrium. The endometrium (uterine mucosa) is the innermost layer that lines the cavity, providing the environment for egg/fetal development and consists of columnar epithelium supported by cellular stroma containing tubular glands. The myometrium is the main bulk of the uterus, which is composed of layers of smooth muscle.

Uterine types of mammals

The morphological diversity of the uterus among mammalian species is reflected by the degree of lateral fusion of the two paramesonephric ducts. For example, a duplex uterus of rabbits and mice (Figure 1.3Ab) lacks the paramesonephric duct fusion in the uterus, creating two separate uterine horns that open into two cervices (two bodies + two cervices). In comparison, a bipartite uterus (in dogs and pigs) consists of two uterine horns that fuse immediately above the common opening to the cervix (two bodies + one cervix). A bicornuate uterus (in cows and horses) also has a pair of uterine horns and one cervix, but the cranially fused paramesonephric ducts form a large uterine body. The complete fusion of the paramesonephric ducts in the uterine segment forms a simplex uterus (in higher primates including human, Figure 1.3Aa), which consists of a single uterine body (one body + one cervix).

MORPHOGENESIS OF THE UTERUS

During female reproductive tract development, the paramesonephric duct undergoes a dynamic transformation from a homogeneous cellular structure into a heterogeneous state via acquisition of defined cell fates and functions in different segments. In both humans and mice, the paramesonephric duct in the late stage of development will differentiate into the oviduct (the fallopian tube), uterus, cervix, and vagina in a cranial to caudal order.

The uterus develops from the middle to upper portion of the paramesonephric duct. The developmental processes of this organ include differentiation of the paramesonephric duct epithelium into luminal and glandular subpopulations and differentiation of the surrounding urogenital ridge mesenchyme into endometrial stroma and myometrium.

Epithelial differentiation in the paramesonephric duct

At the late embryonic stage, the entire paramesonephric duct is uniformly lined by undifferentiated columnar epithelium (Figure 1.4A,E), even though the oviduct, uterus, cervix, and vagina are anatomically distinguishable.[27,46] Notably, in the mouse, the major part of organ-specific epithelial morphogenesis occurs postnatally (see Table 1.1).

In the oviduct development, the undifferentiated columnar epithelial cells of the paramesonephric duct origin differentiate into ciliated and secretory cells of the simple columnar epithelium, which lines the inner wall of the adult oviduct. In the mouse, cilliation of the epithelial cells in the oviduct is first observed at postnatal day 5.[47]

In the mouse uterine epithelium, expression of differentiation markers such as estrogen receptor α (ERα) and progesterone receptor (PR)[46] is established in the first week of its postnatal development[46]

(Figure 1.4), followed by uterine gland differentiation. In the mouse, the uterine epithelium shows a sign of morphogenesis at postnatal day 4–5 (Figure 1.4B,F),[48] and the rudimentary uterine gland is recognized at postnatal day 7[46] (Figure 1.4C,D). The ontogeny of differentiation markers and uterine gland shows slight variation among mouse strains, and the timing of events described above may not match exactly in some strains.[49] In the human, uterine gland formation is also known to occur late in uterine development. Endometrial glands appear in the fetal period; however, they are formed shallow on the surface of the endometrium, and further growth of these glands occurs postnatally.[50] The topic of postnatal development is not covered in this chapter.

In the cervix and vagina, the undifferentiated columnar epithelial cells undergo dramatic morphological changes and are transformed into stratified squamous epithelium.[51] This squamous transformation of the paramesonephric duct epithelium progresses from caudal (vaginal plate) to cranial.[27,52]

Formation of the squamocolumnar junction

Mouse

As a result of organ-specific epithelial differentiation, a boundary termed the squamocolumnar junction forms between columnar and squamous epithelia of the uterus and cervix. In the mouse, the squamocolumnar junction is located in the caudal portion of each uterine horn where the uterine and cervical epithelia meet (Figure 1.3Ab).

The stratified squamous epithelium of the cervix/vagina and the simple columnar epithelium of the uterus are distinctive in their morphology as well as in their gene expression. For example, keratin 14 is essential to maintain the integrity of squamous epithelium[53,54] and is expressed in the vaginal and cervical but not in the uterine epithelium. Progesterone receptor (PR) is also differentially expressed in the epithelial cells of the mouse uterus and vagina (Figure 1.3B). In most estrogen target cells/tissues, PR is up-regulated by estrogen via ERα, as observed in the vaginal epithelial cells.[55] What is interesting in the mouse uterine epithelium, however, is that PR is expressed constitutively, which occurs independently of 17β-estradiol and ERα.[55] In fact, its expression is down-regulated in the mouse uterine epithelium by 17β-estradiol acting through ERα in the stromal cells.[55] This unusual pattern of PR regulation is unique for the uterine epithelial cells of rodents.

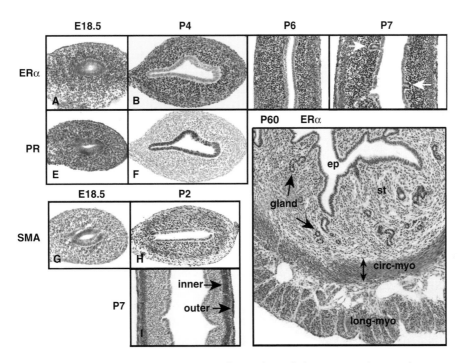

Figure 1.4 Morphogenesis of C57/B6 mouse uterus: ep, luminal epithelium; st, endometrial stroma; circ-myo, circular (inner) myometrium; long-myo, longitudinal (outer) myometrium. Immunohistochemistry (IHC) for estrogen receptor α (ERα) (**A–D, J**), progesterone receptor (PR) (**E,F**) α-smooth muscle actin (SMA) (**G–I**). Epithelial differentiation: at embryonic day 18.5 (E18.5), ERα (**A**) and PR (**E**) are not expressed in the uterine epithelial cells, while the mesenchymal cells show strong immunoreactivity for ERα (**A**). From a late embryonic stage to postnatal day 3 (P3), the uterine epithelium forms a simple tube with an oval-shaped lumen in a transverse view (**H**). At P4, the uterine epithelial tube shows a sign of morphogenesis as several epithelial evaginations protrude into the surrounding mesenchyme (**B,F**). At this stage, epithelial cells are mostly negative for ERα (**B**) but already strongly positive for PR (**F**). Although the epithelial evaginations can be observed as early as P4, uterine glands are totally absent at P6 (**C**) and cannot be observed until P7 (**D**, arrows). In the adult uterus (P60), the uterine epithelium forms an irregular, tubular shape with many folds that protrude into the stroma (**J**). Fully developed uterine glands are projected from the uterine canal deeply into the endometrial stroma (**J**). The entire epithelium is positive for ERα. Stromal differentiation: α-smooth muscle actin (SMA) was undetectable in the embryonic uterine mesenchyme (**G**). At P2, the expression of SMA is detected in the outer layer of the unorganized uterine mesenchyme (**H**). By P7, smooth muscle layers are organized into inner circular and outer longitudinal myometrial layers (**I**). Most inner layer surrounding the epithelium differentiates into endometrial stroma. In the adult uterus (P60), the myometrial layers form a thick circular inner myometrium (circ-myo) and a longitudinal outer myometrium (long-myo) with bundles of smooth muscle (**J**). (See also color plate section.)

Human

In the human, the adult cervix is divided into two regions – endocervix and ectocervix – each of which is covered with a different type of epithelium. The endocervix is lined by simple columnar mucinous epithelium with cervical glands (Figure 1.3Ac), while epithelial cells in the ectocervix and vagina are a stratified squamous type.[56] Therefore, in humans, the squamocolumnar junction forms between the endocervical (columnar) and ectocervical (stratified squamous) epithelia (Figure 1.3Aa).[56]

Mesenchymal induction of epithelial differentiation

The epithelial–mesenchymal interactions play a significant role in organ specification during embryogenesis, as demonstrated in the tooth,[57] lung,[58] and gastrointestinal tracts,[59] as well as in the urogenital tracts.[60] In the paramesonephric duct, epithelial cytodifferentiation is dictated by regional fates of the surrounding mesenchyme.[61] For example, the paramesonephric duct epithelial cells require an instructive induction by the uterine mesenchyme to express uterine epithelial cytodifferentiation.[52] Similarly, the vaginal mesenchyme induces vaginal epithelial differentiation in the paramesonephric duct, and the columnar paramesonephric duct epithelial cells consequently become stratified squamous vaginal cells. Thus, the location of the squamocolumnar junction is ultimately determined by the regional difference in the inductive activity of the uterine and cervical/vaginal mesenchyme.[46,52]

The role of mesenchyme in differentiation of the paramesonephric duct epithelium has been esta lished by a series of tissue recombination studies, in which the mesenchyme and epithelium isolated from the uterus and vagina of newborn mice were recombined.[25,46,61,62] The tissue recombinants were grown as grafts under the renal capsule of adult female hosts. Uterine mesenchyme induced vaginal epithelium to differentiate into a uterine epithelium containing both luminal epithelial cells and glands.[61,62] The induced uterine epithelium expressed a spectrum of differentiation markers characteristic of a normal uterine and not vaginal epithelium such as uterine-type syndecans.[62] PR was also expressed in the uterine pattern in the induced uterine epithelial cells.[46] In the reciprocal tissue recombinants, vaginal mesenchyme induced uterine epithelium to differentiate into stratified squamous epithelium, which showed mucification and cornification as in the host vagina in response to the estrus cycle.[25,61,62] The induced vaginal epithelium expressed vaginal differentiation markers such as the vaginal isoform of syndecan,[62] involucrin, and keratins 1, 10, 14, and 19.[46] In the induced vaginal epithelium, PR was also expressed in the vaginal pattern.[46]

When heterotypic tissue recombinants (uterine epithelium + vaginal mesenchyme and vaginal epithelium + uterine mesenchyme) were made with tissues from mice younger than 5 days old, epithelial cells were uniformly induced by uterine or vaginal mesenchyme to switch their developmental fate.[46,61] However, heterotypic tissue recombinants made with uterine/vaginal tissues from 7-day-old or older neonatal mice exhibited heterogeneous differentiation in response to heterotypic mesenchymal inducers.[46,61] This indicates that the developmental fates of the uterine and vaginal epithelia are determined by the influence of the uterine or vaginal mesenchyme during the first week of postnatal development, and the developmental plasticity of epithelial cells is gradually lost thereafter. Most adult uterine and vaginal epithelial cells, therefore, cannot be re-programmed by newborn uterine or vaginal mesenchyme to express other epithelial phenotypes.[46,52]

Differentiation of uterine stroma

Uterine mesenchymal cells (Figure 1.4G) differentiate into endometrial fibroblasts and myometrial smooth muscle cells of the adult uterus. In the mouse, by postnatal day 3, randomly oriented uterine mesenchymal cells begin to organize into three layers: inner layer; a precursor for the endometrial stroma, and middle and outer layers; precursors for inner and outer myometrium.[48] By this time, the inner circular myometrial layer starts to show positive staining for α-smooth muscle actin (SMA, Figure 1.4H), a marker for smooth muscle cytodifferentiation.[48] The three layers of the uterine stroma become morphologically distinct at postnatal day 5, forming radially oriented endometrial stromal fibroblasts, inner circular myometrial, and outer prospective longitudinal myometrial layers (Figure 1.4I). This differentiation/organization process of the uterine stroma is regulated by uterine epithelium.[48] When undifferentiated uterine mesenchyme from newborn mice is grown by itself for 1 month under the renal capsule of adult female hosts, only a few actin-positive myometrial cells develop in the grafts. In contrast, when the undifferentiated uterine mesenchyme is combined with uterine epithelium and grown as a renal capsule graft for 1 month, a substantial amount of myometrial smooth muscle develops in the graft.[63]

The epithelial factor regulating uterine stromal differentiation appears to be commonly expressed in the mouse and human. This is demonstrated when human endometrial epithelial cells are combined with newborn mouse uterine mesenchyme; the mouse uterine mesenchymal cells are induced to differentiate into endometrial fibroblasts and myometrial smooth muscle cells and organized into layers of endometrium and myometrium.[64] This observation suggests that, similar to the mouse system, stromal differentiation in the human uterus is probably induced by uterine epithelial cells.

Wnt7a, expressed in the developing and adult uterine epithelium, is a candidate involved in the epithelial–mesenchymal interaction during the uterine stromal differentiation.[65] This potential role of Wnt7a is suggested by the observation made in *Wnt7a*[-/-] mice, in which the endometrial stroma layer is hypoplastic and the inner circular myometrium is disorganized.[66]

Genes regulating differentiation of the paramesonephric duct

p63, a homologue of p53 tumor suppressor, plays a key role in cervical/vaginal epithelial differentiation.[52] In the female reproductive tract, p63 is expressed in epithelial cells of the cervix and vagina, but not in the uterus. In the absence of p63, the mouse cervical/vaginal epithelium differentiates into a uterine epithelium.[52] It, therefore, acts as an identity switch for uterine and vaginal/cervical epithelial cells. A tissue recombination study has demonstrated that p63 is induced in the paramesonephric duct epithelial cells by cervical/vaginal mesenchyme. In contrast, uterine mesenchyme turns off its expression and induces uterine epithelial differentiation of originally p63-positive neonatal vaginal epithelium.[52]

Hox (mouse; *HOX* in human) genes provide positional information along the body axis in embryogenesis.[67] *Abdominal B Hox/HOX* genes are expressed in a spatially coordinated pattern through caudal to cranial axis in the developing paramesonephric duct and its derivatives in adulthood.[40,41,68] For example, in the mouse, *Hoxa9* to *Hoxa13* genes are expressed in the following pattern: *Hoxa-9*, from the isthmus of the oviduct to the uterocervical junction; *Hoxa10*, from the future uterotubal junction to the cervix; *Hoxa11*, in the uterus and cervix; and *Hoxa13*, in the cervix and vagina.[40] Upon receiving this positional information, cells become committed to specific cell fates, whereby a female reproductive organ identity is established for each segment of the paramesonephric duct. The significance of this particular special expression pattern of *Hox* genes is shown in the phenotype of *Hoxa10*[-/-] mouse, in which the cranial end of the uterus transforms into an oviduct-like structure.[69]

In the mouse female reproductive tract, *Hoxa* and *Hoxd* genes are expressed predominantly in the mesenchyme. It is believed that the regulatory information encoded by *Hox* genes in the mesenchyme determines the sequential gene expressions in this mesenchymal tissue, which in turn direct organ-specific cytodifferentiation of associated epithelial cells. For example, expression of *Hoxa13/HOXA13* in the vaginal mesenchyme gives this embryonic tissue an ability to induce p63 expression in the paramesonephric duct epithelial cells, which will lead to vaginal epithelial differentiation. The function of *Hoxa13* in cervical/vaginal epithelial differentiation is demonstrated in *A11*[13hd/13hd] mouse, in which the homeobox sequence of *Hoxa11* is replaced with that of *Hoxa13*, and the uterine epithelium is transformed into a vagina-like stratified squamous epithelium.[70]

Expression of *Hoxa10* and *Hoxa11* is lost in the uterine stroma of adult *Wnt7a*[-/-] mice by 16 weeks of age, and stratification of uterine epithelial cells is observed in the adult mutant mouse.[66] This appears to be another example highlighting the importance of proper stromal *Hox* gene expression during epithelial differentiation of the paramesonephric duct. There is also a spontaneous mutant strain of *Wnt7a* called *postaxial hemimelia* (*px*).[71] In this mutant mouse, uterine and vaginal epithelial cells show normal differentiation before puberty, and a normal squamocolumnar junction forms (Figure 1.3B). Therefore, Wnt7a is probably dispensable for specification of the uterine epithelial cell fate during neonatal development. However, 17β-estradiol treatment for young adult *px* mouse induces transformation of the uterine epithelium into stratified squamous epithelium (Figure 1.3Bh), suggesting an essential role of Wnt7a in the maintenance of proper epithelial cytodifferentiation in the adult uterus.

HUMAN CONGENITAL ANOMALIES

The prevalence of congenital uterine anomalies varies significantly among different studies, making it difficult to arrive at an exact estimate. Despite this wide range of prevalence reported, a higher rate of these abnormalities is generally identified in infertile women compared to the general public, implicating a causal association between the anomalies and adverse pregnancy outcome.

Congenital uterine anomalies vary in type and extent of the affected reproductive structures. Whereas the most severe case such as a complete septate uterus[72] may require surgical treatment to restore reproductive capacity, some remain undetected. Regardless of the severity of the disorders, the potential obstetrical complications present a serious health concern to women and create an emotional burden on the family.[73] Therefore, it is crucial to study the mechanism of how such anomalies are derived from developmental inaccuracy, which will be the main focus of this section of the chapter.

Failure in paramesonephric duct formation

If both sides of the paramesonephric ducts are affected (bilateral agenesis), there is a total absence of the uterus, cervix, and upper vagina, or the presence of rudimental paramesonephric duct-derived organs.[74] If only one duct is affected (unilateral agenesis), the unaffected single paramesonephric duct forms a unicornuate (single-horned) uterus with a cervix and vagina. As mentioned earlier in this chapter, normal development of the mesonephric duct is a prerequisite for development of the metanephros as well as for the paramesonephric duct. Therefore, a defect in mesonephric duct development can result in agenesis of both the paramesonephric duct and kidney systems. Indeed, urological disorders are found in 20–30% of women with uterine anomalies.[75] In the case of unilateral agenesis, renal defects are commonly found on the same side that the paramesonephric duct is affected.[76–79] These observations suggest that some conditions with paramesonephric duct agenesis are caused by developmental defects in the mesonephric duct.

Failure in lateral fusion of the paramesonephric duct

Similar to the mechanism creating the marked diversity in uterine types across mammalian species, different degrees of paramesonephric duct fusion during development cause various female reproductive tract abnormalities in human.[80] One example of these congenital anomalies is a didelphic uterus, which is caused by complete failure in lateral fusion of the paramesonephric ducts. Women with this condition have two sets of the uterus, cervix and vagina. In bicornuate and septate uteri, the ducts do fuse together, but the integration point occurs at the uterine segment. Although patients with these disorders develop a single cervix and vagina due to successful paramesonephric duct fusion at the caudal portion, they present an abnormal uterus formation. While a bicornuate uterus has two horns, a septate uterus appears externally normal with one uterine body, but it has remnants of the median septum (see Figure 1.2) protruding down from the cranial wall, dividing the inner chamber into two. Depending on the severity of the protrusion, the inner chamber may be completely or partially separated.[74,80]

Failure in fusion of the paramesonephric duct and the urogenital sinus

Not only failure in lateral fusion of the two paramesonephric ducts leads to congenital defects but also the inability of these ducts to fuse with the sinovaginal bulb seems to cause some reproductive tract anomalies in humans. A transverse vaginal septum is thought to result from failure in the paramesonephric duct and sinovaginal bulb fusion as well as from faulty canalization of epithelial cord.[74] Because the transverse vaginal septum is commonly found at the upper and middle third of the vagina, it has been speculated that the normal duct–bulb fusion may occur at this level of the vagina.[81]

Genetic factors

Some congenital uterine anomalies have a possible hereditary etiology; however, mutations associated with most of these defects have not been identified. Many of the hereditary syndromes with uterine defects show limb/skeletal anomalies,[74] suggesting a mutation may be found in a gene commonly involved for both limb/skeletal and paramesonephric duct development such as HOX genes. Indeed, a mutation in HOXA13 has been identified and linked to an autosomal dominant disorder, hand-foot-genital (HFG) syndrome.[82] However, more studies are needed to discover genes that are responsible for other female uterine disorders.[74,79,80]

Epigenetic factors

Pathogenesis of most congenital uterine anomalies is not very well understood. The sporadic and infrequent nature of some syndromes suggests that epigenetic factors such as exposure to teratogens or exogenous hormones may be involved in the etiology of these conditions.[75]

Ovarian steroids, 17β-estradiol and progesterone, play a critical role in the function of the mature uterus by acting through their receptors. However, knockout mouse studies have revealed that ERα,[83] ERβ,[84] and PR[85] are dispensable for perinatal morphogenesis of the uterus. Although the ERα expression is present throughout the uterine development in the mesenchymal cells,[46] it is only in the late postnatal stage that ERα becomes involved in the maturation process of the uterus, including gland formation.[86] There has not been any report indicating the involvement of the other two receptors in the early uterine development. Due to the constitutive expression of ERα in the developing uterus, an exogenous estrogen such as DES (diethylstilbestrol) can have a significant impact in the uterine morphogenesis.[87]

DES-induced anomalies

DES, a synthetic non-steroidal estrogen, was prescribed largely during the 1940s to 1960s for pregnant women at high risk for miscarriage. It is estimated that more than 2 million mothers, daughters, and sons were exposed to DES in the United States alone.[87] Association of DES with clear cell adenocarcinoma, a rare form of cervical/vaginal cancer, was first established in 1971 by doctors from the Massachusetts General Hospital in Boston.[88] Cervical/vaginal adenosis, characterized by the development of columnar epithelia in the ectocervix/vagina,[89] is commonly found in DES daughters and forms the bed from which clear cell adenocarcinoma develops.[90] The incidences of adenosis and clear cell adenocarcinoma are directly related to the starting time of DES treatment during pregnancy. If it was given before gestational week 8, more than a third of DES daughters developed adenosis. In contrast, adenosis was essentially absent if DES treatment was started at week 22 or later.[90] These findings suggest that the female reproductive system is most vulnerable to DES in the early developmental stage, and the exposure during that particular period disrupts the normal paramesonephric duct development, leading to adenosis. This is confirmed by mouse studies in which animals experienced a perinatal exposure to DES and were later found to have congenital anomalies similar to those observed in DES daughters.[91–93] As in DES daughters, the frequency of cervical/vaginal adenosis in the mouse is also directly related to the timing of DES exposure.[94]

Using the mouse model, mechanisms of DES-induced female reproductive tract abnormalities have been extensively studied.[91–93] In wild-type mice, it was found that DES inhibits expression of p63 in cervical/vaginal epithelium. Although this inhibitory effect of DES on p63 expression is usually transient, it may become permanent if exposed beyond the critical period for epithelial cell fate determination in the paramesonephric duct.[52] This is demonstrated when DES is given from birth to postnatal day 5: some cervicovaginal epithelial cells never regain the ability to express p63, even after discontinuation of the DES treatment.[52] Consequently, p63-negative cervicovaginal epithelial cells differentiate into a uterine epithelium, and the transformed uterine epithelial cells form cervicovaginal adenosis. This is a good example that transient disruption of a developmental process by an exogenous signal can result in an irreversible developmental defect.

The adverse actions of DES are mediated through ERα in the paramesonephric duct derivatives. This explains the absence of obvious congenital anomalies of the female genital tract in the ERα knockout mouse perinatally exposed to DES.[95] It has also been shown that in this knockout mouse, DES elicits no inhibitory effect on p63 expression in the cervicovaginal epithelium.[52]

In the uterus, it has been shown that DES inhibits the expression of Wnt7a,[96] Hoxa10, and Hoxa11[40] via ERα.[95] This down-regulation of Hoxa10 and Hoxa11 in the uterine mesenchyme may cause uterine squamous metaplasia,[40] which is characterized by the development of cervical/vaginal epithelial cells in the uterus.[52] Likewise, down-regulation of Wnt7a, which plays an essential role in differentiation/organization of the uterine stroma, may be the central point in a constellation

of molecular events caused by neonatal DES exposure, leading to disruption of uterine stroma development.[97]

FUTURE DIRECTION IN RESEARCH OF UTERINE DEVELOPMENT

In the last 20 years, our knowledge in molecular/developmental biology has been significantly advanced by mouse studies of targeted mutagenesis. In addition, with the advent of the tissue-specific/conditional gene inactivation, we now have a rare opportunity to study the functions of particular genes in vivo without causing complications such as embryonic lethality. This is of particular importance in studying the development of the uterus because this organ develops late in embryogenesis, and as a result, the phenotypes of many null mutant mice would be impossible to study due to their early embryonic lethality or defects in structures essential for paramesonephric duct development. This novel approach of gene manipulation has certainly led to the identification of key molecules involved in developmental processes of the uterus. The coming years look exciting and promising as such genetic engineering will further broaden our knowledge in understanding normal and abnormal uterine development.

ACKNOWLEDGMENTS

The authors acknowledge Dr Yuzhuo Wang and his laboratory members for kind support with the writing of this chapter, and Dr Gerald R Cunha for providing us with a valuable collection of classic literature on uterine biology.

REFERENCES

1. Ramsey EM. History. In: Wynn RM, ed. Biology of The Uterus. New York: Plenum Press, 1977: 1–18.
2. Bordemer CW. History of the mammalian oviduct. In: Hafez ESE, Blandau RJ, eds. The Mammalian Oviduct. Chicago, IL: The University of Chicago Press, 1969: 3–26.
3. Sadler TW. Langman's Medical Embryology. Baltimore, MD: Lippincott, Williams and Wilkins, 2004.
4. Vize PD, Seufert DW, Carroll TJ et al. Model systems for the study of kidney development: use of the pronephros in the analysis of organ induction and patterning. Dev Biol 1997; 188: 189–204.
5. Ludwig KS, Landmann L. Early development of the human mesonephros. Anat Embryol (Berl) 2005; 209: 439–47.
6. Yu J, McMahon AP, Valerius MT. Recent genetic studies of mouse kidney development. Curr Opin Genet Dev 2004; 14: 550–7.
7. Witschi E. Development and differentiation of the uterus. In: Mack HC, ed. Prenatal Life. Detroit: Wayne State University Press, 1970: 11–34.

8. Koff AK. Development of the vagina in the human fetus. Contrib Embryol 1933; 24: 59–91.

9. O'Rahilly R. The embryology and anatomy of the uterus. In: Wynn RM, ed. The Uterus. Baltimore, MD: Williams & Wilkins, 1973: 17–39.

10. Grünwald P. The relation of the growing tip of the Müllerian duct to the Wolffian duct and its importance for the genesis of malformations. Anat Rec 1941; 81: 1–19.

11. Kobayashi A, Kwan KM, Carroll TJ et al. Distinct and sequential tissue-specific activities of the LIM-class homeobox gene Lim1 for tubular morphogenesis during kidney development. Development 2005; 132: 2809–23.

12. Cornish JA, Etkin LD. The formation of the pronephric duct in Xenopus involves recruitment of posterior cells by migrating pronephric duct cells. Dev Biol 1993; 159: 338–45.

13. Yu J, Carroll TJ, McMahon AP. Sonic hedgehog regulates proliferation and differentiation of mesenchymal cells in the mouse metanephric kidney. Development 2002; 129: 5301–12.

14. Jamin SP, Arango NA, Mishina Y et al. Requirement of Bmpr1a for Müllerian duct regression during male sexual development. Nat Genet 2002; 32: 408–10.

15. Lobe CG, Koop KE, Kreppner W et al. Z/AP, a double reporter for cre-mediated recombination. Dev Biol 1999; 208: 281–92.

16. Brennan J, Capel B. One tissue, two fates: molecular genetic events that underlie testis versus ovary development. Nat Rev Genet 2004; 5: 509–21.

17. Roberts LM, Hirokawa Y, Nachtigal MW et al. Paracrine-mediated apoptosis in reproductive tract development. Dev Biol 1999; 208: 110–22.

18. Wilson JD, George FW, Griffin JE. The hormonal control of sexual development. Science 1981; 211: 1278–84.

19. Hashimoto R. Development of the human Müllerian duct in the sexually undifferentiated stage. Anat Rec A Discov Mol Cell Evol Biol 2003; 272: 514–19.

20. Forsberg JG. Cervicovaginal epithelium: its origin and development. Am J Obstet Gynecol 1973; 115: 1025–43.

21. Forsberg JG. Derivation and differentiation of the vaginal epithelium. Thesis, Lund, 1963.

22. Ludwig KS. The Mayer–Rokitansky–Kuster syndrome. An analysis of its morphology and embryology. Part II: Embryology. Arch Gynecol Obstet 1998; 262: 27–42.

23. Cunha GR. The dual origin of vaginal epithelium. Am J Anat 1975; 143: 387–92.

24. Quigley CA, De Bellis A, Marschke KB et al. Androgen receptor defects: historical, clinical, and molecular perspectives. Endocr Rev 1995; 16: 271–321.

25. Boutin EL, Battle E, Cunha GR. The germ layer origin of mouse vaginal epithelium restricts its responsiveness to mesenchymal inductors: uterine induction. Differentiation 1992; 49: 101–7.

26. Boutin EL, Cunha GR. Does sinus vaginal epithelium persist in the adult mouse vagina? Dev Dyn 1996; 206: 403–11.

27. Kurita T, Cunha GR, Robboy SJ et al. Differential expression of p63 isoforms in female reproductive organs. Mech Dev 2005; 122: 1043–55.

28. Cunha GR. Epithelio–mesenchymal interactions in primordial gland structures which become responsive to androgenic stimulation. Anat Rec 1972; 172: 179–96.

29. Drews U, Sulak O, Schenck PA. Androgens and the development of the vagina. Biol Reprod 2002; 67: 1353–9.

30. Mauch RB, Thiedemann KU, Drews U. The vagina is formed by downgrowth of Wolffian and Müllerian ducts. Graphical reconstructions from normal and Tfm mouse embryos. Anat Embryol (Berl) 1985; 172: 75–87.

31. Kobayashi A, Shawlot W, Kania A et al. Requirement of Lim1 for female reproductive tract development. Development 2004; 131: 539–49.

32. Vainio S, Heikkila M, Kispert A et al. Female development in mammals is regulated by Wnt-4 signalling. Nature 1999; 397: 405–9.

33. Carroll TJ, Park JS, Hayashi S, Majumdar A, McMahon AP. Wnt9b plays a central role in the regulation of mesenchymal to epithelial transitions underlying organogenesis of the mammalian urogenital system. Dev Cell 2005; 9: 283–92.

34. Torres M, Gomez-Pardo E, Dressler GR et al. Pax-2 controls multiple steps of urogenital development. Development 1995; 121: 4057–65.

35. Miyamoto N, Yoshida M, Kuratani S et al. Defects of urogenital development in mice lacking Emx2. Development 1997; 124: 1653–64.

36. Wilson JG, Warakany J. Malformation in the genitourinary tract induced by maternal vitamin A deficiency in the rat. Am J Anat 1948; 83: 357–408.

37. Mendelsohn C, Lohnes D, Decimo D et al. Function of the retinoic acid receptors (RARs) during development (II). Multiple abnormalities at various stages of organogenesis in RAR double mutants. Development 1994; 120: 2749–71.

38. Kastner P, Mark M, Ghyselinck N et al. Genetic evidence that the retinoid signal is transduced by heterodimeric RXR/RAR functional units during mouse development. Development 1997; 124: 313–26.

39. Marshall H, Morrison A, Studer M, Popperl H, Krumlauf R. Retinoids and Hox genes. FASEB J 1996; 10: 969–78.

40. Ma L, Benson GV, Lim H et al. Abdominal B (AbdB) Hoxa genes: regulation in adult uterus by estrogen and progesterone and repression in Müllerian duct by the synthetic estrogen diethylstilbestrol (DES). Dev Biol 1998; 197: 141–54.

41. Izpisua-Belmonte JC, Dolle P, Renucci A et al. Primary structure and embryonic expression pattern of the mouse Hox-4.3 homeobox gene. Development 1990; 110: 733–45.

42. Warot X, Fromental-Ramain C, Fraulob V et al. Gene dosage-dependent effects of the Hoxa-13 and Hoxd-13 mutations on morphogenesis of the terminal parts of the digestive and urogenital tracts. Development 1997; 124: 4781–91.

43. Schnabel CA, Selleri L, Cleary ML. Pbx1 is essential for adrenal development and urogenital differentiation. Genesis 2003; 37: 123–30.

44. Yamaguchi TP, Bradley A, McMahon AP et al. A Wnt5a pathway underlies outgrowth of multiple structures in the vertebrate embryo. Development 1999; 126: 1211–23.

45. Mericskay M, Kitajewski J, Sassoon D. Wnt5a is required for proper epithelial–mesenchymal interactions in the uterus. Development 2004; 131: 2061–72.

46. Kurita T, Cooke PS, Cunha GR. Epithelial–stromal tissue interaction in paramesonephric (Müllerian) epithelial differentiation. Dev Biol 2001; 240: 194–211.

47. Komatsu M, Fujita H. Electron-microscopic studies on the development and aging of the epithelium of mice. Anat Embryol (Berl) 1978; 152: 243–59.

48. Brody JR, Cunha GR. Histologic, morphometric, and immunocytochemical analysis of myometrial development in rats and mice: I. Normal development. Am J Anat 1989; 186: 1–20.

49. Bigsby RM, Li AX, Luo K et al. Strain differences in the ontogeny of estrogen receptors in murine uterine epithelium. Endocrinology 1990; 126: 2592–6.

50. Valdés-Dapena MA. The development of the uterus in late fetal life, infancy, and childhood. In: Norris HJ, Hertig AT, Abell MR, eds. The Uterus. Baltimore, MD: Williams and Wilkins, 1973.

51. Forsberg JG, Norell K. Differentiation of the epithelium in early grafts of the mouse Müllerian vaginal region. Experientia 1966; 22: 402–4.

52. Kurita T, Mills AA, Cunha GR. Roles of p63 in the diethylstilbestrol-induced cervicovaginal adenosis. Development 2004; 131: 1639–49.

53. Chan Y, Anton-Lamprecht I, Yu QC et al. A human keratin 14 "knockout": the absence of K14 leads to severe epidermolysis bullosa simplex and a function for an intermediate filament protein. Genes Dev 1994; 8: 2574–87.

54. Rugg EL, McLean WH, Lane EB et al. A functional "knockout" of human keratin 14. Genes Dev 1994; 8: 2563–73.

55. Kurita T, Lee K, Cooke PS et al. Paracrine regulation of epithelial progesterone receptor by estradiol in the mouse female reproductive tract. Biol Reprod 2000; 62: 821–30.

56. Pixley E. Morphology of the fetal and prepubertal cervico-vaginal epithelium. In: Jordan JA, Singer A, eds. The Cervix. London: WB Saunders, 1976.

57. Jernvall J, Thesleff I. Reiterative signaling and patterning during mammalian tooth morphogenesis. Mech Dev 2000; 92: 19–29.

58. Shannon JM, Hyatt BA. Epithelial–mesenchymal interactions in the developing lung. Annu Rev Physiol 2004; 66: 625–45.

59. Roberts DJ. Molecular mechanisms of development of the gastrointestinal tract. Dev Dyn 2000; 219: 109–20.

60. Cunha GR. Epithelial–stromal interactions in development of the urogenital tract. Int Rev Cytol 1976; 47: 137–94.

61. Cunha GR. Stromal induction and specification of morphogenesis and cytodifferentiation of the epithelia of the Müllerian ducts and urogenital sinus during development of the uterus and vagina in mice. J Exp Zool 1976; 196: 361–70.

62. Boutin EL, Sanderson RD, Bernfield M et al. Epithelial–mesenchymal interactions in uterus and vagina alter the expression of the cell surface proteoglycan, syndecan. Dev Biol 1991; 148: 63–74.

63. Cunha GR, Young P, Brody JR. Role of uterine epithelium in the development of myometrial smooth muscle cells. Biol Reprod 1989; 40: 861–71.

64. Kurita T, Medina R, Schabel AB et al. The activation function-1 domain of estrogen receptor alpha in uterine stromal cells is required for mouse but not human uterine epithelial response to estrogen. Differentiation 2005; 73: 313–22.

65. Miller C, Pavlova A, Sassoon DA. Differential expression patterns of Wnt genes in the murine female reproductive tract during development and the estrous cycle. Mech Dev 1998; 76: 91–9.

66. Miller C, Sassoon DA. Wnt-7a maintains appropriate uterine patterning during the development of the mouse female reproductive tract. Development 1998; 125: 3201–11.

67. Kmita M, Duboule D. Organizing axes in time and space; 25 years of colinear tinkering. Science 2003; 301: 331–3.

68. Taylor HS, Vanden Heuvel GB, Igarashi P. A conserved Hox axis in the mouse and human female reproductive system: late establishment and persistent adult expression of the Hoxa cluster genes. Biol Reprod 1997; 57: 1338–45.

69. Benson GV, Lim H, Paria BC et al. Mechanisms of reduced fertility in Hoxa-10 mutant mice: uterine homeosis and loss of maternal Hoxa-10 expression. Development 1996; 122: 2687–96.

70. Zhao Y, Potter SS. Functional specificity of the Hoxa13 homeobox. Development 2001; 128: 3197–207.

71. Parr BA, Avery EJ, Cygan JA et al. The classical mouse mutant postaxial hemimelia results from a mutation in the Wnt 7a gene. Dev Biol 1998; 202: 228–34.

72. Patton PE, Novy MJ, Lee DM et al. The diagnosis and reproductive outcome after surgical treatment of the complete septate uterus, duplicated cervix and vaginal septum. Am J Obstet Gynecol 2004; 190: 1669–78.

73. Propst AM, Hill JA 3rd. Anatomic factors associated with recurrent pregnancy loss. Semin Reprod Med 2000; 18: 341–50.

74. Simpson JL. Genetics of the female reproductive ducts. Am J Med Genet 1999; 89: 224–39.

75. Lin PC, Bhatnagar KP, Nettleton GS et al. Female genital anomalies affecting reproduction. Fertil Steril 2002; 78: 899–915.

76. Acién P, Acién M, Sánchez-Ferrer M. Complex malformations of the female genital tract. New types and revision of classification. Hum Reprod 2004; 19: 2377–84.

77. Fedele L, Bianchi S, Agnoli B et al. Urinary tract anomalies associated with unicornuate uterus. J Urol 1996; 155: 847–8.

78. Duncan PA, Shapiro LR, Stangel JJ et al. The MURCS association: Müllerian duct aplasia, renal aplasia, and cervicothoracic somite dysplasia. J Pediatr 1979; 95: 399–402.

79. Behera M, Couchman G, Walmer D et al. Müllerian agenesis and thrombocytopenia absent radius syndrome: a case report and review of syndromes associated with Müllerian agenesis. Obstet Gynecol Surv 2005; 60: 453–61.

80. Gell JS. Müllerian anomalies. Semin Reprod Med 2003; 21: 375–88.

81. Rock JA, Zacur HA, Dlugi AM et al. Pregnancy success following surgical correction of imperforate hymen and complete transverse vaginal septum. Obstet Gynecol 1982; 59: 448–51.

82. Mortlock DP, Innis JW. Mutation of HOXA13 in hand-foot-genital syndrome. Nat Genet 1997; 15: 179–80.

83. Lubahn DB, Moyer JS, Golding TS et al. Alteration of reproductive function but not prenatal sexual development after insertional disruption of the mouse estrogen receptor gene. Proc Natl Acad Sci USA 1993; 90: 11162–6.

84. Krege JH, Hodgin JB, Couse JF et al. Generation and reproductive phenotypes of mice lacking estrogen receptor β. Proc Natl Acad Sci USA 1998; 95: 15677–82.

85. Lydon JP, DeMayo FJ, Funk CR et al. Mice lacking progesterone receptor exhibit pleiotropic reproductive abnormalities. Genes Dev 1995; 9: 2266–78.

86. Couse JF, Curtis SW, Washburn TF et al. Disruption of the mouse oestrogen receptor gene: resulting phenotypes and experimental findings. Biochem Soc Trans 1995; 23: 929–35.

87. Giusti RM, Iwamoto K, Hatch EE. Diethylstilbestrol revisited: a review of the long-term health effects. Ann Intern Med 1995; 122: 778–88.

88. Herbst AL, Ulfelder H, Poskanzer DC. Adenocarcinoma of the vagina. Association of maternal stilbestrol therapy with tumor appearance in young women. N Engl J Med 1971; 284: 878–81.

89. Robboy SJ, Szyfelbein WM, Goellner JR et al. Dysplasia and cytologic findings in 4,589 young women enrolled in diethylstilbestrol-adenosis (DESAD) project. Am J Obstet Gynecol 1981; 140: 579–86.

90. Robboy SJ, Young RH, Welch WR et al. Atypical vaginal adenosis and cervical ectropion. Association with clear cell adenocarcinoma in diethylstilbestrol-exposed offspring. Cancer 1984; 54: 869–75.

91. Forsberg JG. Animal model of human disease: adenosis and clear-cell carcinomas of vagina and cervix. Am J Pathol 1976; 84: 669–72.

92. McLachlan JA, Newbold RR, Bullock BC. Long-term effects on the female mouse genital tract associated with prenatal exposure to diethylstilbestrol. Cancer Res 1980; 40: 3988–99.

93. Plapinger L, Bern HA. Adenosis-like lesions and other cervicovaginal abnormalities in mice treated perinatally with estrogen. J Natl Cancer Inst 1979; 63: 507–18.

94. Newbold RR, McLachlan JA. Vaginal adenosis and adenocarcinoma in mice exposed prenatally or neonatally to diethylstilbestrol. Cancer Res 1982; 42: 2003–11.

95. Couse JF, Dixon D, Yates M et al. Estrogen receptor-alpha knockout mice exhibit resistance to the developmental effects of neonatal diethylstilbestrol exposure on the female reproductive tract. Dev Biol 2001; 238: 224–38.

96. Miller C, Degenhardt K, Sassoon DA. Fetal exposure to DES results in de-regulation of Wnt7a during uterine morphogenesis. Nat Genet 1998; 20: 228–30.

97. Brody JR, Cunha GR. Histologic, morphometric, and immunocytochemical analysis of myometrial development in rats and mice: II. Effects of DES on development. Am J Anat 1989; 186: 21–42.

98. MacGregor SN, Tamura RK, Sabbagha RE et al. Underestimation of gestational age by conventional crown–rump length dating curves. Obstet Gynecol 1987; 70: 344–8.

99. Konishi I, Fujii S, Okamura H et al. Development of smooth muscle in the human fetal uterus: an ultrastructural study. J Anat 1984; 139(Pt 2): 239–52.

100. Sasaki C, Yamaguchi K, Akita K. Spatiotemporal distribution of apoptosis during normal cloacal development in mice. Anat Rec A Discov Mol Cell Evol Biol 2004; 279: 761–7.

2 Puberty, menarche and the endometrium

Joseph S Sanfilippo and Mary Anne Jamieson

INTRODUCTION

Puberty is the dynamic process that leads to sexual maturation and the ability to reproduce. It is defined as a period of transition from childhood to adulthood that encompasses physiological, somatic, and constitutional changes associated with further development of the internal and external genitalia and secondary sex characteristics. A host of endocrinological activity is involved with this dynamic process and includes regulation of estrogens, androgens, inhibin, activin, and follistatin, all of which regulate activities related to the hypothalamic–pituitary–gonadal axis. It is during this period of transition that thelarche, adrenarche, pubarche, peak growth velocity, and ultimately menarche occur. The culmination of pubertal development is physical maturity along with the capacity to procreate. The subject of puberty can be subdivided into the somatic or physical changes in association with the external appearance of an adult and the psychological maturational process, both of which are heralded by an efflux of hormones from the adrenal glands and ovaries in girls, and from the testes in boys. It is the culmination of these effects that produces the somatic changes indicative of puberty. This chapter reviews both physiological and pathophysiological pubertal events and conditions that impact on the developing uterus and endometrium.

Correlation exists between Tanner staging and the uterine and ovarian volumes.[1] Initially, there is a 50:50 size ratio between the uterine fundus and the cervix. This association changes during pubertal development, the cervix ultimately becoming one-third the size of the entire uterus. During childhood, the uterus usually lies in the midplane position. Later stages in pubertal development primarily affirm the myometrium, which is a reflection of response to ovarian hormonal stimulation. The endometrium further develops after onset of secondary sex characteristics with resultant menstruation (Table 2.1).

PHYSIOLOGY

Current thinking is that the timing of pubertal development stems from differences in the maturational programming of gonadotropin-releasing hormone

Table 2.1   Organ development.

Infancy	
Uterus	2.5 mm
Ovary	$1.5 \times 3 \times 2.5$ mm

Reproduced with permission of Sanfilippo and Lavery.[2] Uterine length has been evaluated and conveyed in Figure 2.1.[3]

(GnRH). Any discussion of the physiology of puberty must incorporate knowledge and understanding of the neuroendocrinology of the hypothalamic–pituitary–ovarian (HPO) axis. Puberty is but one event in a dynamic process that begins in utero. Overall onset of puberty is determined by genetic factors, but nutrition and environment also play a significant role. This information reflects studies both in humans and in primates.[4–6] GnRH is present, stimulating the release of gonadotropins by 10–18 weeks' gestation.[7–10] Peak levels of gonadotropins and sex steroids occur at 20 weeks' gestation.[11] After this time, negative feedback occurs. Levels continue to rise, which results in increasing gonadal steroid production. In the fetus and term neonate, serum estrogen levels are noted to be approximately 5000 pg/ml at term, but this also reflects the conversion of fetal and maternal C-19 steroid precursors to estrogens by the placenta. The fetal adrenal gland also plays a role in estrogen production throughout fetal life. Marshall and Tanner, astute in their evaluation, took serial photographs every 3 months of British adolescents and noted the pattern as well as rate of development of pubic hair and breasts.[12] They believed the mean age of onset of puberty was 11.2 ± 1.1 years. As noted below, redefinition of the age of precocious puberty was addressed by the Lawson Wilkins Pediatric Endocrine Society (LWPES) who provided the age cut-off of 7 years in white girls and 6 years in Afro-American girls.[13] This information is most important for clinicians dealing with patients in the pediatric-early adolescent age group.

In-utero estrogen levels tend to proliferate in the fetal endometrium, as evidenced by estrogen withdrawal 'menstrual' bleeding often experienced by the female neonate or newborn (Figure 2.2). The HPO axis is suppressed during childhood. The mechanism of this 'central restraint' is unknown. The endometrium is atrophic during these prepubertal

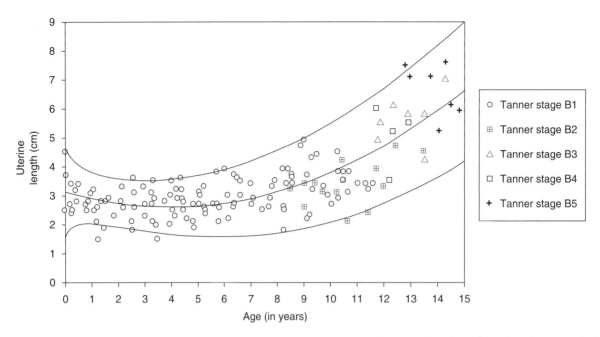

Figure 2.1 Scattergram of uterine length versus age, at different stages of puberty, with 3rd, 50th, and 97th percentile lines superimposed. (Reproduced from Griffin et al,[3] with permission.)

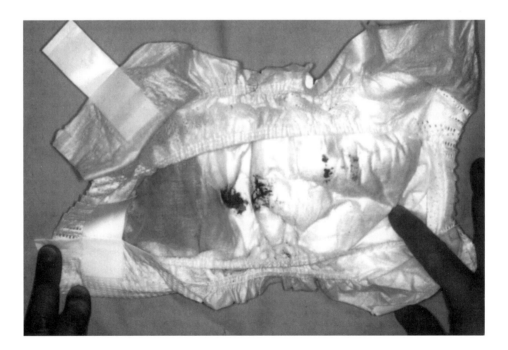

Figure 2.2 Bloodstained diaper from an 8-day-old female, the result of an estrogen-withdrawal bleed.

years. With the onset of puberty, nocturnal and eventually daytime gonadotropin pulses increase; secondarily, gonadal steroids begin to rise, and thelarche occurs.[14–16] Prior to the onset of puberty, mean levels of gonadotropins increase and reflect hypothalamic activity, i.e. pulsatile GnRH secretion. The initial prepubertal level of follicle-stimulating hormone (FSH) secretion undergoes a change in frequency and amplitude of gonadotropin release, initially during sleep. The frequency and amplitude of these gonadotropins being released from the pituitary increases as the pubertal maturation process continues. Continued nocturnal spikes in gonadotropin continue through early pubertal development. Of interest, the luteinizing hormone (LH) increases exceed those of FSH at this point in time. In adults the LH pulses occur every 90 minutes and provide a sustained level of elevation in the circulation for 20 minutes per pulse.[17]

Pubertal development includes adrenarche: i.e. the appearance of pubic and axillary hair, acne, and body odor. This is a reflection of increased adrenal hormone sex steroid production.

Controversy continues regarding the factors responsible for onset of puberty. Leptin, an adipose tissue product, may affect body mass and composition and thus play a role. There appears to be a circadian rhythm to leptin secretion.[18] Inhibin, activin, and follistatin, as well as genetic factors, also play a role. Timing of puberty is affected by exercise, nutrition, and psychiatric related abnormalities, i.e anorexia. With regard to inhibin, the levels of inhibin B correlate with age and FSH concentrations several years before onset of puberty;[19] inhibin A, on the other hand, becomes measurable later in pubertal development.[20] The usual sequence of pubertal development is: accelerated growth, thelarche, adrenarche, and then menarche. A 4.5-year interval (range 1.5–6 years) may be required between the initial sign and menarche.[11]

The Pediatric Research in Office Settings (PROS) study evaluated over 17 000 girls aged 3–12 years. With regard to thelarche, they noted that at age 7, 27% of African-American girls and 6.7% of white girls were Tanner stage 2. At present, concern for precocious onset of breast and/or pubic hair manifests if it occurs before age 7 years in white and 6 years in black girls.[13] Prior to this study, Herman-Giddens et al provided assessment of 17 077 girls in a study that began in 1948 and concluded that onset of menarche in white girls was 12.88 years and in African-Americans 12.16 years. Furthermore, this age of onset of menarche had remained stable for 45 years, i.e. the period of evaluation.[21]

The endometrium is stimulated to proliferate. Menarche will ultimately ensue, but in general it occurs 24 months after thelarche. Menarche usually represents an anovulatory bleed: i.e. unopposed estrogen leads to a thickened proliferative endometrium that cannot sustain itself and 'breaks away' or sloughs erratically. On average, approximately 18 months is required between menarche and the development of regular ovulatory menstrual cycles. In fact, 90% of all menstrual cycles in 'normal adolescents' 12–14 years of age are anovulatory.[22] Presumably this delay represents a maturation process involving the HPO axis, and eventually positive feedback mechanisms develop that give rise to ovarian estradiol-triggered LH surges, ovulation, and the establishment of regular menses.

In this context, the endometrium is converted to its secretory form and then undergoes a synchronized basal slough.

Anovulatory menses of the perimenarche are often problematic or dysfunctional. The patient can present with menometrorrhagia or periods of amenorrhea that cause concern. Reassurance is paramount and often is all that is indicated. However, when anemia, social embarrassment, or school absences result, treatment should be considered.

PATHOPHYSIOLOGY AND CLINICAL CONDITIONS OF RELEVANCE

Persistent ovulatory dysfunction

Many of the features of the 'polycystic ovary syndrome' (PCOS), such as hyperandrogenism, hyperestrogenism, anovulation, and insulin resistance, are in fact physiological during puberty. In 1992, Nobels and Dewailly elegantly hypothesized that many patients who ultimately declare themselves as having PCOS-like chronic anovulation developed their disease during adolescence:[23] i.e. the physiological endocrine 'imbalances' of puberty never spontaneously resolved and ovulatory cycles never ensued. Clinically, patients experience persistent ovulatory dysfunction beyond the perimenarche; they present with menometrorrhagia or periods of amenorrhea and histologically will develop unopposed proliferative endometrium which sloughs erratically, as described above, with regards to perimenarchal dysfunctional bleeding. This subject has been reviewed recently, focusing on PCOS being a heterogeneous endocrine disorder reflected in oligoamenorrhea and signs of hyperandrogenemia. Patients must be reminded of the long-term sequelae of cardiovascular disease and type 2 diabetes mellitus.[24]

Hypothalamic dysfunction: eating disorders and elite athletes

Patients subjected to extremes of diet, stress, and exercise, especially patients with eating disorders and elite athletes, can experience varying degrees of hypothalamic dysfunction.[25–30] Many of these patients are peripubertal. GnRH pulsatility is affected, and this can result in a spectrum of pubertal and menstrual dysfunction. The menstrual manifestations range from luteal phase inadequacy, to oligo-ovulation or anovulation in the presence of continuing gonadal estrogen production and, finally, to anovulation with hypoestrogenization. At the level of the endometrium, these correspond respectively to:

- 'out of phase' histology
- infrequent conversion to secretory endometrium with subsequent slough
- proliferative endometrium and irregular asynchronous shed
- and, finally, endometrial atrophy in the most severe cases.

Although a theoretic concern with all patients in whom there is unopposed estrogen, hyperplasia is extremely rare in adolescents. However, these patients may be at risk in adulthood.

Many etiological theories have been proposed to explain GnRH/hypothalamic dysfunction seen in this population, yet none have accounted for all patients.[29,30] The menstrual complaints or abnormalities improve or resolve when the disease improves or when there is an increase in the dietary intake: exercise ratio.

When menorrhagia results in anemia, and especially when this occurs at menarche, the astute clinician rules out coagulopathy before assuming anovulation. A history of medications known to affect clotting, easy bruising, epistaxis, and past surgeries/transfusions may lend insight. A family history of coagulopathy is also a critical clue. Von Willebrand's disease will often be

diagnosed at menarche. Appropriate diagnostic tests must be obtained. Similarly, in all adolescents who present with abnormal vaginal bleeding, pregnancy or infection (vaginitis, cervicitis, endometriosis, pelvic inflammatory disease [PID]) or trauma must be considered in the differential diagnosis along with endocrinopathy such as thyroid imbalance.

Müllerian anomalies (Figure 2.3) can cause outflow obstruction which may or may not be accompanied by primary amenorrhea. Anomalies such as imperforate hymen, transverse vaginal septum or vaginal agenesis (with a uterus) block all menstrual blood from exiting. Midline fusion defects such as non-communicating rudimentary uterine horn (Figures 2.3–2.5) may trap a focus of active endometrium while the patient experiences normal menses from the contralateral side. These abnormalities present at menarche or in adolescence as cryptomenorrhea or severe dysmenorrhea. Many of these structural anomalies can be diagnosed by ultrasound or computed tomography (CT) scan, but magnetic resonance imaging (MRI) is the gold standard for the more challenging cases (Figures 2.6 and 2.7). At the level of the endometrium, adenomyosis can result presumably from pressure and endometriosis may develop presumably from overwhelming retrograde flow (Figure 2.8). The occluded cavity will contain at least a focus of endometrium and undoubtedly old menstrual blood if menarche (would have) already occurred.

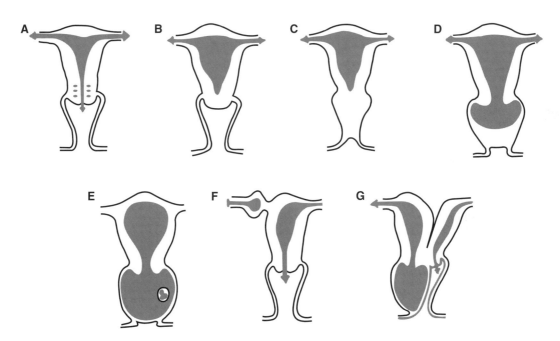

Figure 2.3 Anomalies of the reproductive tract that could result in adolescent endometriosis. (A) Cervical stenosis. (B) Cervical agenesis. (C) Vaginal agenesis. (D) Transverse vaginal septum. (E) Imperforate hymen. (F) Rudimentary uterine horn. (G) Unilateral vaginal obstruction.

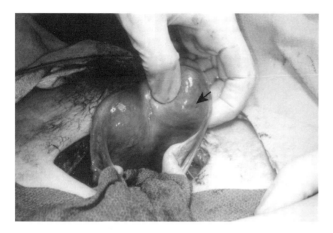

Figure 2.4 Non-communicating right uterine horn at laparotomy (arrow). Patient presented with severe right-sided 'dysmenorrhea' beginning at menarche.

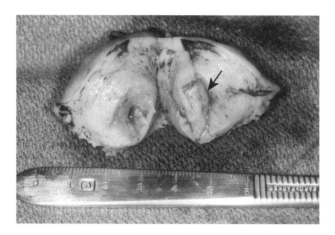

Figure 2.5 Trapped focus of endometrium (arrow) in the non-communicating uterine horn (Figure 2.4). Histology confirmed endometrium, myometrium, and adenomyosis.

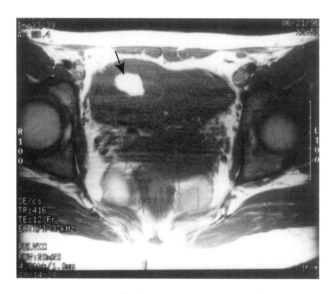

Figure 2.6 MRI of pelvis in same patient photographed in Figures 2.4 and 2.5. Trapped blood within right uterine horn (arrow).

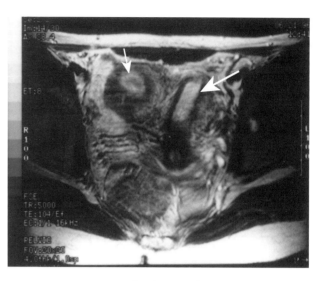

Figure 2.7 T2 MRI of pelvis in the same patient. The endometrial–myometrial (e-m) junction of the right horn is not well defined (top arrow), likely representing adenomyosis (confirmed on specimen histopathology). Note the clarity of the e-m junction of the left uterine horn (non-obstructed) (white arrow).

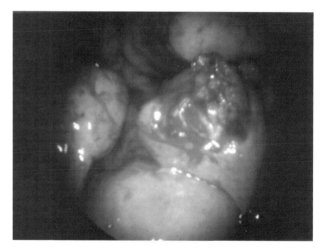

Figure 2.8 Extensive endometriosis in a 16-year-old girl. This was associated with outflow tract obstruction.

SUMMARY

As more scientific information is accrued, it is increasingly more obvious that a well-integrated, well-coordinated series of events leading to onset of puberty occurs beginning in utero. Puberty brings about a series of physiological changes to the uterus and endometrium. With the onset of gonadal estrogen production, the endometrium makes the transition from atrophy to proliferation. With normal pubertal progression, eventually ovulatory cycles ensue and the patient experiences monthly conversion to secretory endometrium followed by the well-known synchronous menstrual shed. The perimenarcheal transition years, however, can cause a spectrum of bleeding problems related to ovulatory inconsistencies as the HPO axis matures. Various clinical conditions experienced by adolescent females can also affect the endometrium and the menstrual pattern in particular.

REFERENCES

1. Ivarsson SA, Nilsson KO, Persson PH. Ultrasonography of the pelvic organs in prepubertal and post-pubertal girls. Arch Dis Child 1983; 58: 352–4.
2. Sanfilippo JS, Lavery JP. The spectrum of ultrasound: antenatal to adolescent years. Semin Reprod Endocrinol 1988; 1: 45.
3. Griffin IJ, Cole TJ, Duncan KA et al. Pelvic ultrasound measurements in normal girls. Acta Paediatr 1995; 84: 536–43.
4. Parent A, Teilmann G, Juul A. The timing of normal puberty and the age limits of sexual precocity: variations around the world, secular trends and changes after migration. Endocr Rev 2003; 24(5): 668–93.
5. Palmert MR, Hirschhorn JN. Genetic approaches to stature, pubertal timing, and other complex traits. Mol Genet Metab 2003; 80: 1–10.
6. Plant T, Barker-Gibb M. Neurobiological mechanisms of puberty in higher primates. Hum Reprod Update 2004; 10(1): 67–77.
7. Rabinovici J. The differential effects of FSH and LH on the human ovary. Baillière's Clin Obstet Gynaecol 1993; 7: 263–81.
8. Beck-Peccoz P, Padmanabhan V, Baggiani A et al. Maturation of hypothalamic–pituitary–gonadal function in normal human fetuses: circulating levels of gonadotropins, their common alpha-subunit and free testosterone, and discrepancy between immunological and biological activities of circulating follicle-stimulating hormone. J Clin Endocrinol Metab 1991; 73: 525–32.
9. Rosenfield RL. The ovary and female sexual maturation. In: Kaplan SA, ed. Clinical Pediatr Endocrinol. Philadelphia, PA: WB Saunders, 1990: 259–324.
10. Kulin HE. Editorial: Puberty: When? J Clin Endocrinol Metab 1993; 76: 24.
11. Lalwani W, Reindollar R, Davis A. Normal onset of puberty. Have definitions of onset changed? Obstet Gynecol Clin N Am 2003; 30: 279–86.
12. Marshall W, Tanner J. Variations in pattern of pubertal changes in girls. Arch Dis Child 1969; 44(239): 291–303.
13. Kaplowitz P, Oberfield S. Re-examination of the age limit for defining when puberty is precocious in girls in the United States: implications for evaluation and treatment. Drug and Therapeutics and Executive Committees of the Lawson Wilkins Pediatric Endocrine Society. Pediatrics 1999; 104: 936–41.
14. Yen SS, Apter D, Butzow T, Laughlin GA. Gonadotrophin releasing hormone pulse generator activity before and during sexual maturation in girls: new insights. Hum Reprod 1993; 8: 66–71.
15. Apter D, Butzow L, Laughlin G, Yen S. Gonadotropin-releasing hormone pulse generator activity during pubertal transition in girls: pulsatile and diurnal patterns of circulating gonadotropins. J Clin Endocrinol Metab 1993; 76: 940–9.
16. Apter D. Ultrasensitive new immunoassays for gonadotropins in the evaluation of puberty. Curr Opin Pediatr 1993; 5: 481–7.
17. Kasa-Vubu J, Padmanabhan V, Kletter G et al. Serum bioactive luteinizing and follicle-stimulating hormone concentrations in girls increase during puberty. Pediatr Res 1993; 23: 829–33.
18. Apter D, Hermanson E. Update of female pubertal development. Curr Opin Obstet Gynecol 2002; 14: 475–81.
19. Crofton P, Evans A, Groome N et al. Dimeric inhibins in girls from birth to adulthood: relationship with age, pubertal stage, FSH and estradiol. Clin Endocrinol (Oxf) 2002; 56: 223–30.
20. Raivio T, Dunkel L. Inhibins in childhood and puberty. Best Pract Res Clin Endocrinol Metab 2002; 16: 43–52.
21. Herman-Giddens M, Slora E, Wasserman R et al. Secondary sexual characteristics and menses in young girls seen in office practice: a study from the Pediatric Research in Office Settings network. Pediatrics 1997; 99(4): 505–12.
22. Wheeler MD. Physical changes of puberty. Endocrinol Metab Clin North Am 1991; 20: 1–14.
23. Nobels F, Dewailly D. Puberty and polycystic ovarian syndrome: the insulin/insulin-like growth factor I hypothesis. Fertil Steril 1992; 58: 655–66.
24. Pfeifer S. Polycystic ovary syndrome in adolescent girls. Semin Pediatr Surg 2005; 14: 111–17.
25. Fisher M, Golden N, Katzman D et al. Eating disorders in adolescents: a background paper. J Adolesc Health 1995; 16(6): 420–37.
26. Carpenter SE. Psychosocial menstrual disorders: stress, exercise and diet's effect on the menstrual cycle. Obstet Gynecol 1994; 6: 536–9.
27. Putukian M. The female triad. Eating disorders, amenorrhea, and osteoporosis. Med Clin North Am 1994; 78: 345–56.
28. Constantini NW, Warren MP. Special problems of the female athlete. Baillière's Clin Rheumatol 1994; 8: 199–219.
29. Eisenberg E. Toward an understanding of reproductive function in anorexia nervosa. Fertil Steril 1981; 36: 543–50.
30. Fruth SJ, Worrell TW. Factors associated with menstrual irregularities and decreased bone mineral density in female athletes. J Orthop Sports Phys Ther 1995; 22: 26–38.

3 Menstrual and estrous cycles

Lois A Salamonsen

INTRODUCTION

The endometrium is a highly dynamic tissue that undergoes cyclical variation with every estrous or menstrual cycle during the reproductive years. Under the influence of the changing hormonal milieu, cellular proliferation, differentiation, and apoptosis occur in association with changes in extracellular matrix (ECM) composition and leukocyte trafficking. Among species, the changes are the most extreme in women, in whom the entire functional layer (functionalis) of the endometrium is shed at menstruation with subsequent regeneration of the tissue from the remaining basal layer (basalis). In other mammals, such renewal occurs only postpartum. The purpose of the remodeling is to provide an environment that is conducive to implantation of the conceptus, but only a time when the conceptus is appropriately developed.[1-3] Because the mechanisms of embryo implantation differ widely between mammalian species, the extent of endometrial preparation or remodeling also varies. Importantly, developmental plasticity that is generally lost in adult tissues is retained in the endometrium since this tissue constantly renews during reproductive life. In this chapter, the focus is on dynamic cyclical changes in women, but comparisons are drawn with mice, the most widely used experimental animals.

In women (Figure 3.1A) the menstrual cycle is broadly divided into three phases – menstrual, proliferative (follicular), and secretory (luteal). The standardized cycle is of 28 days, with day 1 defined as the first day of menstrual bleeding, and ovulation (following the luteinizing hormone [LH] surge) at approximately day 14. Fluctuations of cycle length between 26 and 32 days are common. Normal ovulatory menstrual cycles are associated with consistent morphological changes within the functionalis layer of the endometrium, and classification of the histological changes provides a tool for dating the endometrial biopsy[4] although this is now recognized as having limitations.[5] During menses, most of the functionalis layer is shed; re-epithelialization is initiated during this phase in parallel with the tissue breakdown in adjacent areas.[6] During the proliferative phase and under the influence of estrogen there is rapid cellular

proliferation of all cell types and new ECM is laid down. Following ovulation and under regulation by progesterone, the endometrium undergoes functional differentiation to provide a suitable environment for embryo implantation. Characteristically, the glands become increasingly tortuous with considerable secretory activity. Stromal edema in the mid-secretory phase accompanies the coiling of the specialized spiral arterioles. After day 22, the stromal cells begin a differentiation process, which together with changes in leukocyte content and vasculature (decidualization), is a prerequisite for successful implantation and placentation. In the absence of pregnancy, falling steroid hormone levels in the late secretory phase trigger endometrial regression and menstruation.[7]

The mouse provides an important model for studying endometrial function because of the ability to exploit the vast knowledge of mouse genetics by overexpressing or ablating genes. Therefore it is important to understand its estrous cycle and the endometrial changes driven by this. The mouse has a spontaneous cycle length of only 4–5 days, divided into four phases (proestrus, estrus, metestrus, and diestrus): the LH peak preceding ovulation occurs on the afternoon of proestrus and the mice enter estrus and ovulate in the early hours of the night.[8] The hormonal fluctuations are shown in Figure 3.1B for an outbred strain, but these can differ with strain.[9,10] The stage of the cycle is generally determined by vaginal smear.[11] During proestrus and estrus, there is active mitosis and growth of the genital tract. Metestrus is characterized by some regression of the endometrium and, by late metestrus, degeneration of the epithelium is apparent. Diestrus is a stage of quiescence or slow growth when regeneration begins. Importantly, the mouse cycle, which is dominated by estradiol-17β, is without a true luteal phase since very little progesterone is synthesized unless copulation occurs: what little is present is mostly metabolized to the inactive 20α-hydroxyprogesterone.[12]

The endometrial changes are driven by the ovarian steroid hormones. These elicit their actions primarily by binding to specific high-affinity receptors, which then act as transcription factors and modulate the transcription of a large number and variety of genes. Global

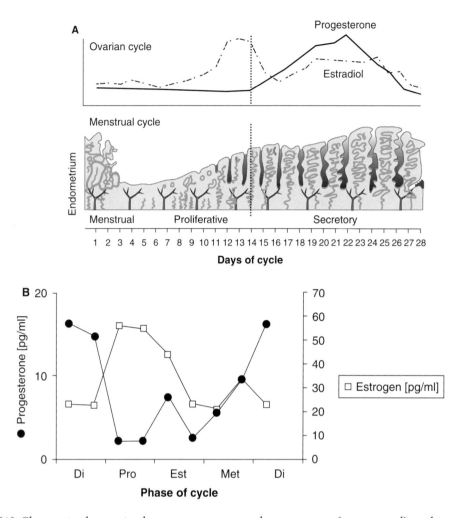

Figure 3.1 (A) Changes in the ovarian hormones, estrogen and progesterone (upper panel), and in endometrial structure (lower panel) during a normalized 28-day menstrual cycle in women. (B) Changes in estrogen and progesterone levels in serum during the mouse estrous cycle. Di, diestrus; Pro, proestrus; Est, estrus; Met, metestrus. (Derived from data in Walmer et al.[10])

gene profiling by microarray analysis, in association with hierarchical clustering, reveals a strong relationship between histopathological dating of human endometrium and molecular profiles across the five major phases of the cycle.[13] Interestingly, the major changes in gene expression occur in the mid-secretory phase with other specific changes being associated with menstruation. Such studies clearly indicate that it is overly simplistic to imagine that a single gene or marker will accurately represent any one phase of the cycle. Likewise in the mouse, specific gene profiles have been identified at estrus and diestrus.[14]

Recent progress in our understanding of daily circadian rhythmicity, its presence in peripheral tissues, and its role in normal physiological functions[15] raises the possibility that major circadian swings in gene activity may occur in the endometrium,[16] making it important that tissue collections are carefully timed. To date there are no published studies on circadian variability in endometrial gene expression.

STEROID HORMONE RECEPTORS

Steroid hormone actions are mediated by genomic and non-genomic signaling. The classical genomic mechanisms of action involve activation of specific nuclear receptors while more rapid biological effects are now thought to be mediated via membrane-bound receptors including G-protein coupled receptors.[17,18] It is not yet known whether the latter are present or functional in the endometrium. The distribution of classical estrogen, progesterone and androgen receptors in the endometrium is detailed elsewhere (see Chapter 4; Salamonsen and Jones[7]) and are summarized only briefly here. Both estrogen receptor α (ERα) and estrogen receptor β (ERβ) are expressed, with ERα being dominant. ERα is present in both epithelial glands and stroma of the functionalis layer. In the human it is maximal during the proliferative phase but declines during the secretory phase. Epithelial ERβ also decreases during the secretory phase: it is not detected in stroma but is the only subtype present in vascular endothelium. Both subtypes are present in the perivascular cells surrounding the blood vessels. Importantly, mice lacking ERα lose uterine estrogen responsiveness, whereas those lacking only ERβ exhibit a relatively normal phenotype and are fertile.[19]

Progesterone receptor A (PR-A) and progesterone receptor B (PR-B) are co-expressed in target cells in human endometrium. PR expression is stimulated by estrogen during the proliferative phase but is down-regulated by its own ligand in the secretory phase. Prior to ovulation, PR-A and PR-B levels are approximately equivalent in glandular epithelium but only PR-B persists in these cells in the mid-secretory phase, suggesting that PR-B is most important for the progesterone-driven phenotypic changes in the glands at this time. In the stroma, PR-A is the dominant isoform throughout the cycle. PRs are also expressed on endothelial cells, although endometrial leukocytes are devoid of PRs.

Androgen receptors (AR)A and ARB are also expressed in the human endometrium, predominantly in the stroma during the proliferative phase. Antiprogestins can induce ARs in the glands and enhance their levels in the stroma: this is of clinical relevance as many of the progestins used in contraceptive preparations, particularly levonorgestrel, exhibit potent androgenic actions.

ENDOMETRIAL PROLIFERATION

Endometrial proliferation and the effects of steroid hormones on this are detailed elsewhere (see Chapters 4 and 9). In brief, in the human, significant epithelial cell mitotic activity and DNA synthesis very early in the cycle indicate the regeneration of epithelium from remaining glands and persisting areas of surface epithelium. From cycle day 5, under the influence of estrogen, mitotic activity is a key feature of all endometrial cellular components. Whereas early proliferative endometrium is thin and contains glands that are narrow, short, straight, and partially collapsed, during the mid-proliferative phase the glands elongate and become more tortuous until they are clearly branched by the late proliferative phase. Tissue recombination studies demonstrate that this pattern of glandular morphogenesis is supported by the stroma. During the secretory phase, the glands increase in diameter but do not proliferate.[20] Insulin-like growth factors (IGF) are likely key candidates for conveying estrogen action

throughout the endometrium, with the balance shifting from the proliferative to the secretory phase, corresponding to the stimulation and inhibition of estrogen-driven proliferation. Other growth factors, including epidermal growth factor (EGF) and transforming growth factor β (TGFβ), are also prevalent in proliferating endometrium. Following ovulation, progesterone plays a key role in regulating endometrial proliferation by suppressing estrogen-driven mitosis in both glands and stroma: mitoses persist at low levels only in surface epithelia and predecidual cells. Specific mechanisms proposed include down-regulation of ER, induction of the enzymes catalyzing estrogen to the less-active estrone (17β-hydroxysteroid dehydrogenase and sulfotransferase), and a decrease in estrogen-induced specific gene expression. Angiogenesis, including proliferative activity in endothelial cells, occurs in three episodes during the menstrual cycle: initial repair during the early proliferative phase; estrogen-driven angiogenesis during the mid-proliferative phase; and progesterone-driven growth of the spiral arterioles during the secretory phase.[21] Dynamic expression of vascular endothelial growth factor (VEGF) and its receptors, as well as other angiogenic and anti-angiogenic factors, throughout the cycle, indicates that complex and distinct mechanisms are involved in blood vessel growth and regeneration (see Chapter 7).

In mice, cellular proliferation is driven largely by the estrus-related estrogen, which acts primarily on luminal and glandular epithelial cells,[22] this is subsequently inhibited by the progesterone that is produced following copulation. Stromal cell proliferation is initiated by this progesterone, and continues as part of the decidual response to the implanting blastocyst.[22,23] These events can be mimicked in ovariectomized mice treated with exogenous hormones.[24] Such effects of steroid hormones on cell proliferation are mediated by paracrine factors, particularly growth factors and cytokines.

ENDOMETRIAL APOPTOSIS

Molecular basis of apoptosis

The term apoptosis was coined in 1972[25] to describe morphologically distinct features of programmed cell death as opposed to the cell death induced by necrosis which results from lethal chemical, biological, or physical events. Necrosis results in the release of cellular contents into the ECM and is followed by an inflammatory response, whereas apoptosis occurs without activation of the immune system. Apoptosis is highly regulated by coordination of gene-directed, energy-dependent biological processes which lead to activation of members of the caspase family of cysteine proteases, whose tightly regulated actions lead to DNA cleavage.[26] Blocking caspases can rescue condemned cells from their apoptotic fate.[27] Two canonical pathways (extrinsic and intrinsic) lead to caspase activation.[28]

The extrinsic pathway begins with ligation of cell surface 'death receptors' which include Fas/CD95, tumor necrosis factor α (TNFα) receptor 1, and two receptors DR4 and DR5 that bind to the TNFα-related apoptosis-inducing ligand (TRAIL). Binding of the appropriate ligand (L) (e.g. Fas-L) to its receptor (e.g. Fas) induces receptor clustering and the formation of a death-inducing signaling complex that recruits multiple procaspase-8 molecules and leads to caspase-8 activation; this in turn activates procaspase-3. Caspase-3 action leads to ordered dismantling, producing the degradation products of actin, DNase, and lamins.

The so-called intrinsic mitochondrial pathway is used extensively for responding to both external and internal stimuli and involves activation of caspase-9. Unlike other caspases, proteolytic processing of caspase-9 has only a minor effect on its catalytic activity, and the key requirement for caspase-9 activity is its association with a dedicated protein cofactor Apaf-1[28] to form a holoenzyme, often known as the apoptosome, which may also contain additional proteins. A critical step towards apoptosome formation is the release of cytochrome c from the mitochondria to the cytosol: this is regulated by members of the Bcl family of apoptotic regulators, which can possess either anti-apoptotic (e.g. Bcl-2 family) or proapoptotic (e.g. Bax family) activity. Cytochrome c is only one of a host of mitochondrial pro-death denizens: these include AIF, Cams/DIABLO, and several procaspases. It is proposed that release of multiple death-promoting molecules might be necessary to ensure swift and certain death.

Under most conditions, the crosstalk between these two pathways is minimal, and they operate largely independently of each other. However, events downstream of caspases are not well understood and there are many other physiological forms of cell death with non-apoptotic morphologies that are not yet adequately classified.

Apoptosis in the human endometrium

Apoptosis in human endometrium appears to be related primarily to the remodeling of this tissue. In 1976, Hopwood and Levison[29] identified apoptotic bodies in glandular epithelial cells through the late secretory to menstrual phases but observed that some were also present during the proliferative phase. Subsequently, apoptotic bodies have been observed as released into the glandular lumen or being engulfed and digested by adjacent glandular cells but not by macrophages.[30] Most apoptosis occurs in the epithelial cells: only very low levels of apoptosis are seen in the stroma.

A number of the components of the two pathways to apoptosis have been identified in human endometrial tissue: their cyclical variation is summarized in Table 3.1. Bcl-2 has a cyclical expression pattern in glandular epithelium, peaking during the late proliferative phase and two candidates for its transcriptional regulators, c-jun and Sp-3, show a similar pattern.[30–33] Bcl-2 expression is low and does not alter cyclically in stromal cells. By contrast, Bax is very low in epithelial cells during the proliferative phase but increases during the secretory phase, being maximal in the late secretory phase.[33] Thus, the Bcl-2/Bax ratio in epithelium alters in favor of apoptosis as the cycle progresses.

Fas and Fas-L are expressed in human endometrium throughout the cycle, but are overall higher in the late secretory phase.[31,32] Interestingly, during the late proliferative phase, both Fas and Fas-L are localized on epithelial cells, mainly on Golgi and in vesicles where they are unable to induce apoptosis. Subsequently, during the secretory phase, they become incorporated into the cell membranes of epithelial cells.[30,32] There are two forms of Fas-L, membrane bound and soluble. Given that conversion from the membrane-bound to the soluble form results from actions of some matrix metalloproteinases (MMPs)[34] it is likely that the increased MMP action during the late secretory/menstrual phases[35] provides soluble Fas-L and hence contributes to apoptosis of the glandular epithelial cells. Fas and Fas-L appear to be absent from endometrial stromal cells.[31,36]

Caspase activities (-3, -8, and -9), along with some cleavage products such as cytokeratin 18 fragments and degradation products of Bid, a member of the Bcl-2 family, which can release cytochrome c from the mitochondrial membrane to the cytosol, are detected during the late secretory phase of the human menstrual cycle.[30,37] Interestingly, caspase-8 has additional roles in proliferation and differentiation:[38] such roles in the endometrium have not been examined.

From these data it appears that both extrinsic and intrinsic pathways are effective in human endometrial epithelial cell apoptosis and that this occurs mainly during the late secretory phase.

Endometrial apoptosis in several mammalian species, including rabbits,[39] hamsters,[40] and monkeys,[41] suggests regulation by steroid hormones, probably acting directly

Table 3.1   Apoptosis and apoptosis-related factors examined in human endometrium

	Phase of cycle				
	P	**ES**	**MS**	**LS**	**Men**
Epithelium					
Apoptotic index	++ to −	+	+	++	+++
Bcl-2	+++	++	+	+	NA
Bax	+/−	++	++	+++	NA
Bcl-x	++	+	++	+++	NA
BAK	+	++	++	+++	NA
Fas	+ to ++	++	ND	+++	NA
Fas-L	+	++	++	++	NA
Stroma					
Apoptotic index	+/−	+/−	+/−	+/−	+
Bcl-2	+	+	+	+	NA
Bax	−	+/−	+/−	+/−	NA
Bcl-x	−	−	−	−	NA
BAK	−	−	−	−	NA
Fas-L	−	−	−	−	NA
Fas	−	−	−	−	NA
Entire endometrium					
Cytochrome c	+	NA	NA	++	NA
Act. caspase-8	+	NA	NA	++	NA
Act. caspase-3	+	NA	NA	++	NA

P, proliferative; S, secretory (E, early; M, mid; L, late), men, menstrual; −, not detectable; +/−, just detectable; +, positive; ++, highly positive; NA, data not available.
Derived from Harada et al,[186] Yamashita et al,[32] Dahmoun et al,[36] Vaskivuo et al,[33] and di Paola et al.[187]

on the promoters of apoptosis-related genes. For example, estrogen–ERα complexes directly regulate Fas-L expression through an estrogen-response element in the Fas-L promoter, whereas Fas is regulated by progesterone.[42] Progesterone also promotes generation of the antiapoptotic $bcl-X_L$ mRNA,[43] consistent with the increase in apoptosis observed in response to withdrawal of progesterone in vitro.[44] Importantly, the trophoblast product, human chorionic gonadotropin (hCG) and progesterone, when administered during the luteal phase, both reduce signs of apoptosis prior to menstruation, providing a mechanism by which epithelial apoptosis is reduced in a fertile cycle.[45] Glycodelin A, a lipocalin secreted by the glands following progesterone stimulation, is apoptotically active,[46] suggesting indirect as well as direct actions of progesterone. Uterine ischemia–reperfusion may be an alternative stimulus in association with menstruation: in a mouse model, it initiated apoptosis in glandular epithelium and in scattered cells in the stroma.[47]

Given that in vivo, apoptosis increases in human endometrium from the mid-secretory phase to a maximum during the menstrual phase, a mechanistic role of apoptosis in the process of endometrial breakdown has been proposed. However, the dissociation between tissue breakdown and apoptosis in endometrial explants[48] suggests that although menstrual-like breakdown and apoptosis can occur at the same time in an endometrial sample, the two processes may not be linked and are probably not mechanistically related. Indeed, apoptosis is seldom if ever seen in massive tissue destruction. It is more likely that the apoptosis is involved in the endometrial remodeling needed to restore normal endometrial architecture following menstruation.

Apoptosis in mouse endometrium

As in the human, the epithelium is the major cellular compartment in which apoptosis is observed during the estrous cycle in the mouse. In mice and rats, estrogen and progesterone both afford protection against apoptosis,[49,50] which occurs primarily at estrus and metestrus.[51] Interestingly, during the transition from proestrus to estrus, there is an increase in the ratio of proapoptotic proteins Bax and Bcl-X_S and a decrease in the antiapoptotic proteins Bcl-2 and Bcl-X_L.[52] Apoptosis is also markedly induced by ovariectomy, through mediation of both Fas and TNFα.[53] However, whereas endometrial apoptosis can be induced in mice lacking functional Fas, it is limited in mice deficient in the TNF-R p55, indicating that TNFα may play a more important role than Fas in apoptosis in this tissue.[47,53]

ENDOMETRIAL DIFFERENTIATION

Following ovulation, during the secretory phase of the human cycle, most of the cells of the endometrium undergo functional differentiation to provide an environment suitable for embryo implantation. This is driven either directly or indirectly by progesterone. Clearly identified changes in the epithelial and stromal cells in the human provide a tool for subdivision of the secretory phase. Histologically, the early secretory phase is characterized by the development of subnuclear vacuoles in the epithelium, resulting in an altered intracellular location of the nuclei. During the early to mid-secretory phase, epithelial glands become increasingly tortuous and have increased secretory activity. After day 22, the process of decidualization is initiated and involves differentiation of stromal cells, observed first in the fibroblast-type cells close to the spiral arterioles, which become noticeably enlarged and rounded: these are characteristic of the late secretory phase. Decidualization also involves changes in the vasculature and ECM, along with infiltration of specific leukocyte subsets. The characteristic morphological changes in the endometrial stroma are not observed during the cycle in the mouse or most other species.

Endometrial receptivity

During most of the cycle, the human endometrium is either hostile (proliferative phase) or non-receptive (early and late secretory phases) to blastocyst implantation. Only for a very short period of time during the mid-secretory phase (postovulatory days 6–10) is the endometrium receptive: this has been coined the 'window of receptivity'.[54] In the mouse, receptivity is strictly determined by the steroidal preparation of the endometrium: progesterone maintains the uterus in a neutral phase and prenidatory estrogen is needed for receptivity.[55]

Much of the emphasis on the secretory phase of the cycle in the human has related to the clinical need for markers of endometrial receptivity. Importantly, histologic endometrial maturation does not necessarily correlate with a functionally mature endometrium.[1] Appropriate markers have proved difficult to identify partly because few morphological or molecular correlates of the receptive state are shared across species.[2,3] No single reliable marker, that appears at the start and then disappears after the receptive phase has yet been identified: it is more likely that a combination of markers will be needed.

Epithelial differentiation

Surface changes

The progesterone-driven differentiative changes in the endometrial epithelium lead to an 'opening' of the 'window of receptivity' for blastocyst implantation. Implantation is a paradox in cell biology: two epithelial apical surfaces, which are normally mutually repulsive, must come together as the trophectoderm becomes apposed to and subsequently adheres to the endometrial epithelium. Therefore, it can be predicted that there must be a modulation of the apicobasal polarity of the luminal epithelium.[56] Morphologically, progesterone-dependent apical cellular protrusions known as pinopods (uterodomes) become visible by scanning electron microscopy on days 20–21 of the human menstrual cycle and are then lost.[57,58] These apparently absorb luminal fluid, and may thus facilitate adhesion of the blastocyst.[59] Their location does not appear to be related to infertility.[60]

Cell surface molecules

The epithelial surface is covered by a protective glycocalyx, made up of complex glycosylated molecules, the composition of which alters during the cycle (see Chapter 19). One component of the glycocalyx in both mouse and humans is the cell-associated mucin, MUC1. Mucins are present on many mucosal surfaces, where they provide resistance to enzyme actions and impair cell–cell and cell–ECM adhesion. MUC1 has both cell surface-associated and secreted isoforms, is hormonally regulated, antiadhesive, and extends above the glycocalyx.[61] Although its expression is highest at the time when the human endometrium is receptive,[61] it is down-regulated in vitro by the human blastocyst[62] and in vivo during the attachment phase of mouse implantation.[63] Intracellular deposits of MUC1 accumulate in the early secretory phase in the human and these are subsequently released into the uterine cavity.[64] Importantly, microheterogeneity of glycoforms of MUC1 could relate to epithelial receptivity.[60] In addition to changes in the protein components of the glycocalyx, changes in the sugar moieties are also observed and appear to be hormonally driven. For example, the enzyme α(1-2)-fucosyltransferase, which regulates the formation of fucosylated H-type-1 sugar on the uterine epithelial surface in the mouse, is stimulated by estrogen and inhibited by progesterone.[65] Other adhesion/antiadhesion molecules on the luminal epithelium that change as uterine receptivity develops include a range of glycoconjugates,[66] trophinin,[67] cadherins,[68] and integrins.

Table 3.2   Some growth factors/cytokines maximally produced by human endometrial glands during the mid-secretory phase of the menstrual cycle

Protein	Human	Mouse	Detected in human uterine fluid	Changed in infertile women
LIF	√	Transient in early pregnancy	√	√
IL-11	√	Decidual cells only	NA	√
IL-6	√	CHECK	NA	NA
Activin A	√	√ Little change	√	√
CSF-1	√	Appears in early pregnancy	NA	
GM-CSF	√	Surge following mating	NA	NA
Fractalkine (CX3CL1)	√	NA	NA	NA
HCC-1 (CCL14)	√	NA	NA	NA
6Ckine (CCL21)	√	NA	NA	NA
Eotaxin (CCL-11)	√	NA	NA	NA
HB-EGF	√	Site of implantation	NA	
Glycodelin A	√	NA	√	√

√, present, NA, no information available.
Derived from Dimitriadis et al,[188] and Lee and DeMayo.[189]

Integrins are transmembrane glycoproteins whose subunits form heterodimers to form cell surface receptors that act as cell adhesion molecules. Certain integrin subunits are present on luminal epithelium in most species and are regulated cyclically in the human but not the mouse[69] with specific alterations during the mid-secretory phase, suggesting a role for α4, β4, and αvβ3 in the establishment of endometrial receptivity. Integrins are also found on uterine stroma. Although integrins have been suggested to play a role in uterine receptivity, studies examining a relationship with infertility are conflicting.[70,71] Interestingly, osteopontin, one of the ligands for αvβ3, is secreted by the uterine epithelium and may form a link with the blastocyst.[72]

Proteins regulating calcium homeostasis

Calcium-binding proteins fall into two functional categories: Ca^{2+} signal transducers, which mediate Ca^{2+} signaling pathways, and Ca^{2+} buffering proteins, which maintain the overall $[Ca^{2+}]$ in a cell. Calmodulin falls into the first of these categories, calbindin d9k into the second, whereas calbindin d28k has both properties. Calbindins d9k and d28 are both expressed on mouse uterine epithelium in a tightly regulated manner, appearing just before implantation and disappearing at implantation sites. Importantly, their dual ablation from the mouse uterus results in complete failure of implantation.[73] Calbindin d9k is not expressed in primate endometrium but calbindin d28k is present in luminal and glandular epithelium with cyclical variation, being maximal in the mid-secretory phase,

suggesting that calcium buffering is also important for uterine receptivity in humans.[74] Calcitonin, which regulates calcium homeostasis and calcium flux across cell membranes, is also present in the epithelium and under progesterone regulation in both rat and human endometrium.[75,76] Antagonism of its synthesis markedly decreases the implantation rate in rats.[77]

Secretory changes

Uterine glands are present in all mammalian uteri and these selectively transport or synthesize and secrete substances into the uterine lumen: collectively, these secretions are known as histotroph. Although the precise components of histotroph are not yet fully defined in any species, they include numerous binding and nutrient transport proteins, ions, glucose, cytokines, enzymes, hormones, growth factors, proteases and their inhibitors, and other substances.[78] The importance of glandular secretions for conceptus survival and development is emphasized in a sheep model in which uterine gland formation is repressed.[79] In rodents, two genes (leukemia inhibitory factor and calcitonin)[77,80] expressed exclusively in endometrial glands are essential for establishment of uterine receptivity and blastocyst implantation, whereas in humans, endometrial glands and their secretions appear to be critical for embryo development throughout the first trimester.[81]

Numerous growth factors and cytokines are produced by endometrial glands (and in most cases also by luminal epithelium). In most instances it is not known whether they are secreted apically into the uterine lumen where they are probably needed for growth and differentiation of the developing blastocyst, or basally for paracrine actions on the underlying stroma. Although many of these factors are produced throughout the cycle, and some have clear functions in the proliferative phase, others such as heparin-binding epidermal growth factor (HB-EGF)[82] and interleukin 11 (IL-11)[83] are produced primarily during the secretory phase, often reaching a maximum during the mid-secretory phase (Table 3.2). Given the pleiotrophy and redundancy within growth factor and cytokine families and the redundancy and different signal transduction pathways utilized by their receptors, it is difficult to define functions, which are known for only a few. Their sites of action are defined in part by the cellular location of their specific receptors. Many growth factors are stored in the ECM after secretion and release by proteolytic action is a critical regulatory step. Other factors undergo post-translational modifications, often by proteolytic processing (which produces either highly active or inactive forms, most of which are not yet well defined). Specificity and diversity can also be determined by the presence of soluble receptors, ligand traps, or binding proteins.

Although many of the same factors are produced by endometrium of different species, the cellular origins and temporal regulation can be different. For example, IL-11 which is produced specifically in decidualizing stromal cells in the mouse during early pregnancy[84] is localized to glandular and luminal epithelium from the early secretory phase in humans, as well as to decidualizing stromal cells.[83] Interestingly, a processing enzyme, proprotein convertase 6 (PC6), is likewise a decidual product only in the mouse, but present in both epithelial and decidual cells in the human.[85,86]

Chemokines, cytokines with known roles in leukocyte trafficking, are also produced by endometrial glands and luminal epithelium. Expression of some chemokines is maximal in the mid-secretory phase and their immunohistochemical location and apical release from polarized epithelial cells suggests release into the uterine lumen[87] where they can act on the trophoblast.[88–90] Endometrial chemokines have been little studied in the mouse.

Stromal differentiation: decidualization

Decidualization can be defined as the process of transformation of the endometrium into the morphologically and functionally distinct decidual tissue of pregnancy. This involves the differentiation and expansion of endometrial stromal fibroblasts, remodeling of the ECM and blood vessels, and influx/proliferation of uterine natural killer (uNK) cells. Unequivocal proof that decidualization is essential for establishment of pregnancy has been provided by a number of genetically modified mice in which decidualization is impaired: these include mice with null mutations of COX-2,[91] LIF,[80] PR-A,[92] steroid receptor coactivator 1,[93] Hoxa-10,[94] Hoxa-11,[95] IL-11 receptor α,[84,96] and components of interferon γ (IFNγ) signaling.[97]

In a narrower sense, the term decidualization is applied to the process whereby endometrial stromal cells differentiate into morphologically distinct decidual cells with a unique biosynthetic and secretory phenotype. These ultimately form the major cellular component of the maternal aspect of the maternal–fetal interface. It is in this context that the term 'decidualization' will be applied here.

Decidualization of endometrial stromal cells occurs only in the presence of progesterone, following estrogen priming of the endometrium. In women, it occurs spontaneously, but to a variable extent during the late secretory phase of every cycle, starting in the cells immediately surrounding the spiral arterioles, approximately 10 days after the postovulatory rise in ovarian progesterone levels.[98] At this time, these cells are often termed 'pre-decidual', and they can be identified by staining for specific markers and by their pavement-like morphology. Once pregnancy is established, and in the presence of continuing progesterone, differentiation progresses throughout the stromal compartment, resulting in a uniformly decidualized tissue that persists throughout gestation (Figure 3.2A). This also occurs when the endometrium is influenced by high levels of continuous progestin (for example, in women using the levonorgestrel intrauterine system). In some non-human primates (rhesus and cynomolgus monkeys) there is enlargement of the stromal cells, especially around the spiral arteries, during the non-fertile luteal phase but not nearly to the extent of that seen in women.[99] Limited spontaneous decidualization is also observed in the functional right horn (in which implantation takes place) in the molossid bat, Molossus ater.[100]

By contrast, in rats and mice decidualization occurs only in the presence of a blastocyst, when it is localized to implantation sites. However, it can be stimulated artificially and, in this situation, the deciduoma develops along the full length of the uterus. At implantation, decidualization begins in the antimesometrial pole of the endometrium where the blastocyst first implants, and later spreads to involve the mesometrial zone. It is not clear why this occurs: there

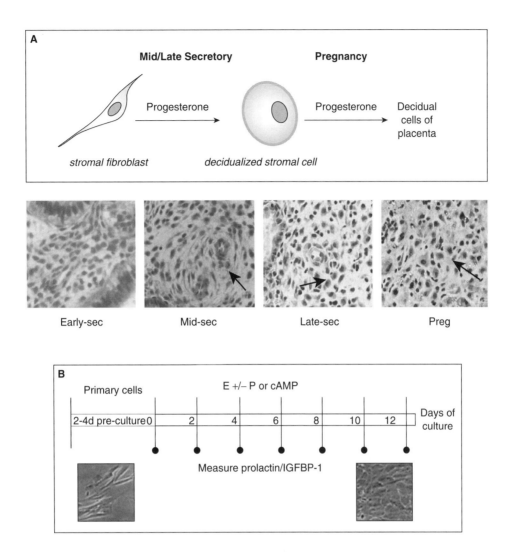

Figure 3.2 Decidualization of human endometrial stromal cells. **(A)** In vivo. During the mid-late secretory (sec) phase of the cycle, under the influence of progesterone, endometrial stromal fibroblasts start to differentiate, initially in areas close to spiral arterioles, to form morphologically and phenotypically distinct decidualized stromal cells. The process continues if pregnancy (Preg) is established and progesterone levels maintained, to provide the decidual cell component of the placenta. Micrographs show this decidual cell development in human endometrial/decidual tissues (arrows). **(B)** In vitro. Stromal fibroblasts isolated from human endometrial samples and established in culture for 2–4 days, can be stimulated to decidualize over 10–12 days by treatment with estrogen plus progesterone (or cyclic AMP). The process can be followed by observation of cell morphology and by measuring the secreted decidual cell markers, prolactin or insulin-like growth factor binding protein 1(IGFBP-1).

may be specific transduction processes from the epithelium only in one location in the lumen or the antimesometrial and mesometrial cells may differ. The latter explanation would be supported by other differences observed between antimesometrial and mesometrial cells, such as the subsequent apoptosis of the antimesometrial cells, and the different expression of certain molecules.[101] Decidual cells in the rodent have a finite life: their death by apoptosis occurs even in artificially induced deciduoma and in spite of maintenance of PR.[102] Decidual regression is tightly controlled and involves a number of factors, including

proteases and members of the TGFβ superfamily, including activin.[103]

Decidualization represents a change from fibroblast to a much more epithelial-like cell, which is surrounded by a basement membrane (characterized by collagen IV and laminins), and which is highly secretory. The process is a continuum, involving synchronized activation of specific genes, resulting in coordinated expression of specific new proteins that appear sequentially as the process proceeds: this was first demonstrated with three well-known markers of the process: relaxin (RLX), prolactin (PRL), and insulin-like growth factor binding protein 1 (IGFBP-1).[104] Up-regulation of cell cycle regulatory genes during decidualization suggests that expansion of the endometrial stromal cells occurs not only by cellular hypertrophy but also by mitosis and endoreduplication.[105]

Decidualization of human endometrial stromal fibroblasts can be recapitulated in culture by continuous treatment of isolated estrogen-primed cells with progesterone over a number of days, providing a physiologically relevant model to study regulatory mechanisms (Figure 3.2B). Morphological change from spindle-like fibroblast to polygonal epithelial-like cells can be readily visualized. Activation of the previously silent prolactin gene is generally used as a biochemical marker of decidualization. Alternatively, decidualization can be driven in vitro by the protein kinase A pathway activator, cyclic AMP (cAMP): this results in a more rapid decidualization response, and a higher level of differentiation.[106,107] Gene microarray analysis of endometrial stromal cells following cAMP stimulation demonstrated responses during the first 48 hours (h) in terms of early (0–6 h), subsequent (12–24 h), and late (24–48 h) events. The early events primarily involve cell cycle regulation, followed by cellular differentiation such as changes in cell morphology and secretory phenotype, while the late events appear to mediate more specialized function and include genes such as those regulating immune modulators.[105] Interestingly, changes induced by 10 days of treatment with the physiological stimuli, estrogen and progesterone, showed considerable concordance with those induced by 48 h of cAMP and included growth factors, neuromodulators, inflammatory cytokines, chemokines, oncogenes, cell adhesion molecules, and transcription factors.[108]

Progesterone receptors and decidualization

Considerable evidence demonstrates that PR-A is the dominant isoform of the PR associated with decidualization. There is lack of decidual response in the uteri of PR-A-deficient mice[109] while in human endometrium in vivo, decidualization is associated with rapid down-regulation of PR-B.[110] Furthermore, the dominant decidual cell gene *IGFBP-1* is more strongly activated by PR-A than PR-B.[111] However, many decidua-specific genes do not have perfect palindromic progesterone response elements in their promoters and it is probable that either regulatory effects of progestins are mediated by degenerate half-sites on the promoters of regulated genes or that there are non-genomic or indirect actions.

Liganded PR can modulate gene expression through protein–protein interactions with other transcription factors, rather than direct interaction with DNA and this may be an important mechanism of PR action in differentiating endometrial stromal cells.[107] Progesterone receptors are necessary for cAMP-induced decidualization in vitro; interestingly, in vitro, progesterone only enhances decidual PRL promoter activity in cells pretreated with cAMP. This suggests that protein kinase A (PKA) signaling may sensitize endometrial stromal cells to progesterone through induction or modification of transcription factors or co-activators capable of modulating PR function; these include the transcription factors C/EBPβ, FOX01a, Stat5, and Stat3.[107,112] The sustained increase in cellular cAMP observed in decidualizing endometrial stromal cells may be at least in part due to inhibition of the activity of its degradative enzymes, the phosphodiesterases.[113] Non-genomic effects of progesterone may also be mediated via membrane (m) PR, at least one of which (mPRα) that has characteristics of a G-protein coupled receptor, is expressed in the uterus and placenta.[114]

Convergence of progesterone with growth factor and cytokine signaling during decidualization

Convergence between progesterone and growth factor/cytokine signaling is known outside the uterus: for example, similar disruptions of mammary gland development are observed in mice lacking PR as in those lacking activin βA, EGF receptor and, two members of the STAT signaling pathway.[115] These same elements are present in decidualized endometrial cells in humans and in the mesometrium of the pregnant rat.[116]

The actions of most of the regulatory molecules that potentiate progesterone-induced decidualization are mediated via their membrane receptors coupled to diverse intracellular signaling pathways (Table 3.3).[117] IL-11 signals by activation of the Jak/Stat pathway,[118] whereas activin A acts via Smad proteins.[119] By contrast, G-protein ligands, including LH/hCG,[120] corticotropin-releasing hormone (CRH),[121] RLX,[122] and prostaglandin E$_2$(PGE$_2$),[123] utilize the cAMP/PKA pathway. Given that cAMP and PKA are necessary for decidualization in vitro by sensitizing endometrial stromal cells to the action of progesterone,[124,125] it is interesting that known generators of cAMP (RLX, PGE$_2$, and HB-EGF) promote IL-11 production and hence enhance progesterone-induced decidualization. IL-11, in turn, regulates a number of the genes associated with decidualization,

Table 3.3 Factors known to enhance decidualization in human endometrium

Factor	Pathway	Action: synergy with P or independent	Reference
HB-EGF	cAMP	Via stim IL-11	Chobotova et al,[129]
LH/hCG	cAMP		Tang et al,[190]
Relaxin	cAMP	Independent	Huang et al,[191]
		Also stim IL-11	Dimitriadis et al,[192]
IL-11	Jak/Stat	Synergy	Dimitriadis et al,[192]
Activin A	Smad	Synergy	Jones et al,[175]
CRH	cAMP	Via CRH-R1	Zoumakis et al,[193]
		Also stim IL-1 and IL-6	Di Blasio et al,[194]
Prostaglandin E_2	cAMP	Synergy	Frank et al,[123]
		Stim IL-11	Dimitriadis et al,[118]

stim, stimulation, P; progesterone.

including those encoding matrix molecules, IGFBP-5 and intracellular IL-1β.[126,127]

Progesterone may sensitize endometrial stromal cells to signaling by cytokines and growth factors, and hence to decidualization, by a number of mechanisms: These include:

1. Up-regulating receptor protein (e.g. EGF-R[128,129])
2. Enhancing cytoplasmic stores of Stat3 protein, thereby providing phosphorylation substrate downstream of EGF and IL-11 receptors[116,118]
3. Formation of direct complexes between Stat3 and PR. Such complexes may act as co-activators for each other in regulating gene expression.[115,116]

Although many molecules enhance progesterone-induced decidualization, only cAMP and RLX can act independently to stimulate decidualization in vitro.[130] Since the RLX-deficient female mouse is fertile, either RLX may not be absolutely required for implantation in the mouse or its role may be to act as a mediator of other factors.[131] Shifts in the steady state between phosphorylation and dephosphorylation (by phosphodiesterase) may favor cAMP accumulation in response to RLX.[132]

Proteases and decidualization

Proteases of a number of classes are involved in decidualization. Blocking MMP action with inhibitors limits decidual development in mice,[133] suggesting a role for MMPs, either by their action on matrix molecules or by release of essential growth factors from binding sites on ECM and/or their cleavage to biologically active forms.[134] A critical role for PC6 in decidualization has also been demonstrated in both mouse and human.[85,135] Since PCs cleave biologically inactive forms of many regulatory molecules (including

growth factors, cytokines, and integrins), to their biologically active forms,[136] the up-regulation of PC6 early during decidualization may be a critical initiating step in the cascade of events that results in widespread endometrial decidualization.

LEUKOCYTES

Cells of lymphomyeloid origin also contribute to endometrial remodeling. Their population within the endometrium is dynamic and in both the human and mouse, trafficking of these cells is regulated with the hormonal cycle. At their most abundant (during the perimenstrual phase in women) they contribute up to 40% of the total cellular content of the tissue. These cells include eosinophils, macrophages, neutrophils, uNK cells, dendritic cells, T cells, B cells, and mast cells.[137,138] Their relative abundance during the menstrual cycle in women (Figure 3.3) is probably a consequence of migration from the blood in response to chemokines,[88] cellular proliferation within the tissue, apoptosis, and cell loss during menstrual shedding. Their phenotypes and state of activation vary and will determine their function. For example, mast cell tryptase and neutrophil elastase are identified extracellularly during menstruation as a result of activation of these cells. It is likely that microenvironmental influences within the tissue determine such phenotypic differences but these are still largely undefined. Uterine NK cells are predominantly associated with decidualization of the tissue; their recruitment and viability are progesterone-dependent. They first appear in human endometrium in the mid-late secretory phase when decidualization is initiated, but in the mouse, they are found only in early pregnancy[138] where they are necessary for blood vessel remodeling.[139]

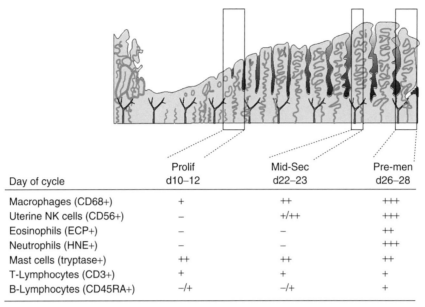

Day of cycle	Prolif d10–12	Mid-Sec d22–23	Pre-men d26–28
Macrophages (CD68+)	+	++	+++
Uterine NK cells (CD56+)	–	+/++	+++
Eosinophils (ECP+)	–	–	++
Neutrophils (HNE+)	–	–	+++
Mast cells (tryptase+)	++	++	++
T-Lymphocytes (CD3+)	+	+	+
B-Lymphocytes (CD45RA+)	–/+	–/+	+

–0,   +1–2,   ++ 3–5,   +++ 6–15% of total endometrial cells

Figure 3.3   Relative abundance of different leukocyte subtypes in the functionalis layer of the human endometrium across the menstrual cycle. Numbers of individual cell types were assessed by counting cells immunostained for specific markers (in brackets) and expressed on a scale of – (0), + (1–2), ++ (3–5) or +++ (6–15)% of total endometrial cells, in biopsies taken during the mid-proliferative (Prolif), mid-secretory (Mid-Sec), or premenstrual (Pre-men) phases of the menstrual cycle. ECP, eosinophil cationic protein; HNE, human neutrophil elastase. (Modified from Salamonsen et al.[137])

MENSTRUATION

Menstruation is the tissue breakdown and induction of endometrial bleeding that occurs at the end of each menstrual cycle. It is initiated by the fall in circulating levels of estrogen and progesterone resulting from the demise of the corpus luteum. The key evidence that menstruation is triggered by loss of steroid support of the tissue is that (1) if the progesterone levels are maintained artificially, menstruation does not occur, (2) administration of the PR antagonist mifepristone during the proliferative and secretory phases of the cycle results in uterine bleeding, and (3) withdrawal of estrogen and progesterone, as in the case of cyclical contraceptive use, results in uterine bleeding. However, the estrogen and progesterone levels fall rapidly with corpus luteum degeneration in all mammals with estrous cycles, whereas only women, some Old-World primates, and some bats menstruate. In these species, decidualization is initiated spontaneously during each cycle, whereas in non-menstruating mammals, decidualization occurs only in response to an implanting blastocyst. Since decidualization is a non-reversible differentiation in preparation for implantation, in a non-conception cycle, the tissue containing these cells must be discarded and new tissue subsequently formed.[140]

During menstruation, most of the functionalis layer of the endometrium is shed, leaving the basalis layer essentially intact. Since the start of the 1990s, there has been a paradigm shift in our view of the mechanisms underlying menstruation.[141] There is no strong evidence to support that hypoxia is a driving factor, as originally proposed by Markee:[142] rather, the process, which is triggered by the withdrawal of progesterone, appears to be initiated and maintained by local expression of proinflammatory and vasoactive mediators, leading to inflammation, tissue destruction, and shedding.

The events that lead to menstrual bleeding are initiated during the late luteal phase of the cycle, when widespread degeneration is observed in the basal lamina supporting the decidualized endometrial cells and the endothelium of blood vessels.[143] Scanning electron microscopy[6] reveals that small lesions are apparent in the luminal epithelium on day 28 of the normal cycle. There is then very rapid but incomplete degeneration of the functionalis layer, exposing open blood vessels and glands. It can therefore be surmised that the primary event initiating menstruation is tissue destruction and that loss of blood vessel integrity is one consequence of this. Ancillary mechanisms have also evolved to ensure that the blood does not clot[144] and that the bleeding stops by the time the tissue destruction has ceased.[141]

Vasoactive mediators

Vasoactive mediators such as prostaglandins (PGs), endothelins, and nitric oxide have integral roles both in regulating blood loss[141] and in augmenting the inflammatory response. Administration of intrauterine prostaglandin $F_{2\alpha}$ ($PGF_{2\alpha}$) causes menses, and increases uterine contraction, as it is overall a vasoconstrictor. Cyclooxygenase 2 (COX-2), the inducible COX isoform, is up-regulated with progesterone withdrawal, coincident with falling expression of the progesterone-dependent metabolizing enzyme prostaglandin dehydrogenase. This results in elevated concentrations of bioactive PGs in the endometrium and menstrual fluid. Endothelin 1 (ET-1), another potent vasoconstrictor, is made and released by human endometrium and can act on both epithelial and endothelial cells. Its production increases around the time of menstruation, suggesting a paracrine role in endometrial bleeding and/or repair.[145]

Inflammatory response

Inflammation is characterized by tissue edema, recruitment of inflammatory cells to an area, and associated release of proinflammatory cytokines. Finn[140] first postulated that menstruation could be regarded as an inflammatory process and considerable data now support this. There is a dramatic increase in the total number of leukocytes in the endometrium immediately prior to menstruation, when they constitute up to 40% of the total cells within the stromal compartment.[146] In particular, cells of the myeloid lineage (neutrophils, eosinophils, macrophages/monocytes) are abundant. Mast cells become highly activated and release granular contents into the local microenvironment, and eosinophil products are also detected extracellularly. Cells of lymphoid origin, particularly uNK cells, are also present in the tissue in substantial numbers, although these appear somewhat earlier during the secretory phase, suggesting a primary role in implantation and establishment of pregnancy.[147] However, their association with decidualized endometrium, and the ultrastructural changes observed in uNK cells following progesterone withdrawal, support a role in menstruation.

Current data suggest that the inflammatory response in the endometrium occurs in response to the withdrawal of progesterone. Inflammatory cells are highly abundant in the uterus of PR-null mice.[92] However, since endometrial and peripheral blood leukocytes do not express PR, it is likely that the recruitment of leukocytes into the endometrium is mediated indirectly via receptor-positive resident cells. The chemokine cohort in late secretory phase endometrium is in accord with the leukocyte subsets recruited at that time.[88] At least one of these (IL-8)[148] is negatively regulated by progesterone. When activated, leukocytes produce a plethora of regulatory molecules, including cytokines, chemokines, and a range of enzymes which are important either directly in matrix degradation, or indirectly by activation of other proteases.

Matrix metalloproteinases

Evidence now supports the concept that endometrial destruction is a consequence of the action of matrix degrading enzymes on ECM, both fibrillar matrix and basal lamina, with resultant loss of blood vessel integrity and shedding of most of the functionalis layer. Immediately prior to and during menstruation, there is induction of the expression, secretion, and activation of MMPs, proteases that together have the capacity to degrade all ECM components. Importantly, these enzymes are secreted in latent forms, which require extracellular activation by a variety of enzymes, including other MMPs (particularly MMP-3, MMP-9, and MT1-MMP) and leukocyte proteases such as tryptase and elastase. If a number of latent enzymes are present within a microenvironment, activation of one enzyme such as MMP-3 can lead to a cascade of subsequent activations. While progesterone is overall inhibitory to expression of many MMPs, local regulators of MMP transcription (predominantly cytokines) are derived from endometrial stromal, epithelial, and vascular cells, as well as leukocytes within the tissue.[149] Such local regulation can explain the very focal nature of the expression of most of the MMPs at menstruation. Important support for a critical role for MMPs in menstruation is that MMP activities (as opposed to immunoreactive protein and mRNA) are significantly increased in endometrium at menstruation compared to other times of the cycle,[35] and that specific inhibitors of MMP can stop the breakdown of endometrial explants in culture.[150] Natural tissue inhibitors of matrix metalloproteinases (TIMPs), which bind active forms of most MMPs with a 1:1 stoichiometry, are also present in human endometrium.[151] For MMP action within any microenvironment, the active form of an MMP must be in excess over the TIMPs, thus providing a very fine balance between a stable tissue and one that is degrading. Figure 3.4 provides a hypothetical scheme for the involvement of leukocytes and MMPs in the tissue destruction at menstruation.

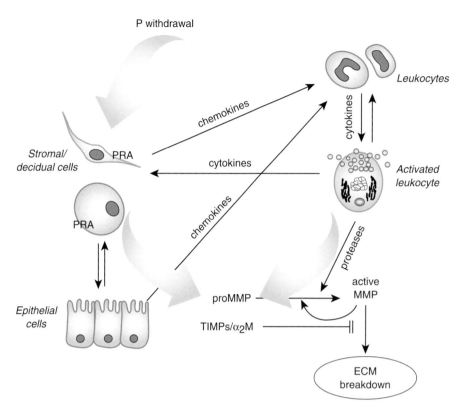

Figure 3.4   Proposed events leading to tissue destruction at menstruation. Withdrawal of progesterone directly affects endometrial stromal cells (which possess progesterone receptors [PR]) and indirectly affects endometrial epithelial/endothelial cells, to stimulate production of chemokines, which act as chemoattractants for leukocytes and stimulate their activation. Activated leukocytes in turn produce cytokines which stimulate local production of latent (pro-) matrix metalloproteinases (MMPs), chemokines, and other mediators. They also produce proteases, which initiate an activation cascade of MMPs. Once active MMPs are present at a focus in the tissue, the change in balance between these and their inhibitors (tissue inhibitors of MMPs [TIMPs] and α_2-macroglobulin [M]), leads to MMP action and breakdown of extracellular matrix (ECM).

Hemostasis

The process of hemostasis in the endometrium is not like that found in other parts of the body and menstrual blood differs from that in the circulation. It appears that the MMP-induced breakdown of tissue results in platelet activation, as platelets found in the endometrial cavity are deactivated.[152] Furthermore, any platelet plugs would be rapidly degraded by the plasminogen activator system, all components of which are present in human endometrium.[144,153] Interestingly, abnormalities of the endometrial fibrinolytic system are associated with increased menstrual blood loss (MBL), whereas antifibrinolytic agents reduce MBL.[154]

ENDOMETRIAL REPAIR

Repair of mucosal surfaces and wounds requires a wealth of growth factors and cytokines, ECM molecules such as fibronectin and hyaluronan and their cellular receptors (including the integrins and CD44), and matrix degrading enzymes such as MMPs. Both the

presence or absence of a factor and the timing of its action are important. For example, IL-1β and TNFα are both beneficial in the early stages of wound repair but deleterious in the later stages.[155] Substantial experimental evidence from studies in mice has shown that blocking key molecules will prevent or seriously impair wound repair. Interestingly, many of these are also important in tissue degradation.

ENDOMETRIAL REPAIR AFTER MENSTRUATION

Endometrial repair is an essential component of the cycle in menstruating animals. Repair of the human uterine surface is complete within 48 h after the first two menstrual days and precedes stromal expansion.[56] ER and PR are detected in the glandular epithelium by day 3, and by day 5, when epithelial reconstruction is complete, strong positive staining for ER and PR is present throughout the endometrium.[157] Studies with tissue recombinations suggest that uterine epithelium is required for stromal responsiveness to hormones, and may explain why re-epithelialization is the first event in restoration.[158] Importantly, even in the absence of all hormonal support (following ovariectomy and endometriotomy), the endometrium stops bleeding and heals, suggesting that normal wound healing mechanisms play a role in the reconstruction of the endometrium during menses and that this is facilitated by proliferative factors other than estrogen.

Interestingly, most wounds heal with scarring and this is not generally seen in endometrial repair in women, although, in mice, postpartum 'nodules' have been reported.[159] The other situation in which scarless wound repair occurs is in fetal skin wounds, particularly at an early developmental age,[160] highlighting the similarities between endometrial remodeling and development.

Repair of mucosal injury in tissues such as the gastrointestinal tract is a biphasic process. Initially, such wounds are resurfaced very rapidly from epithelial cells at the edges of the defect. These appear to redifferentiate towards a migratory phenotype with specialized membrane cytoskeletal and matrix–receptor reorganizations and specialized matrix-dependent signaling patterns.[161,162] The migrating cells require a necrotic layer, consisting of dead cells, plasma exudates, mucus, and fibrin, and if this is removed, restitution is impaired.[163] Following re-epithelialization, maturation of the new epithelium occurs under the influence of numerous peptide and non-peptide regulators. The time course of this repair depends greatly on the severity and tissue depth of the injury.[161] How closely such repair relates to that of endometrium is not yet clear.

Re-epithelialization of the endometrial surface

Scanning electron microscopy[6,164] revealed a dual origin for the restoration of the luminal epithelium, with regeneration beginning in areas in which the mouths of basal glands are free from overlying degenerated tissue. There is then simultaneous and progressive epithelial outgrowth from these, and ingrowth from the intact peripheral surface membrane bordering the denuded basalis. The stromal tissue starts to grow only once the endometrial wound is completely re-epithelialized.

Vascular repair

Within 5 days of menstrual onset, the damaged endometrial vessels have also been repaired.[6] This occurs simultaneously with breakdown, as does re-epithelialization. Subsequent regrowth of vessels occurs

under the influence of estrogen, along with stromal expansion as the proliferative phase progresses.

Stem cells

Any tissue which undergoes self-renewal (e.g. epidermis, hematopoietic system) must establish a lifelong population of relatively pliable stem cells. Stem cells can masquerade behind morphological and biochemical features normally attributed to undifferentiated cell types and it appears that the only infallible traits of stem cells are their robust proliferative capacity and their ability to self-renew.[165] Endometrium is capable of constant mature cell production and post-injury regeneration and it is now clear that genuine multipotential stem cells can be derived from human endometrium.[166] The topic of endometrial stem cells is reviewed in detail elsewhere in this book (see Chapter 10). Whether stem cells are essential for the endometrial repair following menstruation and the site of their origin still remain to be established. Cells of bone marrow origin may contribute to endometrial regeneration following menstruation.[167]

Factors of importance for endometrial repair

Proteolytic enzymes

During wound healing, cells migrate rapidly into the wound site, via proteolytically generated pathways in the provisional matrix, where they produce new ECM and remodel the newly formed matrix. Proteolytic enzymes, including MMPs and serine proteases, are abundant during menstruation but it is difficult to distinguish between roles in breakdown or repair. Limited proteolysis is important for exposing cryptic cell-binding sites on ECM, which are needed for cell migration. Therefore, proteinases that are localized to and activated at the contact areas of the ECM and the plasma membrane are likely to be the best candidate enzymes for regulating cell migration:[168] these include MT-MMPs, MMP-2, and MMP-9, all of which are present in the endometrium during the menstrual phase of the human cycle.[146] Other proteases may be important for release and activation of growth factors needed for endometrial repair (for example, the release of fibroblast growth factor [FGF] from perlecan by the action of MMP-1 and MMP-3[169] and the activation of TGFβ and IL-1β from their precursors by the actions of MMP-2 and MMP-9, respectively).[170,171] MMP-7, which is strongly expressed in endometrial epithelium during the menstrual phase, is important for re-epithelialization following wounding in the trachea;[172] in

MMP-7-null mice, such wounds do not re-epithelialize within the 24h time-frame taken in wild-type animals.[168] Whether MMP-7 is equally important for re-epithelialization of human endometrium remains to be established.

Growth factors

Many growth factors important for wound healing are expressed in endometrial stromal and epithelial cells and leukocytes. Activins are strongly up-regulated during cutaneous wound healing[173] and mice over-expressing their natural inhibitor follistatin show a severe delay in wound healing.[174] Activins, their receptors, and follistatin are all present in human endometrium:[175] during menstruation, activins may be in high concentrations in menstrual fluid and, if so, would be anticipated to play a role in repair mechanisms. Hepatocyte growth factor (HGF) is involved in regeneration of several tissues and promotes proliferation, migration, and lumen formation of endometrial epithelial cells in vitro,[176] but it remains to be established whether these actions occur in vivo. VEGF is important in wound angiogenesis and in both the human and rhesus macaque, VEGF expression peaks during postmenstrual repair in conjunction with TGFβ, IL-1β, or other growth factors.[177,178] Activation of its cognate receptor KDR occurs in the late menstrual and early proliferative phase. The other VEGF receptor, sFLT, is also elevated during menstruation, although its levels peak later than those of KDR. This protein acts as a dominant-negative receptor by sequestering VEGF from KDR, and may thus retard the wave of vascular repair.[177] The vasoconstrictor ET also has marked mitogenic actions and, in the human endometrium, ET-1, the predominant isoform, is maximally expressed during the late secretory and menstrual phase and has been proposed to have roles both in cessation of bleeding and in tissue repair.[145]

Leukocytes

Leukocytes play an important role in cutaneous wound healing, although no one cell type appears absolutely essential for efficient healing.[179] Leukocytes are present in substantial numbers in menstruating endometrium.[146] Although it is difficult to differentiate between the contribution of these cells to endometrial breakdown and their role in repair, certainly during the early stage of repair, regulatory factors derived from leukocytes are likely to be important. For example, interactions between macrophages, eosinophils, and their chemokines clearly contribute to epithelial growth in normal and cancer states,

including mammary gland development.[180] Chemokines may also contribute to tissue repair. For example, IL-8, which is expressed in endometrial vessels,[181] has angiogenic properties[182] and enhances re-epithelialization of skin grafts.[183]

A major difficulty in teasing out which factors are critical for either or both endometrial breakdown or repair has been the lack of availability of readily available animal models: Old-World primates are prohibitively expensive and colonies of menstruating bats are very rare. The recently described modification of a mouse model originally described by Finn and Pope[184] now offers opportunities to examine the importance of individual molecules and cells in these processes.[185]

CONCLUSIONS

Substantial remodeling events occur in the endometrium of all mammals during each menstrual or estrous cycle but these are more extreme in the human than in other species. Differences arise in large part from the necessity to provide a receptive endometrium for embryo implantation in each cycle. Even though hemochorial placentation is common to the human and mouse, because the human goes much further towards preparing the endometrium for implantation even in the absence of a blastocyst, more radical endometrial remodeling is needed. This is likely to be an evolutionary step to facilitate the chance of successful implantation in each cycle, but has meant that women must undergo menstruation throughout their adult lives. Because of the constant remodeling, many molecules normally associated only with developmental biology are found in the endometrium. Many of the major issues of women's health, including abnormal uterine bleeding, endometriosis and infertility, result from disturbances in remodeling, providing a strong case for better understanding of the underlying mechanisms.

ACKNOWLEDGMENTS

The author is supported by the National Health Council and Medical Research Council of Australia (# 143798, #241000). Thanks are due to Dr Guiying Nie and Dr Evdokia Dimitriadis for critical reading of the manuscript.

REFERENCES

1. Swiersz L, Giudice LC. Unexplained infertility and the role of uterine receptivity. Infertil Clin N Am 1997; 8: 523–43.
2. Carson DD, Bagchi I, Dey SK et al. Embryo implantation. Dev Biol 2000; 223(2): 217–37.
3. Sharkey AM, Smith SK. The endometrium as a cause of implantation failure. Best Pract Res Clin Obstet Gynaecol 2003; 17(2): 289–307.
4. Noyes RW, Hertig AT, Rock J. Dating the endometrial biopsy. Fertil Steril 1950; 1: 3–25.
5. Murray MJ, Meyer WR, Zaino RJ et al. A critical analysis of the accuracy, reproducibility, and clinical utility of histologic endometrial dating in fertile women. Fertil Steril 2004; 81(5): 1333–43.
6. Ludwig H, Spornitz UM. Microarchitecture of the human endometrium by scanning electron microscopy: menstrual desquamation and remodeling. Ann N Y Acad Sci 1991; 622: 28–46.
7. Salamonsen LA, Jones RL. Endometrial remodelling. In: Henry HL, Norman AW, eds. Encyclopedia of Hormones. San Diego, CA: Academic Press, 2003: 504–12.
8. Bingel AS. Timing of LH release and ovulation in 4- and 5-day cyclic mice. J Reprod Fertil 1974; 40(2): 315–20.
9. Guttenberg I. Plasma levels of "free" progestin during the estrous cycle in the mouse. Endocrinology 1961; 68: 1006–9.
10. Walmer DK, Wrona MA, Hughes CL, Nelson KG. Lactoferrin expression in the mouse reproductive tract during the natural estrous cycle: correlation with circulating estradiol and progesterone. Endocrinology 1992; 131(3): 1458–66.
11. Rugh R. The mouse. Its Reproduction and Development. New York: Oxford University Press, 1994.
12 Shiota K, Hirosawa M, Hattori N et al. Structural and functional aspects of placental lactogens (Pls) and ovarian 20alpha-hydroxysteroid dehydrogenase in the rat. Endocrine J 1994; 41(Suppl): S43–56.
13. Ponnampalam AP, Weston GC, Trajstman AC, Susil B, Rogers PA. Molecular classification of human endometrial cycle stages by transcriptional profiling. Mol Hum Reprod 2004; 10(12): 879–93.
14. Tan YF, Li FX, Piao YS, Sun XY, Wang YL. Global gene profiling analysis of mouse uterus during the oestrous cycle. Reproduction 2003; 126(2): 171–82.
15. Anonymous. Timing is everything. Nature 2003; 425: 885.
16. Kennaway DJ. The role of circadian rhythmicity in reproduction. Hum Reprod Update 2005; 11(1): 91–101.
17. Boonyaratanakornkit V, Edwards DP. Receptor mechanisms of rapid extranuclear signalling initiated by steroid hormones. Essays Biochem 2004; 40: 105–20.
18. Hewitt SC, Deroo BJ, Korach KS. Signal transduction. A new mediator for an old hormone? Science 2005; 307(5715): 1572–3.
19. Hewitt SC, Harrell JC, Korach KS. Lessons in estrogen biology from knockout and transgenic animals. Annu Rev Physiol 2005; 67: 285–308.
20. Gray CA, Bartol FF, Tarleton BJ et al. Developmental biology of uterine glands. Biol Reprod 2001; 65(5): 1311–23.
21. Girling JE, Rogers PA. Recent advances in endometrial angiogenesis research. Angiogenesis 2005; 8(2): 89–99.
22. Martin L, Finn CA, Stokes J. Refractory period following oestrogenic stimulation of cell division in the mouse uterus. J Endocrinol 1969; 43(1): xl.
23. Moulton BC, Koenig BB. Uterine deoxyribonucleic acid synthesis during preimplantation in precursors of stromal cell differentiation during decidualization. Endocrinology 1984; 115(4): 1302–7.

24. Tong W, Pollard JW. Progesterone inhibits estrogen-induced cyclin D1 and cdk4 nuclear translocation, cyclin E- and cyclin A-cdk2 kinase activation, and cell proliferation in uterine epithelial cells in mice. Mol Cell Biol 1999; 19(3): 2251–64.
25. Kerr JF, Wyllie AH, Currie AR. Apoptosis: a basic biological phenomenon with wide-ranging implications in tissue kinetics. Br J Cancer 1972; 26(4): 239–57.
26. Kaufmann SH, Hengartner MO. Programmed cell death: alive and well in the new millennium. Trends Cell Biol 2001; 11(12): 526–34.
27. Nicholson DW. From bench to clinic with apoptosis-based therapeutic agents. Nature 2000; 407(6805): 810–16.
28. Hengartner MO. The biochemistry of apoptosis. Nature 2000; 407(6805): 770–6.
29. Hopwood D, Levison DA. Atrophy and apoptosis in the cyclical human endometrium. J Pathol 1976; 119(3): 159–66.
30. Otsuki Y. Apoptosis in human endometrium: apoptotic detection methods and signaling. Med Electron Microsc 2001; 34(3): 166–73.
31. Watanabe H, Kanzaki H, Narukawa S et al. Bcl-2 and Fas expression in eutopic and ectopic human endometrium during the menstrual cycle in relation to endometrial cell apoptosis. Am J Obstet Gynecol 1997; 176(2): 360–8.
32. Yamashita H, Otsuki Y, Matsumoto K et al. Fas ligand, Fas antigen and Bcl-2 expression in human endometrium during the menstrual cycle. Mol Hum Reprod 1999; 5(4): 358–64.
33. Vaskivuo TE, Stenback F, Karhumaa P et al. Apoptosis and apoptosis-related proteins in human endometrium. Mol Cell Endocrinol 2000; 165(1–2): 75–83.
34. Tanaka M, Suda T, Haze K et al. Fas ligand in human serum. Nat Med 1996; 2(3): 317–22.
35. Zhang J, Salamonsen LA. In vivo evidence for active matrix metalloproteinases in human endometrium supports their role in tissue breakdown at menstruation. J Clin Endocrinol Metab 2002; 87(5): 2346–51.
36. Dahmoun M, Boman K, Cajander S et al. Apoptosis, proliferation, and sex hormone receptors in superficial parts of human endometrium at the end of the secretory phase. J Clin Endocrinol Metab 1999; 84(5): 1737–43.
37. Otsuki Y. Tissue specificity of apoptotic signal transduction. Med Electron Microsc 2004; 37(3): 163–9.
38. Kang TB, Ben-Moshe T, Varfolomeev EE et al. Caspase-8 serves both apoptotic and nonapoptotic roles. J Immunol 2004; 173(5): 2976–84.
39. Rotello RJ, Hocker MB, Gerschenson LE. Biochemical evidence for programmed cell death in rabbit uterine epithelium. Am J Pathol 1989; 134(3): 491–5.
40. Chen JC, Lin JH, Jow GM et al. Involvement of apoptosis during deciduomal regression in pseudopregnant hamsters effect of progesterone. Life Sci 2001; 68(7): 815–25.
41. Ghosh D, De P, Sengupta J. Effect of RU 486 on the endometrial response to deciduogenic stimulus in ovariectomized rhesus monkeys treated with oestrogen and progesterone. Hum Reprod 1992; 7(8): 1048–60.
42. Mor G, Straszewski S, Kamsteeg M. The Fas/FasL system in reproduction: survival and apoptosis. Scientific World Journal 2002; 2: 1828–42.
43. Viegas LR, Vicent GP, Baranao JL et al. Steroid hormones induce bcl-X gene expression through direct activation of distal promoter P4. J Biol Chem 2004; 279(11): 9831–9.
44. Pecci A, Scholz A, Pelster D, Beato M. Progestins prevent apoptosis in a rat endometrial cell line and increase the ratio of bcl-XL to bcl-XS. J Biol Chem 1997; 272(18): 11791–8.
45. Lovely LP, Fazleabas AT, Fritz MA, McAdams DG, Lessey BA. Prevention of endometrial apoptosis: randomized prospective comparison of human chorionic gonadotropin

versus progesterone treatment in the luteal phase. J Clin Endocrinol Metab 2005; 90(4): 2351–6.

46. Mukhopadhyay D, SundarRaj S, Alok A, Karande AA. Glycodelin A, not glycodelin S, is apoptotically active. Relevance of sialic acid modification. J Biol Chem 2004; 279(10): 8577–84.

47. Okazaki M, Matsuyama T, Kohno T et al. Induction of epithelial cell apoptosis in the uterus by a mouse uterine ischemia-reperfusion model: possible involvement of tumor necrosis factor-alpha. Biol Reprod 2005; 72(5): 1282–8.

48. Li A, Felix JC, Hao J, Minoo P, Jain JK. Menstrual-like breakdown and apoptosis in human endometrial explants. Hum Reprod 2005; 20(6): 1709–19.

49. Finn CA, Publicover M. Hormonal control of cell death in the luminal epithelium of the mouse uterus. J Endocrinol 1981; 91(2): 335–40.

50. Terada N, Yamamoto R, Takada T et al. Inhibitory effect of progesterone on cell death of mouse uterine epithelium. J Steroid Biochem 1989; 33(6): 1091–6.

51. Burroughs KD, Fuchs-Young R, Davis B, Walker CL. Altered hormonal responsiveness of proliferation and apoptosis during myometrial maturation and the development of uterine leiomyomas in the rat. Biol Reprod 2000; 63(5): 1322–30.

52. Mendoza-Rodriguez CA, Monroy-Mendoza MG, Morimoto S, Cerbon MA. Pro-apoptotic signals of the bcl-2 gene family in the rat uterus occurs in the night before the day of estrus and precedes ovulation. Mol Cell Endocrinol 2003; 208(1-2): 31–9.

53. Sato T, Fukazawa Y, Kojima H, Ohta Y, Iguchi T. Multiple mechanisms are involved in apoptotic cell death in the mouse uterus and vagina after ovariectomy. Reprod Toxicol 2003; 17(3): 289–97.

54. Psychoyos A. Endocrine control of egg implantation. In: Greep RO, Astwood EG, Geiger SR, eds. Handbook of Physiology. Washington, DC: American Physiological Society, 1973: 187–215.

55. Dey SK. Implantation. In: Adashi EY, Rock JA, Rosenwaks Z, eds. Reproductive Endocrinology, Surgery, and Technology. Philadelphia, PA: Lippincott-Raven, 1996: 421–34.

56. Thie M, Denker HW. In vitro studies on endometrial adhesiveness for trophoblast: cellular dynamics in uterine epithelial cells. Cells Tissues Organs 2002; 172(3): 237–52.

57. Nikas G, Develioglu OH, Toner JP, Jones HW Jr. Endometrial pinopodes indicate a shift in the window of receptivity in IVF cycles. Hum Reprod 1999; 14(3): 787–92.

58. Psychoyos A, Martel D. Embryo–endometrial interactions at implantation. In: Edwards RG, Purdy JM, Steptoe P, eds. Implantation of the Human Embryo. London: Academic Press, 1985: 195–210.

59. Bentin-Ley U, Sjogren A, Nilsson L et al. Presence of uterine pinopodes at the embryo–endometrial interface during human implantation in vitro. Hum Reprod 1999; 14(2): 515–20.

60. Horne AW, Lalani EN, Margara RA et al. The expression pattern of MUC1 glycoforms and other biomarkers of endometrial receptivity in fertile and infertile women. Mol Reprod Dev 2005; 72(2): 216–29.

61. Hey NA, Graham RA, Seif MW, Aplin JD. The polymorphic epithelial mucin MUC1 in human endometrium is regulated with maximal expression in the implantation phase. J Clin Endocrinol Metab 1994; 78(2): 337–42.

62. Meseguer M, Aplin JD, Caballero-Campo P et al. Human endometrial mucin MUC1 is up-regulated by progesterone and down-regulated in vitro by the human blastocyst. Biol Reprod 2001; 64(2): 590–601.

63. Surveyor GA, Gendler SJ, Pemberton L et al. Expression and steroid hormonal control of Muc-1 in the mouse uterus. Endocrinology 1995; 136(8): 3639–47.

64. Aplin JD, Hey NA, Li TC. MUC1 as a cell surface and secretory component of endometrial epithelium: reduced levels in recurrent miscarriage. Am J Reprod Immunol 1996; 35(3): 261–6.

65. White S, Kimber SJ. Changes in alpha (1-2)-fucosyltransferase activity in the murine endometrial epithelium during the estrous cycle, early pregnancy, and after ovariectomy and hormone replacement. Biol Reprod 1994; 50(1): 73–81.

66. Kimber SJ, Spanswick C. Blastocyst implantation: the adhesion cascade. Semin Cell Dev Biol 2000; 11(2): 77–92.

67. Aoki R, Fukuda MN. Recent molecular approaches to elucidate the mechanism of embryo implantation: trophinin, bystin, and tastin as molecules involved in the initial attachment of blastocysts to the uterus in humans. Semin Reprod Med 2000; 18(3): 265–71.

68. Thie M, Harrach-Ruprecht B, Sauer H et al. Cell adhesion to the apical pole of epithelium: a function of cell polarity. Eur J Cell Biol 1995; 66(2): 180–91.

69. Lessey BA, Damjanovich L, Coutifaris C et al. Integrin adhesion molecules in the human endometrium. Correlation with the normal and abnormal menstrual cycle. J Clin Invest 1992; 90(1): 188–95.

70. Lessey BA, Castelbaum AJ, Sawin SW, Sun J. Integrins as markers of uterine receptivity in women with primary unexplained infertility. Fertil Steril 1995; 63(3): 535–42.

71. Creus M, Ordi J, Fabregues F et al. alphavbeta3 integrin expression and pinopod formation in normal and out-of-phase endometria of fertile and infertile women. Hum Reprod 2002; 17(9): 2279–86.

72. Apparao KB, Murray MJ, Fritz MA et al. Osteopontin and its receptor alphavbeta(3) integrin are coexpressed in the human endometrium during the menstrual cycle but regulated differentially. J Clin Endocrinol Metab 2001; 86(10): 4991–5000.

73. Luu KC, Nie GY, Salamonsen LA. Endometrial calbindins are critical for embryo implantation: evidence from in vivo use of morpholino antisense oligonucleotides. Proc Natl Acad Sci USA 2004; 101(21): 8028–33.

74. Luu KC, Nie GY, Hampton A et al. Endometrial expression of calbindin (CaBP)-d28k but not CaBP-d9k in primates implies evolutionary changes and functional redundancy of calbindins at implantation. Reproduction 2004; 128(4): 433–41.

75. Ding YQ, Zhu LJ, Bagchi MK, Bagchi IC. Progesterone stimulates calcitonin gene expression in the uterus during implantation. Endocrinology 1994; 135(5): 2265–74.

76. Kumar S, Zhu LJ, Polihronis M et al. Progesterone induces calcitonin gene expression in human endometrium within the putative window of implantation. J Clin Endocrinol Metab 1998; 83(12): 4443–50.

77. Zhu L-J, Bagchi MK, Bagchi IC. Attenuation of calcitonin gene expression in pregnant rat uterus leads to a block in embryonic implantation. Endocrinology 1998; 139: 330–9.

78. Kane MT, Morgan PM, Coonan C. Peptide growth factors and preimplantation development. Hum Reprod Update 1997; 3(2): 137–57.

79. Gray CA, Burghardt RC, Johnson GA et al. Evidence that absence of endometrial gland secretions in uterine gland knockout ewes compromises conceptus survival and elongation. Reproduction 2002; 124(2): 289–300.

80. Bhatt H, Brunet LJ, Stewart CL. Uterine expression of leukemia inhibitory factor coincides with the onset of blastocyst implantation. Proc Natl Acad Sci USA 1991; 88(24): 11408–12.

81. Burton GJ, Watson AL, Hempstock J et al. Uterine glands provide histiotrophic nutrition for the human fetus during the first trimester of pregnancy. J Clin Endocrinol Metab 2002; 87(6): 2954–9.

82. Yoo HJ, Barlow DH, Mardon HJ. Temporal and spatial regulation of expression of heparin-binding epidermal growth

factor-like growth factor in the human endometrium: a possible role in blastocyst implantation. Dev Genet 1997; 21(1): 102–8.

83. Dimitriadis E, Salamonsen LA, Robb L. Expression of interleukin-11 during the human menstrual cycle: coincidence with stromal cell decidualization and relationship to leukaemia inhibitory factor and prolactin. Mol Hum Reprod 2000; 6(10): 907–14.

84. Robb L, Li R, Hartley L et al. Infertility in female mice lacking the receptor for interleukin 11 is due to a defective uterine response to implantation. Nat Med 1998; 4(3): 303–8.

85. Nie G, Li Y, Wang M et al. Inhibiting uterine PC6 blocks embryo implantation: an obligatory role for a proprotein convertase in fertility. Biol Reprod 2005; 72(4): 1029–36.

86. Nie GY, Li Y, Minoura H et al. Specific and transient upregulation of proprotein convertase 6 at the site of embryo implantation and identification of a unique transcript in mouse uterus during early pregnancy. Biol Reprod 2003; 68(2): 439–47.

87. Fahey JV, Schaefer TM, Channon JY, Wira CR. Secretion of cytokines and chemokines by polarized human epithelial cells from the female reproductive tract. Hum Reprod 2005; 20(6): 1439–46.

88. Jones RL, Hannan NJ, Kaitu'u TJ et al. Identification of chemokines important for leukocyte recruitment to the human endometrium at the times of embryo implantation and menstruation. J Clin Endocrinol Metab 2004; 89(12): 6155–67.

89. Dominguez F, Pellicer A, Simon C. The chemokine connection: hormonal and embryonic regulation at the human maternal–embryonic interface – a review. Placenta 2003; 24(Suppl B): S48–55.

90. Hannan NJ, Jones RL, White CA, Salamonsen LA. The chemokines, hemofiltrate CC Chemokine (HCC)-1 and macrophage inflammatory protein (MIP) – 1beta CX3CL1, CC14, and CCL4 fractalkine, promote human trophoblast migration at the feto–maternal interface. Biol Reprod 2006; 74(3): 896–904.

91. Lim H, Paria BC, Das SK et al. Multiple female reproductive failures in cyclooxygenase 2-deficient mice. Cell 1997; 91(2): 197–208.

92. Lydon JP, DeMayo FJ, Funk CR et al. Mice lacking progesterone receptor exhibit pleiotropic reproductive abnormalities. Genes Dev 1995; 9(18): 2266–78.

93. Xu J, Qiu Y, DeMayo FJ et al. Partial hormone resistance in mice with disruption of the steroid receptor coactivator-1 (SRC-1) gene. Science 1998; 279(5358): 1922–5.

94. Gendron RL, Paradis H, Hsieh-Li HM et al. Abnormal uterine stromal and glandular function associated with maternal reproductive defects in Hoxa-11 null mice. Biol Reprod 1997; 56(5): 1097–105.

95. Ma L, Benson GV, Lim H et al. Abdominal B (AbdB) Hoxa genes: regulation in adult uterus by estrogen and progesterone and repression in müllerian duct by the synthetic estrogen diethylstilbestrol (DES). Dev Biol 1998; 197(2): 141–54.

96. Bilinski P, Roopenian D, Gossler A. Maternal IL-11Ralpha function is required for normal decidua and fetoplacental development in mice. Genes Dev 1998; 12(14): 2234–43.

97. Ashkar AA, Di Santo JP, Croy BA. Interferon gamma contributes to initiation of uterine vascular modification, decidual integrity, and uterine natural killer cell maturation during normal murine pregnancy. J Exp Med 2000; 192(2): 259–70.

98. de Ziegler D, Fanchin R, de Moustier B, Bulletti C. The hormonal control of endometrial receptivity: estrogen (E2) and progesterone. J Reprod Immunol 1998; 39(1–2): 149–66.

99. Brenner RM, Slayden OV. Cyclic changes in the primate oviduct and endometrium. In: Knobil E, Neill JD, eds. The Physiology of Reproduction, 2nd edn. New York: Raven, 1994: 541–70.

100. Rasweiler JJ 4th. Spontaneous decidual reactions and menstruation in the black mastiff bat, Molossus ater. Am J Anat 1991; 191(1): 1–22.

101. Kennedy TG. Decidualization. In: Henry HL, Norman AW, eds. Encyclopedia of Hormones. San Diego, CA: Academic Press, 2003: 379–85.

102. Gu Y, Soares MJ, Srivastava RK, Gibori G. Expression of decidual prolactin-related protein in the rat decidua. Endocrinology 1994; 135(4): 1422–7.

103. Nie G, Li Y, Salamonsen LA. Serine protease HtrA1 is developmentally regulated in trophoblast and uterine decidual cells during placental formation in the mouse. Dev Dyn 2005; 233(3): 1102–9.

104. Bryant-Greenwood GD, Rutanen EM, Partanen S, Coelho TK, Yamamoto SY. Sequential appearance of relaxin, prolactin and IGFBP-1 during growth and differentiation of the human endometrium. Mol Cell Endocrinol 1993; 95(1–2): 23–9.

105. Tierney EP, Tulac S, Huang ST, Giudice LC. Activation of the protein kinase A pathway in human endometrial stromal cells reveals sequential categorical gene regulation. Physiol Genomics 2003; 16(1): 47–66.

106. Mizuno K, Tanaka T, Umesaki N, Ogita S. Establishment and characterization of in vitro decidualization in normal human endometrial stromal cells. Osaka City Med J 1998; 44(1): 105–15.

107. Gellersen B, Brosens J. Cyclic AMP and progesterone receptor cross-talk in human endometrium: a decidualizing affair. J Endocrinol 2003; 178(3): 357–72.

108. Giudice LC. Elucidating endometrial function in the postgenomic era. Hum Reprod Update 2003; 9(3): 223–35.

109. Mulac-Jericevic B, Mullinax RA, DeMayo FJ et al. Subgroup of reproductive functions of progesterone mediated by progesterone receptor-B isoform. Science 2000; 289 (5485): 1751–4.

110. Mote PA, Balleine RL, McGowan EM, Clarke CL. Colocalization of progesterone receptors A and B by dual immunofluorescent histochemistry in human endometrium during the menstrual cycle. J Clin Endocrinol Metab 1999; 84(8): 2963–71.

111. Gao J, Mazella J, Tang M, Tseng L. Ligand-activated progesterone receptor isoform hPR-A is a stronger transactivator than hPR-B for the expression of IGFBP-1 (insulin-like growth factor binding protein-1) in human endometrial stromal cells. Mol Endocrinol 2000; 14(12): 1954–61.

112. Brosens JJ, Hayashi N, White JO. Progesterone receptor regulates decidual prolactin expression in differentiating human endometrial stromal cells. Endocrinology 1999; 140(10): 4809–20.

113. Bartscha O, Ivell R. Relaxin and phosphodiesterases collaborate during decidualization. Ann N Y Acad Sci 2004; 1030: 479–92.

114. Zhu Y, Bond J, Thomas P. Identification, classification, and partial characterization of genes in humans and other vertebrates homologous to a fish membrane progestin receptor. Proc Natl Acad Sci USA 2003; 100(5): 2237–42.

115. Richer JK, Lange CA, Manning NG et al. Convergence of progesterone with growth factor and cytokine signaling in breast cancer. Progesterone receptors regulate signal transducers and activators of transcription expression and activity. J Biol Chem 1998; 273(47): 31317–26.

116. Liu T, Ogle TF. Signal transducer and activator of transcription 3 is expressed in the decidualized mesometrium of pregnancy and associates with the progesterone receptor through protein–protein interactions. Biol Reprod 2002; 67(1): 114–18.

117. Marinissen MJ, Gutkind JS. G-protein-coupled receptors and signaling networks: emerging paradigms. Trends Pharmacol Sci 2001; 22(7): 368–76.

118. Dimitriadis E, Stoikos C, Baca M et al. Relaxin and prostaglandin E(2) regulate interleukin 11 during human endometrial stromal cell decidualization. J Clin Endocrinol Metab 2005; 90(6): 3458–65.

119. Jones RL, Salamonsen LA, Findlay JK. Activin A promotes human endometrial stromal cell decidualization in vitro. J Clin Endocrinol Metab 2002; 87(8): 4001–4.

120. Tang B, Gurpide E. Direct effect of gonadotropins on decidualization of human endometrial stroma cells. J Steroid Biochem Mol Biol 1993; 47(1–6): 115–21.

121. Ferrari A, Petraglia F, Gurpide E. Corticotropin releasing factor decidualizes human endometrial stromal cells in vitro. Interaction with progestin. J Steroid Biochem Mol Biol 1995; 54(5–6): 251–5.

122. Tseng L, Gao JG, Chen R et al. Effect of progestin, antiprogestin, and relaxin on the accumulation of prolactin and insulin-like growth factor-binding protein-1 messenger ribonucleic acid in human endometrial stromal cells. Biol Reprod 1992; 47(3): 441–50.

123. Frank GR, Brar AK, Cedars MI, Handwerger S. Prostaglandin E2 enhances human endometrial stromal cell differentiation. Endocrinology 1994; 134(1): 258–63.

124. Lane B, Oxberry W, Mazella J, Tseng L. Decidualization of human endometrial stromal cells in vitro: effects of progestin and relaxin on the ultrastructure and production of decidual secretory proteins. Hum Reprod 1994; 9(2): 259–66.

125. Telgmann R, Maronde E, Tasken K, Gellersen B. Activated protein kinase A is required for differentiation-dependent transcription of the decidual prolactin gene in human endometrial stromal cells. Endocrinology 1997; 138(3): 929–37.

126. White CA, Dimitriadis E, Sharkey AM, Salamonsen LA. Interleukin-11 inhibits expression of insulin-like growth factor binding protein-5 mRNA in decidualizing human endometrial stromal cells. Mol Hum Reprod 2005; 11(9): 649–58.

127. White CA, Robb L, Salamonsen LA. Uterine extracellular matrix components are altered during defective decidualization in interleukin-11 receptor alpha deficient mice. Reprod Biol Endocrinol 2004; 2(1): 76.

128. Dai D, Ogle TF. Progesterone regulation of epidermal growth factor receptor in rat decidua basalis during pregnancy. Biol Reprod 1999; 61(1): 326–32.

129. Chobotova K, Karpovich N, Carver J et al. Heparin-binding epidermal growth factor and its receptors mediate decidualization and potentiate survival of human endometrial stromal cells. J Clin Endocrinol Metab 2005; 90(2): 913–19.

130. Mazella J, Tang M, Tseng L. Disparate effects of relaxin and TGFbeta1: relaxin increases, but TGFbeta1 inhibits, the relaxin receptor and the production of IGFBP-1 in human endometrial stromal/decidual cells. Hum Reprod 2004; 19(7): 1513–18.

131. Zhao L, Roche PJ, Gunnersen JM et al. Mice without a functional relaxin gene are unable to deliver milk to their pups. Endocrinology 1999; 140(1): 445–53.

132. Tang M, Mazella J, Zhu HH, Tseng L. Ligand activated relaxin receptor increases the transcription of IGFBP-1 and prolactin in human decidual and endometrial stromal cells. Mol Hum Reprod 2005; 11(4): 237–43.

133. Alexander CM, Hansell EJ, Behrendtsen O et al. Expression and function of matrix metalloproteinases and their inhibitors at the maternal–embryonic boundary during mouse embryo implantation. Development 1996; 122(6): 1723–36.

134. McCawley LJ, Matrisian LM. Matrix metalloproteinases: they're not just for matrix anymore! Curr Opin Cell Biol 2001; 13(5): 534–40.

135. Okada H, Nie G, Salamonsen LA. Requirement for proprotein convertase 5/6 during decidualization of human endometrial stromal cells in vitro. J Clin Endocrinol Metab 2005; 90(2): 1028–34.

136. Seidah NG, Chretien M. Proprotein and prohormone convertases: a family of subtilases generating diverse bioactive polypeptides. Brain Res 1999; 848(1–2): 45–62.

137. Salamonsen LA, Zhang J, Brasted M. Leukocyte networks and human endometrial remodelling. J Reprod Immunol 2002; 57(1–2): 95–108.

138. Hunt JS, Petroff MG, Burnett TG. Uterine leukocytes: key players in pregnancy. Semin Cell Dev Biol 2000; 11(2): 127–37.

139. Croy BA, He H, Esadeg S et al. Uterine natural killer cells: insights into their cellular and molecular biology from mouse modelling. Reproduction 2003; 126(2): 149–60.

140. Finn CA. Implantation, menstruation and inflammation. Biol Rev 1986; 61: 313–28.

141. Salamonsen LA, Kovacs G, Findlay JK. Current concepts of the mechanisms of menstruation. In: Smith SK, ed. Baillière's Clinical Obstetrics and Gynaecology, Dysfunctional Uterine Bleeding. 13 (2) edn. London: Baillière Tyndall, 1999: 161–79.

142. Markee JE. Menstruation in intraocular endometrial transplants in the rhesus monkey. Contrib Embryol 1940; 177: 220–30.

143. Roberts DK, Parmley TH, Walker NJ, Horbelt DV. Ultrastructure of the microvasculature in the human endometrium throughout the normal menstrual cycle. Am J Obstet Gynecol 1992; 166: 1393–406.

144. Schatz F, Aigner S, Papp C et al. Plasminogen activator activity during decidualization of human endometrial stromal cells is regulated by plasminogen activator inhibitor 1. J Clin Endocrinol Metab 1995; 80(8): 2504–10.

145. Salamonsen LA, Marsh MM, Findlay JK. Endometrial endothelin: regulator of uterine bleeding and endometrial repair. Clin Exp Pharm Physiol 1999; 26: 154–7.

146. Salamonsen LA, Woolley DE. Menstruation: induction by matrix metalloproteinases and inflammatory cells. J Reprod Immunol 1999; 44(1–2): 1–27.

147. King A, Burrows T, Verma S et al. Human uterine lymphocytes. Hum Reprod Update 1998; 4(5): 480–5.

148. Kelly RW, Illingworth P, Baldie G et al. Progesterone control of interleukin-8 production in endometrium and choriodecidual cells underlines the role of the neutrophil in menstruation and parturition. Hum Reprod 1994; 9(2): 253–8.

149. Curry TE Jr, Osteen KG. Cyclic changes in the matrix metalloproteinase system in the ovary and uterus. Biol Reprod 2001; 64(5): 1285–96.

150. Marbaix E, Kokorine I, Moulin P et al. Menstrual breakdown of human endometrium can be mimicked in vitro and is selectively and reversibly blocked by inhibitors of matrix metalloproteinases. Proc Natl Acad Sci USA 1996; 93: 9120–5.

151. Zhang J, Salamonsen LA. Tissue inhibitor of metalloproteinases (TIMP)-1, -2 and -3 in human endometrium during the menstrual cycle. Mol Hum Reprod 1997; 3(9): 735–41.

152. Rees MC, Demers LM, Anderson AB, Turnbull AC. A functional study of platelets in menstrual fluid. Br J Obstet Gynaecol 1984; 91(7): 667–72.

153. Casslen B, Nordengren J, Gustavsson B et al. Progesterone stimulates degradation of urokinase plasminogen activator (u-PA) in endometrial stromal cells by increasing its inhibitor and surface expression of the u-PA receptor. J Clin Endocrinol Metab 1995; 80(9): 2776–84.

154. Gleeson N, Devitt M, Sheppard BL, Bonnar J. Endometrial fibrinolytic enzymes in women with normal menstruation and dysfunctional uterine bleeding. Br J Obstet Gynaecol 1993; 100(8): 768–71.

155. Rumalla VK, Borah GL. Cytokines, growth factors, and plastic surgery. Plast Reconstr Surg 2001; 108(3): 719–33.

156. Ferenczy A, Bertrand G, Gelfand MM. Studies on the cytodynamics of human endometrial regeneration. III. In vitro

short-term incubation historadioautography. Am J Obstet Gynecol 1979; 134: 297–304.

157. Okulicz WC, Scarrell R. Estrogen receptor alpha and progesterone receptor in the rhesus endometrium during the late secretory phase and menses. Proc Soc Exp Biol Med 1998; 218(4): 316–21.

158. Bigsby RM. Control of growth and differentiation of the endometrium: the role of tissue interactions. Ann NY Acad Sci 2002; 955: 110–17.

159. Brandon JM. Decidualization in the post-partum uterus of the mouse. J Reprod Fertil 1990; 88(1): 151–8.

160. Samuels P, Tan AK. Fetal scarless wound healing. J Otolaryngol 1999; 28(5): 296–302.

161. Wilson AJ, Gibson PR. Epithelial migration in the colon: filling in the gaps. Clin Sci (Lond) 1997; 93(2): 97–108.

162. Basson MD. In vitro evidence for matrix regulation of intestinal epithelial biology during mucosal healing. Life Sci 2001; 69(25–26): 3005–18.

163. Wallace JL, Whittle BJ. The role of extracellular mucus as a protective cap over gastric mucosal damage. Scand J Gastroenterol Suppl 1986; 125: 79–85.

164. Ferenczy A. Studies on the cytodynamics of human endometrial regeneration. II. Transmission electron microscopy and histochemistry. Am J Obstet Gynecol 1976; 124: 582–95.

165. Fuchs E, Segre JA. Stem cells: a new lease on life. Cell 2000; 100(1): 143–55.

166. Schwab KE, Chan RW, Gargett CE. Putative stem cell activity of human endometrial epithelial and stromal cells during the menstrual cycle. Fertil Steril 2005; 84(Suppl 2): 1124–30.

167. Taylor HS. Endometrial cells derived from donor stem cells in bone marrow transplant recipients. JAMA 2004; 292(1): 81–5.

168. Parks WC. Matrix metalloproteinases in repair. Wound Repair Regen 1999; 7(6): 423–32.

169. Whitelock JM, Murdoch AD, Iozzo RV, Underwood PA. The degradation of human endothelial cell-derived perlecan and release of bound basic fibroblast growth factor by stromelysin, collagenase, plasmin, and heparanases. J Biol Chem 1996; 271(17): 10079–86.

170. Yu Q, Stamenkovic I. Cell surface-localized matrix metalloproteinase-9 proteolytically activates TGF-beta and promotes tumor invasion and angiogenesis. Genes Dev 2000; 14(2): 163–76.

171. Schonbeck U, Mach F, Libby P. Generation of biologically active IL-1 beta by matrix metalloproteinases: a novel caspase-1-independent pathway of IL-1 beta processing. J Immunol 1998; 161(7): 3340–6.

172. Parks WC, Lopez-Boado YS, Wilson CL. Matrilysin in epithelial repair and defense. Chest 2001; 120(1 Suppl): 36–41S.

173. Munz B, Smola H, Engelhardt F et al. Overexpression of activin A in the skin of transgenic mice reveals new activities of activin in epidermal morphogenesis, dermal fibrosis and wound repair. EMBO J 1999; 18: 5205–15.

174. Wankell M, Munz B, Hubner G et al. Impaired wound healing in transgenic mice overexpressing the activin antagonist follistatin in the epidermis. EMBO J 2001; 20(19): 5361–72.

175. Jones RL, Salamonsen LA, Findlay JK. Potential roles for endometrial inhibins, activins and follistatin during human embryo implantation and early pregnancy. Trends Endocrinol Metab 2002; 13(4): 144–50.

176. Sugawara J, Fukaya T, Murakami T et al. Hepatocyte growth factor stimulated proliferation, migration, and lumen formation of human endometrial epithelial cells in vitro. Biol Reprod 1997; 57(4): 936–42.

177. Graubert MD, Ortega MA, Kessel B et al. Vascular repair after menstruation involves regulation of vascular endothelial growth factor-receptor phosphorylation by sFLT-1. Am J Pathol 2001; 158(4): 1399–410.

178. Nayak NR, Brenner RM. Vascular proliferation and vascular endothelial growth factor expression in the rhesus macaque endometrium. J Clin Endocrinol Metab 2002; 87(4): 1845–55.

179. Martin P, Leibovich SJ. Inflammatory cells during wound repair: the good, the bad and the ugly. Trends Cell Biol 2005; 15(11): 599–607.

180. Gouon-Evans V, Lin EY, Pollard JW. Requirement of macrophages and eosinophils and their cytokines/chemokines for mammary gland development. Breast Cancer Res 2002; 4(4): 155–64.

181. Jones RL, Kelly RW, Critchley HOD. Chemokine and cyclooxygenase-2 expression in human endometrium coincides with leukocyte accumulation. Hum Reprod 1997; 12(6): 1300–6.

182. Koch AE, Polverini PJ, Kunkel SL et al. Interleukin-8 as a macrophage-derived mediator of angiogenesis. Science 1992; 258(5089): 1798–801.

183. Rennekampff HO, Hansbrough JF, Kiessig V et al. Bioactive interleukin-8 is expressed in wounds and enhances wound healing. J Surg Res 2000; 93(1): 41–54.

184. Finn CA, Pope M. Vascular and cellular changes in the decidualized endometrium of the ovariectomized mouse following cessation of hormone treatment: a possible model for menstruation. J Endocrinol 1984; 100(3): 295–300.

185. Brasted M, White CA, Kennedy TG, Salamonsen LA. Mimicking the events of menstruation in the murine uterus. Biol Reprod 2003; 69(4): 1273–80.

186. Harada T, Kaponis A, Iwabe T et al. Apoptosis in human endometrium and endometriosis. Hum Reprod Update 2004; 10(1): 29–38.

187. Di Paola M, Loverro G, Caringella AM, Cormioselvaggi GL. Receptorial and mitochondrial apoptotic pathways in normal and neoplastic human endometrium. Int J Gynecol Cancer 2005; 15(3): 523–8.

188. Dimitriadis E, White CA, Jones RL, Salamonsen LA. Cytokines, chemokines and growth factors in endometrium related to implantation. Hum Reprod Update 2005; 11(6): 613–30.

189. Lee KY, DeMayo FJ. Animal models of implantation. Reproduction 2004; 128(6): 679–95.

190. Tang B, Guller S, Gurpide E. Mechanisms involved in the decidualization of human endometrial stromal cells. Acta Eur Fertil 1993; 24(5): 221–3.

191. Huang JR, Tseng L, Bischof P, Janne OA. Regulation of prolactin production by progestin, estrogen, and relaxin in human endometrial stromal cells. Endocrinology 1987; 121(6): 2011–17.

192. Dimitriadis E, Robb L, Salamonsen LA. Interleukin 11 advances progesterone-induced decidualization of human endometrial stromal cells. Mol Hum Reprod 2002; 8(7): 636–43.

193. Zoumakis E, Margioris AN, Stournaras C et al. Corticotrophin-releasing hormone (CRH) interacts with inflammatory prostaglandins and interleukins and affects the decidualization of human endometrial stroma. Mol Hum Reprod 2000; 6(4): 344–51.

194. Di Blasio AM, Pecori Giraldi F, Vigano P et al. Expression of corticotropin-releasing hormone and its R1 receptor in human endometrial stromal cells. J Clin Endocrinol Metab 1997; 82(5): 1594–7.

4 The fine structure of the mature human endometrium

Peter Dockery and Marcella J Burke

Synopsis

Background

- The endometrium undergoes dynamic reorganization during the menstrual cycle in preparation for implantation.
- The mean length of the normal menstrual cycle is just over 28 days, but there is considerable variation.
- It is generally described in three phases: the proliferative phase (days 5–14), the secretory phase (days 14–28), and menses (days 1–4) if no implantation occurs.
- At menstruation the superficial layer is partially or completely shed and remodeled in preparation for the next cycle.

Basic Science

- Histological dating of the endometrial biopsy has been traditionally carried out by the use of the Noyes' criteria.
- The group of descriptors identified provides an excellent overall account of events occurring in the various tissue compartments during the menstrual cycle. However, these criteria are rather subjective and therefore prone to observer bias.
- The use of well-timed biopsies combined with objective morphometric analysis has improved our understanding of the anatomical changes that occur during the normal cycle.
- These methods have revealed the remarkably tight control that exists over certain cellular events during the secretory phase which may be related to a window of uterine receptivity.
- Ultrastructural analysis reveals specific features of early secretory phase gland cells, including giant mitochondria, the nuclear channel system, and subnuclear glycogen deposits.
- The ratio of stromal cells to gland cells is constant during the secretory phase, suggesting tight regulation of cell numbers.
- Recent studies have suggested that environmental endocrine disrupting agents can affect the morphology and the physiology of endometrial epithelial cells and this may affect the implantation window.
- New tools such as non-invasive imaging techniques, confocal microscopy, and functional genomics should shed further light on the mechanisms controlling morphological and functional changes in the endometrium.
- Stereological methods should be used to provide a comprehensive anatomical and structural framework upon which to lay the new physiological and molecular information.

Clinical

- Cycle length has been shown to be variable and periovulatory endocrine relationships are incompletely understood.
- Chronological dating of the endometrial biopsy utilizing the next or the last menstrual period or increase in basal body temperature have been shown to be inaccurate.
- Secretory phase dating based on the time of ovulation or use of the LH surge that precedes ovulation improves the precision of chronological dating.

- An endometrial biopsy should come from a standardized region of the uterus. As the area of interest is generally the commonest site of implantation, the upper part of the uterine corpus is a reasonable choice.
- With advances in clinical imaging, an important challenge is to determine which microscopic method provides the most functionally relevant benchmarks for interpreting clinical images and to bridge the resolution gap both spatially and temporally.

ABSTRACT

This chapter outlines some of the dynamic structural changes that occur in the mature human endometrium during the menstrual cycle. In order to fully interpret our increased knowledge of the underlying physiological and molecular changes in the endometrium, an adequate structural and temporal framework is required. The advantages of adequate dating and mensuration of the endometrial biopsy are highlighted and illustrated with some baseline morphometric data.

INTRODUCTION

The endometrium undergoes dynamic reorganization during the menstrual cycle in preparation for implantation. If no implantation occurs the superficial layer is partially or completely shed and remodeled in preparation for the next cycle.[1] Our understanding of the physiology and molecular biology of the endometrium has increased greatly over the past 20 years.[2–4] The endometrial response to cyclic variations in sex steroids involves a diverse array of mediators, including enzymes, hormones, and bioactive peptides,[2,5–7] exerting local autocrine and paracrine actions that are important in implantation and in maintaining the integrity of the non-pregnant endometrium. The net effect of this interplay is to provide a unique environment which allows or prevents implantation and subsequent nidation.[8] Successful implantation requires synchronization of endometrial maturation and embryonic development.[9] A concept that has become central to our understanding of endometrial function is that of the implantation window, a period of optimal endometrial receptivity.[8] The extent of this window and the physiological, molecular, and anatomical events in the endometrium that frame it are still being defined (see Chapter 21). The recent use of gene expression analysis methodologies is providing an important insight into these complex interactions[10,11] (see Chapter 14).

The lining of the human uterus is a complex mucosa composed of two major compartments: a germinal or basal layer, which persists from cycle to cycle, and a transient superficial functional layer. The function of the latter is to accommodate the implanting blastocyst and provide the maternal component of the placenta.[12] The tissue components of the endometrium are a lining surface epithelium and associated glands with a connective tissue stroma in which is embedded an elaborate vascular tree (Figure 4.1). The nature and control of the dynamic processes occurring in the endometrium are gradually being unraveled, but knowledge of the associated anatomical changes is in places incomplete. This has resulted from a number of factors. Much confusion over the timing and variability of events during the cycle has been caused by elementary shortcomings, such as poor timing of biopsy and selection of subjects.[13,14] To assume a simple link between circulating steroid levels and a morphological feature may be tempting but is essentially naive, because hormonal priming is only one of several influences. The final cellular response is likely to be threshold-dependent with prominent individual variation. Indeed, there is no simple relationship between peripheral hormone levels and morphometric indices.[15] The endometrium must reach a requisite level of development before it can respond in an adequate way to progesterone. Two principal sources of inaccuracy are dating of the biopsy and the sampling procedure.

Dating of the biopsy

Chronological dating of the endometrial biopsy may utilize the next or the last menstrual period or increase in basal body temperature. However, these have been shown to be inaccurate.[14,16] Secretory phase dating based on the time of ovulation or use of the luteinizing hormone (LH) surge that accompanies ovulation improves the precision of chronological dating. Cycle length has been shown to be variable[17] and periovulatory endocrine relationships are incompletely understood. It has been reported that use of the LH peak did not improve the clinical value of endometrial biopsy

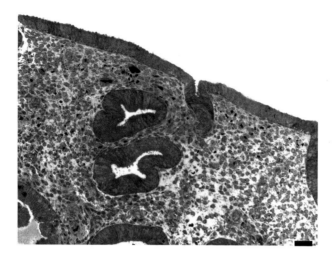

Figure 4.1   Luminal epithelium. A light micrograph showing the main cellular compartments of the endometrium: luminal, glandular epithelium, and stroma (bar = 15 μm).

dating[18] and that midluteal phase endometrial biopsy provides only a crude test of luteal function, which does not precisely distinguish luteal insufficiency.[19] Part of the problem is the simplistic overinterpretation of the histological changes (dating) and the increased tissue heterogeneity during the late secretory phase. These shortcomings can be resolved to some degree by documenting the hormonal events carefully and by noting the provenance of the biopsy combined with an increased objectivity in assessment of tissue differentiation. Much can be gleaned from scientific studies using material obtained under conditions controlled in these respects.

Histological dating of the endometrial biopsy has been traditionally carried out by the use of the Noyes' criteria.[20] The group of descriptors identified provides an excellent overall account of events occurring in the various endometrial compartments throughout the menstrual cycle. However, these criteria are rather subjective and therefore prone to observer bias.[21,22] Greatly improved precision of endometrial dating can be achieved by the use of light microscopical morphometric/stereological methods that remove much of the observer bias.[23,24]

Sampling

In most studies of endometrial structure the whole organ cannot be investigated and so a sample (biopsy) is taken. This should come from a standardized region of the uterus. Many sampling strategies have been developed for complex biological tissues.[25] As the area of

interest is generally the commonest site of implantation, the usual method of taking a biopsy from the fundus and upper part of the body of the uterus is reasonable. If a preferred orientation of the biopsy for sectioning is chosen then this puts certain restrictions on the type of stereological probes that can be applied to the tissue. However, a number of methods enable these constraints to be overcome, allowing greatly enhanced access to the anatomical information contained in the tissue.[25] A characteristic feature of the endometrium is its variability. Certain parameters exhibit considerable variation within the tissue but remarkably low variability between individuals.[26,27] Such tight control of cellular events may reflect biological importance.[28] The great value of adopting a stereological/morphometric approach is that it permits objective quantification of such potentially confusing variation. Sampling strategies have to be specifically designed for each individual study and need to be developed depending on the compartment or feature of interest. If the event is rare, a greater number of blocks/fields have to be examined. The contribution of each level of sampling to the overall observed variation must be taken into account when designing an experimental protocol.[29,30] Pilot studies should examine efficiency and economy of effort for the most productive and scientifically meaningful approach. These costing exercises do not take much time and should form an essential component of any study of endometrial morphology.

THE MENSTRUAL CYCLE

Cyclic changes in endometrial structure have been well described at the light microscopic level.[1] The mean length of the normal human menstrual cycle is just over 28 days, but there is considerable variation. It is generally described in three phases: the proliferative phase (days 5–14), the secretory phase (days 14–28), and menses (days 1–4) if no implantation occurs. The use of improved chronological dating and a number of morphometric methods have improved our appreciation of the anatomical changes within the endometrium.[16,24]

The proliferative phase

The proliferative phase is characterized by postmenstrual re-epithelialization and growth of stromal and glandular elements. This results in an increase in endometrial thickness from about 1 mm to 3–4 mm by the time of ovulation. Ovarian estrogen is the dominant hormone during this part of the cycle. This in turn is dependent on follicle-stimulating hormone (FSH) from the adenohypophysis. The length of this phase can vary from 9 to 23 days.[16] Age seems to affect cycle length: younger women have a longer proliferative phase than older women.[31] Ovulation usually occurs about 16 hours after the surge in LH. This is usually designated as day LH+0 or day 14 of a 28-day cycle.

Histology

The early proliferative phase (days 5–7) is usually characterized by straight, fairly undifferentiated glands with circular cross section lined by a columnar epithelium with basally located nuclei. Their luminal diameter (below 50 μm) changes little in the proliferative phase and the height of the cells remains fairly constant (around 21 μm). Occasional mitotic figures can be seen. The stroma contains spindly cells with relatively large nuclei in which occasional mitoses are seen.

By the mid-proliferative phase (days 8–10) the endometrial glands are longer with slight tortuosity. The cells appear pseudostratified, and mitotic figures are prominent. The late proliferative phase (days 11–14) has glands exhibiting a marked tortuosity, with wider lumena. The gland cells are tall and columnar. At LH−3 there are about 23 mitotic figures per 1000 gland cells. Pseudostratification increases, reaching a maximum between days LH−4/−3 and LH+1/2.[1,16] Variable stromal edema is evident, and mitotic rate in the stroma is highest about 2–3 days before and 1–2 days after ovulation.

The secretory phase

During the secretory phase the endometrium is influenced by progesterone and to a lesser extent estrogen. The length of the secretory phase has been reported to vary between 8 and 17 days.[32] In the early secretory phase (LH+0–LH+7) progesterone rises rapidly and structural changes in the endometrium are also rapid. The length of this part of the menstrual cycle is strictly controlled. The most obvious changes in structure occur in the glands which pass through a series of remarkably coordinated stages of synthesis and secretion.[13,33] By LH+7 the glands have ceased secretion and glycogen-rich material fills their lumina. The nature and composition of these secretory products has been well documented.[34,35]

Histology[1,16,24]

During the early secretory phase (days LH+2/3) there is still a moderate degree of glandular and stromal

mitosis. The proportion (volume fraction %) of the glands at LH+2/3 is about 20%. Initially their epithelium is pseudostratified and their lumina are partially obliterated. Secretory material is generally absent. Nuclei are initially basally located within the gland cells. By day LH+3 subnuclear vacuoles are present in 50% or more of the cells, displacing their nuclei more centrally. Consequently the cells appear taller and less pseudostratified than before. Little secretory material is present. By day LH+4 only occasional mitoses are seen. Sub- and supranuclear vacuoles within the gland cells are maximal on this day. The gland cell volume is also maximal on this day (Table 4.1). Pseudostratification has all but disappeared and secretions appear with luminal diameter beginning to increase. By day LH+5 mitotic activity has ceased in the glands but is still occasionally evident in the stroma. The secretory products within the gland lumina increase as intracellular accumulations decrease, leading to a further increase in glandular diameter. By day LH+6 the glands have become increasingly tortuous. With active secretion into their lumina there is a further diminution of intracellular stores. About 25% of the endometrium is now occupied by glands. On day LH+7 the gland cells contain little secretory material and have acquired a low columnar to cuboidal appearance. This contributes to the saw-tooth appearance of the glands. The amounts of secretory product within the glands and stromal edema are both maximal by day LH+8. The amount of secretory product within the gland lumen remains plentiful. Glandular diameter continues to increase. Edema is less marked and the predecidual reaction has begun around blood vessels which appear to have increased in number.

During the final week of the secretory phase, structural changes occur slowly and mainly involve the stroma and blood vessels. The glands remain full and show little evidence of secretory activity. The late secretory phase is characterized by regression and glandular involution. The epithelium is thrown into dilated tufts, creating a serrated appearance characteristic of the last week of the cycle. The epithelial cells decrease in height, nuclei appear shrunken, and the cytoplasmic borders become ragged and indistinct. There is fraying of the luminal epithelial surface. Infiltration by lymphocytes occurs. By day LH+10 stromal edema has decreased, causing a resultant increase of the gland fraction to about one-third. The proportion of the gland cell occupied by the nucleus increases. On day LH+11 the stromal predecidual reaction (enlargement of stromal cells to resemble the decidual cells of pregnancy) is mainly confined to the perivascular regions, but may also extend to adjacent glands. There is lymphocytic

Table 4.1 Cell and organelle volumes (μm^3) in the human endometrial glandular epithelium during the secretory phase of the menstrual cycle

Feature	LH+2	LH+4	LH+6	LH+8	LH+10
Cell	1127	1486	1115	836	871
Nucleus	275	288	261	213	210
Nucleolus	17	7	5	5	4
Mitochondria	65	112	41	39	40
Rough endoplasmic reticulum	35	25	36	23	18
Secretory apparatus	16	22	42	7	10
Glycogen	31	146	17	20	25

Values represent mean of at least 4 women in each group. Compiled from Dockery et al.[27,36,64,88]

infiltration. The amount of cytoplasm in gland cells continues to increase and the number of apoptotic bodies in the glands increases. By day LH+12 the predecidual reaction extends to beneath the luminal epithelium. There is a continued increase in lymphocyte number. Granulocytes may be found in gland lumina. The predecidual reaction is extensive on days LH+13 and LH+14, with sheet-like formations in the stroma. Disintegration of the stroma and extravasation of erythrocytes are evident.

The morphometric approach

The use of a variety of light microscopical morphometric methods to quantify cellular changes has provided a greater degree of objectivity and precision in the histological dating of the endometrial biopsy and given a clear insight into the complex cellular changes of this dynamic tissue.[23,24,36,37] There are significant differences in the proliferative phase with regard to pseudostratification, stromal and glandular mitoses. In the secretory phase there are differences in nine measured indices, and with the exception of days LH+7 to LH+10, every 48-hour period of the secretory phase can be distinguished statistically. A regression model for dating the endometrial biopsy during the luteal phase[14] used five parameters: the number of mitoses per 1000 gland cells, the amount of secretion in the gland lumen, the proportion of glands occupied by cells, the amount of pseudostratification of gland cells and the amount of predecidual reaction. These methods[37] have been able to identify endometrial defects in certain cases of unexplained infertility which were not identified using Noyes' criteria.[20] Thus, the morphometric approach offers clear advantages.

Menses

If no implantation occurs, shedding of the functional layer of the endometrium ensues. Although the initial trigger comes from rapidly falling levels of progesterone and estrogen, shedding, destruction, and regeneration are largely controlled by local factors. Episodes of spasm and relaxation of the spiral arteries in the functional layer lead to loss of integrity of vascular elements, bleeding into the stroma, accompanied by breakdown, remodeling, and repair.[38] The extent of the loss of the functional layer has been questioned.[39] Tissue shedding is associated with apoptosis, disordered expression of adhesion molecules, loss of filamentous actin from cell borders, and fragmentation of endometrial glands.[5] Microscopic areas of focal necrosis and hemorrhage and lysosomal activity are all evident in the premenstrual endometrium.[40,41] Matrix metalloproteinases (MMPs) and the products of endometrial leukocytes have been implicated in remodeling.[5] Fragmentation of the basal lamina and a marked reduction in cell–cell contact between endothelial cells in the late secretory phase may represent the first signs of vascular compromise.[42] These sites may or may not be associated with hemostatic plugs. Injury to the endothelial cells promotes platelet aggregation, prostaglandin $F_{2\alpha}$ ($PGF_{2\alpha}$) release, and thrombosis and contraction of the vessels.[5] On day 3, surface re-epithelialization is evident. Integrity is restored by day 5. The endothelium exhibits regenerative features.[43]

THE CELLULAR COMPONENTS OF THE ENDOMETRIUM: ULTRASTUCTURE

The luminal epithelium (Figures 4.1–5.5)

The endometrial luminal epithelium is the first maternal interface encountered by the implanting blastocyst. Scanning electron microscopy has revealed important details of its surface but does not allow access to the underlying tissue. The luminal epithelium contains both ciliated and non-ciliated cells. The former increase in number during the proliferative phase. There is an increase in the proportion of

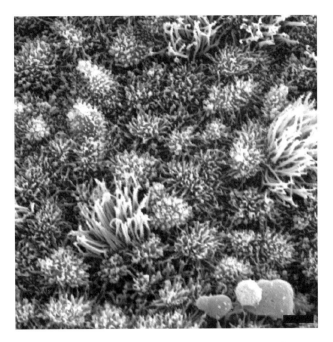

Figure 4.2 Luminal epithelium. A scanning electron micrograph of the luminal epithelium during the receptive phase; note that the surface is covered in microvilli and cilia (bar = 4 μm). (Courtesy of Dr G Nikas.)

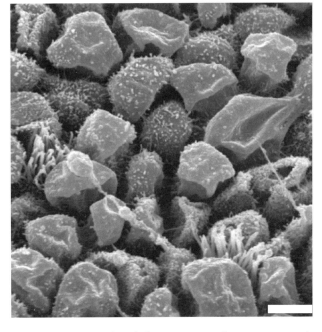

Figure 4.4 Luminal epithelium. Scanning electron micrograph of the luminal epithelium during a receptive phase showing pinopodes and cilia (bar = 4 μm). (Courtesy of Dr G Nikas.)

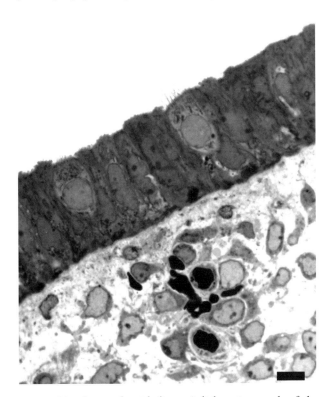

Figure 4.3 Luminal epithelium. A light micrograph of the luminal epithelium during a non-receptive phase (bar = 5 μm).

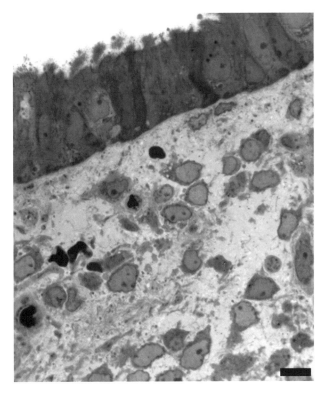

Figure 4.5 Luminal epithelium. A light micrograph of the luminal epithelium during the receptive phase; note the profiles of pinopodes (bar = 5 μm).

non-ciliated to ciliated cells from 30:1 to 15:1 from the early to the late proliferative phase, with a subsequent decrease after day 20 to a final ratio of 50:1.[44,45] Withdrawal of estrogen leads to deciliation.[1]

The morphology of the apical cell membrane of non-ciliated cells alters during the secretory phase.[46] Microvilli decrease and apical protrusions become more prominent. Initially it was suggested that this

Table 4.2   Mean basal lamina thickness (nm) in the human endometrium during the secretory phase of the menstrual cycle

Feature	LH+2	LH+4	LH+6	LH+8	LH+10	LH+13
Luminal epithelium	—	—	60	86	—	83
Glandular epithelium	76	91	90	100	98	—
Small blood vessels	—	—	81	—	105	—

Values represent mean of at least 4 women. Compiled from Dockery et al.[64]

feature represented apocrine secretion. However, Martel et al[47] described surface features called pinopodes and suggested that these play an important role in modulating the uterine environment by actively absorbing material from the uterine lumen. Subsequent studies have confirmed the presence of pinopodes.[48–50] On day 16, cells possess ovoid, long, thick microvilli, and droplet-like deposits are evident on the luminal surface. By days 19–20, the microvilli have diminished and pinopodes are a prominent feature. The pinopodes have regressed by day 22.[8,51,52] Similar changes in the apical surface membranes during the receptive period have been described in the rat. It has been suggested that these features play a key role in the development of a receptive endometrium and could act as a morphological marker for the nidation window in women.[8] Rogers et al[53] found no correlation between the morphology of the uterine luminal epithelium, circulating estrogen and progesterone levels, and subsequent conception rates, but morphology was not assessed during the conception cycle. Psychoyos[8] suggested that the timing of the nidation window (see Chapter 21) appears to be different in normal, stimulated, and artificial cycles. In stimulated cycles (human menopausal gonadotropin [hMG] and chlomiphene) the nidation window is advanced and in artificial cycles delayed by 2 days. Pinopode appearance seems to be associated with other receptivity changes, such as loss of progesterone receptors and peak expression of $\alpha_v\beta_3$ integrin, osteopontin, leukemia inhibitory factor (LIF), and its receptor.[54] The period of formation of uterine pinopodes is short. Its timing varies between different hormonal regimens and exhibits marked interindividual variability. Ovarian hormones seem to affect the depth and geometrical arrangement of tight junctions during different stages of the estrus cycle in rats.[55,56] Freeze fracture techniques revealed tight junctions associated with the luminal epithelial cells in the human endometrium to be deeper and more extensive in the middle of the menstrual cycle (days 14–16) than later (days 24 and 25).[56,57] This suggests that there is a decrease in both area and geometrical complexity of tight junctions around the time of implantation. Similarly, Sarani et al[58] reported a

decrease in the proportion of the cell surface made up of desmosomes around LH+6. Furthermore, a decrease in the expression of connexins and gap junctions occurs during this period in luminal and stromal cells[59,60] (see Chapter 20). Junctional distribution appears to be regulated in a species-specific manner.[55,61,62] In the human uterine luminal epithelium there appears to be an unfastening of junctional complexes around the time of implantation. Marx et al[63] examined the ultrastructure of the basal lamina of the peri-implantation rabbit uterine luminal epithelium and noted loss of the lamina lucida and thickening of the lamina densa during this period. Our findings[64] (Table 4.2) indicate that there may be comparable changes in the human endometrium. We found little evidence of basal laminar disruption during the early secretory phase described by Roberts et al.[65] Changes in polarity and phenotypic expression of epithelial cells in culture can be induced by contact with various matrix molecules added to cell surfaces.[66,67] It has been proposed that a destabilization of the apicobasal polarity of the uterine epithelial cells is important in creating a receptive endometrium for implantation. This priming may be partly steroid directed, but loss of polarity is further stimulated by local factors released during the early embryo–maternal dialogue[66,67] (see Chapters 18 and 19). It is of interest to note that the coefficient of variation between women for the basal lamina thickness at LH+8, around the time when implantation is thought to take place, is only 2%.[64] A low coefficient of variation is often found when the feature it relates to is biologically important for function or survival.[26,28] Some confusion seems to exist over the immunoreactivity of the basal lamina components associated with the luminal epithelium.[68,69] This may reflect methodological differences in the studies. One key feature of the luminal epithelium is its ability to accept or reject an implanting blastocyst, part of which may be due to loss of luminal cell polarity.[70] Pinopodes have been implicated in pinocytosis in rodents (but in humans they appear not to be), which is why Murphy wants to call them uterodomes, and in endocytosis, but an alternative view is that they may represent a manifestation of this altered polarity.

Recent physiological data from our laboratory have suggested that estrogen has the ability to affect microtubule organization via non-genomic mechanisms, which may be important in the conversion of a net secretory cell into a net absorber.[71] This can occur in the presence of progesterone. LIF has been localized to pinopodes, along with biochemical markers of exocytosis, including syntaxin-1, synaptosome-associated protein of 25 kDA (SNAP-25), and vesicle-associated membrane protein 2 (VAMP-2), suggesting a secretory function.[72] There is need for further work to clarify the anatomical and molecular correlates of these events.

The glandular epithelium

The proliferative phase of the menstrual cycle

During this phase, estrogen is the dominant hormone. The gland cells proliferate and assemble the cellular machinery necessary for the dynamic processes that will occur later in the cycle. During the early proliferative phase the luminal surfaces of the cells are covered by microvilli, whose number seems to increase as the cycle progresses.[41] The cells are closely packed, with fairly straight lateral cell membranes.[73] Desmosomes are evident, as are tight junctions which isolate the gland lumen from the internal environment. Gap junctions are present[59,60,74] (see Chapter 20). The nuclei of non-dividing cells are large and ovoid, with a regular profile.[41] They tend to occupy the basal portion of the cell.[73] A thin rim of heterochromatin is present and nucleoli are prominent.[75] In the subnuclear region free ribosomes and polysomes are abundant.[76] Many polysomes are associated with cisternae of rough endoplasmic reticulum (RER). Mitochondrial profiles are numerous and are closely related to one another, but there is nothing unusual about their appearance[1] at this stage. They show no topographic association with RER. Golgi bodies are poorly developed.[41] By the middle of the proliferative phase the cells appear taller with microvilli on the apical membranes.[41] Undulations form in the lateral membranes.[75] Extracellular spaces are present between adjacent cells. The secretory apparatus, including Golgi, smooth endoplasmic reticulum, and secretory vesicles, is poorly developed. However, when present, they tend to be found in the apical cytoplasm. Lipid and lysosome-like bodies have also been reported in the cytoplasm. The number of lysosome-like bodies has decreased.[41] Ciliated cells can be found within the upper portions of the glands. During the late proliferative phase, the glands contain tall columnar cells. Pseudostratification of the epithelium is evident[77]

and mitotic figures are still present. An elaboration of the secretory apparatus is characteristic of the cells at this stage. As ovulation approaches, there is a gradually increasing interdigitation of adjacent lateral cell membranes, slight enlargement of mitochondrial profiles, the cytoplasmic and mitochondrial matrix become more electron dense, free ribosomes, polysomes, and RER decrease in the basal cytoplasm,[41] and occasional glycogen deposits are seen.[76]

The secretory phase

During the early secretory phase, the glandular epithelial cell becomes transformed into a highly polarized cell actively involved in the production and secretion of complex secretory products which are thought to be important in supporting the trophoblast. Characteristic ultrastructural features are associated with this transformation. These include the accumulation of glycogen-rich material in the subnuclear cytoplasm, the formation of giant mitochondrial profiles, and the development of the nuclear channel system (NCS)[33,41,78–85] (Figures 4.6–5.13). Unlike the luminal epithelium, there is remarkable control and maintainance of junctional integrity in the glandular epithelium during the early to mid secretory phase of the menstrual cycle.[86] This would suggest that there is a difference in the regulation of luminal and glandular cells in the human endometrium. This differential regulation makes biological sense; the luminal cells seem to play an important dynamic role in opening or closing of the window while the gland cells function in a more conservative typical epithelial role. The phenomenon of cellular spatial awareness, whereby the same cells respond differently to the same environmental cues, is widespread,[87] and has yet to be fully explored in the human endometrium. Scanning electron microscopic studies show that the openings of the glands become more slit-like as the glands fill up with secretory products. The use of well-timed material has shown that the cellular changes during the early secretory phase are remarkably well controlled between women.[33] A variety of new and traditional stereological probes have been used to quantify these dynamic changes[26,27,64,88] and these are summarized in Table 4.1.

On day LH+2 the nuclei are large, containing little heterochromatin. Nuclear volume decreases as the secretory phase progresses and the proportion of heterochromatin increases. Nucleolar size is maximal at LH+2 and then decreases.[88,89] The cytoplasm at LH+2 shows little polarization. It contains many free ribosomes and small deposits of glycogen-rich material are present. The intracellular glycogen load is maximal at

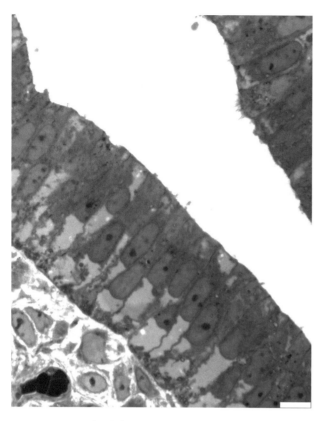

Figure 4.6 Glandular epithelium. A light micrograph showing intracellular accumulation of glycogen-rich material LH+4 (bar=5 μm).

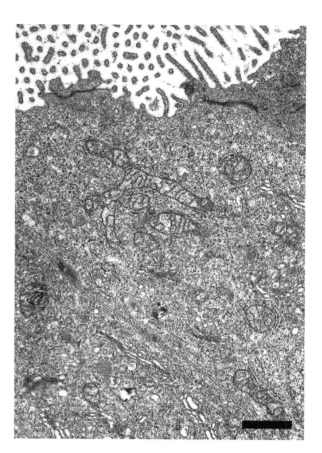

Figure 4.8 Glandular epithelium. Branched mitochondrial profile in glandular epithelial cell at LH+2/3 (bar=0.5 μm).

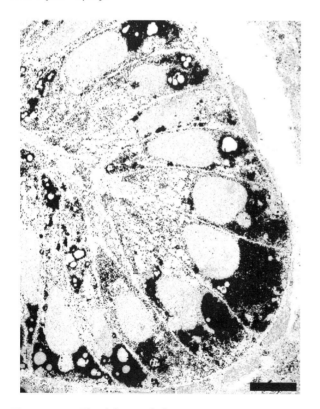

Figure 4.7 Glandular epithelium. A transmission electron micrograph showing the cytochemical localization of glycogen and glycoprotein-rich deposits in human glandular epithelial cells at LH+4/5 (bar=5 μm).

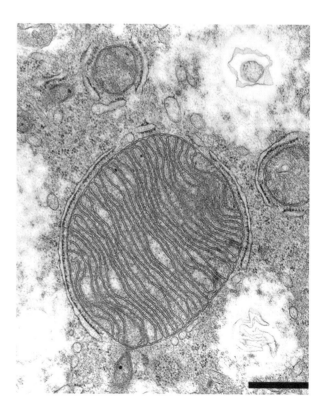

Figure 4.9 Glandular epithelium. Giant mitochondrial profile in glandular epithelial cell at LH+4/5 (bar=0.5 μm).

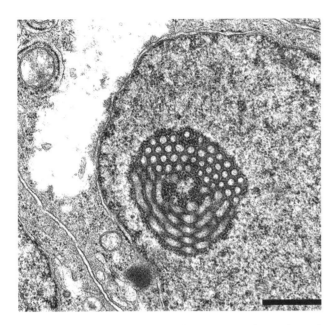

Figure 4.10 Glandular epithelium. Nuclear channel system in the nucleus of glandular epithelial cell at LH+4/5 (bar=0.5 μm).

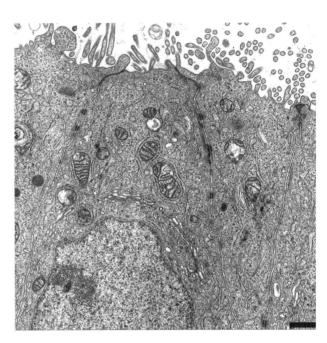

Figure 4.12 Glandular epithelium. Apical portion of glandular epithelial cell at LH+2 showing poorly developed secretory apparatus (bar=0.25 μm).

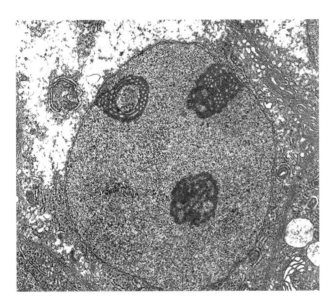

Figure 4.11 Glandular epithelium. Two profiles of nuclear channel systems in glandular epithelial cell at LH+4/5: note no anatomical association with nucleolus (bar=1.0 μm).

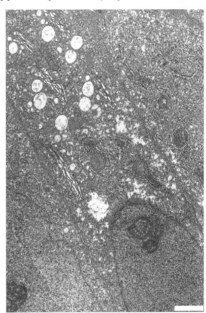

Figure 4.13 Glandular epithelium. Apical portion of glandular epithelial cell at LH+5/6 showing spectacular elaboration of the secretory apparatus (bar=1μm).

LH+4, causing increased cell volume. The volume of secretory apparatus increases to a maximum by LH+6. By day LH+8 the cells have apparently ceased their secretory activity, NCS are uncommon, and the amount of heterochromatin in the nucleus has increased. The interdigitation of lateral membranes is most obvious at this time (see Figure 4.3). During the late secretory phase (days 25–28) the nuclei become deeply indented with aggregation of heterochromatin.[41] Nucleoli are less conspicuous. Remnants of

the nuclear channel system (see below) may be extruded into the cytoplasm and associated with lysosomal elements.[85] The RER is a little more dilated when compared to earlier in the secretory phase. Mitochondrial profiles are numerous and small, while small glycogen deposits are still present in the cytoplasm. Lipid and lysosome-like bodies are present. Giant lysosomes and electron-dense granules are seen, which probably correspond to the apoptotic bodies described in the light microscopic literature.[41]

Giant mitochondria

'Giant' mitochondrial profiles are a characteristic feature of the early secretory phase. Two types of mitochondrial profiles are seen during the early secretory phase: regular (diameter $0.3 \times 1\,\mu m$) and giant (diameter $3–4\,\mu m$)[85,90] (see Figure 4.9). The total mitochondrial volume per cell increases between LH+2 and LH+4 from $65\,\mu m^3$ to $112\,\mu m^3$, then decreases to about $40\,\mu m^3$ between LH+6 and LH+10. Branched mitochondrial profiles have been described in glandular epithelial cells during the secretory phase (see Figure 4.8). Reconstruction studies[90] have suggested that the giant mitochondrial profiles are localized expansions of mitochondria of otherwise normal dimensions. The development of this organelle may be by fusing of small mitochondria or by localized expansion. The presence of the giant mitochondrial profiles during the early luteal phase is perhaps to provide energy for the dynamic changes occurring within the cells at this time. The surface area of the inner mitochondrial membrane may be used as a morphological index of oxidative phosphorylation. We have quantified the surface area changes of the inner and outer mitochondrial membranes during mitochondrial enlargement.[36] The data (Table 4.3) suggest that the enlarged profiles seen at LH+4 are due to a reorganization of existing membrane components already present at LH+2 in agreement with the concept of localized expansion of existing mitochondria.[90] After this time there is a loss of membrane components.[41] Digitate cristae seen within the giant mitochondrial profiles are a feature characteristic of cells where steroids are synthesized or metabolized. Mitochondrial enlargement may be the result of the action of progesterone on mitochondrial DNA.[90] Mitochondrial enlargement has been noted with human chorionic gonadotropin (hCG) treatment.[91] RU486 and R2323, which block progesterone at the receptor level, also have deleterious effects on the development of mitochondrial enlargement.[88,92] Initially there is limited association between the mitochondria and RER, but during enlargement intimate associations develop. There is no substantial change in RER volume between LH+2 and LH+10 (see Table 4.1).

The nuclear channel system

Associated with elaboration of the secretory apparatus within these cells is a spectacular elaboration of the inner nuclear envelope resulting in the feature known as the nuclear (or nucleolar) channel system. When fully developed, the inner nuclear envelope forms a spherical

Table 4.3 The surface area of mitochondria in human endometrial glandular epithelium during the secretory phase of the menstrual cycle

Feature	LH+2	LH+4	LH+6
Surface area outer	744	977	435
Surface area inner	1655	1727	652
Total surface area	2429	2704	1086

Values represent mean of at least 4 women. Compiled from Dockery et al.[97]

or cone-shaped stack of interdigitating membranous tubules each surrounded by a granular intranuclear matrix. There are seven sets of tubules, each containing three rows of coiled tubules which spiral in one and a half turns from the site of origin around a common core[85,93] (see Figures 4.10 and 4.11). The appearance of the NCS is a rapid process; it is seldom seen at LH+3, yet by LH+4 is well developed. The proportion of the structure made up of tubules increases from 12% at LH+4 to about 24% by LH+6. The total volume at LH+4 was found to be $1.22\,\mu m$ $4.74\,\mu m$ at LH+5 and 2.2 by LH+6.[27] The expulsion of the tubular network from the nucleus has been described;[85] however, the timing should be treated with caution due to the lack of adequate chronological dating of biopsies. We found little evidence of this organelle after LH+9. In-vitro and in-vivo studies have demonstrated the progesterone dependence of the NCS,[94,95] its formation being dependent on the 17β position of the D ring of progestational steroids.[83] Progesterone receptor blockade by RU486 before day LH+3 prevents its formation, and administration of the drug later in the cycle causes it to disappear.[88] High levels of estrogen also seem to disrupt the channel systems in vitro and in vivo.[83,96,97] Additional progesterone during the normal secretory phase fails to promote overelaboration of the secretory apparatus or the NCS.[98] However, supraphysiological levels of estrogen followed by high levels of progesterone seem to produce very elaborate channel systems.[97] Exogenous expression of the characteristic repeat domain of the nucleolar chaperone Nopp140 induces the formation of intranuclear structures, termed R-rings, that are apparently identical to the NCS.[99]

The function of the NCS is not known. Some reports link it to elaboration of the secretory apparatus[83,94,95,100,101] (see Figures 4.12 and 4.13). It has been suggested that it facilitates rapid massive transfer of mRNA and ribosomal precursors from nucleus to cytoplasm[102] and, indeed, ribonucleoproteins and nucleoside phosphatases have been localized within the NCS.[103] However, the timing of NCS development and this alleged function are not consistent. Also the mechanisms of transport via such a route and the nature of the the the putative mRNA remain obscure. It is also of interest to note that Ca^{2+} release channels have been reported to be associated with the inner nuclear envelope,[104] which may suggest an alternative role for the NCS in secretory activity. The NCS may not be present in some cases of infertility; this is indeed the case if biopsies are taken at LH+4.[105] However, by LH+5 and +6 the organelle is present and even seems more elaborate than those seen in normal fertile women.[36]

A number of abnormalities, including delay in the development of the secretory apparatus and changes in the expression of a luteal-specific glycoprotein within glandular epithelial cells, have been seen in women classified as unexplained infertile with normal levels of circulating steroids.[88,106] Deviations in nuclear morphology are also observed in these women, including differences in NCS. While there was considerable variation, a basic pattern was identified. This entailed a delay of NCS formation and possible compression of development up to day LH+6 in these 'unexplained' infertile subjects compared with a fertile group.[27]

Cytoskeleton

Rapid (non-genomic) dose-dependent increases in intracellular calcium in response to physiological concentrations of 17β-estradiol and the xenoestrogen BPA occur in human endometrial glandular epithelial cells from both proliferative and secretory phase biopsies.[71,86] Initial qualitative studies have suggested alterations in the patterning of the cytoskeleton.[86] Recent work has demonstrated, for the first time, rapid quantifiable alterations of microtubule patterning in the endometrial epithelial cells in response to these compounds.[71] These changes in calcium ion concentration could also be involved in the modulation of junctional complexes and/or ion channels.[107,108]

Stroma

The endometrial stroma is a connective tissue composed of cells and a complex extracellular matrix containing fibrillar components and ground substance (Figures 4.14 and 4.15). Much is now known about the extracellular matrix of the endometrium[109] (and see Chapter 23), and changes in its composition have shed considerable light on the dynamic nature of the stroma.[2,5] The stromal cell (sometimes referred to as the reticular cell) is a fibroblast-like cell which is responsible for the production of most of the matrix

components.[1] Other cell types present include granulated stromal cells (also known as natural killer [NK] cells – see Chapters 34 and 35) and lymphocytes. In the course of the normal menstrual cycle, the stromal cells undergo morphological changes that correlate with proliferation, differentiation, and maturation.[1,110,111] These vary with time and also with location within the endometrium.[1] The stromal cells of the early proliferative phase resemble undifferentiated fibroblasts with mesenchymal characteristics.[111] As this phase progresses, they become more like fibroblasts. Stromal cells are involved in remodeling the extracellular matrix throughout the menstrual cycle and the first morphological evidence of the activity is seen around ovulation.[41] During the mid to late proliferative period the cells show increased amounts of euchromatin and the formation of prominent nucleoli.[111] The cells contain increasing amounts of RER.[41] In the early secretory phase stromal nuclei contain even more euchromatin and there is an accumulation of glycogen in the cytoplasm. Between LH+2 and LH+8, nuclear diameter increases by around 20% (Table 4.4), representing an increase in volume of 75%.[112] The nuclei also become more rounded during this period, consistent with increased transcriptional activity. Stromal cell density increases from LH+2 to LH+6 and decreases sharply at LH+8. The initial increase in density may be explained by the fact that during this period the glands are filling up with secretory products and their gradual distention pushes the stromal elements closer together. An alternative explanation is increased mitotic activity, but reported mitotic rates for the stromal cells during this period would not account for these changes.[16,24] The dramatic reduction in packing density at LH+8 occurs at a time when stromal edema becomes maximal. These changes are coincident with the increased complexity of basolateral interdigitations between adjacent gland cells and may indicate resorption of water from the gland lumena (Figure 4.16).

An extensive network of junctional complexes, including gap junctions between adjacent stromal cells, has been described, decreasing in extent as the secretory phase progresses.[113] A similar pattern is seen in the glands, where the number and size of gap junctions between adjacent glandular epithelial cells increases during the early proliferative and early secretory phases and subsequently decreases.[65] The findings of both of these studies are in line with the cyclic expression of gap junction connexins[60] (see Chapter 20). Stromal–epithelial interactions[65] include increase in the number and size of lamina densa disruptions, increased complexity of

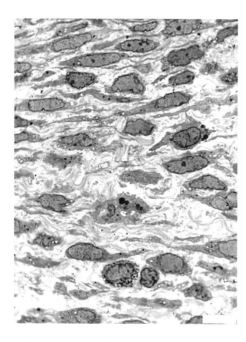

Figure 4.14   Stroma. A light micrograph of endometrial stroma at LH+2/3 (bar = 5 µm).

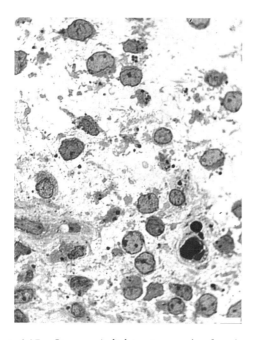

Figure 4.15   Stroma. A light micrograph of endometrial stroma at LH+8 (bar = 5 µm).

epithelial cell projections through the lamina densa, and an increase in close contact between stromal and epithelial cells. These interactions occur principally in the early secretory phase and decrease in frequency thereafter. In a recent study of basal lamina thickness during the secretory phase no obvious disruption to the integrity of the basal lamina was associated with glandular epithelial cells. However, the mean thickness of the basal lamina on day LH+2 was significantly less than any other day of

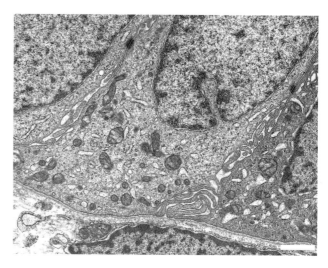

Figure 4.16   Basolateral interdigitation between adjacent glandular epithelial cells (bar = 0.5 µm).

the secretory phase. The basal lamina was thickest at day LH+ 8[64] (see Table 4.2).

The ratio of stromal cells to gland cells seems to be tightly regulated during the secretory phase. The estimation of 'size' for an interconnected non-convex phase such as the connective tissue intercellular space can be expressed using a stereological parameter known as the volume-weighted star volume. This equates to the portion of space that can be 'seen' from a particular position within a tissue. Measurements[114] suggest that from any point in space a distance of 5.5 µm could be traveled before encountering a stromal cell and that this distance remains fairly constant throughout the luteal phase (see Table 4.4).

Endometrial leukocytes

The immunological aspects of implantation are complex and the endometrium contains a wide spectrum of immunocompetent cells[115] (Figure 4.17 and see Chapters 33, 34, and 35). These include T lymphocytes, macrophages, and endometrial granulated lymphocytes. The introduction of monoclonal antibody techniques has allowed their phenotypic characterization.[116–118] There is clear evidence for influence of sex steroids on immune cells in the endometrium.[119] Quantitative studies on well-timed material[120] have provided a valuable insight into the dynamics of these important cells during the secretory phase in normal fertile women.

Leukocytes account for approximately 7% of the stromal cells in the proliferative phase, increasing to 30% in early pregnancy, with alterations occurring in women with unexplained infertility.[121] The granulated lymphocytes (phenotype: CD56+, CD38+, CD2±, CD3–, CD16–) are thought to be important in

Table 4.4 Stromal cell changes in the human endometrium

Feature	LH+2	LH+4	LH+6	LH+8
Number of stromal cells per mm^3	684 000	800 000	102 800	578 000
Stromal cell nuclear diameter (μm)	7.3	8.1	8.1	8.8
Number of stromal cells per gland cell	7	5	5	4
Stromal volume-weighted mean star volume (μm^3)	6000	5500	5800	6200
Diffusion distance (μm)	5.5	5.5	5.5	5.5

Values represent mean of at least 4 women. Compiled from Dockery et al[112] and Treacy et al.[114]

control of trophoblast invasion and also to be involved in transforming growth factor (TGF) production.[117] They increase after LH+7 to make up about 55% of all endometrial leukocytes. The T lymphocytes (phenotype: CD3+, CD8+) are involved in immunosuppression. These cells have been reported in three different locations: intraepithelial, interstitial, and in lymphoid aggregates in the basal region of the endometrium. T lymphocytes (CD8+ T suppressor/cytotoxic cells) increase significantly from LH+4 to LH+7. At LH+7, 22% of stromal leukocytes were CD8+ cells and 8% were CD4+ cells. An interesting study[122] has described a non-genomic mechanism for progesterone-mediated immunosuppression: inhibition of K$^+$ channels, Ca^{2+} signaling, and gene expression in T lymphocytes during pregnancy. Macrophages (phenotype: CD68+, CD14+, Class II MHC+) are also thought to be involved in immunosuppression and antigen presentation and increase from LH+10 to LH+13. Other cells such as B lymphocytes and NK cells are also present.

Blood vessels (Figures 4.18 and 4.19)

Within the myometrium, the arcuate arteries arise from the uterine and ovarian arteries, which in turn give rise to radial arteries. After crossing the endometrial–myometrial junction, they branch to form the basal (anastomosing) and spiral (terminal) arteries. The former supply the basal layer and the latter the functional layer of the endometrium. Branching of the spiral arteries occurs throughout the functional layer. Just below the surface they break up into a prominent subepithelial plexus, which drains into venous sinuses.[12,123] Each spiral arteriole supplies tissue with an approximate endometrial surface area of 4–9 mm^2.[124]

Unlike other vascular beds, the endometrial vasculature undergoes cycles of growth and regression during

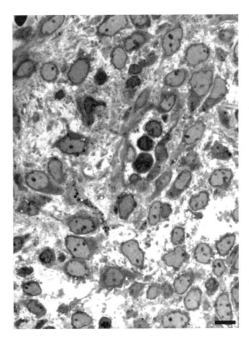

Figure 4.17 A light micrograph of small blood vessel containing circulating leukocytes (bar = 5 μm).

the menstrual cycle.[123] The proliferative phase growth in endometrial thickness is accompanied by growth of the vascular tree. By the middle of the late proliferative phase the sprouting terminal branches of the spiral arteries become somewhat coiled. By the middle of the secretory phase the spiral arteries ascend from the basal to the functional layer.

A variety of methods have been used to document changes in the endometrial vascular bed in the normal menstrual cycle and in various pathologies. The most commonly used is microvascular density, i.e. the number of vascular profiles per unit area. Most quantitative studies using immunocytochemical labeling methods have simply expressed vascular density in terms of number of profiles per unit area of section.[125] More elaborate stereological methods have permitted assessment of the number and lengths of vessel segments.[126–128]

Light microscopic studies of endometrial microvascular density have reported little change throughout the normal menstrual cycle.[125,129] The subepithelial capillary plexus shows significant dilatation of vessels during the late secretory phase.[130] This may be related to the development of edema in the stroma at the time of expected implantation. Due to the disruptive nature of the biopsy and possibility of associated vessel collapse, any comment on vessel diameter should be treated with caution.[13] The possible functional significance of capillary dilatation in terms of implantation needs to be investigated.

Examination of the subepithelial capillary plexus using morphometric methods in endometrial samples

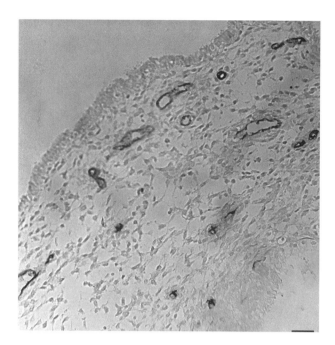

Figure 4.18 A light micrograph of the superficial vascular bed visualized using immunocytochemistry (CD34) (bar = 15 μm).

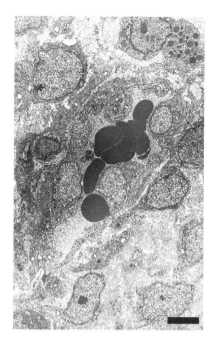

Figure 4.19 An electron micrograph of a small blood vessel and surrounding stroma. (bar = 5 μm).

from 34 fertile women who had a hormonal profile compatible with normal ovarian function[131] in whom biopsies were dated relative to the LH surge, indicated a significant dilatation of the vessels during the postovulatory phase. The area of the capillary lumen and the mean level of progesterone circulating in the plasma 72 hours prior to the biopsy were correlated. Dilatation of the subepithelial capillaries may be related to the development of edema in the mid secretory phase stroma. The possible functional significance of capillary dilatation in terms of implantation, however, needs to be further investigated.

There are two main mechanisms for the formation of new blood vessels: vasculogenesis, de novo development of vessels; and angiogenesis, the creation of new microvessels from pre-existing vessels. Angiogenesis may occur by sprouting/branching, intussusception (i.e. the formation of transcapillary tissue pillars) or elongation; in addition, circulating endothelial cell progenitors may be incorporated into existing vasculature to contribute to these processes (Chapter 7). Angiogenesis is thought to occur in three phases of the menstrual cycle:[127,132] during menses, when vascular repair is occurring; during the proliferative phase, coinciding with the estrogen-driven rapid tissue growth; and during the secretory phase, associated with the elaboration of the spiral arterioles. Until recently there was little evidence of the mechanism involved or their spatial and temporal location.[127,128] Angiogenesis normally involves endothelial cell activation, degradation and breakdown

of the basal lamina, migration and proliferation of endothelial cells, fusion of sprouts, and tube formation.[123,133,134] However, angiogenesis in the human endometrium may not occur via this pathway, as immunohistochemical studies have demonstrated proliferating endometrial endothelial cells at all stages of the cycle within existing vessels rather than associated with vascular sprouts. Other mechanisms, including intussusception and vessel elongation, have been suggested.[123,134,135] Recent evidence has suggested that vessel elongation is a major angiogenic mechanism in mid-late proliferative phase human endometrium. This seems to be followed by a stage of remodeling via intussusception.[127] These findings support organ-specific angiogenesis and are consistent with immunocytochemical studies, which revealed considerable microvascular heterogeneity in the endometrium.[68,123] Steroid hormones play a central role in regulating the endometrial vasculature.[136]

Ultrastructural studies are consistent with these findings. The early proliferative phase endothelial cells contain a small amount of cytoplasm rich in organelles.[42,131] Heterochromatin predominates. Apical and basal surfaces contain pinocytotic vesicles. Two types of pericytes are described. The basal lamina associated with capillaries is loose and discontinuous with cell contact between pericytes and endothelial cells. During the late proliferative period the nuclei enlarge and the amount of euchromatin increases. The complement of cellular organelles also increases with enlargement of mitochondria and dilatation of RER. The basal lamina is more complete than at any other part of the cycle. During the early secretory phase there is a marked degree of heterogeneity in the appearance of the endothelial cells.

The appearance of capillary basal lamina changes during the early proliferative phase of the menstrual cycle. It is loosely formed and discontinuous, becoming more extensive during the late proliferative phase and early secretory phase. It becomes better defined during the mid-secretory phase than at any other time of the menstrual cycle. Fragmentation of the basal lamina is a feature of the late secretory phase.[42] Changes occur in the basal lamina during the secretory phase of the menstrual cycle in well-timed biopsies with a significant increase in its thickness between LH+6 and LH+10.[64] The basal lamina and associated adhesion molecules surrounding blood vessels are important in attaching the endothelial cells to perivascular extracellular matrix.[5] In vascular remodeling and during angiogenesis endothelial cells can alter their complement of cell adhesion molecules and also the nature of the proteolytic enzymes they release to break down the basement membrane, which can alter the fragility of the blood vessel.[123,133] The effect that stromal edema has on angiogenesis and on the changing relationship with the basal lamina in the endometrium is unclear.

A light microscopic study of endometrial vascular anatomy from LH+6 to LH+12[128] (Table 4.5) showed that the proportion of endometrium made up of blood vessel remains constant from LH+6 to LH+12, which is in line with earlier density estimates.[125] The mean proportion of endometrium comprising blood vessel lumen increased between LH+6 and LH+12, but the differences were not significant. The electron microscopical study of endothelial cell profiles in small blood vessels suggests that there was an almost doubling of cell volume and that there were corresponding increases in nuclear volume of around 45% during the period of study (see Table 4.5). The proportion (and volume) of RER, secretory apparatus, and mitochondria also increased between LH+6 and LH +10. These ultrastructural features are compatible with an increase in the activity of the endothelial cells in the late secretory phase but the functional significance of these changes is unclear at present (see Table 4.5). Making estimates based upon these data suggests that there is an increase in the length of individual endothelial cells over the period of study (see Table 4.5). Roberts et al,[42] using material dated by Noyes' criteria,[20] reported that the endometrial capillary basal lamina was loosely formed and discontinuous during the early proliferative phase (days 5–9), becoming more extensive during the

Table 4.5 Endothelial cell features in the human endometrium during the secretory phase of the menstrual cycle

Feature	LH+6	LH+8	LH+10	LH+12
Vv blood vessel lumen: endometrium (%)	1.1	1.1	1.3	1.3
Vv blood vessel: endometrium (%)	3.9	4.1	4.9	4.7
Nuclear diameter (μm)	5.4	5.8	6.1	6.1
Nuclear axial ratio	1.7	1.9	1.8	1.8
Nuclear volume	82	102	119	119
Vv nucleus:cell (%)	60	47	47	44
Cell volume	137	217	253	270
Vv euchromatin: nucleus (%)	85	74	75	79
Volume euchromatin	70	75	89	94
Vv mitochondria: cell (%)	2.5	3.5	3.3	4.7
Volume mitochondria	3	8	8	13
Vv RER:cell (%)	3.1	3.4	5.2	4.8
Volume RER	4	7	13	13
Vv Sec:cell (%)	3.1	4.9	5.7	6.7
Sec volume	4	11	14	18
Length of endothelial cell	77	128	143	156

Values represent mean values for 5 women in each group. Compiled from data by Bulut.[140]

Volume and length estimates have been derived empirically from this data.

late proliferative phase (days 10–14) and early secretory phase (days 15–19). The basal lamina has been reported to be better defined during the mid secretory phase (days 20–22) than at any other time of the menstrual cycle. It increasingly fragments in the late secretory phase (days 23–28). We have also reported changes in the basal lamina during the secretory phase of the menstrual cycle in well-timed biopsies with a significant increase in the thickness between LH+6 and LH+10 (see Table 4.2).[64] Immunochemical studies suggest that the basement membranes of all endometrial blood vessels contain collagen IV and laminin, although heparin sulfate glycoprotein only stains about 55% of vessels.[68] This and other work by Rogers et al[125] indicates there may be some degree of microvascular heterogeneity in the endometrium. Steroid hormones play a central role in regulating endometrial vasculature. These regulatory effects are superimposed on the wide array of regulatory mechanisms that control angiogenesis in this tissue.[134] Bilalis et al[69] noted that immunoreactivity for laminin and fibronectin was reduced at LH+10 compared to other days in the luteal phase of the menstrual cycle. They were also unable to demonstrate any reactivity in a group with unexplained infertility given the same titers of antibodies.

Bleeding disturbances found in users of hormonal contraception seem to be associated with changes in the endometrial vascular bed following abnormal patterns of sex steroid exposure. Endometrial microvascular density is increased in users of Norplant. Other conditions of spontaneous and induced endometrial atrophy showed no significant change in vascular density compared to the control population.[123]

In summary, significant endothelial cell proliferation occurs at all stages of the menstrual cycle. Stereological studies suggest vessel elongation as a major angiogenic mechanism in the mid–late proliferative phase. The mechanisms involved later in the cycle have not yet been elucidated. Sex steroids appear to have the capacity to either promote or inhibit angiogenesis, depending on the actions of local factors, including vascular endothelial growth factor (VEGF) and relaxin.[137–139]

CONCLUSION

The human endometrium undergoes complex and dynamic changes during the menstrual cycle. The use of well-timed biopsies combined with appropriate morphometric analysis has improved our understanding of the anatomical changes occurring in this important tissue. The increased objectivity afforded by the morphometric approach has allowed a clearer definition of the cellular changes in the endometrium. These methods have revealed the remarkably tight control that exists over certain cellular events during the secretory phase of the menstrual cycle which may be related to a window of uterine receptivity. A number of important gaps still exist in our knowledge of the luminal epithelium, stroma, and vasculature. Development and application of appropriate stereological methods[23,124] should provide a clearer anatomical framework to accommodate new physiological, biochemical, and molecular information. While stereology can provide useful quantitative information, other methods will help define the relationships between structure and function. These include modern non-invasive medical imaging technologies, confocal microscopy, and low-temperature electron microscopy techniques such as cryosubstitution.

REFERENCES

1. Wynn RM. The human endometrium: cyclic and gestational changes. In: Wynn RM, Jollie WP, eds. Biology of the Uterus. 2nd edn. New York: Plenum, 1989: 289–332.
2. Edwards R. Physiological and molecular aspects of human implantation. Hum Reprod 1995; 10: 1–11.
3. Horcajadas JA, Riesewijk A, Dominiguez F et al. Determinants of endometrial receptivity. Ann NY Acad Sci 2004; 1034: 166–75.
4. Sivridis E, Giatromanolaki A. New insights into the normal menstrual cycle-regulatory molecules. Histol Histopathol 2004; 19: 511–16.
5. Tabibzadeh S. The signals and molecular pathways involved in human menstruation, a unique process of tissue destruction and remodeling. Mol Hum Reprod 1996; 2: 77–92.
6. Hulboy D, Rudolph L, Matrisian L. Matrix metalloproteinases as mediators of reproductive function. Mol Hum Reprod 1997; 3: 27–45.
7. Kimber SJ. Leukaemia inhibitory factor in implantation and uterine biology. Reproduction 2005; 130: 131–45.
8. Psychoyos A. Nidation window: from basic to clinic. In: Dey Sk, ed. Molecular and Cellular Aspects of Preimplantation Processes, New York: Springer, 1995: 1–14.
9. Beier-Hellwig K, Bonn B, Sterzik K et al. Uterine receptivity and endometrial secretory protein patterns. In: Dey SK, ed. Molecular and Cellular Aspects of Preimplantation Processes. New York: Springer, 1995: 87–98.
10. White CA, Salmonsen LA. A guide to issues in microassay analysis: application to endometrial biology. Reproduction 2005; 130: 1–13.
11. Giudice LC. Elucidating endometrial function in the post-genomic era. Hum Reprod Update 2003; 9: 223–35.
12. Padykula HA. Regeneration in the primate uterus: the role of stem cells. In: Wynn RM, Jollie WP, eds. Biology of the Uterus, 2nd edn. New York: Plenum, 1989: 279–88.
13. Dockery P, Rogers AW. The effects of steroids on the fine structure of the endometrium. Ballieres Clin Obstet Gynaecol 1989; 3: 227–47.
14. Li TC, Rogers AW, Lenton AE et al. A comparison between two methods of chronological dating of endometrial biopsies during the luteal phase and their correlation with histological dating. Fertil Steril 1987; 48: 928–32.
15. Johannisson E, Landgren BM, Rohr HP, Dicsfalusy E. Endometrial morphology and peripheral hormone levels in women with regular menstrual cycles. Fertil Steril 1987; 38: 564–71.
16. Johannisson E. Endocrine responses in the female genital tract. In: Shearman RP, ed. Clinical Reproductive Endocrinology. Edinburgh: Churchill Livingstone, 1985: 127–141.
17. Lenton EA, Langren BM. The normal menstrual cycle. In: Shearman RP, ed. Clinical Reproductive Endocrinology. Edinburgh: Churchill Livingstone, 1985: 81–108.
18. Koninckx P, Brosens JJ, Brosens I. Endometrial dating – still room for controversy. Fertil Steril 2005; 83: 1889–990.
19. Batista MC, Cartledge TP, Merino MJ et al. Midluteal phase endometrial biopsy does not accurately predict luteal function. Fertil Steril 1993; 59: 294–300.
20. Noyes RW, Hertig AT, Rock J. Dating the endometrial biopsy. Fertil Steril 1950; 1: 2–25.
21. Murray MJ, Meyer WR, Zaino RJ et al. A critical analysis of the accuracy, reproducibility, and clinical utility of histologic endometrial dating in fertile women. Fertil Steril 2004; 81: 1333–43.
22. Coutifaris C, Myers ER, Guzick DS et al; NICHD National Cooperative Reproductive Medicine Network. Histological dating of timed endometrial biopsy tissue is not related to fertility status. Fertil Steril 2004; 82: 1264–72.
23. Johannisson E, Parker RA, Landgren BM, Dicsfalusy E. Morphometric analysis of the human endometrium in relation to peripheral hormone levels. Fertil Steril 1982; 38: 564–71.
24. Li TC, Rogers AW, Dockery P et al. A new method of histological dating of human endometrium in the luteal phase. Fertil Steril 1988; 50: 52–60.
25. Mayhew TM. The new stereological methods for interpreting functional morphology from slices of cells and organs. Exp Physiol 1991; 76: 639–65.
26. Dockery P, Li TC, Rogers AW et al. An examination of the variation in the timed endometrial biopsy. Hum Reprod 1988; 3: 715–20.

27. Dockery P, Pritchard K, Warren MA, Li TC, Cooke ID. Changes in nuclear morphology in the human endometrial glandular epithelium in women with unexplained infertility. Hum Reprod 1996; 11: 101–6.

28. Clegg EJ. Morphometric studies of the spleen of the hypoxic mouse. J Microsc 1983; 131: 155–61.

29. Shay J. Economy of effort in electron microscope morphometry. Am J Pathol 1975; 81: 503–11.

30. Gundersen HJG, Østerby R. Optimising sampling efficiency of stereological studies in biology: 'Do more less well'. J Microsc 1981; 121: 65–73.

31. Lenton EA, Langren BM, Sexton L, Harper R. Normal variation in the length of the follicular phase of the menstrual cycle: effect of chronological age. Br J Obstet Gynaecol 1984; 91: 681–4.

32. Lenton EA, Langren BM, Sexton L. Normal variation in the length of the luteal phase of the menstrual cycle: identification of the short luteal phase. Br J Obstet Gynaecol 1984; 91: 685–9.

33. Dockery P, Li TC, Rogers AW, Lenton EA, Cooke ID. The ultrastructure of the glandular epithelium in the timed endometrial biopsy. Hum Reprod 1988; 3: 826–34.

34. Aplin JD. Cellular biochemistry of the endometrium. In: Wynn RM, Jollie WP, eds. Biology of the Uterus, 2nd edn. New York: Plenum, 1989: 89–119.

35. Aplin JD, Mylona P, Kielty C et al. Collagen IV and laminin as markers of differentiation of endometrial stroma. In: Dey SK, ed. Molecular and Cellular Aspects of Preimplantation Processes. New York: Springer, 1995: 331–47.

36. Dockery P, Pritchard K, Taylor A et al. The fine structure of the human endometrium in women with unexplained fertility. Hum Reprod 1993; 8: 667–73.

37. Li TC, Dockery P, Rogers AW, Cooke ID. A quantitative study of endometrial development in the luteal phase: a comparison between women with unexplained fertility and women with normal fertility. Br J Obstet Gynaecol 1990; 97: 576–82.

38. Fraser IS. Mechanisms of endometrial bleeding. Reprod Fertil Dev 1990; 2: 193–8.

39. Wilborn WH, Flowers CE. Cellular mechanisms of endometrial conservation during menstrual bleeding. Semin Reprod Med 1984; 2: 307–41.

40. Henzl MR, Smith RE, Boost G, Tyler ET. Lysosomal concept of menstrual bleeding in humans. J Clin Endocrinol Metab 1972; 34: 860–75.

41. Cornillie FJ, Lauweryns JM, Brosens IA. Normal human endometrium. Gynecol Obstet Invest 1985; 20: 113–29.

42. Roberts DK, Parmley TH, Walker NJ, Horbelt DV. Ultrastructure of the microvasculature in the human endometrium throughout the normal menstrual cycle. Am J Obstet Gynecol 1992; 166: 1393–406.

43. Ferenczy A. Studies on the cytodynamics of human endometrial regeneration. I. Scanning electron microscopy. Am J Obstet Gynecol 1976; 124: 64–74.

44. Ferenczy A. Surface ultrastructural response of the human uterine lining epithelium to hormonal environment. A scanning electron microscopic study. Acta Cytol 1977; 21: 566–72.

45. Masterton R, Armstrong EM, More IAR. The cyclic variation in the percentage of ciliated cells in the normal human endometrium. J Reprod Fertil 1975; 42: 537–40.

46. Johannisson E, Nilsson L. Scanning electron microscopic study of the human endometrium. Fertil Steril 1972; 23: 613–25.

47. Martel D, Malet C, Gautray JP, Psychoyos A. Surface changes of the luminal uterine epithelium during the human menstrual cycle: a scanning electron microscopic study. In: de Brux J, Mortel R, Gautray JP, eds. The Endometrium Hormonal Impacts. New York: Plenum, 1981: 15–29.

48. Nikas G, Drakakis P, Loutradis D et al. Uterine pinopodes as markers of the nidation window in cycling women receiving exogenous oestradiol and progesterone. Hum Reprod 1995; 10: 1208–13.

49. Nikas G, Develioglu OH, Toner JP, Jones HW Jr. Endometrial pinopodes indicate a shift in the window of receptivity in IVF cycles. Hum Reprod 1999; 14: 787–92.

50. Nikas G, Makrigiannakis A. Endometrial pinopides and uterine receptivity. Ann NY Acad Sci 2003; 997: 120–3.

51. Martel D, Frydman R, Glissant M et al. Scanning electron microscopy of postovulatory human endometrium in spontaneous cycles and cycles stimulated by hormone treatment. J Endocrinol 1987; 114: 319–24.

52. Martel D, Frydman R, Sarantis L et al. Scanning electron microscopy of the uterine luminal epithelium as a marker of the implantation window. In: Yoshinaga Y, ed. Blastocyst Implantation. Boston, MA: Adams, 1989: 225–30.

53. Rogers P, Murphy CR, Cameron I et al. Uterine receptivity in women receiving steroid replacement therapy for premature ovarian failure: ultrastructural and endocrinological parameters. Hum Reprod 1989; 4: 349–54.

54. Nikas G, Aghajanova L. Morphological evidence for the 'implantation window' in human luminal endometrium. Hum Reprod 2002; 14: 3101–6.

55. Murphy CR, Swift JG, Mukherjee TM, Rogers AW. The structure of tight junctions between uterine luminal epithelial cells at different stages of pregnancy in the rat. Cell Tissue Res 1982; 223: 281–6.

56. Murphy CR, Swift JG, Need JA et al. A freeze-fracture electron microscopic study of tight junctions of epithelial cells in the human uterus. Anat Embryol (Berl) 1982; 163: 367–70.

57. Rogers PAW, Murphy CR. Morphometric and freeze fracture studies of human endometrium during the peri-implantation period. Reprod Fertil Dev 1992; 4: 265–9.

58. Sarani SA, Ghaffari-Novin M, Warren MA, Dockery P, Cooke ID. Morphological evidence for the 'implantation window' in human luminal endometrium. Hum Reprod 1999; 14: 3101–6.

59. Winterhager E, Grummer R. Cell–cell communication in the endometrium: possible implications for receptivity in the endometrium. In: Glasser SR, ed. The Endometrium. London: Taylor & Francis, 2002: 46–59.

60. Jahn E, Classen-Linke I, Kusche M et al. Expression of gap junction connexins in the human endometrium throughout the menstrual cycle. Hum Reprod 1995; 10: 2666–70.

61. Winterhager E, Kuhnel W. Alterations in intercellular junctions of the uterine epithelium during the preimplantation phase in the rabbit. Cell Tissue Res 1982; 224: 517–26.

62. Johnson SA, Morgan G, Wooding FB. Alterations in uterine epithelial tight junction structure during the oestrous cycle and implantation in the pig. J Reprod Fertil 1988; 83: 915–22.

63. Marx M, Winterhager E, Denker H. Penetration of the basal lamina by processes of the uterine epithelial cells during implantation in the rabbit. In: Denker HW, Aplin JD, eds. Trophoblast Research, Volume 4, Trophoblast Invasion and Endometrial Receptivity, Novel Aspects of the Cell Biology of Embryo Implantation. New York: Plenum, 1990.

64. Dockery P, Khalid J, Sarani SA et al. Changes in basement membrane thickness in the human endometrium during the luteal phase of the menstrual cycle. Hum Reprod Update 1998; 4: 486–95.

65. Roberts DK, Walker NJ, Lavia LA. Ultrastructural evidence of stromal/epithelial interactions in the human endometrial cycle. Am J Obstet Gynecol 1988; 158: 854–61.

66. Denker HW. Trophoblast–endometrial interactions at embryo implantation: a cell biological paradox. In: Denker HW, Aplin JD, eds. Trophoblast Research, Volume 4, Trophoblast Invasion and Endometrial Receptivity, Novel Aspects of the Cell Biology of Embryo Implantation. New York: Plenum, 1990: 3–19.

67. Denker HW. Cell biology of endometrial receptivity and of trophoblast–endometrial interactions. In: Glosser SR, Mulholland J, Psychoyos A, eds. Endocrinology of Embryo–Endometrium Interactions. New York: Plenum, 1994: 17–32.

68. Kelly FD, Tawai SA, Rogers PAW. Immunohistochemical characterization of human endometrial microvascular basement membrane components during the normal menstrual cycle. Hum Reprod 1995; 10: 268–76.

69. Bilalis DA, Klentzeris ID, Fleming S. Immunohistochemical localization of extracellular matrix proteins in luteal phase endometrium of fertile and infertile patients. Hum Reprod 1996; 11: 2713–18.

70. Enders A, Liu IKM, Mead RA, Welsh AO. Active and passive morphological interactions of trophoblasts and endometrium during early implantation. In: Dey SK, ed. Molecular and Cellular Aspects of Preimplantation Processes. New York, Springer, 168–80.

71. Burke MJ, Dockery P, Perret S, Harvey BJ. The effects of xeno-oestrogen on human endometrial cell structure: a physiological and morphological study. J Anat 2002; 200: 209–10.

72. Kabir-Salmani M, Nikzad H, Shiokawa S et al. Secretory role for human uterodomes (pinopods): secretion of LIF. Mol Hum Reprod 2005; 11: 553–9.

73. Cavazos F, Green JA, Hall DG, Lucas FV. Ultrastructure of the human endometrial glandular cell. Am J Obstet Gynecol 1967; 99: 833–54.

74. Davie R, Hopwood D, Levison DA. Intercellular spaces and cell junctions in endometrial glands: their possible role in menstruation. Br J Obstet Gynaecol 1977; 84: 467–76.

75. Verma V. Ultrastructural changes in human endometrium at different phases of the menstrual cycle and their functional significance. Gynecol Obstet Invest 1983; 15: 193–212.

76. Wynn RM, Harris JA. Ultrastructural cyclic changes in the human endometrium I. Normal preovulatory phase. Fertil Steril 1967; 18: 632–48.

77. Fereneczy A, Richart RM. Female Reproductive System: Dynamics of Scan and Transmission Electron Microscopy. New York: John Wiley & Sons, 1974.

78. Dubrauszky V, Pohlmann G. Structurveranderungen am Nukeolus von Korpusendometriumzellen wahrend der Sekretionsphase. Naturwissenschaften 1960; 47: 523–4.

79. Terzakis JA. The nucleolar channel system of the human endometrium. J Cell Biol 1965; 27: 293–304.

80. Wynn RM, Wooley RS. Ultrastructural cyclic changes in the human endometrium. II. Normal postovulatory changes. Fertil Steril 1967; 18: 721–38.

81. Clyman MJ. A new structure observed in the nucleolus of the human endometrial epithelial cell. Am J Obstet Gynecol 1963; 86: 430–2.

82. More IAR, MacSeveney D. The three dimensional structure of the nucleolar channel system in the endometrial glandular cell: serial sectioning and high voltage electron microscopic studies. J Anat 1980; 130: 673–82.

83. Kohorn EI, Rice SI, Hemperly S, Gordon M. The relation and structure of the progestational steroids to nucleolar differentiation in the human endometrium. J Clin Endocrinol Metab 1972; 34: 257–64.

84. Armstrong EM, More IAR, McSeveney D, Chatfield WR. Reappraisal of the ultrastructure of the human endometrial glandular cell. J Obstet Gynaecol Br Commonw 1973; 80: 446–60.

85. Spornitz UM. The functional morphology of the human endometrium and decidua. Advances in Anatomy and Embryology, 124. Berlin: Springer, 1992.

86. Burke MJ. The endometrium: structure function relations. PhD thesis, National University of Ireland, Cork.

87. Shostak S. Embryology: An Introduction to Developmental Biology. New York, Harper Collins.

88. Dockery P, Ismail RMJ, Li TC, Warren MA, Cooke ID. The effect of a single dose of mifepristone (RU486) on the fine structure of the human endometrium during the early luteal phase. Hum Reprod 1997; 12: 1778–84.

89. Roberts DK, Lavia LA, Horbelt DV, Walker NJ. Changes in nuclear and nucleolar areas of endometrial glandular cells throughout the menstrual cycle. Int J Gynecol Pathol 1989; 8: 36–45.

90. Coaker T, Downie T, More IAR. Complex giant mitochondria in the endometrial glandular cell: serial sectioning, high-voltage electron microscopy and three-dimensional reconstruction studies. J Ultrastruct Res 1982; 78: 283–91.

91. Ancla M, Beliasch J, De Brux J. Action of chorionic gonadotrophin on cellular structures in the human endometrium in the secretory phase. J Reprod Fertil 1969; 19: 291–7.

92. Azidian-Boulanger G, Secch J et al. Action of midcycle contraceptive (R2323) on the human endometrium. Am J Gynecol 1976; 15: 1049–56.

93. More IAR, Armstrong EM, MacSeveney D. Observations on the three-dimensional structure of the nucleolar channel system of the human endometrial glandular cell. J Anat 1975; 119: 163–7.

94. Clyman MJ. Electron microscopic changes produced in the human endometrium by norethindrone acetate with ethyl estradiol. Fertil Steril 1963; 14: 352–64.

95. Kohorn EI, Rice SI, Gordon M. In vitro production of nucleolar channel system by progesterone in the human endometrium. Nature 1970; 228: 671–2.

96. Dehou MF, Lejeune B, Airijis C, Leroy F. Endometrial morphology in stimulated in vitro fertilisation cycles and after steroid replacement therapy in cases of primary ovarian failure. Fertil Steril 1987; 48: 995–1000.

97. Dockery P, Tidey R, Li TC, Cooke ID. A morphometric study of the uterine glandular epithelium in women with premature ovarian failure undergoing hormone replacement therapy. Hum Reprod 1991; 6: 1354–64.

98. Li TC, Dockery P, Cooke ID. Effects of exogenous progesterone administration on the morphology of normally developing endometrium in the pre-implantation period. Hum Reprod 1991; 6: 641–4.

99. Isaac C, Pollard JW, Meier UT. Intranuclear endoplasmic reticulum induced by Nopp 140 mimics the nucleolar channel system of human endometrium. J Cell Sci 2001; 114: 4253–64.

100. Luginbuhl WH. Electron microscopic study of the effects of tissue culture on the human endometrium. Am J Obstet Gynecol 1968; 102: 192–201.

101. Gordon M, Kohorn EI, Gore BZ, Rice SI. Effects of postovulatory oestrogens on the fine structure of the epithelial cells in the human endometrium. J Reprod Fertil 1973; 34: 375–8.

102. More IAR, Armstrong EM, MacSeveney D, Chatfield WR. The morphogenesis and fate of the nucleolar channel system in the human endometrial glandular cell. J Ultrastruct Res 1974; 47: 74–85.

103. Buchwalow IB, Belyaeva LA, Zavalshina LE. Localisation of nucleoside phosphatases (ATPase and 5'-nucleotidase) and nuclear ribonucleolar proteins in the human endometrial glandular cells during the secretory phase. Acta Histochemica 1985; 77: 205–8.

104. Gerasimenko OV, Gerasimenko JV, Tepkin AV, Petersen OH. ATP dependent accumulation of inositol triphospate or cyclic ADP-ribose mediated release of Ca^{2+} from the nuclear envelope. Cell 1995; 80: 439–44.

105. Gore BZ, Gordon M. Fine structure of epithelial cell of secretory endometrium in unexplained infertility. Fertil Steril 1974; 25: 103–7.

106. Graham RA, Seif MW, Aplin JD et al. An endometrial factor in unexplained infertility. BMJ 1989; 300: 1428–31.

107. Yoshinaga K. Surges of interest and progress in implantation research in molecular and cellular aspects of preimplantation

Processes. In Dey SK, ed. Molecular and Cellular Aspects of Preimplantation Processes. New York: Springer, 1994.

108. Chan HC, Liu CQ, Fong SK et al. Regulation of Cl⁻ secretion by extracellular ATP in cultured mouse endometrial epithelium. J Membr Biol 1997; 156: 45–52.

109. Aplin JD. Endometrial extracellular matrix. In Glasser SR, Aplin JD, Guidice LC, Tabibzadeh S, eds. The Endometrium. London: Taylor & Francis, 2002: 294–307.

110. Weinke EC, Cavazos F, Hall DG, Lucas FV. Ultrastructure of the human endometrial stroma cell during the menstrual cycle. Am J Obstet Gynecol 1968; 102: 65–77.

111. More IAR, Armstrong EM, Carty M, McSeveney D. Cyclic changes in the ultrastructure of the normal endometrial stromal cell. J Obstet Gynaecol Bri Commonw 1974; 81: 337–47.

112. Dockery P, Warren MA, Li TC et al. A morphometric study of the endometrial stroma during the peri-implantaion period. Hum Reprod 1990; 5: 112–16.

113. Parmley TH, Roberts DK, Emsa NJ, Horbelt DV. Intercellular contacts between stromal cells in the human endometrium throughout the menstrual cycle. Hum Pathol 1990; 21: 1063–6.

114. Treacy J, McGavigan CJ, Cameron IT et al. Human endometrial stroma following exposure to the levonorgestrel intrauterine system (LNG-IUS). J Anat 2002; 201: 432.

115. Warren MA, Li TC, Klentzeris L. Cell biology of the endometrium: histology, cell types and menstrual changes. In: Grundzinskos JG, Simpson JL, Chard T, eds. Cambridge Reviews in Human Reproduction, Uterine Physiology. Cambridge: Cambridge University Press, 1993; 3: 94–124.

116. Bulmer JN, Lunny DP, Hagin SV. Immunohistochemical characterization of stromal leukocytes in non-pregnant human endometrium. Am J Reprod Immunol 1988; 17: 83–90.

117. Bulmer JN, Morrison L, Longfellow M, Ritson T, Pace D. Granulated lymphocytes in human endometrium histochemical and immunohistochemical studies. Hum Reprod 1991; 6: 791–8.

118. King LD, Wellings V, Gardner L, Loke YW. Immunocytochemical characterization of the unusual large granular lymphocytes in human endometrium throughout the menstrual cycle. Hum Immunol 1989; 24: 195–205.

119. Kayisli UA, Guzeloglu-Kayisli O, Arici A. Endocrine–immune interactions in human endometrium. Ann NY Acad Sci 2004; 1034: 50–63.

120. Klentzeris LD, Bulmer JN, Warren MA et al. Endometrial lymphoid tissue in the timed endometrial biopsy: morphometric and immunohistochemical aspects. Am J Obstet Gynecol 1992; 167: 667–74.

121. Klentzeris LD, Bulmer JN, Warren MA et al. Lymphoid tissue in the endometrium of women with unexplained infertility: morphometric immunohistochemical aspects. Hum Reprod 1994; 9: 646–52.

122. Ehring GR, Kerschbaum HH, Eder C et al. A nongenomic mechanism for progesterone-mediated immunosuppression: inhibition of K⁺ channels, Ca²⁺ signaling, and gene expression in T lymphocytes. J Exp Med 1998; 188: 1593–602.

123. Rogers PAW. Structure and function of endometrial blood vessels. Hum Reprod Update 1996; 2: 57–62.

124. Bartelmez GW. Histologic studies on the menstruating mucous membrane during menstruation. Contrib Embryol 1933; 142: 142–57.

125. Rogers PAW, Au CL, Affandi B. Endometrial microvascular density during the normal menstrual cycle and following exposure to long term levonorgestrel. Hum Reprod 1993; 8: 1396–404.

126. Nyengaard JR, Bendtsen TF, Bjugn R et al. A stereological approach to capillary networks in morphometry: In: Sharma AK, ed. Applications to Medical Sciences. Bombay, India: Macmillan India, 1996: 217–31.

127. Gambino LS, Wreford NG, Bertram JF et al. Angiogenesis occurs by vessel elongation in proliferative phase human endometrium. Hum Reprod 2002; 17: 1199–2206.

128. Dockery P, Perret S, Rogers PAW et al. Endometrial morphology and the endometrial vascular bed. In: O'Brien S, Cameron IT, MacLean CI, eds. Disorders of the Menstrual Cycle. London: RCOG Press 2000: 43–55.

129. Hourihan HM, Sheppard BL, Bonnar J. A morphometric study of the effect of oral norethisterone or levonorgestrel on endometrial blood vessel. Contraception 1986; 43: 603–12.

130. Sheppard BL, Bonnar J. The development of vessels of the endometrium during the menstrual cycle. In: Diczfalusy E, Fraser IS, Webb FTG eds. Endometrial Bleeding and Steroidal Contraception. Bath, England: Pitman Press, 1980.

131. Peek M, Landgren BM, Johannisson E. The endometrial capillaries during the normal menstrual cycle; a morphometric study. Hum Reprod 1992; 7: 906–11.

132. Rogers PA, Gargett CE. Endometrial angiogenesis. Angiogenesis 1998; 2: 287–94.

133. Klagsbrun M, D'Amore PA. Regulators of angiogenesis. Ann Rev Physiol 1991; 53: 217–39.

134. Rogers PA, Lederman F, Taylor NI. Endometrial microvascular growth in normal and dysfunctional states. Hum Reprod Update 1998; 5: 503–8.

135. Rogers P. The endometrial vascular bed. In: Cameron IT, Fraser IS, Smith SK eds. Clinical Disorders of the Endometrium and Menstrual Cycle. Oxford: Oxford University Press, 1998: 31–5.

136. Perrot-Applanat M, Ancelin M, Buteau-Lozano H, Meduri G, Bausero P. Ovarian steroids in endometrial angiogenesis. Steroids 2000; 65: 599–603.

137. Girling JE, Rogers PA. Recent advances in endometrial angiogenesis research. Angiogenesis 2005; 8: 89–99.

138. Palejwala S, Tseng L, Wojtczuk A et al. Relaxin gene and protein expression and its regulation of procollagenase and vascular endothelial growth factor in human endometrial cells. Biol Reprod 2002; 66: 1743–8.

139. Unemori EN, Erikson ME, Rocco SE et al. Relaxin stimulates expression of vascular endothelial growth factor in normal human endometrial cells in vitro and is associated with menometrorrhagia in women. Hum Reprod 1999; 14: 800–6.

140. Bulut HE. A morphological study of human endometrial stroma in vivo and in vitro. PhD thesis, Department of Biomedical Science, University of Sheffield, Sheffield, UK.

5 The cytoskeleton of uterine epithelial and stromal cells

Laura A Lindsay and Christopher R Murphy

Synopsis

Background

- In early pregnancy, the morphological and biochemical characteristics of the plasma membrane are altered.
- These changes are regulated by ovarian steroids.
- The loss of microvilli and flattening of the apical plasma membrane is required for implantation and is a common feature across species.

Basic Science

- In the apical plasma membrane, general changes in the glycocalyx, specifically Muc1, are evident at implantation.
- The lateral plasma membrane separates the apical and basolateral membranes and regulates fluid and electrolyte transport.
- Tight junctions on the apical portion of the lateral junctional complex increase dramatically at pregnancy.
- Tight junctions are composed of occludin and a number of claudins which regulate the selectivity and permeability of molecules.
- Adherens junctions are found on the lateral plasma membrane below the tight junctions and express cadherins.
- The terminal web consists of actin filaments that insert into the lateral membrane. It is lost at the time of implantation to facilitate transport through the cytoplasm.
- Desmosomes, the third component of the lateral junctional complex facilities adhesion between cells.
- At the time of implantation, there is a loss of adherens junctions and reduction in desmosome number in the lateral junctional complex.
- At the time of implantation, the depth and complexity of tight junctions increase.
- Decreased permeability of tight junctions at implantation facilitates changes in uterine fluid volume, facilitated by aquaporins.

INTRODUCTION

During early pregnancy there are dramatic changes to all plasma membrane domains of uterine epithelial cells and collectively these changes have been referred to as the 'plasma membrane transformation'.[1-3] Also at this time there are major changes to the uterine fluid which are thought to contribute to blastocyst maturation and nourishment prior to implantation, as well as facilitating the initial interaction between the uterine epithelium and blastocyst. This review will update the general aspects of this concept and in addition will focus on new information on the lateral junctional complex and associated cytoskeleton at the time of implantation. Changes in the tight junctions, the apical-most part of the lateral junctional complex, form the bulk of this chapter, and as tight junctions regulate one potential pathway of fluid and electrolyte transport, the importance and role of luminal fluid are discussed along with recent evidence of transcellular transporter systems.

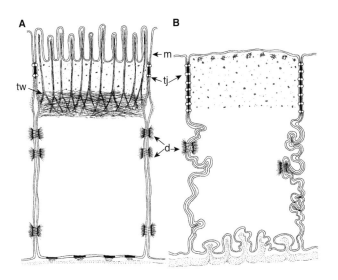

Figure 5.1 Representation of the changes that occur in uterine epithelial cells during the 'plasma membrane transformation'. (**A**) Uterine epithelial cell prior to receptivity (day 1 of pregnancy) showing the apical microvilli (m), the relatively shallow tight junction (tj), and numerous desmosomes (d) down the lateral plasma membrane. (**B**) At the time of uterine receptivity (day 6 of pregnancy) the uterine epithelial cells have undergone the 'plasma membrane transformation' where there is a loss of microvilli (m) and a general flattening of the apical surface. The tight junctions (tj) are deeper and more complex, there is a loss of the terminal web (tw), and fewer desmosomes (d).

THE APICAL PLASMA MEMBRANE

One of the most remarked upon changes during early pregnancy for uterine receptivity, as part of the more general plasma membrane transformation and in response to ovarian hormones, is the dramatic change in morphology and biochemical make-up of the apical plasma membrane.[4-8] On day 1 of pregnancy in the rat, the apical surface of the uterine epithelium is made up of regular microvilli and there is a quite dramatic change in the height and number of these microvilli before attachment. Studies investigating the general morphological changes of the apical plasma membrane found at the time of implantation this surface was indeed flattened, not only in areas around the implanting blastocyst[9-11] but also in inter-implantation sites where opposite sides of the uterus come into contact.[12] The hormonal influence of these changes was also investigated and it was found that changes of the apical plasma membrane, like other aspects of early pregnancy, are tightly regulated by ovarian hormones. Administration of either estrogen or progesterone alone was insufficient for flattening of the plasma membrane.[5,6,13] However, it was found that this flattening could only be mimicked in ovariectomized

animals by the administration of progesterone in combination with estrogen.[14] This was also the minimal hormonal regimen required by ovariectomized rats to enable attachment of transferred blastocysts, hence indicating that this flattening of the apical plasma membrane is a prerequisite for successful implantation. This loss of regular microvilli and general flattening of the apical plasma membrane is a common feature across a variety of species with different placental types. In addition to the common laboratory rodents, similar changes are also observed in other members of the rodent family such as the Chinese hamster[15] and marsupial mice[16] where there are also changes from a regular microvillus apical surface to a flattened or irregular apical plasma membrane. Less-commonly studied species, such as the ungulates (deer,[17] horse,[18] sheep,[19] goats,[20] and camels[21,22]), also demonstrate morphologically similar changes at uterine receptivity. Work on rabbits found a loss of the apical microvilli and a flattening of the apical plasma membrane,[23] and this was also seen in bats,[24] pigs,[25] the cat,[26] and monkeys.[27] Thus, there is a commonality between these wide and varied species at least in regard to the initial stages of implantation where there is a general loss of regular microvilli to produce a relatively flat apical plasma membrane, presumably to facilitate close apposition between the uterine epithelium and trophoblastic cells of the blastocyst. This change in morphology of the apical plasma membrane can be seen in Figure 5.1.

In addition to these morphological changes occurring in the apical plasma membrane of uterine epithelial cells at the time of implantation, a number of biochemical and molecular changes have also been documented. Among these changes, which are common across species, are the general changes in the glycocalyx and more specifically the Muc-1 component of this extracellular glycoprotein network. A 'luminal substance', originally identified in routine electron micrographs on the apical surface of microvilli in mice and rats treated with estradiol,[5,28] was later termed the glycocalyx. Originally, it was shown in the ferret that there was a reduction in the glycocalyx at implantation sites at the early stages of pregnancy[29] and later this was also shown in ovariectomized rats treated with progesterone in combination with estradiol.[30] Similar changes have also been observed in Muc-1 expression on the apical surface of uterine epithelial cells.[31] Muc-1 is a mucin which is thought to cause steric hindrance between the blastocyst and apical surface of the uterine epithelium.[32] In rodents[33] and pigs[34] there is a decrease in Muc-1 expression just

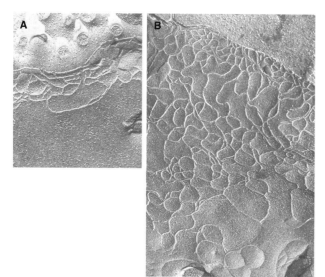

Figure 5.2 Freeze-fracture electron micrographs showing the tight junction region of uterine epithelial cells. (A) On day 1 of pregnancy there are few intersections of the tight junction strands and the tight junctions do not extend very far down the lateral plasma membrane. (B) At the time of uterine receptivity (day 6 of pregnancy) the tight junctions extend further down the lateral plasma membrane and there is an increase in the number of intersections between the strands. Both images are the same magnification.

prior to implantation, while in other species such as humans[35] and rabbits,[36] there is a reduction in Muc-1 locally at sites of implantation. This common loss of Muc-1 from the glycocalyx of the uterine epithelium at the time of implantation presumably allows for closer interaction between uterine epithelium and trophoblast. Furthermore, in the rat the appearance of Muc-1 was shown with immunoelectron microscopy techniques to exist on the external surface of the uterine epithelium, thus being in a unique position to act as an antiadhesive molecule.[37] Other members of the mucin family have also been investigated and a similar reduction in Muc-4 is also seen in the rat at the time of implantation.[38]

Thus it can be seen that there are numerous changes occurring both morphologically and biochemically in the apical plasma membrane of the uterine epithelium in preparation for implantation. The focus of this chapter now shifts to investigating the changes which occur in the lateral plasma membrane during early pregnancy.

THE LATERAL PLASMA MEMBRANE

Even though this membrane domain is not immediately involved with the initial attachment of the blastocyst, it does play an important role in separating apical and basolateral plasma membrane domains and

thus allowing exclusive expression of particular molecules to each membrane domain. In addition to this role, the lateral plasma membrane and the junctional complex contained within is important in adhesion to adjacent cells and underlying stroma, as well as regulating fluid and electrolyte transport, which are discussed later. Even though it has been known for some time that the lateral junctional complex of uterine epithelial cells are regulated by ovarian hormones,[13,15,39,40] recent evidence of the molecular components and hormonal changes induced in these molecules have highlighted the fact that it is the structural as well as molecular changes of these junctions which are important during early pregnancy. The lateral junctional complex, which exists down the lateral plasma membrane between all epithelial cells including the uterine epithelium, consists (from apical to basal) of tight junctions (zonula occludens), adherens junctions (zonula adherens), and one or more desmosomes (macula adherens).

Tight junctions

The tight junction, the most apical part of the lateral junctional complex was originally termed zonula occludentes (occluding junctions) in light of its proposed role in regulation of the paracellular pathway.[41] Initial work on tight junctions involved the use of freeze-fracture electron microscopy techniques to visualize the integral membrane proteins (IMPs), which are seen as strands in replicas using this technique,[42,43] and thus provided a large bank of morphological data for these junctions. The first studies of tight junctions in uterine epithelial cells were from ovariectomized and hormone-treated rats.[44] In ovariectomized rats treated with estradiol alone, the tight junction consisted of strands running parallel to the apical surface with very few intersections of these strands. However, in response to progesterone alone or in combination with estradiol a more complex pattern of tight junctions was seen, with an increase in depth down the lateral plasma membrane and many interconnections of the tight junction strands. On day 1 of pregnancy the appearance of tight junctions was very similar to that seen in response to estradiol: i.e. parallel strands and few interconnections (Figure 5.2A). However, by the time of implantation, there was a dramatic increase in the depth of the tight junctions, which extended to become approximately three times deeper down the lateral plasma membrane when compared to day 1 of pregnancy, as well as an increase in the complexity of the tight junction strands (Figure 5.2B). Similar to ovariectomized animals treated with progesterone alone or in combination with estradiol, there was an increase in the number of interconnections between the strands.[45] This increase in the depth and complexity of tight junctions between uterine epithelial cells at the time of implantation is also seen in a number of species such as rabbits,[46] pigs, where there is an increase in the complexity but not depth of the tight junctions at the time of implantation,[47] and humans, where there is a change in complexity of the tight junction geometry during the menstrual cycle.[48,49] Thus, a common change in tight junction morphology at the time of implantation is seen across species representing another aspect of the 'plasma membrane transformation' of uterine epithelial cells. Figure 5.1 is a diagrammatical representation of the increase in depth and complexity of tight junctions at the time of implantation.

Tight junctions have two main functions: selectivity and permeability of molecules which transverse the paracellular pathway, and providing a physical separation between the apical and basolateral membranes, the so-called fence function.[41,50–53] The components of the tight junction strands, occludin and several members of the claudin family, are thought to convey the permeability and selectivity properties to the tight junction[54] while occludin is suggested to be responsible for the fence function.[55] Recently immunohistochemical studies investigating the changes in the tight junctional strand proteins have shown that occludin is recruited to the tight junction at the time of implantation[56] whereas claudin 4 appears to be one member of the claudin family involved in the tight junction at the time of uterine receptivity (Megan Orchard, University of Sydney, pers comm). In addition, several other proteins associated with tight junctions are also altered during early pregnancy. Zonula occludens-1 (ZO-1), which links the actin cytoskeleton to tight junctional strand molecules, occludin and claudins,[57,58] increases in the apical part of the lateral plasma membrane region at the time of implantation in the rat,[56] suggesting that associated molecules in addition to the junctional strand molecules are altered during early pregnancy.

The changes in tight junctions mentioned above suggest that at the time of implantation, the molecules present on the apical plasma membrane are confined to that part of the membrane where they may play an important role in providing the first interaction with the implanting blastocyst. The change in the distribution in claudins, in addition to freeze-fracture studies, indicates that tight junctions are relatively impermeable at the time of implantation and hence water and solutes must transverse the uterine epithelium via transcellular means; this is expanded upon later.

Adherens junctions

Adherens junctions are found on the lateral plasma membrane just below the tight junction and are inconspicuous in routine electron microscope sections; however, they are visible with specially stained tissue. Visualization of adherens junctions was obtained by developing a staining technique involving the addition of potassium ferrocyanide to standard osmium fixation protocols.[59] Using this technique it was found that on day 1 of pregnancy in the rat prominent densities were seen below the tight junction and these structures disappeared by the time of uterine receptivity (Hyland and Murphy, unpublished observations). Thus, at the time of implantation there is a deepening of the tight junction as well as a disappearance of the adherens junctions. Studies of the molecular components of the adherens junction also support the morphological findings. Cadherins, a molecular component of adherens junctions, has been studied in a number of species and was found to be down-regulated at the time of implantation in mice,[60] rabbits,[31] and humans.[61] Studies have found that calcitonin, which is thought to be essential for normal implantation,[62] could be involved in the down-regulation of E-cadherin and hence the loss of adherens junctions at the time of implantation in the rat.[63]

Terminal web

The terminal web is a layer of actin filaments which inserts into the lateral plasma membrane at the level of the adherens junction and undergoes dramatic change during early pregnancy. In order to visualize this ultrastructurally, a specific staining protocol was developed which included mild membrane permeabilization with Triton follow by labeling of the actin filaments with myosin subfragment 1.[64] Using this technique, the relationship between the terminal web and adherens junctions could be investigated. On day 1 of pregnancy and in ovariectomized animals treated with estradiol a prominent terminal web across the cytoplasm between adherens junctions was seen with bundled microfilaments from microvilli descending into this network (see Figure 5.1A). However, by day 6 of pregnancy when the microvilli are lost, the terminal web dissociated into clumps of filaments in the apical cytoplasm (see Figure 5.1B) as well as in the irregular apical projections.[65] It was also shown that this pattern of disorganized actin filaments could only be mimicked in ovariectomized rats treated with progesterone in combination with estradiol.[66] Hence, at the time of implantation it is suggested that the loss of the terminal web provides a mechanism for the transport of vesicles and molecules through the cytoplasm to enter the apical plasma membrane where they could be involved with the initial attachment reaction with the blastocyst. At the same time, the tight junctions are in effect 'tighter' and hence restrict the movement of molecules from the basolateral to the apical plasma membrane domains, suggesting that introduction of new molecules into the apical plasma membrane could occur through cytoplasmic transport means.

The decreases in the terminal web seen with morphological studies are confirmed with immunohistochemical studies. Actin, the main component of the terminal web, decreases on day 6 of pregnancy in rat uterine epithelial cells.[67] Actin-associated proteins α-actinin and gelsolin were found to be present in the apical cytoplasm on day 6 of pregnancy[67] where they are thought to play a role in the formation of the 'bundles' of actin that are seen near the apical plasma membrane.[65] In-vitro studies have also highlighted a role for the actin cytoskeleton in the change from the non-receptive to receptive states of uterine epithelial cells. RL95-2 cells, derived from a human uterine epithelial cell line, have been shown to have a non-polarized organization of the actin cytoskeleton,[68] and allow trophoblastic cell lines to adhere to the apical surface.[69] In contrast, HEC-1A cells, which exhibit a polarized organization of the cytoskeleton, are repulsive to trophoblast attachment,[68] indicating that it is the disorganized cytoskeleton which is required for attachment and implantation of the blastocyst.

Several molecules have been implicated in the interaction between the actin cytoskeleton and apical surface molecules. The ezrin, radixin, moesin (ERM) protein family members are thought to be such molecules which could possibly act as a potential link between the cytoskeleton and membrane proteins. In the RL95-2 cell line, moesin was found to be absent whereas ezrin levels were reduced.[70] This lack of moesin and reduction in the level of ezrin in human uterine epithelial cell lines capable of adhering to trophoblastic cells suggests that these molecules may play an important role in endometrial receptivity. In-vivo studies indicate that ERM proteins are associated with the uterine epithelium at the time of receptivity in mice.[71] Other structures such as channels are associated with the actin cytoskeleton. A member of the chloride intracellular channel family has been shown to interact with the cortical cytoskeleton in polarized

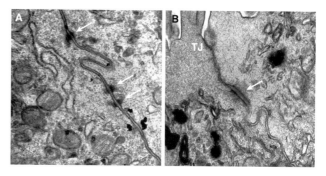

Figure 5.3 Electron micrographs demonstrating the appearance of desmosomes in uterine epithelial cells. (**A**) Prior to uterine receptivity (day 1 of pregnancy) there are several desmosomes (arrows) located along the lateral plasma membrane. (**B**) On day 6 of pregnancy there is a reduction in the number of desmosomes and the formation of a 'giant desmosome' (arrow). The tight junction (TJ) can be seen at the apical part of the lateral plasma membrane. Both images are the same magnification.

epithelial cells in human placental syncytiotrophoblasts.[72] The regulatory cofactor for sodium hydrogen exchanger 3 (NHE-RF) is also thought to play a role linking ion channels and receptors to the actin cytoskeleton and was seen to increase in proliferative when compared to secretory endometrium.[73] Thus, even though morphological evidence of the loss of the terminal web at receptivity has been documented, recent investigation of associated molecules may provide insight into the mechanisms responsible for the removal of the terminal web seen at the time of implantation.

Desmosomes

Desmosomes are the third part of the lateral junctional complex[41] and facilitate adhesion between cells.[74] The desmosome is made up of dense cytoplasmic plaques containing the desmoplakins, plakophilins and plakoglobin,[75] and the intracellular space between the two plaques of the desmosome contains the desmoglea.[76] The desmoglea consist of members of the desmocollin and desmoglein family.[77,78]

Morphological data indicate that there is a decrease in the number of desmosomes between the uterine luminal epithelium at the time of implantation in mice[79] and rats[80] and a similar reduction in morphological desmosomes is seen in humans between the proliferative and mid-luteal phases of the menstrual cycle.[81] A reduction in the number of desmosomes could occur simply as a loss of discrete desmosomes or alternatively desmosomes could aggregate and form structures such as 'giant' desmosomes (Figure 5.3B), which are approximately five times the size of regular desmosomes and are seen on day 6 of pregnancy in the rat.[82] Figure 5.3 demonstrates the reduction in the number of desmosomes between day 1 (see Figures 5.1A and 5.3A) and day 6 of pregnancy (see Figures 5.1B and 5.3B) in the rat. A decrease in desmoplakin mRNA and protein was observed at the time of implantation in mice,[79] while desmoglein protein expression was increased in the apical part of the lateral plasma membrane in the rat on day 6 of pregnancy.[80] A similar increase in the apical part of the lateral plasma membrane was seen with plakoglobin, another desmosomal plaque protein.[67,83]

Desmosomes play an important role in attaching the cytoskeleton to the lateral plasma membrane. Desmoplakin links desmosomes to the intermediate filaments, which in epithelial cells consist of cytokeratin. Studies in the rat uterus showed that during the early stages of pregnancy cytokeratin in seen throughout the cytoplasm while at the time of implantation there is a redistribution of cytokeratin to the apical part of the uterine epithelial cells.[83] This suggests that not only are desmosomes redistributed to the apical part of the lateral plasma membrane but also the associated cytoskeleton is found more apically. A reduction in various members of the cytokeratin family is thought to be important in human reproduction, as a reduction in particular cytokeratin subtypes is seen in conjuction with various contraceptive implants.[84] Studies using colchicine, which disrupts microtubular assembly, in uterine epithelial cells showed a disruption of other cellular systems, including lysosomes, the Golgi apparatus, and in the movement of large vesicles in the apical cytoplasm during early pregnancy.[85–87]

This review of the data surrounding the lateral junctional complex indicates that there is a loss of adherens junctions and reduction in desmosome number, and associated proteins, at the time of implantation and a concomitant increase in the depth and complexity of the tight junction. At the time of implantation the dynamic changes of the lateral junctional complex and associated cytoskeleton suggest that these cells are less adherent to one another and that the paracellular pathway for fluid transport is reduced. This decrease in permeability of the paracellular pathway (i.e. the movement of fluid and solutes between epithelial cells) at the time of implantation, raises the question of how changes in fluid and ion contents of the uterine luminal fluid are regulated.

FLUID TRANSPORT

At the time of implantation in the rat there is a large reduction in the volume of uterine luminal fluid such that the uterine lumen closes down on the implanting blastocyst,[88] thus facilitating the initial attachment reaction. In addition to the decrease in the volume of uterine luminal fluid, there are also changes in electrolyte concentration of the fluid; a decrease in sodium ions,[89] an increase in potassium ions in rats[90–92] and humans,[93] an increase in chloride ions in the rat,[91] as well as an increase in bicarbonate ion concentration and hence pH of the luminal fluid when compared to plasma levels in the rabbit.[94]

Changes in the structure of the apical plasma membrane during early pregnancy may also be linked to the change in luminal fluid volume. The appearance of large, rounded projections at the time of uterine receptivity has been demonstrated in rats and mice and termed 'pinopodes' due to their pinocytotic function.[95,96] The appearance of these structures at the time when there is a reduction in luminal fluid volume suggests that pinopodes could play a role in removal of uterine luminal fluid, at least in rodents. Structures similar to pinopodes have also been identified in other species, such as the hamster,[15] rabbits,[97] cows,[98] deer,[99] camels,[22] pigs,[100] monkeys,[101] and humans.[102–105] Particular clinical interest has followed the discovery of these apical structures in humans, as they are thought to be an indicator of uterine receptivity for blastocyst implantation.[104–107] Functional studies suggested that there is no evidence for pinocytotic activity of these structures in humans and hence they have been termed uterodomes;[108] however, recent evidence suggests that uterodomes may in fact play a secretory role in humans.[3] These uterodomes are clinically significant, as they are thought to be essential for blastocyst implantation and are suggested to be a clinical marker for a receptive endometrium.[109]

Owing to the increase in the depth and complexity of tight junctions at the time of implantation, it is clear that the vast majority of this fluid and electrolyte transport must occur by transcellular means. Investigations are beginning into the cellular mechanisms that underlie these changes in ion concentration of the uterine luminal fluid and it is thought that changes in the chloride ion concentration are due to the cystic fibrosis transmembrane conductance regulator (CFTR) in uterine epithelial cells.[110] Changes in the sodium ion concentration are arguably the most important in regulation of the osmotic gradient, which contributes to the driving force for the movement of water. The presence of claudin 4 in the tight junction at the time of implantation (Megan Orchard, University of Sydney, pers comm), which in other cells is associated with a decrease in paracellular sodium permeability,[111] further suggests that any alteration of sodium ion concentration at the time of implantation is due to transcellular mechanisms. Evidence suggests that the epithelial sodium channel (ENaC) is primarily responsible for the change in the sodium ion concentration[112] and the up-regulation of various sodium–hydrogen exchanger iso-forms at the time of implantation in the rat (Lindsay and Murphy, unpublished observations) may also play a role in the reabsorption of sodium ions at the time of implantation. This reabsorption of sodium ions may lead to the establishment of an osmotic gradient across the uterine epithelium, which could be utilized to transport water through specific water channels.

One mechanism of transcellular water transport is through aquaporin water channels, which have recently been found in the uterus.[113] Investigations into members of the aquaporin family involved in this fluid transport are currently underway, and aquaporin 5 has been demonstrated on the apical surface of uterine epithelial cells at the time of implantation in the rat,[114] where it may play a role in the reabsorption of luminal fluid. There was an increase in aquaporin 5 labeling seen with light and electron microscopy at the time of implantation, and in the rat, an animal which displays asymmetrical implantation, a differential gradient of aquaporin 5 staining across the lumen was demonstrated, suggesting that aquaporin 5 could also play a role in the implantation position.[114] The increase in aquaporin 5 on the apical plasma membrane of uterine epithelial cells could be induced in ovariectomized rats treated with progesterone alone or in combination with estradiol;[115] however, in these animals there was no differential aquaporin 5 staining across the uterine lumen, suggesting that this phenomenon is dependent on the presence of the blastocyst.

SUMMARY

Uterine receptivity is marked by a number of changes of the uterine epithelial cells which are common across species. These changes have been collectively termed the 'plasma membrane transformation', which encompasses changes, both morphological and molecular, of the apical and basolateral membrane domains (see Figure 5.1). Changes of the apical plasma membrane comprise a general flattening of the apical surface and a decrease in various antiadhesive molecules to enable

the intimate attachment of the blastocyst and the uterine epithelium, which is essential for the early stages of implantation. The lateral plasma membrane and its associated junctional complex also undergoes dynamic changes, with an increase in the depth and complexity of tight junctions and a subsequent loss of adherens junctions and a decrease in the number of desmosomes, indicating these cells are less adhesive. The greater complexity and change in molecular composition of the tight junction also prevents the movement of molecules between the apical and basolateral domains, presumably to retain those molecules important for implantation in the apical plasma membrane. The loss of the terminal web at this time, however, provides a mechanism for the addition of components to the apical plasma membrane by transport through vesicles in the cytoplasm. A less-permeable tight junction seen at the time of implantation suggests that changes in the uterine luminal fluid volume and composition occur through transcellular mechanisms, and recent evidence on aquaporins in the apical plasma membrane of uterine epithelial cells at this time provides one such mechanism. There is little doubt that further molecular transcellular mechanisms will be elucidated in the future to further explain the regulation of luminal fluid volume and contents. In the mean time, the concept of a general 'plasma membrane transformation' occurring in these uterine epithelial cells is expanded to include not only morphological changes but also changes in molecular components of the plasma membranes themselves, such as the appearance of transcellular channels, and components of tight junctions which regulate the paracellular pathway.

ACKNOWLEDGMENTS

The authors are grateful to the Australian Research Council who supported aspects of the work described here.

REFERENCES

1. Murphy CR, Shaw TJ. Plasma membrane transformation: a common response of uterine epithelial cells during the peri-implantation period. Cell Biol Int 1994; 18: 1115–28.
2. Murphy CR. Uterine receptivity and the plasma membrane transformation. Cell Res 2004; 14: 259–67.
3. Kabir-Salmani M, Nikzad H, Shiokawa S et al. Secretory role for human uterodomes (pinopods): secretion of LIF. Mol Hum Reprod 2005; 11: 553–9.
4. Nilsson O. Ultrastructure of mouse uterine surface epithelium under different estrogenic influences. 1. Spayed animals and oestrous animals. J Ultrastruct Res 1958; 1: 375–96.

5. Nilsson O. Ultrastructure of mouse uterine surface epithelium under different estrogenic influences. 2. Early effect of estrogen administered to spayed animals. J Ultrastruct Res 1958; 2: 73–95.

6. Nilsson O. Ultrastructure of mouse uterine surface epithelium under different estrogenic influences. 5. Continuous administration of estrogen. J Ultrastruct Res 1959; 2: 342–51.

7. Nilsson O. Ultrastructure of mouse uterine surface epithelium under different estrogenic influences. 6. Changes of some cell components. J Ultrastruct Res 1959; 2: 373–87.

8. Murphy CR. The Plasma Membrane of Uterine Epithelial Cells: Structure and Histochemistry. Stuttgart: Gustav Fischer, 1993: 1–66.

9. Tachi S, Tachi C, Lindner HR. Ultrastructural features of blastocyst attachment and trophoblastic invasion in the rat. J Reprod Fertil 1970; 21: 37–56.

10. Potts DM. The ultrastructure of implantation in the mouse. J Anat 1968; 103: 77–90.

11. Pollard RM, Finn CA. Influence of the trophoblast upon differentiation of the uterine epithelium during implantation in the mouse. J Endocrinol 1974; 62: 669–74.

12. Png FY, Murphy CR. Closure of the uterine lumen and the plasma membrane transformation do not require blastocyst implantation. Eur J Morphol 2000; 38: 122–7.

13. Ljungkvist I. Attachment reaction of rat uterine luminal epithelium. II. The effect of progesterone on the morphology of the uterine glands and the luminal epithelium of the spayed, virgin rat. Acta Soc Med Ups 1971; 76: 110–26.

14. Ljungkvist I. Attachment reaction of rat uterine luminal epithelium. IV. The cellular changes in the attachment reaction and its hormonal regulation. Fertil Steril 1972; 23: 847–65.

15. Blankenship TN, Given RL, Parkening TA. Blastocyst implantation in the Chinese hamster (Cricetulus griseus). Am J Anat 1990; 187: 137–57.

16. Roberts CT, Breed WG. Embryonic–maternal cell interactions at implantation in the fat-tailed dunnart, a dasyurid marsupial. Anat Rec 1994; 240: 59–76.

17. Aitken RJ, Burton J, Hawkins J et al. Histological and ultrastructural changes in the blastocyst and reproductive tract of the roe deer, Capreolus capreolus, during delayed implantation. J Reprod Fertil 1973; 34: 481–93.

18. Allen WR, Hamilton DW, Moor RM. The origin of equine endometrial cups. II. Invasion of the endometrium by trophoblast. Anat Rec 1973; 177: 485–501.

19. Guillomot M, Flechon JE, Wintenberger-Torres S. Conceptus attachment in the ewe: an ultrastructural study. Placenta 1981; 2: 169–82.

20. Wango EO, Wooding FB, Heap RB. The role of trophoblastic binucleate cells in implantation in the goat: a morphological study. J Anat 1990; 171: 241–57.

21. Skidmore JA, Wooding FB, Allen WR. Implantation and early placentation in the one-humped camel (Camelus dromedarius). Placenta 1996; 17: 253–62.

22. Abd-Elnaeim MM, Pfarrer C, Saber AS et al. Fetomaternal attachment and anchorage in the early diffuse epitheliochorial placenta of the camel (Camelus dromedarius). Light, transmission, and scanning electron microscopic study. Cells Tissues Organs 1999; 164: 141–54.

23. Winterhager E, Denker HW. Changes in lipid organisation of uterine epithelial cell membranes at implantation in the rabbit. Trophoblast Res 1990; 4: 323–38.

24. Potts DM, Racey PA. A light and electron microscopic study of early development in the bat Pipistrellus pipistrellus. Micron 1971; 2: 322–48.

25. Dantzer V. Electron microscopy of the initial stages of placentation in the pig. Anat Embryol (Berl) 1985; 172: 281–93.

26. Leiser R, Koob B. Development and characteristics of placentation in a carnivore, the domestic cat. J Exp Zool 1993; 266: 642–56.

27. Enders AC, Hendrickx AG, Schlafke S. Implantation in the rhesus monkey: initial penetration of endometrium. Am J Anat 1983; 167: 275–98.

28. Ljungkvist I. Attachment reaction of rat uterine luminal epithelium. III. The effect of estradiol, estrone and estriol on the morphology of the luminal epithelium of the spayed, virgin rat. Acta Soc Med Ups 1971; 76: 139–57.

29. Enders AC, Schlafke S. Implantation in the ferret: epithelial penetration. Am J Anat 1972; 133: 291–315.

30. Murphy CR, Rogers AW. Effects of ovarian hormones on cell membranes in the rat uterus. III. The surface carbohydrates at the apex of the luminal epithelium. Cell Biophys 1981; 3: 305–20.

31. Denker HW. Endometrial receptivity: cell biological aspects of an unusual epithelium. A review. Ann Anat 1994; 176: 53–60.

32. DeSouza MM, Surveyor GA, Price RE et al. MUC1/episialin: a critical barrier in the female reproductive tract. J Reprod Immunol 1999; 45: 127–58.

33. Surveyor GA, Gendler SJ, Pemberton L et al. Expression and steroid hormonal control of Muc-1 in the mouse uterus. Endocrinology 1995; 136: 3639–47.

34. Bowen JA, Bazer FW, Burghardt RC. Spatial and temporal analyses of integrin and Muc-1 expression in porcine uterine epithelium and trophectoderm in vivo. Biol Reprod 1996; 55: 1098–106.

35. Aplin JD. MUC-1 glycosylation in endometrium: possible roles of the apical glycocalyx at implantation. Hum Reprod 1999; 14: 17–25.

36. Hoffman LH, Olson GE, Carson DD et al. Progesterone and implanting blastocysts regulate Muc1 expression in rabbit uterine epithelium. Endocrinology 1998; 139: 266–71.

37. Isaacs J, Murphy CR. Ultrastructural localisation of Muc-1 on the plasma membrane of uterine epithelial cells. Acta Histochem 2003; 105: 239–43.

38. McNeer RR, Carraway CA, Fregien NL et al. Characterization of the expression and steroid hormone control of sialomucin complex in the rat uterus: implications for uterine receptivity. J Cell Physiol 1998; 176: 110–19.

39. Larsen JF. Electron microscopy of the uterine epithelium in the rabbit. J Cell Biol 1962; 14: 49–64.

40. Murphy CR. Junctional barrier complexes undergo major alterations during the plasma membrane transformation of uterine epithelial cells. Hum Reprod 2000; 15: 182–8.

41. Farquhar MG, Palade GE. Junctional complexes in various epithelia. J Cell Biol 1963; 17: 375–412.

42. Claude P, Goodenough DA. Fracture faces of zonulae occludentes from "tight" and "leaky" epithelia. J Cell Biol 1973; 58: 390–400.

43. Staehelin LA. Structure and function of intercellular junctions. Int Rev Cytol 1974; 39: 191–283.

44. Murphy CR, Swift JG, Mukherjee TM, Rogers AW. Effects of ovarian hormones on cell membranes in the rat uterus. II. Freeze-fracture studies on tight junctions of the lateral plasma membrane of the luminal epithelium. Cell Biophys 1981; 3: 57–69.

45. Murphy CR, Swift JG, Mukherjee TM, Rogers AW. The structure of tight junctions between uterine luminal epithelial cells at different stages of pregnancy in the rat. Cell Tissue Res 1982; 223: 281–6.

46. Winterhager E, Kuhnel W. Alterations in intercellular junctions of the uterine epithelium during the preimplantation phase in the rabbit. Cell Tissue Res 1982; 224: 517–26.

47. Johnson SA, Morgan G, Wooding FB. Alterations in uterine epithelial tight junction structure during the oestrous cycle and implantation in the pig. J Reprod Fertil 1988; 83: 915–22.

48. Murphy CR, Rogers PA, Hosie MJ et al. Tight junctions of human uterine epithelial cells change during the menstrual cycle: a morphometric study. Acta Anat 1992; 144: 36–8.

49. Murphy CR, Swift JG, Need JA et al. A freeze-fracture electron microscopic study of tight junctions of epithelial cells in the human uterus. Anat Embryol (Berl) 1982; 163: 367–70.
50. Balda MS, Matter K. Tight junctions. J Cell Sci 1998; 111: 541–7.
51. Citi S, Cordenonsi M. Tight junction proteins. Biochim Biophys Acta 1998; 1448: 1–11.
52. Kohler K, Zahraoui A. Tight junction: a co-ordinator of cell signalling and membrane trafficking. Biol Cell 2005; 97: 659–65.
53. Miyoshi J, Takai Y. Molecular perspective on tight-junction assembly and epithelial polarity. Adv Drug Deliv Rev 2005; 57: 815–55.
54. Tsukita S, Furuse M, Itoh M. Multifunctional strands in tight junctions. Nat Rev Mol Cell Biol 2001; 2: 285–93.
55. Balda MS, Whitney JA, Flores C et al. Functional dissociation of paracellular permeability and transepithelial electrical resistance and disruption of the apical-basolateral intramembrane diffusion barrier by expression of a mutant tight junction membrane protein. J Cell Biol 1996; 134: 1031–49.
56. Orchard MD, Murphy CR. Alterations in tight junction molecules of uterine epithelial cells during early pregnancy in the rat. Acta Histochem 2002; 104: 149–55.
57. Furuse M, Hirase T, Itoh M et al. Occludin: a novel integral membrane protein localizing at tight junctions. J Cell Biol 1993; 123: 1777–88.
58. Fanning AS, Jameson BJ, Jesaitis LA et al. The tight junction protein ZO-1 establishes a link between the transmembrane protein occludin and the actin cytoskeleton. J Biol Chem 1998; 273: 29745–53.
59. Karnovsky MJ. Use of ferrocyanide-reduced osmium tertoxide in electron microscopy. In: Proceedings of the 14th Annual Meeting of the American Society of Cell Biology. Abstract 294, 1971: 146.
60. Potter SW, Gaza G, Morris JE. Estradiol induces E-cadherin degradation in mouse uterine epithelium during the estrous cycle and early pregnancy. J Cell Physiol 1996; 169: 1–14.
61. Getsios S, Chen GT, Stephenson MD et al. Regulated expression of cadherin-6 and cadherin-11 in the glandular epithelial and stromal cells of the human endometrium. Dev Dyn 1998; 211: 238–47.
62. Zhu LJ, Bagchi MK, Bagchi IC. Attenuation of calcitonin gene expression in pregnant rat uterus leads to a block in embryonic implantation. Endocrinology 1998; 139: 330–9.
63. Li Q, Wang J, Armant DR et al. Calcitonin down-regulates E-cadherin expression in rodent uterine epithelium during implantation. J Biol Chem 2002; 277: 46447–55.
64. Mooseker MS, Tilney LG. Organization of an actin filament–membrane complex. Filament polarity and membrane attachment in the microvilli of intestinal epithelial cells. J Cell Biol 1975; 67: 725–43.
65. Luxford KA, Murphy CR. Reorganization of the apical cytoskeleton of uterine epithelial cells during early pregnancy in the rat: a study with myosin subfragment 1. Biol Cell 1992; 74: 195–202.
66. Luxford KA, Murphy CR. Changes in the apical microfilaments of rat uterine epithelial cells in response to estradiol and progesterone. Anat Rec 1992; 233: 521–6.
67. Png FY, Murphy CR. Cytoskeletal proteins in uterine epithelial cells only partially return to the pre-receptive state after the period of receptivity. Acta Histochem 2002; 104: 235–44.
68. Thie M, Fuchs P, Butz S et al. Adhesiveness of the apical surface of uterine epithelial cells: the role of junctional complex integrity. Eur J Cell Biol 1996; 70: 221–32.
69. John NJ, Linke M, Denker HW. Quantitation of human choriocarcinoma spheroid attachment to uterine epithelial cell monolayers. In Vitro Cell Dev Biol Anim 1993; 29A: 461–8.
70. Martin JC, Jasper MJ, Valbuena D et al. Increased adhesiveness in cultured endometrial-derived cells is related to the absence of moesin expression. Biol Reprod 2000; 63: 1370–6.
71. Matsumoto H, Daikoku T, Wang H et al. Differential expression of ezrin/radixin/moesin (ERM) and ERM-associated adhesion molecules in the blastocyst and uterus suggests their functions during implantation. Biol Reprod 2004; 70: 729–36.
72. Berryman M, Bretscher A. Identification of a novel member of the chloride intracellular channel gene family (CLIC5) that associates with the actin cytoskeleton of placental microvilli. Mol Biol Cell 2000; 11: 1509–21.
73. Stemmer-Rachamimov AO, Wiederhold T, Nielsen GP et al. NHE-RF, a merlin-interacting protein, is primarily expressed in luminal epithelia, proliferative endometrium, and estrogen receptor-positive breast carcinomas. Am J Pathol 2001; 158: 57–62.
74. North AJ, Bardsley WG, Hyam J et al. Molecular map of the desmosomal plaque. J Cell Sci 1999; 112: 4325–36.
75. Garrod DR, Merritt AJ, Nie Z. Desmosomal cadherins. Curr Opin Cell Biol 2002; 14: 537–45.
76. Kitajima Y. Mechanisms of desmosome assembly and disassembly. Clin Exp Dermatol 2002; 27: 684–90.
77. Buxton RS, Cowin P, Franke WW et al. Nomenclature of the desmosomal cadherins. J Cell Biol 1993; 121: 481–3.
78. Burdett ID. Aspects of the structure and assembly of desmosomes. Micron 1998; 29: 309–28.
79. Illingworth IM, Kiszka I, Bagley S et al. Desmosomes are reduced in the mouse uterine luminal epithelium during the preimplantation period of pregnancy: a mechanism for facilitation of implantation. Biol Reprod 2000; 63: 1764–73.
80. Preston AM, Lindsay LA, Murphy CR. Progesterone treatment and the progress of early pregnancy reduce desmoglein 1&2 staining along the lateral plasma membrane in rat uterine epithelial cells. Acta Histochem 2004; 106: 345–51.
81. Sarani SA, Ghaffari-Novin M, Warren MA et al. Morphological evidence for the 'implantation window' in human luminal endometrium. Hum Reprod 1999; 14: 3101–6.
82. Preston AM, Lindsay LA, Murphy CR. Desmosomes in uterine epithelial cells decrease at the time of implantation: an ultrastructural and morphometric study. J Morphol 2005; 267: 103–8.
83. Orchard MD, Shaw TJ, Murphy CR. Junctional plaque proteins shift to the apical surface of uterine epithelial cells during early pregnancy in the rat. Acta Histochem 1999; 101: 147–56.
84. Wonodirekso S, Au CL, Hadisaputra W et al. Cytokeratins 8, 18 and 19 in endometrial epithelial cells during the normal menstrual cycle and in women receiving Norplant. Contraception 1993; 48: 481–93.
85. Parr MB, Kay MG, Parr EL. Colchicine inhibition of lysosome movement in rat uterine epithelium. Cytobiologie 1978; 18: 374–8.
86. Parr M. Apical vesicles in the rat uterine epithelium during early pregnancy: a morphometric study. Biol Reprod 1982; 26: 915–24.
87. Parr M. A morphometric analysis of microtubules in relation to the inhibition of lysosome movement caused by colchicine. Eur J Cell Biol 1979; 20: 189–94.
88. Enders A, Schlafke S. A morphological analysis of the early implantation stages in the rat. Am J Anat 1967; 120: 185–226.
89. Van Winkle LJ, Campione AL, Webster DP. Sodium ion concentrations in uterine flushings from "implanting" and "delayed implanting" mice. J Exp Zool 1983; 226: 321–4.
90. Clemetson CA, Kim JK, Mallikarjuneswara VR et al. The sodium and potassium concentrations in the uterine fluid of the rat at the time of implantation. J Endocrinol 1972; 54: 417–23.
91. Nilsson BO, Ljung L. X-ray micro analyses of cations (Na, K, Ca) and anions (S, P, Cl) in uterine secretions during blastocyst implantation in the rat. J Exp Zool 1985; 234: 415–21.
92. Nordenvall M, Ulmsten U, Ungerstedt U. Influence of progesterone on the sodium and potassium concentrations of rat uterine

fluid investigated by microdialysis. Gynecol Obstet Invest 1989; 28: 73–7.

93. Casslen B, Nilsson B. Human uterine fluid, examined in undiluted samples for osmolarity and the concentrations of inorganic ions, albumin, glucose, and urea. Am J Obstet Gynecol 1984; 150: 877–81.

94. Vishwakarma P. The pH and bicarbonate ion content of the oviduct and uterine fluids. Fertil Steril 1962; 13: 481–5.

95. Enders AC, Nelson DM. Pinocytotic activity of the uterus of the rat. Am J Anat 1973; 138: 277–99.

96. Parr MB, Parr EL. Endocytosis in the uterine epithelium of the mouse. J Reprod Fertil 1977; 50: 151–3.

97. Segalen J, Lescoat D, Chambon Y. Ultrastructural aspects of uterine secretion during the establishment of pregnancy in the rabbit: role of the egg. J Anat 1982; 135: 281–9.

98. Guillomot M, Guay P. Ultrastructural features of the cell surfaces of uterine and trophoblastic epithelia during embryo attachment in the cow. Anat Rec 1982; 204: 315–22.

99. Aitken RJ. Ultrastructure of the blastocyst and endometrium of the roe deer (*Capreolus capreolus*) during delayed implantation. J Anat 1975; 119: 369–84.

100. Keys JL, King GJ. Microscopic examination of porcine conceptus–maternal interface between days 10 and 19 of pregnancy. Am J Anat 1990; 188: 221–38.

101. Bhartiya D, Bajpai VK. Cyclic alterations in rhesus monkey endometrium by scanning electron microscopy. Reprod Fertil Dev 1995; 7: 1199–207.

102. Adams SM, Gayer N, Hosie MJ et al. Human uterodomes (pinopods) do not display pinocytotic function. Hum Reprod 2002; 17: 1980–6.

103. Johannisson E, Nilsson L. Scanning electron microscopic study of the human endometrium. Fertil Steril 1972; 23: 613–25.

104. Nikas G. Pinopodes as markers of endometrial receptivity in clinical practice. Hum Reprod 1999; 14(Suppl 2): 99–106.

105. Nikas G. Cell-surface morphological events relevant to human implantation. Hum Reprod 1999; 14(Suppl 2): 37–44.

106. Adams SM, Murphy CR. A successful pregnancy following SEM fine tuning of hormonal priming. BMC Pregnancy Childbirth 2001; 1: 3.

107. Adams SM, Gayer N, Terry V, Murphy CR. Manipulation of the follicular phase: uterodomes and pregnancy – is there a correlation? BMC Pregnancy Childbirth 2001; 1: 2.

108. Murphy CR. Understanding the apical surface markers of uterine receptivity: pinopods or uterodomes? Hum Reprod 2000; 15: 2451–4.

109. Adams SM, Terry V, Hosie MJ et al. Endometrial response to IVF hormonal manipulation: comparative analysis of menopausal, down regulated and natural cycles. Reprod Biol Endocrin 2004; 2: 21.

110. Chan LN, Tsang LL, Rowlands DK et al. Distribution and regulation of ENaC subunit and CFTR mRNA expression in murine female reproductive tract. J Membr Biol 2002; 185: 165–76.

111. Van Itallie C, Rahner C, Anderson JM. Regulated expression of claudin-4 decreases paracellular conductance through a selective decrease in sodium permeability. J Clin Invest 2001; 107: 1319–27.

112. Yang JZ, Ajonuma LC, Tsang LL et al. Differential expression and localization of CFTR and ENaC in mouse endometrium during pre-implantation. Cell Biol Int 2004; 28: 433–9.

113. Richard C, Gao J, Brown N, Reese J. Aquaporin water channel genes are differentially expressed and regulated by ovarian steroids during the periimplantation period in the mouse. Endocrinology 2003; 144: 1533–41.

114. Lindsay LA, Murphy CR. Redistribution of aquaporins in uterine epithelial cells at the time of implantation in the rat. Acta Histochem 2004; 106: 299–307.

115. Lindsay LA, Murphy CR. Redistribution of aquaporins 1 and 5 in the rat uterus is dependent on progesterone: a study with light and electron microscopy. Reproduction 2005; 131: 369–78.

6 Endometrial angiogenesis, arteriogenesis, and lymphangiogenesis

Jane E Girling and Peter AW Rogers

INTRODUCTION

The human endometrium undergoes regular periods of growth and regression during the menstrual cycle, including concomitant changes in the endometrial vasculature. It therefore provides an excellent model for the study of physiological angiogenesis, arteriogenesis, and lymphangiogenesis. These processes can be considered components of a continuum of vascular development, with considerable overlap and interaction between the mechanisms by which they are controlled. In recent years, a picture of increasing complexity and subtlety is emerging regarding the mechanisms and regulation of endometrial angiogenesis. In contrast, there is a relative paucity of information on endometrial arteriogenesis. Endometrial lymphangiogenesis has also received little attention, due until recently to the lack of adequate tools for identifying lymphatic endothelial cells and accurately distinguishing them from blood vascular endothelial cells.

The aim of this chapter is to bring the reader up to date with current understanding of the processes and regulation of angiogenesis, arteriogenesis, and lymphangiogenesis, and to describe in detail what is known about these subjects in human endometrium and in other model species, including non-human primates and rodents.

ANGIOGENESIS, ARTERIOGENESIS, AND LYMPHANGIOGENESIS

Angiogenesis

There are two main mechanisms of new blood vessel formation: vasculogenesis and angiogenesis. Vasculogenesis occurs during development when the early vascular plexus forms by differentiation of angioblasts, which subsequently form primitive blood vessels.[1] Angiogenesis refers to the formation of new blood vessels from the pre-existing mature vasculature. It may occur by one of several different mechanisms: sprouting, intussusception, elongation/widening, or incorporation of circulating endothelial cells into endometrial vessels[1–3] (Figure 6.1). Sprouting was the first angiogenic mechanism to be described and occurs during neovascularization of avascular tissues or during vascular invasion of growing tumors.[1] It involves a series of steps that include activation of endothelial cells, breakdown of the basement membrane, migration and proliferation of endothelial cells, tube formation, and stabilization of the tube with the formation of new basement membrane and investment in mural cells (pericytes and vascular smooth muscle cells [VSMCs]). In contrast, during intussusception, a vessel is partitioned by the insertion of extracellular matrix (tissue pillars) and endothelial cells. This internal division of a vessel results in the formation of smaller vessels, which may subsequently remodel or enlarge, and it occurs during the formation of vascular structures such as a capillary plexus or vascular arcade.[3,4] Elongation is the lengthways growth of a vessel without formation of new vascular junctions. These different mechanisms of angiogenesis have implications for the functioning of the vascular bed. For instance, during both intussusception and elongation, blood flow is continuous through the growing vessels, in contrast to sprouting where flow only commences once a new patent lumen is formed.

In addition to the proliferation of endothelial cells, growth of new endometrial vessels may require recruitment and incorporation of circulating endothelial progenitor cells into the developing vessel.[2,5] This recruitment of endothelial cells may contribute to angiogenesis by sprouting, intussusception, or elongation.

Arteriogenesis

In addition to angiogenesis, vascular development and remodeling also involves arteriogenesis (arteriole/artery formation). This involves both arterialization and collateral enlargement[4] (see Figure 6.1). Arterialization is the de-novo formation of arterioles and small arterioles from new or pre-existing capillaries, whereas collateral enlargement is the enlargement of pre-existing collateral vessels. Arterialization occurs by the recruitment of pericytes and VSMCs, with the

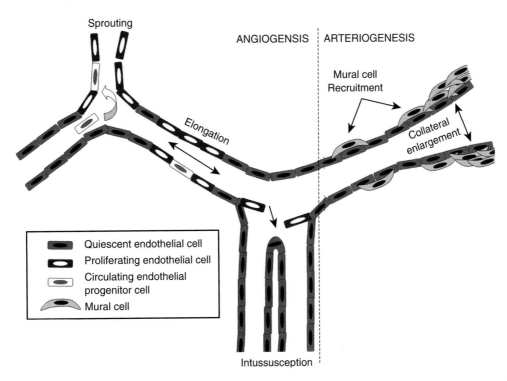

Figure 6.1   Diagram illustrating the mechanisms of angiogenesis and arteriogenesis. Angiogenesis may occur by sprouting, intussusception, or elongation. The relative contribution of proliferating endothelial cells and/or circulating endothelial cells to this process is not known. Arteriogenesis involves both arterialization, which is the de-novo formation of arterioles and small arterioles from new or pre-existing capillaries by the recruitment of pericytes and vascular smooth muscle cells (mural cells), and collateral enlargement, which is the enlargement of pre-existing collateral vessels. Lymphangiogenesis is believed to occur by similar mechanisms to angiogenesis.

vessels gaining the ability to regulate blood flow through rapid alterations in internal diameter. VSMCs and pericytes are believed to belong to the same cell lineage and a continuum of phenotypes is thought to be distributed along the vascular tree.[6] As well as providing mechanical support, these cells are involved in regulating vessel growth and function. Capillaries are supported by pericytes, which are embedded within the vascular basement membrane, whereas arterioles and venules are covered by a coat of VSMCs.[6,7]

Lymphangiogenesis

Lymphangiogenesis is defined as the formation of new lymphatic vessels from pre-existing lymphatic vasculature. With the development of specific lymphatic endothelial cell markers and the interest in the role of lymphatics in the metastatic spread of cancer, research on lymphangiogenesis has increased markedly in recent years. However, this research has focused on the molecular regulation of lymphangiogenesis. Information about the mechanisms of lymphangiogenesis is largely unavailable, although several early studies suggest that

it occurs by similar mechanisms to those observed in the blood vasculature, including sprouting (reviewed in Scavelli et al[8]).

Techniques for measuring angiogensis, arteriogenesis, and lymphangiogenesis

Various techniques are used to measure/detect angiogenesis, arteriogenesis, and lymphangiogenesis. Each has its limitations, and caution is always required in the interpretation of the resulting data. Perhaps the most common measurement made is of vascular density, in which the number of vessel profiles within an area of tissue section are counted. Although this approach has the advantage of being quick and simple, it also has several disadvantages. Any changes noted in vascular density may reflect changes in the vessels, the reference (area), or both. In addition, if overall tissue and vascular growth occur at the same rate, no change in vascular density would be observed. Similar caveats are associated with other common approaches used, such as measuring volume fraction, and neither approach provides information about the mechanisms (e.g. sprouting) of (lymph)angiogenesis. To achieve this, detailed stereological techniques quantifying vessel branch point density and vessel length density are required. Although stereology provides detailed and useful information, it is very time-consuming and requires specialized stereological equipment and knowledge. Another feature commonly measured is cell proliferation, which may be indexed against area or vessel profiles. Ideally, proliferation should be matched with cell death, but this is seldom done. Measuring proliferation also does not take into account cells that may be recruited from surrounding tissue or the bloodstream.

Any vascular bed is a three-dimensional structure, and apart from stereology approaches, this is usually not reflected in the measurements made. Standard histological approaches do not provide information about the resulting vascular bed, its dimensions, or complexity. To obtain such information, techniques using high-resolution three-dimensional reconstructions of microvasculature, either using digitized images of serial sections or confocal microscopy, are required. These techniques enable researchers to consider the distribution, shape, and size of vessels as well as their relationship to other tissue features.

In summary, although no approach is ideal, considerable amounts of useful information have been obtained using one or more of the above techniques. With each study, the choice of approach used should be based on the various pros and cons and the results interpreted with these in mind.

ENDOMETRIAL ANGIOGENESIS, ARTERIOGENESIS, AND LYMPHANGIOGENESIS DURING THE MENSTRUAL CYCLE

Endometrial angiogenesis

Episodes of angiogenesis are associated with all three of the major phases of the menstrual cycle (Figure 6.2). After menstruation, the vessels of the basalis must be repaired following shedding of the functionalis. Markee[9] reported that bleeding did not cease until the arterioles and venules were connected by collateral vessels below the broken surface of the endometrium. During the proliferative phase, growth of new vessels must match the rapid regrowth of the functionalis, which increases in thickness several times within a few days. During the secretory phase, the subepithelial capillary plexus matures and the specialized 'spiral arterioles' grow and coil.[10]

Despite the certainty that angiogenesis must be occurring during the menstrual cycle, it is only recently that objective evidence was obtained to identify the episodes of endometrial angiogenesis, and the mechanisms by which they occurred. Using stereological methods to measure anisotropic structures (structures with specific orientation rather than random distribution) within endometrial tissue sections, it was demonstrated that vessel elongation is a major angiogenic mechanism during the mid–late proliferative phase of the human menstrual cycle.[11] Vessel branch point density (N_v) and vessel length density (L_v) were measured at each stage of the menstrual cycle and used to calculate average vessel length per branch point (L_v/N_v). L_v/N_v remained constant at approximately $100\,\mu m$ throughout the cycle, except during the mid–late proliferative phase when it almost doubled to $190\,\mu m$. As well as demonstrating that vessel elongation is a major angiogenic mechanism during the estrogen-driven proliferative phase, these data also demonstrated that L_v/N_v returns to normal values, through an increase in N_v, in the progesterone-dominated early–mid secretory phase. An increase in N_v could occur by either sprouting or intussusception. However, several lines of evidence suggest that sprouting is not the primary angiogenic mechanism in the endometrium. Structures resembling sprouts have not been identified in endometrial tissue sections (see Girling and Rogers[12] for references), although there was some evidence of sprouts in cytological preparations of endometrium,[13] and proliferating endometrial endothelial cells and the putative marker of sprouting endothelium, $\alpha_v\beta_3$ integrin, were only observed in existing vessel profiles, rather than associated with sprouts.[14] Unfortunately, it will also be difficult to determine whether intussusception is occurring in the endometrium. Ultrastructural techniques can be used to identify features of intussusception; however, definitive proof requires in-vivo observations such as the video/digital recording of developing vessels which was used to observe growing vessels in the chick chorioallantoic membranes.[15] Such techniques cannot currently be replicated in human endometrial tissue, although studies using multiphoton confocal microscopy in animal models may be feasible.

Although the stereological data clearly illustrate that episodes of angiogenesis occur during the menstrual cycle, other commonly used markers of angiogenesis do not provide such evidence. Several studies have examined endometrial endothelial cell proliferation in women at different stages of the menstrual cycle and significant levels of proliferation are observed at all stages, including during phases when tissue growth is

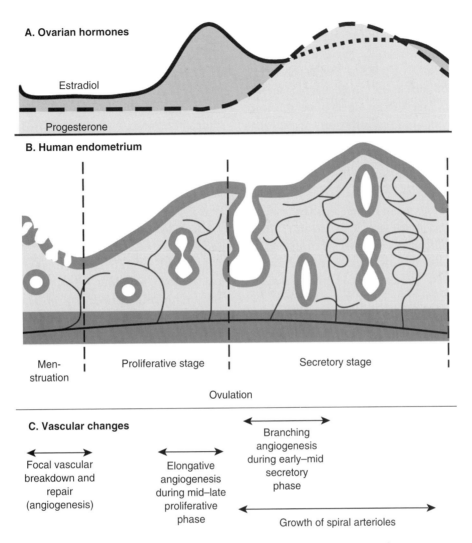

A. Ovarian hormones

Estradiol

Progesterone

B. Human endometrium

Men-
struation

Proliferative stage

Secretory stage

Ovulation

C. Vascular changes

Focal vascular
breakdown and
repair
(angiogenesis)

Elongative
angiogenesis
during mid–late
proliferative
phase

Branching
angiogenesis
during early–mid
secretory
phase

Growth of spiral arterioles

Figure 6.2 Diagram of the human menstrual cycle illustrating changes in (**A**) the circulating estrogen and progesterone concentrations and (**B**) the endometrium. The proposed endometrial vascular changes are outlined in (**C**).

minimal (see Girling and Rogers[12] for references). No consistent changes in proliferation rate are observed and variation in proliferation rates among women, even those at the same stage of the menstrual cycle, is high. It seems unlikely that this variation can be solely explained by individual differences between women, and future studies need to consider methods able to determine the relative contribution of endothelial cell proliferation to endometrial angiogenesis during the menstrual cycle.

Endometrial endothelial cell proliferation has also been examined in ovariectomized, artificially cycling macaques.[16] An artificial menstrual cycle was created by implanting estradiol-containing, and subsequently, progesterone-containing, subcutaneous implants. To stimulate menstruation and the subsequent proliferative phase, the progesterone implant was removed while the estradiol implant remained. A large peak in

endothelial cell proliferation was observed in the macaques 8–10 days after progesterone was withdrawn,[16] which is consistent with the timing of elongative angiogenesis observed in human endometrium. However, no peak in proliferation was observed during the artificial secretory phase, despite the branching angiogenesis observed in human endometrium. This may reflect inherent differences between the menstrual cycle of human and non-human primates, or the particular hormone regimen used in these animals. However, as with the human stereological data, it also raises questions about the relative contribution of endothelial cell proliferation to endometrial angiogenesis. Future studies using stereological measures to examine changes in the endometrial vasculature in this primate model will be of considerable interest.

The concept that circulating cells have an important role in angiogenesis has received considerable attention in the recent vascular biology literature.[2,5] However, the role of circulating endothelial progenitor cells (EPCs) in endometrial function has not yet been addressed in detail, although initial studies indicate their potential importance in endometrial angiogenesis. In immunodeficient mice receiving a bone marrow transplant from donor mice constitutively expressing β-galactosidase under the transcriptional regulation of an endothelial cell-specific promoter, EPCs were detected in various tissues, including the uterus.[2] When ovarian cycling was hormonally induced in these mice, X-gal staining was observed in the endometrial vasculature, as well as in isolated cells in the stroma.[2] It is also interesting to note that ovariectomized mice treated with estrogen had significantly increased numbers of bone marrow-derived circulating EPCs and significantly accelerated re-endothelialization with increased numbers of EPCs at a site of arterial injury in comparison to control animals.[17,18] Increased numbers of circulating EPCs have also been observed in women with high estrogen plasma concentrations due to ovarian hyperstimulation (prior to in-vitro fertilization[18]). It will be interesting to determine if a relative increase in circulating EPCs is also observed in women during the estrogen-dominant proliferative stage of the menstrual cycle and whether these circulating cells are pivotal to endometrial angiogenesis.

Endometrial arteriogenesis

Despite the regular cyclic regrowth of human endometrial vasculature providing an ideal model for the study of arteriogenesis, little is known of the temporal or spatial changes in endometrial arteriolar structure or function (see Rogers and Abberton[19] and references therein). Two types of arteriole are present in the primate endometrium: straight arterioles and the specialized 'spiral' arterioles distinctive to the menstruating primate. The spiral arterioles differ from other arterioles as they are heavily coiled, have larger than normal VSMCs, and, in the human, have no internal elastic lamina. (By contrast, in rhesus monkeys, a thick inner elastic membrane or lamina was described.[10]) The spiral arterioles develop during the secretory phase of the menstrual cycle, arising from the radial artery at the endometrial/myometrial border and supplying the subepithelial capillary plexus. The straight arterioles also arise from the radial artery. A proportion of the straight arterioles supply the basalis, whereas others run alongside the endometrial spiral arterioles in the functionalis. Using immunohistochemical techniques,

Abberton et al[20] quantified an average of 8–10 straight arterioles/mm² in human endometrial cross sections; this compared with less than 1 spiral arteriole/mm.[2]

Alpha smooth muscle actin (α-SMA) is a contractile cytoskeletal protein. It is one of the earliest differentiation markers of VSMC and is also found in pericytes. In the human endometrium, α-SMA is expressed in both large and small vessels of the vascular tree, in pericytes, and in the myofibroblasts scattered throughout the endometrial stroma.[20–22] Abberton et al[20,21] did not observe any significant change in the α-SMA expression on either straight or spiral arterioles across the menstrual cycle. In contrast, Kohnen et al[22] reported an increase in α-SMA around the spiral arterioles during the secretory phase.

Other VSMC differentiation markers have also been considered, including myosin heavy chain, smooth muscle myosin, and γ-SMA.[21,22] These markers show a more restricted distribution in the endometrial vasculature, suggesting spatially organized differences in the VSMC phenotype (reviewed in Rogers and Abberton[19]). It is not yet known whether the different phenotypes reflect the level of VSMC differentiation or whether they reflect functional differences at different vascular locations.

VSMC proliferation can be demonstrated by immunohistochemistry using antibodies directed against α-SMA and the proliferating cell nuclear antigen (PCNA). Abberton et al[23] illustrated that total endometrial VSMC proliferation was low during the early stages of the menstrual cycle (2–2.5% of VSMCs were PCNA-positive), increasing significantly during the mid–late secretory stages to approximately 4%. When straight and spiral arterioles were considered separately, the pattern of PCNA-positive VSMC in the spiral arterioles across the menstrual cycle matched total PCNA-positive VSMC, presumably reflecting the growth and coiling of spiral arterioles during the secretory phase. In contrast, the number of PCNA-positive VSMCs surrounding straight arterioles was consistent across the menstrual cycle. The mechanism(s) for the differential proliferation rates among vessel types is unknown, although it may reflect variations in expression of key receptors.

Endometrial lymphangiogenesis

While the location of various blood vessel types has been well characterized in the endometrium, the scientific literature on uterine lymphatics is not extensive; even the presence or absence of lymph vessels has been controversial. Only two studies (one in

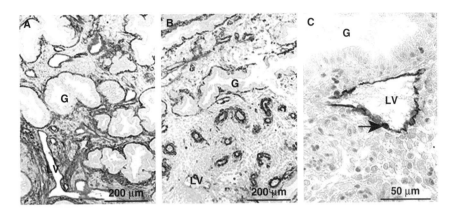

Figure 6.3   Photomicrographs illustrating lymphatic vessels immunostained with antibodies against D2-40 (stained blue) and α-smooth muscle actin (α-SMA, stained brown) in (**A**) functionalis and (**B**) basalis from human endometrium during the late secretory phase of the menstrual cycle. (**C**) Example of a proliferating lymphatic endothelial cell (arrow) immunostained brown using an antibody against PCNA. (See also color plate section.)

the rat and one in humans) have considered the functional role of lymphatic vessels, and both illustrated rapid lymphatic drainage of India ink from the myometrium, but no or minimal drainage when the ink was delivered to the endometrium.[24,25] The few histological studies available have focused on rodents, although one study by Blackwell and Fraser[26] observed lymphatic vessels in the functionalis region in approximately two-thirds of human endometrial samples examined. Most rodent studies report numerous lymphatic vessels in the myometrium, with minimal/absent lymphatics in the endometrium.[27,28] In contrast, a Japanese study using three different morphological/histological techniques found numerous endometrial lymphatics in the rat, particularly in the basal, antimesometrial portion of the endometrium during diestrus.[29]

Recently, specific markers for lymphatic endothelial cells have been identified, enabling detailed studies of lymphatic growth and function[30] (Figure 6.3). Using the specific lymphatic endothelial cell marker D2-40 (antibody against podoplanin), the location and density of lymphatic vessels in human uterine tissues across the menstrual cycle has been described.[31] The basalis exhibited the highest lymphatic vascular length density, with similar densities to that observed in the myometrium. In contrast, very few lymphatic vessels were present in the functionalis. There was no significant change in lymphatic vascular length density across the menstrual cycle in any region. The proliferation of endometrial lymphatic endothelial cells was also considered. Despite the low density of lymphatic vessels in the functionalis, the proportion of lymphatic vessel profiles containing proliferating endothelial cells was significantly higher in the functionalis in comparison to the basalis; levels of proliferation were not cycle dependent.

REGULATION OF ANGIOGENESIS, ARTERIOGENESIS, AND LYMPHANGIOGENESIS

Regulation of angiogenesis

Promotors

The blood vascular system appeared relatively early in evolutionary history and develops early during the ontogeny of all vertebrates. It is a complex system with critical roles in functions, including oxygen transport, nutrition, excretion, fluid balance, homeostasis, and immune defense. As such, it is associated with a long list of hormones, growth factors, and cytokines, as well as adhesion, cytoskeletal, and extracellular proteins. These have been shown to have various direct and indirect effects on angiogenesis.[7] The list includes pleiotropic growth factors such as fibroblast growth factor (FGF), transforming growth factors α (TGF-α) and β (TGF-β), and epidermal growth factor (EGF). However, the most well-known growth factors in regard to angiogenesis belong to the vascular endothelial growth factor (VEGF) family. This is a family of angiogenic and lymphangiogenic peptides, including VEGF-A, VEGF-B, VEGF-C, VEGF-D, and placental growth factor.[7,30,32] The family member that has received the most attention is VEGF-A. It has four common splice variants ($VEGF_{121}$, $VEGF_{165}$, $VEGF_{189}$, and $VEGF_{206}$ [$VEGF_{120}$, $VEGF_{164}$, $VEGF_{188}$, and $VEGF_{205}$ in mice]) with different solubilities, binding affinities for heparin and extracellular matrix, and interactions with VEGF receptor. The properties of the blood vasculature may vary depending on which VEGF-A isoform is prominent. This can be illustrated with data from research using a mouse tumor model. When transfected cells expressing only one VEGF-A isoform were injected into immune-compromised mice, only $VEGF_{164}$ was able to fully rescue tumor growth.[33] $VEGF_{120}$, which is a freely diffusible protein, induced fewer, less-branched vessels that did not pervade the entire tumor mass. The vascular density of $VEGF_{188}$ (which is almost completely sequestered in the extracellular matrix) -expressing tumors was significantly greater than wild-type tumors, but most of the vessels were of small caliber and failed to connect the tumor vessels to the systemic vasculature.

VEGF-A signals via two tyrosine kinase receptors, VEGFR-1 (Flt-1) and VEGFR-2 (KDR/Flk-1), which are both expressed on endothelial cells. VEGFR-2 mediates VEGF-A-stimulated endothelial cell proliferation, whereas VEGFR-1 may be a negative regulator of VEGF-A activity and appears to signal some of the more subtle effects of VEGF, such as endothelial cell migration and modulation of immune function. In contrast, VEGF-C and VEGF-D can induce both angiogenesis and lymphangiogenesis through binding and activating VEGFR-2 and VEGFR-3, which in the adult are found predominantly on blood and lymphatic endothelial cells, respectively. VEGF-C and VEGF-D differ from other members of the mammalian VEGF family because of the presence of propeptides at both the N- and C-termini of the conserved VEGF homology domain. Proteolytic cleavage of the propeptides by plasmin modulates bioactivity of both molecules, increasing affinity for both VEGFR-2 and -3. VEGF signaling may be further modified through the association of VEGFR-1 and -2 with the co-receptors neuropilin (Nrp)-1 and -2.[7,30,32]

In addition to the growth factors described above, a number of other factors play a critical role in angiogenesis. One such factor is adrenomedullin, a 52-amino acid peptide hormone with similarities to the calcitonin gene-related peptide, which is expressed by many tissues in the body. Adrenomedullin is involved with various physiological and pathological pathways, including cell growth, differentiation, vasodilation, angiogenesis, and vascular remodeling. Its actions are mediated by paracrine, autocrine, and potentially endocrine mechanisms.[34]

Extracellular proteolysis is implicated in the initial stages of angiogenesis, including matrix remodeling, basement membrane degradation, migration of endothelial cells, and activation of cytokines and release of growth factors.[35] This process involves various proteinases, including the plasminogen system and matrix metalloproteinases (MMPs). Urokinase-type plasminogen (uPA) and tissue-type PA convert the inactive proenzyme PA into the serine protease plasmin, which is able to degrade matrix proteins as well as activate several MMPs.[35]

Inhibitors

Blood vessel growth, maintenance, and regression are believed to occur as a result of a balance between both promotors and inhibitors of angiogenesis. In addition to the promotors discussed above, various endogenous inhibitors of angiogenesis have been identified, including molecules such as endostatin and tumstatin, which are derived from collagen XVIII and IV, respectively, and another extracellular matrix-associated protein, thrombospondin 1 (Tsp-1) (see Folkman[36] and Nyberg et al[37] for reviews and primary literature). Other molecules include angiostatin, which is formed after protease-induced cleavage of plasminogen, tissue inhibitor of MMP-2 (TIMP-2), which has antiangiogenic effects independent of MMP inhibition, and the soluble version of VEGFR-1, soluble Fms-like tyrosine kinase 1 (sFlt-1). The research about these molecules is fuelled by their potential use in clinical settings to reduce solid tumor growth, or in the treatment of disease such as macular degeneration or diabetic retinopathy. Angiogenic inhibitors can act at various levels. They may block the production of, or neutralize, an angiogenic promoter, or interfere with receptor interaction. An inhibitor may also act directly on endothelial cells, preventing migration or proliferation.

Regulation of arteriogenesis

Several molecular pathways are involved with arteriogenesis, including platelet-derived growth factor B (PDGF-B) and its receptor PDGFR-β. PDGF-B is secreted by endothelial cells and is important in the recruitment of mural cells (particularly pericytes), which express PDGFR-β (see Jain[7] and Banfi et al[38] for review and primary literature). The tyrosine kinase receptor Tie-2 and its ligands, angiopoietin-1 (Ang-1) and angiopoietin-2 (Ang-2), are also important during arteriogenesis. These factors have been reported to regulate the recruitment of VSMC precursors during arteriolization in other systems (see Rogers and Abberton[19] and Jain[7] for review). While Ang-1 is believed to play a role in VSMC recruitment and vessel maturation, Ang-2 is a partial antagonist of Ang-1 and is thought to have a role in destabilizing vessels prior to remodeling. TGF-β1 is a pleiotrophic cytokine that has roles in both angiogenesis and arteriogenesis via its receptors, which include endoglin and down-stream signaling molecules such as ALK1 and Smad5.[7] TGF-β1 has various roles, including stimulating endothelial cell proliferation, stimulating extracellular matrix and protease production, and in the differentiation of mesenchymal cells to mural cells.

Regulation of lymphangiogenesis

In addition to the vital signaling via VEGF-C, VEGF-D, and VEGFR-3 (discussed above), the homeobox transcription factor Prox-1 and the forkhead transcription factor FOXC2 are both thought to have roles in lymphangiogenesis.[39,40] Prox-1 is an early marker of lymphatics and is expressed by a subpopulation of endothelial cells that give rise to lymphatic vessels. FOXC2 is thought to be involved in the maturation of lymphatics, particularly of the vessel valves. In developing lymphatic vessels, FOXC2 is expressed by all endothelial cells, whereas in adults, the highest expression is observed in endothelial cells of the lymphatic valves. Molecules and pathways already known to have roles in angiogenesis and arteriogenesis have also been linked with lymphangiogenesis. This includes the angiopoietin-Tie and the ephrin-Eph pathways. Mice deficient in Ang-2 have defects in their lymphatic vessels and develop subcutaneous edema and chylous ascites shortly after birth. In mice with a deletion in the last residue of ephrinB2, normal vasculature developed; however, maturation of lymphatic vessels was abnormal. Defects were noted in the lymphatic valves and the lymphatic capillaries were covered by VSMCs (lymphatic capillaries normally lack mural cells) (see Baldwin et al[39] and Tammela et al[40] for reviews and primary literature).

REGULATION OF ENDOMETRIAL ANGIOGENESIS, ARTERIOGENESIS, AND LYMPHANGIOGENESIS

Endometrial growth and differentiation is under the overall control of estrogen and progesterone. However, it is not clear how these steroids specifically regulate growth and maturation of endometrial vasculature. Rapid tissue growth and elongation of endometrial vessels occur during the proliferative phase of the menstrual cycle as circulating estrogen concentrations increase. Growth and coiling of the spiral arterioles occur during the secretory phase as progesterone concentrations increase. In contrast, vascular regression and breakdown of endometrial tissue occur at the end of the secretory phase with the withdrawal of steroid hormones. Detailed research is still required to determine not only the mechanisms of vascular growth at different menstrual cycle stages but also the regulatory factors involved.

Direct regulation by estrogen and progesterone

Much of the work concerning the endometrial vasculature has focused on the effects of estrogen on angiogenesis. Conventionally, estrogen is thought to be uterotropic and a promoter of angiogenesis; however, recent data suggest that estrogen may also be anti-angiogenic, depending on the hormonal milieu in the model being examined. Whether estrogen also has a role in pericyte recruitment, arteriogenesis, or lymphangiogenesis has yet to be examined. Currently there is evidence that estrogen acts on the endometrial vasculature directly via the endothelial or mural cells, but also indirectly via other endometrial cell types. Using immunohistochemical techniques, estrogen receptor α (ERα) and estrogen receptor β (ERβ) have both been detected in human endometrial VSMCs.[41,42] In contrast, only ERβ mRNA and protein were detected in human endometrial endothelial cells, and both in-vitro and in-vivo.[41–44] ERα was only expressed at very low levels, if at all.[43,44] In the rhesus macaque (*Macaca mulatta*), only ERβ was present on VSMCs and endothelial cells.[45] The presence of ER on endometrial pericytes has not been considered, nor have studies considered variations in receptor distribution between endometrial lymphatic and blood endothelial cells.

Evidence to support the proangiogenic activities of estrogen are provided by both in-vitro and in-vivo studies in human and non-human primates. In in-vitro assays, estradiol treatment stimulated an increase in human endometrial endothelial cell proliferation within 48 hours and capillary formation and branching within 8 days,[43] and also increased the proliferative response of human endometrial endothelial cells to VEGF.[46] Using full-thickness hysterectomy samples, elongative angiogenesis has been demonstrated during the estrogen-dominant proliferative stage of the human menstrual cycle.[11] In ovariectomized, artificially cycling macaques, a peak of endothelial cell proliferation was observed in animals classified as mid-proliferative (8–10 days after progesterone implant withdrawal, estradiol implant remaining). A similar peak did not occur in those macaques in which both the progesterone and estradiol implants were removed, indicating that the endothelial cell proliferation was estradiol dependent.[16] Estrogen also stimulates an increase in uterine blood flow and vasodilation within the endometrium. In baboons, estrogen treatment significantly increased the paracellular cleft width between endometrial endothelial cells within 6 hours of treatment.[47] The estrogen-induced increase in vascular permeability was believed to be due to the increase in cleft width and apparent opening of the tight junctions between endothelial cells.

In contrast to the above evidence in primate species suggesting that estrogen can be angiogenic, recent data from rodent models suggest more complicated interactions. In two separate studies in which ovariectomized mice were treated with estrogen, a reduction in blood endometrial vascular density was observed.[48,49] Based in part on these observations, the authors of the first study concluded that estrogen promotes vascular permeability, but 'profoundly inhibits' endometrial angiogenesis. Measures of vascular density, however, do not take into account the edema and resulting tissue expansion that is induced by estrogen. In the second study, a reduction in stromal cell density (cells/mm^2) was observed in addition to the reduced vascular density. This illustrated the tissue edema that had occurred in response to estrogen. In addition, the ratio of vascular density to stromal cell density increased, suggesting an estrogen-induced increase in vessels relative to the stromal compartment. A significant increase in endothelial cell proliferation 24 hours following estrogen treatment was also observed, and it was concluded that estrogen promotes angiogenesis.[49,50] In a third study, which also used estrogen-treated ovariectomized mice, no change in the volume fraction of total or proliferating endometrial endothelial cells was observed after 24 hours, despite the edema and an increase in uterine mass and endometrial area.[51] The discrepancy among these studies is due in part to the different approaches that were used to examine endometrial vasculature, and careful interpretation will be necessary in future studies. Detailed stereological studies identifying changes in vessel length and branching (such as those used in human studies outlined earlier[11]) are required to clarify the effects of estrogen on angiogenesis in the rodent endometrium.

Less work has focused on the effects of progesterone on endometrial angiogenesis and arteriogenesis, although there is a large body of work concerning long-term progestin contraceptive therapy and the endometrial vasculature. The effects of progesterone on lymphangiogenesis have yet to be considered. It is not yet known whether progesterone acts directly via receptors on the endometrial vasculature, or indirectly via other cell types. Results from various studies examining progesterone receptors (PRs) in human and non-human endometrial endothelial cells and VSMCs have not produced consistent results. Using immunohistochemistry, PRs have either been reported as being absent from endometrial endothelium or VSMCs of humans,[22,52] or present on only a proportion of arterioles.[53] PRs were not detected in endothelial cells or VSMCs in rhesus macaques (*Macaca mulatta*), although PRs were strongly expressed in the perivascular stroma.[45] In contrast, in in-vitro studies, functional nuclear PRs were identified on approximately 25–30% of endothelial cells from a wide variety of tissue types, including endometrium.[54] Progesterone inhibited endothelial cell proliferation in vitro, and arrested the cell cycle in the G_0/G_1 phase in human dermal endothelial cells.[54] Further studies also identified PRs in human endometrial endothelial cells[44,45] and found that progesterone inhibited VEGF-induced endothelial cell proliferation in vitro.[46] In contrast, PRs were not identified on endothelial cells in vitro by Kayisli et al.[43] Despite not finding receptors, progesterone treatment stimulated proliferation of human endometrial endothelial cells in vitro within 48 hours of treatment and capillary formation and branching within 8 days of treatment.[43]

In addition to the variable results, the majority of the studies discussed above did not differentiate between the progesterone receptor isoforms, PR-A and PR-B, which are known to function in different ways. PR-B is typically a strong activator of target genes; in contrast, PR-A represses PR-B activity when both proteins are co-expressed in cultured cells.[55] Future studies will need to confirm the presence/absence of the two PR isoforms in endometrial endothelial cells (blood and lymphatic), pericytes, and VSMCs, and determine how receptor distribution varies during the menstrual cycle.

Despite several in-vitro studies suggesting inhibitory effects of progesterone, endometrial angiogenesis and arteriogenesis have been observed in response to progesterone in vivo in primate endometrium. During the secretory phase of the human menstrual cycle, there was an increase in the vessel branch point density, suggesting some form of branching angiogenesis.[11] This is also the phase when growth and coiling of the endometrial spiral arterioles occurred, with a significant increase in proliferation of the VSMCs surrounding spiral arterioles.[23] Unlike estrogen, the angiogenic effects of progesterone are believed to occur without concurrent vasodilation.[48] There was no change in endometrial endothelial paracellular cleft width 6 hours after progesterone treatment in baboons.[47]

Vascular changes are also noted in response to progesterone in rodents. In both the rat and mouse, considerable endothelial cell proliferation was observed during early pregnancy, correlating with increasing progesterone production by the corpora lutea.[56,57] Several vascular changes were also observed following progesterone treatment in ovariectomized mice. A significant increase in vascular density[48] and the number of proliferating endothelial and α-SMA positive cells[57,58] was observed following progesterone treatment, and the proportion of endometrial capillaries associated with pericytes also increased.[59] Progesterone treatment of ovariectomized mice caused a significant increase in the percentage of vessels with minimal or extensive α-SMA coverage in comparison to the vehicle-treated mice.[58] Progesterone obviously has multiple actions on the endometrial vasculature and its actions deserve greater attention. Future research will need to elucidate the mechanism of progesterone activity and the interactions between angiogenesis, pericyte recruitment, and arteriogenesis.

The activity of estrogen and progesterone are often considered in isolation in both in-vivo and in-vitro studies. However, during a normal menstrual cycle, the actions of estrogen modify the endometrial vasculature prior to an increase in circulating progesterone. Thus, the actions of estrogen will modulate the subsequent actions of progesterone. Recent research using estrogen- and progesterone-treated mice suggests that estrogen may restrict the angiogenic activity of progesterone. In ovariectomized mice, progesterone-induced endothelial cell proliferation was significantly reduced by estrogen priming prior to progesterone treatment,[57] although estrogen priming had no influence on the progesterone-induced changes in mural cell proliferation or recruitment.[58] Conversely, during early pregnancy in rodents, circulating progesterone increases during before a nidatory estrogen surge to initiate implantation. Using electron microscopy and a hormonal regimen designed to mimic pregnancy, the percentage of capillary profiles with pericytes increased from 6% in ovariectomized mice to 15% following 3 days of progesterone injections. The percentage of capillaries with pericytes increased further if an estradiol injection was given at the same time as the last progesterone injection (69%).[59] During pregnancy, the percentage of vessel profiles with pericytes increased from 5% on day 4 to 74% on day 5, dropping to 14% on day 6. As well as illustrating the potential for rapid changes in pericyte coverage, these results highlight the need for carefully designed models

taking into account temporal changes in ovarian steroids for studies of particular hormonal and reproductive events.

Regulation of angiogenic factors by estrogen and progesterone

Promotors

Although the endometrium is under the overall control of estrogen and progesterone, these hormones act indirectly via various growth factors, including the potent endothelial cell mitogen VEGF-A. VEGF-A is expressed by both the epithelium and stroma of the primate and rodent endometrium, with changes noted in the intensity of staining through the menstrual cycle. Estrogen and progesterone are known to affect VEGF-A mRNA and protein levels both in vitro and in vivo; however, the details of how estrogen and progesterone and VEGF-A affect angiogenesis are still to be described in detail (see Girling and Rogers[12] for review).

Estrogen stimulates endometrial VEGF-A production in vitro and in vivo in both primates and rodents. In cultured human endometrial cells, estrogen stimulated VEGF-A protein expression,[60,61] and in baboons and rhesus monkeys, endometrial stromal and epithelial VEGF-A mRNA levels were restored by estrogen following a reduction after ovariectomy.[16,62] In ovariectomized estrogen-treated mice, VEGF-A and VEGFR-2 mRNA increased in endometrial stromal cells within 2 and 6 hours, respectively.[48] By 24 hours post administration, there was no stromal VEGF-A or VEGFR-2 mRNA and VEGF-A expression was restricted to the luminal epithelium. These last results highlight the temporal and spatial variation in the endometrial response to steroid hormones. Future studies will need to carefully elucidate the interactions between specific cell types and VEGF-A and their role in controlling endometrial vascular development.

In both primates and rodents, the strongest expression of VEGF-A is observed in the endometrial epithelium. However, an in-vitro study has illustrated that most epithelial VEGF-A is secreted apically into the uterine lumen.[63] Based on these observations, it was hypothesized that epithelial VEGF is unlikely to have a role in endometrial angiogenesis. However, this hypothesis was not supported by further research in which endometrial epithelial and stromal cells were co-cultured with human myometrial microvascular endothelial cells.[64] Myometrial microvascular endothelial cell tube formation increased by approximately 65% over culture in media only when endothelial cells were cultured in either media supplemented with human recombinant VEGF-A or co-cultured with endometrial epithelial cells. A further increase occurred when endothelial cells were treated with estrogen and co-cultured with endometrial epithelial cells. The observed tube formation was similar to that in media only when the endothelial cells were co-cultured with endometrial stromal cells (with or without estrogen).[64] These results suggest that estrogen regulates endometrial angiogenesis by regulating the production and secretion of angiogenic factors such as VEGF-A by endometrial epithelial cells. It must be noted, however, that in in-vitro culture, the directional secretion (from the apical surface) that is observed in vivo does not occur and additional experimental models will be required to determine whether any epithelial VEGF-A is normally secreted into the endometrial stromal and whether this is sufficient to have a role in endometrial angiogenesis.

Although VEGF-A is predominant in endometrial epithelium, foci of intense VEGF-A staining have also been observed within the human endometrium.[65] Many of these foci were within blood vessels and were found to correlate both temporally and spatially with endometrial endothelial cell proliferation.[66] The greatest percentage of focal VEGF-expressing blood vessels were observed during the estrogen-dominant proliferative stage of the menstrual cycle, with the greatest numbers of positive vessels in the subepithelial capillary plexus. These foci were found to correspond to adherent neutrophils within the endometrialmicrovessels and it was hypothesized that leukocytes may provide a source of VEGF directly to the proliferating vessels.[66,67] It has also been hypothesized that VEGF may modulate neutrophil migration into the endometrium, creating an autocrine amplification mechanism that may have a role in VEGF-induced angiogenesis and inflammation.[68]

Following from the detailed observations in human endometrium, estrogen treatment was found to cause a significant increase in the number of VEGF-positive intravascular endometrial neutrophils in ovariectomized mice.[69] If neutropenia was induced at the same time as mice were treated with estrogen, endometrial neutrophils were reduced to basal levels and estrogen-induced endothelial cell proliferation was reduced by 30–40%. These results support a role of neutrophils in estrogen-induced angiogenesis. The study also identified a population of VEGF-positive intravascular leukocytes that were not reduced by neutropenia. Potential candidates for these additional leukocytes are the monocytes/macrophages, which constitute around 10% of all endometrial cells.[70] Future studies will need to carefully address the role of various leukocytes in endometrial blood vessel growth and remodeling.

Considerably less attention has been paid to the interactions between progesterone and VEGF-A, although VEGF-A is hypothesized to have an important role in progesterone-induced endometrial angiogenesis. In ovariectomized mice, progesterone-induced endothelial cell proliferation was significantly reduced when mice were concurrently treated with a VEGF antiserum.[57] In comparison to the relatively rapid effects of estrogen on VEGF-A production and endothelial cell proliferation, the effects of progesterone are slower and of a lower magnitude. In the study by Ma et al,[48] VEGF-A and VEGFR-2 increased steadily within the endometrial stroma over a 24-hour period in response to a single progesterone injection.

Few studies have yet to play close attention to where and when the specific VEGF-A isoforms are located within the endometrium and what implications this may have for how endometrial angiogenesis is controlled. In the human endometrium, $VEGF_{121}$ and $VEGF_{165}$ predominate and estrogen increases VEGF-A expression, possibly of all isoforms.[71] Progesterone selectively increases the expression of $VEGF_{189}$ in the human uterus: this isoform is secreted in vitro by decidualized endometrial stromal cells. In mice, VEGF isoforms have only been examined in uteri during pregnancy. $VEGF_{164}$ was found to be the dominant isoform.[72]

The FGF family is a group of heparin-binding growth factors that have multiple biological functions, including cell proliferation, migration, embryogenesis, and tumorigenesis.[73] There are over 20 structurally related peptides in this family and they exert their effects via tyrosine kinases FGF receptors 1–4 (FGFR1–4). FGF-2 is just one example of several FGFs that have been identified in the endometrium. It has been detected in both the primate and rodent endometrium.[74,75] In the human endometrium, FGF-2 was detected in both the glandular and luminal epithelium, and to a lesser extent in the stroma.[76] Staining was also observed in the endothelial cells. A similar pattern of FGF-2 immunostaining was observed in the rhesus monkey.[77] FGFR-1 and -2 were also detected in the human and rhesus monkey endometrium, with variations in staining pattern across the menstrual cycle.[77] FGFs are pleiotropic growth factors and, because of this, their specific role in endometrial angiogenesis is difficult to determine and any change in the endometrial expression pattern of FGF or its receptors will not necessarily indicate changes in angiogenesis. Although difficult to quantify, the activity of FGFs will contribute to the balance of angiogenic promotors and inhibitors in various ways. This includes interactions with factors such as VEGF-A[78] and the MMPs.[79]

Another hormone linked with angiogenesis that has activity in the endometrium is adrenomedullin. Immunostaining for adrenomedullin has been observed in both the endometrial epithelium and stroma, although the highest degree of immunostaining was seen in the stromal macrophages.[80] Adrenomedullin is also expressed by endometrial endothelial cells both in vitro and in vivo.[81] It promotes endometrial endothelial cell proliferation in vitro, and induces cyclic AMP production, showing that it acts as an autocrine growth factor for human endometrial endothelial cells.[81]

Human endometrial microvascular endothelial cells are known to express various molecules important in extracellular proteolysis, including uPA, tissue-type PA, PA inhibitor-1 or uPA receptor expression.[82] Production of uPA by human endometrial microvascular endothelial cells increased when VEGF, basic fibroblast growth factor (bFGF), or a combination of these factors with TNF-α, was added to the culture.[82] The enhanced uPA/plasmin activity, in combination with the increased VEGFR-2 expression, may enhance the angiogenic capacity of endometrial endothelial cells.[82] Endometrial endothelial cells also express various MMPs, including MMP-1, MMP-2, MMP-10, membrane-type (MT) 1-MMP, MT3-MMP, and MT4-MMP mRNA under basal conditions, as well when stimulated with VEGF.[83,84] The VEGF-enhanced capillary tube formation in fibrin and/or collagen matrices was reduced in the presence of the MMP inhibitor BB94 or uPA blocking antibodies. Tube formation was also reduced when TIMP-1 or TIMP-3 was overexpressed.[83]

Inhibitors

There is still very little information about specific angiogenic inhibitors in the endometrium. Molecules such as endostatin and Tsp-1 are produced by endometrial stromal cells in vitro.[85–87] Hypoxia was found to significantly reduce endostatin production by cultured human endometrial stromal cells;[86] however, information about endostatin production in vivo

through the menstrual cycle is not available. Tsp-1 mRNA expression in the human endometrium is higher in the secretory phase in comparison to the proliferative phase.[85] In in-vitro experiments, Tsp-1 MRNA and protein expression by endometrial stromal cells increased with progesterone treatment, but not following estrogen treatment. Conditioned media from progesterone-treated stromal cells inhibited FGF-2-mediated migration of bovine aortic endothelial cells; the inhibition was blocked in the presence of an antibody against Tsp-1. Comparable inhibition of migration was observed if bovine aortic endothelial cells were incubated in media containing Tsp-1 at a similar concentration to that in media from progesterone-treated endothelial cells. The authors suggest that Tsp-1 may be linked to the inhibition of vessel formation during the later stages of the menstrual cycle and that Tsp-1 is a progesterone-dependent protein in the endometrium.

As discussed above, the MMPs and their inhibitors (the TIMPs) have an important role in the endometrium, with both angiogenic and antiangiogenic activities. The soluble VEGF receptor sFlt-1 has also been detected in the human endometrium. sFlt-1 was immunoprecipitated from endometrial samples with the greatest expression in the early menstrual samples, but also in tissues from the late secretory phase.[88] A broader picture of angiogenic regulation will be developed as research continues to examine the interaction between inhibitors and promotors in the human endometrium through the menstrual cycle.

Regulation of arteriogenic factors by estrogen and progesterone

Several studies have examined Ang-1, Ang-2, and Tie-2 expression in the human endometrium[89] (reviewed in Rogers and Abberton[19]). Results have varied considerably, with staining reported variously in the epithelium, stroma, and uterine natural killer cells. In the most recent study, staining for Ang-1 was observed in stroma, and luminal and glandular epithelial cells, as well as in endothelial cells in both secretory and proliferative endometrial samples, whereas Ang-2 was detected in the stroma and in glandular epithelial cells.[89] Tie-2 was observed in glandular epithelium, as well as in endometrial endothelium, an observation that is at least consistent among studies as well as with staining patterns observed in other tissues.

Regulation of lymphangiogenic factors by estrogen and progesterone

Studies of immunostaining for VEGF-C and VEGF-D in normal human endometrium report variable levels of VEGF-C in stroma, glands, and blood vessels,[90,91] and little or no evidence for VEGF-D in any tissue compartment.[92] VEGF-C and VEGF-D protein were also detected in human endometrium using sodium dodecyl sulfate–polyacrylamide gel electrophoresis (SDS–PAGE).[31] Significantly lower levels of these proteins were detected in the endometrium in contrast to the myometrium, despite the high density of lymphatic vessels present in the basalis region. Protein expression of VEGF-D increased significantly in the secretory phase in contrast to the proliferative phase. There are also recent publications investigating the immunohistochemical expression of VEGFR-3 in human endometrium.[90–92] Immunostaining was observed in endometrial blood endothelial cells in two of the studies,[90,91] but the third reported no immunostaining in endometrial tissues.[92] VEGFR-3 is often used as a specific marker of lymphatic vessels, so it is somewhat surprising that studies identifying the protein on blood vessels made no mention of staining in lymphatic vessels. Although the above data suggest that the lymphatic growth factors are regulated by steroid hormones, considerably more research is required to determine their specific interactions between estrogen and progesterone.

Regulation of angiogenesis, arteriogenesis, and lymphangiogenesis during menstruation

Menstruation occurs at the end of the menstrual cycle as a result of estrogen and progesterone withdrawal following corpus luteal regression. The primary mechanism that initiates menstruation is believed to be tissue destruction within the functionalis, with associated vascular breakdown and bleeding (see Salamonsen[93] for review). Each bleeding event is focal and is halted by vasoconstriction of spiral arterioles in the basalis. Regeneration of the endometrium and its vasculature begins while menstruation is still in progress. This means that vascular breakdown and repair are occurring simultaneously at different foci within the endometrium.

Our understanding of the mechanisms controlling the repair of endometrial microvessels following menstruation is perhaps the least understood of the endometrial angiogenic episodes. It has been thought that menstrual angiogenesis is a hypoxia-related process. Support for this comes from Markee's[9] classic study in which endometrial explants were transplanted into the anterior chamber of the eye in rhesus macaques. Vasoconstriction followed by vasodilation of the spiral arterioles was observed following progesterone withdrawal. If such vasoconstriction occurred in the endometrium in situ, it would provide a possible mechanism for vessel repair through hypoxia-induced up-regulation of VEGF-A. Considerably more VEGF-A mRNA and GLUT-1, a glucose transporter and marker of anaerobic metabolism that is induced by ischemia, was found in endometrium collected from menstruating women in comparison to tissues from women in the proliferative or secretory phase.[88] High levels of VEGF-A mRNA were also observed in the glands and necrotic areas of menstrual phase endometrium.[60] In the rhesus macaque, VEGF-A mRNA was up-regulated in the glands and stroma of superficial endometrial tissues 1–2 days following progesterone withdrawal during artificially induced menstruation.[16]

However, despite Markee's[9] observations in macaques and the high VEGF-A levels that have been observed in the endometrium from menstruating women, there is no direct evidence for vasoconstriction or hypoxia during menstruation.[93,94] Perimenstruation, no significant changes in blood flow were observed[95] and no ischemia/reperfusion episodes have been detected.[96] Only very low levels of the hypoxia-inducible factors HIF-1α and HIF-2α, early markers of hypoxia, have been observed in the human endometrium.[97] Instead of vasoconstriction and hypoxia, current theory now considers menstruation to be an inflammatory-type process.[93,94] Future studies will need to examine various inflammatory mediates and factors and their interaction with endometrial angiogenesis.

Regulation of angiogenesis, arteriogenesis, and lymphangiogenesis during early pregnancy/implantation

For a successful pregnancy, a blastocyst must implant into a receptive endometrium. The process is complex, with interactions between numerous molecules from both the mother and embryo. Angiogenesis and increased vascular permeability are believed to be central to the formation of a receptive endometrium, although for obvious ethical reasons, very little is known about these processes during the earliest stages of pregnancy in the human endometrium. Even less information is available concerning endometrial arteriogenesis or lymphangiogenesis during early pregnancy.

Key angiogenic and arteriogenic factors have been identified in the endometrium during early pregnancy in non-human primates and rodents, including VEGF-A, the angiopoietins, and their associated receptors (see Wang et al[98] and Liu et al[99] and references therein). Angiogenic factors are also produced by the trophoblast, which will have localized effects at the site of implantation. In rodents, increasing numbers of proliferating endometrial endothelial cells are observed in the early days of pregnancy (prior to implantation).[56,57] Inhibition or blocking of VEGF, or treatment with other compounds that block angiogenesis, has been shown to reduce/prevent implantation in rodents.[99–101]

USE OF EXPERIMENTAL IN-VIVO AND IN-VITRO MODELS

To appropriately investigate the multiple angiogenic, arteriogenic, and lymphangiogenic mechanisms that occur in the human endometrium, research with both in-vivo and in-vitro models is required. Because of their close evolutionary relationship and a similar menstrual cycle, non-human primates provide the most appropriate model for the study of endometrial function relevant to humans. In addition to studying changes during the menstrual cycle of these animals, various hormone manipulations that allow careful examination of individual variables have provided useful results. However, various ethical and economic factors restrict the use of primate models and other animal systems are also required. Despite the major differences between the menstrual cycle in humans/primates and the estrus cycle in rodents, mouse models are invaluable in this regard. Studies using such mouse models have contributed greatly to our understanding of the endometrial vasculature. Although caution has to be taken when extrapolating information to humans, these models provide systems that can be easily manipulated in a relatively short time span. Future studies may also make use of the extensive and ever-developing range of transgenic mice to increase our understanding of vascular function in the endometrium.

In addition to in-vivo studies, detailed in-vitro studies are an essential component of studies examining endometrial vascular development and function. Techniques have now been developed to culture endometrial endothelial cells and are being used to characterize their activity (e.g. Kookwijk et al[82]). This is important as endothelial cells from different tissues/organs often exhibit specific characteristics. For example, human endometrial microvascular

endothelial cells are much more sensitive to stimulation by VEGF than are human foreskin microvascular endothelial cells, which respond better to bFGF.[82] VEGF or bFGF increased the formation of capillary-like structures by human endometrial microvascular endothelial cells cultured in 2% human serum on top of three-dimensional fibrin matrices. In contrast, human foreskin microvascular endothelial cells only formed tubes when they were stimulated with both tumor necrosis factor α (TNF-α) and an additional growth factor. This differing response is thought to be due to greater VEGFR-2 expression in endometrial microvascular endothelial cells in comparison to human foreskin microvascular endothelial cells.[82]

Research using cultured endometrial endothelial cells can be extended when co-cultures of other cell types are included in the experimental system, such as in the studies discussed earlier by Albrecht et al.[64] An alternative in-vitro system was also used by Print et al.[102] Supernatants collected from cultured endometrium were found to contain soluble factors. These supernatants were able to stimulate proliferation in human umbilical endothelial cells in vitro, as well as angiogenesis. VEGF-A was found to be a component of the supernatant and the proliferative effects of endometrial supernatants decreased if an antibody against VEGF-A was included in culture. The effects of supernatants on gene expression in human umbilical vein endothelial cells were analyzed using gene array technology and increased expression of several angiogenic promoters (e.g. CXC receptor-4, VE-cadherin, endoglin, PECAM-1) was observed.[102] Gene array technology has also been used to examine gene expression in estrogen- or progestin-treated human endometrial endothelial cells.[84] A wide variety of genes were affected by the hormones and cluster analysis, indicating that many were involved in intracellular signaling pathways. Several angiogenic factors were also detected (e.g. VEGF-A, VEGFR-2, angiopoietin-2). Continued development and design of innovative in-vitro systems will be invaluable in future studies of endometrial vasculature.

CONCLUSIONS

Growth and regression of the vasculature is a fundamental component of the cyclic changes occurring in the human endometrium during the menstrual cycle. This requires angiogenesis, arteriogenesis, and lymphangiogenesis. Multiple mechanisms of angiogenesis have been identified in the endometrium, depending on the stage of the menstrual cycle. Elongative angiogenesis has been observed in the proliferative stage of the cycle, whereas some form of branching angiogenesis is believed to occur during the secretory phase. Proliferation of both endometrial endothelial and mural cells have been observed during the menstrual cycle; however, it has not yet been possible to elucidate the relative contribution of cell proliferation and/or recruitment (from adjacent tissues or the circulation) to the vascular growth and remodeling.

Endometrial angiogenesis, arteriogenesis, and lymphangiogenesis are regulated by many different factors, although the ovarian steroids estrogen and progesterone are the overall regulators of endometrial growth and function. Estrogen is generally thought to promote growth of endometrial vasculature, although studies using rodent models have produced conflicting results, relating in part to the different experimental techniques used. Less attention has focused on the actions of progesterone, although studies do indicate that this hormone has multiple and essential actions on the endometrial vasculature.

Multiple regulators of vascular development have been identified in the endometrium. Of these, the VEGF family of growth factors is the most well known, although the details of how the family members and their receptors interact to control angiogenesis, arteriogenesis, and lymphangiogenesis are still to be elucidated in full. This includes determining which endometrial cell types are responsible for VEGF production and, in the case of VEGF-A, which isoforms are present.

Animal models provide an invaluable resource for the study of the endometrial vasculature. However, study using non-human primate models is costly. This means the use of rodent models is useful, despite the differences between a primate menstrual cycle and the rodent's estrous cycle. Care will always be required when translating information gained from animal models to the study of the human endometrium, particularly as the number of studies using transgenic mice increases. Despite the difficulties, continuing research will not only increase our understanding of angiogenesis, arteriogenesis, and lymphangiogenesis in general and during the normal menstrual cycle but may lead to knowledge relevant to the various blood-vessel associated disorders and pathologies of the endometrium, including menorrhagia, breakthrough bleeding, endometriosis, and endometrial cancer.

REFERENCES

1. Risau W. Mechanisms of angiogenesis. Nature 1997; 386: 671–4.
2. Ashara T, Masuda H, Takahashi T et al. Bone marrow origin of endothelial progenitor cells responsible for postnatal vasculogenesis in physiological and pathological neovascularization. Circ Res 1999; 85: 221–8.
3. Burri PH, Djonov V. Intussusceptive angiogenesis – the alternative to capillary sprouting. Mol Aspects Med 2002; 23: S1–27.
4. Peirce SM, Skalak TC. Microvascular remodeling: a complex continuum spanning angiogenesis to arteriogenesis. Microcirculation 2003; 10: 99–111.
5. Khakoo AY, Finkel T. Endothelial progenitor cells. Ann Rev Med 2005; 56: 79–101.
6. Armulik A, Abramsson A, Betsholtz C. Endothelial/pericyte interactions. Circ Res 2005; 97: 512–23.
7. Jain RK. Molecular regulation of vessel maturation. Nat Med 2003; 9: 685–93.
8. Scavelli C, Weber E, Aglianò M et al. Lymphatics at the crossroads of angiogenesis and lymphangiogenesis. J Anat 2004; 204: 433–49.
9. Markee JE. Menstruation in intraocular endometrial transplants in the rhesus monkey. Contrib Embryol 1940; 177: 220–30.
10. Kaiserman-Abramof IR, Padykula HA. Angiogenesis in the postovulatory primate endometrium: the coiled arteriolar system. Anat Rec 1989; 224: 479–89.
11. Gambino LS, Wreford NG, Bertram JF et al. Angiogenesis occurs by vessel elongation in proliferative phase human endometrium. Hum Reprod 2002; 17: 1199–206.
12. Girling JE, Rogers PAW. Recent advances in endometrial angiogenesis. Angiogenesis 2005; 8: 89–99.
13. Ono M, Shiina Y. Cytological evaluation of angiogenesis in endometrial aspirates. Cytopathology 2001; 12: 37–43.
14. Hii LLP, Rogers PAW. Endometrial vascular and glandular expression of integrin $\beta_v\alpha_3$ in women with and without endometriosis. Hum Reprod 1998; 13: 1030–5.
15. Djonov VG, Galli AB, Burri PH. Intussusceptive arborization contributes to vascular tree formation in the chick chorio-allantoic membrane. Anat Embryol 2000; 202: 347–57.
16. Nayak NR, Brenner RM. Vascular proliferation and the vascular endothelial growth factor expression in the rhesus macaque endometrium. J Clin Endocrinol Metab 2002; 87: 1845–55.
17. Iwakura A, Luedemann C, Shastry S et al. Estrogen-mediated, endothelial nitric oxide synthase-dependent mobilization of bone marrow-derived endothelial progenitor cells contributes to reendothelialization after arterial injury. Circulation 2003; 108: 3115–21.
18. Strehlow K, Werner N, Berweiler J et al. Estrogen increases bone marrow-derived endothelial progenitor cell production and diminishes neointima formation. Circulation 2003; 107: 3059–65.
19. Rogers PAW, Abberton KM. Endometrial arteriogenesis: vascular smooth muscle cell proliferation and differentiation during the menstrual cycle and changes associated with endometrial bleeding disorders. Microsc Res Tech 2003; 60: 412–19.
20. Abberton KM, Taylor NH, Healy DL et al. Vascular smooth muscle α-actin distribution around endometrial arterioles during the menstrual cycle; increased expression during the perimenopause and lack of correlation with menorrhagia. Hum Reprod 1996; 11: 204–11.
21. Abberton KM, Healy DL, Rogers PAW. Smooth muscle alpha actin and myosin heavy chain expression in the vascular smooth muscle cells surrounding endometrial arterioles. Hum Reprod 1999; 14: 3095–100.
22. Kohnen G, Campbell S, Jeffers MD, Cameron IT. Spatially regulated differentiation of endometrial vascular smooth muscle cells. Hum Reprod 2000; 15: 284–92.
23. Abberton KM, Taylor NH, Healy DL et al. Vascular smooth muscle cell proliferation in arterioles of the human endometrium. Hum Reprod 1999; 14: 1072–9.
24. Head JR, Lande IJM. Uterine lymphatics: passage of ink and lymphoid cells from the rat's uterine wall and lumen. Biol Reprod 1983; 28: 941–55.

25. Ueki M. Histologic study of endometriosis and examination of lymphatic drainage in and from the uterus. Am J Obstet Gynecol 1991; 165: 201–9.

26. Blackwell PM, Fraser IS. Superficial lymphatics in the functional zone of normal human endometrium. Microvasc Res 1981; 21: 142–52.

27. Lauweryns JM, Cornillie FJ. Topography and ultrastructure of the uterine lymphatics in the rat. Eur J Obstet Gynec Reprod Biol 1984; 18: 309–27.

28. Head JR, Seelig Jr LL. Lymphatic vessels in the uterine endometrium of virgin rats. J Reprod Immunonol 1984; 6: 157–66.

29. Uchino S, Ichikawa S, Okubo M et al. Methods of detection of lymphatics and their changes with oestrous cycle. Int Angiol 1987; 6: 271–8.

30. McColl BK, Stacker SA, Achen MG. Molecular regulation of the VEGF family – inducers of angiogenesis and lymphangiogenesis. APMIS 2004; 112: 463–80.

31. Donoghue JF, Lederman FL, Susil BJ, Rogers PAW. Lymphangiogenesis of normal endometrium and endometrial adenocarcinoma. Hum Reprod 2007; 22: 1705–13.

32. Hoeben A, Landuyt B, Highley MS et al. Vascular endothelial growth factor and angiogenesis. Pharmacol Rev 2004; 56: 549–80.

33. Grunstein J. Isoforms of vascular endothelial growth factor act in a coordinate fashion to recruit and expand tumor vasculature. Mol Cell Biol 2000; 20: 7282–91.

34. Ribatti D, Nico B, Spinazzi R et al. The role of adrenomedullin in angiogenesis. Peptides 2005; 26: 1670–5.

35. Rakic JM, Maillard C, Bajou K et al. Role of plasminogen activator–plasmin system in tumor angiogenesis. Cell Mol Life Sci 2003; 60: 463–73.

36. Folkman J. Endogenous angiogenesis inhibitors. APMIS 2004; 112: 496–507.

37. Nyberg P, Xie L, Kalluri R. Endogenous inhibitors of angiogenesis. Cancer Res 2005; 65: 3967–79.

38. Banfi A, von Degenfeld G, Blau H. Critical role of microenvironmental factors in angiogenesis. Curr Atheroscler Rep 2005; 7: 227–34.

39. Baldwin ME, Stacker SA, Achen MG. Molecular control of lymphangiogenesis. Bioessays 2002; 24: 1030–40.

40. Tammela T, Petrova TV, Alitalo K. Molecular lymphangiogenesis: new players. Trends Cell Biol 2005; 15: 434–41.

41. Critchley HOD, Brenner RM, Henderson TA et al. Estrogen receptor β, but not estrogen receptor α, is present in the vascular endothelium of the human and nonhuman primate endometrium. J Clin Endocrinol Metab 2001; 86: 1370–8.

42. Leece G, Meduri G, Ancelin M et al. Presence of estrogen receptor β in the human endometrium through the cycle: expression in glandular, stromal, and vascular cells. J Clin Endocrinol Metab 2001; 86: 1379–86.

43. Kayisli UA, Luk J, Guzeloglu-Kayisli O et al. Regulation of angiogenic activity of human endometrial endothelial cells in culture by ovarian steroids. J Clin Endocrinol Metab 2004; 89: 5794–802.

44. Krikun G, Schatz F, Taylor R et al. Endometrial endothelial cell steroid receptor expression and steroid effects on gene expression. J Clin Endocrinol Metab 2005; 90: 1812–18.

45. Brenner RM, Slayden OD. Steroid receptors in blood vessels of the rhesus macaque endometrium: a review. Arch Histol Cytol 2004; 5: 411–16.

46. Iruela-Arispe ML, Rodriguez-Manzaneque JC, Abu-Jawdeh G. Endometrial endothelial cells express estrogen and progesterone receptors and exhibit a tissue specific response to angiogenic growth factors. Microcirculation 1999; 6: 127–40.

47. Albrecht ED, Aberdeen GW, Niklaus AL et al. Acute temporal regulation of vascular endothelial growth/permeability factor expression and endothelial morphology in the baboon endometrium by ovarian steroids. J Clin Endocrinol Metab 2003; 88: 2844–52.

48. Ma W, Tan J, Matsumoto B et al. Adult tissue angiogenesis: evidence for negative regulation by estrogen in the uterus. Mol Endocrinol 2001; 15: 1983–92.

49. Heryanto B, Rogers PAW. Regulation of endometrial endothelial cell proliferation by estrogen and progesterone in the ovariectomized mouse. Reproduction 2002; 123: 107–13.

50. Heryanto B, Lipson KE, Rogers PAW. Effect of angiogenesis inhibitors on estrogen-mediated endometrial endothelial cell proliferation in the ovariectomized mouse. Reproduction 2003; 125: 337–46.

51. Hastings JM, Licence DR, Burton GJ et al. Soluble vascular endothelial growth factor receptor 1 inhibits edema and epithelial proliferation induced by 17β-estradiol in the mouse uterus. Endocrinology 2003; 144: 326–34.

52. Press MF, Udove JA, Greene GL. Progesterone receptor distribution in the human endometrium. Am J Pathol 1988; 131: 112–24.

53. Rogers PAW, Lederman F, Kooy J et al. Endometrial vascular smooth muscle estrogen and progesterone receptor distribution in women with and without menorrhagia. Hum Reprod 1996; 11: 2003–8.

54. Vaquez F, Rodríguez-Manzaneque JC, Lydon JP et al. Progesterone regulates proliferation of endothelial cells. J Biol Chem 1999; 274: 2185–92.

55. Mulac-Jericevic B, Conneely OM. Reproductive tissue selective actions of progesterone receptors. Reproduction 2004; 128: 139–46.

56. Goodger AM, Rogers PAW. Uterine endothelial cell proliferation before and after embryo implantation in rats. J Reprod Fertil 1993; 99: 451–7.

57. Walter LM, Rogers PAW, Girling JE. The role of progesterone in endometrial angiogenesis in pregnant and ovariectomized mice. Reproduction 2005; 129: 765–77.

58. Girling JE, Lederman FL, Walter LM, Rogers PAW. Progesterone, but not estrogen, stimulates vessel maturation in the mouse endometrium. Endocrinology 2007; Epub ahead of print.

59. Lunan C, Rogers PAW. Pericytes in the stroma of the rat uterus. J Reprod Fertil 1981; 63: 267–70.

60. Charnock Jones DS, Sharkey AM, Rajput-Williams J et al. Identification and localization of alternatively spliced mRNAs for vascular endothelial growth factor in human uterus and estrogen regulation in endometrial carcinoma cell lines. Biol Reprod 1993; 48: 1120–8.

61. Huang JC, Kiu DY, Dawood MY. The expression of vascular endothelial growth factor isoforms in cultured human endometrial stromal cells and its regulation by 17β-estradiol. Mol Hum Reprod 1998; 4: 603–7.

62. Niklaus AL, Aberdeen GW, Babischkin JS et al. Effect of estrogen on vascular endothelial growth factor/permeability factor expression by glandular epithelial and stromal cells in the baboon endometrium. Biol Reprod 2003; 68: 1997–2004.

63. Hornung D, Lebovic DI, Shifren JL et al. Vectorial secretion of vascular endothelial growth factor by polarized human endometrial epithelial cells. Fertil Steril 1998; 69: 909–15.

64. Albrecht ED, Babischkin JS, Lidor Y et al. Effect of estrogen on angiogenesis in co-cultures of human endometrial cells and microvascular endothelial cells. Hum Reprod 2003; 18: 2039–47.

65. Gargett CE, Lederman F, Lau TM et al. Lack of correlation between vascular endothelial growth factor production and endothelial cell proliferation in the human endometrium. Hum Reprod 1999; 14: 2080–8.

66. Gargett CE, Lederman F, Heryanto B et al. Focal vascular endothelial growth factor correlates with angiogenesis in human endometrium. Role of intravascular neutrophils. Hum Reprod 2001; 16: 1065–75.

67. Mueller MD, Lebovic DI, Garrett E et al. Neutrophils infiltrating the endometrium express vascular endothelial growth

factor: potential role in endometrial angiogenesis. Fertil Steril 2000; 74: 107–12.

68. Ancelin M, Chollet-Martin S, Hervé MA et al. Vascular endothelial growth factor VEGF189 induces human neutrophil chemotaxis in extravascular tissue via an autocrine amplification mechanism. Lab Invest 2004; 84: 502–12.

69. Heryanto PAW, Girling JE, Rogers PAW. Intravascular neutrophils partially mediate the endometrial endothelial cell proliferative response to estrogen in ovariectomized mice. Reproduction 2004; 127: 613–20.

70. Wood GW, Hausmann E, Choudhuri R. Relative role of CSF-1, MCP-1/JE, and RANTES in macrophage recruitment during successful pregnancy. Mol Reprod Dev 1997; 46: 62–70.

71. Ancelin M, Buteau-Lozano H, Meduri G et al. A dynamic shift of VEGF isoforms with a transient and selective progesterone-induced expression of VEGF189 regulates angiogenesis and vascular permeability in human uterus. Proc Natl Acad Sci USA 2002; 99: 6023–8.

72. Halder JB, Zhao X, Soker S et al. Differential expression of VEGF isoforms and VEGF(164)-specific receptor neuropilin-1 in the mouse uterus suggests a role for VEGF(164) in vascular permeability and angiogenesis during implantation. Genesis 2000; 26: 213–14.

73. Ornitz DM, Itoh N. Fibroblast growth factors. Genome Biol 2001; 2(3): reviews: 3005.

74. Wordinger RJ, Moss AE, Lockard T et al. Immunohistochemical localization of basic fibroblast growth factor within the mouse uterus. J Reprod Fert 1992; 96: 141–52.

75. Samathanam CA, Adesanya OO, Zhou J et al. Fibroblast growth factors 1 and 2 in the primate uterus. Biol Reprod 1998; 59: 491–6.

76. Möller B, Rasmussen C, Lindblom B et al. Expression of angiogenic growth factors VEGF, FGF-2, EGF and their receptors in normal human endometrium during the menstrual cycle. Mol Hum Reprod 2001; 7: 65–72.

77. Wei P, Chen X-L, Song X-X et al. VEGF, bFGF and their receptors in the endometrium of rhesus monkey during menstrual cycle and early pregnancy. Mol Reprod Dev 2004; 68: 456–62.

78. Stavri GT, Zachery IC, Baskerville PA et al. Basic fibroblast growth factor upregulates the expression of vascular endothelial growth factor in vascular smooth muscle cells. Synergistic interaction with hypoxia. Circulation 1995; 92: 11–14.

79. Nuttall RK, Kennedy TG. Epidermal growth factor and basic fibroblast growth factor increase the production of matrix metalloproteinases during in vitro decidualization of rat endometrial stromal cells. Endocrinology 2000; 141: 629–36.

80. Zhao Y, Hague S, Manek S et al. PCR display identifies tamoxifen induction of the novel angiogenic factor adrenomedullin by a non estrogenic mechanism in the human endometrium. Oncogene 1998; 16: 409–15.

81. Nikitenko LL, MacKenzie IZ, Rees MCP et al. Adrenomedullin is an autocrine regulator of endothelial growth in human endometrium. Mol Hum Reprod 2000; 6: 811–19.

82. Kookwijk P, Kapiteijn K, Molenaar B et al. Enhanced angiogenic capacity and urokinase-type plasminogen activator expression by endothelial cells isolated from human endometrium. J Clin Endocrinol Metab 2001; 86: 3359–67.

83. Plaisier M, Kapiteijn K, Koolwijk P et al. Involvement of membrane-type matrix metalloproteinases (MT-MMPs) in capillary tube formation by human endometrial microvascular endothelial cells: role of MT3-MMP. J Clin Endocrinol Metab 2004; 89: 5828–36.

84. Krikun G, Mor G, Huan J et al. Metalloproteinase expression by control and telomerase immortalized human endometrial endothelial cells. Histol Histopathol 2005; 20: 719–24.

85. Iruela-Arispe ML, Porter R, Bornstein P et al. Thrombospondin-1, an inhibitor of angiogenesis, is regulated by progesterone in the human endometrium. J Clin Invest 1996; 97: 403–12.

86. Nasu K, Nishida M, Fukuda J et al. Hypoxia simultaneously inhibits endostatin production and stimulates vascular endothelial growth factor production by cultured human endometrial stromal cells. Fert Steril 2004; 82: 756–9.

87. Kawano Y, Nakamura S, Nasu K, et al. Expression and regulation of thrombospondin-1 by human endometrial stromal cells. Fertil Steril 2005; 83: 1056–9.

88. Graubert MD, Ortega MA, Kessel B et al. Vascular repair after menstruation involves regulation of vascular endothelial growth factor-receptor phosphorylation by sFLT-1. Am J Pathol 2001; 158: 1399–410.

89. Hirchenhain J, Huse I, Hess A et al. Differential expression of angiopoietins 1 and 2 and their receptor Tie-2 in human endometrium. Mol Hum Reprod 2003; 9: 663–9.

90. Möller B, Lindblom, Olovsson M. Expression of the vascular endothelial growth factors B and C and their receptors in human endometrium during the menstrual cycle Acta Obstet Gynecol Scand 2002; 81: 817–24.

91. Mints M, Blomgren B, Falconer C et al. Expression of the vascular endothelial growth factor (VEGF) family in human endometrial blood vessels. Scand J Clin Lab Invest 2002; 62: 167–76.

92. Yokoyama Y, Charnock-Jones DS, Licence D et al. Expression of vascular endothelial growth factor (VEGF)-D and its receptor, VEGF receptor 3, as a prognostic factor in endometrial carcinoma. Clin Cancer Res 2003; 9: 1361–9.

93. Salamonsen LA. Tissue injury and repair in the female reproductive tract. Reproduction 2003; 125: 301–11.

94. Salamonsen LA, Lathbury LJ. Endometrial leukocytes and menstruation. Hum Reprod 2000; 6: 16–27.

95. Fraser IS, Peek MJ. Effects of exogenous hormones on endometrial capillaries. In: Alexander NJ, d'Arcangues C, eds. Steroid Hormones and Uterine Bleeding. Washington, DC: AAAS Publications, 1992: 65–79.

96. Gannon BJ, Carati CJ, Verco CJ. Endometrial perfusion across the normal human menstrual cycle assessed by laser Doppler fluxmetry. Hum Reprod 1997; 12: 132–9.

97. Zhang J, Salamonsen LA. Expression of hypoxia-inducible factors in human endometrium and suppression of matrix metalloproteinases under hypoxic conditions do not support a major role for hypoxia in regulating tissue breakdown at menstruation. Hum Reprod 2002; 17: 265–74.

98. Wang H, Li Q, Lin H et al. Expression of vascular endothelial growth factor and its receptors in the rhesus monkey (*Macaca mulatta*) endometrium and placenta during early pregnancy. Mol Hum Reprod Dev 2003; 65: 123–31.

99. Liu Y-X, Gao F, Wei P et al. Involvement of molecules related to angiogenesis, proteolysis and apoptosis in implantation in rhesus monkey and mouse. Contraception 2005; 71: 249–62.

100. Rockwell LC, Pillai S, Olson CE et al. Inhibition of vascular endothelial growth factor/vascular permeability factor action blocks estrogen-induced uterine edema and implantation in rodents. Biol Reprod 2002; 67: 1804–10.

101. Rabbani MM, Rogers PAW. Role of vascular endothelial growth factor in endometrial vascular events before implantation in rats. Reproduction 2001; 122: 85–90.

102. Print C, Valtoa R, Evans A et al. Soluble factors from human endometrium promote angiogenesis and regulate the endothelial cell transcriptome. Hum Reprod 2004; 19: 2356–66.

7 Endometrial imaging

Julie Lukic and Seang Lin Tan

INTRODUCTION

Embryo implantation is one of the main limiting factors to achieving a higher success rate in in-vitro fertilization (IVF). Successful implantation depends on many parameters, particularly the maturity of oocytes, the morphological quality of embryos, and (of most recent interest to researchers) uterine receptivity. Rogers et al[1] performed a mathematical analysis and estimated the relative contribution of uterine receptivity to conception as being 31–64%. This agrees with the earlier estimation by Walters et al[2] in 1985 that the relative contribution of the embryo quality and uterine receptivity to successful IVF pregnancy is 45–55%, respectively.

There is no doubt that over the past decade considerable advances have been made in the field of assisted reproductive technology (ART). However, despite the many successes, there still remains a large group of couples for whom there is no identifiable cause for their failure in establishing or maintaining a pregnancy. Although there have been a large number of advances in ovarian stimulation protocols[3,4] and improvements in culture media,[5] there has been relatively little research into improving uterine receptivity. Subsequent research may well prove that a lack of uterine receptivity and defects in implantation may be responsible for the majority of cases of failed IVF cycles. At present, such studies have been mostly concentrated in the field of molecular research; however, the clinical applications from this research are yet to be delineated.

An optimum method for investigating uterine receptivity should be non-invasive, easy to perform, and yield immediate results to the clinician. Ultrasound imaging fulfills all these criteria. Recent advances in ultrasound imaging include transvaginal scanning, three-dimensional (3D) ultrasound, sonohysterography, and color Doppler ultrasound.

The standard method of endometrial dating has traditionally been by histological assessment of an endometrial biopsy.[6] However, due to the invasive nature of this method, it is not acceptable in an ART cycle. Likewise, estrogen and progesterone levels, although initially thought to be correlated with endometrial thickness,[7,8] have since proven to be inaccurate at assessing uterine receptivity[9–11] as normal endometrial development occurs over a wide range of serum hormonal concentrations.[12]

ENDOMETRIAL THICKNESS

Since the introduction of transvaginal scanning, there have been many attempts to establish a relationship between endometrial thickness and endometrial receptivity. Endometrial thickness is defined as the minimal distance between the two echogenic interfaces of the myometrium and endometrium measured through the central longitudinal axis of the uterine body.[13] It is important when measuring endometrial thickness that the entire length of the uterus is imaged to avoid taking an oblique section of the uterus, which would make the measurement inaccurate. The measurement is performed just below the fundus and incorporates any tissue but should exclude any intracavity fluid.[14]

Endometrial thickness tends to be maximal around ovulation and reflects endometrial growth during the cycle. There is no consensus on the ideal endometrial thickness for implantation in natural or stimulated cycles or on the exact timing of the ultrasound examination that best predicts pregnancy to occur. Most reports have evaluated the role of ultrasound on the day of human chorionic gonadotropin (hCG) administration, or during the early luteal phase. Gonen et al[15] suggested that endometrial thickness is significantly greater in those women that achieve pregnancy but other studies[10,16] suggest that endometrial thickness does not reliably predict the probability of pregnancy. Khalifa et al[17] found no statistically significant difference in endometrial pattern or thickness on day of hCG or day of embryo transfer between conception and non-conception cycles. On the other hand, Isaacs et al[18] had no pregnancies when the endometrial thickness was less than 7 mm but 91% of conception cycles had an endometrial thickness of equal to or greater than 10 mm. Friedler et al[13] reviewed 25 reports, comprising 2665 ART cycles, and found that 8 reports found a difference in mean endometrial thickness between conception and non-conception cycles as being statistically significant whereas 17 reports found no significant difference. Values between 6 mm and

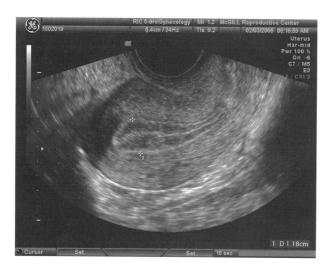

Figure 7.1   Triple line multilayered endometrium.

10 mm have been touted as discriminating between conception and non-conception cycles. Irrespective of whether there is an ideal endometrial thickness for pregnancy to occur, an endometrial thickness less than 6 mm has a strong negative predictive value (NPV) for pregnancy.[19] Nonetheless, pregnancies have occurred exceptionally with levels as low as 4 mm.[20]

If the endometrium is very thin during an ART cycle, the patient should be monitored during a natural menstrual cycle to determine the maximum thickness of the endometrium when not under the effect of ovarian stimulation. A hysteroscopy would be usefully performed to exclude the presence of endometrial adhesions, which should be divided, if present.

ENDOMETRIAL PATTERN

Endometrial pattern is defined as the relative echogenicity of the endometrium and adjacent myometrium.[13] Forrest et al[21] demonstrated that in the early follicular phase the endometrium appears as a central linear echo representing the uterine cavity. The thickness as well as the sonographic appearance change throughout the menstrual cycle, but by the mid-follicular phase, it becomes defined as three hyperechogenic lines separated by two hypoechoic layers. By the mid-luteal phase, the endometrium is hyperechoic and the triple lines are no longer distinguishable.

Several classifications exist for endometrial patterns. In 1984 Smith et al[22] postulated four grades of endometrium and labeled them A–D. Gonen and Casper[23] later simplified this to three types: type A describes an entirely homogeneous hyperechogenic pattern without a central echogenic line; type B is an

intermediate isoechogenic pattern with the same reflectivity as the surrounding myometrium and an absent central echogenic line; and type C is a multilayered 'triple line' endometrium consisting of a prominent outer and central hyperechogenic line and inner hypoechogenic black region (Figure 7.1). The classification was further simplified by Sher et al[24] to two grades: non-multilayered and multilayered. The non-multilayered is a homogeneous hyperechogenic endometrium and the multilayered is a triple line multilayered pattern or 'halo' pattern.

A homogeneous hyperechogenic endometrium is associated with low pregnancy rates[25] but its presence does not completely preclude a pregnancy. Shapiro et al[26] reported a pregnancy rate of 62.5% if the endometrial thickness was equal or greater than 6 mm with a triple line pattern. Friedler et al[13] reviewed 22 reports on endometrial patterns, comprising 3736 ART cycles. He concluded that a non-multilayered endometrial pattern on the day of hCG administration had a NPV of 85.7% for conception. However, a multilayered pattern proved to have a low positive predictive value (PPV) of 33.1% and a low specificity of 13.7% to predict a clinical pregnancy.

Hence, even though the endometrial pattern may be related to uterine receptivity, it is a non-specific parameter for the prediction of conception following ART.[13]

ENDOMETRIAL VOLUME

Volume estimation of the endometrium can be made easily because of good contrast between endometrial tissue and myometrium by 3D transvaginal ultrasound. Raga et al[27] measured endometrial volume in 71 women. They found that an endometrial volume of greater than 2 ml is a prerequisite for good endometrial receptivity. No pregnancy was achieved when the endometrial volume was less than 1 ml. However, once an endometrial volume of 2 ml was reached, there did not appear to be any further increase in endometrial receptivity as the volume increased above 2 ml. This is in agreement with Schild et al,[28] who also showed no relationship between mean endometrial volume measured by 3D ultrasound and IVF outcome.

Child et al[29] performed transvaginal ultrasound measurement of endometrial volume on 144 women in 164 cycles and found that 3D volume estimation was better than endometrial thickness for screening for failure of pituitary suppression in an IVF cycle; however, the two had similar sensitivity and specificity if used to just predict pituitary suppression. They

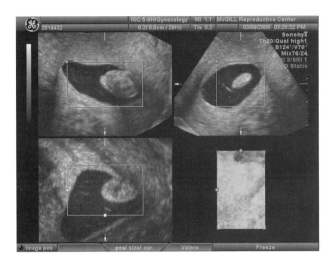

Figure 7.2 Two-dimensional saline sonohysterogram of a uterine fibroid.

concluded that endometrial volume or thickness could replace routine measurement of serum estradiol as a predictor of the state of pituitary suppression.

SONOHYSTEROGRAPHY

Diagnostic hysteroscopy has long been the definitive method for assessing the uterine cavity. However, two-dimensional (2D) B-mode transvaginal ultrasound, along with the instillation of sterile saline through the cervical canal, can provide just as clear a view of the uterine cavity as that obtained with hysteroscopy. This method is simple, reliable, cost-effective, and usually well tolerated by the patient.

Cicinelli et al[30] found that conventional transvaginal sonography was the most accurate technique for detecting submucous myomas and evaluating their size, intracavity growth, and location (see Figure 7.2). They found a 90% sensitivity and 98% specificity of the technique, and that it measured tumor size more accurately than did hysteroscopy. De Kroon et al[31] also had excellent results. They examined 214 saline contrast hysterosalpingograms and found 180 cases (84.1%) were conclusive, 12 (5.6%) failed, and 22 (10.3%) were inconclusive. A uterine size of above 600 cm^3 was the best predictor for failure and or inconclusiveness.

Where 2D transvaginal ultrasonography falls short is that the probe can only provide images of the lower pelvis in the sagittal and coronal planes. Henceforth, 3D transvaginal sonography has been favored increasingly in the field of ART to allow us to have a view of the coronal plane. Three-dimensional ultrasound allows more detailed evaluation of pelvic organs by collecting a series of sequential ultrasound images and converting them into an ultrasound volume. It facilitates the demonstration of transverse planes in addition to the sagittal and coronal views, thus allowing for more precise volumetric determinations. Kyei-Mensah et al[32,33] found that 3D transvaginal ultrasound produced highly reproducible ovarian and endometrial volume estimations as well as being able to more accurately measure ovarian follicle volume for IVF cycles compared to 2D ultrasound.

The longitudinal coronal view is the one most favored for the detection of uterine anomalies, masses, and irregularities, as the entire endometrium, and, in particular, the cornual regions, can be displayed. Data are stored and can be accessed at any time for later analysis. It can be reconstructed to allow visualization of an organ from any chosen angle and in any arbitrary plane. In this manner, a normal uterus can be distinguished from an arcuate uterus, a septate uterus, and a bicornuate uterus, and any uterine polyps can be assessed as well (Figures 7.3, 7.4).

Salim et al[34] compared 3D transvaginal ultrasound combined with saline instillation into the uterine cavity to diagnostic hysteroscopy for the assessment of submucous fibroids. A total of 61 submucous fibroids were identified. There was an overall agreement of classification in 54 fibroids, or 89% of cases. The best level of agreement was achieved in the women with fibroid polyps, but the level of agreement decreased with increasing degree of myometrial involvement. Sylvestre et al[35] performed 3D sonohysterography on 209 infertile patients found to have a suspected intrauterine lesion on 2D ultrasound. Ninety-two patients were found to have an actual lesion. Compared to hysteroscopy, the 3D sonohysterogram was found to have a sensitivity of 100% and a PPV of 92%, and 2D sonohysterograms had a sensitivity of 98% and a PPV of 95%.

Hence, a sonohysterogram is an excellent tool to determine if there is any growth in the uterus, which can distort the endometrial lining. This is important since such growths have been noted to impair implantation of embryos.[36] If a submucous fibroid or polyp is visualized at the time of a sonohysterogram, a hysteroscopy should be performed to excise the growth before assisted conception is undertaken.

MAGNETIC RESONANCE IMAGING

Dueholm et al[37] compared the accuracy of magnetic resonance imaging (MRI), non-enhanced transvaginal

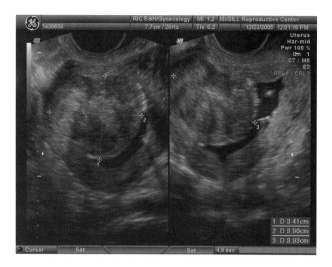

Figure 7.3 Three-dimensional saline sonohysterogram of an intrauterine polyp.

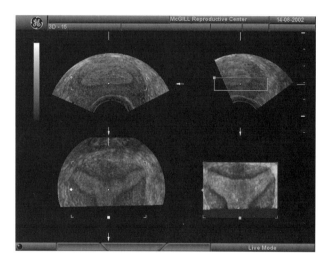

Figure 7.4 Septate uterus.

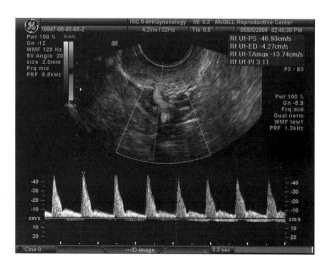

Figure 7.5 Uterine artery Doppler.

ultrasound, saline infusion sonography, and hysteroscopy in the evaluation of abnormalities of the uterine cavity using hysterectomy specimens as the gold standard. They found that all methods performed well in detecting uterine lesions, but that MRI and saline infusion sonography were superior to hysteroscopy for the assessment of submucous fibroids. They concluded that MRI rather than hysteroscopy should be used for the preoperative assessment of submucous fibroids; however, its availability and high cost puts it currently out of the realm of routine investigation.

Doppler ultrasound

Color Doppler ultrasound determines the presence or absence of blood flow and provides information about the direction, velocity, and character of that flow. The uterine artery was the first vessel investigated in relation to implantation. Steer et al[38] studied the uterine arterial blood flow in 82 women undergoing IVF on the day of embryo transfer. The pulsatility index (PI; an index of resistance to blood flow) was calculated and the patients grouped as to whether the PI was low (1–1.99), medium (2–2.99) (Figure 7.5), or high (≥3.0). There were no pregnancies in the high PI group and those patients that became pregnant had a considerably lower PI compared with those who did not. Zaidi et al[39] showed that an elevated PI of the uterine arteries is associated with a similarly poor bad prognostic value, even if it is performed on the day of hCG administration. It should be noted that there is dirunal variation in uterine artery blood flow[40–42] and it is therefore important to measure the blood flow about the same time each day. It is also important to take into account any minor reversals of flow, as this has a significant effect on the values of the PI measured. Steer's and Zaidi's studies have been confirmed by a number of groups.[43,44] Failure to take into account diurnal variation in blood flow may account for some studies that have failed to confirm that Doppler uterine artery blood flow is able to predict pregnancy rates.[45]

It has been postulated that local vascularization at the site of implantation is probably more important than global vascularization of the uterus measured by resistance in uterine arteries. Endometrial blood flow can be non-invasively evaluated by color and power Doppler ultrasound. Power Doppler ultrasound is more sensitive than color Doppler imaging at detecting low-velocity flow and hence improves the visualization of small vessels.[46] Thus, with more sensitive color Doppler machines and with the addition of 3D subendometrial and endometrial blood flow can be measured and its potential as a predictor of implantation assessed. There is no standard consensus on where the subendometrial region resides, ranging from 5 mm[31,32] to 10 mm,[33] which may account for the differences in study results.

Zaidi et al[47] studied 96 women undergoing IVF treatment on the day of hCG using power Doppler with 2D ultrasound. They observed no pregnancies in the group of women where subendometrial color flow and intraendometrial vascularization were absent. This was supported by similar findings by Battaglia et al.[48] However, a recent study by Ng et al[45] has not supported these findings. Because poor blood flow may be important in determining results, administration of hCG may be delayed by 1 or 2 days until uterine artery and subendometrial blood flow indices improve. Another alternative is to use low-dose aspirin. Rubinstein et al[49] performed a randomized controlled trial to show that the administration of low-dose aspirin in patients with poor uterine perfusion significantly improved results. This study has been validated by other studies.[50,51]

Another method to improve blood flow is to administer nitroglycerin (NTG) patches as a vasodilator. Cacciatore et al[52] demonstrated its usefulness in a small cohort of 17 women. However, in our experience, tachyphylaxis causes the need for an increasing dose of medication, which leads to a high incidence of unacceptable side effects in patients. Similarly, vaginal sildenafil has been postulated to improve uterine receptivity[53] but it has proven valueless in our hands.

A recent advance in oocyte vitrification may allow a new therapeutic option in these cases. There have been a few small series reporting the successful use of vitrification.[54,55] We have successfully achieved about a 90% survival rate in vitrifying human oocytes using a McGill Cryoleaf system[56] in over 40 women in whom we have vitrified over 400 oocytes. When these oocytes were thawed and the fertilized oocytes transferred, we have achieved a greater than 40% clinical pregnancy rate per cycle. We have used this technique to preserve fertility in a number of women with various cancers who wish to preserve their fertility before chemotherapy.[57,58] Oocyte vitrification with fertilization and transfer in a subsequent hormonally supported cycle, where there is better endometrial thickness and appearance and uterine perfusion, may prove a useful way to rescue these cycles in future.

REFERENCES

1. Rogers P, Milne B, Trounson A. A model to show uterine receptivity and embryo viability following ovarian stimulation for in vitro fertilization. J In Vitro Fertil Embryo Transf 1986; 3: 93–8.

2. Walters DE, Edwards RG, Meistrich ML. A statistical evaluation of implantation after replacing one or more human embryos. J Reprod Fertil 1985; 74: 557–61.

3. Tan SL, Balen A, Husseing EL et al. A prospective randomised study of the optimum timing of human chorionic gonadotropin administration after pituitary desensitisation in in-vitro fertilization. Fertil Steril 1992; 57: 1259–64.

4. Biljan MM, Mahutte NG, Dean N et al. Effects of pretreatment with an oral contraceptive on the time required to achieve pituitary suppression with gonadotropin-releasing hormone analogues and subsequent implantation and pregnancy rates. Fertil Steril 1998; 6: 1063–9.

5. Gardner DK, Pool TB, Lane M. Embryo nutrition and energy metabolism and its relationship to embryo growth, differentiation, and viability. Semin Reprod Med 2000; 18: 205–18.

6. Noyes RW, Hertig AT, Rock J. Dating the endometrial biopsy. Fertil Steril 1950; 1: 23.

7. Hall DA, Hann LE, Ferruci JT et al. Sonographic morphology of the normal menstrual cycle. Radiology 1979; 133: 185–92.

8. Fleischer AC, Pittaway DE, Beard LA et al. Sonographic depiction of endometrial changes occurring with ovulation induction. J Ultrasound Med 1984; 3: 341–6.

9. Ben Nun I, Less A, Kaneti H et al. Lack of correlation between hormonal blood levels and endometrial maturation in agonadal women with repeat implantation failure following embryo transfer from donated eggs. J Assist Reprod Genet 1992; 2: 102–5.

10. Glissant A, de Mouzon J, Frydman R. Ultrasound study of the endometrium during in vitro fertilisation cycles. Fertil Steril 1985; 44: 786–90.

11. Oliveira JBA, Baruffi RLR, Maun A et al. Endometrial ultrasonography as a predictor of pregnancy in an in vitro fertilization programme. Hum Reprod 1993; 8: 1312–15.

12. Li TC, Nutall L, Klentsens L et al. How well does ultrasonographic measurement of endometrial thickness predict the results of histological dating? Hum Reprod 1992; 7: 1–5.

13. Friedler S, Schenker JG, Herman A et al. The role of ultrasonography in the evaluation of endometrial receptivity following assisted reproductive treatment: a critical review. Hum Reprod Update 1996; 2: 323–35.

14. Bourne T, Hamberger L, Hahlin S, Granberg S. Ultrasound in gynecology: endometrium. Int J Gynaecol Obstet 1997; 56: 115–27.

15. Gonen Y, Casper RF, Jacobsen W et al. Endometrial thickness and growth during ovarian stimulation: a possible predictor of implantation in in vitro fertilization. Fertil Steril 1989; 52: 446–50.

16. Welker BG, Gembruch U, Diedrich K et al. Transvaginal sonography of the endometrium during ovum pickup in stimulated cycles for in vitro fertilization. J Ultrasound Med 1989; 8: 549–53.

17. Khalifa G, Brzyski RG, Oehninger S et al. Sonographic appearance of the endometrium. The predictive value for the outcome of in vitro fertilisation in stimulated cycles. Hum Reprod 1992; 7: 677–80.

18. Isaacs JD Jr, Wells CS, Williams DB et al. Endometrial thickness is a valid monitoring parameter in cycles of ovulation induction with menotropin alone. Fertil Steril 1996; 65: 262–6.

19. Coulam CB, Bustillo M, Soenksen DM, Britten S. Ultrasonographic predictors of implantation after assisted reproduction. Fertil Steril 1994; 62: 1004–10.

20. Sundstrom P. Establishment of a successful pregnancy following in-vitro fertilization with an endometrial thickness of no more than 4 mm. Hum Reprod 1998; 13: 1550–2.

21. Forrest TS, Elyaderani MK, Muilenburg MI et al. Cyclic endometrial changes: ultrasound assessment with histologic correlation. Radiology 1988; 167: 233–7.

22. Smith B, Porter R, Ahuja K, Craft I. Ultrasonic assessment of endometrial changes in stimulated cycles in an in vitro

fertilization and embryo transfer program. J In Vitro Fertil Embryo Transf 1984; 1: 233–8.

23. Gonen Y, Casper RF. Prediction of implantation by the sonographic appearance of the endometrium during controlled ovarian stimulation for IVF. J In Vitro Fertil Embryo Transf 1990; 7: 146–52.

24. Sher G, Herbert C, Maassarani G et al. Assessment of the later proliferative phase endometrium by ultrasonography in patients undergoing in-vitro fertilization and embryo transfer (IVF/ET). Hum Reprod 1991; 6: 232–7.

25. Check JH, Lurie D, Dietterich C et al. Adverse effect of a homogeneous hyperechogenic endometrial sonographic pattern, despite adequate endometrial thickness on pregnancy rates following in-vitro fertilization. Hum Reprod 1993; 8: 1293–6.

26. Shapiro H, Cowell C, Casper RF. The use of vaginal ultrasound for monitoring endometrial preparation in a donor oocyte program. Fertil Steril 1993; 59: 1055–8.

27. Raga F, Bonilla-Musoles F, Casan EM et al. Assessment of endometrial volume by three-dimensional ultrasound prior to embryo transfer: clues to endometrial receptivity. Hum Reprod 1999; 14: 2851–4.

28. Schild RL, Indefrei D, Eschweiler S et al. Three-dimensional endometrial volume calculation and pregnancy rate in an in-vitro fertilization programme. Hum Reprod 1999; 14: 1255–8.

29. Child T, Sylvestre C, Tan SL. Endometrial volume and thickness measurements predict pituitary suppression and non-suppression during IVF. Hum Reprod 2002; 17: 3110–13.

30. Cicinelli E, Romano F, Silvio AP et al. Transabdominal sonohysterography, transvaginal sonography and hysteroscopy in the evaluation of submucous myomas. Obstet Gynecol 1995; 85: 42–7.

31. de Kroon CD, Willem Jansen F, Louve LA et al. Technology assessment of saline contrast hysterosonography. Am J Obstet Gynecol 2003; 188: 945–9.

32. Kyei-Mensah A, Zaidi J, Pitroff R et al. Transvaginal three-dimensional ultrasound: accuracy of follicular volume measurements. Fertil Steril 1996; 65: 371–6.

33. Kyei-Mensah A, Maconochie N, Zaidi J et al. Tansvaginal three-dimensional ultrasound: reproducibility of ovarian and endometrial volume measurements. Fertil Steril 1996; 66: 718–22.

34. Salim R, Lee C, Davies A et al. A comparative study of three-dimensional saline infusion sonohysterography and diagnostic hysteroscopy for the classification of submucous fibroids. Hum Reprod 2005; 20: 253–7.

35. Sylvestre C, Child T, Tulandi T et al. A prospective study to evaluate the efficacy of two and three dimensional sonohysterography in women with intrauterine lesions. Fertil Steril 2003; 79: 1222–5.

36. Eldar-Geva T, Meagher S, Healey DI et al. Effect of intramural, subserosal, and submucosal uterine fibroids on the outcome of assisted reproductive treatment. Fertil Steril 1998; 70: 687–91.

37. Dueholm M, Lundorf E, Hansen ES et al. Evaluation of the uterine cavity with MRI, transvaginal sonography, hysteroscopic examination and diagnostic hysteroscopy. Fertil Steril 2001; 76: 350–7.

38. Steer CV, Campbell S, Tan SL. The use of transvaginal colour flow imaging after in vitro fertilization to identify optimum uterine conditions before embryo transfer. Fertil Steril 1992; 57: 372–6.

39. Zaidi J, Pittrof R, Shaker A et al. Assessment of uterine artery blood flow on the day of human chorionic gonadotrophin administration by transvaginal color Doppler ultrasound in an in vitro fertilization program. Fertil Steril 1996; 65: 377–81.

40. Tan SL, Zaidi J, Campbell S et al. Blood flow changes in the ovarian and uterine arteries during the normal menstrual cycle. Am J Obstet Gynecol 1996; 175: 625–31.

41. Zaidi J, Jurkovic D, Campbell S et al. Description of circadian rhythm in uterine artery blood flow during the peri-ovulatory period. Hum Reprod 1995; 10: 1642–6.

42. Zaidi J, Jurkovic S, Campbell S et al. Circadian variation in uterine artery blood flow indices during the follicular phase of the menstrual cycle. Ultrasound Obstet Gynecol 1995; 5: 406–10.

43. Ng EHY, Chan CCW, Tang OS et al. Endometrial and subendometrial blood flow measured during early luteal phase by three-dimensional power Doppler ultrasound in excessive ovarian responders. Hum Reprod 2004; 19: 924–31.

44. Schild RL, Knobloch C, Dorn C et al. Endometrial receptivity in an in vitro fertilization program as assessed by spiral artery blood flow, endometrial thickness, endometrial volume, and uterine artery blood flow. Fertil Steril 2001; 75: 361–6.

45. Ng EHY, Chan CCW, Tang OS et al. The role of endometrial and subendometrial blood flows measured by three dimensional power Doppler ultrasound in the prediction of pregnancy during IVF treatment. Hum Reprod 2006; 21: 164–70.

46. Guerriero S, Ajossa S, Lai MP et al. Clinical applications of colour Doppler energy imaging in the female reproductive tract and pregnancy. Hum Reprod Update 1999; 5: 515–29.

47. Zaidi J, Campbell S, Pittrof R, Tan SL. Endometrial thickness, morphology, vascular penetration and velocimetry in predicting implantation in an in vitro fertilization program. Ultrasound Obstet Gynecol 1995; 6: 191–8.

48. Battaglia C, Artini PG, Giulini S et al. Colour Doppler changes and thromboxane production after ovarian stimulation with gonadotrophin-releasing hormone agonist. Hum Reprod 1997; 12: 2477–82.

49. Rubinstein M, Marazzi A, Polak de Fried E. Low-dose aspirin treatment improves ovarian responsiveness, uterine and ovarian blood flow velocity, implantation, and pregnancy rates in patients: a prospective, randomized, double-blind placebo-controlled assay. Fertil Steril 1999; 71(5): 825–9.

50. Weckstein LN, Jacobson A, Galen D et al. Low-dose aspirin for oocyte recipients with a thin endometrium: prospective, randomised study. Fertil Steril 1997; 68(5): 927–30.

51. Wada I, Hsu CC, Williams G et al. The benefits of low-dose aspirin therapy in women with impaired uterine perfusion during assisted conception. Hum Reprod 1994; 9: 1954–7.

52. Cacciatore B, Halmesmaki E, Kaaja R et al. Effects of transdermal nitroglycerin on impedence to flow in the uterine, umbilical, and fetal middle cerebral arteries in pregnancies complicated by preeclampsia and intrauterine growth retardation. Am J Obstet Gynecol 1998; 179: 140–5.

53. Sher G, Fisch JD. Effect of vaginal sildenafil on the outcome of in vitro fertilization (IVF) after multiple IVF failures attributed to poor endometrial development. Fertil Steril 2002; 78(5): 1073–6.

54. Kuleshova L, Lopata A. Vitrification can be more favourable than slow cooling. Fertil Steril 2002; 78(3): 449–54.

55. Kuwayama M, Vajta G, Kato O, Leibo SP. Highly efficient vitrification method for cryopreservation of human oocytes. Reprod Biomed Online 2005; 1: 300–8.

56. Chian RC, Son WY, Huang J et al. High survival rates and pregnancies of human oocytes following vitrification: preliminary report. 61st Annual Meeting American Society for Reproductive Medicine, Montreal, Canada, 2005.

57. Rao GD, Chian RC, Son WS et al. Fertility preservation in women undergoing cancer treatment. Lancet 2004; 363: 1829–30.

58. Holzer HEG, Tan SL. Fertility preservation in oncology. Minerva Ginecol 2005; 56: 99–109.

8 Estrogen and progesterone regulation of cell proliferation in the endometrium of muridae and humans

Wei Tong, Andrea Niklaus, Liyin Zhu, Haiyan Pan, Bo Chen,
Mira Aubuchon, Nanette Santoro, and Jeffrey W Pollard

Synopsis

Background

- Two extremes of hormonal control over uterine cell proliferation can be seen in humans (and Old-World primates) and laboratory rodents.
- Adult rats and mice have an estrous cycle that is without a true luteal phase and is dominated by estradiol-17β (E_2).
- In these rodents only very small amounts of progesterone (P_4) are synthesized following ovulation and the uterine lining is remodeled but not shed.
- Humans have a luteal phase that follows ovulation, progesterone (P_4) continues to be synthesized, and endometrial stromal cells decidualize.
- If pregnancy does not occur, chorionic gonadotropin is not available to maintain P_4 synthesis, and the uterine lining is sloughed off during menstruation.
- This is followed by cell proliferation under the influence of E_2 to replenish the lost functionalis layer.
- Thus, rodent models are useful for dissecting the mechanisms whereby E_2 stimulates uterine cells to proliferate and P_4 inhibits proliferation and triggers differentiation.

Basic Science

- In the adult mouse, the estrogen produced at proestrus stimulates cell proliferation, which is restricted to the luminal and glandular epithelium.
- E_2 exerts its effects primarily through a dramatic shortening of the G_1 period, although the duration of the S phase is also diminished.
- E_2 activates two signaling pathways in epithelial cells that run in parallel.
- The canonical cell cycle regulatory machinery results in phosphorylation of RB, with the consequent activation of downstream gene transcription.
- The licensing of DNA replication occurs through the activation of MCM protein binding to the origins of DNA replication.
- Every estrous cycle stimulates an approximately four-fold increase in epithelial cell number followed by a return to the basal state by apoptosis. Cell viability is directly related to estrogen receptor (ER) occupancy and, providing occupancy is maintained, apoptosis is prevented.
- Many tissue actions of sex steroid hormones are mediated by growth factors synthesized locally.
- IGF, Wnt, VEGF, and EGF family ligands are implicated in local control of cell proliferation.
- The first wave of epithelial proliferation is followed by another wave in the luminal and glandular epithelium on pregnancy day 2 that is independent of E_2.
- P_4 then inhibits further epithelial cell proliferation, blocking both the canonical pathway and replication licensing, and causes the cells to differentiate in preparation to accept a blastocyst.
- P_4 also enhances stromal cell proliferation and primes these cells to respond to E_2 with a single round of DNA synthesis that involves 30–40% of the cells, and occurs immediately before implantation.

- Proliferation begins in the periluminal stromal cells immediately adjacent to the implanting blastocyst, and rapidly expands circumferentially. The inner cells of the primary decidual zone fail to undergo cytokinesis and become polyploid.
- This stromal proliferative response occurs in LIF nullizygous mice in which implantation fails.
- The growth factor Indian hedgehog (IHH) is essential for P_4E_2-induced stromal cell proliferation prior to decidualization.
- There are several transcription factors, including EMX2, C/EBP-β, and BETB1.
- Stromal cells become refractory to further proliferative signals from E_2.
- Differentiation occurs rapidly so that the embryo is completely surrounded by decidual cells. The stromal cells that proliferated in response to E_2 before implantation are the ones that differentiate into decidual cells.

Clinical

- Edometrial hyperplasia, polyps, and adenocarcinoma increase dramatically with reproductive aging, suggesting that control over proliferation is relaxed in older women.
- Fifty percent of women seek medical consultation at some point in their lives for bleeding disorders.
- Untreated endometrial hyperplasia poses a significant risk for progression to endometrial cancer.
- Unopposed estrogen is the major risk factor for developing endometrial cancer.
- Progesterone is still used in the treatment of endometrial cancer.

INTRODUCTION

In an adult mammal, the uterus undergoes waves of cell proliferation, differentiation, and remodeling in preparation to receive a blastocyst. These processes are under the overall regulation of ovarian sex steroid hormones that act through their transcription factor receptors. In the most commonly studied species, rats and mice, adult animals have an estrous cycle that is without a true luteal phase and is, therefore, dominated by estradiol-17β (E_2). Only very small amounts of progesterone (P_4) are synthesized before ovulation and much of what is synthesized is largely converted in situ to 20α-hydroxyprogesterone, an inactive metabolite.[1] Nevertheless, the small increase in circulating P_4 levels is required to enhance the positive feedback of E_2 in the hypothalamus to cause the luteinizing hormone (LH) surge that induces ovulation, thereby synchronizing fertilization with the uterine preparation for implantation that, in the mouse, occurs 4.5 days later. If copulation occurs, the corpora lutea are maintained and P_4 synthesis continues, causing differentiation of the uterus and a switch in sensitivity to E_2-stimulated cell proliferation from the epithelium to the stroma in preparation for blastocyst implantation. In contrast to species with estrous cycles, Old-World primates have a luteal phase that follows ovulation, P_4 continues to be synthesized, and the stromal cells begin to decidualize.[2] If pregnancy does not occur, chorionic gonadotropin is not available to maintain P_4 synthesis, and the uterine lining is sloughed off during menstruation followed by cell proliferation to replenish the lost functionalis layer. These two extremes of hormonal control over uterine cell proliferation are discussed in this chapter.

CELL PROLIFERATION IN THE MURID UTERUS

Figures 8.1 and 8.2 show the pattern of DNA synthesis in the adult mouse uterus from ovulation through to implantation. Initially, the estrogen produced at proestrus stimulates cell proliferation that is restricted to the luminal and glandular epithelium.[3] This drops at estrus and reaches the lowest point at metestrus when some stromal cell proliferation is detected. If the mice have copulated, there is little cell proliferation on day 1, but this is followed by another wave of proliferation in the luminal and glandular epithelium on day 2 that is presumably independent of E_2 since this hormone has by and large disappeared at this time. P_4 synthesized from the newly formed corporea lutea, beginning on day 2, inhibits further epithelial cell proliferation and causes differentiation of these cells to accept the blastocyst. It also slightly enhances stromal cell proliferation while preparing these cells to respond to E_2 with a single round of DNA synthesis that occurs immediately before implantation[3] (see Figure 8.2). This E_2 synthesis is required for blastocyst

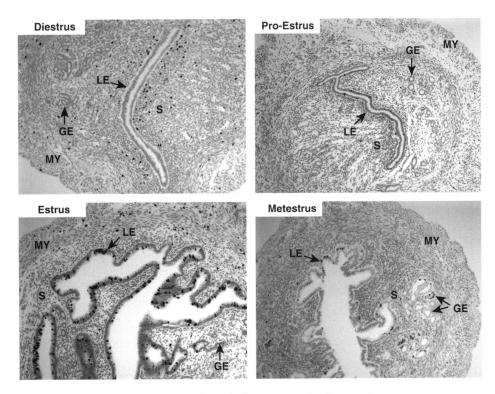

Figure 8.1   Cell proliferation in the mouse uterus through the estrus cycle, showing 5 μm transverse sections of mouse uteri isolated from mice at the phases of the estrus cycle indicated and given bromodeoxyuridine (BrdU) 2 hours before killing to mark cells undergoing DNA synthesis. The sections shown with the mesometrial area at the top were immunostained with an anti-BrdU antibody followed by identification of positive cells with a vector stain kit and brief staining with hematoxylin. Black stains indicate proliferating cells whose number peaks in the luminal and glandular epithelium at estrus. There is also a small amount of stromal cell proliferation at diestrus. LE, luminal epithelium; GE, glandular epithelium; S, stroma; MY, myometrium.

implantation, thereby again coordinating uterine responses with implantation. This stromal DNA synthesis appears to be necessary for the stromal cells to respond to the implanting blastocyst with a decidual response which itself is characterized by rapid cell proliferation.[4] This proliferation begins in the periluminal stromal cells immediately adjacent to the implanting blastocyst, and rapidly expands in an outward and circular zone so that the embryo is completely surrounded by decidual cells (see Figure 8.2). In addition, the inner cells of the primary decidual zone fail to undergo cytokinesis and become polyploid.[5–7]

The events occurring during the estrous cycle and early pregnancy can be exactly mimicked in ovariectomized mice given exogenous hormones.[8–13] This has allowed controllable systems to study the mechanism of action of these hormones. Thus, in the ovariectomized mouse, E_2 stimulates a round of DNA synthesis in the luminal and glandular epithelium, beginning at approximately 6 hours after administration and peaking at 12–15 hours. This is followed by a wave of cell division and a second round of DNA synthesis and cell division such that the epithelial cell number increases approximately four-fold.[12] It has

been proposed that these cells are not arrested in G_0, but instead are slowly cycling in the absence of E_2. This hormone therefore, exerts its effects primarily through a dramatic shortening of the G_1 period, although the duration of the S phase is also diminished.[12,14–17] Later, at around 21 hours after E_2 administration, there is also proliferation of endothelial cells.[12] Low-potency estrogens that do not cause true uterine growth but do induce the early wet weight responses also stimulate this endothelial cell proliferation. It has been suggested that this proliferation replenishes the endothelial cells that become fenestrated during the uterine vascular response.[15] It is likely, however, that this non-estrogen-regulated stromal endothelial cell proliferation is largely responsible for much of the increase in DNA content measured by Mueller at 24 hours after E_2 administration.[9]

P_4 pretreatment of ovariectomized mice for at least 2 days completely inhibits both the luminal and glandular epithelial proliferative response to E_2.[10,11,13,18] In addition, it also suppresses the basal rate of cell proliferation observed in these cells in the absence of ovarian steroid hormones.[13] P_4 also inhibits apoptosis in the E_2-primed uterine epithelium.[19] An argument can

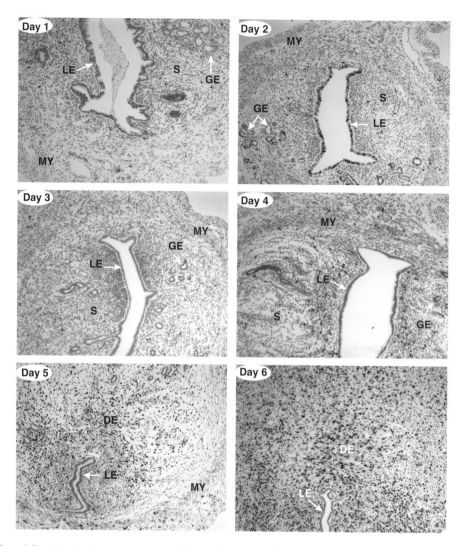

Figure 8.2   Cell proliferation in the mouse uterus during the pre- and peri-implantation periods, showing 5 μm transverse sections of mouse uteri, orientated with the mesometrial side on top, isolated on the days of pregnancy shown (day 1 in the morning of plug detection) and given bromodeoxyuridine (BrdU) 2 hours before killing. Proliferating cells were detected as described in Figure 8.1 and are shown by the black stain. There is a burst of epithelial cell proliferation on day 2, followed by a complete suppression from day 3 onwards under the influence of progesterone. There is stromal proliferation on day 4, followed by extensive proliferation on days 5 and 6 as the decidua forms in response to the implanting embryo that occurs midway through day 4. Shown here for days 5 and 6 are the antimesometrial areas. DE, decidua; LE, luminal epithelium; GE, glandular epithelium; S, stroma; MY, myometrium.

therefore be made that P_4 treatment results in the removal of cells from the cell cycle into the G_0 phase. In this state, the epithelial cells become differentiated and are morphologically distinct from the cycling cells with characteristically aligned nuclei with subnuclear vacuolation.[13] P_4 treatment does slightly elevate stromal cell proliferation and primes these cells to respond to E_2 with a single wave of DNA synthesis that involves 30–40% of the cells, particularly those in the periluminal region. Once completed, these cells then become refractory to further proliferative signals from E_2.[13,20,21]

To achieve complete suppression of uterine epithelial cell proliferation, P_4 must be administered for at least 2 days prior to E_2 administration, a regimen that replicates pregnancy.[3,22] P_4 administered coincidentally with E_2 reduces DNA synthesis by 40% for the first round but completely suppresses the second round of E_2-induced cell proliferation. Studies in which the timing of P_4 addition relative to E_2 was varied indicated that cells were only susceptible to this P_4 inhibition during the first 3 hours of G_1, after which they became irreversibly committed to cell division.[23,24]

At every estrous cycle, the approximate four-fold increase in epithelial cell number is followed by a return to normal levels. Similarly, in the hormone-treated mouse following metabolism of E_2 and its loss from the tissue, apoptotic cell death intervenes and the cell number returns to the basal state.[12,15] In early experiments using low-potency estrogens, the E_2 regulation of cell viability was shown to be directly related to estrogen receptor (ER) occupancy and, providing occupancy is maintained, apoptosis is prevented.[15,25] By varying the timing of administration of these low-potency estrogens, it was determined that at least 9 hours of ER occupancy were necessary for a full proliferative response.[15,26] Based on these data, it was suggested that there are critical transition points early and, at 6–9 hours after E_2 administration. In fact, Stack and Gorski,[27] in their ratchet model of the E_2 response in immature uteri, have argued for several step-like transitions in a full estrogenic response. However, it is still uncertain if there is a requirement for continuous ER occupancy or whether there are distinct events that require critical levels of occupancy. These timing experiments have been repeated with large-scale gene expression analysis.[28] The chaperone protein BIP, whose synthesis is E_2-regulated, is required for the transition between the early and late phase at 6 hours after E_2, since its activity appears to be required for sustained ERα activity.[29] An interesting phenomenon occurs following continuous estrogen exposure where epithelial cell density is further increased over that attained with a single injection but, thereafter, the cell number enters a stable state characterized by intrinsic small waves of cell death followed by compensatory waves of cell proliferation.[30]

Cell proliferation in the immature uterus in response to exogenous sex hormones has been well studied in rodents. This is rather different from the adult response because, physiologically, although responsive to E_2, the uterus will develop even in the absence of E_2 although after puberty it needs E_2 to reach adult size. In the immature rat uterus, there is a high rate of cell proliferation in all cell layers until day 15 postpartum (pp).[31] Until this age, these cells are not fully responsive to E_2 even though they contain ER. In the mouse uterus, cell proliferation is independent of estrogen until days 25–30 pp since ovariectomy does not influence the rate of cell proliferation until this age.[32] Similar conclusions can be drawn from the fact that mice that have a fully formed, although atrophic, uterus even in the absence of ERα.[33] Cell proliferation in the immature uterus is instead regulated by pituitary factors and locally synthesized growth factors.[34] The acquisition of true E_2 responsiveness is coincident with puberty and this is quantitatively different from the immature uterus, because the acute proliferation response to E_2 is restricted to the epithelium and does not require hypothalamic, pituitary, or adrenal factors.[34] After day 15 of age, in rats, the intrinsic rate of cell proliferation drops and the cells gain the ability to respond to E_2. In ovariectomized animals this is characterized by an induced wave of cell proliferation of most cell types in both the endometrium and myometrium.[31,35] Interestingly, however, only the epithelial cells respond to P_4 by an inhibition of cell proliferation.[36] This immature uterine experimental system, in response to E_2, has been used extensively to study E_2 regulation of cell proliferation, since essentially all cells participate, but it may be non-physiological and not representative of the true estrogenic response in adult.

CELL PROLIFERATION IN THE HUMAN ENDOMETRIUM

Sex steroid effects on cell proliferation in the human uterus are similar to the rodent but have the additional complication that the uterus is divided into differentially responsive areas, the upper and lower functionalis and basalis regions. Furthermore, because of the luteal phase and the induction of decidualization in the absence of pregnancy, cells are shed at menstruation. Replacement of the epithelial layer is seeded from the basalis,[2,37] perhaps suggesting a population of stem cells in this zone.[38,39] In humans, cell proliferation has been measured indirectly using markers such as the proliferating cell nuclear antigen (PCNA), a subunit of DNA polymerase, or by phospho-histone H3, and Ki67, a growth-related antigen detected by a monoclonal antibody, or by the ex-vivo incorporation of [^{3}H]-thymidine or bromodeoxyuridine (BrdU). Because direct kinetic studies cannot be performed, caution needs to be exercised in interpreting the results.

The human cycle is dominated by a proliferative phase where E_2 exerts its action, and a secretory phase where P_4 causes differentiation of the epithelial cells and stromal cells undergo predecidual changes (Figure 8.3). The proliferative responses to hormones vary according to region and, although they are broadly similar to the mouse, they differ in important respects. The luminal and glandular epithelium proliferate during the 'proliferative phase', presumably in response to E_2, and this continues at high levels until the third postovulatory day.[40–42] It is greatest in the upper functionalis layer in both the luminal and glandular epithelium and gradually declines as the glands penetrate into the basalis layer. The latter is proliferatively inactive although it may contain progenitor cells that seed the regenerating glandular

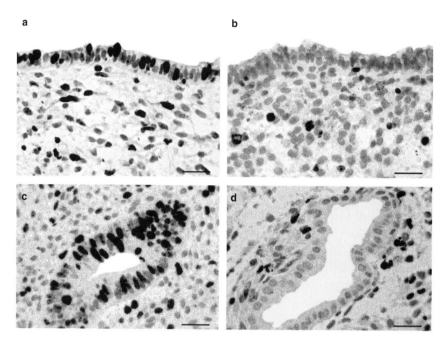

Figure 8.3 Cell proliferation in the human uterus. Endometrial biopsies were taken from normal reproductive-age women with no apparent abnormalities at either proliferative or secretory stage of the menstrual cycle. Biopsies were fixed, sectioned at 5 μm, and immunostained for the cell proliferation marker Ki67, followed by staining with hematoxylin. Black staining indicates positive cells. Panels show luminal (a,b) and glandular (c,d) epithelial areas from proliferative (a,c) and areas from secretory, mid-luteal phase 5–9 days post the LH surge (b,d) phases. Both the luminal and glandular epithelium show extensive cell proliferation during the proliferative phase and this is completely suppressed during the secretory phase. Stromal proliferation, however, is detected at both phases of the menstrual cycle. Data from Niklaus et al[44] (bar = 20 μm).

structures after menstruation.[39] Immunostaining revealed that epithelial cells were ER positive and about 30% of the upper functionalis layer were Ki67 positive at the mid-proliferative phase,[43] a number that was increased slightly to 45% by the analysis of endometrial biopsies from mid-reproductive age women without any uterine pathologies.[44] This study also showed that the rates in luminal and glandular epithelium were comparable, with the glands showing slightly higher numbers of cells in cycle. Similar results were found with BrdU or [³H]-thymidine labeling of tissue explants.[40,41] This epithelial proliferation declines as the secretory phase is reached and P_4 concentrations are elevated until no proliferative activity can be detected in the luminal or glandular epithelium.[42,44] Although the extent of epithelial proliferation varies according to the region, the pattern of response to hormones is similar.[18,41,45] In contrast to the mouse, however, during the early dominance of E_2 in the proliferative phase, there is substantial stromal cell proliferation with labeling indexes similar to that found in the epithelium,[41,44] probably reflecting the repair of the uterus following the previous menstruation since it is largely confined to the upper functionalis region. Proliferation is slightly diminished during the secretory phase with a decline at mid-secretory phase but a

significant increase at the end of the cycle. Proliferation in late cycle seems to be largely accounted for by blood-derived cells (CD45+), including T cells, macrophages, and possibly granulocytes.[40] Notable, too, is the substantial endothelial cell proliferation throughout the cycle, probably representing angiogenesis associated with the tissue growth.[41] Further details can be found in Chapter 5.

E_2, P_4, AND GROWTH FACTORS IN THE REGULATION OF UTERINE CELL DYNAMICS

There has been a long debate over whether sex steroid hormones act directly on the uterus and, if so, whether their actions on one cell type are mediated indirectly through another cell type (paracrine action). Early experiments administering very small concentrations of E_2 into the uterine lumen on only one side, indicated a direct action of this hormone on cell proliferation in that horn of the uterus, since the contralateral horn did not respond.[46] This indicates that the action of E_2 in the uterus is not mediated through systemic factors. E_2 and P_4 act through their cognate receptors since their actions on cell proliferation can be completely abrogated by receptor antagonists,[34,47] results that were confirmed by gene targeting in mice of the ER (estrogen receptor knockout; ERKO) or PR (progesterone receptor knockout; PRKO). In the former, there is a hypoplastic but completely formed uterus that is unresponsive to E_2, as assessed by classical response such as water imbibition and cell proliferation.[33] These data showed the lack of requirement for E_2 signaling during uterine development and the complete requirement for E_2 in the adult. The PRKO mouse has a normally structured but hyperplastic uterus and in ovariectomized PRKO mice, P_4 could not antagonize E_2 induction of epithelial cell proliferation.[48]

The cell specificity of responses to sex steroid hormones can be assessed using receptor-null mutant tissues. Tissue recombinants between stroma and epithelium were derived from immature (immediately postpartum) uterine tissue from mice with or without steroid hormone receptors, grafted under the kidney capsule. The actions of both E_2 and P_4 on cell proliferation are mediated through the stroma and the cognate receptors are not required in uterine epithelial cells,[49-51] strongly suggesting that sex steroid action on the epithelium is mediated through paracrine factors synthesized or released from the uterine stroma. However, caution does need to be exercised in the interpretation of these results, since embryological development of organs usually requires stromal–epithelial interactions and the uterus appears to be no exception. Thus, given the non-cell type-restricted proliferative response to E_2 in the developing uterus and the observed high level of proliferation in the stroma of the tissue recombinants,[49] it may be that an immature phenotype is maintained to some degree and that the adult pattern of restricted cell proliferation does not develop fully. Such a suggestion is given some credence by recent experiments using heterotypic recombinants between mouse and human uterine cell types, which indicated in the adult human that the ER is required in the epithelial cells for E_2-induced cell proliferation.[52] These issues will only be resolved by gene targeting of steroid hormone receptors in a cell type and developmentally restricted manner. It is interesting, however, that epithelial proliferation was not inhibited but the stromal response to E_2 in a progestinized uterus was ablated using a knockin mutation that ablated the DNA binding of the ER to the classic estrogen response element.[53] This indicated that the epithelial cell proliferation was regulated by a non-classical receptor pathway perhaps by binding to the DNA through a tethered mechanism using Sp1 or indeed via an ER-mediated membrane signal transduction mechanism[54] and that the regulation of epithelial and stromal proliferation is different.

The conclusions of the above tissue-recombinant experiments are that steroid hormone actions in mouse are mediated by paracrine factors. The paradigm that hormone action is mediated by locally synthesized growth factors was established by the direct sex steroid hormonal regulation of colony-stimulating factor 1 (CSF-1) in the uterus.[55] It has become apparent over the last decade that many local actions of sex steroid hormones are mediated by growth factors synthesized locally in response to these hormones.[56-59] Many such factors have been described, with the striking feature that the uterine epithelium appears to be a potent cytokine producer.[56,60] Cytokines can be targeted to the embryo, regulate local immune function, influence angiogenesis, and modulate uterine cell proliferation[58,61-69] (see Chapter 35). In the latter case, considerable attention has fallen upon the epidermal growth factor (EGF) class of ligands because, at different stages, EGF, transforming growth factor α (TGFα), heparin-binding (HB) EGF, and amphiregulin are synthesized in the uterus.[70-74] For example, EGF and the EGF receptor (EGFR) are synthesized in response to E_2 in the uterus of ovariectomized mice.[73,75-77] EGF or TGFα administered to ovariectomized, adrenalectomized, hypothectomized mice from slow-release pellets implanted in the kidney capsule causes cell proliferation in the uterine epithelium, and antibodies to EGF attenuate the mitogenic response to E_2.[78,79] However, both EGF- and TGF null mutant mice appear to be fertile and, therefore, most likely have normal proliferative responses to the steroid hormones.[80] Indeed, triple null mutants of EGF, TGFα, and amphiregulin are fertile even in the presence of only one active allele of the EGFR, suggesting normal uterine cell proliferation.[81] Unfortunately, EGFR null mutant mice, even upon the most permissive genetic background, do not survive more than a few days.[82] Nevertheless, using tissue recombinants of embryonic EGFR null and wild-type uterus similar to those described above, uterine cell proliferation rates were reduced in the grafts even though cell differentiation was overtly normal.[50] This suggests that EGFR signaling is important for growth but not cell commitment in the uterus. However, tissue recombinants in which the epithelium lacked the EGFR and the stroma was wild type, showed normal epithelial proliferative responses to E_2. This suggests that the proliferative signal to E_2 derives from the stroma and is not provided by the EGF family of ligands, although members could be required for full development of the stroma. These data contrast with the administration in vivo of EGF and the direct action of EGF on uterine epithelial cells cultured in vitro.[78,83]

Interestingly, EGF can transactivate the ER and stimulate its transcriptional activity even in the absence of ligand.[84] Furthermore, EGF does not have a mitogenic effect on the uterine epithelium in the ERKO mice.[85] These data strongly suggest a cross-talk between sex steroid hormone receptor and growth factor signaling, ideas that are consistent with ER activation by the MAP kinase, protein kinase C and A pathways in the absence of ligand.[86] Thus, there may be independent signaling pathways that can stimulate uterine epithelial cell proliferation involving both steroid hormones and growth factors. It remains to be determined how these interact in the adult mouse in vivo.

Other important growth factors are the insulin-like growth factors (IGF-1 and II). IGF-1 mRNA and protein are expressed in the uterine epithelium at day 1 and 2 of pregnancy in mice, and expression is potentiated by E_2 in ovariectomized mice.[87–92] However, in ovariectomized rats treated with E_2, IGF-1 mRNA appears restricted to the stroma and myometrium with lower expression in the epithelium,[87] data that we have confirmed in mice (unpublished observations). Once P_4 is synthesized during pregnancy, IGF-1 expression in mice is detectable only in the stroma.[93] [^{125}I]-IGF-1 binding was restricted principally to the myometrium, although, given the sensitivity of this technique, it seems likely that most cells express receptors.[88] The expression of these receptors is potentiated by E_2 in ovariectomized mice. Using organ culture of immature uterus, IGF-1 was shown to potentiate the proliferative response, principally in the myometrium but also in the stroma.[91] Studies with the IGF-1 null mutant mouse have confirmed the importance of IGF-1 in uterine biology. These mice have a hypotrophic uterus with minimal development of the myometrium, showing that IGF-1 is required for uterine development.[94] In wild-type adult mice, E_2 was shown to induce IGF-1 receptor activation in the uterine epithelium[95,96] and this required ER.[97] Furthermore, exogenous IGF-1 stimulated the IGF-1 receptor and induced the cell proliferation marker PCNA, although only a small increase, if any, in DNA synthesis was reported.[97] IGF-1 also activated ER, suggesting a direct requirement for this receptor in the epithelial cells in contradistinction to the chimera experiments described above.[97] However, we have recently found definitive evidence for the requirement of IGF-1R signaling in the E_2 stimulation of uterine epithelial DNA synthesis in adult mice, showing that this is, at least, one essential factor for this cell proliferation.[97a]

The data regarding IGF-1 signaling in the uterus are perplexing, however, because analysis of IGF-1 null mutant mice in tissue grafting experiments shows that systemic but not local IGF-1 is required for E_2 induced uterine epithelial cell proliferation.[98] Furthermore, in IGF-1 null mutant mice with hypotrophic uteri, IGF-1 was necessary for the epithelial cells to progress through G_2 and not for their traverse through G_1.[99] Furthermore, as described above, treatment of rat uteri with IGF-1 stimulated myometrial and, to a lesser degree stromal, but not epithelial DNA synthesis.[91] These contradictory data probably reflect a number of mitigating factors, including redundancy between systemic and locally produced IGF-1, adult vs neonatal tissues, and developmental compensation in null mutant mice. There is also a cross-regulation between IGF-1 and EGF in the uterus,[100] adding further complexity to the inter-relationships between growth factors and steroid hormone receptors in the regulation of uterine cell proliferation. These data strongly suggest cross-talk between sex steroid hormone receptor and growth factor signaling, ideas that are consistent with ER activation by the MAP kinase, protein kinase C and A pathways in the absence of ligand.[86]

IGF-1 appears to be the major insulin-like growth factor in the uterus, but IGF-1 is also expressed in adult mouse uterus. Furthermore, many of the IGF-binding proteins are expressed under the regulation of E_2, suggesting a complex interplay of activators and regulators of IGF action.[91] Keratinocyte growth factor (KGF) may also have an important role in the development of the uterus. KGF and KGFR is expressed in the neonatal mouse uterus, and KGF administration to newborn mice resulted in proliferation and extensive invagination of the uterine epithelium.[101]

The Wnt signaling pathway is important for the regulation of cell proliferation in the uterus. Gene ablation of Wnt5a significantly perturbs uterine development, with loss of the glandular epithelium (using grafting of neonatal tissue). The loss of Wnt5a also affects responses to the potent estrogen agonist diethylstilbestrol (DES).[102] In adult mice, E_2 induces expression of Wnt4, Wnt5a, and the Wnt receptor, Frizzled 2, but in an ER-independent manner.[103] This early induction of Wnt4 and Wnt5a by E_2 appears to be critical for DNA synthesis since in-vivo delivery by adenovirus of SFRP-2, a Wnt antagonist, inhibited epithelial DNA synthesis.[103] The physiological relevance of these data, however, has recently been called into question because a Wnt-reporter mouse (Tcf-Lef-LacZ) failed to show Wnt activity at estrus although substantial activity was detected at implantation, particularly in the myometrium and in the luminal epithelium upon embryo attachment.[104,105] These data are also somewhat at odds with the data from nuclear β-catenin staining (a downstream transcriptional activator of Wnt signaling) since this was largely detected in the uterine stroma and not the epithelium.[106] This suggests that the Wnt pathway is important in the regulation of uterine function but that more research needs to be done to clarify the roles of the various Wnts in this process.

There are many other growth factors whose expression is influenced by E_2 and P_4.[37,57,58,60,107,108] Several of these are candidates for regulating cell proliferation. For example, both the (generally) inhibitory cytokines TGFβ1 and tumor necrosis factor α (TNFα) are expressed in the uterus under hormonal regulation.[109,110] However, unfortunately, the TGFβ1 null mutant, even on a permissive SCID background, has profound defects in ovulation and embryo development and uterine cell proliferation has not been studied.[111] TGFβ1 is delivered in seminal plasma at mating[112] and may play some role in the suppression of cell proliferation at this time. However, this inhibition of proliferation still occurs even in ovariectomized P_4E_2-treated mice that have not been exposed to seminal fluid, suggesting that it plays only a minor role if any.[113] TNF receptor null mutants display normal fertility.[114] Consequently, roles for these and other growth factors have yet to be assigned in the regulation of cell proliferation in the uterus.[57]

Several workers have suggested that E_2 acts through other mechanisms. For example, uterine distention induces epithelial cell proliferation. This led to the suggestion that edema might be responsible for regulating proliferation, presumably through the access of serum growth factors to uterine cells.[115] However, there is a lack of correlation between uterine edema in response to various estrogens and cell proliferation.[116,117] This being said, stromal synthesis of the potent angiogenic factor VEGF (vascular endothelial growth factor) is regulated by E_2 in the uterus and its inhibition with a soluble form of the VEGF-R1 receptor (s-Flt1) caused a reduction in edema, vascular permeability, and an inhibition of epithelial cell proliferation by ~50%.[118] This suggests that VEGF-A either had a direct effect on the epithelial cell, or acts via a serum growth factor such as IGF-1, or indirectly stimulates endothelial cells to synthesize a paracrine factor. Alternatively, the loss of vascular permeability might simply starve proliferating cells of essential nutrients.

It has been suggested that E_2 causes the loss of an inhibitor of cell proliferation[119] synthesized either locally or systemically. The efficacy of local administration into the uterine lumen of low dosages of E_2 and the lack of contralateral effects when E_2 is administered to only one uterine horn[46] strongly argues against a systemic mediator (estromedin) but instead indicates local regulation of cell proliferation. However, until the molecular mechanisms of E_2 are known, it cannot be completely ruled out that E_2 inhibits the local expression of an inhibitor of cell proliferation such as an IGF-binding protein. Indeed, recent studies suggest that the ERβ has a negative regulatory role in uterine cell proliferation, although the mechanism is unknown.[120] Furthermore, estrogen may regulate the expression of receptors that enable the uterus to respond to circulating growth factors.

E_2 not only stimulates proliferation of resident cells but also controls the uterine populations of blood-borne cells, of which mononuclear phagocytes and eosinophils are the most abundant. The former cells are recruited into the stroma in abundance during estrus, a situation that can be mimicked by E_2 in ovariectomized mice. Studies with the osteopetrotic mouse, which carries a null mutation in the major macrophage growth factor CSF-1 gene, together with the intraluminal installation of CSF-1, has provided compelling evidence that CSF-1 is the major (although not the only) regulator of macrophage populations in the uterus.[66,121,122] Uterine CSF-1 expression is restricted to the epithelium and is under the regulation of E_2 and P_4.[25] Since CSF-1 is not only chemotactic for macrophages but also promotes their survival and proliferation, it seems likely that the increase in their cell number is a mix of recruitment and proliferation.[123,124] Thus, in this case, there is indisputable evidence that female sex steroid hormones regulate a particular uterine cell population through the mediation of a growth factor that involves epithelial to mesenchymal interactions. Although the uterine macrophage recruitment coincides with the peak of E_2-induced DNA synthesis, it seems unlikely that these cells are mediators of this response since uterine cell proliferation is unaffected in the CSF-1 null mutant.[125]

Eosinophil recruitment appears to be regulated through the E_2 induction of a chemoattractant for these cells[126] that has now been identified as eotaxin.[127] It has been suggested that these eosinophils play an important role in the E_2 induction of cell proliferation. However, acute glucocorticoid treatment of mature ovariectomized mice inhibits the local uterine 'inflammatory' response, including the recruitment of eosinophils, without significantly inhibiting E_2-induced cell division.[128] Furthermore, mice homozygous for a null mutation in the eotaxin gene have no uterine eosinophils but display a normal cell proliferation response to the female sex steroid hormones.[127]

In addition to locally synthesized growth factors, circulating hormones can influence uterine cell proliferation, particularly in the immature uterus. These include thyroid hormone, glucocorticoids, and insulin.[129] Furthermore, the vitamin A metabolite, retinoic acid, can inhibit E_2-induced uterine stromal and myometrial cell proliferation without influencing epithelial responses in the immature uterus.[130] Both thyroid hormone and retinoic acid receptors (RARs) can interact with estrogen receptor half sites and, consequently, alter ER occupancy at these sites.[131] RARs are expressed in the uterus and their concentration varies through the estrus cycle; this cyclical interference with E_2–ER signaling could provide a potential mechanism for the effects of retinoic acid. Alternatively, retinoic acid RAR complexes could act on downstream genes. These pathways and their physiological relevance remain to be established.

There are a number of quantitative trait genetic loci (QTL) in both the rat and mouse that affect responsiveness to estrogens.[132–134] In the mouse, these traits affect the classical uterine wet weight response, but variations in cell proliferation in the different strain backgrounds have not been determined. None of the QTL map to the ER locus, so elucidation of the mechanism whereby the estrogen response is modulated is still lacking. Intriguingly, one of the QTL in the mouse maps to a chromosomal region that also contains the RAR and the thyroid receptor.[132]

Just as in the rodent uterus, several growth factors are expressed through the menstrual cycle in humans, including EGF, IGF-1, TGFα, TNFα, and CSF-1.[57,58,107,135–137] Indeed, it has also been suggested that E_2 stimulates epithelial cell proliferation through a paracrine mediator in the human uterus since there is a dissociation of receptor expression and proliferative response.[2] Despite this suggestion as discussed above, heterotypic recombinants show that the ER is required in the human epithelium for cell proliferation.[52] Nevertheless, it seems likely that growth factors are also involved in regulating human endometrial proliferation. Interestingly, in the basalis region, there are large lymphoid aggregates at the base of the glands comprised mainly of active T cells which produce the growth-inhibiting molecule IFNγ (interferon γ), and may thus restrain cell proliferation in this region[40,136,138] (see Chapter 33). This is completely different from the mouse, where T cells are essentially excluded. Interestingly, the IFNγ promoter has been shown to contain functional estrogen response elements (EREs)

and endometrial T cells contain ER,[136] suggesting a direct regulatory role of E_2 acting through IFNγ to limit the epithelial proliferation to the upper layer of endometrium. TNFα is also synthesized abundantly at this stage, suggesting an inhibitory role for this molecule as well.

In humans, progesterone directly inhibits uterine epithelial cell proliferation in a manner analogous to the Muridae.[42] However, unlike in Muridae, it also induces 17β-hydroxysteroid dehydrogenase-2, an enzyme that metabolizes E_2 to its less active derivative estrone. Thus, part of its action is to reduce the potency of the mitogen in the uterus.[139] Following removal of P_4, menstruation occurs and this involves apoptosis in the glands, infiltration of lymphoid cells, sloughing, and repair of the tissue. This in many ways parallels an inflammatory response. A major cytokine synthesized at this time is TNFα and this may regulate cell death.[140,141] Consistent with this, TNFα introduced into the mouse uterine lumen induced endothelial cell death.[142] Given the dramatic remodeling that occurs in the uterus, it is highly likely that many growth factors are all involved in these processes. These include those that mediate cell death (TNFα, TGFβ), together with those that influence remodeling, such as angiogenic factors (VEGF), cell proliferation (IGFs, hepatocyte growth factor [HGF], EGF-like ligands, KGF, FGF), and lymphoid recruitment (interleukins IL-1, IL-6, TNFα, CSF-1).[37,58,141,143]

STROMAL CELL PROLIFERATION

The second dramatic cell proliferative response of the endometrium occurs during the decidualization of the uterine stroma in response to an invading blastocyst into a suitably hormonally primed uterus (see Figure 8.2). In Muridae, implantation occurs at the antimesometrial pole of the uterus during a limited period of receptivity that occurs in the progestinized uterus in response to E_2.[5] In mice, at least, this E_2 signal is mediated by leukemia inhibitory factor (LIF) since implantation is inhibited in LIF nullizygous mice and, even in hormonally primed uteri of LIF–/– mice, an artificial stimulus does not induce decidualization.[144] LIF is synthesized in response to E_2 in the progestinized uterus and acts through its receptor residing on the luminal epithelial surface.[145] The epithelial signal induces a number of events in the stroma, including rapid vascularization, probably exerted through the action of eicosanoids, and rapid cell proliferation.[6,146,147] Initially, however, the immediate subepithelial cells are stimulated to enter into rounds of DNA synthesis but without a corresponding mitosis.[6] These cells, therefore, become polyploid and form the primary decidual zone that eventually surrounds the implanting embryo.[6] Distal cells also undergo DNA synthesis but these cells enter mitosis and this wave of cell proliferation moves in a crescent to surround the invading blastocyst and produce a secondary decidual zone.[6] The mesometrial cells continue to proliferate and differentiate into the maternal portion of the placenta. The early decidual response requires the transcription factor C/EBPβ since no decidualization occurs in mice homozygous for a null mutation in this gene.[148] Careful studies of uterine cells, pulse-labeled prior to decidualization, indicate that the stromal cells that proliferated in response to E_2 before implantation are the ones that differentiate into decidual cells.[4] This initial stromal proliferative response in the progestinized uterus in preparation for decidualization has long been thought to be essential for embryo implantation. It occurs even in LIF nullizygous mice, thus temporally separating two actions of E_2.[149] Another growth factor found to be essential for this process is the P_4-regulated Indian hedgehog (IHH), since decidualization does not occur in mice homozygous for a null mutation in *Ihh*. In these null mutant mice, the P_4E_2-induced stromal cell proliferation did not occur, indicating that IHH is an essential mediator of the synergistic action of these hormones.[150] Studies have shown that the P_4E_2-induced stromal proliferation requires a systemic mediator that is likely to be upstream of IHH.[151]

Cell proliferation during decidualization does not require estrogen but absolutely needs progesterone, without which the decidual reaction stops and regression occurs.[152] For the maximal decidual response, however, the uteri need to be primed with E_2 6 days earlier, and this is one of the functions of estrous estrogen.[153] The rate of cell division at the peak of the decidual response is extremely rapid, with doubling times estimated at 5 hours with essentially all cells being involved.[6] Although LIF binding to its receptor together with blastocyst attachment seem to be the activating signals, little is known about the regulation of this proliferation. 'Inert' mediators such as arachis oil are as effective as the blastocyst in providing an apical epithelial stimulus.[153] The mechanism of this epithelial to stromal signal transduction is still unknown, although early data suggested that it may involve the removal of an inhibitor.[154] Similarly, little is known about the control of proliferation in decidual cells, although candidate growth factors have been identified.[57,155] TGFβ1 is found intracellularly in the

primary decidua and is associated with the extracellular matrix in the secondary decidua; TGFβ2 is in the secondary decidua while activin β is expressed more mesometrially by day 8.5 of pregnancy.[109,156–158] Similarly, TGFα and HB-EGF are expressed in the decidua surrounding the invading blastocyst[70,159,160] and their receptor, the EGFR, is coincidentally expressed.[161] Members of the fibroblast growth factor (FGF) family, FGF itself and KGF, are both expressed in the decidua.[162] Receptors for many of these factors are expressed[57] together with those for CSF-1 and steel factor (SF), but little is known about their functions.[163] Decidualization, however, is amenable to manipulation since in the rat and human, stromal cells exposed to P_4 in vivo can be cultured and decidualization induced.[164,165] In this system, FGF is a mitogen.[164,166]

A null mutation in the Il-11α receptor gene is compatible with normal differentiation of the antimesometrial decidua but, over time, the mesometrial decidua thins and disappears, indicating that mesometrial decidualization (not proliferation) is regulated by IL-11.[167,168] Local trophoblast invasion is increased. IL-11 is also required for the differentiation of the uterine natural killer (uNK) cell progenitors that proliferate in the mesometrial decidua.[169] The loss of uNK cells in IL-15 deficient mice does not block pregnancy, although the decidua is hypoplastic, suggesting that uNK cells may have an effect on proliferation and/or differentiation.[170]

Decidualization not only involves substantial cell proliferation but also considerable cell death either during the rapid invasion and remodeling caused by the embryo or if the pregnancy fails. Initially, the uterine epithelium adjacent to the embryo dies away by apoptosis, resulting ultimately in a denuded cavity.[7] Later, the antimesometrial decidua also becomes 'crushed' and cells die away in response to the growing embryo. TGFβ1 induces apoptotic cell death of this population in vitro.[171]

Little is known about the cellular dynamics of decidualization in the human uterus. Large glycogen-containing cells are present, reminiscent of the mouse. The human decidua is populated by many lymphoid cells, particularly macrophages and eosinophils, and it is likely that proliferation of lymphoid cells, observed at the end of the secretory phase, continues if pregnancy occurs.[40,172–174] Just as in the mouse, it is probable that CSF-1 is responsible for the increase in macrophage number.[175,176] LIF is expressed in the luminal and glandular epithelium while the LIFR is also found in these cells with elevated levels through the secretory phase.[177,178] This suggests that similar signaling mechanisms might occur in the human uterus. There is abundant VEGF synthesized by decidual cells, suggesting that this may be an important angiogenic factor at this time, stimulating endothelial cell proliferation and migration.[179] IHH is expressed in the human endometrium during the secretory phase.[180]

MOLECULAR MECHANISM OF E$_2$ AND P$_4$ ACTION ON UTERINE CELL PROLIFERATION

In cultured cells, peptide growth factors stimulate cell proliferation by activating a cascade of intracellular mediators, such as the RAS/RAF, phosphoinositide 3-kinase (PI3K), and mitogen-activated protein kinase (MAPK) pathways and by initially turning on the expression of proto-oncogene transcription factors, such as c-fos, c-jun, and c-myc. Rapid and transient expression of these 'immediate-early' genes renders cells competent to progress through the cell cycle; thus, they are also called 'competence' factors. Other genes encoding 'progression' factors must be turned on by immediate-early transcription factors or through receptor-mediated signal transduction pathways, in order to complete the cell cycle. Both 'competence' and 'progression' phase factors are required for entry to the DNA synthesis (S) phase of the cell cycle. The final commitment of cells to enter into the S phase occurs at the restriction point (R point),[181,182] after which mitogens are no longer required for cells to complete the cell cycle.

E$_2$ and P$_4$ act at the G$_1$ phase of the cell cycle, as already described. E$_2$ reduces the long G$_1$ phase in the unstimulated epithelium (>72 hours) to approximately 6–8 hours.[12,17,183] P$_4$ exerts its inhibitory effect on the cell cycle of uterine epithelial cells early in G$_1$, because P$_4$ has to be given no later than 3 hours after E$_2$ treatment in order to antagonize the E$_2$ effect.[24] This action in adult mice is not through stimulation of E$_2$ catabolism or the inhibition of E$_2$ binding to the ER in the uterus.[184–186] Furthermore, P$_4$ does not inhibit the overall stimulation of protein synthesis and rRNA synthesis in the epithelium,[187] or the induction of edema in the stroma.[21] In the adult, only epithelial cells respond acutely to E$_2$ treatment by proliferation. Because the epithelial cells only represent 5% of the total, data derived from whole uterine homogenates are unlikely to reveal the mechanism of estrogen control over cell proliferation. Methods are available to

achieve purification of at least the luminal epithelial compartment.[188,189] In contrast, in the immature uterus, essentially all cell types respond to E$_2$ by proliferation with similar kinetics, and biochemical analysis of total uterine homogenates can reveal information about the regulation of cell proliferation. Nevertheless, there is an assumption implicit in these studies that all cells respond similarly to E$_2$, which may not be the case.

In ovariectomized immature rats and mice, E$_2$ induces all uterine cell types to undergo cell division.[31,32] Initially, E$_2$ stimulates c-fos mRNA and protein levels 1 hour after administration in all cell types, with the most prominent expression in the epithelium.[190–192] E$_2$ also differentially regulates members of the jun family of transcription factors. While E$_2$ up-regulates jun-B and jun-D in the luminal and glandular epithelium at 2 hours after treatment, it represses the constitutively expressed c-jun in the luminal epithelium.[193] E$_2$ also induces mRNA expression for N-myc at 1 hour, c-myc at 4 hours, and c-Ha-ras at 8 hours, as determined by analysis of total uterine RNA by Northern blotting.[194,195] In mature rodents, E$_2$ specifically stimulates cell proliferation in the luminal and glandular epithelium.[10,12,15] Correlated with this, E$_2$ stimulates c-fos, jun-B, and jun-D mRNA and protein levels rapidly and transiently only in the epithelium,[196–198] while it represses c-jun mRNA levels in these cells.[192,197] E$_2$ also upregulates c-Ha-ras mRNA and c-myc protein level in the epithelium, peaking at 12 hours.[199–201] The induction of these immediate-early genes is not blocked by protein synthesis inhibitors, suggesting a direct transcriptional effect.[196,202,203] Indeed, EREs have been found in some of their promoters.[204,205] Therefore, E$_2$ induces these immediate-early genes directly in a characteristic temporal sequence prior to DNA synthesis in its target cells of the uterus in a fashion strikingly similar to the response pattern induced by growth factors in cultured cells.

Further studies have shown that the expression of these immediate-early genes is not strictly correlated with cell proliferation. The short-acting estrogen, 16α-E$_2$, while not capable of promoting DNA synthesis, does induce the early uterotropic responses and also stimulates these early response genes.[196,201] P$_4$, which antagonizes E$_2$ action by specifically blocking E$_2$-induced cell proliferation in the epithelial cells in both immature and mature rodents,[13,23,24] does not inhibit c-fos, jun-B, c-myc, or c-Ha-ras expression, at least at the mRNA level, in these cells,[64,192,199] data that are confirmed on a more global scale by microarray analysis.[206] Pretreatment with P_4 even induces c-fos protein earlier in the epithelium and the stroma.[64,207] Furthermore, tamoxifen, a weak estrogen in the uterus that induces cell proliferation inthe epithelium with similar kinetics to E_2, only up-regulates *c-fos* and *jun-B* mRNA expression in a late and persistent fashion.[208,209] However, among all the immediate-early genes, a correlation with cell prolifer-ation can best be drawn with repression of *c-jun* expression in the epithelial cells, since P_4 concurrently administered with E_2 can block the repression of *c-jun* in the epithelium of mature rats.[210] Despite this, 16α-E_2 can also repress *c-jun* mRNA expression without promoting DNA synthesis.[210] To solve this contradic-tion will require measuring the duration of this *c-jun* repression by E_2 and 16α-E_2, respectively. Perhaps sus-tained depletion of *c-jun* mRNA is essential to permit cell proliferation. This remains to be determined. Furthermore, the studies performed so far cannot rule out the possibility that translational regulation or post-translational modification of these immediate-early proteins is important in the regulation of cell prolifer-ation in the uterus.

Since the proto-oncogene transcription factors studied so far may not be the key mediators of sex steroid hormones' action on cell proliferation in the endometrium, the progression factors have recently drawn more attention. This is also the situation for growth factor stimulation of cells in culture and it may be in the uterus that these progression factors are under the regulation of an E_2-induced growth factor. It is believed that the principal regulators of the G_1 to S transition are the cyclin-dependent kinases (CDKs). Binding of their cyclin partners regulates CDKs. The D-type cyclins, together with their partners CDK4 and 6, are G_1 phase cyclins, while cyclin E and A, with their partner CDK2, are thought to function at the G_1–S transition. This is a simplified view, since cyclin C together with its partner CDK3 appears to be required for exit from G_0 and cyclin Ds can interact with CDK2 and cyclin E with CDK1 and CDK3.[211,212] Furthermore, cyclin A, the only essential cyclin as shown by gene ablation studies, is also involved in the regulation of the degradation of important cell cycle regulatory molecules through its binding to the ubiquitin ligase SKP2.[213] Cyclin–CDK complexes are subjected to negative and positive regulation by phosphorylation. CDK-activating kinase (CAK) can phosphorylate a conserved threonine residue (Thr[160] in CDK2, Thr[161] in CDC2). Full CDK activation however, also requires dephosphorylation of a conserved threonine–tyrosine pair near the amino

terminus (Thr[14] and Tyr[15] in CDK2 and CDC2), which is completed by a dual-specificity phosphatase, CDC25a. Another major regulation of CDK activity involves two families of small proteins, termed cyclin-dependent kinase inhibitors (CKIs). The Ink4 family includes p15[Ink4b], p16[Ink4a], p18[Ink4c], and p19[Ink4d] that specifically inactivate cyclin D/CDK4, 6, while the cip/kip family includes p21[Cip1/Waf1], p27[Kip1], and p57[Kip2], which bind and inhibit both cyclin D/CDK4, 6 and cyclin E, A/cdk2 complexes (Figure 8.3;[211,214–216]). Finally, a less well-studied regulation is the subcellular localization of cyclins and CDKs, that in turn, regulates their access to substrates.[217,218]

The restriction point where cells lose their depen-dence on mitogens occurs in late G_1 phase. This transition is thought to be controlled by the retinoblas-toma (RB) family proteins, pRB, p107, and p130. In their hypophosphorylated state, RB members bind to transcription factors such as E_2F1–5 and inhibit their activities. Mitogens can stimulate D-type cyclin syn-thesis and assembly with catalytic partners CDK4 and CDK6. Activated CDK4 and CDK6 trigger initial phosphorylation of pRB. Phosphorylated pRB releases E2Fs, enabling them to transactivate S phase genes, such as thymidine kinase, DNA-polymerase-α, etc. Also, E2Fs turn on cyclin E gene expression, and cyclin E in complex with its partner CDK2 further phosphorylates pRB, promoting G_1–S phase progres-sion. Therefore, a positive feedback loop ensures the hyperphosphorylation of RB proteins, facilitating irreversible G_1 to S progression. The level of cyclin A is dramatically increased at the G_1–S boundary by the transcriptional activity of E2Fs. In concert with all the above, the CDK2 inhibitors p27 or p21 are sequestered into complexes with excess cyclin D–CDK 4/6 complexes, thereby, releasing the repression of cyclin E/CDK2 and cyclin A/CDK2 activities. Cyclin E, A/CDK2 can also phosphorylate proteins at replica-tion origins, and this activity might also promote DNA synthesis (Figure 8.4;[211,214–216]).

In addition to the canonical cell cycle regulatory machinery, DNA needs to be licensed for replication. DNA synthesis is initiated by the formation of the pre-replicative complex (pre-RC) at origins of replica-tion during early G_1.[219–221] Pre-RC formation involves the sequential assembly of more than 20 replication factors. The origin of DNA replication is first marked by the origin recognition complex (ORC), a hetero-hexameric complex, which serves as a scaffold for the loading of additional proteins. The binding of CDC6 and CDT1 to the ORC facilitates the loading of the minichromosome maintenance proteins (MCM 2–7)

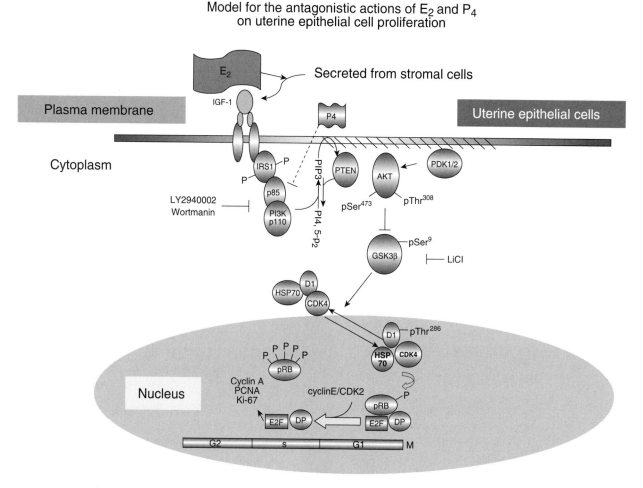

Figure 8.4   Regulation of the canonical cell cycle machinery by estrogens and progesterone in the mouse uterus. E_2 stimulates the canonical cyclin-dependent cell cycle machinery through the nuclear translocation of cyclin D1/CDK4 complexes. This is effected by the stimulation of the PI 3-kinase pathway from IGF-1 responding to IGF-1. Once activated, PI 3-kinase causes a signaling cascade to AKT to GSK-3β, whose activity is inhibited by an AKT-induced phosphorylation on Ser[9]. Cyclin D1, whose nuclear egress is regulated by GSK-3β-induced phosphorylation of Thr[286], is thus not phosphorylated and is therefore retained in the nucleus, together with its catalytic CDK4 partner. P_4 blocks the activation of PI 3-kinase by an unknown mechanism and thereby maintains the activity of GSK-3β, with the resultant loss of nuclear cyclin D_1. The points of regulation by P_4 are indicated, as are the activities of the various inhibitors (Wortmanin, LY2940002, LiCl) used to establish this pathway in vivo.

on the replication origins in stochiometric amounts to form the pre-RC. The loading of the hexameric MCM complex leads to the loss of the requirement for ORC, CDC6, and CDT1 for subsequent DNA replication.[222,223] Once loaded, origin firing can be activated by two kinases, CDC7-DBF4 kinase (DDK) and CDK, to commence DNA synthesis. This involves the orderly recruitment of additional replication factors, including CDC45, PCNA, and DNA polymerase α, the latter of whose primase activity initiates DNA replication. Pre-RC formation confers competence on the origins to replicate only once in S phase.

Studies on ovariectomized animals have shown in both the immature mouse uterus and the mature rat uterine epithelium that E_2 up-regulates cyclin D1

mRNA level two to three-fold, starting at 8 hours after administration.[224,225] Consistent with this, in mature mouse uterine epithelial cells, E_2 gradually stimulates cyclin D_1 protein level by ~two-fold at 12 hours.[218] Cyclin D1 is thought to act early in G_1; therefore it is unclear how important this late induction (8–12 hours) of cyclin D1 level is for the regulation of the first cycle of cell proliferation. It could solely be due to the general effect of estrogen to increase mRNA and protein levels by two–four-fold.[187] The ability to isolate the uterine epithelium in a pure state after hormone administration in adult mice allows biochemical analysis of the cell cycle machinery and comparison with immunohistochemical localization of the various proteins. Using these methods it was shown in the adult uterine epithelium that E_2 does not elevate the overall activity of cyclin D1/CDK4 or cyclin D1/CDK6 activity over the first 12 hours of treatment,[218] in contrast to findings in cultured estrogen-responsive mammary epithelial cells.[226–228] However, E_2 does cause a significant redistribution of cyclin D1 and, to a lesser extent, CDK4 from the cytoplasm to the nucleus.[218] This process begins within 2 hours of E_2 administration at the peak of uterine ER occupancy and is maximal within 3–5 hours, coincident with significantly enhanced phosphorylation of RB and p107, before returning to the basal level by 15 hours when DNA synthesis is maximal. The nuclear association of cyclin D1 and CDK4 makes the nuclear substrates, such as RB and p107, accessible to this complex. Furthermore, translocation may also activate other cyclin D1-dependent functions such as the ligand-independent transcriptional activation of the ER and SRC-1 by cyclin D1 association.[229–231] Following cyclin D1/CDK4 nuclear translocation, E_2 induces, in an orderly manner, a small but significant elevation in cyclin E protein concentration, increased cyclin E/CDK2 activity, further phosphorylation of RB and p107, and elevated cyclin A/CDK2 activity, resulting in hyperphosphorylation of the RB family proteins.[218] This presumably releases the transcriptional repression of E_2F family members, which results in activation of S-phase genes, including nuclear translocation of PCNA, a DNA polymerase δ component.[218] In another study, E_2 treatment of mature rats was reported to have no effect on CDK2 activity in total uterine cell lysates.[232] However, it is likely that other non-responsive cell types obscured the E_2-induced CDK2 activity in luminal epithelium in these experiments. In mature rats, the cyclin B1 mRNA level is elevated at 16–24 hours after E_2 administration, which corresponds to the G_2–M transition of the uterine epithelial cell cycle.[225] In decidual cells, however, cyclin D3 appears to be the dominant D-type cyclin and this is at least in part regulated by HB-EGF. Cyclin D3 activity also appears to be required for DNA replication in the polyploid cells of the inner decidual zone.[233,234]

Pretreatment with P_4, which completely inhibits E_2-induced cell proliferation in mature mouse uterine epithelium, does not reduce overall protein levels of cyclin D1, CDK4, or CDK6, nor does it inhibit cyclin D1/CDK4 or cyclin D1/CDK6 activities in total epithelial cell lysates. However, P_4 causes nuclear exclusion of cyclin D1 and CDK4, although not CDK6. Thus, the access of cyclin D1/CDK4 to nuclear substrates or targets following E_2 treatment is inhibited

by P_4. This results in the absence of phosphorylation of pRB and p107. Hypophosphorylated RB tightly binds to the nucleus, preventing E_2F transcriptional activation following P_4 pretreatment and, consequently, an inhibition of cyclin A expression. In contrast, p107 protein decreases and the majority disappears from the nucleus. P_4 pretreatment does not alter cyclin E protein concentration significantly, but reduces its associated activities below the control level. This is probably due to the inactivation of its kinase partner, CDK2, shown by the absence of the activated form of CDK2 after P_4 treatment. P_4 also abrogates cyclin A protein synthesis and cyclin A/CDK2 activities. All of the above result in complete absence of phosphorylation of RB and p107 over the entire 12-hour time course and the complete suppression of DNA synthesis[218] (see Figure 8.1).

The activity of CDKs is regulated by their association with the CKIs. Among all the known CKIs, only $p27^{Kip1}$ is significantly expressed in mouse uterine epithelial cells. However, the E_2-induced down-regulation of $p27^{Kip1}$ in uterine epithelial cells is not reversed by P_4 treatment. P_4 also down-regulates E_2-induced elevation in CDK2 activity in $p27^{Kip1}$ nullizygous mice. E_2 and P_4 regulation of cell proliferation is normal in $p27^{Kip1 -/-}$ mouse uterus, indicating that $p27^{Kip1}$ is not required for E_2 or P_4 action.[235]

The expression of cell cycle regulators has also been studied in normal human endometrial glands and stroma during the menstrual cycle and in endometrial carcinomas by immunohistochemistry and by real-time polymerase chain reaction (PCR) measurements in laser-captured endometrial epithelial fractions.[44,236] In one set of studies, cyclin D1 is restricted to a few cells of the normal endometrium.[236] In contrast, cyclin E, CDK2, and CDK4 are present in a substantially higher percentage of the gland cells during the proliferative phase. This number declines during the secretory phase, and these proteins become undetectable in the gland cells by the end of the secretory phase, but they do not decline in the stroma.[237] It is intriguing that cyclin E, CDK2, CDK4, and $p16^{Ink4a}$ are more apparent in the cytoplasm of the gland and stromal cells than the nucleus.[238] Cyclin A is highly expressed in the glands and lumen of the proliferative phase and this expression is absent in the secretory phase.[44] In the lumen and glandular epithelial cells of the normal endometrium, $p27^{Kip1}$ is negligible during the proliferative phase, whereas it is markedly increased in the secretory phase.[44] Stromal cells exhibit a constant expression of $p27^{Kip1}$ throughout the cycle.[239] Progesterone and synthetic progestins can significantly reduce endometrial gland proliferation.[240] In correlation, medroxyprogesterone acetate (MPA) greatly increases p27[Kip1] expression in hyperplastic epithelia.[239] Therefore, it seems that the cell cycle regulatory machinery is modulated in a similar fashion to mouse epithelium, with the exception that p27[Kip1] is possibly involved in the P_4-induced growth suppression of normal and hyperplastic endometrium in humans.

In mice, at least, the nuclear translocation of cyclin D1 appears to be a central point in the regulation of uterine epithelial cell proliferation. It is therefore perplexing that cyclin D1 null mutant mice exhibit normal uterine cell proliferation in response to both E_2 and P_4. Analysis of the cell cycle machinery in the cyclin D1 null mutant mice showed that CDK4 activity was almost at the wild-type level and, consequently, that pRB and p107 phosphorylation were normal. Immunodepletion experiments indicated that this CDK4 activity was entirely dependent upon cyclin D2 in the D1[-/-] mice but that the cyclin D2 did not significantly contribute to the CDK4 activity in wild-type mice. In cyclin D1 null mutant mice, the cyclin D2 complex also normally associated with p27[kip1], thereby removing its inhibition from cyclin E/CDK2 complexes. Indeed, this action of cyclin D1/CDK4 titering P27[kip1] was an essential function, since crosses between cyclin D1 and P27 null mutant mice resulted in reciprocal correction of the mutant phenotypes.[241] Fascinatingly, in the uterine epithelium of D1[-/-] mice, cyclin D2 is now transported to the nucleus in response to E_2 and this was inhibited by P_4.

All these studies suggest that the cellular localization of a D-type cyclin is essential in the hormonal regulation of uterine cell proliferation. Glycogen synthase kinase (GSK)-3β phosphorylates cyclin D1 on Thr[286] and this results in its export from the nucleus by the nuclear exportin, chromosome region maintenance 1 (CRM1). In the uterine epithelium, E_2 treatment causes an inhibitory phosphorylation at Ser[9] on GSK-3β that inhibits this subsequent Thr[286] phosphorylation. P_4 completely suppresses this inhibitory phosphorylation, giving a constitutively active GSK-3β that phosphorylates cyclin D1 and therefore causes its egress from the nucleus. The GSK-3β inhibitor, LiCl, applied in a pleurionic gel in the uterine lumen of P_4E_2-treated mice reversed the P_4-induced nuclear exclusion of cyclin D1. Nuclear localization of cyclin D1 resulted in sequential phosphorylation of pRB induction of cyclin E and cyclin A/CDK2 activity and the expression of the proliferation markers Ki67 and PCNA. However, BrdU incorporation could not be detected. This indicated that true DNA synthesis was not initiated even though

many components of the pathway were activated.[242] These data suggest that there must be another parallel pathway independent of pRB, whose activity is stimulated by E_2 and inhibited by P_4.

Ser[9] phosphorylation of GSK-3β is effected by the AKT kinase, that in turn is activated by phosphorylation on Thr[308] and Ser[473] through the PI3K pathway. E_2 caused phosphorylation of Thr[308] and Ser[473] detected at 2 hours post-treatment, reaching a maximum at 8 hours, in parallel with Ser[9] phosphorylation on GSK-3β. P_4 pretreatment, significantly, though not entirely, inhibited this effect. To confirm that this E_2 induction of AKT phosphorylation was through the PI3K pathway and to test the hypothesis that this pathway regulated the E_2-induced accumulation of cyclin D1, we inhibited PI3K in the luminal epithelial cells by an intraluminal injection of the PI3K inhibitors, wortmanin or LY2940002 immediately before E_2 treatment. This significantly reduced the phosphorylation of Ser[473] in response to E_2, and, especially with LY2940002, essentially abolished the Ser[9] inhibitory phosphorylation of GSK-3β. Immunohistochemical analysis showed that these treatments blocked the E_2-induced accumulation of cyclin D1 in the uterine luminal epithelial cells. This confirmed the activation by E_2 of the PI3K pathway that results in the nuclear accumulation of cyclin D1 and that this pathway is inhibited by P_4 with the consequent inhibition of cell cycle progression.[242] This PI3K pathway appears to be stimulated by IGF-1,[97a] as suggested by previous observation of the E_2-induced tyrosine phosphorylation of the IGF-1R.[97]

The failure in the reversal of the PI3K kinase pathway in P_4E_2-treated uteri to stimulate DNA synthesis suggested that another pathway might be activated to complete this process. A candidate would be the replication licensing machinery that is required for initiation of DNA synthesis. Indeed, in uterine luminal epithelial cells, E_2 induces loading of the MCM complex onto chromatin in a temporal fashion, starting at 2 hours and peaking at 8–11 hours in a fashion that parallels the induction of DNA synthesis. In most species this loading is regulated by the CDC6 level or localization. However, E_2 neither changed CDC6 concentration nor its localization. Instead, CDT1 protein concentration was dramatically elevated by E_2 in parallel with MCM complex binding to chromatin. This suggested that CDT1 is the limiting factor for pre-replication licensing in the uterine luminal epithelium. P_4 inhibits this MCM complex binding to chromatin in response to E_2. This is achieved at several different levels. First, MCM 2, 3, 4, 5, and 6 transcripts are down-regulated by P_4. Secondly,

MCM 2, 3, and 4 protein levels are reduced. Since a small reduction in the concentration of any one MCM protein is sufficient in other systems to inhibit DNA synthesis, this down-regulation would appear to be a major reason for the P_4 block of DNA synthesis. It is important to note that MCM2 and 3 mRNA protein are down-regulated in human luminal and glandular epithelial cells during the secretory phase. However, in addition, P_4 inhibits the induction of CDT1 by E_2. The net result of all these levels of regulation is that P_4 inhibits replication licensing through inhibiting pre-replication complex binding to origins of replication.[243]

Analysis of other mouse mutants has revealed a role for the Krüppel-like factor-9/basic transcription element binding protein-1 (*Klfp/Bteb1*) (a member of the Sp-1 family) in the regulation of uterine cell proliferation. This transcription factor interacts with the PR and enhances its transcriptional activation in cooperation with CREB-binding protein (CBP).[244] Gene ablation of *Bteb1*[245] resulted in uterine hypoplasia and reduced fertility due to decreased implantation rates.[246,247] There were perturbations in uterine proliferation, with luminal epithelial proliferation delayed by 1 day to day 3 during pregnancy and glandular epithelial proliferation being significantly depressed and also mistimed.[248] Hormone reconstitution experiments showed that the inhibition of endometrial proliferation in all compartments in response to a combined P_4E_2 injection was affected by the loss of *Bteb1*.[248] Thus, it can be concluded that PR signaling to cell division is perturbed by loss of *Bteb1*. Similarly, the transcription factor C/EBPβ (CCAAT enhancer binding protein β) is required for E_2-induced epithelial cell proliferation.[148,249] Overexpression of another transcription factor, *Emx2*, a target of Hoxa10 in the uterus,[250] inhibited glandular epithelial cell proliferation.[251] This was accompanied by a reduced rate of implantation. However, the molecular basis of the actions of these transcription factors in controlling epithelial cell proliferation and the relationship of them to the canonical cell cycle machinery has not yet been described.

In other epithelia such as in the skin or crypt of the colon, reduction of DNA synthesis and subsequent differentiation is accompanied by down-regulation of genes associated with RNA splicing and transport and protein synthesis. Conversely upon stimulation of cell proliferation, cellular growth is initiated through an increase in ribosomal transcription, and therefore ribosome number per cell, together with an increase in translational initiation rates, results in protein accumulation. The rate of protein accumulation is a determinant of the rate of cell proliferation.[252,253] Thus, E_2 stimulates protein and rRNA synthesis in the uterine epithelium early in G_1, while cell growth, as defined by protein and rRNA content per cell, increases to a similar extent.[187] In other cell types, reduction of DNA synthesis during cell differentiation is usually accompanied by down-regulation of transcripts encoding proteins involved in RNA splicing and transport and protein synthesis. However, in the uterus, these processes, as assessed by expression analysis in a large-scale 27 000 cDNA microarray experiment, were unaffected by treatment for 3 days with P_4, although coincidental P_4 and E_2 treatment did lower the rate of protein synthesis.[243] This was consistent with earlier studies where P_4 was shown not to down-regulate E_2-induced protein and rRNA synthesis nor proto-oncogenes such as *c-fos*, *c-myc*, and c-Ras^{Ha}.[187,199] Therefore, induction of the immediate-early genes correlates better with cell growth than DNA synthesis, which suggests that these genes are required for the growth response. P_4 specifically targets pathways that regulate cell cycle progression, including the pRB and the entire DNA replication process, which includes DNA replication complex assembly, DNA replication elongation, and nucleosome assembly and modification. Thus, the regulations by P_4 of hyperplasia and hypertrophy are distinct.

SUMMARY

Cellular proliferation in the uterus is regulated by a complex interplay between E_2 and P_4. These interactions can be synergistic or antagonistic. E_2 acts via its receptor, and continuous occupancy through the G_1 phase of the cell cycle is required for cell proliferation. Loss of receptor binding partway through the cell cycle triggers apoptosis. E_2, at least in mice, appears to act via paracrine signaling from the stroma that activates two signaling pathways in the epithelial cells that run in parallel. The first pathway is the canonical cell cycle regulatory machinery that results in phosphorylation of RB, with the consequent activation of downstream gene transcription. The second pathway causes the licensing of DNA replication through the activation of MCM protein binding to the origins of DNA replication. These pathways intersect at the G_1–S phase boundary (Figure 8.5). This, together with the activation of rRNA and protein synthesis and the consequent epithelial cell hypertrophy, results in cells entering the S phase and undergoing division. In the epithelium of both mice and humans, P_4 inhibits E_2 action on cell proliferation. In mice, P_4 inhibits both of the E_2-induced cell cycle regulatory pathways without influencing cellular hypertrophy, although there are

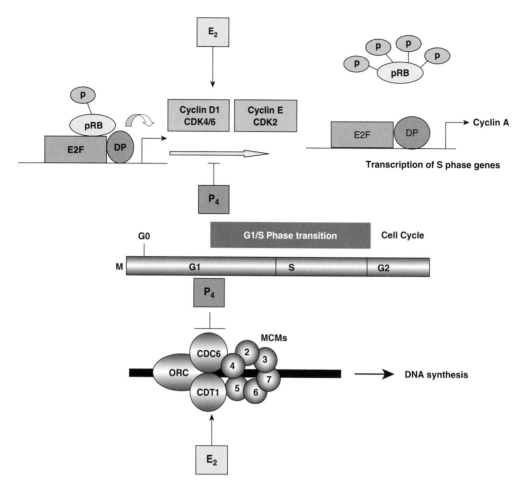

Figure 8.5   Progesterone antagonizes two estrogen-induced cell cycle regulatory pathways in the mouse uterine epithelium. In adult uterine epithelial cells, E_2 stimulates two pathways that appear to run in parallel: the cyclin-dependent cell cycle regulatory machinery and DNA replication licensing. These two pathways converge at the G_1–S transition to activate DNA synthesis. P_4 blocks both these pathways and thereby completely inhibits the E_2-induced DNA synthesis.

many genes whose transcriptional abundance is altered by P_4. E_2-induced cell proliferation is blocked, allowing for the differentiation of a receptive epithelium for blastocyst attachment and implantation. The identification of the molecular basis for the action of these hormones should lead to new therapeutic strategies for reproductive medicine and contraception. E_2 exposure is a major risk factor for endometrial and breast cancer, and understanding the mechanisms of its action will lead to new insights into the deregulation that occurs in these diseases.

REFERENCES

1. Bazer FW, Ott TL, Spender TE. Endocrinology of the transition from recurring estrous cycles to establishment of pregnancy in subprimate mammals. Endocrinol Pregnancy 1998; 134: 206–12.
2. Brenner RM, Slayden OD. Cyclic changes in the primate oviduct and endometrium. Physiol Reprod 1994; 1: 541–69.
3. Martin L, Finn CA. Hormone secretion during early pregnancy in the mouse. J Endocrinol 1969; 45: 57–65.
4. Moulton BC, Koenig BB. Uterine deoxyribonucleic acid synthesis during preimplantation in precursors of stromal cell differentiation during decidualization. Endocrinology 1984; 115: 1302–7.
5. Finn CA. In: Bishop MWH, ed. Ad. Reprod Physiol New York: Academic Press, 1971: 1–26.
6. Das RM, Martin L. Uterine DNA synthesis and cell proliferation during early decidualization induced by oil in mice. J Reprod Fertil 1978; 53: 125–8.
7. Finn CA, Porter DG. Handbooks in Reproductive Biology. The Uterus. London: Elek Science, 1975; 1.
8. Allen E, Smith CM, Gardner WU. Accentuation of the growth effect of theelin on genital tissues of the ovariectomized mouse by arrest of mitotis with colchicine. Am J Anat 1937; 61: 321–41.
9. Mueller GC. Estrogen action: a study of the influence of steroid hormones on genetic expression. Biochem Soc Symp 1971; 3: 1–29.
10. Clark BF. The effects of oestrogen and progesterone on uterine cell division and epithelial morphology in spayed, adrenalectomized rats. J Endocrinol 1971; 50: 527–8.
11. Martin L, Finn CA. In: Hubinont PO, Leroy F, Galand P eds. Basic Actions of Sex steroids on Target Organs Basel, Switzerland: S Karger, 1971: 172–88.
12. Martin L, Finn CA, Trinder G. Hypertrophy and hyperplasia in the mouse uterus after oestrogen treatment: an autoradiographic study. J Endocrinol 1973; 56: 133–44.

13. Martin L, Finn CA, Trinder G. DNA synthesis in the endometrium of progesterone-treated mice. J Endocrinol 1973; 56: 303–7.

14. Epifanova OI. Mitotic cycles in estrogen treated mice; a radioautographic study. Expl Cell Res 1966; 42: 562–77.

15. Martin L, Pollard JW, Fagg B. Oestriol, oestradiol-17β and the proliferation and death of uterine cells. J Endocrinol 1976; 69: 103–15.

16. Das RM. The effects of oestrogen on the cell cycle in epithelial and connective tissues of the mouse uterus. J Endocrinol 1972; 55: 21–30.

17. Galand P, de Maertelaer V. Models of oestrogen action: a cell kineticist's view. Epithelial Cell Biol 1992; 1: 177–88.

18. Clarke CL, Sutherland RL. Progestin regulation of cellular proliferation. Endocr Rev 1990; 11: 266–301.

19. Terada N, Yamamoto R, Takada T et al. Inhibitory effect of progesterone on cell death of mouse uterine epithelium. J Steroid Biochem 1989; 33: 1091–6.

20. Finn CA, Martin L, Carter J. A refractory period following oestrogenic stimulation of cell division in the mouse uterus. J Endocrinol 1969; 44: 121–6.

21. Martin L, Finn CA. Interactions of oestradiol and progestins in the mouse uterus. J Endocrinol 1970; 48: 109–15.

22. Finn CA, Martin L. The onset of progesterone secretion during pregnancy in the mouse. J Reprod Fertil 1971; 25: 299–300.

23. Das RM, Martin L. Progesterone inhibition of mouse uterine epithelial proliferation. J Endocrinol 1973; 59: 205–6.

24. Martin L, Das RM, Finn CA. The inhibition by progesterone of uterine epithelial proliferation in the mouse. J Endocrinol 1973; 57: 549–54.

25. Pollard JW, Pacy J, Cheng SVY, Jordan EG. Estrogens and cell death in the mouse uterine luminal epithelium. Cell Tissue Res 1987; 249: 533–40.

26. Harris JA, Gorski J. Evidence for a discontinuous requirement for estrogen in stimulation of deoxyribonucleic acid synthesis in the immature rat uterus. Endocrinology 1978; 103: 240–4.

27. Stack G, Gorski J. Estrogen-stimulated deoxyribonucleic acid synthesis: a ratchet model for the prereplicative period. Endocrinology 1985; 117: 2017–23.

28. Hewitt SC, Deroo BJ, Hansen K et al. Estrogen receptor-dependent genomic responses in the uterus mirror the biphasic physiological response to estrogen. Mol Endocrinol 2003; 17: 2070–83.

29. Ray S, Hou X, Zhou HE et al. Bip is a molecular link between the phase I and phase II estrogenic responses in uterus. Mol Endocrinol 2006; 20: 1825–37.

30. Lee AE. Cell division and DNA synthesis in the mouse uterus during continuous oestrogen treatment. J Endocrinol 1972; 55: 507–13.

31. Kaye AM, Sheratzky D, Lindner HR. Kinetics of DNA synthesis in immature rat uterus: age dependence and estradiol stimulation. Biochim Biophys Acta 1972; 261: 475–86.

32. Ogasawara Y, Okamoto S, Kitamura Y, Matsumoto K. Proliferative pattern of uterine cells from birth to adulthood in intact, neonatally castrated, and/or adrenalectomized mice, assayed by incorporation of [^{125}I]iododeoxyuridine. Endocrinology 1983; 113: 582–7.

33. Korach KS. Insights from the study of animals lacking functional estrogen receptor. Science 1994; 266: 1524–7.

34. Quarmby VE, Fox-Davies C, Korach KS. Estrogen action in the mouse uterus: the influence of the neuroendocrine-adrenal axis. Endocrinology 1984; 114: 108–15.

35. Kirkland JL, LaPointe L, Justin E, Stancel GM. Effects of estrogen on mitosis in individual cell types of the immature rat uterus. Biol Reprod 1979; 21: 269–72.

36. Sakamoto S, Abe A, Kudo H et al. Effects of estrogen and progesterone on thymidine kinase activity in the immature rat uterus. Am J Obstet Gynecol 1983; 145: 711–15.

37. Tabibzadeh, S. Cytokines and the hypothalamic–pituitary–ovarian–endometrial axis. Hum Reprod Update 1994; 9: 947–67.

38. Kato K, Yoshimoto M, Kato K et al. Characterization of side-population cells in human normal endometrium. Hum Reprod 2007; 22: 1214–23.

39. Gargett CE. Uterine stem cells: what is the evidence? Hum Reprod Update 2007; 13: 87–101.

40. Tabibzadeh S. Proliferative activity of lymphoid cells in human endometrium throughout the menstrual cycle. J Clin Endocrinol Metab 1990; 70: 437–43.

41. Ferenczy A, Bertrand G, Gelfand MM. Proliferation kinetics of human endometrium during the normal menstrual cycle. Am J Obstet Gynecol 1979; 133: 859–67.

42. Brenner RM, Slayden OD, Rodgers WH et al. Immunocytochemical assessment of mitotic activity with an antibody to phosphorylated histone H3 in the macaque and human endometrium. Hum Reprod 2003; 18: 1185–93.

43. Shiozawa T, Li Sf, Nakayama K, Nikaido T, Fujii S. Relationship between the expression of cyclins/cyclin-dependent kinases and sex-steroid receptors/Ki67 in normal human endometrial glands and stroma during the menstrual cycle. Mol Hum Reprod 1996; 2: 745–52.

44. Niklaus AL, Aubuchon M, Zapantis G et al. Assessment of the proliferative status of epithelial cell types in the endometrium of young and menopausal transition women. Hum Reprod 2007; 22: 1778–88.

45. Felix JC, Farahmand S. Endometrial glandular proliferation and estrogen receptor content during the normal menstrual cycle. Contraception 1997; 55: 19–22.

46. Stack G, Gorski J. Direct mitogenic effect of estrogen on the prepubertal rat uterus: studies on isolated nuclei. Endocrinology 1984; 115: 1141–50.

47. Cullingford TE, Pollard JW. RU 486 completely inhibits the action of progesterone on cell proliferation in the mouse uterus. J Reprod Fertil 1988; 83: 909–14.

48. Lydon JP, DeMayo FJ, Funk CR et al. Mice lacking progesterone receptor exhibit pleiotropic reproductive abnormalities. Genes Dev 1995; 9: 2266–78.

49. Cooke PS, Buchanan DL, Young P et al. Stromal estrogen receptors mediate mitogenic effects of estradiol on uterine epithelium. Proc Natl Acad Sci USA 1997; 94: 6535–40.

50. Cooke PS, Buchanan DL, Kurita T et al. In: Bazer FW, ed. Endocrinol Pregnancy. Totowa, NJ: Humana Press, 1998: 491–506.

51. Kurita T, Young P, Brody JR et al. Stromal progesterone receptors mediate the inhibitory effects of progesterone on estrogen-induced uterine epithelial cell deoxyribonucleic acid synthesis. Endocrinology 1998; 139: 4708–13.

52. Kurita T et al. The activation function-1 domain of estrogen receptor alpha in uterine stromal cells is required for mouse but not human uterine epithelial response to estrogen. Differentiation 2005; 73: 313–22.

53. O'Brien JE, Peterson TJ, Tong MH et al. Estrogen-induced proliferation of uterine epithelial cells is independent of estrogen receptor alpha binding to classical estrogen response elements. J Biol Chem 2006; 281: 26683–92.

54. Pedram A, Razandi M, Levin ER. Nature of functional estrogen receptors at the plasma membrane. Mol Endocrinol 2006; 20: 1996–2009.

55. Pollard JW, Bartocci A, Arceci R et al. Apparent role of the macrophage growth factor, CSF-1, in placental development. Nature 1987; 330: 484–6.

56. Pollard JW. Regulation of polypeptide growth factor synthesis and growth factor-related gene expression in the rat and mouse uterus before and after implantation. J Reprod Fertil 1990; 88: 721–31.

57. Pollard JW. In: Bazer FW, ed. Endocrinology of Pregnancy. Totowa, NJ: Humana Press, 1998: 59–82.

58. Rider V, Piva M. In: Bazer FW, ed. Endocrinology of Pregnancy. Totowa, NJ: Humana Press, 1998: 83–124.

59. Hunt JS. Immunobiology of pregnancy. Cur Opin Immunol 1992; 4: 591–6.

60. Robertson SA, Mau VJ, Hudson SN, Tremellen KP. Cytokine–leukocyte networks and the establishment of pregnancy. Am J Reprod Immunol 1997; 37: 438–42.

61. Pampfer S, Arceci RJ, Pollard JW. Role of colony stimulating factor-1 (CSF-1) and other lympho-hematopoietic growth factors in mouse preimplantation development. Bioessays 1991; 13: 535–40.

62. Hunt JS, Pollard JW. Macrophages in the uterus and placenta. Curr Prog Microbiol Immunol 1992; 181: 39–63.

63. Pollard JW. Lymphohematopoietic cytokines in the female reproductive tract. Curr Opin Immunol 1991; 3: 772–7.

64. Cullingford TE, Pollard JW. In: Khan SA, Stancel GM eds. Protooncogenes and Growth Factors in Steroid Hormone-Induced Growth Differentiation. Boca Raton, FL: CRC Press, 1994: 13–30.

65. Gouon-Evans V, Pollard JW. Eotaxin is required for eosinophil homing into the stroma of the pubertal and cycling uterus. Endocrinology 2001; 142: 4515–21.

66. Pollard JW, Lin EY, Zhu L. Complexity of uterine macrophage responses to cytokines in mice. Biol Reprod 1998; 58: 1469–75.

67. Robertson SA. Control of the immunological environment of the uterus. Rev Reprod 2000; 5: 164–74.

68. Chakraborty I, Das SK, Dey SK. Differential expression of vascular endothelial growth factor and its receptor mRNAs in the mouse uterus around the time of implantation. J Endocrinol 1995; 147: 339–52.

69. Hyder SM, Stancel GM, Chiappetta C et al. Uterine expression of vascular endothelial growth factor is increased by estradiol and tamoxifen. Cancer Res 1996; 56: 3954–60.

70. Wang XN, Das SK, Damm D et al. Differential regulation of heparin-binding epidermal growth factor-like growth factor in the adult ovariectomized mouse uterus by progesterone and estrogen. Endocrinology 1994; 135: 1264–71.

71. Das SK, Tsukamura H, Paria BC et al. Differential expression of epidermal growth factor receptor (EGF-R) gene and regulation of EGF-R bioactivity by progesterone and estrogen in the adult mouse uterus. Endocrinology 1994; 134: 971–81.

72. Han VKM, Hunter ESI, Pratt RM et al. Expression of rat transforming growth factor alpha mRNA during development occurs predominately in the maternal decidua. Mol Cel Biol 1987; 7: 2335–43.

73. Gardner RM, Verner G, Kirkland JL, Stancel GM. Regulation of uterine epidermal growth factor (EGF) receptors by estrogen in the mature rat and mouse during estrous cycle. J Steroid Biochem 1989; 32: 339–43.

74. Zhang Z, Funk C, Glasser SR, Mulholland J. Progesterone regulation of heparin-binding epidermal growth factor-like growth factor gene expression during sensitization and decidualization in the rat uterus: effects of the antiprogestin, ZK 98.299. Endocrinology 1994; 135: 1256–63.

75. Mukku VR, Stancel GM. Receptors for epidermal growth factors in the rat uterus. Endocrinology 1985; 117: 149–54.

76. Loose-Mitchell DS et al. In: Schomberg DW, ed. Growth Factors in Reproduction. Berlin: Springer Verlag, 1991: 185–95.

77. Lingham RB, Stancel GM, Loose-Mitchell DS. Estrogen regulation of epidermal growth factor receptor messenger ribonucleic acid. Mol Endocrinol 1988; 2: 230–5.

78. Nelson KG, Takahashi T, Bossert NL et al. Epidermal growth factor replaces estrogen in the stimulation of female genital-tract growth and differentiation. Proc Natl Acad Sci USA 1991; 88: 21–5.

79. Nelson KG, Takahashi T, Lee D et al. Transforming growth factor-α is a potential mediator of estrogen action in the mouse uterus. Endocrinology 1992; 131: 1657–64.

80. Luetteke NC, Qiu TH, Peiffer RL et al. TGF α deficiency results in hair follicle and eye abnormalities in targeted and waved-1 mice. Cell 1993; 73: 263–78.

81. Luetteke NC, Qiu TH, Fenton SE et al. Targeted inactivation of the EGF and amphiregulin genes reveals distinct roles for EGF receptor ligands in mouse mammary gland development. Development 1999; 126: 2739–50.

82. Threadgill DW, Dlugosz AA, Hansen LA et al. Targeted disruption of mouse EGF receptor: effect of genetic background on mutant phenotype. Science 1995; 269: 230–4.

83. Tomooka Y, DiAugustine RP, McLachlan JA. Proliferation of mouse uterine epithelial cells in vitro. Endocrinology 1986; 118: 1011–18.

84. Ignar-Trowbridge DM, Nelson KG, Bidwell MC et al. Coupling of dual signaling pathways: Epidermal growth factor action involves the estrogen receptor. Proc Natl Acad Sci USA 1992; 89: 4658–62.

85. Curtis SW, Washburn T, Sewall C et al. Physiological coupling of growth factor and steroid receptor signaling pathways: estrogen receptor knockout mice lack estrogen-like response to epidermal growth factor. Proc Natl Acad Sci USA 1996; 93: 12626–30.

86. Smith CL. Cross-talk between peptide growth factor and estrogen receptor signaling pathways. Biol Reprod 1998; 58: 627–32.

87. Ghahary A, Murphy LJ. Uterine insulin-like growth factor-I receptors: regulation by estrogen and variation throughout the estrous cycle. Endocrinology 1989; 125: 597–604.

88. Ghahary A, Chakrabarti S, Murphy LJ. Localization of the sites of synthesis and action of insulin-like growth factor-I in the rat uterus. Mol Endocrinol 1990; 4: 191–5.

89. Murphy LJ, Bell GI, Friesen HG. Tissue distribution of insulin-like growth factor 1 and 2 messenger ribonucleic acid in the adult rat. Endocrinology 1987; 120: 1279–82.

90. Murphy LJ, Murphy LC, Friesen HG. Estrogen induces insulin-like growth factor-I expression in the rat uterus. Mol Endocrinol 1987; 1: 445–50.

91. Murphy LJ, Ghahary A. Uterine insulin-like growth factor-I: Regulation of expression and its role in estrogen-induced uterine proliferation. Endocr Rev 1990; 11: 443–53.

92. Murphy LJ. Estrogen induction of insulin-like growth factors and myc proto-oncogene expression in the uterus. J Steroid Biochem Mol Biol 1991; 40: 223–30.

93. Kapur S, Tamada H, Dey SK, Andrews GK. Expression of insulin-like growth factor-I (IGF-1) and its receptor in the peri-implantation mouse uterus, and cell-specific regulation of IGF-1 gene expression by estradiol and progesterone. Biol Reprod 1992; 46: 208–19.

94. Baker J, Hardy MP, Zhou J et al. Effects of an Igf1 gene null mutation on mouse reproduction. Mol Endocrinol 1996; 10: 903–18.

95. Richards RG, DiAugustine RP, Petrusz P et al. Estradiol stimulates tyrosine phosphorylation of the insulin-like growth factor-1 receptor and insulin receptor substrate-1 in the uterus. Proc Natl Acad Sci USA 1996; 93: 12002–7.

96. Richards RG, Walker MP, Sebastian J, DiAugustine RP. Insulin-like growth factor-1 (IGF-1) receptor-insulin receptor substrate complexes in the uterus. Altered signaling response to estradiol in the IGF-1(m/m) mouse. J Biol Chem 1998; 273: 11962–9.

97. Klotz DM, Hewitt SC, Ciana P et al. Requirement of estrogen receptor-alpha in insulin-like growth factor-1 (IGF-1)-induced uterine responses and in vivo evidence for IGF-1/estrogen receptor cross-talk. J Biol Chem 2002; 277: 8531–7.

97a. Zhu L, Pollard JW. Estradiol-17β regulates mouse uterine epithelial cell proliferation through insulin like growth factor-1 signaling. Proc Natl Acad Sci USA 2007; 104 : 15847–50.

98. Sato T, Wang G, Hardy MP et al. Role of systemic and local IGF-1 in the effects of estrogen on growth and epithelial proliferation of mouse uterus. Endocrinology 2002; 143: 2673–9.

99. Adesanya OO, Zhou J, Samathanam C et al. Insulin-like growth factor 1 is required for G2 progression in the estradiol-induced mitotic cycle. Proc Natl Acad Sci USA 1999; 96: 3287–91.

100. Hana V, Murphy LJ. Interdependence of epidermal growth factor and insulin-like growth factor-I expression in the mouse. Endocrinology 1994; 135: 107–12.

101. Hom YK, Young P, Thomson AA, Cunha GR. Keratinocyte growth factor injected into female mouse neonates stimulates uterine and vaginal epithelial growth. Endocrinology 1998; 139: 3772–9.

102. Mericskay M, Kitajewski J, Sassoon D. Wnt5a is required for proper epithelial–mesenchymal interactions in the uterus. Development 2004; 131: 2061–72.

103. Hou X, Tan Y, Li M et al. Canonical Wnt signaling is critical to estrogen mediated uterine growth. Mol Endocrinol 2004; 18: 3035–4.

104. Mohamed OA, Jonnaert M, Labelle-Dumais C et al. Uterine Wnt/beta-catenin signaling is required for implantation. Proc Natl Acad Sci USA 2005; 102: 8579–84.

105. Mohamed OA, Dufort D, Clarke HJ. Expression and estradiol regulation of Wnt genes in the mouse blastocyst identify a candidate pathway for embryo–maternal signaling at implantation. Biol Reprod 2004; 71: 417–24.

106. Li J, Zhang JV, Cao YJ et al. Inhibition of the beta-catenin signaling pathway in blastocyst and uterus during the window of implantation in mice. Biol Reprod 2005; 72: 700–6.

107. Brigstock DR. In: Bailliere's Clinical Endocrinology and Metabolism. Bailliere Tindall, 1991: 791–808.

108. Lee DS, Yanagimoto Ueta Y, Xuan X et al. Expression patterns of the implantation-associated genes in the uterus during the estrous cycle in mice. J Reprod Dev 2005; 51: 787–98.

109. Tamada H, McMaster MT, Flanders KC et al. Cell type-specific expression of transforming growth factor-b1 in the mouse uterus during the peri-implantation period. Mol Endocrinol 1990; 4: 965–72.

110. Hunt JS, Chen HL, Hu XL, Pollard JW. Analysis of tumor necrosis factor-alpha gene expression in virgin and pregnant normal and osteopetrotic (op/op) mice. Biol Reprod 1993; 49: 441–52.

111. Ingman WV, Robker RL, Woittiez K, Robertson SA. Null mutation in transforming growth factor beta1 disrupts ovarian function and causes oocyte incompetence and early embryo arrest. Endocrinology 2006; 147: 835–45.

112. Tremellen KP, Seamark RF, Robertson SA. Seminal transforming growth factor beta1 stimulates granulocyte-macrophage colony-stimulating factor production and inflammatory cell recruitment in the murine uterus. Biol Reprod 1998; 58: 1217–25.

113. Martin L, Finn CA, Carter J. Effects of progesterone and oestradiol-17 beta on the luminal epithelium of the mouse uterus. J Reprod Fertil 1970; 21: 461–9.

114. Hunt JS, Robertson SA. Uterine macrophages and enviromental programming for pregnancy success. J Reprod Immunol 1996; 32: 1–25.

115. Leroy F, Bogaert C, Van Hoeck J. Stimulation of cell division in the endometrial epithelium of the rat by uterine distention. J Endocrinol 1976; 70: 517–18.

116. Galand P, Tchernitchin N, Tchernitchin AN. Dissociation of uterine eosinophilia and water imbibition from other estrogen-induced responses by nafoxidine pretreatment. Mol Cell Endocrinol 1985; 42: 227–33.

117. Grunert G, Porcia M, Tchernitchin AN. Differential potency of oestradiol-17 beta and diethylstilboestrol on separate groups of responses in the rat uterus. J Endocrinol 1986; 110: 103–14.

118. Hastings JM, Licence DR, Burton GJ et al. Soluble vascular endothelial growth factor receptor 1 inhibits edema and epithelial proliferation induced by 17beta-estradiol in the mouse uterus. Endocrinology 2003; 144: 326–34.

119. Soto AM, Sonnenschein C. Cell proliferation of estrogen-sensitive cells: the case for negative control. Endocrin Rev 1987; 8: 44–51.

120. Wada-Hiraike O, Hiraike H, Okinaga H et al. Role of estrogen receptor beta in uterine stroma and epithelium: insights from estrogen receptor beta-/- mice. Proc Natl Acad Sci USA 2006; 103: 18350–5.

121. Pollard JW, Hunt JS, Wiktor-Jedrzejczak W, Stanley ER. A pregnancy defect in the osteopetrotic (op/op) mouse demonstrates the requirement for CSF-1 in female fertility. Dev Biol 1991; 148: 273–83.

122. De M, Sanford T, Wood GW. Relationship between macrophage colony-stimulating factor production by uterine epithelial cells and accumulation and distribution of macrophages in the uterus of pregnant mice. J Leukocyte Biol 1993; 53: 240–8.

123. Webb SE, Pollard JW, Jones GE. Direct observation and quantification of macrophage chemoattraction to the growth factor CSF-1. J Cell Sci 1996; 109: 793–803.

124. Stanley ER, Guilbert LT, Tushinski RJ, Bartelmez SH. CSF-1–a mononuclear phagocyte lineage-specific hemopoietic growth factor. J Cell Biochem 1983; 21: 151–9.

125. Cohen PE, Zhu L, Pollard JW. The absence of CSF-1 in osteopetrotic (csfm^op/csfm^op) mice disrupts estrous cycles and ovulation. Biol Reprod 1997; 56: 110–18.

126. Xu Q, Leiva MC, Fischkoff SA, Handschumacher RE, Lyttle CR. Leukocyte chemotactic activity of cyclophilin. J Biol Chem 1992; 267: 11968–71.

127. Gouon-Evans V, Lin EY, Pollard JW. Requirement of macrophages and eosinophils and their cytokines/chemokines for mammary gland development. Breast Cancer Res 2002; 4: 155–64.

128. Tchernitchin AN, Mena MA, Soto J, Unda C. The role of eosinophils in the action of estrogens and other hormones. Med Sci Res 1989; 17: 5–10.

129. Bigsby RM, Cunha GR. Effects of progestins and glucocorticoids on deoxyribonucleic acid synthesis in the uterus of the neonatal mouse. Endocrinology 1985; 117: 2520–6.

130. Boettger-Tong HL, Stancel GM. Retinoic acid inhibits estrogen-induced uterine stromal and myometrial cell proliferation. Endocrinology 1995; 136: 2975–83.

131. Zhu YS, Yen PM, Chin WW, Pfaff DW. Estrogen and thyroid hormone interaction on regulation of gene expression. Proc Natl Acad Sci USA 1996; 93: 12587–92.

132. Roper RJ, Griffith JS, Lyttle CR et al. Interacting quantitative trait loci control phenotypic variation in murine estradiol-regulated responses. Endocrinology 1999; 140: 556–61.

133. Griffith JS, Jensen SM, Lunceford JK et al. Evidence for the genetic control of estradiol-regulated responses. Implications for variation in normal and pathological hormone-dependent phenotypes. Am J Pathol 1997; 150: 2223–30.

134. Wendell DL, Gorski J. Quantitative trait loci for estrogen-dependent pituitary tumor growth in the rat. Mamm Genome 1997; 8: 823–9.

135. Tabibzadeh S. Human endometrium: an active site of cytokine production and action. Endocr Rev 1991; 12: 272–90.

136. Tabibzadeh S. Role of cytokines in endometrium and at the fetomaternal interface. Reprod Med Rev 1994; 3: 11–28.

137. Dimitriadis E, White CA, Jones RL, Salamonsen LA. Cytokines, chemokines and growth factors in endometrium related to implantation. Hum Reprod Update 2005; 11: 613–30.

138. Stewart CJR, Maura A, Farquharson A, Foulis AK. The distribution and possible function of gamma-interferon immunoreactive cells in normal endometrium and myometrium. Virchows Arch A Pathol Anat 1992; 420: 419–24.

139. Tseng L, Gurpide E. Induction of human endometrial estradiol dehydrogenase by progestins. Endocrinology 1975; 97: 825–33.

140. Tabibzadeh S, Zupi E, Babaknia A et al. Site and menstrual cycle-dependent expression of proteins of the tumour necrosis factor (TNF) receptor family, and BCL-2 oncoprotein and phase-specific production of TNF α in human endometrium. Hum Reprod 1995; 10: 277–86.

141. Hunt JS. Expression and regulation of the tumour necrosis factor-α gene in the female reproductive tract. Reprod Fertil Dev 1993; 5: 141–53.

142. Shalaby MR, Laegreid WW, Ammann AJ, Liggitt HD. Tumor necrosis factor-alpha-associated uterine endothelial injury in vivo. Influence of dietary fat. Lab Invest 1989; 61: 564–70.

143. Sugawara J, Fukaya T, Murakami T, Yoshida H, Yajima A. Hepatocyte growth factor stimulates proliferation, migration, and lumen formation of human endometrial epithelial cells in vitro. Biol Reprod 1997; 57: 936–42.

144. Stewart CL, Kaspar P, Brunet LJ et al. Blastocyst implantation depends on maternal expression of leukaemia inhibitory factor. Nature 1992; 359: 76–9.

145. Bhatt H, Brunet LJ, Stewart CL. Uterine expression of leukemia inhibitory factor coincides with the onset of blastocyst implantation. Proc Natl Acad Sci USA 1991; 88: 11408–12.

146. Kennedy TG. In: Hillier K, ed. Eicosanoids and Reproduction. Lancaster: MTP Press, 1996: 73–88.

147. Lim H, Paria BC, Das SK et al. Multiple female reproductive failures in cyclooxygenase 2-deficient mice. Cell 1997; 91: 197–208.

148. Bagchi MK, Mantena SR, Kannan A, Bagchi IC. Control of uterine cell proliferation and differentiation by C/EBPbeta: functional implications for establishment of early pregnancy. Cell Cycle 2006; 5: 922–5.

149. Cheng JG, Shatzer T, Sewell L et al. Leukemia inhibitory factor can substitute for nidatory estrogen and is essential to inducing a receptive uterus for implantation but is not essential for subsequent embryogenesis. Endocrinology 2000; 141: 4365–72.

150. Lee K, Jeong J, Kwak I et al. Indian hedgehog is a major mediator of progesterone signaling in the mouse uterus. Nat Genet 2006; 38: 1204–9.

151. Bigsby RM, Caperell-Grant A, Berry N et al. Estrogen induces a systemic growth factor through an estrogen receptor-alpha-dependent mechanism. Biol Reprod 2004; 70: 178–83.

152. Ogle TF, George P, Dai D. Progesterone and estrogen regulation of rat decidual cell expression of proliferating cell nuclear antigen. Biol Reprod 1998; 59: 444–50.

153. Finn CA. Oestrogen and the decidual cell reaction of implantation in mice. J Endocrinol 1965; 32: 223–9.

154. Pollard JW, Martin L, Finn CA. Actinomycin D and uterine epithelial protein synthesis. J Endocrinol 1976; 69: 161–2.

155. Clark DA. Cytokines, decidua and early pregnancy. Oxf Rev Reprod Biol 1992; 16: 83–111.

156. Manova K, Paynton BV, Bachvarova RF. Expression of activins and TGF beta 1 and beta 2 RNAs in early postimplantation mouse embryos and uterine decidua. Mech Dev 1992; 36: 141–52.

157. Lea RG, Flanders KC, Harley EB et al. Release of transforming growth factor (TGF)-beta 2-related suppressor factor from postimplantation murine decidual tissue can be correlated with the detection of a subpopulation of cells containing RNA for TGF-beta 2. J Immunol 1992; 148: 778–87.

158. Cheng HL, Schneider SL, Kane CM et al. TGF-beta 2 gene and protein expression in maternal and fetal tissues at various stages of murine development. J Reprod Immunol 1993; 25: 133–48.

159. Tamada H, Das SK, Andrews GK, Dey SK. Cell-type-specific expression of transforming growth factor-a in the mouse uterus during the peri-implantation period. Biol Reprod 1991; 45: 365–72.

160. Zhang Z, Funk C, Roy D et al. Heparin-binding epidermal growth factor-like growth factor is differentially regulated by progesterone and estradiol in rat uterine epithelial and stromal cells. Endocrinology 1994; 134: 1089–94.

161. Brown MJ, Zogg JL, Schultz GS, Hilton FK. Increased binding of epidermal growth factor at preimplantation sites in mouse uteri. Endocrinology 1989; 124: 2882–8.

162. Wordinger RJ, Smith KJ, Bell C, Chang IFC. The immunolocalization of basic fibroblast growth factor in the mouse uterus during the initial stages of embryo implantation. Growth Factors 1994; 11: 175–86.

163. Arceci RJ, Pampfer S, Pollard JW. Role and expression of colony-stimulating factor-1 and steel factor receptors and their ligands during pregnancy in the mouse. Reprod Fertil Dev 1992; 4: 619–32.

164. Piva M, Flieger O, Rider V. Growth factor control of cultured rat uterine stromal cell proliferation is progesterone dependent. Biol Reprod 1996; 55: 1333–42.

165. Irwin JC, Utian WH, Eckert RL. Sex steroids and growth factors differentially regulate the growth and differentiation of cultured human endometrial stromal cells. Endocrinology 1991; 129: 2385–92.

166. Rider V, Kimler BF, Justice WM. Progesterone–growth factor interactions in uterine stromal cells. Biol Reprod 1998; 59: 464–9.

167. Bilinski P, Roopenian D, Gossler A. Maternal IL-11Ralpha function is required for normal decidua and fetoplacental development in mice. Genes Dev 1998; 12: 2234–43.

168. Bao L, Devi S, Bowen-Shauver J et al. The role of interleukin-11 in pregnancy involves up-regulation of alpha2-macroglobulin gene through janus kinase 2-signal transducer and activator of transcription 3 pathway in the decidua. Mol Endocrinol 2006; 20: 3240–50.

169. Ain R, Trinh ML, Soares MJ. Interleukin-11 signaling is required for the differentiation of natural killer cells at the maternal–fetal interface. Dev Dyn 2004; 231: 700–8.

170. Barber EM, Pollard JW. The uterine NK cell population requires IL-15 but these cells are not required for pregnancy nor the resolution of a Listeria monocytogenes infection. J Immunol 2003; 171: 37–46.

171. Moulton BC. Transforming growth factor-beta stimulates endometrial stromal apoptosis in vitro. Endocrinology 1994; 134: 1055–60.

172. Bulmer JN, Johnson PM. Macrophage populations in the human placenta and amniochorion. Clin Exp Immunol 1984; 57: 393–403.

173. Bulmer JN, Ritson A, Pace D. In: Denker HW, Aplin JD eds. Trophoblast Research. New York: Plenum, 1996: 431–51.

174. Bulmer JN. In: Bronson RA, Alexander NJ, Anderson D, Branch DW, Kutteh WH, eds. Reproductive Immunology. Oxford: Blackwell Sciences, 1996: 212–39.

175. Daiter E, Pampter S, Yeung YG et al. Expression of colony stimulating factor-1 in the human uterus and placenta. J Clin Endocrinol Metab 1992; 74: 850–8.

176. Daiter E, Pollard JW. Colony stimulating factor-1 (CSF-1) in pregnancy. Reprod Med Rev 1992; 1: 83–97.

177. Charnock-Jones DS, Sharkey AM, Fenwick P, Smith SK. Leukaemia inhibitory factor mRNA concentration peaks in human endometrium at the time of implantation and the blastocyst contains mRNA for the receptor at this time. J Reprod Fertil 1994; 101: 421–6.

178. Cullinan EB, Abbondanzo SJ, Anderson PS et al. Leukemia inhibitory factor (LIF) and LIF receptor expression in human endometrium suggests a potential autocrine/paracrine function

in regulating embryo implantation. Proc Natl Acad Sci USA 1996; 93: 3115–20.

179. Sharkey AM, Charnock-Jones DS, Boocock CA et al. Expression of mRNA for vascular endothelial growth factor in human placenta. J Reprod Fertil 1993; 99: 609–15.

180. Kao LC, Tulac S, Lobo S et al. Global gene profiling in human endometrium during the window of implantation. Endocrinology 2002; 143: 2119–38.

181. Pardee AB. G$_1$ events and regulation of cell proliferation. Science 1989; 246: 603–8.

182. Smith JA, Martin L. Do cells cycle? Proc Natl Acad Sci USA 1973; 70: 1263–7.

183. Quarmby VE, Korach KS. The influence of 17 beta-estradiol on patterns of cell division in the uterus. Endocrinology 1984; 114: 694–702.

184. Clark BF. Absence of oestradiol-17 beta dehydrogenase from the progesterone-dominated mouse uterus. J Endocrinol 1980; 85: 155–9.

185. Quarmby VE, Martin L. Effects of progesterone on uptake and metabolism of 17 beta-estradiol by mouse uterine luminal epithelium. Mol Cell Endocrinol 1982; 27: 317–30.

186. Quarmby VE, Martin L. Qualitative effects of progesterone on estrogen binding in mouse uterine luminal epithelium. Mol Cell Endocrinol 1982; 27: 331–42.

187. Cheng SV, MacDonald BS, Clark BF, Pollard JW. Cell growth and cell proliferation may be dissociated in the mouse uterine luminal epithelium treated with female sex steroids. Exp Cell Res 1985; 160: 459–70.

188. Fagg B, Martin L, Rogers L et al. A simple method for removing the luminal epithelium of the mouse uterus for biochemical studies. J Reprod Fertil 1979; 57: 335–9.

189. Mani SK, Decker GL, Glasser SR. Hormonal responsiveness by immature rabbit uterine epithelial cells polarized in vitro. Endocrinology 1991; 128: 1563–73.

190. Loose-Mitchell DS, Chiappetta C, Stancel GM. Estrogen regulation of c-fos messenger ribonucleic acid. Mol Endocrinol 1988; 2: 946–51.

191. Boettger-Tong HL, Murthy L, Stancel GM. Cellular pattern of c-fos induction by estradiol in the immature rat uterus. Biol Reprod 1995; 53: 1398–406.

192. Nephew KP, Peters GA, Khan SA. Cellular localization of estradiol-induced c-fos messenger ribonucleic acid in the rat uterus: c-fos expression and uterine cell proliferation do not correlate strictly. Endocrinology 1995; 136: 3007–15.

193. Nephew KP, Tang M, Khan SA. Estrogen differentially affects c-jun expression in uterine tissue compartments. Endocrinology 1994; 134: 1827–34.

194. Travers MT, Knowler JT. Oestrogen-induced expression of oncogenes in the immature rat uterus. FEBS Letts 1987; 211: 27–30.

195. Murphy LJ, Murphy LC, Friesen HG. Estrogen induction of N-myc and c-myc proto-oncogene expression in the rat uterus. Endocrinology 1987; 120: 1882–8.

196. Webb DK, Moulton BC, Khan SA. Estrogen induces expression of c-jun and jun-B protooncogenes in specific rat uterine cells. Endocrinology 1993; 133: 20–8.

197. Yamashita S, Takayanagi A, Shimizu N. Temporal and cell-type specific expression of c-fos and c-jun protooncogenes in the mouse uterus after estrogen stimulation. Endocrinology 1996; 137: 5468–75.

198. Papa M, Mezzogiorno V, Bresciani F, Weisz A. Estrogen induces c-fos expression specifically in the luminal and glandular epithelia of adult rat uterus. Biochem Biophy Res Comm 1991; 175: 480–5.

199. Cheng SV, Pollard JW. c-rasH and ornithine decarboxylase are induced by oestradiol-17 beta in the mouse uterine luminal epithelium independently of the proliferative status of the cell. FEBS Lett 1986; 196: 309–14.

200. Huet-Hudson YM, Andrews GK, Dey SK. Cell type-specific localization of c-myc protein in the mouse uterus: modulation by steroid hormones and analysis of the periimplantation period. Endocrinology 1989; 125: 1683–90.

201. Persico E, Scalona M, Cicatiello L et al. Activation of 'immediate-early' genes by estrogen is not sufficient to achieve stimulation of DNA synthesis in rat uterus. Biochem Biophy Res Comm 1990; 171: 287–92.

202. Kirkland JL, Murphy L, Stancel GM. Progesterone inhibits the estrogen-induced expression of c-fos messenger ribonucleic acid in the uterus. Endocrinology 1992; 130: 3223–30.

203. Weisz A, Bresciani F. Estrogen induces expression of c-fos and c-myc protooncogenes in rat uterus. Mol Endocrinol 1988; 2: 816–24.

204. Weisz A, Rosales R. Identification of an estrogen response element upstream of the human c-fos gene that binds the estrogen receptor and the AP-1 transcription factor. Nucleic Acids Res 1990; 18: 5097–106.

205. Hyder SM, Nawaz Z, Chiappetta C et al. The protooncogene c-jun contains an unusual estrogen-inducible enhancer within the coding sequence. J Biol Chem 1995; 270: 8506–13.

206. Pan H, Zhu L, Deng Y, Pollard JW. Microarray analysis of uterine epithelial gene expression during the implantation window in the mouse. Endocrinology 2006; 147: 4904–16.

207. Baker DJ, Nagy F, Nieder GL. Localization of c-fos-like proteins in the mouse endometrium during the peri-implantation period. Biol Reprod 1992; 47: 492–501.

208. Nephew KP, Polek TC, Khan SA. Tamoxifen-induced proto-oncogene expression persists in uterine endometrial epithelium. Endocrinology 1996; 137: 219–24.

209. Nephew KP, Polek TC, Akcali KC, Khan SA. The antiestrogen tamoxifen induces c-fos and jun-B, but not c-jun or jun D, protooncogenes in the rat uterus. Endocrinology 1993; 133: 419–22.

210. Bigsby RM, Li A. Differentially regulated immediate early genes in the rat uterus. Endocrinology 1994; 134: 1820–6.

211. Murray AW. Recycling the cell cycle: cyclins revisited. Cell 2004; 116: 221–34.

212. Landis MW, Pawlyk BS, Li T et al. Cyclin D1-dependent kinase activity in murine development and mammary tumorigenesis. Cancer Cell 2006; 9: 13–22.

213. Ji P, Golden L, Ren H et al. Skp2 contains a novel cyclin A binding domain that directly protects cyclin A from inhibition by p27Kip1. J Biol Chem 2006; 281: 24058–69.

214. Sherr CJ. G1 phase progression: cycling on cue. Cell 1994; 79: 551–5.

215. Sherr CJ, Roberts JM. Inhibitors of mammalian G1 cyclin-dependent kinases. Genes Dev 1995; 9: 1149–63.

216. Sherr CJ. Cancer cell cycles. Science 1996; 274: 1672–7.

217. Diehl JA, Cheng M, Roussel MF, Sherr CJ. Glycogen synthase kinase-3B regulates cyclin D1 proteolysis and subcellular localization. Genes Dev 1998; 12: 3499–511.

218. Tong W, Pollard JW. Progesterone inhibits estrogen-induced cyclin D1 and cdk4 nuclear translocation, cyclin E,A-cdk2 kinase activation and cell proliferation in uterine epithelial cells in mice. Mol Cell Biol 1999; 19: 2252–64.

219. Tye BK. MCM proteins in DNA replication. Annu Rev Biochem 1999; 68: 649–86.

220. Forsburg SL. Eukaryotic MCM proteins: beyond replication initiation. Microbiol Mol Biol Rev 2004; 68: 109–31.

221. Kearsey SE, Cotterill S. Enigmatic variations: divergent modes of regulating eukaryotic DNA replication. Mol Cell 2003; 12: 1067–75.

222. Hua XH, Newport J. Identification of a preinitiation step in DNA replication that is independent of origin recognition complex and cdc6, but dependent on cdk2. J Cell Biol 1998; 140: 271–81.

223. Donovan S, Harwood J, Drury LS, Diffley JF. Cdc6p-dependent loading of Mcm proteins onto pre-replicative chromatin in budding yeast. Proc Natl Acad Sci USA 1997; 94: 5611–16.

224. Geum D, Sun W, Paik SK et al. Estrogen-induced D1 and D3 gene expressions during mouse uterine cell proliferation in vivo: differential induction mechanism of cyclin D1 and D3. Mol Reprod Dev 1997; 46: 450–8.

225. Zhang Z, Laping J, Glasser S et al. Mediators of estradiol-stimulated mitosis in the rat uterine luminal epithelium. Endocrinology 1998; 139: 961–6.

226. Musgrove EA, Lee CSL, Buckley MF, Sutherland RL. Cyclin D1 induction in breast cancer cells shortens G1 and is sufficient for cells arrested in G1 to complete the cell cycle. Proc Natl Acad Sci USA 1994; 91: 8022–6.

227. Prall OWJ, Sarcevic B, Musgrove EA et al. Estrogen-induced activation of cdk4 and cdk2 during G1–S phase progression is accompanied by increased cyclin D1 expression and decreased cyclin-dependent kinase inhibition association. J Biol Chem 1997; 272: 10882–94.

228. Planas-Silva M, Weinberg RA. Estrogen-dependent cyclin E-cdk2 activation through p21 redistribution. Mol Cell Biol 1997; 17: 4059–69.

229. Zwijsen RML, Wientjens E, Kolmpmaker R et al. CDK-independent activation of estrogen receptor by cyclin D1. Cell 1997; 88: 405–15.

230. Zwijsen RML, Buckle RS, Hijmans EM et al. Ligand-independent recruitment of steroid receptor coactivators to estrogen receptor by cyclin D1. Genes Deve 1998; 12: 3488–98.

231. Neuman E, Ladha MH, Lin N et al. Cyclin D1 stimulation of estrogen receptor transcriptional activity independent of cdk4. Mol Cell Biol 1997; 17: 5338–47.

232. Altucci L, Addeo R, Cicutiello L et al. Estrogen induces early and timed activation of cyclin-dependent kinases 4, 5, and 6 and increases cyclin messenger ribonucleic acid expression in rat uterus. Endocrinology 1997; 138: 978–84.

233. Tan J, Raja S, Davis MK et al. Evidence for coordinated interaction of cyclin D3 with p21 and cdk6 in directing the development of uterine stromal cell decidualization and polyploidy during implantation. Mech Dev 2002; 111: 99–113.

234. Tan Y, Li M, Cox S et al. HB-EGF directs stromal cell polyploidy and decidualization via cyclin D3 during implantation. Dev Biol 2004; 265: 181–95.

235. Tong W, Kiyokawa H, Soos TJ et al. The absence of p27[Kip1], an inhibitor of G1 cyclin-dependent kinases, uncouples differentiation and growth arrest during the granulosa→luteal transition. Cell Growth Differ 1998; 9: 787–94.

236. Nikaido T, Li Sf, Shiozawa T, Fujii S. Coabnormal expression of cyclin D1 and p53 protein in human uterine endometrial carcinomas. Cancer 1996; 78: 1248–53.

237. Shiozawa T, Li SF, Nakayama K, Nikaido T, Fujii S. Relationship between the expression of cyclins/cyclin-dependent kinases and sex-steroid receptors/Ki67 in normal human endometrial glands and stroma during the menstrual cycle. Mol Hum Reprod 1996; 2: 745–52.

238. Shiozawa T, Nikaido T, Shimizu M et al. Immunohistochemical analysis of the expression of cdk4 and p16INK4 in human endometrioid-type endometrial carcinoma. Cancer 1997; 80: 2250–6.

239. Shiozawa T, Nikaido T, Nakayama K et al. Involvement of cyclin-dependent kinase inhibitor p27Kip1 in growth inhibition of endometrium in the secretory phase and of hyperplastic endometrium treated with progesterone. Mol Hum Reprod 1998; 4: 899–905.

240. Moyer DL, Felix JC. The effects of progesterone and progestins on endometrial proliferation. Contraception 1998; 57: 399–403.

241. Tong W, Pollard JW. Genetic evidence for the interactions of cyclin D1 and p27(Kip1) in mice. Mol Cell Biol 2001; 21: 1319–28.

242. Chen B, Pan H, Zhu L et al. Progesterone inhibits the estrogen-induced phosphoinositide 3-kinase→AKT→GSK-3beta→cyclin D1→pRB pathway to block uterine epithelial cell proliferation. Mol Endocrinol 2005; 19: 1978–90.

243. Pan H, Deng Y, Pollard JW. Progesterone blocks estrogen-induced DNA synthesis through inhibition of replication licensing. Proc Natl Acad Sci USA 2006; 103: 14021–6.

244. Simmen RC, Zhang XL, Zhang D et al. Expression and regulatory function of the transcription factor Sp1 in the uterine endometrium at early pregnancy: implications for epithelial phenotype. Mol Cell Endocrinol 2000; 159: 159–70.

245. Morita M, Kobayashi A, Yamashita T et al. Functional analysis of basic transcription element binding protein by gene targeting technology. Mol Cell Biol 2003; 23: 2489–500.

246. Zhang XL, Zhang D, Michel EJ et al. Selective interactions of Kruppel-like factor 9/basic transcription element-binding protein with progesterone receptor isoforms A and B determine transcriptional activity of progesterone-responsive genes in endometrial epithelial cells. J Biol Chem 2003; 278: 21474–82.

247. Simmen RC, Eason RR, McQuown et al. Subfertility, uterine hypoplasia, and partial progesterone resistance in mice lacking the Kruppel-like factor 9/basic transcription element-binding protein-1 (Bteb1) gene. J Biol Chem 2004; 279: 29286–94.

248. Velarde MC, Geng Y, Eason RR et al. Null mutation of kruppel-like factor9/basic transcription element binding protein-1 alters peri-implantation uterine development in mice. Biol Reprod 2005; 73: 472–81.

249. Mantena SR, Kannan A, Cheon YP et al. C/EBPbeta is a critical mediator of steroid hormone-regulated cell proliferation and differentiation in the uterine epithelium and stroma. Proc Natl Acad Sci USA 2006; 103: 1870–5.

250. Taylor HS, Daftary GS, Selam B. Endometrial HOXA10 expression after controlled ovarian hyperstimulation with recombinant follicle-stimulating hormone. Fertil Steril 2003; 80(Suppl 2): 839–43.

251. Taylor HS, Fei X. Emx2 regulates mammalian reproduction by altering endometrial cell proliferation. Mol Endocrinol 2005; 19: 2839–46.

252. Stanners CP, Adams ME, Harkins JL, Pollard JW. Transformed cells have lost control of ribosome number through their growth cycle. J Cell Physiol 1979; 100: 127–38.

253. Brooks RF, Shields R. Cell growth, cell division and cell size homeostasis in Swiss 3T3 cells. Exp Cell Res 1985; 156: 1–6

9 Progesterone antagonists and the non-human primate endometrium

Robert M Brenner and Ov D Slayden

INTRODUCTION

The importance of progesterone (P) in reproductive physiology cannot be overestimated. Progesterone prepares the uterus for implantation and is key to the maintenance of pregnancy.[1–3] Like other steroid hormones, the genomic effects of P are mediated through interactions with specific intracellular progesterone receptors (PRs). Because PRs play key roles in so many aspects of human reproduction, numerous PR ligands with either agonist or antagonist actions have been synthesized by pharmaceutical companies to modulate the actions of this key hormone. Compounds with mixed agonist and antagonist effects, known as selective progesterone receptor modulators (SPRMs),[4,5] are the most recently developed ligands, and these are reviewed in Chapter 38. A recent, very thorough review of the human endometrium has been published in Endocrine Reviews, with extensive coverage of normal physiology, angiogenesis, steroid receptors, cytokines, and menstruation.[6] In this chapter, we focus on strongly antagonistic ligands (antiprogestins, PR antagonists; abbreviated here as PAs) and their effects on the non-human primate endometrium. For preclinical studies of endometrial effects of PAs, non-human primates are the animal model of choice. First, their reproductive tracts closely resemble those of women. Secondly, in these species, unlike most other laboratory animals, PAs can block the effects of estrogens on endometrial proliferation in addition to blocking the action of P on progestational differentiation.[7] Thirdly, ovariectomized macaques can be treated sequentially with implants of estradiol (E2) and P to induce artificial menstrual cycles that provide a controlled hormonal environment in which to test various doses and modalities of PA treatments. Hodgen[8] was the first to report that development of a fully functional endometrium that could sustain pregnancy could be established in ovariectomized monkeys treated sequentially with Silastic implants of E2 and P. In such an artificial cycle, the withdrawal of P at the end of the cycle results in menstruation identical to natural menses. Because they allow such precise control of hormonal states, we used induced cycles to assess the effects of several PAs, including mifepristone (RU 486; Roussel UCLAF) ZK 137 316, and ZK 230 211 (Schering AG).[9–11]

CYCLIC CHANGES IN THE ENDOMETRIUM

Our review begins with a survey of the normal parameters of the primate endometrial cycle as background for comparison with the effects of PAs. Figure 9.1 shows a rhesus macaque uterus cut along the longitudinal axis from fundus to cervix. The dotted line indicates the plane of all the histological sections presented in this review. Figure 9.2 illustrates the histology of the rhesus macaque endometrium at the end of the induced

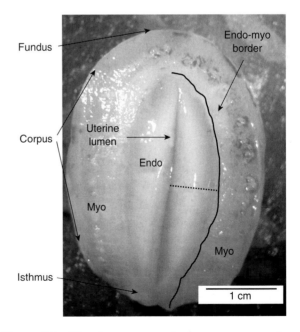

Figure 9.1 The rhesus uterus. A rhesus macaque uterus is shown after being cut in half along the fundus to cervical axis. A black line has been drawn to delineate the endometria–myometrial border and a dashed line drawn to indicate the plane along which all histological sections were cut. Endo = endometrium, Myo = myometrium. Magnification: see 1 cm bar. (Modified with permission from reference 56).

proliferative phase (14 days of E_2 alone) and at the end of the induced secretory phase (14 additional days of E_2+P). After 14 days of E_2 treatment the upper endometrial layers contain relatively straight tubular glands. Most of the proliferating cells are in the mid and upper functionalis zones, not the basalis[12] (Figure 9.2c; Figure 9.3a–c). Stromal cell proliferation occurs in all zones. The upper zones also contain abundant apoptotic cells (Figure 9.2c), suggesting that during the proliferative phase there is a balance of cell birth and cell death. New growth of small blood vessels in the upper functionalis zone peaks on day 8 of the proliferative phase.[13] In the proliferative phase, spiral arteries begin to grow but are confined to the basalis zone.

The effects of P on the epithelium become evident by day 3 of the artificial secretory phase. At this time, P suppresses cell proliferation in the glandular epithelium of the functionalis and induces secretory changes, including hypertrophy and accumulation of glycogen in the basal portions of the cells. In macaques and other non-human primates (though not in women) P stimulates a burst of proliferation in the basalis glands during the early luteal phase (Figure 9.2f and Figure 9.3d). When P declines at the end of the cycle, the basalis regresses due to apoptosis and atrophy, but does not undergo menstrual breakdown.[12,14,15]

By day 7 of E_2+P treatment, the endometrial stroma becomes highly edematous and the spiral arteries begin to enlarge (Figure 9.2g,h). Spiral artery growth is associated with a striking P-dependent increase in cell proliferation in endothelial, smooth muscle, and perivascular stromal cells. In rhesus macaques, decidualization does not occur during the cycle, but pregnancy or treatment for 5 months with E_2+P will induce a highly decidualized endometrium with enlarged stromal cells, enlarged spiral arteries, and atrophied or absent glands. Decidualization of the endometrial stroma and glandular atrophy has also been reported in macaques treated for 14 weeks with intrauterine devices that released levonorgestrel, a synthetic progestin.[16]

Cyclic changes in endometrial steroid receptors

Estrogen receptors, at both the mRNA[17] and protein levels,[18] are increased by E_2 and decreased by P. During the proliferative phase, staining for estrogen receptor α (ERα) is strongly positive in the nuclei of glandular epithelial and stromal cells in all zones, and subsequent P treatment suppresses this staining much more in the functionalis than the basalis (Figure 9.4a–d).

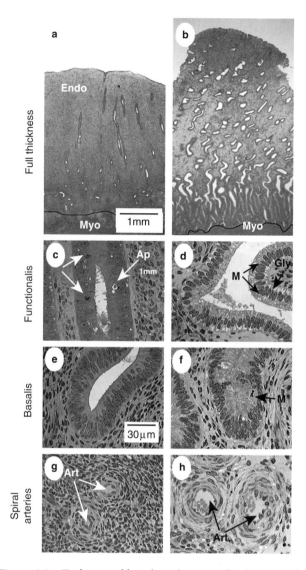

Figure 9.2   Endometrial histology during artificial cycle. Left column – 2 weeks of E. E_2 induces a typical proliferative phase appearance, with straight tubular glands (a), mitoses evident in the functionalis (c), but not the basalis zone (e), and small spiral arteries (g). Right column – 2 additional weeks of E_2+P. E_2+P induces a typical secretory appearance with sacculated glands (b) gland cells with basal glycogen vacuolation (d) mitosis in the basalis (f) and enlarged spiral arteries (h). Endo = endometrium. Myo = myometrium. M = mitotic figure, Ap = apoptotic figure, Gly = glycogen, Art = spiral artery. Original magnifications: a–b see 1 mm bar; c–h, see 30 μm bar). (Modified with permission from reference 56).

Estrogen receptor β (ERβ) and ERα are both present in the glands and stroma of the endometrium, but ERβ is the only ER isoform that was detectable in the vascular endothelial cells of both the human and primate endometrium.[19] ERβ may play a key role in endometrial vascular physiology, but its role in endometrial growth has not been established, and ERβ knockout mice show no endometrial phenotype.[20]

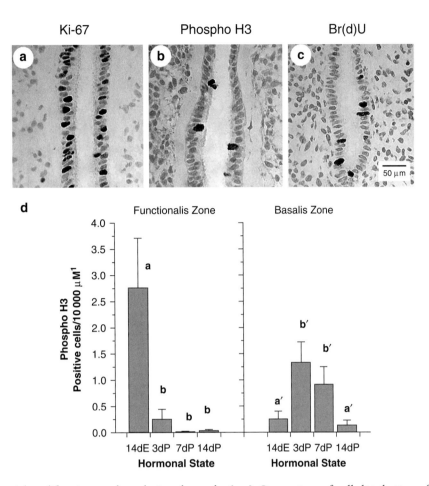

Figure 9.3 Endometrial proliferation markers during the cycle. (a–c) Comparison of cell distribution of Ki-67, Phospho H3 markers and Br(d)U labeling of DNA synthesis in glands during the proliferative phase. All three markers provide valid proliferative indices, but Ki-67 marks cells in all stages of the cell cycle, Phopho H3 marks only mitotic figures and Br(d)U marks only cells during DNA synthesis. Magnifications: see 50 μm bar. (d) Quantitative comparison of Phospho H3 labeling in the functionalis versus the basalis zone after treatment with 14 days of E_2 followed by 3, 7 and 14 days of E_2+P. In the functionalis zone, Phospho H3 label is elevated by E_2 and suppressed by P treatment. In the basalis zone, Phospho H3 labeling is low after 14 days of E_2, elevated by 3–7 days of E_2+P, and low after 14 days E_2+P. Data were first analyzed by one-way ANOVA then Fisher's Protected LSD (FPLSD 6). Bars with different letters are significantly different ($P < 0.05$). (Modified with permission from reference 57).

Two functional PRs (PR-A and PR-B) have been identified. PR-B is a larger molecule than PR-A due to the presence of an additional 165 amino acids in the *N*-terminal domain, and these two isoforms appear to be differentially expressed in the human endometrium, with PR-A dominating over PR-B.[21] Radioligand binding studies show that E_2 increases and P treatment decreases total PR binding in the macaque endometrium. Immunocytochemistry (ICC) with antibodies that recognize both PR isoforms shows that E_2 treatment increases PR nuclear staining in the glandular epithelium and stroma in all zones. Sequential P treatment dramatically suppresses PR staining in the glandular cells but *not* in the stromal cells of the functionalis zone, and only slightly suppresses PR staining in the glands and stroma of the basalis (Figure 9.4e–h). During the luteal phase, P induces dramatic morphological and

biochemical changes in the glands of the functionalis, even though these cells lack detectable PR. These effects are either mediated indirectly through P-dependent factors secreted by the underlying stromal cells (which retain PR) or by non-genomic mechanisms within the glands themselves. New research approaches to discriminate between these possibilities are needed.

Androgen receptor (AR) is also present in the macaque and human endometrium.[22,23] Receptor binding and ICC studies show that AR expression is increased by E_2 and suppressed by P treatment[23] and is normally restricted to the stroma. As with ERα and PR, P suppresses AR staining much more in the functionalis than the basalis (Figure 9.4i–l). Although the role of endometrial AR has not been established, it is hormonally influenced, as it increases dramatically during treatment with progesterone antagonists

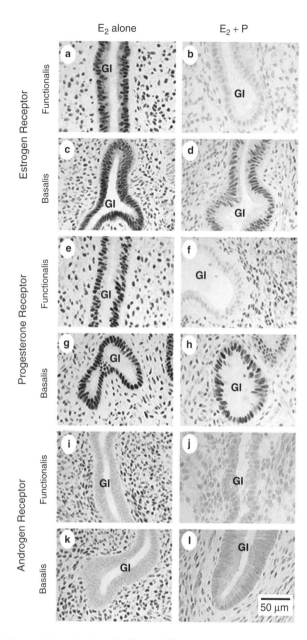

Figure 9.4 Zonal and cellular differences in steroid receptors during the artificial cycle. Left column – 2 weeks of E_2. After E_2 treatment, in both functionalis and basalis, ERα and PR are strongly stained in glands and stroma, while AR is only stained in stroma (ERα a–c; PR e–g; AR i–k). Right Column – 2 additional weeks of $E_2 + P$. After $E_2 + P$ treatment P suppresses ERα strongly in the glands and stroma of the functionalis but only weakly in the basalis (ER b–d). P also suppresses PR strongly in the the functionalis, but only in the glands, not the stroma, and only weakly in the basalis (PR f–h). P suppresses stromal AR strongly in the functionalis and weakly in the basalis (AR j–l). Gl = gland. Magnification: bar = 50 μm for all. (Modified with permission from reference 56).

(see further) and in women with polycystic ovarian disease.[24] Recent reports indicate that the human endometrium also expresses glucocorticoid receptors (GRs). GRs are completely non-detectable in the glands but are expressed by stromal fibroblasts, lymphocytes, endothelial cells,[25] and uterine natural killer (NK) cells.[26] The physiological role of GRs in the endometrium remains to be determined.

In sum, there are marked differences in receptor expression, hormonal responsiveness, and proliferative rates between the functionalis and basalis zones of the endometrium and between the glandular and stromal compartments. The basalis zone is unique in that the steroid receptors in this zone are resistant to P suppression. Moreover, the basalis, which contains ERα and PR, fails to grow under E_2 influence but undergoes a proliferative spurt during P treatment. Under normal conditions, AR and GR are only expressed by the stroma. The physiological significance of these regulatory differences, and the specific cell signaling pathways involved, deserve further investigation.

THE ENDOMETRIAL EFFECTS OF PROGESTERONE ANTAGONISTS

Ovulatory cycles

PAs can inhibit ovulation during the natural menstrual cycle, and this was first described in cycling cynomolgus monkeys. In that study, RU 486 (5 mg/day) administered on days 10–12 of the menstrual cycle, delayed the midcycle LH surge and lengthened the intermenstrual interval from the typical ~30 days to 61 days, effectively blocking one menstrual cycle.[27] Similar results were reported for women treated with RU 486 during the follicular phase; RU 486 disrupted follicle maturation and delayed progression of the menstrual cycle.[28] A single high dose of RU 486 administered to women during the midluteal phase of the cycle also suppressed serum LH pulse amplitude and frequency, was luteolytic, and induced menstruation.[29] Hypothalamic–hypophyseal PR were likely key sites of action for these effects, although ovarian and endometrial PR may also have been affected.

We used naturally cycling rhesus macaques to evaluate chronic administration of various PAs, particularly those from Schering AG (specifically ZK 137 316 and ZK 230 211). Low doses (0.03 mg/kg) of ZK 137 316 inhibited endometrial development but still allowed menstrual and ovarian cyclicity in half of the animals treated, whereas higher doses inhibited menstrual cyclicity in all animals.[30,31] Daily administration of a subthreshold dose (0.005 mg/kg) of ZK 230 211 to naturally cycling macaques had no effect on either menstrual cyclicity or menstruation, but increasing the dose to 0.05 mg/kg blocked ovulation, prevented the

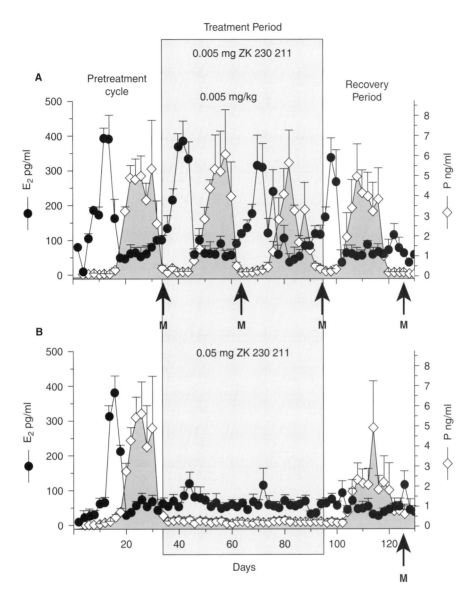

Figure 9.5 Effects of ZK 230 211 on ovulatory cycles in rhesus macaques. Cycling macaques were treated daily for 60 days with ZK 230 211 at doses of either 0.005 or 0.05 mg/kg. Daily serum E_2 and P levels were measured and menstruation (M) was recorded. Panel A: Effects of 0.005 mg/kg dose. Ovarian steroid secretion of E_2 and P were unaffected and menstruation occurred at appropriate intervals. This dose has no antiproliferative effects. Panel B: Effects of 0.05 mg/kg dose. Preovulatory E_2 surges, ovulatory cycles, secretion of P and menstrual bleeding were all inhibited, and there was an endometrial antiproliferative effect. Basal serum E_2 levels were maintained at follicular phase levels of 80–100 pg/ml. All inhibitory effects were reversed when treatment was stopped. (Modified with permission from reference 56).

development of a luteal phase, and induced amenorrhea while serum E_2 concentrations remained at midfollicular phase levels (Figure 9.5). These effects were fully reversible.[11]

In a long-term (1 year) study of chronic administration of RU 486 to naturally cycling cynomolgus macaques, atrophic changes in both the eutopic endometrium and in endometriotic lesions were noted.[32] In the animals with endometriosis, tonic ovarian estradiol secretion was maintained, suggesting that PA could be used to treat endometriosis long term without the sequelae of

hypoestrogenism, specifically bone density loss, as had typically been seen with gonadotropin agonist therapy. In the same animals, chronic mifepristone treatment also induced amenorrhea and suppressed the number of ovulations compared to controls.[33]

Also, low doses of RU 486 administered chronically to ovarian intact, fertile women as a contraceptive strategy inhibited glandular mitosis and induced stromal compaction in the endometrium.[34] These data indicate that PAs can act centrally to block P action at the hypothalamic and/or hypophyseal level and suppress luteinizing hormone (LH), inhibit ovulation, and block luteal P secretion. The amenorrhea that accompanies such treatment in ovarian intact women or macaques is therefore partly due to inadequate luteal P production and partly due to blockade of any residual effects of P in the endometrium by the PA. Experiments in ovariectomized animals, to be discussed below, indicate clearly that PAs can act directly on the endometrium to suppress its growth and menstrual cyclicity.

Artificial cycles: endometrial antiproliferative effects

The most surprising finding in the field of PA research was Hodgen's report[35] that mifepristone (RU 486) had an antiestrogenic effect on the endometrium. Hodgen's group treated ovariectomized cynomolgus macaques with E_2 plus mifepristone in the absence of P and found that the typical effects of E_2 on endometrial proliferation and growth were strongly inhibited. Because mifepristone binds only weakly to ERα, Hodgen's group called this action a 'noncompetitive antiestrogenic effect'. We confirmed Hodgen's report in a study of ovariectomized rhesus macaques treated with E_2 plus mifepristone compared to E_2 alone (Figure 9.6). Although mifepristone could indeed block the ability of E_2 to stimulate endometrial proliferation, it did not

block E_2 action in the oviduct or the vagina.[9] Consequently, we use the term 'endometrial antiproliferative effect' rather than 'antiestrogenic effect' because of the endometrial-specific nature of the response.

Other PAs had similar, specific, endometrial antiproliferative effects. For example, in endometria from ovariectomized animals treated for 28 days with either E_2 alone or E_2+ZK 230 211, PA treatment suppressed the effects of E_2 on endometrial thickness and mitotic activity, induced stromal compaction accompanied by stromal cell atrophy, and produced hyalinizing degeneration of the spiral arteries, all in the presence of high serum E_2 levels, without blocking E_2 action in the oviduct[11] (Figure 9.7). These and other data indicated that continuous treatment with an adequate dose of ZK 230 211 in ovariectomized rhesus macaques artificially cycled with sequential administration of E_2 and P inhibited both the overall proliferative growth of the endometrium attributable to E_2 action and the progestational differentiation typically induced by P. Surprisingly, PA treatment was associated with normal or increased endometrial ERα and PR levels (see Figure 9.7). Indeed, all the antiproliferative, suppressive effects of the PAs we have studied occurred in the presence of physiologically adequate serum E_2 levels (80–100 pg/ml) and elevated ERα and PR.[9,11,30,36]

Mechanisms underlying the antiproliferative effect

The failure of E_2 to act as a proliferative hormone in the presence of elevated levels of ERα during PA treatment is counterintuitive. Several hypotheses have been proposed to explain this conundrum. For example, direct antiproliferative and apoptotic effects of RU 486 have been observed in vitro in various breast cancer[37] and human endometrial[38] cell lines, and these effects have been referred to as receptor-mediated cytostatic and cytotoxic effects.[37] The antioxidant properties of RU 486, rather than its receptor-binding properties, are cited as responsible for these cytostatic and antiproliferative effects.[38,39] Although RU 486 can induce apoptosis in the endometrial cell line EM42 by increasing the Bax/Bcl-2 ratio,[40] RU 486 does not induce apoptosis or have antiproliferative or antidifferentiative effects in the macaque oviduct, nor does it block estrogen action in bone.[32] Two of the most potent PAs, ZK 137 316 and ZK 230 211, lack antioxidant properties (Kristof Chwalisz, pers comm) but have strong antiproliferative effects in the macaque endometrium.[11,30] Moreover, in rodents treated with various PAs, E_2 action in the endometrium is enhanced

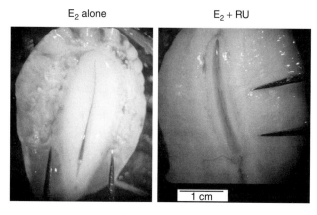

E_2 alone E_2 + RU

1 cm

Figure 9.6 RU 486 (RU) can suppress the effects of E_2 on endometrial growth. Ovariectomized animals were treated for either 28 days with E_2 alone or 28 days with E_2+RU 486 (1 mg/kg daily). The uteri were removed at necropsy, halved longitudinally and photographed fresh through a stereomicroscope. A Dumont #5 forceps was included for scale. E_2 alone: The endometrium:myometrium ratio is approximately 1:3, normal for the proliferative phase, and the lumen is slit-like. E_2+RU 486: The endometrium:myometrium ratio is approximately 1:5 due to extreme shrinkage of the endometrium, and the lumen is no longer slit-like. Magnification: Bar = 1 cm. (Modified with permission from reference 9; Copyright 1994, The Endocrine Society).

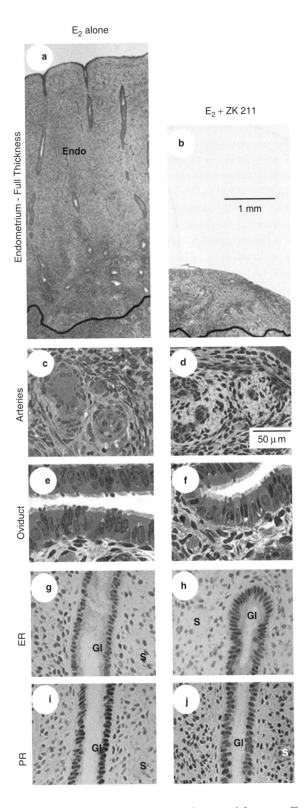

Figure 9.7 Histology and immunocytochemistry of the endometrial antiproliferative effect. Ovariectomized animals were treated for 28 days with either E_2 alone or E_2+ZK 230 211 (0.032 mg/kg IM daily) (ZK 211). E_2 alone: E_2 treatment induces proliferative growth in the endometrium marked by straight tubular glands (a) and arteries with normal muscular walls (c). The oviductal epithelium is in a fully ciliated-secretory state (e). ICC of endometrial ERα (g) and PR (i) show strong staining in glands and stroma. E_2+ZK 230 211: PA treatment induced overall endometrial shinkage (b) and degenerating arteries (d) but did not inhibit oviductal differentiation, which is known to require estrogen action. ICC of endometrial ERα (h) and PR (j) showed that these receptors were maintained or slightly increased. Magnification is marked with bars. Endo = endometrium. Gl = gland. S = stroma. Arrows point to ciliated cells. A dark line was drawn to indicate the endometrial–myometrial border. (Modified with permission from reference 11).

(not suppressed), as indicated by increases in cell height and mitotic activity of the uterine luminal epithelium.[41] Consequently, it is unlikely that the antiproliferative effects of PAs are due completely to their antioxidant properties.

There is evidence that RU 486 can bind to ERβ in vitro and act as an estrogen antagonist;[42] these data raise the possibility that the endometrial antiproliferative effect induced by RU 486 is mediated by ERβ. However, several other PAs, with different molecular structure, have similar endometrial antiproliferative effects, and it is not known whether any or all of these can antagonize ERβ. McDonnell's laboratory has screened for PAs with ERβ-sparing ability and isolated an ERβ-sparing PA that, like RU 486, can inhibit ovulation in mice.[43] These results indicate that the antiovulatory effect of PA does not require ERβ, at least in mice. A test is needed to determine whether an ERβ-sparing PA can induce endometrial antiproliferative effects in non-human primates.

Another line of evidence indicates that androgens, which are known to inhibit estrogen action in the endometrium, may be involved in the antiproliferative effect. For example, in menopausal women treated with an estrogen–androgen combination, the endometrium showed severe stromal compaction and glandular atrophy[44] remarkably similar to that seen in the macaque endometrium after treatment with PA. Women with recurrent miscarriages show elevated androgens that are thought to antagonize estrogen action directly in the endometrium.[45] Testosterone and danazol directly inhibit human endometrial cell proliferation in tissue culture when the medium contains estrogenic levels of phenol red.[46] Androstenedione inhibits the growth of human endometrial epithelial cells in culture, and this effect can be blocked by an AR antagonist, cyproterone acetate.[47] Long-term treatment with androgenic progestogens (e.g. levonorgestrel) induces endometrial atrophy.[48]

In view of the above, we evaluated the effects of PA on endometrial AR in macaques and women. In the macaque studies, we treated ovariectomized macaques for 14 days with either E_2 or E_2+RU 486. RU 486 significantly increased AR steroid-binding capacity above that of the animals treated with E_2 alone (Figure 9.8a). In E_2-treated animals, ICC showed that the glands were negative and AR was only expressed in the stroma. However, after E_2 + RU 486, glandular AR became strongly positive and AR staining in the stroma was enhanced (Figure 9.8b, c). Similar results were obtained in animals treated with ZK 137 316 and ZK 230 211.[23]

In the human studies, we evaluated endometria from women during normal cycles,[19] after treatment for 30

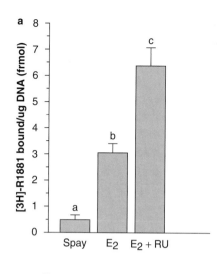

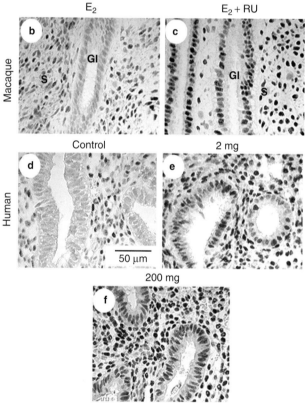

Figure 9.8 Endometrial AR is elevated by treatment with RU 486. (a) Receptor binding assay with ^{3}H-R1881 as the androgenic ligand. AR binding is low in an untreated ovariectomized animal (spay), elevated by E_2 treatment and significantly elevated by E_2+RU 486 (RU) treatment. Bars marked with different letters are significantly different ($P<0.05$, FPLSD). (b–c) ICC for endometrial AR in ovariectomized rhesus macaque. E_2 treatment increases AR staining only in the stroma (b). E_2+RU 486 treatment increases staining in the glands as well as the stroma (c). (d–f) ICC for AR in the human endometrium. During the normal proliferative phase, AR is only seen in stromal cells (d). After RU 486 treatment, AR staining is increased in the glands and the stroma (e–f). Gl = Glands, S = stroma. Magnification bar = 50 μm for all images. (Modified with permission from reference 7).

days with 2 mg mifepristone daily,[49] or after treatment with a single oral dose of 200 mg mifepristone around the time of the ovulatory LH surge.[50] During the normal cycle, AR staining predominated in the endometrial stroma and was absent from the glands.[23] As in macaques, mifepristone treatment (both chronic and acute) dramatically increased AR staining in the glands as well as the stroma (Figure 9.8d–f). In a separate study in which women were treated for 5 months with low doses (2–5 mg/day) of mifepristone, there were also strong increases in AR staining in the endometrial glands and stroma as compared to controls.[51]

A working hypothesis

On the basis of the above findings, we developed the following working hypothesis: the increases in endometrial AR that result from PA treatment lead to increased binding of endogenous androgens in both the stroma and glands. This increase enhances the ability of endogenous androgens to antagonize estrogen-driven endometrial proliferation. To test this hypothesis, we administered the antiandrogen flutamide (FLU) to ovariectomized rhesus macaques treated with E_2 + PA.[10] Animals were treated for 28 days with either E_2 alone, E_2 + ZK 137 316, or E_2 + ZK 137 316 + FLU at doses known to be effective.

Figure 9.9 shows the effects of these treatments on the macaque endometrium. As expected, treatment with E_2 + ZK 137 316 suppressed endometrial thickness, increased stromal compaction, and caused hyalinizing degeneration of the spiral arteries compared to E_2 alone. Consistent with our hypothesis, treatment with FLU prevented these effects. We also found that if FLU was administered along with ZK 137 316 near the end of the luteal phase, menstruation was induced as expected, indicating that FLU had no ability to compete with PA at the PR level. We concluded that FLU inhibited the endometrial antiproliferative effects of ZK 137 316 by acting as an antiandrogen.

PA treatment elevates AR in both glands and stroma, but the relative roles of these two cell types in the antiproliferative effect is not clear. Conceivably, any stimulatory effects of E_2 on mitosis that are mediated directly by glandular ER might be counteracted by direct, antagonistic effects of androgens through glandular AR. However, in many species, E_2 regulates endometrial glandular mitosis *indirectly* through stromally derived growth factors.[52,53] By elevating stromal AR levels, PAs may indirectly cause androgenic suppression of stromally derived, estrogen-dependent growth factors essential to glandular mitosis. Additional research is needed to distinguish between these possibilities.

In sum, the endometrial antiproliferative effect induced by PA treatment is clearly associated with enhanced expression of the endometrial androgen receptor, as it can be prevented by concurrent treatment with an antiandrogen. However, we lack a clear, mechanistic understanding of several aspects of this hypothesis, including (1) the nature of any endometrial androgens involved, (2) how androgens affect stromal–epithelial interactions, and (3) whether AR can be activated in a ligand-independent manner. More information on the nature, synthesis, and metabolism of endogenous endometrial androgens would be helpful.

Glandular hyperplasia

There are a number of reports that long-term, daily treatment with low doses of a PA may induce a form of benign glandular hyperplasia in the human endometrium. For instance, in Baird's laboratory, women treated for 120 days with 2 or 5 mg/day of mifepristone showed evidence of glandular dilation and simple endometrial hyperplasia. However, the epithelium lining the glands was low and mitotically inactive compared to control samples from the proliferative phase, when measured with the mitotic marker, antiphosphorylated histone H3.[51] Baird's laboratory concluded that the simple hyperplasia induced by mifepristone treatment consisted of dilated glands lined by an atrophic, inactive, and nonmitotic epithelium quite unlike the pseudostratified, proliferative epithelium typical of true cystic glandular hyperplasia.[51] In ovariectomized rhesus macaques treated for 5 months with E_2 plus the strong antagonist ZK 230 211, we observed similar, mitotically inactive, dilated glands without atypia.[54]

In another study, long-term treatment (6 months) of a female cushingoid patient with a very high dose of mifepristone (400 mg daily) induced an extensive, benign endometrial hyperplasia which was fully reversible when treatment was stopped.[55] Interpretation of these findings is complicated by the fact that mifepristone at such high doses has antiglucocorticoid effects, and these may have affected endometrial glucocorticoid receptors with unknown consequences.

A full explanation of the mechanism through which PAs cause cystic, glandular dilation is not at hand. Presumably, the endometrial glands, like other epithelial systems, continually pump fluid (primarily a serum transudate) across the basement membrane into the glandular lumen. If fluid egress is blocked, fluids would dilate the glands and flatten the epithelial lining as in any cyst. In the macaque endometrium, degeneration of the upper portions of the glands and loss of contact

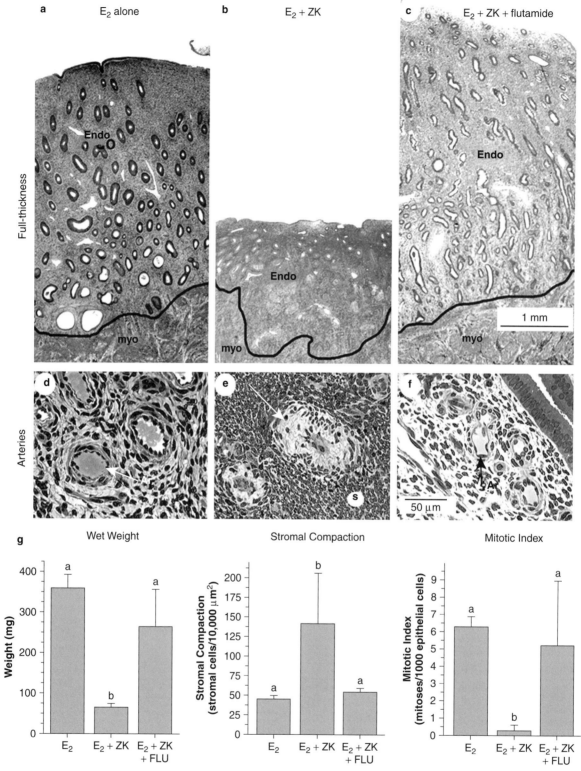

Figure 9.9   Flutamide can prevent the endometrial antiproliferative effect. Ovariectomized animals were treated for 28 days with either E_2 alone, $E_2+0.10$ mg/kg ZK 137 316 or $E_2+0.10$ mg/kg ZK 137 316+2 mg/kg Flutamide (FLU)[10]. (a–f) Histological effects. E_2 treatment induced a normal, proliferative endometrium (a) with normal spiral arteries (d); E_2+ZK 137 316 caused severe endometrial shrinkage (b) and induced degenerative changes in arteries (e); concurrent treatment with E_2+ZK 137 316+FLU prevented these suppressive effects of ZK 137 316. Endo=endometrium; Myo=myometrium. Arrows point to artery wall. Magnification shown as bar. (g) Morphometric analysis of the histological effects. Histograms depicting how the above treatments affected endometrial wet weight, stromal compaction (stromal cells/mm²) and mitotic index are shown. Bars with different letters are significantly different ($P<0.05$; FPLSD). These quantitative data indicate that FLU can prevent the endometrial antiproliferative effects of ZK137 316. (Modified with permission from reference 56).

with the lumen is sometimes observed, which could result in such increases in intraglandular pressures.

CONCLUSIONS

Non-human primates, because of their human-like menstrual cycles, are important model animals for the development and assessment of PAs. In cycling primates, PAs can be applied acutely during the late luteal phase to block P and induce menstruation. Indeed, such acute PA administration provides a sensitive in vivo bioassay for PAs. We found, for example, that ZK 137 316 required a dose of 0.15 mg/kg (IM) to induce menstruation, whereas ZK 230 211 achieved the same effect at 0.03 mg/kg, a fivefold difference in potency.[11] When applied chronically at low doses that do not block ovulation, the ability of a particular PA to suppress the progestational effects of P can be evaluated. When applied chronically at higher doses that block ovulation, the ovary continues to secrete E_2 at follicular phase levels, and PAs can then be assessed for their ability to inhibit E_2-dependent endometrial proliferation, induce spiral artery degeneration, suppress breakthrough bleeding, and affect glandular dilation.

PAs are extremely valuable gynecological therapeutics that can provide contraception, inhibit endometriosis, control menorrhagia, relieve irregular bleeding, and, conceivably, allow the safe use of estrogens for relief of menopausal symptoms. Chronic administration of an effective PA may allow women to avoid or delay their menstrual periods and give them more control over their reproductive lives. However, a certain degree of 'endometrial vigilance' is essential because the mechanism underlying the glandular dilation and simple hyperplasia that is sometimes evident in both the human and macaque uterus is not fully understood. Hopefully, clinical, basic, and pharmaceutical scientists will continue to collaborate, as they have in the past, toward development of new, safe, and effective PAs to enhance women's health.

ACKNOWLEDGMENTS

We gratefully acknowledge the Animal Care Technicians in the Division of Laboratory Animal Medicine for care of the animals during this study and Kunie Mah for superb immunocytochemistry. This study was supported by NIH grants HD43209 (RMB), HD07675 (ODS), HD19182 (RMB), and RR00163.

REFERENCES

1. Ghosh D, Sengupta J. Endometrial responses to a deciduogenic stimulus in ovariectomized rhesus monkeys treated with oestrogen and progesterone. J Endocrinol 1989; 120: 51–8.
2. Navot D, Laufer N, Kopolovic J et al. Artificially induced endometrial cycles and establishment of pregnancies in the absence of ovaries. N Engl J Med 1986; 314: 806–11.
3. Hodgen GD, Tullner WW. Plasma estrogens, progesterone and chorionic gonadotropin in pregnant rhesus monkeys (*Macaca mulatta*) after ovariectomy. Steroids 1975; 25: 275–82.
4. Giannoukos G, Szapary D, Smith CL et al. New antiprogestins with partial agonist activity: potential selective progesterone receptor modulators (SPRMs) and probes for receptor- and coregulator-induced changes in progesterone receptor induction properties. Mol Endocrinol 2001; 15: 255–70.
5. Chwalisz K, Garg R, Brenner RM et al. Selective progesterone receptor modulators (SPRMs): a novel therapeutic concept in endometriosis. Ann N Y Acad Sci 2002; 955: 373–88.
6. Jabbour HN, Kelly RW, Fraser HM, Critchley HO. Endocrine regulation of menstruation. Endocr Rev 2006; 27: 17–46.
7. Brenner RM, Slayden OD, Critchley HO. Anti-proliferative effects of progesterone antagonists in the primate endometrium: a potential role for the androgen receptor. Reproduction 2002; 124: 167–72.
8. Hodgen GD. Surrogate embryo transfer combined with estrogen-progesterone therapy in monkeys. Implantation, gestation, and delivery without ovaries. JAMA 1983; 250: 2167–71.
9. Slayden OD, Hirst JJ, Brenner RM. Estrogen action in the reproductive tract of rhesus monkeys during antiprogestin treatment. Endocrinology 1993; 132: 1845–56.
10. Slayden OD, Brenner RM. Flutamide counteracts the antiproliferative effects of antiprogestins in the primate endometrium. J Clin Endocrinol Metab 2003; 88: 946–9.
11. Slayden OD, Chwalisz K, Brenner RM. Reversible suppression of menstruation with progesterone antagonists in rhesus macaques. Hum Reprod 2001; 16: 1562–74.
12. Brenner RM, Slayden OD, Rodgers WH et al. Immunocytochemical assessment of mitotic activity with an antibody to phosphorylated histone H3 in the macaque and human endometrium. Hum Reprod 2003; 18: 1185–93.
13. Nayak NR, Brenner RM. Vascular proliferation and vascular endothelial growth factor expression in the rhesus macaque endometrium. J Clin Endocrinol Metab 2002; 87: 1845–55.
14. Padykula HA, Coles LG, Okulicz WC et al. The basalis of the primate endometrium: a bifunctional germinal compartment. Biol Reprod 1989; 40: 681–90.
15. Okulicz WC, Balsamo M, Tast J. Progesterone regulation of endometrial estrogen receptor and cell proliferation during the late proliferative and secretory phase in artificial menstrual cycles in the rhesus monkey. Biol Reprod 1993; 49: 24–32.
16. Wadsworth PF, Heywood R, Allen DG et al. Treatment of rhesus monkeys (*Macaca mulatta*) with intrauterine devices loaded with levonorgestrel. Contraception 1979; 20: 177–84.
17. Koji T, Brenner RM. Localization of estrogen receptor messenger ribonucleic acid in rhesus monkey uterus by nonradioactive in situ hybridization with digoxigenin-labeled oligodeoxynucleotides. Endocrinology 1993; 132: 382–92.
18. Brenner RM, West NB, McClellan MC. Estrogen and progestin receptors in the reproductive tract of male and female primates. Biol Reprod 1990; 42: 11–19.
19. Critchley HOD, Brenner RM, Henderson TA et al. Estrogen receptor beta, but not estrogen receptor alpha, is present in the vascular endothelium of the human and nonhuman primate endometrium. J Clin Endocrinol Metab 2001; 86: 1370–8.
20. Hewitt SC, Korach KS. Oestrogen receptor knockout mice: roles for oestrogen receptors alpha and beta in reproductive tissues. Reproduction 2003; 125: 143–9.

21. Mangal RK, Wiehle RD, Poindexter AN III, Weigel NL. Differential expression of uterine progesterone receptor forms A and B during the menstrual cycle. J Steroid Biochem Mol Biol 1997; 63: 195–202.
22. Adesanya OO, Zhou J, Wu G, Bondy C. Location and sex steroid regulation of androgen receptor gene expression in rhesus monkey uterus. Obstet Gynecol 1999; 93: 265–70.
23. Slayden OD, Nayak NR, Burton KA et al. Progesterone antagonists increase androgen receptor expression in the rhesus macaque and human endometrium. J Clin Endocrinol Metab 2001; 86: 2668–79.
24. Apparao KB, Lovely LP, Gui Y et al. Elevated endometrial androgen receptor expression in women with polycystic ovarian syndrome. Biol Reprod 2002; 66: 297–304.
25. Bamberger AM, Milde-Langosch K, Loning T, Bamberger CM. The glucocorticoid receptor is specifically expressed in the stromal compartment of the human endometrium. J Clin Endocrinol Metab 2001; 86: 5071–4.
26. Henderson TA, Saunders PT, Moffett-King A et al. Steroid receptor expression in uterine natural killer cells. J Clin Endocrinol Metab 2003; 88: 440–9.
27. Collins RL, Hodgen GD. Blockade of the spontaneous midcycle gonadotropin surge in monkeys by RU 486: a progesterone antagonist or agonist? J Clin Endocrinol Metab 1986; 63: 1270–6.
28. Liu JH, Garzo G, Morris S et al. Disruption of follicular maturation and delay of ovulation after administration of the antiprogesterone RU 486. J Clin Endocrinol Metab 1987; 65: 1135–40.
29. Garzo VG, Liu J, Ulmann A et al. Effect of an antiprogesterone (RU486) on the hypothalamic–hypophyseal–ovarian–endometrial axis during the luteal phase of the menstrual cycle. J Clin Endocrinol Metab 1988; 66: 508–17.
30. Slayden OD, Zelinski-Wooten MB, Chwalisz K et al. Chronic treatment of cycling rhesus monkeys with low doses of the antiprogestin ZK 137 316: morphometric assessment of the uterus and oviduct. Hum Reprod 1998; 13: 269–77.
31. Zelinski-Wooten MB, Slayden OD, Chwalisz K et al. Chronic treatment of female rhesus monkeys with low doses of the antiprogestin ZK 137 316: establishment of a regimen that permits normal menstrual cyclicity. Hum Reprod 1998; 13: 259–67.
32. Grow DR, Williams RF, Hsiu JG, Hodgen GD. Antiprogestin and/or gonadotropin-releasing hormone agonist for endometriosis treatment and bone maintenance: a 1-year primate study. J Clin Endocrinol Metab 1996; 81: 1933–9.
33. Grow DR, Reece MT, Hsiu JG et al. Chronic antiprogestin therapy produces a stable atrophic endometrium with decreased fibroblast growth factor: a 1-year primate study on contraception and amenorrhea. Fertil Steril 1998; 69: 936–43.
34. Baird DT, Brown A, Critchley HO et al. Effect of long-term treatment with low-dose mifepristone on the endometrium. Hum Reprod 2003; 18: 61–8.
35. Wolf JP, Hsiu JG, Anderson TL et al. Noncompetitive antiestrogenic effect of RU 486 in blocking the estrogen-stimulated luteinizing hormone surge and the proliferative action of estradiol on endometrium in castrate monkeys. Fertil Steril 1989; 52: 1055–60.
36. Slayden OD, Brenner RM. RU 486 action after estrogen priming in the endometrium and oviducts of rhesus monkeys (Macaca mulatta). J Clin Endocrinol Metab 1994; 78: 440–8.
37. Bardon S, Vignon F, Montcourrier P, Rochefort H. Steroid receptor-mediated cytotoxicity of an antiestrogen and an antiprogestin in breast cancer cells. Cancer Res 1987; 47: 1441–8.
38. Murphy AA, Zhou MH, Malkapuram S et al. RU486-induced growth inhibition of human endometrial cells. Fertil Steril 2000; 74: 1014–19.
39. Parthasarathy S, Morales AJ, Murphy AA. Antioxidant: a new role for RU-486 and related compounds. J Clin Invest 1994; 94: 1990–5.
40. Han S, Sidell N. RU486-induced growth inhibition of human endometrial cells involves the nuclear factor-kappaB signaling pathway. J Clin Endocrinol Metab 2003; 88: 713–19.
41. Chwalisz K, Stöckemann K, Fritzemeier K-H, Fuhrmann U. Modulation of oestrogenic effects by progesterone antagonists in the rat uterus. Hum Reprod Update 1998; 4: 570–83.
42. Zou A, Marschke KB, Arnold KE et al. Estrogen receptor beta activates the human retinoic acid receptor alpha-1 promoter in response to tamoxifen and other estrogen receptor antagonists, but not in response to estrogen. Mol Endocrinol 1999; 13: 418–30.
43. Sathya G, Jansen MS, Nagel SC et al. Identification and characterization of novel estrogen receptor-beta-sparing antiprogestins. Endocrinology 2002; 143: 3071–82.
44. Grody MH, Lampe EH, Masters WH. Estrogen-androgen substitution therapy in the aged female. Obstet Gynecol 1953; 2: 36–45.
45. Okon MA, Laird SM, Tuckerman EM, Li T-C. Serum androgen levels in women who have recurrent miscarriages and their correlation with markers of endometrial function. Fertil Steril 1998; 69: 682–90.
46. Rose GL, Dowsett M, Mudge JE et al. The inhibitory effects of danazol, danazol metabolites, gestrinone, and testosterone on the growth of human endometrial cells in vitro. Fertil Steril 1988; 49: 224–8.
47. Tuckerman EM, Okon MA, Li T-C, Laird SM. Do androgens have a direct effect on endometrial function? An in vitro study. Fertil Steril 2000; 74: 771–9.
48. Critchley H, Wang H, Jones R et al. Morphological and functional changes in human endometrium following intrauterine levonorgestrel delivery. Hum Reprod 1998; 13: 1218–24.
49. Cameron ST, Critchley HOD, Thong KJ et al. Effects of daily low dose mifepristone on endometrial maturation and proliferation. Hum Reprod 1996; 11: 2518–26.
50. Cameron ST, Critchley HOD, Buckley CH et al. Effect of two antiprogestins (mifepristone and onapristone) on endometrial factors of potential importance for implantation. Fertil Steril 1997; 67: 1046–53.
51. Narvekar N, Cameron S, Critchley H et al. Low-dose mifepristone inhibits endometrial proliferation and up-regulates androgen receptor. J Clin Endocrinol Metab 2004; 89: 2491–7.
52. Cooke PS, Buchanan DL, Young P et al. Stromal estrogen receptors mediate mitogenic effects of estradiol on uterine epithelium. Proc Natl Acad Sci USA 1997; 94: 6535–40.
53. McClellan MC, Rankin S, West NB, Brenner RM. Estrogen receptors, progestin receptors and DNA synthesis in the macaque endometrium during the luteal–follicular transition. J Steroid Biochem Mol Biol 1990; 37: 631–41.
54. Slayden OD, Zelinski MB, Chwalisz K et al. Chronic progesterone antagonist–estradiol therapy suppresses breakthrough bleeding and endometrial proliferation in a menopausal macaque model. Hum Reprod 2006; 21: 3081–90.
55. Newfield R, Spitz I, Isacson C, New M. Long-term mifepristone (RU486) therapy resulting in massive benign endometrial hyperplasia. Clin Endocrinol (Oxf) 2001; 54: 399–404.
56. Slayden OD, Brenner RM. Role of progesterone in the structural and biochemical remodelling of the primate endometrium. Ernst Schering Res Found Workshop 2005; 52: 89–118.
57. Slayden OD, Brenner RM. Hormonal regulation and localization of estrogen, progestin and androgen receptors in the endometrium of nonhuman primates: effects of progesterone receptor antagonists. Arch Histol Cytol 2004; 67: 883–91.

10 Endometrial stem cells

Caroline E Gargett

INTRODUCTION

The endometrium of humans and some primates undergoes cyclical processes of regeneration, differentiation, and shedding as part of the menstrual cycle. Endometrial regeneration also follows parturition, almost complete curettage, and in postmenopausal women taking estrogen replacement therapy. Although physical shedding of endometrial tissue does not occur in non-menstruating species, there are cycles of endometrial growth and apoptosis.

The concept that endometrial stem/progenitor cells are responsible for the remarkable regenerative capacity of endometrium was proposed some 35 years ago. However, attempts to isolate, characterize, and locate endometrial stem cells have only been undertaken in the last few years as experimental approaches to identify somatic or adult stem cells in other adult tissues have been developed. This latter endeavor has been fueled by the enormous interest in the clinical potential of human embryonic stem cells (hESCs) as the new therapeutic for regenerating tissues damaged or lost by injury and the aging process. The controversy surrounding the use of embryos to generate hESCs has encouraged the exploration of other sources of stem cells from adult human tissues.

This chapter reviews the evidence available to date for the existence of somatic stem/progenitor cells in human and mouse endometrium, and describes the emerging concepts relating to somatic stem cell behavior in other tissues that have relevance to the endometrium, including the stem cell niche, somatic stem cell plasticity, and molecular pathways involved in regulating stem cell activity. Approaches used in other tissues provide direction for future studies in endometrium that have the potential to significantly improve our understanding of endometrial regeneration. Application of these fundamental studies to the current knowledge on the pathophysiology of a variety of common gynecological diseases associated with abnormal endometrial proliferation, including endometriosis, adenomyosis, endometrial hyperplasia, and endometrial cancer, is also discussed. The possible use of endometrial stem/progenitor cells in tissue engineering applications relevant to urogynaecology are also mentioned.

SOMATIC STEM CELLS

Definitions and concepts

Stem cells are a rare subset of undifferentiated cells with no distinguishing morphological features that identify their location in tissues. They are defined by their functional properties, which include high proliferative potential, substantial self-renewal capacity, and ability to differentiate along specific molecular pathways to produce large numbers of at least one type of differentiated functional progeny[1–3] (Figure 10.1). Self-renewal or the ability to produce identical daughter stem cells is necessary for maintenance of the stem cell pool in tissues. Asymmetric cell division is one mechanism for producing an identical daughter cell and a more differentiated daughter. However stem cells also undergo symmetric divisions either producing two daughter stem cells or two transit amplifying (TA) progenitors. Differentiation is defined as a change in cell phenotype due to expression of different genes usually associated with the function of the cell and not associated with cell division.[4] Stem cells exhibit a wide range of differentiation potential. The zygote is totipotential, producing all cell types in the embryo and extraembryonic tissues. Human embryonic stem cells are pluripotent stem cells found in the inner cell mass of the blastocyst which have capacity to differentiate into all cell types of the three embryonic layers: ectoderm, mesoderm, and endoderm. The differentiation potential of these cells becomes increasingly restricted in lineage potential as embryonic development proceeds.[3] Arising from their progeny are the multipotent stem cells or somatic stem cells found in adult tissues that differentiate into several cell lineages, usually component cells of the tissue in which they reside. Progenitor cells derived from somatic stem cells are committed to a particular differentiation pathway and have limited ability to self-renew.[5,6] Tissue specific stem cells may be considered progenitors. Unipotent

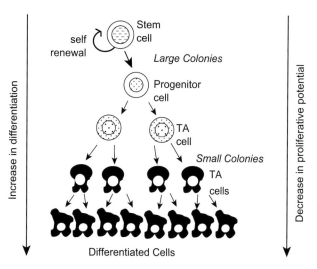

Figure 10.1 Hierarchy of stem cell differentiation. Stem cells undergo asymmetric cell divisions, which enable them to self-renew and replace themselves, or differentiate to give rise to committed progenitors. These proliferate and give rise to more differentiated transit amplifying (TA) cells, which rapidly proliferate and finally differentiate to produce a large number of terminally differentiated functional cells with no capacity for proliferation. The possible relationship of colonies initiated by human endometrial epithelial and stromal cells to the hierarchical model is shown. We postulate that the large colonies are initiated by putative stem/progenitor cells and the small colonies initiated by putative TA cells. (Reproduced with permission from Chan et al.[34])

stem cells are those with capacity to differentiate into a single, mature end stage cell type. A classical example is the germ stem cell of the testis that produces sperm.[7] TA cells have properties intermediate between stem cells and end-stage differentiated cells, with limited proliferative potential, and inability to self-renew, but they undergo several rounds of cell division, progressively acquiring differentiation markers as part of the cellular amplification process, to produce numerous terminally differentiated cells[2,8] (see Figure 10.1).

There is recent evidence to suggest that the dogma of hierarchical differentiation of stem cells and their progeny is more flexible than shown in Figure 10.1. Studies with hemopoietic stem cells have shown that there is a continuum of stem cell and progenitor capacity to self-renew and differentiate that is dependent on cell cycle phase and the specific microenvironment, suggesting that stem cells and progenitors are the same cell with different phenotypes under different conditions.[9] Similarly, epidermal stem cells, TA cells, and early differentiating keratinocytes all have the capacity to regenerate a fully stratified epidermis with appropriate spatial and temporal expression of differentiation markers in vitro and in vivo.[10]

The stem cell niche

In 1978 Schofield first proposed that stem cells were regulated by a specific physiological microenvironment, which he termed the niche.[11] Much of our current knowledge on the structure, function, and operation of the germ stem cell and somatic stem cell niches has been derived from elegant studies in model organisms, in particular the *Drosophila melanogastor* ovary and testis and *Caenorhabditis elegans* gonad, where the location of each cell is well characterized.[12] Far less is known about mammalian somatic stem cell niches, which are anatomically more complex in comparison and more difficult to study. However, there are common features between the *Drosophila* stem cell niche and those of mammalian somatic stem cells. Each has a precise location, with the stem cells in close relationship to one or more surrounding differentiated somatic cells, and together with the extracellular matrix and other secreted molecules, the niche cells provide a microenvironment that regulates key somatic stem cell functions.[7,8] Thus, signals from the niche microenvironment impinge on intrinsic somatic stem cell signaling to regulate stem cell proliferation and cell fate decisions.[3]

Stem cell niches vary in their cellular composition, structure, and location for somatic stem cells in different tissues. They have been identified and well characterized for epidermal stem cells in the hair follicle bulge of epidermis,[13] for epithelial stem cells in the intestinal crypts,[14,15] the periosteum for hemopoietic stem cells,[16] and neural stem cells in the subventricular zone and subgranular zone of the central nervous system.[17] Niche cells have been identified as osteoblasts lining the surface of trabecular bone[18] in the hemopoietic stem cell niche, as endothelial cells in the neural stem cell niche,[17] and possibly subepithelial mesenchymal cells in the intestinal stem cell niche.[19] Adhesion molecules and niche cells anchor the somatic stem cell in place during periods of stem cell inactivity and manage the asymmetric stem cell divisions to allow the controlled release of stem cells destined for proliferation and differentiation out of the stem cell niche.[7,8] Adhesion molecules identified as having a role in stem cell niches include the cadherins and integrins.[13,18] The niche cells maintain the somatic stem cell in a state of proliferative quiescence for much of the time through signaling pathways inhibitory for growth and differentiation, often involving transforming growth factor-β (TGFβ) and bone morphogenetic protein (BMP) family members.[7]

One of the key functions of niche cells is to sense the need for tissue replacement, and communicate proliferative and cell fate determining signals to the resident stem cell. While these mechanisms have been best characterized for *Drosophila* germ stem cell niches, the signaling pathways appear to be conserved across species from fly to man and from germ stem cell to somatic stem cell niches.[3] These include the Wnt/β-catenin and BMP pathways.[3,7] Other pathways involved include Notch and Hedgehog, while growth factors such as fibroblast growth factor 2 (FGF-2), insulin-like growth factor, and vascular endothelial growth factor also have roles in certain niches. For example, the Notch pathway is important in regulating self-renewal of hemopoietic stem cells, while the Wnt/β-catenin signaling maintains hemopoietic stem cells in an undifferentiated state,[20] promotes intestinal stem cell activation and self-renewal,[15] and acts on bulge epidermal stem cells to regulate hair follicle development and regeneration.[8]

Somatic stem cell plasticity

An area of considerable controversy in the stem cell field is the concept of somatic stem cell plasticity. There is a substantial body of literature suggesting that somatic stem cell fates are not limited to the tissue in which they reside or within embryonic germ layer boundaries.[3,21–23] Transdifferentiation describes the conversion of cells of one tissue lineage into cells of a different lineage, with concomitant loss of original tissue-specific markers and function, and acquisition of markers and function of the new cell type, without an intervening cell division.[21,24] It involves nuclear reprogramming and represents a form of metaplasia or alteration of key developmental genes.[24,25] This plasticity is the capacity of somatic stem cells to differentiate into lineages in response to different microenvironmental cues, particularly tissue damage.[9,22,24] Experiments have shown that bone marrow stem cells traffic via the bloodstream and incorporate into damaged tissues, changing into skeletal muscle cells, neurons and glia, hepatocytes, endothelial cells, myocardial cells, and epithelial cells of gut, skin, and lung, while neuronal cells produce blood cells and skeletal muscle cells.[22,23] This plasticity has been detected in tissues of gender-mismatched bone marrow transplant recipients by their coexpression of newly acquired tissue-specific antigens in Y-chromosome containing cells, or by tracking genetically tagged (e.g. green fluorescent protein [GFP]) transplanted cells. In the clinical setting, chimerism has been detected in the liver, gut, and endometrium[26] of bone marrow transplant recipients

and, in studies of solid organ transplantation, where circulating recipient cells have colonized donor hearts and kidneys.[27] These surprising findings suggest that somatic stem cells are more ES cell-like than originally thought and have major implications for therapeutics, providing hope that these cells can be used for cell-based therapies without the ethical problems posed by the use of hESC derivatives.[23] The concept of stem cell plasticity, however, has been refuted and in many studies it is a rare event.[21] Alternative explanations for these phenomena include the transplantation of multiple stem cell types, especially if the source is bone marrow or skeletal muscle, cell fusion, de-differentiation after in-vitro culture, or the presence of truly pluripotent cells residing in the adult.[3,5] Some elegant studies using transgenic mice have demonstrated that fusion is a rare event and occurs in some cases and not others.[5] In many cases somatic stem cells showing plasticity were substantially amplified in vitro prior to transplantation. In particular, a new and extremely rare multipotential adult progenitor cell (MAPC) isolated from mouse and human bone marrow,[5] with properties similar to ES cells, requires prolonged culture at low density. It is not known if MAPC exist in vivo. As a result of these uncertainties, several leading stem cell scientists have advocated for greater rigor for claiming stem cell plasticity, insisting that engraftment is robust and persistent in the regenerating tissue and that functional capacity is demonstrated, since many studies have relied on morphology and immunostaining alone.[5,21]

Role in tissue homeostasis, repair, and regeneration

Somatic stem cells have a key role in tissue homeostasis, providing replacement cells in regenerating tissues and cells lost by apoptosis or when a tissue is injured.[7,28] The function of somatic stem cells is highly regulated to ensure an appropriate balance in stem cell replacement and provision of sufficient differentiated mature cells for tissue and organ function. To undertake this key function, a balance between self-renewal and differentiation is imperative and appears to be regulated by the stem cell niche.

Recently it has become apparent that somatic stem cells not only reside and function in highly regenerative tissues like the bone marrow, intestine, and epidermis where they produce a steady supply of differentiated cells to maintain blood cell numbers and replace shed intestinal epithelial cells and skin cells but are also found in tissues of low cell turnover, such as neural, liver, prostate, and pancreas. In all these tissues, somatic stem cells function to maintain tissue homeostasis by replenishing functional tissue cells lost by apoptosis.[29,30] Following injury, normally quiescent somatic stem cells undergo cell division, producing TA cells that undergo rapid proliferation and expansion to eventually repair the lost tissue with sufficient numbers of functional end-stage cells. In some cases, such as liver and pancreas, it appears that fully mature cells have the capacity to revert to a proliferative phenotype to effect tissue replacement.[31] These processes are not fully understood and it is not clear if mature cells can de-differentiate into stem-like cells with a concomitant change in epigenetic and transcriptional profiles or if fully mature cells have latent stem cell capacities.[32]

GLOSSARY

Stem cell terminology

Cancer stem cells. Rare cells present in tumors with stem cell properties that may arise when somatic stem or progenitor cells undergo genetic damage and are responsible for growth and spread of the tumor. The proliferation of cancer stem cells is no longer under control of the stem cell niche.

Differentiation. Process whereby stem cells produce more specialized functional cells that constitute the tissue or organ in which they reside.

Label retaining cell (LRCs). measures stem cell quiescence, and are those cells which retain a DNA synthesis label for a prolonged period of time because they rarely proliferate. LRCs have been demonstrated to behave as somatic stem cells.

Progenitor cells. They are derived from somatic stem cells and are committed to a particular differentiation pathway. They are less differentiated than TA cells.

Prospective isolation. The ability to predict which freshly dissociated cells are stem cells and separate them from their more differentiated progeny. This is usually done on the basis of surface marker expression by FACS or magnetic bead sorting.

Self-renewal. The ability of a stem cell to give rise to one or two daughter cells with equivalent stem cell properties.

Somatic stem cells. Undifferentiated cells that reside in adult tissues, which have high proliferative potential, capacity to self-renew, and generate one or more types of differentiated cells to replace tissue cells that die or are lost.

Stem cell niche. One or more cells in direct contact with a somatic stem cell that control its fate, in particular whether to self-renew or differentiate.

Stem cell plasticity. The capacity of somatic stem cells to differentiate into lineages of a different embryonic germ layer in response to different microenvironmental cues, in particular tissue damage.

IDENTIFICATION OF SOMATIC STEM CELLS AND STEM CELL ASSAYS

Identification and characterization of somatic stem cells is a major challenge because of the paucity of these cells in tissues and the lack of defining cell surface markers that enable their isolation for study. The approaches used to identify somatic stem cells in tissues and a number of surrogate assays that have been developed to assess stem cell function are briefly reviewed. Their relevance to approaches that have or could be informative in the quest to identify endometrial stem cells is also mentioned.

Stem cell assays have been developed and are well characterized for identifying the hierarchies of hemopoietic stem cells. These cells are much easier to analyze than other somatic stem cells due to their nonadherent growth, circulation in the bloodstream, albeit in low numbers, and capacity to home to bone marrow and reconstitute blood-forming tissue for each of their eight lineages. Moreover, a number of surface markers have been identified in man and mouse that make identification of hemopoietic stem cells and their their differentiating progeny relatively easy to investigate in in-vivo models. Although adaptation of these assays to assess the various functions of somatic stem cells in tissues with a very different architecture of adherent cells is rapidly developing, it is proving to be a difficult task.[33] There is a real challenge to develop predictive surrogate assays for tissue stem cell activity in cell populations removed from their natural microenvironment.[33]

This is particularly the case for endometrial stem cells, for which there are no phenotypic markers or, until recently, assays of their function.[34]

Stem cell markers

There are no specific phenotypic markers of somatic stem cells. A great deal of research activity has been devoted to the identification of stem cell markers for the purpose of prospectively obtaining pure populations of freshly isolated stem cells for further characterization, identification of stem cell location in situ, and eventually for their use in the clinic as cell-based therapies. There are many studies that have simply designated a population of cells as stem cells based on marker expression. The danger of this approach is that many markers currently used to identify somatic stem cells are also present on other mature cells: e.g. CD34 is a hemopoietic stem cell marker and a mature endothelial cell marker and CD90 is a hemopoietic stem cell marker and a marker of endometrial functionalis stromal cells (CE Gargett and KE Schwab, unpublished work). Furthermore, cells alter their phenotype in culture, and marker expression of cultured stem cells may not reflect the in-vivo situation.[33] This becomes particularly important in studies examining the plasticity of stem cells. Expression of a stem cell marker does not imply stem cell activity. Before claiming that a population of cells are stem cells based on phenotypic marker expression, it is therefore necessary to validate stem cell function using at least one surrogate stem cell assay.[33] Studies on endometrial stromal cells have demonstrated that cell populations sorted by fluorescence-activated cell sorting (FACS) on the basis of expression of a mesenchymal stem cell marker, Stro-1,[35] do not correlate with colony-forming efficiency.[36]

In-vitro assays of stem cell activity

There are a range of assays that examine the functions of somatic stem cells, including in-vitro assays of clonogenicity, proliferative potential, self-renewal, and differentiation, and in-vivo self-renewal and tissue reconstitution. Clonogenicity is the ability of single cells to initiate colonies of cells when seeded at extremely low seeding densities on cloning plates or by limiting dilution. These colony-forming assays have been extensively used for characterizing hemopoietic stem cells and their progenitors and provide a useful

read-out assay for assessing potential stem cell markers as an initial approach in uncharacterized tissues.[33,37] This approach has been used for a range of epithelial and stromal tissues.[34,38–40] Proliferative potential is examined by determining the total number of progeny or total cell output from a single cell or population of putative stem cells by serial passage until senescence, and usually results in the total production of billions of cells.[38,41] This assay has been used to assess the proliferative potential of fresh human cells, FACS or magnetic bead sorted for putative stem cell markers, for the purpose of identifying potential markers of keratinocyte, mammary epithelial and mesenchymal stem cells.[40,42,43] Assays for self-renewal can be investigated both in vitro in serial cloning assays[44] and in vivo by serial transplantation methods.[45] In-vitro serial cloning assays rely on the ability of the initial colony-forming cell to undergo a self-renewing division during colony formation and that the resultant cell has the same colony-initiating capacity on replating the harvested clone at limiting dilution. Ideally, somatic stem cells should have capacity to self-renew multiple times and hence undergo multiple rounds of serial cloning. These techniques will identify somatic stem cells and progenitor cells, the difference being the extent to which they can undergo self-renewal.[41]

The differentiation potential of isolated populations of candidate stem cells is evaluated after culturing the cells in differentiation-inducing media, or transplanting them and analyzing the tissue formed by immunohistochemical identification of phenotypic differentiation markers or expression of tissue-specific transcription factors. Mesenchymal stem cells isolated from bone marrow, adipose tissue, and dental pulp have been characterized for their capacity to differentiate into a number of mesenchymal lineages, including adipocytic, smooth muscle, chondrocytic, and osteoblastic lineages.[39,46,47]

Tissue reconstitution assays of stem cell activity

The gold standard assay of somatic stem cell activity involves in-vivo reconstitution of the tissue from which the putative stem cell population was derived.[33,37,48] These techniques require the use of congenic strains of mice or immunocompromised mice (e.g. NUDE and NOD/SCID)[49] as hosts for the engraftment of putative stem cell populations, the latter essential for xenotransplanting human somatic stem cell populations. An important issue is the ability to track transplanted cells and identify their progeny. The use of transgenic mice ubiquitously expressing either β-galactosidase (ROSA26) or GFP to derive putative stem cell populations is an excellent approach for tracking these cells transplanted into recipient mice of the same genetic background.[50] Other approaches are to tag cells with membrane intercalating dyes such as PKH26 or similar molecules, although these will dilute as the cells proliferate. The value of these approaches is that the transplanted cells and their derivatives can be identified immunohisto-chemically within the architecture of the newly derived tissue. Alternatives include using genetic tagging of putative stem cell populations with markers[45] or capitalizing on the specificity of antibodies to detect species differences.[39] A key issue for tissue reconstitution assays is the requirement to provide a numerical or qualitative advantage for the transplanted cells over the resident endogenous stem cells.[37] Usually this is achieved by the prior induction of significant tissue damage or ablation of the organ or tissue to be reconstituted. For example, irradiation is used to ablate the bone marrow for hemopoietic stem cell assays and cleared mammary fat pads are used for reconstitution of mammary glands.[45] Competitive repopulation is used to quantitate the numbers of repopulating hemopoietic stem cells for bone marrow reconstitution, but this approach is more difficult for other somatic stem cells. Yet another approach is to transplant putative stem cell populations into an ectopic tissue site. The kidney capsule is particularly useful, as it provides a rich vascular supply and contains the transplanted cells in a local region.[50] While this environment does not recapitulate the tissue environment important for provision of suitable stem cell niches and inductive cues, it has been used successfully to obtain intestinal crypts from intestinal epithelial cells transplanted into NOD/SCID recipient mice.[51] A challenge is to demonstrate that a single cell can regenerate all the lineages of the tissue from which it was derived, and this has been achieved for mammary epithelial stem cells.[45] Ideally, several approaches need to be used, as there are technical limitations of each assay type. There is a range of possibilities for endometrial reconstitution from putative stem cell populations. Endometrium does grow ectopically, as endometriosis in the peritoneal cavity, and there are numerous models of endometriosis[52] using transplantation of endometrial tissue that suggest an ectopic site may work. Furthermore, there is a model of endometrial breakdown and repair that could be adapted for examining tissue reconstitution potential of putative

endometrial stem cells.[53] Self-renewal capacity of putative stem cell populations extends the above approaches and is examined by harvesting the reconstituted tissue, obtaining single cell suspensions, and retransplanting them back into another host for evaluation of their ability to reconstitute the appropriate tissue a second time. Serial tissue reconstitution indicates that the original transplanted stem cell underwent a self-renewing cell division in vivo. This has been done extensively for hemopoietic stem cells and more recently for other somatic stem cell populations.[37,45]

Label-retaining cell approach to identify somatic stem cells

Another in-vivo approach for identification of somatic stem cells in their stem cell niche is to capitalize on their infrequent cycling characteristics relative to TA cells. This label-retaining cell (LRC) approach involves labeling the majority of tissue cells with a DNA synthesis label such as bromodeoxyuridine (BrdU) or tritiated thymidine followed by a chase period of weeks to months during which time the label is diluted with each cell division to undetectable levels as the tissue grows or regenerates. Putative stem cells retain the label for prolonged periods of time, whereas the more mature, proliferating TA cells rapidly dilute the label. LRCs have been identified in epidermis, mammary gland, prostate, and endometrium.[29,54–56] More recently, a number of elegant studies using conditional activation of fluorescently tagged transgenes under the control of tissue-specific promoters have been used to identify and characterize LRCs in epidermis.[13,32]

EVIDENCE FOR SOMATIC STEM/PROGENITOR CELLS IN HUMAN ENDOMETRIUM

Indirect evidence for endometrial stem cells

The human endometrium is a highly regenerative tissue and the concept that this regeneration is mediated by stem cells located in the basalis layer was first postulated 35 years ago[57] and reiterated by Padykula in 1984.[58] Evidence from early kinetic studies of endometrial cell proliferation show zonal differences that predict an orderly replacement of endometrial epithelial and stromal cells from rarely proliferating putative stem/progenitors residing in the basalis near

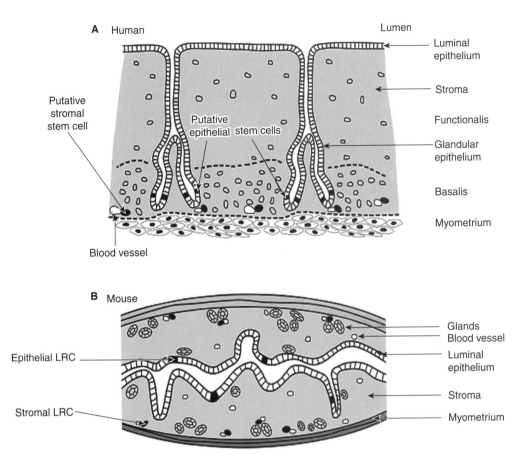

A Human

Lumen

Luminal epithelium

Stroma

Functionalis

Glandular epithelium

Basalis

Myometrium

Putative stromal stem cell

Putative epithelial stem cells

Blood vessel

B Mouse

Glands
Blood vessel

Luminal epithelium

Stroma

Myometrium

Epithelial LRC

Stromal LRC

Figure 10.2 Schematic showing the possible location of putative endometrial stem/progenitor cells in (**A**) human and (**B**) mouse endometrium. In human endometrium, it is predicted that candidate epithelial stem/progenitors will be located in the basalis in the base of the glands and stromal stem/progenitors near blood vessels. In mouse endometrium, the location of epithelial and stromal LRCs (candidate stem/progenitor cells) that have the capacity to rapidly proliferate during estrogen-stimulated growth of regressed endometrium are shown in the luminal epithelium and mainly near blood vessels at the endometrial–myometrial junction, respectively.

the endometrial–myometrial junction whose progeny are the rapidly proliferating TA cells observed in the functionalis[59,60] (Figure 10.2). More recently, a disjunction between the proliferative index of endometrial glands in the basalis and functionalis has been observed in both the proliferative and secretory stages of artificially cycled macaques using phosphorylated histone H3 as a proliferation marker.[61] Further support for this hypothesis comes from primate studies and clinical practice, where endometrium completely regenerated and supported pregnancy after surgical removal of almost all endometrial tissue by curettage.[62,63] In another clinical situation, pockets of endometrial tissue are observed to regenerate in a minority of women treated with electrosurgical ablation for menorrhagia.[64]

Further clinical evidence suggesting the presence of somatic stem cells in endometrium comes from observations that human endometrium has the propensity to undergo ossification, often after termination of

pregnancy, and while the calcified tissue is not of fetal origin, it is usually associated with chronic inflammation and trauma,[65] conditions known to promote incorporation of mesenchymal stem cells into regenerating tissues.[37] In addition, tissues such as smooth muscle, bone, and cartilage can also be found in the endometrium.[66,67] Mesenchymal stem cells have the capacity to differentiate into smooth muscle, fat, bone, and cartilage in vivo and in vitro,[68] and together these observations suggest that under certain circumstances resident endometrial or bone marrow-derived multipotent mesenchymal stem cells may undergo an inappropriate differentiation.

More recent evidence indicates that endometrial glands are monoclonal in origin, suggesting that they arise from a single progenitor or stem cell. In almost half of histologically normal proliferative endometrial samples, rare glands have been observed that fail to express PTEN protein (PTEN null glands) because

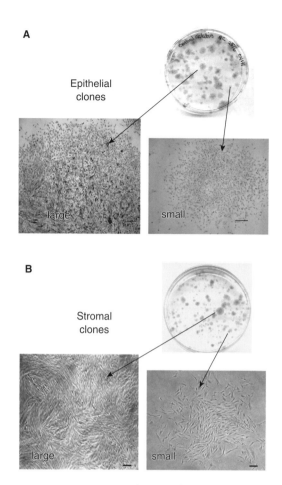

Figure 10.3 Human endometrial (**A**) epithelial and (**B**) stromal colonies formed when single cell suspensions are seeded at cloning density and cultured for 15 days in serum-containing medium. The cells in the rare large clones were small and densely packed with a high nuclear–cytoplasmic ratio and the clones typically contained >4000 cells, whereas those in small clones were large, loosely arranged, and contained between 50 and 3500 cells (scale bars =200 μm). (Adapted from Chan et al.[34])

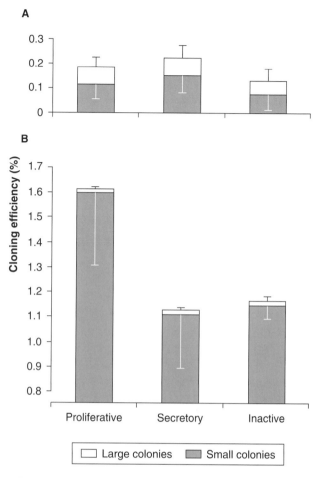

Figure 10.4 Cloning efficiency of human endometrial (**A**) epithelial and (**B**) stromal cells from proliferative, secretory, and inactive endometrium cultured in serum-containing medium. Each bar consists of the cloning efficiency for small (black bars) and large (white bars) colonies, which together represent the total cloning efficiency observed. Results shown are means±SEM of 4–7 samples. Inactive endometrium was from 4 samples, which included perimenopausal women and women taking oral contraceptives. (Adapted with permission from Schwab et al.[71])

of a mutation and/or deletion in the *PTEN* gene.[69] These PTEN-mutant glandular clones persist in the basalis region between menstrual cycles to regenerate their respective glands in the functional layer in subsequent cycles. PTEN null glands are increased in the endometrium of women in conditions of unopposed estrogen, particularly endometrial hyperplasia, a monoclonal epithelial proliferative disorder. In a separate study, monoclonality was detected in carefully dissected individual endometrial glands using a polymerase chain reaction (PCR)-based assay for nonrandom X chromosome inactivation of the androgen receptor gene.[70] Furthermore, adjacent glands up to 1 mm in distance shared clonality, indicating that well-circumscribed regions of endometrium were derived from the same precursor cell. These studies suggest

that several glands share the same stem cell, which raises questions on the locality of candidate human epithelial stem/progenitor cells.

Evidence from functional studies

Despite the likelihood that the amazing regenerative potential of human endometrium is mediated via resident stem/progenitor cells, it was only very recently that the first evidence based on functional assays was published.[34,71,72,79] Besides the glandular and luminal epithelium of human endometrium, there is also a substantial stromal component supporting these glands, indicating that stromal or mesenchymal stem cells may also be found in human endometrium.[72] Using purified single cell suspensions obtained from hysterectomy tissues, it was demonstrated that 0.22±0.07% of endometrial epithelial cells and 1.25 ±0.18% of stromal cells formed individual colonies of >50 cells/colony within 15 days when seeded at clonal density.[34] Two types of colony formed for both epithelial and stromal cells (Figure 10.3). The large colonies were rare (0.09% of epithelial and 0.02% of stromal cells) containing >4000 cells and comprised small, densely packed cells with high nuclear:cytoplasmic ratio that were postulated to be initiated by candidate endometrial stem/progenitor cells. The more common, small colonies were composed of large, loosely arranged cells with low nuclear:cytoplasmic ratio initiated by more mature cells, probably TA cells (see Figure 10.1). Further work has shown that the percentage of clonogenic epithelial and stromal cells in human endometrium does not vary significantly across the menstrual cycle[71] (Figure 10.4). This contrasts with a cloning study on endometrial stromal cells derived from Pipelle biopsy tissues at various stages across the menstrual cycle, which demonstrated very high levels of cloning, ranging from 27% in the early proliferative stage to 45% in the late proliferative stage, using a limiting dilution assay and plating at 0.2 cells/well.[73] However, in this study the average size of the clones after 14 days was only 12 cells and the proliferative output of these clones bore no relationship to the original colony size. It would appear that the putative stem/progenitor cells may have been overlooked in this study, since a total of 25 000 wells would be required to isolate one large colony-initiating stromal cell. This would also explain the inability to detect a relationship between proliferative potential and colony size. In another cloning study, 13% of 6-month cultured endometrial cells from a single sample were clonogenic by limiting dilution.[74] The resulting clones exhibited high proliferative potential as they continued to proliferate in culture for another 24 months. It would appear that the culture conditions favored self-renewing cell divisions of putative endometrial stem/progenitor cells present in the original sample.

A number of growth factors required for epithelial and stromal cell colony formation in serum-free medium have also been identified. Clonogenic epithelial cells require either epidermal growth factor (EGF) or transforming growth factor α (TGFα) or platelet derived growth factor BB (PDGF-BB).[34] These cultures also required fibroblast feeder layers to establish clonal

growth, indicating the need for stromal–epithelial cell signaling and the importance of stem cell niche for endometrial epithelial stem/progenitor cells. Thus it is likely that colony-forming endometrial epithelial cells express EGF receptors and receive proliferative signals from feeder cells expressing PDGF receptor β. Clonogenic stromal cells also required either, EGF, TGFα or PDGF-BB but were also clonogenic in FGF-2- containing serum-free medium,[34,71] indicating that clonally derived stromal cells express EGF receptors, PDGF receptor β, and FGF receptors. Whether combinations of these growth factors further enhance growth of clonogenic endometrial cells has not been determined. Cell-type specific markers were used to characterize the cellular phenotype of the endometrial colonies.[34] While small epithelial clones expressed epithelial cell adhesion molecule (Ep-CAM) and cytokeratin, the large colonies did not express Ep-CAM and either weakly or failed to express cytokeratin. However, they expressed α_6-integrin subunits (CD49f), a marker expressed on the basal membrane of endometrial epithelium in tissue, but epithelial clones did not express the stromal cell marker, collagen I. Both large and small stromal clones expressed CD90, a fibroblast marker. A significant proportion of stromal clones contained α-smooth muscle actin-expressing cells indicative of myofibroblast or smooth muscle cell differentiation. Since it is had been hypothesized that endometrial stem cells would reside in the basalis, it is not surprising that clonally derived stromal cells differentiated into myofibroblast or smooth muscle cell lineages, as there are considerable numbers of myofibroblasts in the basalis,[75] and myometrium develops from undifferentiated Müllerian duct mesenchyme.[66]

Current studies examining stem cell attributes of the rare epithelial and stromal cells initiating large colonies have demonstrated their high proliferative potential as they undergo 30–32 population doublings before senescence or transformation.[76] These clonally derived endometrial cells also undergo self-renewing cell divisions in vitro as demonstrated by their serial cloning ability. This high proliferative potential of endometrial stromal cells has been noted earlier in kinetic growth studies of serially passaged bulk cultures (as opposed to clonally derived cells) where 50% of specimens underwent more than 24 population doublings, and several between 60 and 100.[77] It is likely that a number of stromal stem/progenitor cells present in these cultures were responsible for this enormous proliferative capacity. Large secondary stromal clones expanded in culture also exhibit multilineage differentiation, and, similar to bone marrow and adipose tissue mesenchymal stem cells, they differentiated into four mesenchymal lineages in vitro, specifically, adipocytes, smooth muscle cells, chondrocytes, and osteoblasts.[76] In contrast, epithelial and stromal cells initiating the small colonies failed to serially clone or undergo substantial proliferation, indicating they are more differentiated endometrial cells with limited proliferative potential and self-renewal capacity.[76] Their differentiation capacity could not be examined, as these small clones could not be sufficiently expanded in culture. These data suggest that the rare epithelial and stromal cells initiating large colonies, but not small colonies, have characteristic properties of somatic epithelial and mesenchymal stem/progenitor cells and are probably responsible for the remarkable, cyclical, regenerative capacity of human endometrium. These initial findings lay the groundwork for further studies to characterize stem cell properties in vivo and for the discovery of specific endometrial stem/progenitor cell markers. A schematic showing the possible location of putative human endometrial stem/progenitor cells in the basalis is shown in Figure 10.2A.

In a separate unique study, endometrial epithelial stem cell kinetics was investigated by examining epigenetic errors encoded in methylation patterns of individual glands in human endometrium.[78] This approach depends on endogenous DNA sequences that become polymorphic as epigenetic variants arise during cell division when methylation at CpG sites alters within a particular gene. In a cyclically, remodeling tissue such as human endometrium, a persistent polymorphism indicates heritable epigenetic variants in the stem cells, since those variants or mutations that occur in TA or mature cells are lost during shedding. Thus, the total number of stem cell divisions may be inferred from the numbers of somatic errors accumulated within individual glands.[79] Methylation sites of the CSX gene, which is not expressed in human endometrium, were examined to ensure that any changes in methylation patterns would have no functional consequences, and are probably due to a random process associated with aging.[78] The extent of methylation of endometrial glands increased with age until menopause, after which it remained relatively constant, indicating that the number of epigenetic errors was a reflection of the mitotic activity of endometrial stem cells.[78] Mathematical modeling of the data was more consistent with the concept that an individual gland contains a stem cell niche with an unknown number of long-lived stem cells rather than a single immortal stem cell that always divides asymmetrically.

It would appear that a stochastic model of stem cell kinetics operates, where a population of epithelial stem cells exist in the endometrial gland niche that undergo symmetric and asymmetric cell divisions to maintain a constant number of stem cells in the niche.[78] There was no evidence for a reduction in stem cell number with aging because gland diversity remained constant after menopause, consistent with the finding of clonogenic epithelial cells in inactive perimenopausal endometrium.[71] These random replication errors that accumulate in a clock-like manner provide a record of endometrial stem cell replication history which may be useful to investigate the role that putative endometrial stem/progenitor cells may have in proliferative disorders of the endometrium.

Markers of endometrial stem/progenitor cells

Currently there are no known markers for endometrial epithelial stem/progenitor cells that distinguish them from their mature progeny. However, sorting endometrial stromal cells by magnetic beads or FACS and examining the sorted populations for clonogenic activity have now excluded several potential markers. These include Stro-1, a mesenchymal stem cell marker, which did not enrich for endometrial stromal cells with clonogenic activity, and CD133, a hemopoietic stem cell marker (unpublished observations). However coexpression of two perivascular cell markers CD146 and PDGF receptor-β does give a significant 15-fold enrichment of multipotent, clonogenic stromal cells from human endometrium.[80] This rare population of candidate endometrial stromal stem/progenitor cells are postulated to reside in the basalis (see Figure 10.2A), although co-expression of these 2 markers also occurs in functionalis vessels.[80] At this stage no progress has been made in identifying markers that will recognize endometrial epithelial stem/progenitor cells.

There have been a number of expression studies examining endometrial tissues using antibodies to stem cell markers. Bearing in mind the caveats outlined previously, these studies may assist in determining which markers might be worth examining for prospective isolation and subsequent testing in stem cell assays. Many of the classical stem cell markers have been examined in human endometrium for other purposes, but few have examined the basalis, making them less informative. The expression of hemopoietic stem cell markers, CD34, c-kit/CD117, and the survival marker, bcl-2, has been examined in hysterectomy tissues. Basically, this study found immunostaining for all three markers in basalis glands and stroma, with CD34 specific for basalis stroma.[81] Flow cytometric analysis of fresh and cultured decidual stromal cells showed that some expressed Stro-1, a mesenchymal stem cell marker, and also CD34, a hemopoietic stem cell marker, although their co-expression was not determined.[82] CD44 (hyaluronin receptor), a well-known non-specific stem cell marker immunostains basalis glandular epithelium during the secretory stage of the menstrual cycle, and may have potential as one marker to enrich for endometrial epithelial stem/progenitor cells.[83] Whether any of these markers have value in identifying endometrial epithelial or stromal stem/progenitor cells has yet to be determined.

Source of endometrial stem/progenitor cells

The embryonic female reproductive tract has its origins in the intermediate mesoderm, which begins to form soon after gastrulation. As this embryonic tissue proliferates, it is thought that some cells undergo mesenchymal to epithelial transition to give rise to the coelomic epithelium that later invaginates to form the paramesonephric ducts.[84] These ducts, also known as Müllerian ducts, comprise surface epithelium and underlying urogenital ridge mesenchyme. During fetal life, the glands commence developing as the undifferentiated uterine surface epithelium invaginates into the underlying mesenchyme and smooth muscle differentiation of the mesenchyme commences to form the myometrium.[85] It would be expected that a small number of fetal epithelial and mesenchymal stem cells remain in the fully developed adult endometrium and contribute to tissue replacement associated with its cyclic regeneration.[72] Whether there is an ultimate uterine stem cell that has the capacity to replace all endometrial and myometrial cell types, including epithelial, stromal, vascular, and smooth muscle, or whether there are separate epithelial and mesenchymal stem cells is not currently known. The differences in phenotypes, growth factor dependence, and frequency of clonogenic endometrial epithelial and stromal cells suggest that there are at least two types of endometrial progenitor cell. However, this does not exclude the possibility that an as-yet unidentified, more primitive precursor to

these clonogenic cells exists in human endometrium. Sophisticated studies examining the relative reconstitution capacity of endometrial cells separated using lineage specific and differentiation stage markers that have yet to be elucidated are required to distinguish these possibilities.

Another possible source of endometrial stem cells is the bone marrow. Increasingly, it is being recognized that bone marrow stem cells circulate, albeit in low numbers, and populate various organs. A significant level of chimerism, ranging from 0.2% to 52%, was detected by reverse transcriptase-polymerase chain reaction (RT-PCR) and immunohistochemistry in the endometrium of four women who received single antigen HLA-mismatched bone marrow transplants, 2–13 years earlier.[26] It appears that the level of chimerism increased with time elapsed since transplantation, although the number of cases was small. The high level of chimerism may also be related to the original degree of endometrial damage and to loss of endogenous endometrial stem/progenitor cell populations, resulting from pretransplant conditioning or ongoing graft vs host disease in chimeric tissues. The patient with 52% chimerism had received both total body irradiation and chemotherapy and had moderate graft vs host disease, while the other three patients had only received chemotherapy. The degree of endometrial chimerism observed is similar to that in other organs of bone marrow transplant recipients,[27] and it appears that cell turnover and inflammatory stimuli have a role. The donor-derived cells in endometrium were in focal areas of the glands and stroma, suggesting local proliferation of the incorporated cells.[26] This observation, together with the similar percentage of donor-derived epithelial and stromal cells in each patient, suggests that there may be a single endometrial stem cell responsible for production of both glands and stroma. While most gland profiles observed were exclusively of the donor or host type, there was some chimerism within individual glands, suggesting that not all were monoclonal,[26] which contrasts with monoclonality described for non-transplanted women.[70] Polyclonal glands containing only a few donor cells could result from fusion of bone marrow-derived cells with endometrial cells, but this possibility was excluded after examining tissues stained with a DNA complexing dye.[26] The endometrial epithelial and some stromal cells did not express CD45, a leukocyte marker, which distinguished them from donor endometrial leukocytes, although these would have been detected in the RT-PCR products. These interesting preliminary observations rely solely on marker expression. It raises a number of questions that require further research to determine whether transdifferentiation of bone marrow stem cells into functional endometrial cells actually occurs. Bone marrow contains at least three different stem cells – hemopoietic stem cells, mesenchymal stem cells, and endothelial progenitors – and all have been demonstrated to circulate. Just which bone marrow stem cells, or even myeloid cells, contribute to endometrial regeneration needs to be determined. Whether bone marrow-derived cells regularly engraft the endometrium with each menstrual cycle or at the time of the bone marrow transplant, or subsequently on the resumption of endometrial cycling, is not known. Does this engraftment of endometrium with bone marrow stem cells occur under normal physiological conditions? Certainly, large numbers of mature bone marrow-derived cells traverse the endometrium on a regular basis, particularly perimenstrually. Whether the local tissue damage associated with menstruation is sufficient to attract bone marrow stem cells into the endometrium for permanent residence remains to be determined. Just where bone marrow-derived stem cells incorporate into endometrial tissue is another interesting question. Is it the basalis, functionalis, or both regions of the endometrium? Vascular cells were not examined in the Taylor study, but, given the involvement of circulating endothelial progenitors in pathological tissues undergoing angiogenesis, it is expected that they may contribute to endometrial neovascularization during the menstrual cycle. The studies required to answer some of these questions are not possible in humans and will rely on animal studies using transgenic reporter mice.

EVIDENCE FOR SOMATIC STEM/PROGENITOR CELLS IN MOUSE ENDOMETRIUM

The mouse is a well-established animal model for investigating endometrial function, despite the fact that mice do not menstruate. However, mouse endometrium undergoes cycles of cellular proliferation and apoptosis during its 4-day estrus reproductive cycle and can be induced to undergo substantial regeneration on administration of estrogen following ovariectomy (see Chapter 9). Futhermore, mouse and human endometrium have a similar structure, although defined functionalis or basalis layers are not present in the mouse. Another similarity is the monoclonality of endometrial glands, as demonstrated in chimeric mice,[86] providing indirect evidence suggesting that single putative epithelial stem/progenitor cells are responsible for production of individual glands. One advantage of using mouse endometrium to investigate a role for endometrial stem/progenitor cells in endometrial growth is that glandular development is a postnatal event. The power of transgenic animals in dissecting molecular pathways also makes the mouse an attractive model.

A reliable way to identify somatic stem cells and their location in the stem cell niche in vivo is to use pulse chase experiments, otherwise known as the LRC technique. LRCs are defined as cells which retain a DNA synthesis label after a prolonged chase period of weeks to months, where label retention gives an indication of the proliferative history of the cells. Thus, the LRC approach discriminates between somatic stem cells and their more differentiated progeny based on their relative frequencies of undergoing cell division. LRCs have been identified as somatic stem cells in the epidermis by demonstrating their clonogenic properties.[54] An advantage of using this approach for identifying somatic stem/progenitor cells in endometrium is that the precise location of these rare cells can be established, and their phenotype and that of the neighboring cells that form the stem cell niche identified when there are no known stem cell markers. Several important technical considerations when establishing the LRC technique in a tissue for the first time include determining the optimal timing for labeling all tissue cells with BrdU, dosage of BrdU, how long to chase prior to LRC analysis, and defining an LRC in immunostained sections, as a reduced intensity is observed after 1–2 cell divisions before BrdU becomes undetectable (3–4 divisions). Furthermore, confocal microscopy is essential for detecting co-localization of phenotypic markers and BrdU (Figure 10.5).

In studies on C57BL/6J mice, the optimal window for labeling was postnatal days 3–6 at the time when the undifferentiated uterine epithelium begins to invaginate into the mesenchyme to form the glands.[56] Optimal chase periods for detection of epithelial and stromal LRCs differed, with 4–8 weeks optimal for epithelial LRCs and 8–12 weeks for stromal LRCs. At these times, approximately 3% of epithelial and 6% of stromal cells were LRCs.[56] Endometrial LRCs were generally well separated rather than in clusters and epithelial LRCs were located in the luminal epithelium rather than in the glands, although the occasional LRC was observed in the necks of glands (see Figure 10.2B). This unusual finding suggests that putative stem cells in luminal epithelium are responsible for the growth of glands, as is the case during development. Perhaps the lack of epithelial LRCs in individual glands indicates the technical difficulties in

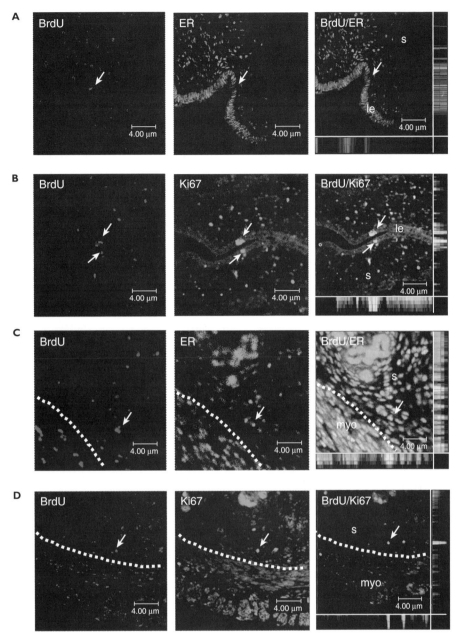

Figure 10.5 Confocal microscopy images showing (**A, B**) epithelial label-retaining cells (LRCs) and (**C, D**) stromal LRCs in mouse endometrium. Postnatal bromodeoxyuridine (BrdU)-labeled mouse endometrium double immunofluorescent stained for BrdU (red) and ERα (green), showing (**A**) lack of co-expression in a single epithelial LRC in the luminal epithelium at 8 weeks chase (blue arrows) but ERα expression in mature epithelial cells, and (**C**) co-localization of BrdU and ERα in some stromal LRCs near the endometrial–myometrial junction at 12-weeks chase (white arrows). Endometrium from postnatal BrdU-labeled, (**B**) 4- and (**D**) 8-weeks chased, ovariectomized mice double immunofluorescent stained for BrdU (red) and proliferation marker, Ki-67 (green) to visualize estrogen-stimulated proliferation of (**B**) epithelial LRC (blue arrows) and of (**D**) stromal LRCs (white arrows). The x/z and y/z planes are shown on the far right and underneath the merged pictures, demonstrating true co-localization of the two markers within individual whole nuclei. Dotted line indicates endometrial–myometrial junction; le, luminal epithelium; s, stroma; myo, myometrium (scale bars = 40 μm). (See also color plate section.)

finding rare cells in two-dimensional tissue sections. It also suggests that luminal LRCs have an important role in regenerating luminal epithelium, which undergoes substantial proliferation and apoptosis during the estrous cycle (see Chapter 9), and that glandular cells may be regenerated from luminal epithelium, or that perhaps glandular epithelium has the capacity to self-duplicate as do pancreatic β cells,[31] obviating the need for epithelial stem/progenitors. Stromal LRCs were observed in a variety of locations: near the endometrial–myometrial border (see Figure 10.5C,D), adjacent to luminal and glandular epithelium, and near blood vessels (Figure 10.2B). Double immunolabeling and confocal microscopy demonstrated that epithelial and stromal LRCs did not express CD45, indicating that murine endometrial LRCs were neither leukocytes nor derived from bone marrow cells.[56] Approximately 40% of stromal LRCs located near the endometrial–myometrial junction or gland profiles either co-expressed α-smooth muscle actin or were in close association with CD31-positive endothelial cells, but the LRCs themselves did not express CD31.[56] Thus, some mouse stromal LRCs are perivascular cells, similar to bone marrow[68] and human endometrial mesenchymal stem/progenitor cells.[80] In a similar study using CD1 mice, 2–5% of stromal LRCs were detected between 9 and 16 weeks chase, but no epithelial LRCs were detected, even after a 1-week chase. One-third of these stromal LRCs co-expressed c-kit (CD117), the stem cell factor receptor found on hemopoietic stem cells.[87]

Estrogen receptor α (ERα) was differentially expressed in endometrial epithelial and stromal LRCs.[56] Epithelial LRCs did not express (ERα), although they were adjacent to ERα-expressing luminal epithelium (see Figure 10.5A), and, although the majority of stromal LRCs also did not express ERα, 16% had ERα-positive nuclei (see Figure 10.5C).[56] Despite the lack of ERα expression, all epithelial LRCs in BrdU-labeled pulse-chased ovariectomized mice underwent proliferation within 8 hours of 17β-estradiol administration, as detected by co-localization of BrdU and the proliferation marker, Ki-67 (see Figure 10.5B). In contrast, only some stromal LRCs proliferated 8 hours after the 17β-estradiol injection and these were mainly located near the endometrial–myometrial junction (see Figure 10.5D). These data indicate that epithelial and some stromal LRCs are recruited into the cell cycle by estrogen, suggesting that they have the capacity to act as stem/progenitor cells and proliferate during physiological endometrial growth. The purpose and function of stromal LRCs that do not proliferate in response to estrogen stimulation is currently unknown, but it is unlikely that they are endometrial mesenchymal stem/progenitor cells. Endometrial epithelium is known to respond indirectly to estrogen via cell–cell interaction involving ERα-expressing stromal cells,[88] which also appears to be recapitulated for epithelial LRCs. The exact nature of the neighboring stromal niche cells that instruct epithelial LRCs to undergo cell division is currently unknown. In contrast, estrogen appears to have a direct proliferative effect on stromal LRCs, and just what role neighboring vascular cells have in regulating stromal LRC function is yet to be determined. These initial studies provide new insights and define a new approach to investigating the role of putative endometrial stem/progenitor cells in regulating epithelial and stromal growth in mouse endometrium.[72]

GLOSSARY

Gynecological diseases

Adenomyosis. Extensive growth and invasion of basalis endometrium into the myometrium with associated smooth muscle hyperplasia.

Endometrial carcinoma. Malignant tumor of endometrial epithelial cells. Type 1, the common form, is associated with estrogen stimulation and endometrial hyperplasia and occurs in younger and perimenopausal women. Type 2 tumors are high-grade, poorly differentiated endometroid endometrial carcinomas, serous and clear cell endometrial carcinomas not associated with estrogen and occur in the older postmenopausal women.

Endometrial hyperplasia. An irregular, non-invasive, non-physiological proliferation of endometrial glands with a variable amount of stroma. Some are premalignant lesions that progress to endometrial carcinoma.

Endometriosis. Growth of endometrial tissue outside the uterine cavity commonly in the peritoneal cavity, resulting in inflammation, pain, and infertility.

Pelvic floor prolapse. The downward descent of pelvic organs into the vagina, resulting in herniation of the uterus, rectum, bowel, bladder, or any combination of these. It is due to weakening of muscles and ligaments of the vagina and pelvic floor supporting the pelvic organs, most commonly from childbirth and aging.

ENDOMETRIAL STEM/PROGENITOR CELLS – CLINICAL PERSPECTIVE

Gynecological disease

A number of gynecological conditions are associated with abnormal endometrial proliferation and it is possible that putative endometrial stem/progenitor cells may play a role in the pathophysiology of diseases such as endometriosis, endometrial hyperplasia, endometrial cancer, and adenomyosis.[72] For example, alterations in the number, function, regulation, and location of epithelial and/or stromal endometrial stem/progenitor cells may be responsible for any one of these endometrial diseases. Furthermore, clonogenic epithelial and stromal cells are present in non-cycling and perimenopausal endometrium[71] and may be responsible for regenerating endometrium in women given estrogen replacement therapy.

Endometriosis, defined as the growth of endometrium outside the uterine cavity, is a common gynecological disorder affecting 6–10% of women (see Chapter 46). It is a major clinical problem, causing inflammation, pain, and infertility. Despite its common occurrence, little is known about its pathogenesis. The most commonly held theory on the etiology of endometriosis is that viable endometrial cells reach the peritoneal cavity through retrograde menstruation.[89] However, it is well known that menstrual debris is present in the peritoneal cavity of 90% of menstruating women, suggesting that only some endometrial cells from some women are capable of establishing endometriotic implants. Several theories have been suggested, including abnormal endometrium, genetic factors, altered peritoneal environment, reduced immune surveillance, and increased angiogenic capacity.[89] It is possible that in 6–10% of women who develop endometriosis, endometrial stem/progenitor cells are inappropriately shed during menstruation and reach the peritoneal cavity where they adhere and establish endometriotic implants.[72] While long-term endometriotic lesions may develop from endometrial stem/progenitor cells, those that resolve may have been established by more mature TA cells. The monoclonality of some endometriotic lesions and the increasing evidence indicating that endometriosis can develop into ovarian clear cell and endometroid carcinomas[90] are consistent with the concept that endometriosis could have a stem cell origin. This is further supported by the demonstration of clonogenic cells in a long-term culture derived from a sample of endometriosis tissue.[74] If bone marrow stem cells have the capacity to seed the endometrium and transdifferentiate into functional endometrial cells, it is possible that they may have the capacity to behave similarly outside the endometrial environment, particularly in sites other than the peritoneal cavity.[26] Alternatively, it has been postulated that some forms of endometriosis may arise from remnant fetal Müllerian cells, which have characteristic stem cell properties of high proliferative potential, multipotency, and self-renewal. Adenomyosis, a condition affecting 1% of women, results from basal endometrium undergoing extensive invasion of the myometrium and is associated with smooth muscle hyperplasia; it is also considered to arise from fetal Müllerian cells.[91] It is possible that endometrial stem/progenitor cells or their niche cells demonstrate abnormal behavior in adenomyosis, and these putative stem cells have an abnormally orientated niche such that their differentiating progeny move toward the myometrium rather than functionalis to produce pockets of endometrial tissue deep in the myometrium.[72] Alterations in the putative endometrial stem cell niche, particularly in the partner cells that regulate stem cell fate decisions, may result in excessive smooth muscle differentiation of putative endometrial stem/progenitor cells, producing the observed myometrial hyperplasia. Much research needs to be undertaken to establish a role for endometrial or bone marrow stem cells or endometrial progenitors in the pathogenesis of endometriosis or adenomyosis.

There is an increasing interest amongst researchers and oncologists in the concept that cancers contain small numbers of cells with stem cell properties that are responsible for their growth and spread.[92,93] There is considerable similarity in the properties of adult stem cells in normal tissues and cancer stem cells. Cancer stem cells have a long life span, enormous proliferative potential, and self-renewal capacity, enabling them to maintain and expand the cancer cell population, although they themselves are quiescent and rarely proliferate.[94] Many features of carcinoma can be explained by the stem cell concept, including clonal origin and heterogeneity of tumors, some associated with TA cells or progenitors, the mesenchymal influence on cancer behavior, the local formation of precancerous lesions, and the plasticity of tumor cells.[93] Only a small proportion of the tumor actually comprises cancer stem cells, ~2–5% in breast cancer. Thus, cancer stem cells act as precursor cells that produce the proliferating more-differentiated cancer cells killed by chemotherapy or radiation. Cancer stem cells differ from normal tissue stem cells in that their proliferation is no longer controlled by the neighboring niche cells in the stem cell niche.[92] It is likely that cancer stem cells arise from somatic stem cells that have accumulated multiple genetic and epigenetic changes over a period of time, giving them selective proliferative advantage that allows their clonal expansion and succession in the stem cell niche.[93] Thus, cancer stem cells are likely to be the key tumor cells involved in the initiation, progression, metastasis, and recurrence of tumors after treatment. The key role of cancer stem cells in these processes has been established in acute myeloid leukemia, and in solid tumors such as breast cancer and glioblastoma.[92] Key genes involved in the self-renewal pathways that regulate somatic stem cells, such as Wnt/β-catenin, sonic hedgehog, and PTEN tumor suppressor gene, are associated with a range of cancers. Microsatellite instability or mutations in the *PTEN* gene are known to be involved in endometrial hyperplasia and endometrioid endometrial carcinoma, but whether endometrial cancer stem cells are involved is not currently known. Furthermore, the Wnt-β-catenin signaling pathway is involved in endometrial carcinoma and endometrial stromal sarcomas.[95,96] Endometrial carcinoma is the commonest female genital tract malignancy and the incidence of new cases is increasing (see Chapters 55 and 56). Based on epidemiological data, there are two distinct types of endometrial carcinoma.[97] Type 1, which accounts for ~80% of all endometrial cancers, occurs in younger and perimenopausal women in a setting of estrogenic stimulation and endometrial hyperplasia. Type 2 tumors include high-grade, poorly differentiated endometrioid endometrial carcinoma and the aggressive serous and clear cell carcinomas that occur in older postmenopausal women and are not associated with estrogen.[97] It is currently unknown whether cancer stem cells have a role in endometrial cancers, or in endometrial hyperplasia, but this is an area open for future research. Surgery is the main treatment for endometrial cancer;[97] however, possible future therapies targeting cancer stem cells, perhaps blocking molecules regulating asymmetric cell division, may improve the prospects for those women with advanced or Type 2 tumors.

Tissue engineering applications

There is great interest in the use of both embryonic and somatic stem cells in tissue engineering applications for restoring function to aging or diseased tissues and organs. Medical advances have ensured increasing longevity, and the aging population has many tissues in need of repair.[98] The failure of artificial implants to last longer than 10–15 years and the problems associated with non-degradable synthetic materials make cell-based therapies for tissue replacement attractive.[99] There is now a focus on using a combination of temporary biological scaffold materials to provide initial support and stem cells to promote appropriate tissue genesis and regeneration of functional tissue.[99] This is particularly important for the provision of supportive tissues and could be adapted for tissue engineering support of the female reproductive tract.

Pelvic floor prolapse is a major problem that results in 10% of women requiring surgery, with an alarming 30% of these requiring repeat surgery.[100] The use of artificial and biological scaffolds for pelvic floor prolapse surgery has improved outcomes to a limited degree. Thus, the use of tissue constructs comprising scaffolds and autologous endometrial mesenchymal stem/progenitor cells may provide a possible solution for treatment of pelvic floor prolapse in the future.

CONCLUSIONS AND FUTURE DIRECTIONS FOR ENDOMETRIAL STEM/PROGENITOR CELL RESEARCH

Endometrial stem cell research is in its infancy but major advances have already been made that have identified rare populations of epithelial and stromal cells with progenitor activity in human and mouse endometrium that are likely responsible for its remarkable regenerative capacity. Whether there is a single more primitive endometrial stem cell that produces all endometrial cell types is yet unknown and whether the endometrial stromal progenitor has full mesenchymal stem cell activity in vivo is yet to be determined. Much still needs to be done to fully identify and characterize endometrial epithelial and mesenchymal stem/progenitor cells. There is a need to identify specific markers of both cell types to allow their prospective isolation for molecular characterization and determination of their location in tissue. Animal xenotransplantation models are needed to examine key stem cell properties of self-renewal and tissue reconstitution in vivo. Whether the bone marrow is a source of endometrial stem/progenitor cells needs confirmation under physiological conditions, and whether bone marrow-derived cells are major or minor contributors to endometrial regeneration is yet to be determined. The putative endometrial stem cell niches for epithelial and stromal stem/progenitors need further characterization. How estrogen and progesterone interact with endometrial stem/progenitor cells or their neighboring niche cells needs clarification. The signaling pathways that regulate endometrial stem/progenitor cell activity have yet to be investigated and candidate pathways involving the Wnt, hedgehog, BMP pathways, and the *HOX* genes should be investigated, as these molecules or pathways have already been detected in endometrium or have important roles during endometrial development.

As endometrial stem/progenitor cells become better characterized, their role in gynecological disorders associated with abnormal endometrial proliferation can be assessed. This will not only increase understanding of the pathogenesis of endometriosis, adenomyosis, endometrial hyperplasia, and endometrial cancer but also has the potential to change the way these diseases may be treated in the future, particularly as therapeutic agents that target key stem cell functions are developed.

ACKNOWLEDGMENTS

The author thanks the National Health and Medical Research Council (ID 284344), the Royal Australian and New Zealand College of Obstetricians and Gynaecologists, and the Australian and New Zealand Charitable Trusts for financial support; Rachel Chan, Kjiana Schwab, and Rachel Zillwood for their contributions to these studies; and Nancy Taylor and Nicki Sam for collection of human tissues.

REFERENCES

1. Weissman IL. Stem cells – Scientific, medical, and political issues. N Engl J Med 2002; 346: 1576–9.
2. Potten CS, Loeffler M. Stem cells: attributes, cycles, spirals, pitfalls and uncertainties. Lessons for and from the crypt. Development 1990; 110: 1001–20.
3. Eckfeldt CE, Mendenhall EM, Verfaillie CM. The molecular repertoire of the 'almighty' stem cell. Nat Rev Mol Cell Biol 2005; 6: 726–37.
4. Bach SP, Renehan AG, Potten CS. Stem cells: the intestinal stem cell as a paradigm. Carcinogenesis 2000; 21: 469–76.
5. Lakshmipathy U, Verfaillie C. Stem cell plasticity. Blood Rev 2005; 19: 29–38.
6. McCulloch EA, Till JE. Perspectives on the properties of stem cells. Nat Med 2005; 11: 1026–8.
7. Li L, Xie T. Stem cell niche: structure and function. Annu Rev Cell Dev Biol 2005; 21: 605–31.
8. Fuchs E, Tumbar T, Guasch G. Socializing with the neighbors: stem cells and their niche. Cell 2004; 116: 769–78.
9. Quesenberry PJ, Dooner G, Colvin G, Abedi M. Stem cell biology and the plasticity polemic. Exp Hematol 2005; 33: 389–94.
10. Li A, Pouliot N, Redvers R, Kaur P. Extensive tissue-regenerative capacity of neonatal human keratinocyte stem cells and their progeny. J Clin Invest 2004; 113: 390–400.
11. Schofield R. The relationship between the spleen colony-forming cell and the haemopoietic stem cell. Blood Cells 1978; 4: 7–25.
12. Ohlstein B, Kai T, Decotto E et al. The stem cell niche: theme and variations. Curr Opin Cell Biol 2004; 16: 693–9.
13. Tumbar T, Guasch G, Greco V et al. Defining the epithelial stem cell niche in skin. Science 2004; 303: 359–63.
14. Booth C, Potten CS. Gut instincts: thoughts on intestinal epithelial stem cells. J Clin Invest 2000; 105: 1493–9.
15. Sancho E, Batlle E, Clevers H. Signaling pathways in intestinal development and cancer. Annu Rev Cell Dev Biol 2004; 20: 695–723.
16. Nilsson SK, Simmons PJ. Transplantable stem cells: home to specific niches. Curr Opin Hematol 2004; 11: 102–6.
17. Doetsch F. A niche for adult neural stem cells. Curr Opin Gen Devel 2003; 13: 543–50.
18. Zhang JW, Niu C, Ye L et al. Identification of the haematopoietic stem cell niche and control of the niche size. Nature 2003; 425: 836–41.
19. Mills JC, Gordon JI. The intestinal stem cell niche: there grows the neighborhood. Proc Natl Acad Sci USA 2001; 98: 12334–6.
20. Reya T, Duncan AW, Ailles L et al. A role for Wnt signaling in self-renewal of haematopoietic stem cells. Nature 2003; 423: 409–14.
21. Wagers AJ, Weissman IL. Plasticity of adult stem cells. Cell 2004; 116: 639–48.
22. Blau HM, Brazelton TR, Weimann JM. The evolving concept of a stem cell: entity or function? Cell 2001; 105: 829–41.
23. Raff M. Adult stem cell plasticity: fact or artifact? Annu Rev Cell Dev Biol 2003; 19: 1–22.
24. Tosh D, Slack JMW. How cells change their phenotype. Nat Rev Mol Cell Biol 2002; 3: 187–94.
25. Pomerantz J, Blau HM. Nuclear reprogramming: a key to stem cell function in regenerative medicine. Nat Cell Biol 2004; 6: 810–16.
26. Taylor HS. Endometrial cells derived from donor stem cells in bone marrow transplant recipients. JAMA 2004; 292: 81–5.
27. Korbling M, Estrov Z. Adult stem cells for tissue repair – a new therapeutic concept? N Engl J Med 2003; 349: 570–82.
28. Snyder EY, Loring JF. A role for stem cell biology in the physiological and pathological aspects of aging. J Am Geriatr Soc 2005; 53: S287–91.
29. Tsujimura A, Koikawa Y, Salm S, et al. Proximal location of mouse prostate epithelial stem cells: a model of prostatic homeostasis. J Cell Biol 2002; 157: 1257–65.
30. Clarke RB, Smith GH. Stem cells and tissue homeostasis in mammary glands. J Mammary Gland Biol Neoplasia 2005; 10: 1–3.
31. Dor Y, Brown J, Martinez OI et al. Adult pancreatic beta-cells are formed by self-duplication rather than stem-cell differentiation. Nature 2004; 429: 41–6.
32. Guasch G, Fuchs E. Mice in the world of stem cell biology. Nat Genet 2005; 37: 1201–6.
33. Kaur P, Li A, Redvers R et al. Keratinocyte stem cell assays: an evolving science. J Investig Dermatol Symp Proc 2004; 9: 238–47.
34. Chan RWS, Schwab KE, Gargett CE. Clonogenicity of human endometrial epithelial and stromal cells. Biol Reprod 2004; 70: 1738–50.
35. Simmons PJ, Torok-Storb B. Identification of stromal cell precursors in human bone marrow by a novel monoclonal antibody, STRO-1. Blood 1991; 78: 55–62.
36. Schwab KE, Gargett CE. Indentifying markers for stromal stem/progenitors in human endometrium. Reprod Fertil Develop 2004; 16(Suppl): 98, P268.
37. van Os R, Kamminga LM, de Haan G. Stem cell assays: something old, something new, something borrowed. Stem Cells 2004; 22: 1181–90.
38. Pellegrini G, Golisano O, Paterna P et al. Location and clonal analysis of stem cells and their differentiated progeny in the human ocular surface. J Cell Biol 1999; 145: 769–82.
39. Gronthos S, Mankani M, Brahim J et al. Postnatal human dental pulp stem cells (DPSCs) in vitro and in vivo. Proc Natl Acad Sci USA 2000; 97: 13625–30.
40. Stingl J, Eaves CJ, Zandieh I et al. Characterization of bipotent mammary epithelial progenitor cells in normal adult human breast tissue. Breast Cancer Res Treat 2001; 67: 93–109.
41. Reynolds BA, Rietze RL. Neural stem cells and neurospheres – re-evaluating the relationship. Nat Methods 2005; 2: 333–6.
42. Li A, Simmons PJ, Kaur P. Identification and isolation of candidate human keratinocyte stem cells based on cell surface phenotype. Proc Natl Acad Sci USA 1998; 95: 3902–7.

43. Gronthos S, Zannettino ACW, Hay SJ et al. Molecular and cellular characterisation of highly purified stromal stem cells derived from human bone marrow. J Cell Sci 2003; 116: 1827–35.

44. Loeffler M, Roeder I. Conceptual models to understand tissue stem cell organization. Curr Opin Hematol 2004; 11: 81–7.

45. Kordon EC, Smith GH. An entire functional mammary gland may comprise the progeny from a single cell. Development 1998; 125: 1921–30.

46. Pittenger MF, Mackay AM, Beck SC et al. Multilineage potential of adult human mesenchymal stem cells. Science 1999; 284: 143–7.

47. Zuk PA, Zhu M, Ashjian P et al. Human adipose tissue is a source of multipotent stem cells. Mol Biol Cell 2002; 13: 4279–95.

48. Joseph NM, Morrison SJ. Toward an understanding of the physiological function of mammalian stem cells. Dev Cell 2005; 9: 173–83.

49. Greiner DL, Hesselton RA, Shultz LD. SCID mouse models of human stem cell engraftment. Stem Cells 1998; 16: 166–77.

50. Xin L, Lawson DA, Witte ON. The Sca-1 cell surface marker enriches for a prostate-regenerating cell subpopulation that can initiate prostate tumorigenesis. Proc Natl Acad Sci USA 2005; 102: 6942–7.

51. Booth C, O'Shea JA, Potten CS. Maintenance of functional stem cells in isolated and cultured adult intestinal epithelium. Exp Cell Res 1999; 249: 359–66.

52. Hull ML, Prentice A, Wang DY et al. Nimesulide, a COX-2 inhibitor, does not reduce lesion size or number in a nude mouse model of endometriosis. Hum Reprod 2005; 20: 350–8.

53. Kaitu'u TJ, Shen J, Zhang J et al. Matrix metalloproteinases in endometrial breakdown and repair: functional significance in a mouse model. Biol Reprod 2005; 73: 672–80.

54. Morris RJ, Potten CS. Slow cycling (label-retaining) epidermal cells behave like clonogenic stem cells in vitro. Cell Prolif 1994; 27: 279–89.

55. Welm BE, Tepera SB, Venezia T et al. Sca-1(pos) cells in the mouse mammary gland represent an enriched progenitor cell population. Dev Biol 2002; 245: 42–56.

56. Chan RWS, Gargett CE. Identification of label-retaining cells in mouse endometrium. Stem Cells 2006; 24: 1529–38.

57. Prianishnikov VA. On the concept of stem cell and a model of functional-morphological structure of the endometrium. Contraception 1978; 18: 213–23.

58. Padykula HA, Coles LG, McCracken JA et al. A zonal pattern of cell proliferation and differentiation in the rhesus endometrium during the estrogen surge. Biol Reprod 1984; 31: 1103–18.

59. Ferenczy A, Bertrand G, Gelfand MM. Proliferation kinetics of human endometrium during the normal menstrual cycle. Am J Obstet Gynecol 1979; 133: 859–67.

60. Padykula HA, Coles LG, Okulicz WC et al. The basalis of the primate endometrium: a bifunctional germinal compartment. Biol Reprod 1989; 40: 681–90.

61. Brenner RM, Slayden OD, Rodgers WH et al. Immunocytochemical assessment of mitotic activity with an antibody to phosphorylated histone H3 in the macaque and human endometrium. Hum Reprod 2003; 18: 1185–93.

62. Hartman C. Regeneration of monkey uterus after surgical removal of endometrium and accidental endometriosis. West J Surg Obstet Gynecol 1944; 52: 87–102.

63. Wood C, Rogers PAW. Pregnancy after planned partial endometrial resection. Aust NZ J Obstet Gynaecol 1993; 33: 316–18.

64. Tresserra F, Grases P, Ubeda A et al. Morphological changes in hysterectomies after endometrial ablation. Hum Reprod 1999; 14: 1473–7.

65. Biervliet FP, Maguiness SD, Robinson J, Killick SR. A successful cycle of IVF-ET after treatment of endometrial ossification; case report and review. J Obstet Gynaecol 2004; 24: 472–3.

66. Bird CC, Willis RA. The production of smooth muscle by the endometrial stroma of the adult human uterus. J Pathol Bacteriol 1965; 90: 75–81.

67. Roth E, Taylor HB. Heterotopic cartilage in the uterus. Obstet Gynecol 1966; 27: 838–44.

68. Short B, Brouard N, Occhiodoro-Scott T et al. Mesenchymal stem cells. Arch Med Res 2003; 34: 565–71.

69. Mutter GL, Lin MC, Fitzgerald JT et al. Changes in endometrial PTEN expression throughout the human menstrual cycle. J Clin Endocrinol Metab 2000; 85: 2334–8.

70. Tanaka M, Kyo S, Kanaya T et al. Evidence of the monoclonal composition of human endometrial epithelial glands and mosaic pattern of clonal distribution in luminal epithelium. Am J Pathol 2003; 163: 295–301.

71. Schwab KE, Chan RW, Gargett CE. Putative stem cell activity of human endometrial epithelial and stromal cells during the menstrual cycle. Fertil Steril 2005; 84: 1124–30.

72. Gargett CE. Uterine stem cells; what is the evidence? Hum Reprod Update 2007; 13: 87–101.

73. Loughney AD, Redfern CP. Menstrual cycle related differences in the proliferative responses of cultured human endometrial stromal cells to retinoic acid. J Reprod Fertil 1995; 105: 153–9.

74. Tanaka T, Nakajima S, Umesaki N. Cellular heterogeneity in long-term surviving cells isolated from eutopic endometrial, ovarian endometrioma and adenomyosis tissues. Oncol Rep 2003; 10: 1155–60.

75. Fujii S, Konishi I, Mori T. Smooth muscle differentiation at the endometrio-myometrial junction. An ultrastructural study. Virchows Archiv A Pathol Anat Histopathol 1989; 414: 105–12.

76. Gargett CE, Zillwood R, Schwab KE. Characterising the stem cell activity of human endometrial cells. Hum Reprod 2005; 20 (Suppl 1): i95.

77. Holinka CF, Gurpide E. Proliferative potential and polymorphism of human endometrial stromal cells. Gynecol Endocrinol 1987; 1: 71–81.

78. Kim JY, Tavare S, Shibata D. Counting human somatic cell replications: methylation mirrors endometrial stem cell divisions. Proc Natl Acad Sci USA 2005; 17739–44.

79. Ro S, Rannala B. Methylation patterns and mathematical models reveal dynamics of stem cell turnover in the human colon. Proc Natl Acad Sci USA 2001; 98: 10519–21.

80. Schwab KE, Gargett CE. Co-expressions of two perivascular cell markers isolates mesenchymal stem-like cells from human endometrium. Hum Reprod 2007; 22: 2903–11.

81. Cho NH, Park YK, Kim YT et al. Lifetime expression of stem cell markers in the uterine endometrium. Fertil Steril 2004; 81: 403–7.

82. Garcia-Pacheco JM, Oliver C, Kimatrai M et al. Human decidual stromal cells express CD34 and STRO-1 and are related to bone marrow stromal precursors. Mol Hum Reprod 2001; 7: 1151–7.

83. Hamilton AE, Nayak NN, Vo KC et al. Analysis of stem cell markers in human endometrium reveals cell-specific expression. Proc Int Soc Stem Cell Res 2005; 3: 67–P154.

84. Kobayashi A, Behringer RR. Developmental genetics of the female reproductive tract in mammals. Nat Rev Genet 2003; 4: 969–80.

85. Spencer TE, Hayashi K, Hu J et al. Comparative developmental biology of the mammalian uterus. Curr Top Dev Biol 2005; 68: 85–122.

86. Lipschutz JH, Fukami H, Yamamoto M et al. Clonality of urogenital organs as determined by analysis of chimeric mice. Cells Tiss Organs 1999; 165: 57–66.

87. Cervello I, Martinez-Conejero JA, Escobedo C et al. Identification, characterisation and colocalisation of the label

retaining cell population in the murine endometrium. Hum Reprod 2007; 22: 45–51.

88. Cooke PS, Buchanan DL, Young P et al. Stromal estrogen receptors mediate mitogenic effects of estradiol on uterine epithelium. Proc Natl Acad Sci USA 1997; 94: 6535–40.

89. Giudice LC, Kao LC. Endometriosis. Lancet 2004; 364: 1789–99.

90. Van Gorp T, Amant F, Neven P et al. Endometriosis and the development of malignant tumors of the pelvis. A review of literature. Best Pract Res Clin Obstet Gynaecol 2004; 18: 349–71.

91. Ferenczy A. Pathophysiology of adenomyosis. Hum Reprod Update 1998; 4: 312–22.

92. Pardal R, Clarke MF, Morrison SJ. Applying the principles of stem-cell biology to cancer. Nat Rev Cancer 2003; 3: 895–902.

93. Miller SJ, Lavker RM, Sun TT. Interpreting epithelial cancer biology in the context of stem cells: tumor properties and therapeutic implications. Biochim Biophys Acta 2005; 1756: 25–52.

94. Reya T, Morrison SJ, Clarke MF et al. Stem cells, cancer, and cancer stem cells. Nature 2001; 414: 105–11.

95. Latta E, Chapman WB. PTEN mutations and evolving concepts in endometrial neoplasia. Curr Opin Obstet Gynecol 2002; 14: 59–65.

96. Moreno-Bueno G, Hardisson D, Sanchez C et al. Abnormalities of the APC/beta-catenin pathway in endometrial cancer. Oncogene 2002; 21: 7981–90.

97. Amant F, Moerman P, Neven P et al. Endometrial cancer. Lancet 2005; 366: 491–505.

98. Vats A, Bielby RC, Tolley NS et al. Stem cells. Lancet 2005; 366: 592–602.

99. Rahaman MN, Mao JJ. Stem cell-based composite tissue constructs for regenerative medicine. Biotechnol Bioeng 2005; 91: 261–84.

100. Delancey JO. The hidden epidemic of pelvic floor dysfunction: achievable goals for improved prevention and treatment. Am J Obstet Gynecol 2005; 192: 1488–95.

11 Transgenic models of uterine biology

Indrani C Bagchi and Milan K Bagchi

INTRODUCTION

In adult mammals, the principal function of the uterus is to support the development of the embryo during pregnancy. The uterine tissue consists of the luminal and glandular epithelia, stroma, and myometrium. During development, the Müllerian duct differentiates to form the luminal and glandular epithelia of the uterus. The urogenital ridge that surrounds the Müllerian duct gives rise to the connective tissue stroma and the myometrium. The luminal epithelium and the stroma together constitute the endometrium. Waves of cell proliferation, differentiation, and remodeling in the pubertal animals prepare the endometrium for embryo implantation and establishment of pregnancy. Although the cellular events that regulate various phases of uterine biology during the reproductive cycles and pregnancy are well described, the molecular pathways that underlie these processes are largely unknown. However, during the past several years, with the advent and continued refinement of the gene knockout and knockin technologies, transgenic mice have become extremely useful tools for determining the functional roles of molecules involved in various aspects of uterine physiology. Creation of several mouse models by gene targeting and homologous recombination in embryonic stem cells and extensive analysis of the reproductive phenotypes of the mutant mice have generated an initial blueprint of the pathways that are involved in normal uterine development and establishment of pregnancy. In this chapter, we provide a brief description of these transgenic models.

GENES INVOLVED IN EARLY UTERINE DEVELOPMENT

The development of the uterine tissue involves differentiation of Müllerian duct epithelium into the luminal and glandular epithelial cells and its surrounding urogenital ridge mesenchyme into stroma and muscle layers. Recent development of a number of knockout mouse models has contributed to our understanding of the factors that play an essential role in early uterine development (Table 11.1). These models are described below.

Wnt pathways

The mammalian *Wnt* genes are homologues of the *Drosophila* segment polarity gene *Wingless*. They encode secreted signaling glycoproteins that influence multiple processes during development.[1] Recent research using knockout mice has shown that members of the *Wnt* family of proteins play a critical role in female reproductive tract development. Mutant mice lacking *Wnt-7a* allele are viable but exhibit various malformations in the uterus. The uterus is hypoplastic with a marked reduction in the stromal compartment, a lack of uterine glands, and a disorganized myometrium.[2,3] In addition, *Wnt-7a* mutant uterine epithelium fails to maintain a normal columnar phenotype and becomes stratified upon puberty. Thus, in the absence of *Wnt-7a*, both epithelial and mesenchymal differentiation are disrupted in the uterus.[2,3] Another member of the *Wnt* family, *Wnt-5a*, is also important for the development of the uterus. *Wnt-5a* mutants die at birth due to a failure to complete anteroposterior body axis development.[4] In the absence of *Wnt-5a*, the uterus fails to form glands.[5]

Homeobox genes

Homeobox or *Hox* genes encode a family of transcription factors sharing a highly conserved 61 amino acid helix–loop–helix domain or homeodomain.[6] In the developing Müllerian duct, a number of posterior *Abdominal B Hox* genes are expressed in nested patterns. For example, *Hoxa-9* expression is detected in the future isthmus region of the oviduct, while *Hoxa-10* and *Hoxa-11* are expressed at the uterotubal junction and uterus, respectively.[7,8] Consistent with these observations, targeted mutagenesis of these genes has led to region-specific defects along the female reproductive tract. Mutation of the *Hoxa-11* gene produced sterility in females.[9] The *Hoxa-11* mutant uteri are significantly smaller than wild-type littermates and display abnormal stromal and glandular differentiation.[10] Histological analysis demonstrated normal uterine morphology in *Hoxa-11* mutants as compared with

Table 11.1   Gene knockouts that affect uterine development and function

Gene	Phenotype	Reference
Genes involved in early uterine development		
Wnt-7a (*Wnt-7a*)	Abnormal development of uterus	2, 3
Wnt-5a (*Wnt-5a*)	Absence of uterine glands	5
Homeobox A11 (*Hoxa11*)	Abnormal stromal and glandular differentiation	10, 11
Homeobox A10 (*Hoxa10*)	Homeotic transformation of the uterus	12
Genes involved in uterine growth in adult mice		
Estrogen receptor α (*Esr1*)	Hypoplastic uteri	14, 16
Centromere protein B (*Cenpb*)	Defects in uterine epithelium	20
25-Hydroxyvitamin D-1α-hydroxylase (*Cyp27b1*)	Hypoplastic uteri	23
Vitamin D receptor (*Vdr*)	Hypoplastic uteri	24
Insulin-like growth factor 1 (*Igf1*)	Hypoplastic uteri	26
Genes involved in uterine receptivity and embryo implantation		
Progesterone receptor (*Pgr*)	Defects in uterine receptivity and decidualization	31
Basic transcription element-binding protein 1 (*BTEB1*)	Impaired uterine growth and embryo implantation	36
FK506 binding protein (*FKBP52*)	Defects in uterine receptivity	38
Leukemia inhibitory factor (*Lif*)	Blastocyst fail to implant	42
Interleukin-11 receptorA (*IL11ra*)	Defects in decidualization	44, 45
Common signal transducing receptor Gp130 (*Gp130*)	Blastocyst fail to implant	48
Homeobox A10 (*Hoxa10*)	Defects in decidualization	50
Cyclooxygenase-2 (*Ptgs2*)	Defects in implantation and decidualization	52
	Delay in the onset of decidualization	54
12/15 Lipoxygenase (*Alox12*)	Impairment in embryo implantation	55
Phospholipase A$_2$ (*Pla2g4a*)	Delayed implantation, aberrant embryo spacing	58
Lysophosphatidic acid receptor 3 (*LPA3*)	Delayed implantation, aberrant embryo spacing	59
CCAAT/enhancer binding protein β (*C/EBPβ*)	Defects in decidualization	61

controls at the newborn stage. However, by day 14 after birth, a significant reduction in the stromal tissues was observed in the *Hoxa-11* mutants, which decreased further by day 21 after birth. This was accompanied by a decrease in cell proliferation and an increase in apoptosis in the *Hoxa-11* mutant uterus, suggesting that *Hoxa-11* is involved in controlling cellular proliferation and apoptotic responses in the neonatal uterus.[11]

Hoxa-10 deficiency causes homeotic transformation of the anterior part of the uterus into oviduct-like structure and reduced fertility in females.[12] To address the role of this developmental defect in female infertility, wild-type blastocysts were transferred into *Hoxa-10* mutant uteri distal to the transformed region. Interestingly, this procedure did not result in successful implantation, suggesting that in addition to its role in proper patterning of the reproductive tract *Hoxa-10* is also required in the adult uterus for embryo implantation.[13] The functional role of *Hoxa-10* in embryo implantation and establishment of pregnancy is described later.

GENES INVOLVED IN UTERINE GROWTH IN ADULT MICE

The functional status of hormone-primed epithelium and underlying stroma is important for the establishment of pregnancy. In pubertal mice, the hormonal changes that occur immediately before ovulation lead to well-characterized physiological and biochemical alterations in the uterus in preparation for potential pregnancy. The luminal and the glandular epithelial cells of the uterus undergo multiple rounds of mitotic divisions. In mice, the estrous cycle is without a true luteal phase since only a small amount of progesterone is synthesized following ovulation. It is believed that, during the normal reproductive cycle, this low level of progesterone controls the estrogen-mediated proliferative activity of uterine epithelial cells. Dysregulated uterine growth can create a hypoplastic or hyperplastic epithelium, leading to non-productive interactions with the embryo and failure of pregnancy. The analysis of transgenic mouse models over the last few years has led to the identification of an array of molecules that regulate uterine growth in adult mice (see Table 11.1).

Estrogen receptor alpha

The cellular actions of estrogen are mediated by its intracellular receptors. There are two isoforms of the estrogen receptor, estrogen receptor α (ERα) and estrogen receptor β (ERβ). In the uterus, ERα is the predominant form of ER. Mutant mouse models lacking ERα and ERβ have been developed.[14,15] Analysis of these mutant mouse models provided insights into the isoform-specific receptor-mediated effects of estrogen in the regulation of uterine function. The ERα null mice were impaired in the growth and function of the female reproductive tract. The uterine epithelia of these null mice were hypoplastic and failed to support blastocyst attachment.[14,16,17] In contrast, the ERβ null females did not have any detectable uterine defect and were able to carry pregnancies successfully to term.[15,17]

Centromere protein B

The centromere is essential for proper chromosome movement during mitosis and meiosis.[18,19] A number of centromere proteins have been identified but little is known about their roles in whole animals. Interestingly, generation of Centromere protein B (Cenpb) null mice indicated that Cenpb deficiency leads to severe female reproductive dysfunction resulting from abnormality of uterine epithelium.[20] The Cenpb null females show significantly reduced uterine weights compared to wild-type littermates. The mice are found to be initially reproductively competent but show age-dependent reproductive deterioration, leading to a complete breakdown at or before 9 months of age.[20] Histology of the uterus reveals severe disruption in luminal and glandular epithelium but normal stroma and myometrium.[20] These disruptions are expected to influence the proper functioning of the uterine epithelium, and this, in turn, can cause problems in establishment of pregnancy.

25-hydroxyvitamin D-1 α-hydroxylase and VDR

Studies with transgenic animals showed that vitamin D, a major regulator of mineral ion homeostasis, plays a significant role in the growth and differentiation of the uterus. 1α, 25-Dihydroxyvitamin D is the most potent metabolite of vitamin D and is believed to exert most of its actions via the vitamin D receptor (VDR), a member of the nuclear receptor superfamily.[21,22] The mitochondrial cytocrome P450 enzyme 25-hydroxyvitamin D-1 α-hydroxylase catalyzes the generation of this metabolite. Mice deficient in 25-hydroxyvitamin D-1 α-hydroxylase were generated by gene targeting.[23] The mutant female mice are infertile, with significantly smaller uteri compared to wild-type littermates. Histological analysis revealed uterine hypoplasia at 7 weeks of age with a poorly developed endometrium.[23] Not surprisingly, the VDR null female mice also exhibited similar uterine phenotype.[24] Although normal uterine development was observed in these mice until 4–5 weeks, the uterus failed to mature at 7 weeks, resulting in a hypoplastic uterus.[24]

Insulin-like growth factor I

Insulin-like growth factors (IGFs) are multifunctional regulators involved in various biological processes.[25] Loss of IGF1 in mice leads to a dramatic hypoplastic uterine phenotype demonstrating its critical role in uterine growth and differentiation.[26] On an average, the weight of IGF1 null uterus is about 13% of that of wild-type. Although the luminal epithelial cells morphologically appeared normal, the abundance and complexity of secretory glandular elements is significantly reduced in IGF1 null uteri.[26]

GENES INVOLVED IN UTERINE RECEPTIVITY AND EMBRYO IMPLANTATION

During early pregnancy, estrogen and progesterone act in concert to induce changes in the uterine epithelium and stroma, creating an endometrium that is receptive for blastocyst implantation.[27,28] Subsequently, progesterone induces the undifferentiated stromal cells to proliferate and then undergo terminal differentiation to form the 'decidua', a unique and transient tissue that helps maintain an environment conducive for the growth and development of the implanting embryo.[29,30] In accordance with the functional roles attributed to these hormones during early pregnancy, mice lacking ERα and progesterone receptor (PR) exhibited defects in uterine receptivity and failed to initiate implantation.[16,31] Additionally, the transgenic technology has resulted in the development of other mouse models, which led to the identification of several novel factors that play important roles in the regulation of uterine receptivity and decidual response during implantation (see Table 11.1).

Progesterone receptors

The biological activities of progesterone are mediated by the PR isoforms, PR-A and PR-B. The PR knockout (PRKO) mice lacking both receptor isoforms are infertile and display hyperplastic luminal and glandular epithelial cells due to unopposed estrogen action. The PRKO mice also exhibit defects in implantation and decidualization.[31] They exhibit a refractory uterus that does not respond to an artificial deciduogenic stimulus.[31] Similar phenotypic deficiencies were recapitulated in mice lacking PR-A.[32,33] In contrast, the PR-B null mice showed no abnormal uterine phenotype.[32,33] The known progesterone-mediated responses in the uterus are therefore mediated via PR-A.

Basic transcription element-binding protein 1

The transcriptional activity of PR is influenced by co-regulatory proteins expressed in a tissue- and cell-specific fashion.[34] Previous studies have shown that basic transcription element-binding protein 1 or BTEB1, a member of the Sp/Kruppel-like family of transcription factors, interacts with PR isoforms to mediate progestin sensitivity of target genes in endometrial epithelial cells in vitro.[35] A recent report showed that ablation of the *BTEB1* gene in female mice results in uterine growth retardation, fewer number of implantation sites, decreased litter size, and partial or total resistance to progesterone.[36] In contrast, the ovarian function is essentially unaltered in these null mice. Since PR-A rather than PR-B is thought to mediate the majority of progesterone-dependent responses in the uterus, the observed uterine phenotypes of BTEB1 null females might arise from an impaired PR-A activity resulting from the loss of BTEB1 in the uteri of mutant mice.

FKBP52

FKBP52, a co-chaperone for progesterone receptor, is important for receptor folding and functional maturation of the ligand-binding domain.[37] Since progesterone and its receptor critically regulate uterine function during pregnancy, it is not surprising that mice lacking FKBP52 are infertile and exhibit a defect in implantation and decidualization.[38] It was reported that hormone-binding activity of PR is compromised in FKBP52 null females. This leads to an impairment in the PR-dependent pathways that regulate uterine receptivity and decidual response.[38]

Leukemia inhibitory factor

Leukemia inhibitory factor (LIF), a member of the interleukin-6 (IL-6) family of cytokines, is expressed at low levels in many different tissues and exhibits a multitude of biological actions, including cell proliferation and differentiation.[39] In mice, LIF expression is up-regulated in the uterine glandular epithelium prior to implantation and is also expressed in subluminal stromal cells surrounding the blastocyst at the time of the attachment reaction.[40,41] The role of LIF in implantation was revealed by the generation of a LIF-deficient mouse model by Stewart and coworkers.[42] Homozygous females lacking a functional *LIF* gene produced viable blastocysts but the embryos did not attach, and implantation failed to occur, presumably due to uterine defects.

Although the LIF null mouse was the first genetically engineered model of implantation defect, the pathway that mediates the function of this cytokine in the pregnant uterus still eludes us. In a recent study, subtractive hybridization of uterine RNA from wild-type and LIF null mice has led to the identification of cochlin, an extracellular matrix protein, as a potential downstream target of LIF signaling.[43] Although cochlin is expressed in the luminal epithelium at the time of implantation, mice lacking cochlin are fertile and do not exhibit a defect in implantation.[43] Further work is needed to uncover the signaling pathway that mediates LIF action in the uterus during early pregnancy.

Interleukin-11 receptor α

The IL-6 family of cytokines includes IL-6 and IL-11, among others. Recent studies have shown that IL-11 plays a key role in the uterine response to implantation. Female mice harboring null mutation of interleukin-11 receptor α (IL-11Rα) are infertile.[44,45] This was due to a post-implantation defect in the decidualization process.[44,45] In IL-11Rα null uteri, embryo attachment occurred and a primary decidual zone formed in the underlying stroma. However, the formation of secondary decidual zone in the mutant uteri was markedly reduced in comparison with wild-type littermates.[44,45] The limited decidua that was formed in the IL-11Rα null uteri degenerated progressively, leading to abnormal placenta formation and embryonic lethality.[44,45]

Gp130

LIF and IL-11 both act via a heterodimeric receptor complex composed of a ligand-specific α chain and a signaling component termed gp130.[46] In the uterus, gp130 transduces activities of the LIF/IL-6 family of cytokines through the signal transducer and activator of transcription (STAT) pathway.[47] To define STAT-dependent physiological responses during LIF/IL-6 signaling, a knockin mouse was created in which the endogenous gp130 was replaced by a mutant lacking all STAT-binding sites. These mutant mice phenocopied mice deficient in LIF.[48] As in the female LIF null mice, histological analysis of uteri of mutant gp130 females revealed the presence of blastocysts but showed no signs of implantation. Blastocysts recovered from gp130 null mice developed to term when transferred to pseudopregnant wild-type recipient mice, while no signs of pregnancy were observed when transferred to gp130 recipient mice. These results pointed to a uterine deficiency at the time of embryo implantation that is similar to the defect described in mice lacking LIF.[48]

Hoxa-10

In addition to its function during uterine development, *Hoxa-10* plays an essential role in adult females during embryo implantation. *Hoxa-10* is induced in the stromal cells in response to progesterone during early pregnancy.[49] The stromal cell proliferation is impaired in *Hoxa-10* null uteri, which leads to implantation and decidualization failures without affecting epithelial cell functions.[50] A recent study explored the downstream targets of Hoxa-10 during decidualization using gene expression profiling of uteri of wild-type and *Hoxa-10* null mice.[51] This study showed that *Hoxa-10* deficiency compromised natural killer (NK) cell differentiation without altering trafficking of NK precursor cells during decidualization.[51]

These data suggested that *Hoxa-10* is necessary for maintaining normal decidual development during the post-implantation period.

Lipid signaling pathways

It has been thought for a long time that prostaglandins (PGs) play an important role during embryo implantation.[28] The cyclooxygenase enzymes COX-1 and COX-2 mediate PG synthesis and are expressed in the mouse uterus during early pregnancy.[28] Of primary interest is the expression of COX-2, which is induced in the luminal epithelum and underlying stromal cells at the site of blastocyst attachment.[52] Studies from SK Dey's laboratory have shown that COX-2 null females are infertile, with defective ovulation, fertilization, implantation, and decidualization.[52] COX-2-derived prostacyclin (PGI$_2$) is the primary PG that is produced at the implantation site and the implantation defects in the COX-2 null mice are partially rescued by administration of PG.[53] This group also proposed that the COX-2-derived prostacyclins function via the nuclear receptor (peroxisome proliferator-activated receptor δ; PPARδ[53]). In another study, Stewart and co-workers have shown that COX-2 is not absolutely required for blastocyst implantation and decidualization in the mouse.[54] In the latter study, loss of COX-2 in the null mouse retarded the rate at which decidualization proceeds during the first 24 hours of implantation. Thereafter, both decidual and embryonic development proceeded apparently normally and resulted in the birth of viable offspring.[54] The basis of the discrepancy between the Dey and Stewart studies is unclear, since mice of the same genetic background were used in both cases.

It was observed that, besides cyclooxygenase, an alternate arachidonic acid metabolizing pathway via lipoxygenase (LOX) enzymes is active in preimplantation mouse uterus.[55] The leukocyte-12/15-LOX (L-12/15-LOX) and epidermal-12/15-LOX (E-12/15-LOX) enzymes are markedly induced in response to progesterone in the uterine surface epithelium immediately prior to implantation.[55] Mice bearing null mutation in the *L-12/15-LOX* gene showed significantly reduced uterine levels of the arachidonic acid metabolites 12- and 15-HETEs and 13-HODE. These mice also displayed a partial impairment in implantation. This partial phenotype is not surprising, as the E-12/15-LOX pathway, which produces lesser amounts of similar metabolites, remained intact in these mutant mice. It has been postulated that the

12/15-LOX-derived arachidonic acid metabolites function by acting as activating ligands of PPARγ, another member of the nuclear receptor family.[55]

Arachidonic acid, the substrate for the COX and LOX pathways, is generated by phospholipase A_2 (PLA_2). In response to a variety of stimuli, PLA_2 hydrolyzes the ester bonds of fatty acids in membrane phospholipids, producing free fatty acids, including arachidonic acids. Female mice carrying a null mutation in the gene coding for cytosolic $PLA_2\alpha$ have been developed.[56,57] These mice produced small litters and frequently exhibited pregnancy failures.[56,57] Using embryo transfer experiments, it was shown that the initiation of implantation is delayed in the null females for about 24 hours, leading to retarded fetoplacental development.[58] Furthermore, loss of $PLA_2\alpha$ resulted in aberrant embryo spacing in the uterus. Surprisingly, decidualization was not affected in $PLA_2\alpha$ knockout animals.[58] It is believed that retarded embryonic development and their resorption in $PLA_2\alpha$ null females contributed to the observed small litter size.

A phenotype similar to that displayed by the $PLA_2\alpha$ null mice was observed in mice lacking the receptor for lysophosphatidic acid (LPA).[59] LPAs are small bioactive phospholipids that exhibit a variety of biological functions via at least four G-protein-coupled receptors LPA_{1-4}.[60] Deletion of LPA_3 in mice resulted in significantly reduced litter size, which is attributed to delayed implantation and altered embryo spacing.[59] These events, in turn, led to delayed embryonic development, defective placenta shared by multiple embryos, and embryonic death.

CCAAT/enhancer-binding protein β

In a recent study, the CCAAT/enhancer-binding proteinβ (C/EBPβ), a transcription factor that regulates cell proliferation and differentiation in a variety of tissues, has emerged as a critical regulator of implantation.[61] The expression of C/EBPβ is rapidly induced in pregnant uterus in response to nidatory estrogen at the time of blastocyst attachment and increased further during the decidualization phase of pregnancy.[61] This expression was localized in the proliferating as well as the decidualized stromal cells surrounding the implanted embryo. The female C/EBPβ null mice are infertile.[62] To determine the function of this gene during implantation, uterine response to an artificial decidual stimulus was measured in wild-type and C/EBPβ null mice. While a dramatic decidual response was observed in the uteri of wild-type mice, the uteri of

C/EBPβ knockout mice failed to exhibit any decidual response.[61] Blastocysts transferred to the uteri of C/EBPβ knockout mice failed to grow, presumably due to a defect in decidualization. Further analysis revealed defects in steroid-induced stromal cell proliferation and differentiation in C/EBPβ null uteri, establishing C/EBPβ as a key mediator of steroid responsiveness of the uterine stroma during decidualization.[61]

SUMMARY AND PERSPECTIVES

Starting with the generation of the LIF knockout mouse in 1992, continued development of genetically engineered mouse models keeps adding to our knowledge of the molecules that critically regulate the functions of the female reproductive tract. Certain of these models were useful in detailed clarification of the roles of known regulators of uterine functions such as the estrogen and progesterone receptors. In most other cases, however, they have led to the identification of novel regulatory factors involved in uterine growth and embryo–endometrial interaction during early pregnancy. During the past 5 years, DNA microarray technology has been used extensively to compare the uterine gene expression profiles of wild-type and mutant mice. These experiments have revealed hitherto unknown pathways downstream of critical regulatory molecules and provided important insights into the cellular mechanisms by which the functions of the female reproductive tract are controlled. In the coming years, continued refinement of the transgenic methodology is likely to generate stage-specific, tissue-specific, and inducible knockout models, which will allow further analysis of molecules that control endometrial functions during the reproductive cycle and pregnancy.

REFERENCES

1. Nelson WJ, Nusse R. Convergence of Wnt, β-catenin, and cadherin pathways. Science 2004; 303: 1483–7.
2. Parr BA, McMahon AP. Sexually dimorphic development of the mammalian reproductive tract requires Wnt-7a. Nature 1998; 395: 707–10.
3. Miller C, Sassoon DA. Wnt-7a maintains appropriate uterine patterning during the development of the mouse female reproductive tract. Development 1998; 125: 3201–11.
4. Yamaguchi TP, Bradley A, McMahon AP et al. A Wnt5a pathway underlies outgrowth of multiple structures in the vertebrate embryo. Development 1999; 126: 1211–23.
5. Mericskay M, Kitajewski J, Sassoon D. Wnt5a is required for proper epithelial–mesenchymal interactions in the uterus. Development 2004; 131: 2061–72.

6. Kmita M, Duboule D. Organizing axes in time and space; 25 years of collinear tinkering. Science 2003; 301: 331–3.

7. Dolle P, Izpisua-Belmonte JC, Brown JM et al. HOX-4 genes and the morphogenesis of mammalian genitalia. Genes Dev 1991; 5: 1767–77.

8. Taylor HS, Van den Heuvel GB, Igarashi P. A conserved Hox axis in the mouse and human female reproductive system: late establishment and persistent adult expression of the Hoxa cluster genes. Biol Reprod 1997; 57: 1338–45.

9. Hsieh-Li HM, Witte DP, Weinstein M et al. Hoxa 11 structure, extensive antisense transcription, and function in male and female fertility. Development 1995; 121: 1373–85.

10. Gendron RL, Paradis H, Hsieh-Li HM et al. Abnormal uterine stromal and glandular function associated with maternal reproductive defects in Hoxa-11 null mice. Biol Reprod 1997; 56: 1097–105.

11. Wong KHH, Wintch HD, Capecchi MR. Hoxa11 regulates stromal cell death and proliferation during neonatal uterine development. Mol Endocrinol 2004; 18: 184–93.

12. Satokata I, Benson GV, Maas RL. Sexually dimorphic sterility phenotypes in Hoxa-10-deficient mice. Nature 1995; 374: 460–63.

13. Benson GV, Lim H, Paria BC et al. Mechanisms of reduced fertility in Hoxa-10 mutant mice: uterine homeosis and loss of maternal Hoxa-10 expression. Development 1996; 122: 2687–96.

14. Lubahn DB, Moyer JS, Golding TS et al. Alteration of reproductive function but not prenatal sexual development after insertional disruption of the mouse estrogen receptor gene. Proc Natl Acad Sci USA 1993; 90: 11162–6.

15. Krege JH, Hodgin JB, Couse JF et al. Generation and reproductive phenotypes of mice lacking estrogen receptor beta. Proc Natl Acad Sci USA 1998; 95: 15677–82.

16. Hewitt SC, Goulding EH, Eddy EM et al. Studies using the estrogen receptor alpha knockout uterus demonstrate that implantation but not decidualization-associated signaling is estrogen dependent. Biol Reprod 2002; 67: 1268–77.

17. Hewitt SC, Korach KS. Oestrogen receptor knockout mice: roles for oestrogen receptors α and β in reproductive tissues. Reproduction 2003; 125: 143–9.

18. Craig JM, Earnshaw WC, Vagnarelli P. Mammalian centromere: DNA sequence, protein composition, and role in cell cycle progression. Exp Cell Res 1998; 246: 249–62.

19. Dobie KW, Hari KL, Maggert KA et al. Centromere proteins and chromosome inheritance: a complex affair. Curr Opin Genet Dev 1999; 9: 206–17.

20. Fowler KJ, Hudson DF, Salamonsen LA et al. Uterine dysfunction and genetic modifiers in centromere protein-B deficient mice. Genome Res 2000; 10: 30–41.

21. Bouillon R, Okamura WH, Norman AW. Structure–function relationships in the vitamin D endocrine system. Endocr Rev 1995; 16: 200–57.

22. Mangelsdorf DJ, Evans RM. The RXR heterodimers and orphan receptors. Cell 1995; 83: 841–50.

23. Panda DK, Miao D, Tremblay ML et al. Targeted ablation of the 25-hydroxyvitamin D 1α-hydroxylase enzyme: evidence for skeletal, reproductive, and immune dysfunction. Proc Natl Acad Sci USA 2001; 98: 7498–503.

24. Yoshizawa T, Handa Y, Uematsu Y et al. Mice lacking the vitamin D receptor exhibit impaired bone formation, uterine hypoplasia and growth retardation and weaning. Nat Genet 1997; 16: 391–6.

25. Jones JI, Clemmon DR. Insulin-like growth factors and their binding proteins: biological actions. Endocr Rev 1995; 16: 3–34.

26. Baker J, Hardy MP, Zhou J et al. Effects of an Igf1 gene null mutation on mouse reproduction. Mol Endocrinol 1996; 10: 903–18.

27. Carson DD, Bagchi I, Dey SK et al. Embryo implantation. Dev Biol 2000; 223: 217–37.

28. Dey SK, Lim H, Das SK et al. Molecular cues to implantation. Endocr Rev 2004; 25: 341–73.

29. Irwin JC, Giudice L. Decidua. In: Knobil E, Neill JD, eds. Encyclopedia of Reproduction. New York: Academic Press, 1999: 823–35.

30. Gu Y, Gibori G. Deciduoma. In: Knobil E, Neill JD, eds. Encyclopedia of Reproduction. New York: Academic Press, 1999: 836–42.

31. Lydon JP, DeMayo FJ, Funk CR et al. Mice lacking progesterone receptor exhibit pleiotropic reproductive abnormalities. Genes Dev 1995; 9: 2266–78.

32. Mulac-Jericevic B, Mullinax RA, DeMayo FJ et al. Subgroup of reproductive functions of progesterone mediated by progesterone receptor-B isoform. Science 2000; 289: 1751–4.

33. Conneely OM, Mulac-Jericevic B, Lydon JP et al. Reproductive functions of the progesterone receptor isoforms: lessons from knock-out mice. Mol Cell Endocrinol 2001; 179: 97–103.

34. McKenna NJ, Lanz RB, O'Malley BW. Nuclear receptor coregulators: cellular and molecular biology. Endocr Rev 1999; 20: 321–44.

35. Zhang D, Zhang X-L, Michel FJ et al. Direct interaction of the Kruppel-like family (KLF) member, BTEB1, and PR mediates progesterone-responsive gene expression in endometrial epithelial cells. Endocrinology 2002; 140: 2517–25.

36. Simmen RCM, Eason RR, McQuown JR et al. Subfertility, uterine hypoplasia, and partial progesterone resistance in mice lacking the Kruppel-like factor 9/basic transcription element-binding protein-1 (Bteb1) gene. J Biol Chem 2004; 279: 29286–94.

37. Pratt WB, Toft DO. Regulation of signaling protein function and trafficking by the hsp90/hsp70-based chaperone machinery. Exp Biol Med 2003; 228: 111–33.

38. Tranguch S, Cheung-Flynn J, Daikoku T et al. Cochaperone immunophilin FKBP52 is critical to uterine receptivity for embryo implantation. Proc Natl Acad Sci USA 2005; 102: 14326–31.

39. Hilton DJ. LIF: lots of interesting functions. Trends Biochem Sci 1992; 17: 72–6.

40. Bhatt H, Brunet LJ, Stewart CL. Uterine expression of leukemia inhibitory factor coincides with the onset of blastocyst implantation. Proc Natl Acad Sci USA 1991; 88: 11408–12.

41. Song H, Lim H, Das SK et al. Dysregulation of EGF family of growth factors and COX-2 in the uterus during the preattachment and attachment reactions of the blastocyst with the luminal epithelium correlates with implantation failure in LIF-deficient mice. Mol Endocrinol 2000; 14: 1147–61.

42. Stewart CL, Kaspar P, Brunet LJ et al. Blastocyst implantation depends on maternal expression of leukaemia inhibitory factor. Nature 1992; 359: 76–9.

43. Rodriguez CI, Cheng JG, Liu L, Stewart CL. Cochlin, a secreted von Willebrand factor type a domain-containing factor, is regulated by leukemia inhibitory factor in the uterus at the time of embryo implantation. Endocrinology 2004; 145: 1410–18.

44. Robb L, Li R, Hartley L et al. Infertility in female mice lacking the receptor for interleukin 11 is due to a defective uterine response to implantation. Nat Med 1998; 4: 303–8.

45. Bilinski P, Roopenian D, Gossler A. Maternal IL-11R alpha function is required for normal decidua and fetoplacental development in mice. Genes Dev 1998; 12: 2234–43.

46. Taga T, Kishimoto T. Gp130 and the interleukin-6 family of cytokines. Annu Rev Immunol 1997; 15: 797–819.

47. Cheng JG, Chen JR, Hernandez L et al. Dual control of LIF expression and LIF receptor function regulate Stat3 activation at the onset of uterine receptivity and embryo implantation. Proc Natl Acad Sci USA 2001; 98: 8680–5.

48. Ernst M, Inglese M, Waring P et al. Defective gp130-mediated signal transducer and activator of transcription (STAT) signaling results in degenerative joint disease, gastrointestinal ulceration, and failure of uterine implantation. J Exp Med 2001; 194: 189–203.

49. Ma L, Benson GV, Lim H et al. Abdominal B (AbdB) Hoxa genes: regulation in adult uterus by estrogen and progesterone and repression in Müllerian duct by the synthetic estrogen diethylstilbestrol (DES). Dev Biol 1998; 197: 141–54.

50. Lim H, Ma L, Ma W et al. Hoxa-10 regulates uterine stromal cell responsiveness to progesterone during implantation and decidualization in the mouse. Mol Endocrinol 1999; 13: 1005–17.

51. Rahman MA, Li M, Li P et al. Hoxa-10 deficiency alters region-specific gene expression and perturbs differentiation of natural killer cells during decidualization. Dev Biol 2006; 290: 105–17.

52. Lim, H, Paria BC, Das SK et al. Multiple female reproductive failures in cyclooxygenase 2-deficient mice. Cell 1997; 91: 197–208.

53. Lim H, Gupta RA, Ma W et al. Cyclo-oxygenase-2-derived prostacyclin mediates embryo implantation in the mouse via PPARδ. Genes Dev 1999; 13: 1561–74.

54. Cheng JG, Stewart CL. Loss of cyclooxygenase-2 retards decidual growth but does not inhibit embryo implantation or development to term. Biol Reprod 2003; 68: 401–4.

55. Li Q, Cheon YP, Kannan A et al. A novel pathway involving progesterone receptor, 1215 lipoxygenase-derived eicosanoids, and peroxisome proliferator-activated receptor gamma regulates implantation in mice. J Biol Chem 2004; 279: 11570–81.

56. Bonventre JV, Huang Z, Taheri MR et al. Reduced fertility and postischaemic brain injury in mice deficient in cytosolic phospholipase A2. Nature 1997; 390: 622–5.

57. Uozumi N, Kume K, Nagase T et al. Role of cytosolic phospholipase A2 in allergic response and parturition. Nature 1997; 390: 618–22.

58. Song H, Lim H, Paria BC et al. Cytosolic phospholipase A2a deficiency is crucial for 'on-time' embryo implantation that directs subsequent development. Development 2002; 129: 2879–89.

59. Ye X, Hama K, Contos JJA et al. LPA3-mediated lysophosphatidic acid signaling in embryo implantation and spacing. Nature 2005; 435: 104–8.

60. Ishii I, Fukushima N, Ye X et al. Lysophospholipid receptors; signaling and biology. Annu Rev Biochem 2004; 73: 321–54.

61. Mantena SR, Kannan A, Cheon YP et al. C/CBPbeta is a critical mediator of steroid hormone-regulated cell proliferation and differentiation in the uterine epithelium and stroma. Proc Natl Acad Sci USA 2006; 103: 1870–5.

62. Sterneck E, Tessarollo L, Johnson PF. An essential role for C/EBPbeta in female reproduction. Genes Dev 1997; 11: 2153–62.

12 Estrogen-regulated genes in the endometrium

Sylvia C Hewitt and Kenneth S Korach

ESTROGEN RECEPTORS

Estrogen's effects on endometrial tissue are mediated by the hormone-regulated transcription factor, the estrogen receptor (ER). Ligand-modulated nuclear transcription factors, including the ER, share a general domain structure, domains A–F[1–3] (Figure 12.1). The C domain encodes the ER's DNA-binding domain (DBD), which includes two zinc finger motifs responsible for recognition and binding to specific DNA sequences (estrogen responsive elements [EREs]). ER primarily binds as a symmetrical homodimer to ERE sequences, with each ER molecule contacting one arm of the 5 base pair inverted repeat.[4–6] The consensus ERE sequence is a 13 base pair inverted repeat sequence, GGTCAnnnTGACC;[5] however the majority of response element sequences contain one or more variations from the consensus. In addition, ER can interact with ERE half-sites when there is a nearby Sp1 site.[7]

The ligand-binding domain (LBD, domain E) is the segment of the receptor protein that binds specifically to the agonist or antagonist ligands. This is accomplished through an arrangement of 12 α-helical regions that forms a binding 'pocket' accommodating the appropriate ligand.[1,8] Ligand binding induces a more compact arrangement of the LBD structure in which the position of the C-terminal α-helix, termed helix 12, is altered by the binding mode (unliganded, agonist, or antagonist), thereby determining the capacity to recruit transcriptional co-activators, proteins that modulate the transcriptional activity of the receptors.

The AF-1 region in the amino terminus and the AF-2 region within the ligand-binding domain of the ER are involved in ligand-independent and ligand-dependent transcriptional activation, respectively, as deletion or mutations of these regions result in a diminished ability to regulate genes.[9,10]

Two different ER genes, Esr1 and Esr2, are distinct gene loci that encode receptors ERα and ERβ, respectively, which share the ability to bind estrogens and regulate similar genes. High homology (98%) exists in the DBD of these ERs (see Figure 12.1), whereas there is poor homology in the N-terminal region and low

homology (54%) in the LBDs, despite the similar affinities of ERα and ERβ for endogenous estrogens such as estradiol, estrone, or estriol.

TRANSCRIPTIONAL REGULATION BY ESTROGEN RECEPTORS

The mechanism by which ERs mediate transcription involves interaction of the AFs with a complex of molecules that assembles and ultimately results in synthesis of mRNA.[11,12] Much is now known about RNA polymerase II and the enzymes and factors involved in transcription, as discussed in several recent reviews.[11,13,14]

In the most generalized models of ER action, agonist binds to the receptor, which interacts with DNA regulatory sequences in target genes (Figure 12.2). The ligand–ER complex then recruits the transcriptional co-modulators and, consequently, regulates transcription. However, numerous variations in this mechanism have been described. For example, many estrogen responsive genes lack the canonical ERE sequence, and interact with estrogen receptors via a tethering mechanism whereby ER recruits other transcription factors such as SP1 or AP1, which then directly interact with AP1 or Sp1 binding motifs (see Figure 12.2).[7,15–17]

Steroid receptor co-activators are numerous and diverse,[18,19] but have in common a nuclear receptor interaction motif, LXXLL, that interacts with helix 12 in the AF-2 domain of agonist-activated nuclear receptors. Transcriptional co-regulators vary in their specific functions;[20] in the case of co-activators, some, such as the steroid receptor co-activators (SRCs; also called p160s) modify histones via associated histone acetyltransferase (HAT) activities, which allow access of transcriptional enzymes to the DNA. Others, such as the thyroid receptor activating protein (TRAP) complex, act as a scaffold to assemble other co-regulators and RNA polymerase. A third type of co-regulator, for example BRG-1, possesses chromatin remodeling activity that increases transcriptional efficiency. CAPERa is an ER co-activator which also interacts with the transcriptional co-activator ASC2 and may

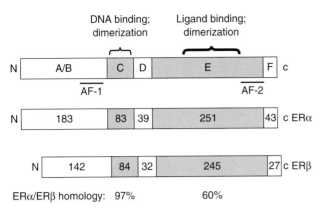

DNA binding; dimerization   Ligand binding; dimerization

ERα/ERβ homology: 97%   60%

(ERβ domains from SeqWeb GAP analysis of mouse ERα
amino acids 1–599 compared to mouse ERβ 1–530)

Figure 12.1 Schematic representation of estrogen receptor domains and comparison of homology between ERα and ERβ. The estrogen receptors can be divided into six domains, A–F. The C domain encodes the region of the ER that directly interacts with ERE DNA sequences of target genes. It includes two zinc finger chelating motifs. The E domain encodes the ligand binding domain. In addition, two AF or activation function domains are located in the A/B and E domains, respectively. Both are involved in regulating gene transcription. The N-terminal AF-1 activity is independent of ligand binding, while the activity of AF-2 is regulated by agonist binding. The D domain is described as a linker domain, and the F domain is not essential in some contexts. The A/B domain also contains phosphorylation sites. The ERs function as homodimers, and sequences important for dimerization are found in the C and E domains.

serve to integrate transcriptional and splicing activities.[21,22] Co-regulators are thought to undergo dynamic association with the promoters; p160 and TRAP220 complexes are cyclically exchanged on and off of estrogen responsive genes in a process of repeated chromatin remodeling/transcriptional initiation and transcriptional re-initiation/maintenance, respectively. These mechanisms are more fully discussed elsewhere.[14,18,19,23–26] Co-repressors, such as Nrip-1, often have associated histone deacetylase (HDAC) activity, which generally decreases DNA accessibility.[23]

The best characterized ER co-regulators (p160s) interact with the AF-2 domain, although co-regulators that interact with the N-terminus or both AFs have also been described. The co-activator p68 interacts with the AF-1 region of ERα, possesses RNA helicase activity, and associates with SRA, a RNA molecule with co-activator activity.[27–29] The co-repressor RTA interacts with ER AF-1 to inhibit tamoxifen activity.[30] Additionally, interaction between HDAC4 and the N-terminal region of ERα inhibits transcriptional activity.[31] Similarly, SPBP interacts with phosphoserine 118 in the AF-1 region and decreases ERα-mediated transcription,

possibly by recruiting the co-repressor NCor.[32] Splicing Factor 3ap120 has also been shown to interact with phosphoserine 118 in ERα, but increases transcription and potentiates splicing of ER target genes.[33]

'Non-genomic' signaling by ERs

In addition to those discussed above, several mechanisms to account for very rapid (within minutes or seconds) 'non-genomic' responses to estrogens (see Figure 12.2), indicate that receptors, either distinct or identical to the nuclear ER, interact with and activate signal cascades at the cell membrane.[34–36] Some estrogen-initiated rapid effects are mediated through a G-protein-coupled mechanism and are inhibited by adrenergic receptor signaling antagonists but not by ER antagonists.[35] These rapid effects can be initiated by BSA-conjugated steroids, which cannot enter the cell but can interact with the surface, indicating that extracellular components are sufficient to initiate response. Examples of these extracellular receptors have been difficult to isolate or identify. One potential candidate is GPR30, a G-protein-coupled receptor that has been shown to bind to estrogen, resulting in activation of Src/Shc and MAPK activity as well as adenylate cyclase activity through a Gα protein.[35,37,38] Many studies have focused on a model of membrane-bound ERα. In these models, approximately 2% of cellular ER is localized to the membrane, concentrated in caveolar structures, which act as scaffolds to assemble signaling molecules. ER and AR have been shown to interact with caveolin in an agonist-dependent manner, leading to the suggestion that caveolae might function to translocate ER to the plasma membrane.[35] Although data suggestive of a rapid estrogen response are accumulating in many models, the presence of or biological role for non-genomic estrogen responses in the endometrium remains to be determined.

Cross-talk mechanisms

Finally, activators of other non-ER membrane receptor pathways can also result in agonist-independent activation of ER-mediated transcription.[34,39] For example, increasing intracellular cAMP can lead to increased ER-mediated transcription,[34,39–41] and epidermal growth factor (EGF) or insulin-like growth factor 1 (IGF-1) receptor signaling can result in ERα-mediated activity.[34] These responses might result from interaction between signaling pathways and the ERs or associated co-regulators. The ER-growth factor 'cross-talk'

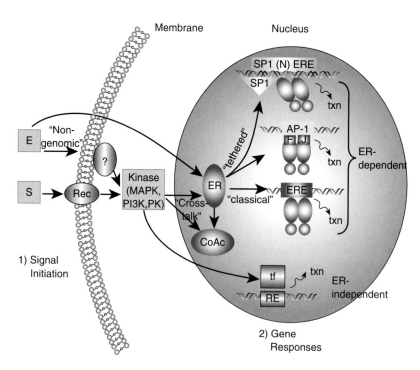

Figure 12.2   Mechanisms of gene regulation in response to estrogen. Estrogen (E), due to its lipophilic properties, can enter cells through the membrane and interact with the estrogen receptor (ER). Agonist binding alters the conformation of the ER, enabling recruitment of co-activators (CoAc). In the classical mechanism, the transcriptionally active ER complex can interact with genes containing estrogen responsive enhancer (ERE) DNA sequences through direct binding, resulting in gene transcription (txn). Alternatively, the transcriptionally active ER complex can recruit other transcription factors, such as SP1 or AP1 (F, fos: J, jun) which then interact with target genes. In this 'tethered' mechanism, ER is tethered to the target gene DNA, rather than binding directly with ERE sequences. Molecules that signal through membrane receptors, such as growth factors (S), can initiate signaling cascades, such as MAP kinase (MAPK) or PI3 kinase signaling cascades, which can regulate ER or its co-activators in a cross-talk mechanism, or can result in ER-independent direct regulation of other transcription factors (tf) and thus their target genes. The 'non-genomic' mechanism involves interaction of E with receptors on the cell surface. This receptor is depicted by '?' in this diagram because there is evidence both for a non-ER receptor, such as GPR30, or ERα associated with membrane structures. Regardless of the receptor utilized, resulting signals initiate cascades that can regulate activities of the ER or other transcription factors.

mechanisms (see Figure 12.2) were demonstrated in vivo by an increase in uterine weight and proliferation of the uterine epithelial cells in ovariectomized mice following EGF or IGF-1 treatment.[42–44] The lack of these responses in similarly tested αERKO mice indicated that the ERα is downstream of the growth factor receptor signaling in this response and that ERα is required.[43–45] Additionally, IGF-1 treatment increases expression of an estrogen-responsive luciferase reporter gene in the uterus of transgenic mice,[44] indicating direct activation of ER by IGF-1 signaling.

ESTROGEN RESPONSE IN THE ENDOMETRIUM

Although the mechanistic details of endometrial biology and the intricacies of their processes vary in different species, properly timed and coordinated events in response to the fluctuations in ovarian hormone levels

are universally critical to development and maintenance of an endometrium competent for embryo implantation and nurturing early embryonic gestation. Other chapters in this book describe the details leading to and the mechanisms that underlie endometrial growth, development, and embryo implantation. Here, we focus on a rapidly growing body of knowledge relating to the uterine genes that have been identified as targets of estrogen regulation during these processes. In Chapter 13 the uterine genes regulated by progesterone are described.

Early studies focused on identification of estrogen-regulated genes by measuring their expression through the estrous cycle or in response to exogenously administered estrogens or ER antagonists. These approaches yielded a modest number of genes in comparison to the more recent profusion of data produced from microarray approaches; however, in contrast to the numerous genes identified by genomic approaches, many of the genes identified prior to the availability of global microarray analysis have been thoroughly

Table 12.1 Estrogen-related uterine genes

Gene	Reference	Model	Method	Time	Peak time on 24 hours array (see Figure 12.3)
Ckb	49	Ovex rat	Northern blot	2 hours	2 hours
Dtr (Hbegf)	50	Ovex mouse	Northern blot	2 hours	2 hours
Fos	46	Ovex mouse uterus Ovex rat uterus	Northern blot IHC in situ	1–2 hours	2 hours
G6pd	51, 52	Rat uterus Ovex mouse	Enzyme activity Northern blot	12 hours	24 hours
Gapd	53	Ovex ewe	Slot blot	12–24 hours	24 hours
Gja1 (connexin 43) Gjb2 (connexin 26)	54	Ovex rat uterus	Northern blot	7 days	6 hours (Gja1)
Hras	55	Endom fibrobl	RT-PCR	12–24 hours	12–24 hours
Hsf	56	Ovex mouse	Northern blot Western blot	6 hours	6 hours
Igf1	57	Ovex rat	Northern blot	6 hours	12 hours
Jun	58	Ovex rat uterus	Northern blot IHC	1–2 hours	2 hours
Ltf	59	Ovex mouse uterus	Northern blot	24–36 hours	24 hours
Myc	60, 61	Ovex rat Ovex mouse	Northern blot, IHC	6 hours	6 hours
Odc1	52, 62, 63	Immature mouse Ovex mouse	Enzyme activity Northern blot	12–24 hours	12–24 hours
Oxtr	64, 65	Ovex rat	Binding site assay; Northern blot	2 hours	2 hours
Pgr	66, 67	Ovex G pig; Ovex rat (dec epi, inc stroma)t	Binding assay; IHC	24 hours	6–12 hours
Rab11	68	Ovex rat, delayed implantation rat	Northern blot IHC in situ	4 days	24 hours
Sfrp4	69	Ovex rat	Northern blot	48 hours	12–24 hours
Ski	70	Ovex rat	RT-PCR IHC in situ	3–24 hours	2 hours
Wisp2 (Ccn5)	71	Ovex rat	RT-PCR Western blot IHC	48 hours	2 hours

characterized in terms of their expression patterns in uterine cells and the identification of DNA elements and promoter sequences underlying their regulation (Table 12.1, Figure 12.3). Examples of these genes include *Fos*, *Lactoferrin*, and *Pgr*.[46–48]

ENDOMETRIAL MODELS

A cycling female provides an environment in which uterine responses to ovarian sex hormones occur in a biologically relevant manner; however, for many studies, this system is inappropriate as it is difficult to discern estrogen-specific effects, and in the

case of humans, it is often not feasible to conduct such studies. Several models have been successfully used to isolate and study estrogen-specific responses in the endometrium. One of the most commonly utilized experimental systems is the ovariectomized rodent. This system allows the administration of test compounds without a need to consider the estrous hormonal fluctuations. The acute physiological response of the rodent uterine tissue to ER agonist has been described in detail, and includes effects that occur in two phases.[72,73] Initial (early) responses that occur within several hours include transcription of 'early' genes such as *Fos*, increase in tissue weight due to water uptake, and infiltration of the tissue by

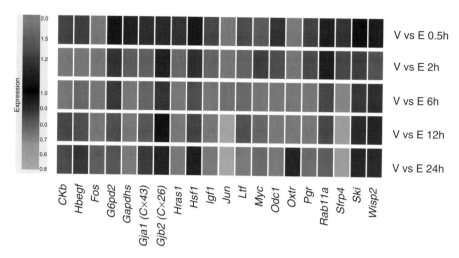

Figure 12.3 Heat map display of estrogen-regulated uterine genes from Table 12.1 showing values from microarray analysis. Ovariectomized animals were treated with E and sampled after 0.5, 2, 6, 12, and 24 hours. Each comparison is a pair of samples (vehicle compared to E_2 treatment at that time point) with red indicating higher transcript level in E_2 compared to vehicle and green indicating lower transcript level in E_2 treated compared to vehicle. *Ckb*, creatine kinase b; *Hbegf*, heparin-binding EGF-like growth factor; *Fos*, FBJ osteosarcoma oncogene; *G6pd2*, glucose-6-phosphate dehydrogenase 2; *Gapdhs*, glyceraldehyde-3-phosphate dehydrogenase, spermatogenic; *Gja1*, gap junction membrane channel protein alpha 1 (connexin 43); *Gjb2* gap junction membrane channel protein beta 2 (connexin 26); *Hras1*, Harvey rat sarcoma virus oncogene 1; *Hsf1*, heat shock transcription factor 1; *Igf1*, insulin-like growth factor 1; *Jun*, Jun oncogene; *Ltf*, lactotransferrin; *Myc*, myelocytomatosis oncogene; *Odc1*, ornithine decarboxylase, structural 1; *Oxtr*, oxytocin receptor; *Pgr*, progesterone receptor; *Rab11a*, RAB11a, member RAS oncogene family; *Sfrp4*, secreted frizzled-related sequence protein 4; *Ski*, Sloan-Kettering viral oncogene homolog; *Wisp2*, WNT1 inducible signaling pathway protein 2. (See also color plate section.)

immune system cells including eosinophils. Later responses that peak 16–24 hours after the ER agonist is administered include transcription of 'late' genes such as lactoferrin and coordinated waves of mitosis of the epithelial cells (described in greater detail in Chapter 9). This experimental model has been and continues to be a valuable and productive approach for the identification of and characterization of estrogen-regulated endometrial genes.

A second mouse model that is employed to highlight estrogen-regulated aspects of uterine function as it relates to embryo implantation is the 'delayed implantation' model. This model makes use of the observation that mouse implantation occurs in a very specific hormonal environment with precise temporal restrictions (see Section V of this book). In this design, females are mated, and then ovariectomized to remove ovarian sex steroids just prior to implantation on the morning of day 4 of pregnancy. They are then given exogenous progesterone to maintain the endometrium in an estrogen-deficient state, which prevents embryo implantation until the estrogen is replaced.[74] Thus, the uterine responses to estrogen that are essential to implantation can be examined. However, this approach has several limitations, including the complexity of responses due to progesterone signaling as well as signals from the implanting embryo that make it difficult to identify estrogen- and endometrial-specific events.

Both types of rodent models are complemented by the availability of transgenic and knockout mice, which can be employed in these well-established models, yielding greater understanding of components involved in endometrial estrogen responses. For example, mice lacking estrogen or progesterone receptors,[75–77] as well as mice expressing mutated forms of the ER,[78] have been engineered and utilized to complement studies of uterine gene regulation mechanisms.

In addition to the rodent models, endometrial gene regulation has also been studied in domestic agricultural animal models, including bovine, ovine, and pig.[79] Although these models are more difficult to manipulate experimentally because of their large sizes and longer reproductive cycles, characterization of endometrial responses might lead to identification of factors crucial in maximizing reproductive output. Primate models, including baboon and rhesus monkey, have also been used as more representative of human reproductive processes.[80,81] Studies of human endometrium utilize endometrial biopsy samples or samples obtained at hysterectomy.[82,83] Additionally, primary endometrial cultures grown from biopsy samples as well as endometrial cell lines are utilized as in-vitro experimental models for human endometrium.[84,85]

Microarray analysis of estrogen regulation

The development and increasing availability of microarray technology has led to an enormous body of data regarding estrogen regulation of uterine genes. Not only has the number of identified uterine genes increased but also comparison of temporal patterns of expression has become possible, as has analysis of sensitivity and range of responses to potentially estrogenic compounds. Numerous studies have now been published detailing genomic responses of endometrial models.[82,83,86–98] These reports have generated an enormous body of data regarding literally thousands of genes. What remains are the enormous tasks of:

- Determining which of these responses are direct results of estrogen regulation, and which are secondary responses to primary estrogen targets, or which might reflect biological changes rather than gene regulation,
- Building an understanding of how genomic patterns of expression underlie resulting biological responses.

Tools for these tasks are continuously being developed to integrate and analyze these datasets. Software packages (Table 12.2A) that allow comparison and analysis of microarray datasets, and central repositories of microarray datasets are increasingly available (Table 12.2B).

Additional novel technologies have the potential to identify estrogen responsive endometrial genes. One approach is mathematical analysis of available gene sequences for canonical transcription factor regulatory sequences.[110–112] This approach, although promising and fruitful, is limited by the availability of gene sequences, especially in the rodent models. Additionally, this approach identifies possible estrogen targets, but does not account for tissue selectivity. However, these computer models have the potential to prove quite useful in combination with microarray studies. A second novel technology is chromatin immunoprecipitation combined with microarray, termed 'ChIP on chip', which probes for recruitment of proteins to gene regulatory sequences,[113–117] and aids in identification of responses that are a direct result of ER activity as opposed to secondary responses resulting from regulation of other transcription factors.

Analysis of mouse uterine gene regulation

The remainder of this chapter focuses on microarray analysis using the ovariectomized mouse uterine model. This model lends itself to evaluation of how gene responses might underlie biological events. Additionally, due to the experimental nature of the model, exogenous compounds can be evaluated and compared to known ER agonists, to indicate whether responses might utilize ER-mediated mechanisms. Similarly, transgenic mice expressing ER mutants or mutations in other genes with important uterine function can by utilized in microarray studies in this model. Evaluation of gene regulation in transgenic models in comparison to wild-type mice can reveal altered gene responses that elucidate mechanisms that underlie biological responses.

Initially, uterine gene expression was evaluated during a time course of estradiol administered to an ovariectomized adult mouse[88] (Figure 12.4). As described above, the biological events occurring within 24 hours have been divided into early and late events. It was interesting, then, that the endogenous uterine gene responses throughout this time could be categorized as early or late as well (see Figure 12.4): i.e. in general, the genomic pattern mirrored the biological processes, and in addition, some gene regulation was distinct and observed only at early and late time points, while others occurred throughout the time course. A significant proportion of the transcripts exhibited decreased expression, indicating transcriptional repression or other mechanisms that decrease transcript levels are occurring in response to estrogen. In the initial study, 8000 clones were included on the microarray chip, and several hundred genes were identified as estrogen regulated. Considering the many biological events occurring (fluid uptake, immune infiltration, transcription, protein synthesis, metabolism, proliferation), it is not surprising that the genomic pattern represents a wide array of processes and signaling pathways. Most interesting was the observation that genes induced early included those that might hamper cell cycle progression, such as Cdkn1a (p21) and Mad2l1, while genes appearing later included those expected for proliferation, such as cyclins B and G and Cdc2a, suggesting the timing of the regulation of these gene products controls the synchronous epithelial cell proliferation at the proper time.[88]

Subsequently, we have repeated this study using a more comprehensive chip (Agilent Mouse Chip), which included 20 000 features. In this analysis, 2000–3000 genes were significantly ($p < 0.001$) regulated by at least two-fold. Again, numerous functions and pathways were represented. Functional analysis using Ingenuity Pathway Analysis indicated that at the 2-hour time point the top five functions of regulated uterine genes were:

Table 12.2A   Examples of software packages for analysis of microarray datasets

FREE

AMIADA (Analyzing MIcroArray DAta)
http://dambe.bio.uottawa.ca/amiada.asp 99

ArrayTrack (FDA) http://www.fda.gov/nctr/science/centers/
toxicoinformatics/ArrayTrack/index.htm

BioConductor http://www.bioconductor.org/

BRB Array Tools, Biometric Research Branch, NCI
http://linus.nci.nih.gov/BRB-ArrayTools.html

Cluster tools Michael Eisen's lab; Lawrence Berkeley
National Lab (LBNL) http://rana.lbl.gov/EisenSoftware.htm[100]

GEPAS (Gene Expression Pattern Analysis Suite)
http://gepas.bioinfo.cipf.es/

DAVID/EASE (NIAID) http://david.niaid.nih.gov/david/
ease.htm

DNA–Chip Analyzer (dChip) Wong Lab Department of
Statistics, Harvard University http://biosun1.harvard.edu/
complab/dchip/101

**Engene (Gene-Expression Data Processing and
Exploratory Data Analysis)** http://www.engene.cnb.uam.es/

Expression Profiler, European Bioinformatics Institute EBI
http://ep.ebi.ac.uk/EP/

Gene Expression Data Analysis Tool (GEDA) UPCI, Center
for Pathology Informatics
http://bioinformatics.upmc.edu/GE2/GEDA.html

GenePattern Broad Institute, MIT http://www.broad.mit.
edu/cancer/software/genepattern/index.html

Genesis Bioinformatics Group, Institute of Biomedical
Engineering, Graz University of Technology http://genome.
tugraz.at/genesisclient/genesisclient_description.shtml[102]

GeneXPress Stanford University http://genexpress.
stanford.edu/

GoMiner (NCI) http://discover.nci.nih.gov/gominer/

J Express Pro MolMine http://www.molmine.com/

MicroArray Explorer http://maexplorer.sourceforge.net/

XCluster, Stanford http://genetics.stanford.edu/~sherlock/
cluster.html

COMMERCIAL

Acuity, Molecular Devices
http://www.moleculardevices.com/pages/software/gn_acuity.html

ArrayStat, Imaging Research Inc.
http://www.imagingresearch.com/products/AST.asp

Avadis, Strand Life Science http://avadis.strandls.com/

ExpressionSieve, BioSieve
http://www.biosieve.com/product.html

GeneLinker, Improved Outcomes Software
http://www.improvedoutcomes.com/

GeneMaths Applied Maths http://www.applied-maths.com/
genemaths/genemaths.htm

GeneSifter http://www.genesifter.net/web/

GeneSight Biodiscovery http://www.biodiscovery.com/
index/genesight

Genespring, Agilent http://www.chem.agilent.com/
scripts/pds.asp?lpage=27881

Ingenuity Pathway Analysis http://www.ingenuity.com/
index.html

JMP Microarray (JMP Genomics) http://www.jmp.com/
software/genomics/microarray.shtml

Metacore (GeneGo) http://www.genego.com/
metacore.php

Partek Software http://www.partek.com/html/products/
products.html

Rosetta Resolver http://www.rosettabio.com/products/
resolver/default.htm

SilicoCyte http://www.silicocyte.com/dis/index.htm

Vector Xpression http://register.informaxinc.com/solutions/
xpression/main.html Invitrogen Lifescience

PATHWAYS DATABASES

Biobase http://www.biobase-international.com/pages/
index.php

BioCyc Knowledge Library; MetaCyc – Metabolic Encyclopedia
http://biocyc.org/ (SRI International)

Biomolecular Interaction Network Database http://www.
bind.ca/Action[103, 104] (Unleashed Informatics)

Cytoscape http://www.cytoscape.org/

Database of Quantitative Cellular Signaling (DOQCS)
http://doqcs.ncbs.res.in/[105]

(EMP) Enzymes and Metabolic Pathways database
http://www.empproject.com/

ExPASy – Biochemical Pathways http://www.expasy.ch/
cgi-bin/search-biochem-index

GenMAPP http://www.genmapp.org/

KEGG (Kyoto Encyclopedia of Genes and Genomes)
http://www.genome.jp/kegg/

Kinase Pathway Database http://kinasedb.ontology.ims.
u-tokyo.ac.jp:8081/

Pathway Studio (Ariadne Genomics)
http://www.ariadnegenomics.com/products/pathway/

---

1. Gene expression (113 associated genes).
2. Cell death (122 associated genes).
3. Cellular growth and proliferation (156 associated genes).
4. Cellular development (99 associated genes).
5. Tissue development (69 associated genes).

The top five functions associated with estrogen-regulated genes at 24 hours were:

1. DNA replication, recombination, and repair (56 associated genes).
2. Lipid metabolism (54 associated genes).

Table 12.2B Microarray data repositories

ArrayExpress – European Bioinformatics Institute
http://www.ebi.ac.uk/arrayexpress/

ChipDB – http://staffa.wi.mit.edu/chipdb/public/index.html

Gene Expression Atlas; GNF SymAtlas Genomics
Institute of the Novartis Research Foundation
http://symatlas.gnf.org/SymAtlas/

Gene Expression Database (GXD) – Mouse Genome
Informatics, Jackson Laboratory. http://www.informatics.jax.org/
mgihome/GXD/aboutGXD.shtml

Gene Expression Omnibus (GEO), NCBI
http://www.ncbi.nlm.nih.gov/geo/

Human Gene Expression Index (HuGE Index).
http://www.biotechnologycenter.org/hio/databases/index.html

List Of Lists Annotated (LOLA) – McCormick Genomics
Center, Gorge Washington University http://www.lola.gwu.edu/

MUSC DNA Microarray Database – Medical University of
South Carolina http://proteogenomics.musc.edu/ma/musc_
madb.php?page=home&act=manage

READ (RIKEN cDNA Expression Array Database) –
RIKEN (The Institute of Physical and Chemical Research),
Japan. http://read.gsc.riken.go.jp/[106]

RNA Abundance Database (RAD)
http://www.cbil.upenn.edu/RAD/php/index.php[107]

Stanford Microarray Database (SMD)
http://genome-www5.stanford.edu/[108]

Yale Microarray Database (YMD)
http://info.med.yale.edu/microarray/[109]

3. Small molecule biochemistry (67 associated genes).
4. Cell cycle (85 associated genes).
5. Cell death (119 associated genes).

The shift in gene functions as the estrogen response progresses reflects the observed cellular changes, with increasing gene expression early, as the uterus recovers from its quiescent ovariectomized state, followed by the cellular changes that must occur to enable the later proliferation. The predominance of genes associated with DNA replication and metabolism at 24 hours reflects the cellular division and differentiation that occur.

In this experimental analysis of estrogen responsive uterine genes, it is apparent that samplings at 2- or 24-hour time points will represent most of the observed gene responses (see Figure 12.4); therefore, subsequent studies have used these time points to give a 'snapshot' of early and late gene regulation patterns.

To evaluate the ER dependence of the uterine genes, the ER antagonist ICI 182–780 was used and was shown to prevent changes in transcript levels.[88] To assess the ERα or ERβ specificity for regulation of the uterine genes, WT, αERKO (which lacks ERα), and βERKO (lacking ERβ) were compared.[88] These studies confirmed the dominant role for ERα in this model, as regulation of uterine genes in βERKO and WT samples

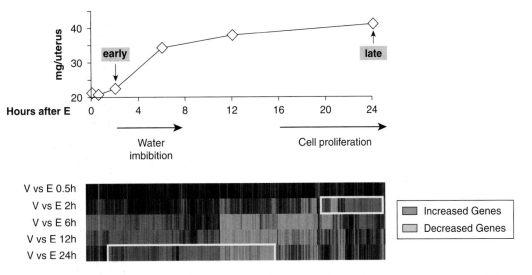

Figure 12.4 Analysis of uterine gene responses by microarray. The top panel is a schematic representation of the experimental design. It shows the trend in increasing uterine weight in an ovariectomized mouse following a single injection of estradiol (E). The initial weight increase is a result of water imbibition: cell proliferation begins and continues after 16–24 hours. Uteri were collected after 0.5, 2, 6, 12, or 24 hours, and the gene profiles relative to vehicle treated samples were obtained by microarray. The bottom panel is a heat map representation of the transcripts significantly different from corresponding vehicle control by at least two-fold at $p < 0.001$ showing the increases in red and the decreases in green. The yellow and gray boxes highlight transcripts that are characteristic of early and late time points, respectively. In subsequent studies the 2- and 24-hour time points were sampled as representative of early and late responses, as they appear to include most uterine responses and can provide a 'snapshot' from minimal sampling. (See also color plate section.)

did not differ significantly, while the αERKO lacked nearly all of the gene responses. Interestingly, both increased and decreased uterine transcripts required ERα, indicating that even mechanisms that lead to decreased transcript levels are mediated by ERα.

Others have assessed uterine gene regulation in this or similar models and have further evaluated xenoestrogenic compounds.[87,91,118,119] Additionally, similar studies have been carried out with prepubertal models.[120,121]

As described at the start of the chapter, the growth factors EGF and IGF-1 can mimic estrogens in eliciting epithelial proliferation and nuclear translocation of the ERα in the uterus.[122] Similarly, EGFR blocking antibodies can prevent uterotropic response to estrogen.[42] As growth factor and ER signaling pathways seem to be linked, we have examined the gene profiles of EGF and IGF-1 in our microarray study.[123] Previous in-vitro reporter gene studies had indicated an ER requirement for growth factor-initiated gene regulation;[124] therefore, we expected both overlap and ERα dependence of growth factor and estrogen gene regulation. The changes in transcript following administration of growth factors or estrogen were similar in identity and intensity; however, genes that were selectively regulated by estrogen were apparent (Figure 12.5A). In addition, the gene regulation resulting from growth factors was ERα-independent. Given the clear ERα dependence of the biological responses to growth factors, this result was unexpected. An accepted rationale for microarray analysis is that the observed changes in transcript levels underlie biological endpoints and will yield an understanding of the mechanisms controlling biological processes. In this case, however, a considerable genomic response is seen despite the clear absence of resulting biology. If the proliferation is not a culmination of the events mediated by regulation of critical genes, then one might ask what leads to proliferation. The changes in transcript observed by microarray were verified by reverse transcriptase-polymerase chain reaction (RT-PCR), and the following conclusions were made:[123]

1. Some genes (e.g. *Cdkn1a (p21)* [see Figure 12.5B], *Cyr61, Fos, Igfbp3, Igfbp5, Sox 4, Txnip*) can be regulated by either E_2 or by growth factors. However, regulation by growth factors is ERα-independent, as it occurs in the αERKO and is not inhibited by the ER antagonist ICI.
2. Some genes (e.g. *Mad2l1* [see Figure 12.5B], *Inhbb, Ramp3, Igf1, Ltf*) are exclusively regulated by E_2, and not by growth factors. These genes require the presence of ERα, but since they are not regulated

by growth factors, and growth factors can induce proliferation, they are not necessarily required for proliferation.
3. Some genes (e.g. *Klf9 (Bteb1)* [Figure 12.5B], *Baiap*) are selectively regulated by growth factors.

These findings have caused us to re-evaluate the original cross-talk hypothesis. Rather than a linear progression (E_2 or growth factors to ER to gene), we feel our results indicate a convergence of signals: i.e. each signal (E_2 or growth factors) independently initiates its associated pathway and resulting downstream events. Some of these downstream modulators overlap; thus, similar outcomes are observed from distinct signals (see Figure 12.2). Ultimately, we need to understand how these signals are able to result in an ER-dependent biological response.

Tethered pathway analysis

Our microarray study design has proven useful in evaluation of ER-mediated mechanisms such as the tethered pathway shown in Figure 12.2. Mutation of the first zinc finger of the DNA-binding domain of the ERα prevents ER–ERE binding, this mutated ERα retains the ability to regulate genes via the tethered pathway.[17] This mutation has been 'knocked in' to a mouse, replacing the ERα gene and resulting in a mouse model referred to as the 'nonclassical ER knock in' (Nerki).[78] Female mice heterozygous for this mutation are infertile due to ovarian and uterine pathologies;[78] however, by intercrossing with the αERKO line, a mouse with one copy each of the Nerki ERα and one copy of the null ERα has been generated.[125] The Nerki/αERKO uterus resembles the αERKO in that it lacks increased uterine weight when challenged with estrogen. Interestingly, Nerki/αERKO mice lack the E_2-mediated induction of *Aqp5*, consistent with the lack of weight increase due to water imbibition (Figure 12.6). Additionally, the cell cycle regulator, *Cdkn1a* is increased by E_2, indicating it is regulated by the tethered mechanism (Figure 12.6).

These microarray studies, in combination with other emerging tools and technologies, will allow future integration of gene regulatory mechanisms, identification of critical components in uterine biology, and possibly lead to identification of novel pathways that previously escaped investigation. For example, in the future we hope to utilize ChIP on chip technologies to identify uterine genes that are direct targets of ER binding to discern which uterine genes identified by microarray

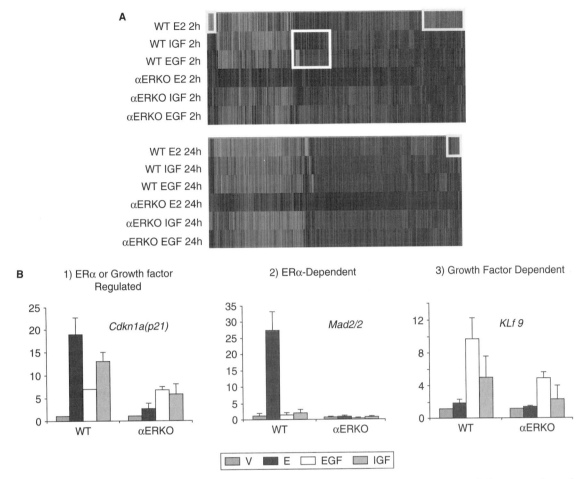

Figure 12.5 (A) Microarray comparison of WT and αERKO uterine gene responses to E_2 or growth factors epidermal growth factor (EGF) or insulin-like growth factor 1 (IGF) for 2 or 24 hours. Growth factor responses are ERα independent. Examples of ERα-dependent (yellow boxes) and growth factor-dependent (white box) clusters are highlighted. (B) Examples of regulatory modes observed by microarray. (1) ERα or growth factor regulated: RT-PCR analysis of *Cdkn1a* (p21) or shows it is increased by either E_2 or growth factors; the E_2 induction requires ERα, as E_2-mediated increase is attenuated in the αERKO, whereas the growth factors increase them in both WT and αERKO, indicating the growth factor regulation is independent of ERα. (2) ERα dependent: RT-PCR analysis of *Mad2l1* (MAD2 [mitotic arrest deficient, homolog]-like 1 [yeast]) indicates it is increased by E, not by growth factors, and is dependent on ERα. (3) Growth factor-dependent: RT-PCR analysis of KLf9 (Kruppel-like factor 9) shows it is increased by growth factors and is not dependent on ERα. (See also color plate section.)

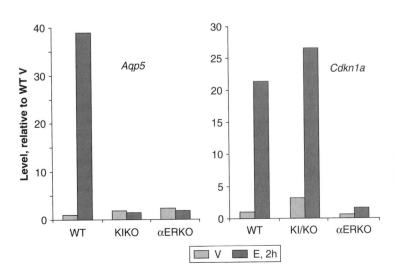

Figure 12.6 Gene responses in tethered selective mutant mouse reflect biological observations. RT-PCR analysis of *Aqp5* (aquaporin 5) indicates ERE-dependent transcriptional regulation, as regulation is only seen in the WT samples. Analysis of *Cdkn1a* indicates the tethered mode is utilized for this gene, as the response is preserved in the tethered-selective KI/KO sample.

analysis are directly regulated by ER signaling and which reflect changes secondary to initial events or changes in the tissue. Additionally, we hope to pinpoint the uterine cell types (luminal and glandular epithelium, stroma, myometrium, immune response cells, vascular cells) in which genes are expressed. It is clear the estrogen's effects on the endometrium are critical to successful reproduction; additionally, the uterine model is a sensitive one in which to study estrogen responses. The greatly increased numbers of identified estrogen-regulated uterine genes has complicated and expanded the focus of uterine studies, but also promises future novel revelations regarding uterine biology.

REFERENCES

1. Renaud JP, Moras D. Structural studies on nuclear receptors. Cell Mole Life Sci 2000; 57(12): 1748–69.
2. Robinson-Rechavi M, Escriva Garcia H, Laudet V. The nuclear receptor superfamily. J Cell Sci 2003; 116(Pt 4): 585–6.
3. Tsai MJ, O'Malley BW. Molecular mechanisms of action of steroid/thyroid receptor superfamily members. Annu Rev Biochem 1994; 63: 451–86.
4. Glass CK. Differential recognition of target genes by nuclear receptor monomers, dimers, and heterodimers. Endocr Rev 1994; 15(3): 391–407.
5. Verrijdt G, Haelens A, Claessens F. Selective DNA recognition by the androgen receptor as a mechanism for hormone-specific regulation of gene expression. Mol Genet Metab 2003; 78(3): 175–85.
6. Klinge CM. Estrogen receptor interaction with estrogen response elements. Nucleic Acids Res 2001; 29(14): 2905–19.
7. O'Lone R, Frith MC, Karlsson EK, Hansen U. Genomic targets of nuclear estrogen receptors. Mol Endocrinol 2004; 18(8): 1859–75.
8. Nagy L, Schwabe JWR. Mechanism of the nuclear receptor molecular switch. Trends Biochem Sci 2004; 29(6): 317–24.
9. Metzger D, Ali S, Bornert JM, Chambon P. Characterization of the amino-terminal transcriptional activation function of the human estrogen receptor in animal and yeast cells. J Biol Chem 1995; 270(16): 9535–42.
10. Parker MG. Structure and function of estrogen receptors. Vitam Horm 1995; 51: 267–87.
11. Edwards DP. The role of coactivators and corepressors in the biology and mechanism of action of steroid hormone receptors. J Mammary Gland Biol Neoplasia 2000; 5(3): 307–24.
12. Carroll JS, Brown M. Estrogen receptor target gene: an evolving concept. Mol Endocrinol 2006; 20(8): 1707–14.
13. McKenna NJ, Lanz RB, O'Malley BW. Nuclear receptor coregulators: cellular and molecular biology. Endocr Rev 1999; 20(3): 321–44.
14. Smith CL, O'Malley BW. Coregulator function: a key to understanding tissue specificity of selective receptor modulators. Endocr Rev 2004; 25(1): 45–71.
15. Kushner PJ, Agard DA, Greene GL et al. Estrogen receptor pathways to AP-1. J Steroid Biochem Mol Biol 2000; 74(5): 311–17.
16. Safe S. Transcriptional activation of genes by 17 beta-estradiol through estrogen receptor-Sp1 interactions. In: Litwack G,

Begley T, eds. Vitamins and Hormones – Advances in Research and Applications, Vol 62. San Diego, CA: Academic Press, 2001: 231–52.
17. Jakacka M, Ito M, Weiss J et al. Estrogen receptor binding to DNA is not required for its activity through the nonclassical AP1 pathway. J Biol Chem 2001; 276(17): 13615–21.
18. McKenna NJ, O'Malley BW. Minireview: nuclear receptor coactivators – an update. Endocrinology 2002; 143(7): 2461–5.
19. McKenna NJ, O'Malley BW. Combinatorial control of gene expression by nuclear receptors and coregulators. Cell 2002; 108(4): 465–74.
20. Hall JM, McDonnell DP. Coregulators in nuclear estrogen receptor action: from concept to therapeutic targeting. Mol Interv 2005; 5(6): 343–57.
21. Jungbauer A, Beck V. Yeast reporter system for rapid determination of estrogenic activity. J Chromatogr B Analyt Technol Biomed Life Sci 2002; 777(1–2): 167–78.
22. Dowhan DH, Hong EP, Auboeuf D et al. Steroid hormone receptor coactivation and alternative RNA splicing by U2AF65-related proteins CAPERalpha and CAPERbeta. Mol Cell 2005; 17(3): 429–39.
23. Spiegelman BM, Heinrich R. Biological control through regulated transcriptional coactivators. Cell 2004; 119(2): 157–67.
24. Glass CK, Rosenfeld MG. The coregulator exchange in transcriptional functions of nuclear receptors. Genes Dev 2000; 14(2): 121–41.
25. Hermanson O, Glass CK, Rosenfeld MG. Nuclear receptor coregulators: multiple modes of modification. Trends Endocrinol Metab 2002; 13(2): 55–60.
26. Helvering LM, Adrian MD, Geiser AG et al. Differential effects of estrogen and raloxifene on messenger RNA and matrix metalloproteinase 2 activity in the rat uterus. Biol Reprod 2005; 72(4): 830–41.
27. Lanz RB, McKenna NJ, Onate SA et al. A steroid receptor coactivator, SRA, functions as an RNA and is present in an SRC-1 complex. Cell 1999; 97(1): 17–27.
28. Endoh H, Maruyama K, Masuhiro Y et al. Purification and identification of p68 RNA helicase acting as a transcriptional coactivator specific for the activation function 1 of human estrogen receptor alpha. Mol Cell Biol 1999; 19(8): 5363–72.
29. Watanabe M, Yanagisawa J, Kitagawa H et al. A subfamily of RNA-binding DEAD-box proteins acts as an estrogen receptor alpha coactivator through the N-terminal activation domain (AF-1) with an RNA coactivator, SRA. EMBO J 2001; 20(6): 1341–52.
30. Norris JD, Fan D, Sherk A, McDonnell DP. A negative coregulator for the human ER. Mol Endocrinol 2002; 16(3): 459–68.
31. Leung KC, Doyle N, Ballesteros M et al. Estrogen inhibits GH signaling by suppressing GH-induced JAK2 phosphorylation, an effect mediated by SOCS-2. Proc Natl Acad Sci USA 2003; 100(3): 1016–21.
32. Gburcik V, Bot N, Maggiolini M, Picard D. SPBP is a phospho-serine-specific repressor of estrogen receptor alpha. Mol Cell Biol 2005; 25(9): 3421–30.
33. Masuhiro Y, Mezaki Y, Sakari M et al. Splicing potentiation by growth factor signals via estrogen receptor phosphorylation. Proc Natl Acad Sci USA 2005; 102(23): 8126–31.
34. Coleman KM, Smith CL. Intracellular signaling pathways: nongenomic actions of estrogens and ligand-independent activation of estrogen receptors. Front Biosci 2001; 6: D1379–D91.
35. Cato AC, Nestl A, Mink S. Rapid actions of steroid receptors in cellular signaling pathways. Sci STKE 2002; 2002(138): RE9.
36. Levin ER. Integration of the extranuclear and nuclear actions of estrogen. Mol Endocrinol 2005; 19(8): 1951–9.

37. Filardo EJ, Quinn JA, Frackelton AR Jr, Bland KI. Estrogen action via the G protein-coupled receptor, GPR30: stimulation of adenylyl cyclase and cAMP-mediated attenuation of the epidermal growth factor receptor-to-MAPK signaling axis. Mol Endocrinol 2002; 16(1): 70–84.

38. Thomas P, Pang Y, Filardo EJ, Dong J. Identity of an estrogen membrane receptor coupled to a G protein in human breast cancer cells. Endocrinology 2005; 146(2): 624–32.

39. Li XT, O'Malley BW. Unfolding the action of progesterone receptors. J Biol Chem 2003; 278(41): 39261–4.

40. Sadar MD. Androgen-independent induction of prostate-specific antigen gene expression via cross-talk between the androgen receptor and protein kinase A signal transduction pathways. J Biol Chem 1999; 274(12): 7777–83.

41. Nazareth LV, Weigel NL. Activation of the human androgen receptor through a protein kinase A signaling pathway. J Biol Chem 1996; 271(33): 19900–7.

42. Nelson KG, Takahashi T, Bossert NL, Walmer DK, McLachlan JA. Epidermal growth factor replaces estrogen in the stimulation of female genital-tract growth and differentiation. Proc Natl Acad Sci USA 1991; 88(1): 21–5.

43. Curtis SW, Washburn T, Sewall C et al. Physiological coupling of growth factor and steroid receptor signaling pathways: estrogen receptor knockout mice lack estrogen-like response to epidermal growth factor. Proc Natl Acad Sci USA 1996; 93(22): 12626–30.

44. Klotz DM, Hewitt SC, Ciana P et al. Requirement of estrogen receptor-alpha in insulin-like growth factor-1 (IGF-1)-induced uterine responses and in vivo evidence for IGF-1/estrogen receptor cross-talk. J Biol Chem 2002; 277(10): 8531–7.

45. Klotz DM, Hewitt SC, Korach KS, Diaugustine RP. Activation of a uterine insulin-like growth factor I signaling pathway by clinical and environmental estrogens: requirement of estrogen receptor-alpha. Endocrinology 2000; 141(9): 3430–9.

46. Boettger-Tong HL, Murthy L, Stancel GM. Cellular pattern of c-fos induction by estradiol in the immature rat uterus. Biol Reprod 1995; 53(6): 1398–406.

47. Liu Y, Teng CT. Estrogen response module of the mouse lactoferrin gene contains overlapping chicken ovalbumin upstream promoter transcription factor and estrogen receptor-binding elements. Mol Endocrinol 1992; 6(3): 355–64.

48. Kraus WL, Montano MM, Katzenellenbogen BS. Cloning of the rat progesterone receptor gene 5'-region and identification of two functionally distinct promoters. Mol Endocrinol 1993; 7(12): 1603–16.

49. Pentecost BT, Mattheiss L, Dickerman HW, Kumar SA. Estrogen regulation of creatine kinase-B in the rat uterus. Mol Endocrinol 1990; 4(7): 1000–10.

50. Wang XN, Das SK, Damm D et al. Differential regulation of heparin-binding epidermal growth factor-like growth factor in the adult ovariectomized mouse uterus by progesterone and estrogen. Endocrinology 1994; 135(3): 1264–71.

51. Ringler MB, Hilf R. Effect of estrogen on synthesis of glucose-6-phosphate dehydrogenase in R3230AC mammary tumors and uteri. Biochim Biophys Acta 1975; 411(1): 50–62.

52. Curtis SW, Shi H, Teng C, Korach KS. Promoter and species specific differential estrogen-mediated gene transcription in the uterus and cultured cells using structurally altered agonists. J Mol Endocrinol 1997; 18(3): 203–11.

53. Zou K, Ing NH. Oestradiol up-regulates oestrogen receptor, cyclophilin, and glyceraldehyde phosphate dehydrogenase mRNA concentrations in endometrium, but down-regulates them in liver. J Steroid Biochem Mol Biol 1998; 64(5–6): 231–7.

54. Grummer R, Chwalisz K, Mulholland J, Traub O, Winterhager E. Regulation of connexin26 and connexin43 expression in rat endometrium by ovarian steroid hormones. Biol Reprod 1994; 51(6): 1109–16.

55. Katzenellenbogen BS, Montano MM, Le Goff P et al. Antiestrogens: mechanisms and actions in target cells. J Steroid Biochem Mol Biol 1995; 53(1–6): 387–93.

56. Zhang WH, Andersson S, Cheng GJ et al. Update on estrogen signaling. FEBS Lett 2003; 546(1): 17–24.

57. Murphy LJ, Murphy LC, Friesen HG. Estrogen induces insulin-like growth factor-I expression in the rat uterus. Mol Endocrinol 1987; 1(7): 445–50.

58. Nephew KP, Webb DK, Akcali KC et al. Hormonal regulation and expression of the jun-D protooncogene in specific cell types of the rat uterus. J Steroid Biochem Mol Biol 1993; 46(3): 281–7.

59. Escribano J, Hernando N, Ghosh S et al. cDNA from human ocular ciliary epithelium homologous to beta ig-h3 is preferentially expressed as an extracellular protein in the corneal epithelium. J Cell Physiol 1994; 160(3): 511–21.

60. Murphy LJ, Murphy LC, Friesen HG. Estrogen induction of N-myc and c-myc proto-oncogene expression in the rat uterus. Endocrinology 1987; 120(5): 1882–8.

61. Huet-Hudson YM, Andrews GK, Dey SK. Cell type-specific localization of c-myc protein in the mouse uterus: modulation by steroid hormones and analysis of the periimplantation period. Endocrinology 1989; 125(3): 1683–90.

62. Lavia LA, Stohs SJ, Lemon HM. Polyamine biosynthetic decarboxylase activities following estradiol-17 beta or estriol stimulation of the immature rat uterus. Steroids 1983; 42(6): 609–18.

63. Levy C, Glikman P, Vegh I et al. Estradiol, progesterone and tamoxifen regulation of ornithine decarboxylase (ODC) in rat uterus and chick oviducts. Prog Clin Biol Res 1984; 142: 133–44.

64. Soloff MS. Uterine receptor for oxytocin: effects of estrogen. Biochem Biophys Res Commun 1975; 65(1): 205–12.

65. Zingg HH, Rozen F, Breton C et al. Gonadal steroid regulation of oxytocin and oxytocin receptor gene expression. Adv Exp Med Biol 1995; 395: 395–404.

66. Milgrom E, Thi L, Atger M, Baulieu EE. Mechanisms regulating the concentration and the conformation of progesterone receptor(s) in the uterus. J Biol Chem 1973; 248(18): 6366–74.

67. Parczyk K, Madjno R, Michna H et al. Progesterone receptor repression by estrogens in rat uterine epithelial cells. J Steroid Biochem Mol Biol 1997; 63(4–6): 309–16.

68. Chen D, Ganapathy P, Zhu LJ et al. Potential regulation of membrane trafficking by estrogen receptor alpha via induction of rab11 in uterine glands during implantation. Mol Endocrinol 1999; 13(6): 993–1004.

69. Fujita M, Ogawa S, Fukuoka H et al. Differential expression of secreted frizzled-related protein 4 in decidual cells during pregnancy. J Mol Endocrinol 2002; 28(3): 213–23.

70. Yamanouchi K, Soeta C, Harada R, Naito K, Tojo H. Endometrial expression of cellular protooncogene c-ski and its regulation by estradiol-17beta. FEBS Lett 1999; 449(2–3): 273–6.

71. Mason HR, Grove-Strawser D, Rubin BS, Nowak RA, Castellot JJ Jr. Estrogen induces CCN5 expression in the rat uterus in vivo. Endocrinology 2004; 145(2): 976–82.

72. Clark JH, Peck EJ, Jr. Female Sex Steroids. Berlin: Springer-Verlag, 1979.

73. Katzenellenbogen BS, Bhakoo HS, Ferguson ER et al. Estrogen and antiestrogen action in reproductive tissues and tumors. Recent Prog Horm Res 1979; 35: 259–300.

74. Yoshinaga K, Adams CE. Delayed implantation in the spayed, progesterone treated adult mouse. J Reprod Fertil 1966; 12(3): 593–5.

75. Couse JF, Korach KS. Estrogen receptor null mice: what have we learned and where will they lead us? Endocr Rev 1999; 20(3): 358–417.

76. Dupont S, Krust A, Gansmuller A et al. Effect of single and compound knockouts of estrogen receptors alpha (ERalpha) and beta (ERbeta) on mouse reproductive phenotypes. Development 2000; 127(19): 4277–91.

77. Lydon JP, DeMayo FJ, Funk CR et al. Mice lacking progesterone receptor exhibit pleiotropic reproductive abnormalities. Genes Develop 1995; 9: 2266–78.

78. Jakacka M, Ito M, Martinson F et al. An estrogen receptor (ER)alpha deoxyribonucleic acid-binding domain knock-in mutation provides evidence for nonclassical ER pathway signaling in vivo. Mol Endocrinol 2002; 16(10): 2188–201.

79. Spencer TE, Bazer FW. Temporal and spatial alterations in uterine estrogen receptor and progesterone receptor gene expression during the estrous cycle and early pregnancy in the ewe. Biol Reprod 1995; 53(6): 1527–43.

80. Fazleabas AT. A baboon model for simulating pregnancy. Methods Mol Med 2006; 121: 101–10.

81. Dwivedi A, Gupta G, Keshri G, Dhar JD. Changes in uterine ornithine decarboxylase activity and steroid receptor levels during decidualization in the rat induced by CDRI-85/287. Eur J Endocrinol 1999; 141(4): 426–30.

82. Mirkin S, Arslan M, Churikov D et al. In search of candidate genes critically expressed in the human endometrium during the window of implantation. Hum Reprod 2005; 20(8): 2104–17.

83. Yanaihara A, Otsuka Y, Iwasaki S et al. Differences in gene expression in the proliferative human endometrium. Fertil Steril 2005; 83(Suppl 1): 1206–15.

84. Paszkiewicz-Gadek A, Porowska H, Pietruczuk M et al. Effect of estradiol and raloxifene on MUC1 expression and adhesive properties of Ishikawa cells. Oncol Rep 2005; 14(2): 583–9.

85. Ylikomi T, Wurtz JM, Syvala H et al. Reappraisal of the role of heat shock proteins as regulators of steroid receptor activity. Crit Rev Biochem Mol Biol 1998; 33(6): 437–66.

86. Reese J, Das SK, Paria BC et al. Global gene expression analysis to identify molecular markers of uterine receptivity and embryo implantation. J Biol Chem 2001; 276(47): 44137–45.

87. Watanabe H, Suzuki A, Kobayashi M et al. Analysis of temporal changes in the expression of estrogen-regulated genes in the uterus. J Mol Endocrinol 2003; 30(3): 347–58.

88. Hewitt SC, Deroo BJ, Hansen K et al. Estrogen receptor-dependent genomic responses in the uterus mirror the biphasic physiological response to estrogen. Mol Endocrinol 2003; 17(10): 2070–83.

89. Fertuck KC, Zacharewski TR. Temporal responses to estrogen in the uterus. Pure Appl Chem 2003; 75(11–12): 2415–18.

90. Bethin KE, Nagai Y, Sladek R et al. Microarray analysis of uterine gene expression in mouse and human pregnancy. Mol Endocrinol 2003; 17(8): 1454–69.

91. Watanabe H, Suzuki A, Mizutani T et al. Genome-wide analysis of changes in early gene expression induced by oestrogen. Genes Cells 2002; 7(5): 497–507.

92. Ho Hong S, Young Nah H, Yoon Lee J et al. Analysis of estrogen-regulated genes in mouse uterus using cDNA microarray and laser capture microdissection. J Endocrinol 2004; 181(1): 157–67.

93. Kao LC, Tulac S, Lobo S et al. Global gene profiling in human endometrium during the window of implantation. Endocrinology 2002; 143(6): 2119–38.

94. Kao LC, Germeyer A, Tulac S et al. Expression profiling of endometrium from women with endometriosis reveals candidate genes for disease-based implantation failure and infertility. Endocrinology 2003; 144(7): 2870–81.

95. Wu Y, Kajdacsy-Balla A, Strawn E et al. Transcriptional characterizations of differences between eutopic and ectopic endometrium. Endocrinology 2006; 147(1): 232–46.

96. Matsuzaki S, Canis M, Pouly JL et al. Differential expression of genes in eutopic and ectopic endometrium from patients with ovarian endometriosis. Fertil Steril 2006; 86(3): 548–53.

97. Punyadeera C, Dassen H, Klomp J et al. Oestrogen-modulated gene expression in the human endometrium. Cell Mol Life Sci 2005; 62(2): 239–50.

98. Maxwell GL, Chandramouli GV, Dainty L et al. Microarray analysis of endometrial carcinomas and mixed mullerian tumors reveals distinct gene expression profiles associated with different histologic types of uterine cancer. Clin Cancer Res 2005; 11(11): 4056–66.

99. Xia X, Xie Z. AMADA: analysis of microarray data. Bioinformatics 2001; 17(6): 569–70.

100. Eisen MB, Spellman PT, Brown PO, Botstein D. Cluster analysis and display of genome-wide expression patterns. Proc Natl Acad Sci USA 1998; 95(25): 14863–8.

101. Zhong S, Li C, Wong WH. ChipInfo: software for extracting gene annotation and gene ontology information for microarray analysis. Nucleic Acids Res 2003; 31(13): 3483–6.

102. Sturn A, Mlecnik B, Pieler R et al. Client-server environment for high-performance gene expression data analysis. Bioinformatics 2003; 19(6): 772–3.

103. Bader GD, Donaldson I, Wolting C et al. BIND – The Biomolecular Interaction Network Database. Nucleic Acids Res 2001; 29(1): 242–5.

104. Alfarano C, Andrade CE, Anthony K et al. The Biomolecular Interaction Network Database and related tools: 2005 update. Nucleic Acids Res 2005; 33(Database issue): D418–24.

105. Sivakumaran S, Hariharaputran S, Mishra J, Bhalla US. The Database of Quantitative Cellular Signaling: management and analysis of chemical kinetic models of signaling networks. Bioinformatics 2003; 19(3): 408–15.

106. Bono H, Kasukawa T, Hayashizaki Y, Okazaki Y. READ: RIKEN Expression Array Database. Nucleic Acids Res 2002; 30(1): 211–13.

107. Stoeckert C, Pizarro A, Manduchi E et al. A relational schema for both array-based and SAGE gene expression experiments. Bioinformatics 2001; 17(4): 300–8.

108. Sherlock G, Hernandez-Boussard T, Kasarskis A et al. The Stanford Microarray Database. Nucleic Acids Res 2001; 29(1): 152–5.

109. Cheung KH, White K, Hager J et al. YMD: a microarray database for large-scale gene expression analysis. Proc AMIA Symp 2002; 140–4.

110. Kamalakaran S, Radhakrishnan SK, Beck WT. Identification of estrogen-responsive genes using a genome-wide analysis of promoter elements for transcription factor binding sites. J Biol Chem 2005; 280(22): 21491–7.

111. Jin VX, Sun H, Pohar TT et al. ERTargetDB: an integral information resource of transcription regulation of estrogen receptor target genes. J Mol Endocrinol 2005; 35(2): 225–30.

112. Bourdeau V, Deschenes J, Metivier R et al. Genome-wide identification of high-affinity estrogen response elements in human and mouse. Mol Endocrinol 2004; 18(6): 1411–27.

113. Jin VX, Leu YW, Liyanarachchi S et al. Identifying estrogen receptor alpha target genes using integrated computational genomics and chromatin immunoprecipitation microarray. Nucleic Acids Res 2004; 32(22): 6627–35.

114. Laganiere J, Deblois G, Giguere V. Functional genomics identifies a mechanism for estrogen activation of the retinoic acid receptor alpha1 gene in breast cancer cells. Mol Endocrinol 2005; 19(6): 1584–92.

115. Bray JD, Jelinsky S, Ghatge R et al. Quantitative analysis of gene regulation by seven clinically relevant progestins suggests a highly similar mechanism of action through progesterone receptors in T47D breast cancer cells. J Steroid Biochem Mol Biol 2005; 97(4): 328–41.

116. Carroll JS, Liu XS, Brodsky AS et al. Chromosome-wide mapping of estrogen receptor binding reveals long-range regulation requiring the forkhead protein FoxA1. Cell 2005; 122(1): 33–43.

117. DeNardo DG, Kim HT, Hilsenbeck S et al. Global gene expression analysis of estrogen receptor transcription factor cross talk in breast cancer: identification of estrogen-induced/activator protein-1-dependent genes. Mol Endocrinol 2005; 19(2): 362–78.

118. Watanabe H, Suzuki A, Goto M et al. Comparative uterine gene expression analysis after dioxin and estradiol administration. J Mol Endocrinol 2004; 33(3): 763–71.

119. Moggs JG. Molecular responses to xenoestrogens: mechanistic insights from toxicogenomics. Toxicology 2005; 213(3): 177–93.

120. Fertuck KC, Eckel JE, Gennings C, Zacharewski TR. Identification of temporal patterns of gene expression in the uteri of immature, ovariectomized mice following exposure to ethynylestradiol. Physiol Genom 2003; 15(2): 127–41.

121. Moggs JG, Ashby J, Tinwell H et al. The need to decide if all estrogens are intrinsically similar. Environ Health Perspect 2004; 112(11): 1137–42.

122. Ignar Trowbridge DM, Nelson KG, Bidwell MC et al. Coupling of dual signaling pathways: epidermal growth factor action involves the estrogen receptor. Proc Natl Acad Sci USA 1992; 89(10): 4658–62.

123. Hewitt SC, Collins J, Grissom S, Deroo B, Korach KS. Global uterine genomics in vivo: microarray evaluation of the estrogen receptor alpha-growth factor cross-talk mechanism. Mol Endocrinol 2005; 19(3): 657–68.

124. Ignar Trowbridge DM, Teng CT, Ross KA et al. Peptide growth factors elicit estrogen receptor-dependent transcriptional activation of an estrogen-responsive element. Mol Endocrinol 1993; 7(8): 992–8.

125. O'Brien JE, Peterson TJ, Tong MH et al. Estrogen-induced proliferation of uterine epithelial cells is independent of estrogen receptor alpha binding to classical estrogen response elements. J Biol Chem 2006; 281(36): 26683–92.

13   Progesterone-regulated genes in the endometrium

Kevin Lee, Jinrong Wang, and Francesco DeMayo

INTRODUCTION

The ovarian steroid hormone progesterone (P_4) is a critical regulator of reproductive events associated with all aspects of the establishment and maintenance of pregnancy. Well-characterized functions of P_4 include regulating uterine receptivity for blastocyst attachment, controlling the progression of uterine and embryonic interactions, inducing stromal cell differentiation, and regulating epithelial cell proliferation. Most of the physiological affects of P_4 are mediated through its receptor, the progesterone receptor (PGR). PGR is a transcription factor that belongs to the nuclear receptor superfamily. This superfamily represents the largest family of transcription factors that share structural similarities and key functional domains.[1,2] The three major functional domains of PGR, like all nuclear receptors, are the ligand-binding domain (LBD), the DNA-binding domain (DBD), and an activation domain (AF). The LBD confers specificity to the receptor for a particular ligand or molecule that regulates its transcriptional activation. The DBD determines which DNA sequences the receptor will recognize, while the AFs link the transcriptional activity of the receptors to the core transcriptional complexes.[3] As shown in Figure 13.1, PGR is encoded in one gene and exists as several isoforms with the most well characterized being PRA, PRB, and PRC. These isoforms arise from the alternate translation start sites in the *PGR* gene. The human PRA isoform differs from the PRB isoform in that it lacks the first 164 amino acids contained in PRB, whereas the PRC isoform contains a truncated DBD and a full-length LBD.[4]

MECHANISM OF ACTION

The molecular mechanisms by which the PGR regulates the transcription of target genes has long been an area of active research. As shown in Figure 13.2, the steroid hormone receptors can be activated by several mechanisms. The first, traditional ligand-dependent mechanism by which receptors can be activated is by

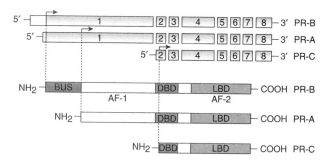

Figure 13.1 Diagram of transcript and protein structure of PGR isoforms.

the binding of P_4 to the LBD of PGR. In the absence of ligand, the PGRs are associated with chaperone proteins in the cytoplasm and are transcriptionally inactive. Upon ligand binding, the receptors are phosphorylated, released from the chaperones, and free to translocate into the nucleus.[1] Another mechanism by which PGR can be activated is through a ligand-independent mechanism.[5] The ligand-independent activation of the receptor is a result of the integration of other signaling pathways, usually membrane receptor signaling that results in the activation of kinases and ultimately the phosphorylation of the receptor. The ligand-independent transcription of PGR can be due to a variety of different factors. The first study that demonstrated the ligand independent transcription of PGR showed that cAMP (8-bromocAMP) addition can phosphorylate the receptor, dependent on protein kinase A (PKA), and activate gene transcription.[6] Dopamine can also activate PGR in a lig-and-independent manner, both in cell transfection systems,[7] as well as in vivo in the mouse brain.[8] Cyclin A/cyclin-dependent kinase-2 (Cdk2) have also been shown to phosphorylate PGR and potentiate ligand-independent signaling.[9,10] Since P_4 is known to stimulate proliferation of the endometrium, these results may be important in elucidating PGR action in the uterus.

Through either ligand-dependent or ligand-independent mechanisms, phosphorylated PGR undergoes a conformational change and attains the ability to bind progesterone response elements (PREs) to stimulate expression of target genes. The progesterone–PGR

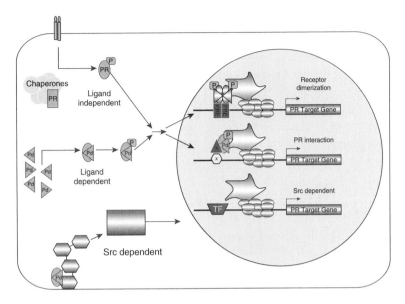

Figure 13.2   Mechanisms of PGR action.

complex forms a homodimer that binds to cis-acting PREs in the regulatory regions of the target genes. The PREs for transcription activators are usually present in the 5'-flanking region of specific genes. Although the perfect inverted repeat consensus sequence was identified as AGGACA(nnn)TGTCCT, most progesterone-responsive genes have imperfect palindromes or do not have recognizable PREs. To date, only a handful of genes containing full inverted repeat PRE elements have been found.[11–16] Many in-vitro studies have shown that the PGR may also regulate genes through cross-talk with other transcription factors or half-sites of the palindromic sequence. For example, several genes, including mouse prostaglandin E receptor, human glycodelin, and its own promoter in the human have been shown to be regulated through a cooperative interaction of PGR with Sp1.[17–19] PGR interacts with the RelA-p65 subunit to activate nuclear factor-κB (NF-κB), leading to immunosuppression necessary for a successful pregnancy outcome.[20] Human prolactin is regulated by PGR cooperatively with C/EBP-β,[21] while other important molecules such as vascular endothelial growth factor (VEGF) have been shown to be regulated through a series of half-sites.[22]

Upon the binding of the receptor to the PRE, the activated receptor then interacts with coactivators, which will link the steroid hormone receptor to the basal transcriptional machinery of the cell. The coactivators not only link the receptor to the transcription machinery but also either possess themselves, or recruit other nuclear proteins that possess enzymatic activities that are necessary for efficient gene expression. These include a number of acetyltransferase

proteins, such as CBP/p300, pCAF, p160s (including the steroid receptor coactivator [SRC] members, SRC1, SRC2, and SRC3), the ATP-coupled chromatin-remodeling SWI-SNF complex; methyltransferases, such as coactivator-associated arginine (R) methyltransferase-1 (CARM1), and PRMT-1/2; and ubiquitin ligases, such as E6-AP and Rsp5.[23] Non-liganded receptors can repress basal transcription of target genes through corepressors N-CoR (nuclear receptor corepressor) and SMRT (silencing mediator of repressed transcription).[24] The coactivators of the steroid receptor (SRC) family were the first identified coactivators. In a yeast two-hybrid system, SRC-1 was identified as a protein that interacts with and enhances PGR transcriptional activity, as well as, other nuclear receptors, without altering the basal activity.[25] Subsequently, two more SRC family members – SRC-2 [transcriptional intermediary factor 2 (TIF2)/GR-interacting protein 1 (GRIP-1)] and SRC-3 [(ACTR/pCIP/receptor associated coactivator (RAC3)/TRAM-1/amplified in breast cancer 1 (AIB1)] – have been identified.[26] This family of coactivators is able to bind to a coactivator-binding groove within the LBD of PGR via an NR box motif (LxxLL, where L = leucine and x is any amino acid).[27] The mechanism of action, physiological affects, and identification of new coactivators remains an active area of research.

The most recently discovered mechanism by which PGR can activate gene transcription is through its hormone-dependent ability to mediate activation of the Src/Ras/Raf/mitogen-activated protein kinase signaling cascade. Cytoplasmic PGR interacts directly with the Src homology 3 (SH3) domain of Src tyrosine kinase through a proline-rich motif located at the N-terminus of the receptor.[28] This mechanism of action is independent of transcription, and may contribute to the central role Src kinases regulation of cellular proliferation, differentiation, and motility. This mechanism shows that PGR has a dual function: it is not only capable of acting as a transcription factor but is also capable of directly activating signaling pathways from the cytoplasm.

REGULATION OF PGR AND COACTIVATOR EXPRESSION

Regulation of PGR in the mouse endometrium

The level of PGR expression in the uterus is largely steroid hormone regulated. During normal pregnancy in mice, PGR expression is low on 0.5 day postcoitum (dpc) (day 0.5 = vaginal plug) and beings to rise in the epithelium at 1.5 dpc. During 2.5–3.5 dpc, PGR is significantly up-regulated in both the epithelium and the subepithelial stroma. After implantation on 4.5 dpc, PGR is no longer detectable in the luminal epithelium, but up-regulated in the subepithelial stroma at the site of implantation. As implantation proceeds, PGR levels continue to increase until 6.5 dpc in the decidual cells.[29]

PGR and estrogen receptor α (ERα) are involved in a complex and compartmental specific reciprocal regulation. Tibbetts and coworkers investigated the effects of exogenous estrogen and progesterone on the expression of PGR and ERα in the compartments of the uterus of ovariectomized mice. They demonstrated exogenous estradiol (E_2) decreased PGR levels in luminal epithelium, while increasing levels of PGR in the stroma and myometrium. When E_2 administration was supplemented with P_4, ERα expression was increased in the glandular epithelium, but reduced in the myometrium. P_4 repressed PGR expression in all compartments.[30] The complex relationship between ERα and PGR in the different uterine compartments can also be seen in numerous tissue reconstitution experiments. Tissue recombination experiments have shown that the primary action of P_4 is coordinating stroma regulation of epithelial function.[31] In experiments utilizing wild-type and PRKO tissues, it was demonstrated that stromal P_4-PGR controls E_2-induced epithelial cell proliferation and gene expression.[32] Complementary tissue recombination studies have implicated that mitogenic effects of steroid hormones on the uterine stroma may be dependent upon epithelial signals.[33] Additional studies using wild-type and ERα knockout tissue show that uterine epithelial cell proliferation and repression of the uterine epithelial PGR are mediated by stroma ERα.[34] Therefore, both P_4 and E_2 regulate the expression of growth factor(s) that can coordinate the expression of genes between the epithelium and the stroma.

Likewise, receptivity of the mouse endometrium is steroid dependent, largely due to the combined actions of both E_2 and P_4. In adult mice, E_2 causes epithelial cell proliferation, while the combined action of E_2 and P_4 is necessary to drive proliferation in stromal cells. During normal pregnancy in mice, preovulatory estrogen surge stimulates uterine epithelial cell proliferation on 0.5 dpc. At 1.5 dpc, with the withdrawal of E_2, a large number of epithelial cells undergo apoptosis. The formation of the corpora lutea at 2.5 dpc causes rising P_4 levels that initiate uterine stromal cell proliferation. With P_4 priming of the uterus, preimplantation ovarian E_2 secretion on 3.5 dpc further enhances uterine stromal proliferation and differentiation, rendering the uterus to the receptive state for implantation.[35]

Regulation of PGR in the human endometrium

Like the mouse, the expression of PGR in the human endometrium is under the control of E_2 and P_4, which positively and negatively regulate PGR expression, respectively. In the proliferative phase of the endometrial cycle, occurring before ovulation, the uterus is primarily under the control of E_2, which is secreted in increasing quantities by the ovary. The stromal cells and the epithelial cells proliferate rapidly at the first stage. During the proliferative phase of the cycle, high levels of PGR are present in the nuclei of epithelial and stromal cells of the human endometrium and in myometrial smooth muscle cells. The secretory phase of the endometrial cycle begins after ovulation. Continued E_2 causes slight additional cellular proliferation in the endometrium, while P_4 from the newly formed corpus luteum causes marked swelling and secretory development. The glands increase in tortuosity; an excess of secretory substances accumulates in the glandular epithelial cells. Also, the cytoplasm of the stromal cells increases; lipid and glycogen deposits increase greatly in the stromal cells; and the blood supply to the endometrium further increases in proportion to the developing secretory activity. During this stage, detection of PGR in the luminal and glandular epithelium declines markedly, to undetectable levels. On the other hand, stromal and myometrial cells continue to express high levels of PGR despite the high levels of circulating P_4 and low E_2.[36-38] Ribonuclease protection assay (RPA) shows PGR mRNA expression in the myometrium is higher in most of the proliferative phase compared with the secretory phase, and total PGR mRNA expression significantly decreases during the normal secretory phase.[39] There is no significant difference between PGR regulation in the endometrium and myometrium.[40] Immunostaining studies also show that PGR in normal human endometrium decreases rapidly in stromal and glandular cells during the progression of the secretory phase.[41] Menstruation is caused by the sudden reduction of the E_2 and P_4, especially P_4, at the end of the monthly ovarian cycle, followed by rapid involution of the endometrium. Decreased stimulation of the endometrial cells by progesterone triggers the menstruation. Therefore, PGR is required to produce a highly secretory endometrium, containing large amounts of stored nutrients that can provide appropriate conditions for implantation of a fertilized ovum during the latter half of the menstrual cycle.

PRA and PRB are coexpressed in target cells of the human uterus. In the glands, PRA and PRB were expressed before subnuclear vacuole formation and glycogenolysis implicating both isoforms in this process, whereas persistence of PRB during the midsecretory phase suggested its significance in glandular secretion. In the stroma, the predominance of PRA throughout the cycle implicates this isoform in postovulatory progesterone-mediated events.[42] Given the opposing proliferative effects of the PGR isoforms in this tissue, we would predict that the relative expression levels of PGR isoforms in the uterus would be expected to play an important role in determining appropriate hormone responsiveness. Functional PGR also promotes quiescence in the pregnant uterus. This prevention of uterine contractions is necessary to prevent spontaneous abortion. Recent evidence has suggested a role for PRC in parturition. The up-regulation of this inhibitory PGR isoform by NF-κB on the PGR promoter may inhibit PGR activity and lead to a loss of uterine quiescence.[43]

Regulation of co-factors in the human endometrium

Cofactors N-CoR, SMRT, PCAF, CBP, SRC-1, SRC-2, SRC-3, and p300 mRNA are all expressed in the human endometrium and myometrium. In the myometrium, the levels of these cofactors are not cycle dependent. However, in the cycling endometrium, SRC-1, N-CoR, and SRC-3 levels are dependent upon cycle stage. Immunohistochemistry studies show that SRC-1 and N-CoR stain positive in the glandular epithelium and stroma in menstrual phase endometrium and are weakly expressed in the proliferative and secretory stages.[44] SRC-3 is expressed in the glandular epithelium and is increased in the late secretory phase,[45] while p300 and CBP levels are relatively constant throughout the cycle.[41] Protein and mRNA levels for CBP, SRC-2, and SRC-3 are decreased at term in fundal myometrium. These decreased levels of coactivators may diminish PGR ability to maintain uterine quiescence, and, therefore, contribute to the initiation of parturition.[46]

PGR and cofactor expression in endometrial cancer

Since the coactivators are important in activating steroid hormone function, it is reasonable to assume that aberrant levels of coactivators could lead to inappropriate hormonal response. Although endometrial cancers are often PGR positive, in a comparison of normal and malignant human endometrium, there was no significant difference in PGR mRNA expression by quantitative reverse transcriptase-polymerase chain reaction (RT-PCR). Only a trend toward significance between different grades of carcinoma, with intermediate stages, could be found.[39] However, aberrant ratios between PRA and PRB, as well as abnormal expression of coactivators, have been well studied in many different cancers.

In endometrial cancers, the loss of expression of either PRA or PRB is a common event. This loss is associated with higher clinical grade, which suggests a relationship between the loss of PGR isoform expression and features of poorer prognosis.[47] A binary transgenic system in which the GAL-4 gene, driven by the murine cytomegalovirus (CMV) promoter (CMV-GAL-4 mice), served as the transactivator of the PR-A gene, carrying four GAL-4 binding sites (UAS; UAS-PR-A mice) yields a three-fold increase of PRA over PRB. This ratio of PGR isoforms results in a dramatic mammary gland phenotype that includes extensive epithelial cell hyperplasia, excessive ductal branching, and a disorganized basement membrane, which are all features associated with neoplasia.[48] In contrast, overexpression of PRB in the mammary gland leads to premature ductal growth arrest and inadequate lobulo-alveolar differentiation.[49] Collectively, these data suggest that PRA and PRB have physiologically different functions in different tissues and that alterations in their ratios carry different consequences depending on the tissue.

SRC2 and SRC3 protein levels are increased significantly in the endometrium, in both the epithelium and the stroma of polycystic ovary syndrome (PCOS) women, a group that have a higher likelihood of developing estrogen-induced endometrial hyperplasia and cancer.[45] In addition, N-CoR, SMRT, SRC-1, SRC-2, and SRC-3 are up-regulated in malignant endometrium.[39] The up-regulation of these cofactors presumably affects steroid-dependent action, and has obvious clinical relevance in the treatment of steroid hormone-regulated cancers.[50,51] Further investigation of the molecular and phenotypic affects of abnormal levels of these cofactors in cancers is an active field of research.

ANIMAL MODELS OF PGR SIGNALING

The generation of animal models has greatly facilitated the ability of researchers to investigate the PGR signaling axis. These animals have served to define the role of PGR in uterine biology and have also served as tools to identify the pathways that are regulated by PGR.

PGR knockout models

Genetic ablation of both PRA and PRB in mice (PRKO) leads to pleiotropic reproductive abnormalities, including defects in female reproductive behavior, failure to ovulate, failure of the uterus to support embryo implantation (as seen by a lack of a decidual response), and defects in branching and glandular development in the mammary glands.[52] The selective ablation of PRA in mice (PRAKO) demonstrates that PRA is the major mediator of P_4 signaling in the mouse uterus regulating uterine function. Like the PRKO mice, these mice fail to ovulate or undergo a decidual reaction from the administration of exogenous hormones.[53] The PRB isoform regulates uterine epithelial cell proliferation. Selective activation of PRB in the uterus resulted in an abnormal P-dependent induction of epithelial proliferation, in contrast to its ability to inhibit E-induced proliferation in the normal uterus. This gain of PRB-dependent proliferative activity by removal of PRA indicates that PRA is required not only to inhibit E-induced hyperplasia of the uterus, but also to limit potentially adverse proliferative effects of the PRB. Surprisingly, the PRB knockout

(PRBKO) mouse showed no overt uterine phenotype, but a clear mammary gland phenotype.[54] PRA and PRB are clearly the predominant forms of PGR in the uterus and mammary gland, respectively. Therefore, it will be important to identify molecular markers of the opposing proliferative activities of PRA and PRB that can be used to assess the conservation of these signaling responses in the human setting.

Progesterone receptor activity indicator mouse model

To investigate the relationship between PR and steroid receptor coactivators (SRCs) in vivo, the Progesterone Receptor Activity Indicator (PRAI) system that monitors PGR transcription was developed. The PRAI system consists of a modified bacterial artificial chromosome (BAC) clone that contains the PGR locus. The DBD of the PGR was replaced with the yeast Gal4 DNA-binding domain, and a humanized green fluorescent protein (hrGFP) reporter under the control of Upstream Activating Sequences for the Gal4 gene (UAS_G) was inserted in tandem with the modified PGR gene. Therefore, expression of hrGFP in the uterus is indicative of PGR activity. This model has been shown to faithfully mirror endogenous PGR signaling under various endocrine states. SRC-1$^{-/-}$ PRAI mice reveal that SRC-1 modulates PGR activity in the uterus in a cell-specific fashion. In response to $E_2 + P_4$, SRC-1 is involved in PGR gene activation in stroma and myometrium. In contrast, after chronic P_4 treatment, SRC-1 was involved in the down-regulation of PGR target genes in the luminal and glandular epithelium.

Uterine gland knock out model

The pleitropic effects of ovarian steroids have also been used to create additional animal models to study implantation. In the first month after birth, the sheep endometrium develops from a simple tubular lumen to its adult morphology that includes intercaruncular regions filled with uterine glands.[55] Since the developmental cue for gland formation is the withdrawal of P_4 from the prenatal environment, by ovariectomizing newborn ewes and implanting a 19-norprogestin implant, the developmental cue of P_4 withdrawal was removed and uterine glands failed to develop.[56] This approach of prolonged P_4 exposure into neonatal ewes has led to the development of the ovine uterine gland knockout (UGKO) animal.[57] This model has been useful in rapidly identify genes expressed by the endometrial epithelium.[58]

Coactivator knockout models

Mice homozygous for the ablation of SRC-1 were fertile and viable. This was not surprising, considering the overlap in function and expression patterns among these coactivators. Expression of RNA encoding SRC-2 was increased in the SRC-1 null mutant, perhaps compensating partially for the loss of SRC-1 function in target tissues. However, the SRC-1-null mice exhibit partial hormone resistance in progesterone target tissues. The SRC-1$^{-/-}$ mouse uterus showed a decreased growth in response to decidual stimuli when stimulated with E_2 and P_4. Thus, this coactivator is responsible for modulating the actions of PGR in the mouse uterus.

SRC-2 is required during pregnancy. Although the SRC-2 null females are able to implant and the decidual reaction appears histologically normal, litter size of SRC-2 null females is drastically reduced. The reduction is presumably due to the marked increase of in-utero embryonic resorptions observed between E12.5 and E18.5 during pregnancies of SRC-2-null females. SRC-2 null females often displayed a marked placental hypoplasia with decreased numbers of trophoblastic trabeculae and embryonic capillaries in the labyrinthine region.[59]

Knockout studies of other coactivators have given inconclusive results on their necessity for P_4-mediated action in the uterus. The SRC-3 mouse has no apparent defects in uterine phenotype. Other coactivator knockouts, such as CBP, P300, and CARM-1, are embryonic or perinatal lethal, thus precluding further study.[60] Disruption of the maternal copy of E6-AP is correlated with Angelman syndrome, a genetic neurological disorder.[61] Although E6-AP ablation has been shown to impair the response of the uterus to exogenous estrogen, the effect on P_4-mediated action has yet to be shown.[62]

FKBP52

As previously stated, in the absence of P_4, PGR interacts with molecular chaperones in the cytoplasm. This interaction maintains the receptors in functional and competent to bind hormone and subsequently activates gene transcription. One of these molecular chaperones, FKBP52, belongs to a subclass of immunophillin proteins, FK506-binding proteins (FKBPs), due to its ability

to bind FK506, an immunosuppressive drug. It was originally discovered as a component of the unliganded steroid receptor heterocomplex. Heat shock protein 90 (Hsp90) serves as an adaptor protein that binds both to PGR and the FKBPs. Although the role of Hsp90 for maintenance of receptor function has been established, until recently very little was known about the role of other chaperones. FKBP52 catalyzes conformational changes in protein structure via a peptidyl-prolyl cis–trans isomerase domain.[63] In-vitro evidence from cell culture assays showed that FKBP52 strongly potentiates PGR transcriptional activity.[64] In the mouse, uterus FKBP52 is highly up-regulated during the peri-implantation period. At 0.5 dpc, it is primarily expressed in the uterine epithelium, with expression expanding into the stroma by 3.5 dpc. During implantation, FKBP52 is localized in the decidualizing stroma cells surrounding the newly formed implantation sites. In Hoxa10$^{-/-}$ mice, which are known to have endometrial defects, FKBP52 is decreased.[65] FKBP52 null females are completely infertile due to the inability to attain uterine receptivity and, therefore, have implantation failure. These mice exhibit reduced PGR transcriptional activity, and the expression of known targets of PGR target genes is not induced.[66] Further work has demonstrated that the FKBP52$^{-/-}$ uterus showed a normal growth response to estradiol, and unaltered expression of genes controlled by ER and PRB. In contrast, two known PRA-regulated genes amphiregulin (Areg) and calcitonin were not induced in the FKBP52$^{-/-}$, suggesting that FKBP52 specifically regulates PRA transactivation.[67]

Src knockout mice

As previously mentioned, PGR can directly activate signaling pathways in the cytoplasm by interaction with Src kinase. Therefore, Src null mice can be utilized as a tool to study PGR action. The first member of the Src family of protein tyrosine kinases was originally identified as the transforming protein (v-Src) of the oncogenic retrovirus Rous sarcoma virus (RSV).[68] Viral v-Src is an activated version of a normal cellular protein (c-Src) with intrinsic tyrosine kinase activity.[69] Src protein tyrosine kinases are 52–62 kDa proteins composed of six distinct functional regions: the Src homology (SH) 4 domain, the unique region, the SH3 domain, the SH2 domain, the catalytic domain, and a short negative regulatory. The SH3 and SH2 domains are protein-binding domains present in lipid kinases, protein and lipid phosphatases, cytoskeletal proteins, adaptor molecules, transcription factors, and other proteins, and the catalytic domain possesses tyrosine-specific protein kinase activity. Src has been shown to regulate multiple signaling pathways, including proliferation, differentiation, survival, metastasis, and angiogenesis.[70]

It is known that Src has an essential role in bone formation, since its mutation induces defects in bone remodeling of mice, including impaired osteoclast function and the development of osteopetrosis.[71] Since Src kinases are directly involved in proliferation, differentiation, and angiogenesis, all critical prerequisites for decidualization, the effect of Src ablation was looked at during this decidualization in the mouse uterus. Immunohistochemical studies revealed that active Src kinase is strongly expressed in the decidua and markedly increased in an artificially stimulated horn. Src null mice showed no apparent decidual response, and the uterus lacked expression of known decidual markers. This result clearly demonstrates that Src activity is indispensable for an appropriate P_4-induced decidualization.[72] Additionally, in human endometrial stromal cells, the kinase activity of c-Src was increased during in-vitro decidualization. These effects are clearly hormone dependent, as withdrawal of E_2 and P_4 reduced c-Src kinase activity to the basal level and also changed the pattern of tyrosine phosphorylation to the unstimulated state. These results corroborate the mouse results that the activation of c-Src kinase is mediated by ovarian hormone stimulation and plays an important role in decidualization.[73]

IDENTIFICATION OF PGR-REGULATED GENES

Through candidate gene approaches and differential library screenings, until recently, only a few P_4-PGR-regulated genes have been identified. Some of these include the genes encoding amphiregulin (Areg),[74] histidine decarboxylase (Hdc) (13), Hoxa-10 and -11 (14), calcitonin,[75] calbindin-D9K,[16] Indian hedgehog[76,77] (18), hypoxia-inducible factor 1 (HIF1A),[78] and immune-responsive gene.[79] High-density DNA microarray technology has immensely improved the ability to identify PGR-regulated genes in the uterus.

Yoshioka et al provided one of the first microarray-based investigations of gene expression around the time of implantation by attempting to identify genes with differential expression between preimplantation (day 3.5) and postimplantation (day 5.0) stages. Of the 6500 genes examined, they detected changes in mRNA level in 399 genes. The expression of 192 genes increased and that of 207 genes decreased in the transition from the preimplantation to the postimplantation phase. The relatively large percentage of genes changed in this microarray is presumably due to not only genes directly responsible for implantation but also to changes in decidual tissue.[80]

Reese et al further refined the microarray performed by Yoshioka et al. This group compared gene expression profiles between implantation and interimplantation sites on 3.5 dpc, as well as the differences in uterine gene expression profile of P_4 treated, delayed implanting mice against those in which delayed implantation was terminated by E_2 treatment. In this manner, they sought to determine which genes are expressed specifically at implantation sites, and under maternal hormonal control. They reported 36 up-regulated and 27 down-regulated genes at the implantation site. However, since the implanting blastocysts were in the implantation sites, but not in the inter-implantation sites, these genes may be of embryonic origin. However, physical disruption of the uterine epithelium would likely result in different gene expression profiles. They identified 128 up-regulated and 101 down-regulated genes upon termination of delayed implantation by E_2. A combined analysis of these experiments showed specific up-regulation of 27 genes both at the implantation site and during implantation.[81]

Cheon et al. used high-density DNA microarray technology to identify PGR-responsive genes in the mouse uterus by treating female mice at 2.5 dpc of pregnancy with the antiprogestin RU486 and investigating changes in gene expression 24 hours later. This approach identified PGR-regulated genes by inhibiting PGR action at a time when PGR levels were elevated in all compartments. This approach identified the impact of withdrawal of P_4-PGR signaling on axis on gene expression and identified 148 possible P_4-PGR target genes. Although RU486 is mostly known as an antiprogestin, it is also an antagonist of glucocorticoid and androgen receptors. Therefore, in order to validate these results, the PRKO mouse was utilized.[82]

Jeong et al utilized oligonucleotide arrays to define the molecular pathways regulated by the P_4-PGR signaling axis. PRKO and wild-type mice were ovariectomized and then treated with vehicle or 1 mg P_4 every 12 hours. Mice were killed either 4 hours after the first injection or after the fourth injection of P_4 (40 hours). In this experiment, the effect of P_4 and PGR both alone and in combination could be measured. The 4 hour time point was chosen in order to identify genes that are directly regulated by the P_4-PGR axis. Genes that are separately affected by either PGR ablation or P_4 treatment may be the result of several mechanisms. Genes solely regulated by PGR ablation may be due to developmental differences between the PRKO and the wild-type uterus, or ligand-independent activation of the PGR. On the other hand, genes regulated by P_4 solely may be due to a P_4 effect on other PGR isoforms, such as PRC, or activation of other nuclear receptors. However, since the majority of the genes identified were regulated both by P_4 and PGR suggests that in the mouse uterus the majority of PRA and PRB are the conduit for the majority of P_4 action. At the 4 hour time point, 139 genes were found up-regulated by P_4 and PGR, while 96 genes were found to be down-regulated. Conversely, the major change in gene expression after chronic P_4 treatment was a down-regulation of genes.[83]

In general, investigation of the adult mouse uterus has been involved in dissecting the factors and molecular mechanisms by which the uterus is able to support implantation. However, as with other mammals, the mouse uterus of a mature female undergoes a cyclic trophy–atrophy alternation called the estrous cycle. This steroid-driven event is the equivalent of the menstrual cycle in humans and reflects the cyclic change of the uterine endometrium in preparation for embryo implantation. The estrous cycle can be divided into four stages – proestrus, estrus, metestrus, and diestrus – in accordance with the typical characteristics of uterine structure and function. Proestrous is characterized by gradually increasing E_2 concentrations and proliferation of endometrial cells. The estrus stage is when ovulation and sexual receptivity occur, and E_2 levels peak and P_4 levels start to rise. If no conceptus exists, the uterus regresses because serum E_2 concentrations decrease and P_4 concentrations continue to increase. E_2 levels remain low through metestrous and diestrous, while P_4 levels remain high. Tan and co-workers performed cDNA microarray to investigate genes that were differentially expressed at estrus and diestrus. Of the 8192 genes examined, 51 were up-regulated and 51 were down-regulated. Although the function of many of the differentially expressed genes they found are still unknown, these genes may be important for understanding the mechanisms of the estrous cycle and eventual endometrial receptivity after copulation.[84]

Although the window of implantation in the human uterus has been temporally defined as cycle days 20–24, the molecular definition of this window has been difficult to define.[85] Kao et al used high-density oligonucleotide microarray to identify genes that were differentially expressed in late proliferative stage at the peak of circulating (E_2) and the mid-secretory phase (peak E_2 and P_4 and timed to 8–10 days after the luteinizing hormone [LH] surge) of human endometrial biopsies. Timing to the LH surge assured that the uteri were in the window of implantation. This study reported significant up-regulation of 156 genes and down-regulation of 377 genes within the putative window of implantation.[86]

Although the various microarray approaches were taken in these studies, including pregnancy, antagonist treatment, exogenous P_4 treatment, and during the cycle both in mice and humans, a number of genes were found in common between many of the arrays, including those encoding the known P_4-regulated genes – amphiregulin (Areg), mucin-1 (Muc-1), and follistatin (Fst) – as well as new targets such as glutathione S-transferases, immune response gene 1, CCAAT/ enhancer-binding protein β, and interleukin-13Ra2 were found in the majority of the arrays. This amount of mutually overlapping information between the arrays, especially with known P_4 target genes such as Areg, Muc-1, and Fst, serves to validate the differential approaches taken by these investigators. Elucidating the spatiotemporal expression and function of these targets will help resolve the molecular pathways.

PROGESTERONE REGULATED TARGET GENES

Calcium-binding proteins

Calcium-binding protein (CaBP)-d9k and CaBP-d28k are members of a large family of intracellular proteins with similar structural characteristics called EF-hand motifs that are responsible for binding free calcium. Both are thought to act as cytosolic calcium buffers.[87] In the mouse uterus, CaBP-d9k is expressed in the endometrial luminal and glandular epithelium at the time of implantation. At 4.5 dpc it was detected in the luminal epithelium, but not in the glandular epithelium. Upon embryo implantation, CaBP-d9k disappears at implantation sites following embryo attachment. CaBP-d9k expression in vivo is increased by P_4, but not E_2 and a consensus PRE has been found in its promoter.[16,88] CaBP-28k, a closely related family member, shows an almost identical expression pattern to CaBP-d9k.[89] Hong et al performed intrauterine injection of morpholino oligonucleotides (MO) against CaBP-d9k into WT and CaBP-d28k null mice just before implantation to determine if CaBP-d9k is necessary for implantation. Implantation was only blocked in the CaBP-d28k null background when CaBP-d9k MOs were injected, thus demonstrating the necessity for CaBPs in implantation.[89]

In the human uterus, CaBP-d9k is not detectable, while CaBP-d28k is found during all stages of the menstrual cycle. During the human menstrual cycle, CaBP-d28k protein is detected predominantly in the luminal and glandular epithelium, with low expression in the stroma. In both the epithelium and the stroma, the expression peaks in the mid-secretory phase, when the endometrium is receptive to implantation.[90]

CCAAT/enhancer-binding protein β

CCAAT/enhancer-binding protein β (C/EBPβ) is a transcription factor that belongs to the basic region-leucine zipper class DNA-binding proteins that bind to DNA as a homodimer and a heterodimer. Numerous functions of this gene include the ability to regulate cellular proliferation, differentiation, and apoptosis. C/EBPβ is intronless and yields multiple protein isoforms due to alternative translational start sites or cleavage of the full-length C/EBPβ protein, including dominant negatives (as reviewed in Zahnow[91]).

Mice with a targeted deletion of the C/EBPβ gene exhibit reproductive defects. Although these animals develop normally and males are fertile, adult females are sterile. Transplantation of normal ovaries into mutant females partially restored fertility. Therefore, the primary reproductive defect is due to ovarian origin. Further transplantation experiments proved that although C/EBPβ null ovaries produce functional oocytes, the ovary fails to form corpora lutea, the major source of P_4 in early implantation.[92] C/EBPβ is rapidly induced in the pregnant uterus at the time of blastocyst attachment and has been identified by microarray analysis.[81,82] The expression of C/EBPβ increased further during the decidualization phase of pregnancy and was localized in the proliferating, as well as, the decidualized stromal cells surrounding the implanted embryo. In order to study the uterus of the C/EBPβ null animals, the defect in ovarian function and, therefore, alteration in hormone levels, had to be circumvented by treatment with exogenous hormones. The C/EBPβ null animals failed to respond to an artifical deciduogenic stimulus and were shown to have a defect in stromal cell proliferation and differentiation. In addition, E_2-induced proliferation of uterine epithelial cells is decreased in C/EBPβ null animals.[93]

In the human endometrium during the proliferative phase, C/EBPβ is expressed in the epithelium, with occasional stromal expression. Expression also appeared to be increased in endometrial carcinoma.[94] The specific functions of C/EBPβ have also been studied in human endometrial stromal cells. C/EBPβ regulates the promoters of well-known decidual markers, including inducing prolactin and cyclooxygenase 2 (COX-2), and inhibiting P450arom promoter activity.[21,95,96]

Homeobox (Hox) genes

Homeobox (Hox) genes were first described in the fruit fly, *Drosophila melanogaster*, as genes that are important for establishing segment identity during development. Mutation or misexpression of Hox genes leads to the development of one body segment in place of another.[97] When Hox genes are ablated in the fruit fly, the body segment in which it is normally expressed develops the characteristics of an adjacent segment, usually anterior, but occasionally posterior.[98] This phenomenon is known as anterior or posterior transformation. Hox genes are characterized by a well-conserved 183 base pair that encodes a homeodomain which binds DNA through a helix–loop helix motif to alter gene transcription.[99,100] To date, all research into the role of Hox genes in uterine development and implantation has occurred solely in mice and humans.

Taylor et al characterized the Hox genes and their expression necessary for the development of the mouse reproductive tract. These genes are Hoxa9, Hoxa10, Hoxa11, and Hoxa13. In Müllerian tract development before differentiation into the fallopian tube, uterus, cervix, and vagina, all four Hoxa genes are found throughout the tube. However, during structural differentiation that occurs from birth to 2 weeks, the expression pattern of the Hox genes becomes restricted and leads to the development of distinct structures. Hoxa9 is expressed in the presumptive fallopian tube, Hoxa10 is expressed in the developing uterus, Hoxa11 is in the posterior uterine segment and the cervix, and Hoxa13 is found in the primordial vagina.[101] In the adult mouse uterus, both Hoxa10 and Hoxa11 are regulated by progesterone acting through its cognate receptor, PGR. These data correspond to previous data that, in Hoxa10 null mice, only progesterone-dependent stromal, and not estrogen-dependent epithelial, cell proliferation is abrogated.[102] Gene targeting experiments to ablate specific Hox genes have elucidated their developmental and reproductive function. Mice null for either Hoxa10 or

Hoxa11 show implantation failure.[98,103] However, this phenotype is confounded by subtle developmental phenotypes. The anterior 25% of Hoxa10 null mice uteri undergo anterior transformation into an oviduct-like structure,[104] and the Hoxa11 null mice exhibit decreased stromal development and expression of leukemia inhibitory factor (LIF).[105] To eliminate developmental effects, intrauterine transfection of antisense oligonucleotides to Hoxa10 into the uterine lumen on day 2 of pregnancy was undertaken. This treatment greatly reduced the number of implantation sites, thus supporting the role of adult maternal Hox proteins for implantation.[106] Additionally, the ablation of another homeobox gene, Hmx3, has also been shown to be important for implantation in mice. Although an exploration of its infertility has yet to be done, a perturbation of the Wnt and LIF gene expression in the female null uterus may be contributing factors.[107]

HoxA10 and 11 have also been implicated to have a role in human reproduction. Cell culture experiments have shown that expression of both Hox genes is regulated by E_2 and P_4, and that HoxA10 and 11 are expressed in the glandular epithelia and the stroma of human uteri.[108,109] Although Hox expression is expressed throughout the menstrual cycle, there is a significant increase in expression during the mid and late luteal phases.[108,109] In patients with endometriosis, there is no mid-luteal increase of HoxA10 and 11,[109] and similar patterns are seen for HoxA10 in patients diagnosed with leiomyomas.[110]

Colony-stimulating factor 1

Colony-stimulating factor 1 (CSF-1), or macrophage CSF (m-CSF), is a glycosylated homodimer with essential disulfide linkage that has a molecular size of 47–76 kDa.[111] The human CSF-1 gene is alternatively spliced, leading to three major transcripts, all with biological activity.[112] CSF-1 is a P_4-regulated gene in endometrial stromal cells and modulates differentiation, survival, and proliferation in numerous cell types.[113]

CSF-1 increases approximately 1000-fold during pregnancy, with a concomitant increase in CSF-1 mRNA in the luminal and glandular epithelium.[114,115] In mice, CSF-1 is first expressed at 2.5 dpc, and increases throughout pregnancy, reaching a peak at 14–15 dpc.[116] The biological significance of CSF-1 in the uterus was found in the osteopetrotic op/op mice, in which a frameshift mutation forms a knockout of the CSF-1 gene.[117] Mice with the op/op allele have pleiotropic reproductive abnormalities. Females have a low ovulation rate, decreased implantation, and fetal survival rates. Treatment of op/op mice with human recombinant CSF-1 fails to rescue the reproductive phenotype, suggesting that local synthesis of CSF-1 is necessary for uterine function.[118]

CSF-1 is expressed in the human endometrial tissue during normal cycling, with high levels during the proliferative phase. Also, first trimester decidual tissue has higher levels of CSF-1 than non-pregnant controls.[119] In addition to the expression of CSF-1 in human pregnancy, several correlative links have been made between abnormal CSF-1 expression and infertility. Low circulating levels of CSF-1 in both preconceptional and 8-week gestational stages are associated with recurrent spontaneous abortion.[120] Additionally, a comparison between CSF-1 levels in follicular fluid and blood plasma that included fertile and infertile women demonstrated an elevation in the follicular fluid/plasma ratio of CSF-1 levels in the infertile group.[121]

Vascular endothelial growth factor

An important stage in embryo implantation in all mammals is the connection of the fetal and maternal blood supplies. For this connection to occur, there must be dramatic growth and remodeling of the endometrial vasculature. VEGF-A, a homodimeric glycoprotein first discovered as an endothelial cell mitogen and also known as vascular permeability factor (VPF) due to its ability to induce vascular leakage in guinea pig skin,[122] is a factor that may be important in this process. Five human VEGF-A isoforms – $VEGF_{121}$, $VEGF_{145}$, $VEGF_{165}$, $VEGF_{189}$, and $VEGF_{206}$ (denoted by number of amino acids) – are generated through alternative splicing of a single gene.[123] The mouse VEGF-A gene undergoes similar splicing, leading to the generation of $VEGF_{120}$, $VEGF_{164}$, and $VEGF_{188}$. The murine VEGFs are shorter than the respective human VEGFs by one amino acid. The different isoforms of VEGF have distinctive properties due to this molecular heterogeneity. Native VEGF ($VEGF_{165}$) is a secreted protein that remains largely bound to the cell surface and extracellular matrix that is able to bind heparin. $VEGF_{121}$ does not bind heparin and is freely soluble, while $VEGF_{189}$ and $VEGF_{206}$ remain almost completely bound to the cellular membrane. $VEGF_{165}$ and $VEGF_{121}$ are the dominant forms in humans, although it has been shown that the human endometrium synthesizes all the splice variants of VEGF-A.[124] VEGF-A effects are predominantly mediated through two tyrosine kinase receptors: VEGFR-1 (fms-like tyrosine kinase [Flt-1]) and VEGFR-2 (also known as fetal liver kinase-1 [Flk-1] in the human or kinase domain region [KDR] in the mouse). VEGFR-2 is the major positive regulator of VEGF signaling to affect an increase in angiogenesis, vascularization, and vasodilation. Ablation of the specific components of the VEGF signal transduction cascade shows their necessity for vascular development, as demonstrated in VEGF-A heterozygous, VEGFR-1 null, and VEGFR-2 null mice which are all lethal, early in embryonic life.[125–127]

The uterine expression of VEGF has been well characterized. The human VEGF promoter has been shown to be regulated by ER through a variant response element[128] and PGR through a series of half-sites.[22] In the mouse, VEGF RNA expression is induced in the luminal epithelium on days 1 and 2, presumably due to high E_2 levels. On day 3, a low level of VEGF can be visualized in the stroma. On days 4–5, VEGF can be seen in the luminal epithelial cells and in the periepithelial stroma. After the blastocyst attaches, the luminal epithelium and periepithelial stroma at the implantation site strongly express VEGF, with increasing expression on both the mesometrial and antimesometrial poles.[129] More recent evidence suggests that, in the mouse uterus, the $VEGF_{164}$ is the dominant isoform in mouse decidualization and that regulation of VEGFR-2 shows an appropriate spatiotemporal regulation to transduce VEGF signaling in the decidual response.[130]

The expression of VEGF-A and its receptors has been well characterized in the human uterus. Several studies have shown that VEGF is expressed throughout the human cycle, with the highest expression in glandular epithelium at the secretory phase,[131,132] and that E_2 treatment increases levels of the $VEGF_{121}$, $VEGF_{165}$, and $VEGF_{189}$ isoforms.[133] In addition, in the endometrial stroma, E_2 when combined with P_4 induces expression of $VEGF_{189}$ specifically, suggesting that $VEGF_{189}$ may have an important role in the human uterus.[134] Surprisingly, in the array performed by Kao et al, VEGF levels are decreased during the window of implantation.[86]

VEGF-A levels have also been found to be correlated with several uterine disease states that negatively impact fertility. In women with moderate to severe endometriosis, peritoneal fluid concentrations of VEGF-A were significantly higher in controls.[132] Also, the presence of VEGF-A in the majority of uterine leiomyoma suggests that this factor is important for the local angiogenesis and growth of these tumors.[135] Decreased cytoblastic expression of VEGF-A and VEGFR-1 have also been associated with increased incidence of severe preeclampsia.[136]

Mucin 1

Mucin 1 (Muc1), a negative regulator of cellular adhesion, is a heavily glycosylated high-molecular-weight membrane protein whose large extracellular domain consists of a variable number of tandem repeats of 20 conserved amino acids, each of which contains five potential O-linked glycosylation sites.[137] The variable number of these tandem repeats (16 in mice; 20–125 in humans) leads to substantial polymorphic variation in the final gene product.[138] These tandem repeats seem to sterically hinder adhesion-promoting molecules and have the net effect of inhibiting cell–cell adhesion.

Muc1 expression is regulated by P_4 in all species studied so far.[139–142] In the uterus, Muc1 is restricted to the epithelium, and high expression of Muc1 is inhibitory to blastocyst attachment. In addition, there have been numerous reports that Muc1 is regulated by steroid hormones across species. However, the expression pattern of Muc1 in the endometrium shows species-to-species variation. In mice, Muc1 is greatly reduced in luminal epithelium during the window of implantation. However, in humans, expression of Muc1 is increased during the receptive phase.[142,143] However, in-vitro studies have shown that during the adhesion phase of implantation, the blastocyst induces a paracrine signal to cleave the Muc1 extracellular domains at the site of attachment.[142,144] Although mice null for Muc1 are fertile when isolated in pathogen-free environments, under normal housing conditions, chronic infection and inflammation of the lower reproductive tract occurs as common flora leads to opportunistic infection. These chronic infections then lead to reduced fertility rates, which shows the necessity of the Muc1 in natural environments.[145]

In the human uterus, studies have correlated Muc1 levels to fertility. The concentrations of Muc1 proteins in uterine flushings in women suffering from recurrent spontaneous miscarriages were significantly lower than in the controls throughout the luteal phase and most drastically at the time of implantation.[146] In addition, the polymorphic variation due to the number of tandem repeats that range from 20 to 125 in humans has also been implicated in infertility. Women with idiopathic infertility have a median allele size that is significantly smaller than control groups.[138]

Immune response gene 1

Immune responsive gene 1 (Irg1) is a recently found gene in macrophages that is induced following lipopolysaccharide (LPS) stimulation. The induction of Irg1 by LPS is mediated by the tyrosine kinase and protein kinase C (PKC) pathway.[147] Irg1 was shown to be regulated by several of the previously cited arrays.[80–82] In adult mice, Irg1 expression was limited to the uterine luminal epithelium, where it is expressed only during pregnancy, with a peak coinciding with implantation. Irg1 mRNA expression is regulated synergistically by P_4 and E_2. As in cultured macrophages, the regulation of Irg1 is due to an induced PKC pathway in the uterine epithelium.[148] To investigate the function of Irg1 during implantation, antisense oligodeoxynucleotides were injected into preimplantation mouse uteri. This treatment led to suppression in Irg1 mRNA expression and caused an impairment of embryo implantation.[79]

Indian hedgehog

Indian hedgehog (Ihh) is a member of the Hh family of diffusible morphogens that have been shown to be critical regulators of *Drosophila* and vertebrate development.[149,150] All Hh proteins undergo autocatalytic cleavage to form an amino terminal peptide, which is modified by the addition of a cholesterol moiety and palmitoylation, and participates in both short- and long-range paracrine signaling.[151,152] The amino terminal Hh ligand interacts with a 12-span transmembrane receptor protein, Patched (Ptch).[150] The interaction between the Hh and Ptch relieves Ptch-mediated inhibition of the activity of a G protein-coupled seven-span transmembrane protein, Smoothened (Smo). Upon the loss of inhibition by Ptch, Smo begins a signaling cascade that allows the Gli family of transcription factors to translocate to the nucleus and activate the transcription of target genes.[153] Another Hh-regulated pathway, independent of Gli transcription factors, works through dephosphorylation of a transcription factor, yet to be defined, to regulate COUP-TFII expression.[154]

Ihh was shown to be induced by P_4 in the murine uterus. Ihh expression is restricted to the epithelium, while the established effectors of Ihh, Ptch1, Gli transcription factors, and COUP-TFII are coordinately expressed in the endometrial stroma.[76,77] Conditional ablation of Ihh, specifically in PGR-positive uterine cells of the mouse, shows that Ihh is an essential mediator of PGR action in the mouse uterus that regulates the window of receptivity. Its ablation leads to complete infertility, as the endometrium is refractory to embryo attachment, is unable to support the formation of implantation sites, and demonstrates a complete lack of a progesterone-mediated stromal proliferative, angiogenic, and decidual response.[155]

Other P_4 target genes to have functional significance in implantation include calcitonin[75] and Areg.[74] Intraluminal injection of antisense oligonucleotides to calcitonin into the rat uterus leads to drastically reduced numbers of implantation sites.[156] Treatment with Areg antisense oligonucleotides delays blastocyst formation in vitro.[157]

CONCLUSIONS

Progesterone is a critical transcription factor in the uterus that is associated with all aspects of the establishment and maintenance of pregnancy. In the pregenomic era, candidate gene approaches to identify P_4 target genes led to many of the well-characterized genes in the uterus. The recent identification of additional PGR isoforms, as well as mPGR involved in membrane signaling, has emphasized the growing complexity of understanding PGR actions. However, our recent ability to examine large numbers of genes simultaneously by microarray analysis has not only led to an expansion of the number of P_4 target genes but also to our ability to scrutinize entire pathways.

Although gene ablation studies have been instrumental in understanding uterine gene function, a number of the progesterone target genes implicated in implantation, including Ihh, VEGF, and Hif-1,[76,78,130] are lethal at early developmental stages due to perturbation of bone morphogenesis or vascular development.[125,158,159] Additionally, coactivator knockouts, such as CBP, P300, and CARM-1, are embryonic or perinatal lethal, thus precluding further study of how these genes affect P_4 signaling. Although exogenous treatments, such as intraluminal infusions of oligodeoxynucleotides, antibodies, or chemical antagonists designed to block specific proteins, have often been utilized, these studies often led to results that are incompatible with the null mutations of genes, as reviewed in Lee and DeMayo.[160] Additional genetic mouse models will provide valuable tools to elucidate the molecular mechanisms of PGR signaling and its regulated genes in the endometrium.

ACKNOWLEDGMENTS

The manuscript for this chapter was prepared with the assistance of Janet DeMayo MS and John Ellsworth. The work was supported in part by the NICHD/NIH, as part of the Cooperative Program on Trophoblast–Maternal Tissue Interactions (U01HD042311), and the Reproductive Biology Training Grant (T32HD07165).

REFERENCES

1. Tsai MJ, O'Malley BW. Molecular mechanisms of action of steroid/thyroid receptor superfamily members. Annu Rev Biochem 1994; 63: 451–86.
2. Evans RM. The steroid and thyroid hormone receptor superfamily. Science 1988; 240: 889–95.
3. Ribeiro RC, Kushner PJ, Baxter JD. The nuclear hormone receptor gene superfamily. Annu Rev Med 1995; 46: 443–53.
4. Wei LL, Hawkins P, Baker C et al. An amino-terminal truncated progesterone receptor isoform, PRc, enhances progestin-induced transcriptional activity. Mol Endocrinol 1996; 10: 1379–87.
5. Power RF, Conneely OM, O'Malley BW. New insights into activation of the steroid hormone receptor superfamily. Trends Pharmacol Sci 1992; 13: 318–23.
6. Denner LA, Weigel NL, Maxwell BL et al. Regulation of progesterone receptor-mediated transcription by phosphorylation. Science 1990; 250: 1740–3.
7. Power RF, Mani SK, Codina J et al. Dopaminergic and ligand-independent activation of steroid hormone receptors. Science 1991; 254: 1636–9.
8. Mani SK, Allen JM, Clark JH et al. Convergent pathways for steroid hormone- and neurotransmitter-induced rat sexual behavior. Science 1994; 265: 1246–9.
9. Zhang Y, Beck CA, Poletti A et al. Phosphorylation of human progesterone receptor by cyclin-dependent kinase 2 on three sites that are authentic basal phosphorylation sites in vivo. Mol Endocrinol 1997; 11: 823–32.
10. Pierson-Mullany LK, Lange CA. Phosphorylation of progesterone receptor serine 400 mediates ligand-independent transcriptional activity in response to activation of cyclin-dependent protein kinase 2. Mol Cell Biol 2004; 24: 10542–57.
11. Cheng KW, Cheng CK, Leung PC. Differential role of PR-A and -B isoforms in transcription regulation of human GnRH receptor gene. Mol Endocrinol 2001; 15: 2078–92.
12. Gao J, Mazella J, Tang M, Tseng L. Ligand-activated progesterone receptor isoform hPR-A is a stronger transactivator than hPR-B for the expression of IGFBP-1 (insulin-like growth factor binding protein-1) in human endometrial stromal cells. Mol Endocrinol 2000; 14: 1954–61.
13. Matsui D, Sakari M, Sato T et al. Transcriptional regulation of the mouse steroid 5alpha-reductase type II gene by progesterone in brain. Nucleic Acids Res 2002; 30: 1387–93.
14. Moore MR, Zhou JL, Blankenship KA et al. A sequence in the 5' flanking region confers progestin responsiveness on the human c-myc gene. J Steroid Biochem Mol Biol 1997; 62: 243–52.
15. Slater EP, Cato AC, Karin M et al. Progesterone induction of metallothionein-IIA gene expression. Mol Endocrinol 1988; 2: 485–91.
16. Lee KY, Oh GT, Kang JH et al. Transcriptional regulation of the mouse calbindin-D9k gene by the ovarian sex hormone. Mol Cells 2003; 16: 48–53.
17. Tsuchiya S, Tanaka S, Sugimoto Y et al. Identification and characterization of a novel progesterone receptor-binding element in the mouse prostaglandin E receptor subtype EP2 gene. Genes Cells 2003; 8: 747–58.
18. Gao J, Mazella J, Seppala M, Tseng L. Ligand activated hPR modulates the glycodelin promoter activity through the Sp1 sites in human endometrial adenocarcinoma cells. Mol Cell Endocrinol 2001; 176: 97–102.
19. Tang M, Mazella J, Gao J, Tseng L. Progesterone receptor activates its promoter activity in human endometrial stromal cells. Mol Cell Endocrinol 2002; 192: 45–53.
20. Leonhardt SA, Boonyaratanakornkit V, Edwards DP. Progesterone receptor transcription and non-transcription signaling mechanisms. Steroids 2003; 68: 761–70.
21. Christian M, Pohnke Y, Kempf R et al. Functional association of PR and CCAAT/enhancer-binding protein beta isoforms: promoter-dependent cooperation between PR-B and liver-enriched inhibitory protein, or liver-enriched activatory protein and PR-A in human endometrial stromal cells. Mol Endocrinol 2002; 16: 141–54.
22. Mueller MD, Vigne JL, Pritts EA et al. Progestins activate vascular endothelial growth factor gene transcription in endometrial adenocarcinoma cells. Fertil Steril 2003; 79: 386–92.
23. Smith CL, O'Malley BW. Coregulator function: a key to understanding tissue specificity of selective receptor modulators. Endocr Rev 2004; 25: 45–71.
24. Wagner BL, Norris JD, Knotts TA et al. The nuclear corepressors NCoR and SMRT are key regulators of both ligand- and 8-bromo-cyclic AMP-dependent transcriptional activity of the human progesterone receptor. Mol Cell Biol 1998; 18: 1369–78.
25. Onate SA, Tsai SY, Tsai MJ, O'Malley BW. Sequence and characterization of a coactivator for the steroid hormone receptor superfamily. Science 1995; 270: 1354–7.
26. McKenna NJ, Xu J, Nawaz Z et al. Nuclear receptor coactivators: multiple enzymes, multiple complexes, multiple functions. J Steroid Biochem Mol Biol 1999; 69: 3–12.
27. Heery DM, Kalkhoven E, Hoare S, Parker MG. A signature motif in transcriptional co-activators mediates binding to nuclear receptors. Nature 1997; 387: 733–6.
28. Boonyaratanakornkit V, Scott MP, Ribon V et al. Progesterone receptor contains a proline-rich motif that directly interacts with SH3 domains and activates c-Src family tyrosine kinases. Mol Cell 2001; 8: 269–80.
29. Tan J, Paria BC, Dey SK, Das SK. Differential uterine expression of estrogen and progesterone receptors correlates with uterine preparation for implantation and decidualization in the mouse. Endocrinology 1999; 140: 5310–21.
30. Tibbetts TA, Mendoza-Meneses M, O'Malley BW, Conneely OM. Mutual and intercompartmental regulation of estrogen receptor and progesterone receptor expression in the mouse uterus. Biol Reprod 1998; 59: 1143–52.
31. Cooke PS, Uchima FD, Fujii DK et al. Restoration of normal morphology and estrogen responsiveness in cultured vaginal and uterine epithelia transplanted with stroma. Proc Natl Acad Sci USA 1986; 83: 2109–13.
32. Kurita T, Young P, Brody JR et al. Stromal progesterone receptors mediate the inhibitory effects of progesterone on estrogen-induced uterine epithelial cell deoxyribonucleic acid synthesis. Endocrinology 1998; 139: 4708–13.
33. Bigsby RM, Aixin L, Everett L. Stromal–Epithelial Interactions Regulating Cell Proliferation in the Uterus. New York: Raven Press, 1993.
34. Kurita T, Lee K, Saunders PT et al. Regulation of progesterone receptors and decidualization in uterine stroma of the estrogen receptor-alpha knockout mouse. Biol Reprod 2001; 64: 272–83.
35. Huet-Hudson YM, Andrews GK, Dey SK. Cell type-specific localization of c-myc protein in the mouse uterus: modulation by steroid hormones and analysis of the periimplantation period. Endocrinology 1989; 125: 1683–90.
36. Garcia E, Bouchard P, De Brux J et al. Use of immunocytochemistry of progesterone and estrogen receptors for endometrial dating. J Clin Endocrinol Metab 1988; 67: 80–7.

37. Lessey BA, Killam AP, Metzger DA et al. Immunohistochemical analysis of human uterine estrogen and progesterone receptors throughout the menstrual cycle. J Clin Endocrinol Metab 1988; 67: 334–40.

38. Press MF, Udove JA, Greene GL. Progesterone receptor distribution in the human endometrium. Analysis using monoclonal antibodies to the human progesterone receptor. Am J Pathol 1988; 131: 112–24.

39. Kershah SM, Desouki MM, Koterba KL, Rowan BG. Expression of estrogen receptor coregulators in normal and malignant human endometrium. Gynecol Oncol 2004; 92: 304–13.

40. Vienonen A, Miettinen S, Blauer M et al. Expression of nuclear receptors and cofactors in human endometrium and myometrium. J Soc Gynecol Investig 2004; 11: 104–12.

41. Shiozawa T, Shih HC, Miyamoto T et al. Cyclic changes in the expression of steroid receptor coactivators and corepressors in the normal human endometrium. J Clin Endocrinol Metab 2003; 88: 871–8.

42. Mote PA, Balleine RL, McGowan EM, Clarke CL. Colocalization of progesterone receptors A and B by dual immunofluorescent histochemistry in human endometrium during the menstrual cycle. J Clin Endocrinol Metab 1999; 84: 2963–71.

43. Condon JC, Hardy DB, Kovaric K, Mendelson CR. Up-regulation of the progesterone receptor (PR)-C isoform in laboring myometrium by activation of NF-κB may contribute to the onset of labor through inhibition of PR function. Mol Endocrinol 2006; 20: 764–75.

44. Wieser F, Schneeberger C, Hudelist G et al. Endometrial nuclear receptor co-factors SRC-1 and N-CoR are increased in human endometrium during menstruation. Mol Hum Reprod 2002; 8: 644–50.

45. Gregory CW, Wilson EM, Apparao KB et al. Steroid receptor coactivator expression throughout the menstrual cycle in normal and abnormal endometrium. J Clin Endocrinol Metab 2002; 87: 2960–6.

46. Condon JC, Jeyasuria P, Faust JM et al. A decline in the levels of progesterone receptor coactivators in the pregnant uterus at term may antagonize progesterone receptor function and contribute to the initiation of parturition. Proc Natl Acad Sci USA 2003; 100: 9518–23.

47. Arnett-Mansfield RL, deFazio A, Wain GV et al. Relative expression of progesterone receptors A and B in endometrioid cancers of the endometrium. Cancer Res 2001; 61: 4576–82.

48. Shyamala G, Yang X, Silberstein G et al. Transgenic mice carrying an imbalance in the native ratio of A to B forms of progesterone receptor exhibit developmental abnormalities in mammary glands. Proc Natl Acad Sci USA 1998; 95: 696–701.

49. Shyamala G, Yang X, Cardiff RD, Dale E. Impact of progesterone receptor on cell-fate decisions during mammary gland development. Proc Natl Acad Sci USA 2000; 97: 3044–9.

50. Shang Y, Brown M. Molecular determinants for the tissue specificity of SERMs. Science 2002; 295: 2465–8.

51. Wu H, Chen Y, Liang J et al. Hypomethylation-linked activation of PAX2 mediates tamoxifen-stimulated endometrial carcinogenesis. Nature 2005; 438: 981–7.

52. Lydon JP, DeMayo FJ, Funk CR et al. Mice lacking progesterone receptor exhibit pleiotropic reproductive abnormalities. Genes Dev 1995; 9: 2266–78.

53. Mulac-Jericevic B, Lydon JP, DeMayo FJ, Conneely OM. Defective mammary gland morphogenesis in mice lacking the progesterone receptor B isoform. Proc Natl Acad Sci USA 2003; 100: 9744–9.

54. Mulac-Jericevic B, Mullinax RA, DeMayo FJ et al. Subgroup of reproductive functions of progesterone mediated by progesterone receptor-B isoform. Science 2000; 289: 1751–4.

55. Wiley AA, Bartol FF, Barron DH. Histogenesis of the ovine uterus. J Anim Sci 1987; 64: 1262–9.

56. Bartol FF, Wiley AA, Coleman DA et al. Ovine uterine morphogenesis: effects of age and progestin administration and withdrawal on neonatal endometrial development and DNA synthesis. J Anim Sci 1988; 66: 3000–9.

57. Spencer TE, Stagg AG, Joyce MM et al. Discovery and characterization of endometrial epithelial messenger ribonucleic acids using the ovine uterine gland knockout model. Endocrinology 1999; 140: 4070–80.

58. Gray CA, Burghardt RC, Johnson GA et al. Evidence that absence of endometrial gland secretions in uterine gland knockout ewes compromises conceptus survival and elongation. Reproduction 2002; 124: 289–300.

59. Gehin M, Mark M, Dennefeld C et al. The function of TIF2/GRIP1 in mouse reproduction is distinct from those of SRC-1 and p/CIP. Mol Cell Biol 2002; 22: 5923–37.

60. Yadav N, Lee J, Kim J et al. Specific protein methylation defects and gene expression perturbations in coactivator-associated arginine methyltransferase 1-deficient mice. Proc Natl Acad Sci USA 2003; 100: 6464–8.

61. Jiang YH, Armstrong D, Albrecht U et al. Mutation of the Angelman ubiquitin ligase in mice causes increased cytoplasmic p53 and deficits of contextual learning and long-term potentiation. Neuron 1998; 21: 799–811.

62. Smith CL, DeVera DG, Lamb DJ et al. Genetic ablation of the steroid receptor coactivator-ubiquitin ligase, E6-AP, results in tissue-selective steroid hormone resistance and defects in reproduction. Mol Cell Biol 2002; 22: 525–35.

63. Davies TH, Sanchez ER. Fkbp52. Int J Biochem Cell Biol 2005; 37: 42–7.

64. Barent RL, Nair SC, Carr DC et al. Analysis of FKBP51/FKBP52 chimeras and mutants for Hsp90 binding and association with progesterone receptor complexes. Mol Endocrinol 1998; 12: 342–54.

65. Daikoku T, Tranguch S, Friedman DB et al. Proteomic analysis identifies immunophilin FK506 binding protein 4 (FKBP52) as a downstream target of Hoxa10 in the periimplantation mouse uterus. Mol Endocrinol 2005; 19: 683–97.

66. Tranguch S, Cheung-Flynn J, Daikoku T et al. Cochaperone immunophilin FKBP52 is critical to uterine receptivity for embryo implantation. Proc Natl Acad Sci USA 2005; 102: 14326–31.

67. Yang Z, Wolf IM, Chen H et al. FK506-binding protein 52 is essential to uterine reproductive physiology controlled by the progesterone receptor A isoform. Mol Endocrinol 2006; 20: 2682–94.

68. Brugge JS, Erikson RL. Identification of a transformation-specific antigen induced by an avian sarcoma virus. Nature 1977; 269: 346–8.

69. Collett MS, Brugge JS, Erikson RL. Characterization of a normal avian cell protein related to the avian sarcoma virus transforming gene product. Cell 1978; 15: 1363–9.

70. Thomas SM, Brugge JS. Cellular functions regulated by Src family kinases. Annu Rev Cell Dev Biol 1997; 13: 513–609.

71. Soriano P, Montgomery C, Geske R, Bradley A. Targeted disruption of the c-src proto-oncogene leads to osteopetrosis in mice. Cell 1991; 64: 693–702.

72. Shimizu A, Maruyama T, Tamaki K et al. Impairment of decidualization in SRC-deficient mice. Biol Reprod 2005; 73: 1219–27.

73. Maruyama T, Yoshimura Y, Yodoi J, Sabe H. Activation of c-Src kinase is associated with in vitro decidualization of human endometrial stromal cells. Endocrinology 1999; 140: 2632–6.

74. Das SK, Chakraborty I, Paria BC et al. Amphiregulin is an implantation-specific and progesterone-regulated gene in the mouse uterus. Mol Endocrinol 1995; 9: 691–705.

75. Ding YQ, Zhu LJ, Bagchi MK, Bagchi IC. Progesterone stimulates calcitonin gene expression in the uterus during implantation. Endocrinology 1994; 135: 2265–74.

76. Takamoto N, Zhao B, Tsai SY, DeMayo FJ. Identification of Indian hedgehog as a progesterone-responsive gene in the murine uterus. Mol Endocrinol 2002; 16: 2338–48.

77. Matsumoto H, Zhao X, Das SK, Hogan BL, Dey SK. Indian hedgehog as a progesterone-responsive factor mediating epithelial–mesenchymal interactions in the mouse uterus. Dev Biol 2002; 245: 280–90.

78. Daikoku T, Matsumoto H, Gupta RA et al. Expression of hypoxia-inducible factors in the peri-implantation mouse uterus is regulated in a cell-specific and ovarian steroid hormone-dependent manner. Evidence for differential function of HIFs during early pregnancy. J Biol Chem 2003; 278: 7683–91.

79. Cheon YP, Xu X, Bagchi MK, Bagchi IC. Immune-responsive gene 1 is a novel target of progesterone receptor and plays a critical role during implantation in the mouse. Endocrinology 2003; 144: 5623–30.

80. Yoshioka K, Matsuda F, Takakura K et al. Determination of genes involved in the process of implantation: application of GeneChip to scan 6500 genes. Biochem Biophys Res Commun 2000; 272: 531–8.

81. Reese J, Das SK, Paria BC et al. Global gene expression analysis to identify molecular markers of uterine receptivity and embryo implantation. J Biol Chem 2001; 276: 44137–45.

82. Cheon YP, Li Q, Xu X et al. A genomic approach to identify novel progesterone receptor regulated pathways in the uterus during implantation. Mol Endocrinol 2002; 16: 2853–71.

83. Jeong JW, Lee KY, Kwak I et al. Identification of murine uterine genes regulated in a ligand-dependent manner by the progesterone receptor. Endocrinology 2005; 146: 3490–505.

84. Tan YF, Li FX, Piao YS et al. Global gene profiling analysis of mouse uterus during the oestrous cycle. Reproduction 2003; 126: 171–82.

85. Adams EC, Hertig AT, Rock J. A description of 34 human ova within the first 17 days of development. Am J Anat 1956; 98: 435–93.

86. Kao LC, Tulac S, Lobo S et al. Global gene profiling in human endometrium during the window of implantation. Endocrinology 2002; 143: 2119–38.

87. Thomasset M, Dupret JM, Brehier A, Perret C. Calbindin-D9K (CaBP9K) gene: a model for studying the genomic actions of cacitriol and calcium in mammals. Adv Exp Med Biol 1990; 269: 35–6.

88. Tatsumi K, Higuchi T, Fujiwara H et al. Expression of calcium binding protein D-9k messenger RNA in the mouse uterine endometrium during implantation. Mol Hum Reprod 1999; 5: 153–61.

89. Luu KC, Nie GY, Salamonsen LA. Endometrial calbindins are critical for embryo implantation: evidence from in vivo use of morpholino antisense oligonucleotides. Proc Natl Acad Sci USA 2004; 101: 8028–33.

90. Luu KC, Nie GY, Hampton A et al. Endometrial expression of calbindin (CaBP)-d28k but not CaBP-d9k in primates implies evolutionary changes and functional redundancy of calbindins at implantation. Reproduction 2004; 128: 433–41.

91. Zahnow CA. CCAAT/enhancer binding proteins in normal mammary development and breast cancer. Breast Cancer Res 2002; 4: 113–21.

92. Sterneck E, Tessarollo L, Johnson PF. An essential role for C/EBPbeta in female reproduction. Genes Dev 1997; 11: 2153–62.

93. Mantena SR, Kannan A, Cheon YP et al. C/EBPbeta is a critical mediator of steroid hormone-regulated cell proliferation and differentiation in the uterine epithelium and stroma. Proc Natl Acad Sci USA 2006; 103: 1870–5.

94. Arnett B, Soisson P, Ducatman BS, Zhang P. Expression of CAAT enhancer binding protein beta (C/EBP beta) in cervix and endometrium. Mol Cancer 2003; 2: 21.

95. Lee YS, Terzidou V, Lindstrom T et al. The role of CCAAT/enhancer-binding protein β in the transcriptional regulation of COX-2 in human amnion. Mol Hum Reprod 2005; 11: 853–8.

96. Yang ZM, Le SP, Chen DB et al. Expression patterns of leukaemia inhibitory factor receptor (LIFR) and the gp130 receptor component in rabbit uterus during early pregnancy. J Reprod Fertil 1995; 103: 249–55.

97. McGinnis W, Levine MS, Hafen E et al. A conserved DNA sequence in homoeotic genes of the Drosophila Antennapedia and bithorax complexes. Nature 1984; 308: 428–33.

98. Hunt P, Whiting J, Nonchev S et al. The branchial Hox code and its implications for gene regulation, patterning of the nervous system and head evolution. Development 1991; Suppl 2: 63–77.

99. McGinnis W, Krumlauf R. Homeobox genes and axial patterning. Cell 1992; 68: 283–302.

100. Affolter M, Percival-Smith A, Muller M et al. Similarities between the homeodomain and the Hin recombinase DNA-binding domain. Cell 1991; 64: 879–80.

101. Taylor HS, Van den Heuvel GB, Igarashi P. A conserved Hox axis in the mouse and human female reproductive system: late establishment and persistent adult expression of the Hoxa cluster genes. Biol Reprod 1997; 57: 1338–45.

102. Lim H, Ma L, Ma WG et al. Hoxa-10 regulates uterine stromal cell responsiveness to progesterone during implantation and decidualization in the mouse. Mol Endocrinol 1999; 13: 1005–17.

103. Satokata I, Benson G, Maas R. Sexually dimorphic sterility phenotypes in Hoxa10-deficient mice. Nature 1995; 374: 460–3.

104. Benson GV, Lim H, Paria BC et al. Mechanisms of reduced fertility in Hoxa-10 mutant mice: uterine homeosis and loss of maternal Hoxa-10 expression. Development 1996; 122: 2687–96.

105. Gendron RL, Paradis H, Hsieh-Li HM et al. Abnormal uterine stromal and glandular function associated with maternal reproductive defects in Hoxa-11 null mice. Biol Reprod 1997; 56: 1097–105.

106. Bagot CN, Troy PJ, Taylor HS. Alteration of maternal Hoxa10 expression by in vivo gene transfection affects implantation. Gene Ther 2000; 7: 1378–84.

107. Wang W, Van De Water T, Lufkin T. Inner ear and maternal reproductive defects in mice lacking the Hmx3 homeobox gene. Development 1998; 125: 621–34.

108. Taylor HS, Arici A, Olive D, Igarashi P. HOXA10 is expressed in response to sex steroids at the time of implantation in the human endometrium. J Clin Invest 1998; 101: 1379–84.

109. Taylor HS, Bagot C, Kardana A et al. HOX gene expression is altered in the endometrium of women with endometriosis. Hum Reprod 1999; 14: 1328–31.

110. Cermik D, Arici A, Taylor HS. Coordinated regulation of HOX gene expression in myometrium and uterine leiomyoma. Fertil Steril 2002; 78: 979–84.

111. Das SK, Stanley ER. Structure–function studies of a colony stimulating factor (CSF-1). J Biol Chem 1982; 257: 13679–84.

112. Ladner MB, Martin GA, Noble JA et al. Human CSF-1: gene structure and alternative splicing of mRNA precursors. EMBO J 1987; 6: 2693–8.

113. Kariya M, Kanzaki H, Hanamura T et al. Progesterone-dependent secretion of macrophage colony-stimulating factor by human endometrial stromal cells of nonpregnant uterus in culture. J Clin Endocrinol Metab 1994; 79: 86–90.

114. Pollard JW, Bartocci A, Arceci R et al. Apparent role of the macrophage growth factor, CSF-1, in placental development. Nature 1987; 330: 484–6.

115. Arceci RJ, Pampfer S, Pollard JW. Expression of CSF-1/c-fms and SF/c-kit mRNA during preimplantation mouse development. Dev Biol 1992; 151: 1–8.

116. Arceci RJ, Shanahan F, Stanley ER, Pollard JW. Temporal expression and location of colony-stimulating factor 1 (CSF-1) and its receptor in the female reproductive tract are consistent with CSF-1-regulated placental development. Proc Natl Acad Sci USA 1989; 86: 8818–22.

117. Pollard JW, Hunt JS, Wiktor-Jedrzejczak W, Stanley ER. A pregnancy defect in the osteopetrotic (op/op) mouse demonstrates the requirement for CSF-1 in female fertility. Dev Biol 1991; 148: 273–83.

118. Wiktor-Jedrzejczak W, Urbanowska E, Aukerman SL et al. Correction by CSF-1 of defects in the osteopetrotic op/op mouse suggests local, developmental, and humoral requirements for this growth factor. Exp Hematol 1991; 19: 1049–54.

119. Kauma SW, Aukerman SL, Eierman D, Turner T. Colony-stimulating factor-1 and c-fms expression in human endometrial tissues and placenta during the menstrual cycle and early pregnancy. J Clin Endocrinol Metab 1991; 73: 746–51.

120. Katano K, Matsumoto Y, Ogasawara M et al. Low serum M-CSF levels are associated with unexplained recurrent abortion. Am J Reprod Immunol 1997; 38: 1–5.

121. Shinetugs B, Runesson E, Bonello NP et al. Colony stimulating factor-1 concentrations in blood and follicular fluid during the human menstrual cycle and ovarian stimulation: possible role in the ovulatory process. Hum Reprod 1999; 14: 1302–6.

122. Ferrara N, Davis-Smyth T. The biology of vascular endothelial growth factor. Endocr Rev 1997; 18: 4–25.

123. Tischer E, Mitchell R, Hartman T et al. The human gene for vascular endothelial growth factor. Multiple protein forms are encoded through alternative exon splicing. J Biol Chem 1991; 266: 11947–54.

124. Charnock-Jones DS, Sharkey AM, Rajput-Williams J et al. Identification and localization of alternately spliced mRNAs for vascular endothelial growth factor in human uterus and estrogen regulation in endometrial carcinoma cell lines. Biol Reprod 1993; 48: 1120–8.

125. Ferrara N, Carver-Moore K, Chen H et al. Heterozygous embryonic lethality induced by targeted inactivation of the VEGF gene. Nature 1996; 380: 439–42.

126. Fong GH, Rossant J, Gertsenstein M, Breitman ML. Role of the Flt-1 receptor tyrosine kinase in regulating the assembly of vascular endothelium. Nature 1995; 376: 66–70.

127. Shalaby F, Rossant J, Yamaguchi TP et al. Failure of blood-island formation and vasculogenesis in Flk-1-deficient mice. Nature 1995; 376: 62–6.

128. Mueller MD, Vigne JL, Minchenko A et al. Regulation of vascular endothelial growth factor (VEGF) gene transcription by estrogen receptors alpha and beta. Proc Natl Acad Sci USA 2000; 97: 10972–7.

129. Chakraborty I, Das SK, Dey SK. Differential expression of vascular endothelial growth factor and its receptor mRNAs in the mouse uterus around the time of implantation. J Endocrinol 1995; 147: 339–52.

130. Halder JB, Zhao X, Soker S et al. Differential expression of VEGF isoforms and VEGF(164)-specific receptor neuropilin-1 in the mouse uterus suggests a role for VEGF(164) in vascular permeability and angiogenesis during implantation. Genesis 2000; 26: 213–24.

131. Torry DS, Holt VJ, Keenan JA et al. Vascular endothelial growth factor expression in cycling human endometrium. Fertil Steril 1996; 66: 72–80.

132. Shifren JL, Tseng JF, Zaloudek CJ et al. Ovarian steroid regulation of vascular endothelial growth factor in the human endometrium: implications for angiogenesis during the menstrual cycle and in the pathogenesis of endometriosis. J Clin Endocrinol Metab 1996; 81: 3112–18.

133. Bausero P, Cavaille F, Meduri G et al. Paracrine action of vascular endothelial growth factor in the human endometrium: production and target sites, and hormonal regulation. Angiogenesis 1998; 2: 167–82.

134. Ancelin M, Buteau-Lozano H, Meduri G et al. A dynamic shift of VEGF isoforms with a transient and selective progesterone-induced expression of VEGF189 regulates angiogenesis and vascular permeability in human uterus. Proc Natl Acad Sci USA 2002; 99: 6023–8.

135. Gentry CC, Okolo SO, Fong LF et al. Quantification of vascular endothelial growth factor-A in leiomyomas and adjacent myometrium. Clin Sci (Lond) 2001; 101: 691–5.

136. Zhou Y, McMaster M, Woo K et al. Vascular endothelial growth factor ligands and receptors that regulate human cytotrophoblast survival are dysregulated in severe preeclampsia and hemolysis elevated liver enzymes, and low platelets syndrome. Am J Pathol 2002; 160: 1405–23.

137. Gendler SJ, Lancaster CA, Taylor-Papadimitriou J et al. Molecular cloning and expression of human tumor-associated polymorphic epithelial mucin. J Biol Chem 1990; 265: 15286–93.

138. Horne AW, White JO, Margara RA et al. MUC 1: a genetic susceptibility to infertility? Lancet 2001; 357: 1336–7.

139. Surveyor GA, Gendler SJ, Pemberton L et al. Expression and steroid hormonal control of Muc-1 in the mouse uterus. Endocrinology 1995; 136: 3639–47.

140. Bowen JA, Bazer FW, Burghardt RC. Spatial and temporal analyses of integrin and Muc-1 expression in porcine uterine epithelium and trophectoderm in vivo. Biol Reprod 1996; 55: 1098–106.

141. Hild-Petito S, Fazleabas AT, Julian J, Carson DD. Mucin (Muc-1) expression is differentially regulated in uterine luminal and glandular epithelia of the baboon (*Papio anubis*). Biol Reprod 1996; 54: 939–47.

142. Hoffman LH, Olson GE, Carson DD, Chilton BS. Progesterone and implanting blastocysts regulate Muc1 expression in rabbit uterine epithelium. Endocrinology 1998; 139: 266–71.

143. Hey NA, Graham RA, Seif MW, Aplin JD. The polymorphic epithelial mucin MUC1 in human endometrium is regulated with maximal expression in the implantation phase. J Clin Endocrinol Metab 1994; 78: 337–42.

144. Meseguer M, Aplin JD, Caballero-Campo P et al. Human endometrial mucin MUC1 is up-regulated by progesterone and down-regulated in vitro by the human blastocyst. Biol Reprod 2001; 64: 590–601.

145. DeSouza MM, Surveyor GA, Price RE et al. MUC1/episialin: a critical barrier in the female reproductive tract. J Reprod Immunol 1999; 45: 127–58.

146. Hey NA, Li TC, Devine PL et al. MUC1 in secretory phase endometrium: expression in precisely dated biopsies and flushings from normal and recurrent miscarriage patients. Hum Reprod 1995; 10: 2655–62.

147. Lee CG, Jenkins NA, Gilbert DJ et al. Cloning and analysis of gene regulation of a novel LPS-inducible cDNA. Immunogenetics 1995; 41: 263–70.

148. Chen B, Zhang D, Pollard JW. Progesterone regulation of the mammalian ortholog of methylcitrate dehydratase (immune response gene 1) in the uterine epithelium during implantation through the protein kinase C pathway. Mol Endocrinol 2003; 17: 2340–54.

149. Lee JJ, von Kessler DP, Parks S, Beachy PA. Secretion and localized transcription suggest a role in positional signaling for

products of the segmentation gene hedgehog. Cell 1992; 71: 33–50.

150. Ingham PW, Taylor AM, Nakano Y. Role of the *Drosophila* patched gene in positional signaling. Nature 1991; 353: 184–7.

151. Pepinsky RB, Zeng C, Wen D et al. Identification of a palmitic acid-modified form of human Sonic hedgehog. J Biol Chem 1998; 273: 14037–45.

152. Porter JA, Young KE, Beachy PA. Cholesterol modification of hedgehog signaling proteins in animal development. Science 1996; 274: 255–9.

153. Alcedo J, Ayzenzon M, Von Ohlen T et al. The *Drosophila* smoothened gene encodes a seven-pass membrane protein, a putative receptor for the hedgehog signal. Cell 1996; 86: 221–32.

154. Krishnan V, Pereira FA, Qiu Y et al. Mediation of Sonic hedgehog-induced expression of COUP-TFII by a protein phosphatase. Science 1997; 278: 1947–50.

155. Lee K, Jeong J, Kwak I et al. Indian hedgehog is a major mediator of progesterone signaling in the mouse uterus. Nat Genet 2006; 38: 1204–9.

156. Zhu LJ, Bagchi MK, Bagchi IC. Attenuation of calcitonin gene expression in pregnant rat uterus leads to a block in embryonic implantation. Endocrinology 1998; 139: 330–9.

157. Tsark EC, Adamson ED, Withers GE 3rd, Wiley LM. Expression and function of amphiregulin during murine preimplantation development. Mol Reprod Dev 1997; 47: 271–83.

158. St-Jacques B, Hammerschmidt M, McMahon AP. Indian hedgehog signaling regulates proliferation and differentiation of chondrocytes and is essential for bone formation. Genes Dev 1999; 13: 2072–86.

159. Iyer NV, Kotch LE, Agani F et al. Cellular and developmental control of O_2 homeostasis by hypoxia-inducible factor 1 alpha. Genes Dev 1998; 12: 149–62.

160. Lee KY, DeMayo FJ. Animal models of implantation. Reproduction 2004; 128: 679–95.

14 Transcriptomics

Linda C Giudice, Said Talbi, Amy Hamilton, and Bruce A Lessey

INTRODUCTION

The transcriptome is composed of all mRNA molecules that are transcribed from genes in a given tissue, cell, or organism, under a specified set of conditions.[1] The study of transcriptomics examines mRNA levels, usually using high-throughput techniques based on DNA microarray technology.[2] With sequencing of the human genome and major technological advances in simultaneously analyzing large data sets and large numbers of genes and their products, the post-genomic era has heralded a revolution in global gene expression analysis and sophisticated bioinformatic approaches to mine data and enable understanding of biological processes, key regulators, biochemical pathways, and subcellular constituents involved in the expression of specific genes and gene families.[3] Several reviews on the application of these technologies to reproductive medicine have recently been published.[4–9] Application to the endometrium is presented herein.

The endometrium is a complex tissue composed of a multitude of cell types, including luminal and glandular epithelium, stromal fibroblasts, lymphocytes, and endothelial and smooth muscle cells in the vasculature.[10] These cells respond to estradiol and progesterone directly or indirectly by paracrine communications via secreted products from nearby cells that are mostly steroid hormone-responsive. The tissue undergoes dynamic growth under the influence of estradiol, and under the influence of progesterone undergoes glandular secretory transformation, stromal fibroblast differentiation (decidualization), and immune cell proliferation and functional changes. In the presence of an embryo, additional cell–cell interactions occur, and in the absence of successful embryonic implantation, the tissue is shed during the menses.[10] Cyclic changes in the endometrium are shown in Figure 14.1 which reflects changes in thickness, cellularity, and phases and stages of the cycle.

Several approaches have been used, clinically, to assess the health and normalcy of the endometrium.[5] These include:

- direct visualization using the hysteroscope to assess the presence of polyps, fibroids, and cancer
- ultrasound evaluation to assess thickness and pattern (relevant to infertility) and sonohysterography and magnetic resonance imaging to evaluate endometrial abnormalities (e.g. submucous fibroids, intracavitary masses)
- histological assessment of biopsied endometrium or endometrial tissue in hysterectomy specimens.

The last assessment is used to evaluate cellular normalcy in the setting of abnormal uterine bleeding, suspicion of hyperplasia and cancer, appropriate development of the endometrium at specific times of the cycle (for fertility), and evidence of inflammation and/or infection, especially in the setting of abnormal uterine bleeding and/or unusual findings on ultrasound or at hysteroscopy and hysterectomy. Recent studies have questioned the utility of the endometrial biopsy as a clinical tool for fertility ('dating' the endometrium[11,12]) because of significant inter- and intra-observer variability and because histological delay fails to distinguish between fertile and infertile couples.[13] Also, histological features fail to distinguish reliably specific menstrual cycle days or narrow intervals of days,[14] in contrast to the evaluation originally reported over half a century ago.[11]

In the research setting, endometrial gene products have been investigated using reverse transcriptase-polymerase chain reaction (RT-PCR) and in-situ hybridization analysis, and detection of specific proteins has been investigated using immunohistochemistry, Western blotting, and immunoassays of products secreted by endometrial cells and explant cultures. After sequencing of the human genome and in the era of functional genomics, simultaneous analysis of multiple genes and gene products using array platforms has been pursued. This 'molecular phenotyping' of human endometrium has focused on distinguishing among the phases of the cycle, defining receptivity to embryonic implantation, investigating endometrial disorders, and studying molecular events occurring dynamically throughout the cycle.[5,6] In addition, similar studies have been performed in the mouse and some large animals. This chapter describes the transcriptome of whole endometrial tissue from women, non-human primates, and rodents, and endometrial cells in culture in response to steroid hormones and trophoblast secreted products. In addition, the transcriptomes of endometrium from women undergoing

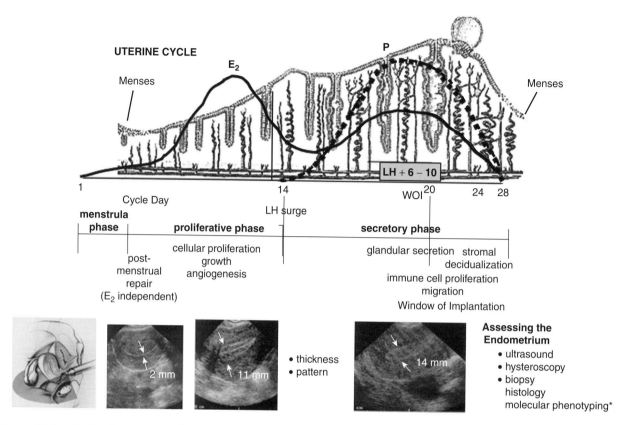

Figure 14.1 Cyclic changes in endometrium across the cycle. Shown are hormonal profiles, cycle phases and stages, and ultrasonographic appearance of the endometrium in early proliferative, late proliferative, and mid-secretory phases. (Adapted from Giudice.[5])

infertility treatment and those with endometriosis are presented. The transcriptome of endometrial hyperplasia and cancer is presented in Chapter 55.

ENDOMETRIAL TRANSCRIPTOME, BIOLOGICAL PROCESSES, AND BIOCHEMICAL PATHWAYS

General comments

Several investigators have recently reported results of cDNA and oligonucleotide array analyses and subtractive hybridization and differential display of endometrial gene expression in human and non-human primate endometrium and endometrial cells and explants in culture or after laser capture microdissection. The sections below focus on global gene expression profiling of primate endometrium across the menstrual cycle, select pair-wise comparisons of different phases, and laser capture microdissection of glands and stromal fibroblasts, as well as during the estrus cycle of wild-type mice, ovariectomized and estradiol (E2)/estrogen analogue-treated wild-type mice, and estrogen and progesterone receptor (ERKO and PRKO) knockout mice.

Global analyses across the menstrual cycle

There are two major studies of human endometrial gene expression across the menstrual cycle by two different groups, using different platforms.[15,16] In addition, several groups have analyzed specific stages of the cycle compared to other stages (pair-wise comparisons). A schematic of when samples in humans and non-human primates have been obtained during the menstrual cycle and which groups conducted these across the cycle[15-24] is shown in Figure 14.2. The variability of human tissue, quality of RNA, and robustness of the data underscore the challenges in these types of translational studies. In the study by Talbi et al,[16] samples from various times across the menstrual cycle were analyzed using high-density oligonucleotide microarrays (whole genome) containing 54 600 probe sets. "Forty-six subjects were recruited, but only 22 had endometrial samples that yielded sufficient and good-quality RNA for subsequent microarray analysis and had agreement among pathologists regarding cycle stage. Six samples had different histological readings from two or more pathologists or were evaluated by only one pathologist, and these were considered 'ambiguous' or unknown. This study

Microarray Studies Comparing Cycle Phases in Women and Non-Human Primates

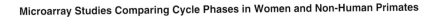

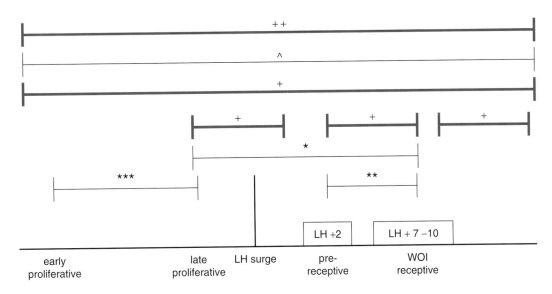

* Kao et al, 2002[17], 2003[59]; Borthwick et al, 2003[19]; Ace & Oculicz, 2004[21]

** Carson et al 2002[18]; Riesewijk et al, 2003[20]; Mirken et al, 2004[24]; Horcajadas et al, 2004[22]

*** Punyadeera et al, 2005[23]

∧ Ponnampalan et al, 2004[15]

+ Talbi, Hamilton et al, 2006[16]

++ Burney et al, 2006[60]

Figure 14.2   Schematic representation of microarray studies comparing cycle phases in women and non-human primates (see text). Symbols correspond to citations. (Adapted from Giudice.[5])

provided the first, whole genome-wide gene, gene ontology, and gene clustering analyses across the entire menstrual cycle in normo-ovulatory women. Different data analyses were conducted to determine how samples clustered together (Figure 14.3)".[5] Principal component analysis (PCA, Figure 14.3A), a completely unbiased approach, used the entire gene set (54 600 probe sets). In contrast, hierarchical clustering analysis (Figure 14.3B) used a more limited gene set (7231 probe sets derived from pair-wise comparisons of early-secretory epithelium [ESE] vs proliferative epithelium [PE], mid-secretory epithelium [MSE] vs ESE, and late-secretory epithelium [LSE] vs [MSE]). Several important observations derive from these studies:[5] (a) samples with known histology cluster into cycle phases and cluster into the same cycle phases in both analyses; (b) hierarchical clustering analysis (see Figure 14.3B) reveals two major branches and several sub-branches. PE and ESE cluster together in the first major branch and MSE and LSE in the second major branch; (c) 'ambiguous' or unknown samples cluster into cycle phases that are the same by both PCA and hierarchical clustering; (d) hierarchical clustering reveals that samples have

unique molecular profiles; and (e) samples cluster independently of how they were obtained (biopsy or curetting) or for the clinical indication for which they were obtained (e.g. uterine fibroids, pelvic floor prolapse). Importantly, this study demonstrates that assignment of menstrual cycle stage is based on gene expression profiles and cluster grouping, and that samples have unique molecular signatures that preclude a priori knowledge of histologically determined cycle phase, providing a powerful adjunct to the 'gold standard' of histological assessment of the endometrium.[11,12] While unique gene signatures lead to clustering in groups (phases), the molecular signatures are not identical (see Figure 14.3B). This may be the result of, for example, different complements of cell types in a specimen. Furthermore, samples may cluster in phases but have unique molecular 'fingerprints' that distinguish them, as in women who have endometriosis (see 'Endometrial transcriptomes in women with endometriosis' section below).

In the study of Ponnampalam et al[15] endometrial samples were analyzed using a cDNA array with 13 600 probe sets. This was the first study on clustering of samples by gene array analysis. Initial hierarchical

A

Principal Component Analysis Reveals Clustering of Samples into Cycle Phases

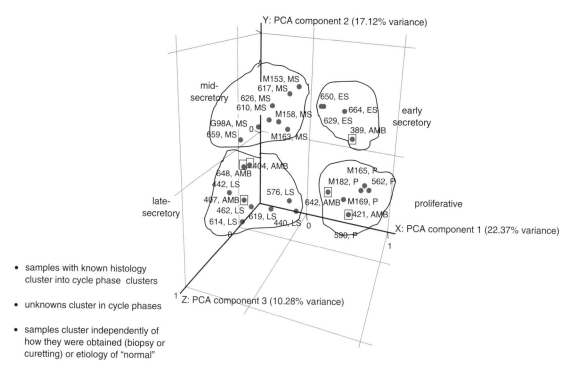

- samples with known histology cluster into cycle phase clusters

- unknowns cluster in cycle phases

- samples cluster independently of how they were obtained (biopsy or curetting) or etiology of "normal"

B

Hierarchical Clustering Analysis: Samples Cluster into Cycle Phases and Unique Molecular Profiles

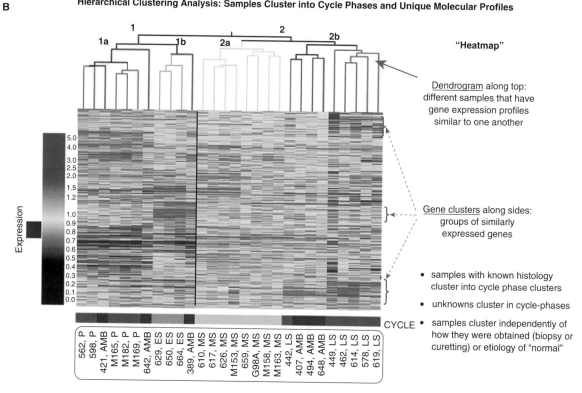

"Heatmap"

Dendrogram along top: different samples that have gene expression profiles similar to one another

Gene clusters along sides: groups of similarly expressed genes

- samples with known histology cluster into cycle phase clusters

- unknowns cluster in cycle-phases

- samples cluster independently of how they were obtained (biopsy or curetting) or etiology of "normal"

Figure 14.3 Gene clustering in the endometrium. (**A**) Principal component analysis (PCA) of human endometrium across the menstrual cycle. PCA was applied to all samples; numbers refer to individual sample labels. 'Ambiguous' (or unknown) samples (see text) are labeled AMB (dots in squares). Analysis reveals clustering of samples into cycle phases. (**B**) Hierarchical clustering analysis. The 'Heatmap' represents relative gene expression levels in the endometrial samples across the menstrual cycle. Each horizontal line represents a single gene, and each column represents a single sample. Samples cluster by cycle phase (bar at bottom of the Heatmap: proliferative (red), early-secretory (light blue), mid-secretory (olive), late secretory (purple), and ambiguous samples (dark blue). Relative expression of each gene is color-coded: high (red) or low (blue), as indicated in the color legend on the left side of the figure. Hierarchical clustering reveals sample clustering into cycle phases and unique molecular profiles. (Adapted from Talbi et al,[16] with permission.)

clustering analysis of 43 samples revealed two main branches: one containing menstrual (M), early-proliferative epithelium (EPE)–mid-proliferative epithelium (MPE), late-proliferative epithelium (LPE), and ESE–MSE, and the second containing M, M–EPE, MSE, LSE, and LSE–M. After removing six outliers for disagreement between two pathologists or for poor hybridization, two main branches resulted for 37 samples. One branch contained M, EPE–MPE, LPE–ESE, and ESE–MSE and the other contained M, MSE–LSE, and LSE–M. Because of too few samples for analysis, MSE and LSE were then merged. Thus, it is difficult to compare directly gene expression profiles between the data of Ponnampalam et al[15] and Talbi et al,[16] due to these different approaches for data analysis, as well as different platforms for hybridization.

The endometrial transcriptome under the influence of estrogen

In the proliferative phase and under the influence of E_2, cellular constituents of the endometrium undergo proliferation, as evidenced by high cellular mitotic indices[25] and increasing tissue thickness (see Figure 14.1). DNA synthesis and cellular mitoses increase dramatically in the epithelium, stroma, and vascular endothelium in the late proliferative phase, compared to the mid-proliferative phase, and are nearly absent in the early proliferative phase. In LPE, the straight glands become more voluminous and tortuous, resulting in the development of a glandular network, and cell proliferation also results in an elaborate system of blood vessels, as well as an increase in the fibroblast population in the stromal compartment (see Giudice and Ferenczy[26] for review). The tissue grows from approximately 2 mm in the postmenstrual repair phase to about 11–14 mm just before ovulation[11,25] and inappropriate growth of the endometrium (too thin or too thick) may be associated with infertility, miscarriage, and pregnancy disorders (see Giudice[4] for review). Gene ontology analyses by Talbi et al[16] reveal high expression of genes in the proliferative phase that are involved in cell adhesion, cell–cell signaling, cell cycle regulation, and cell division. Included in the latter are genes involved in DNA replication, strand elongation, DNA metabolism, chromatin cycle and segregation, mitosis, G_1/S and G_2M transitions, and response to DNA damage. Other genes/families include collagen metabolism and extracellular matrix (ECM) regulation that probably participate in ECM remodeling accompanying tissue growth. Others include genes involved in signal transduction and ion channels, the latter of which await further investigation for potential roles in the endometrium during this phase of the cycle and perhaps as targets for drug development in the future. Molecular functions highly represented in the late proliferative phase are related to cell cycle regulation and DNA synthesis, steroid binding, receptor-mediated events, and ECM structural constituents.[16] The cellular components active in events in LPE, identified by gene ontology analysis, include primarily the chromosomes, the replication fork, DNA polymerase/primer complexes, microtubule skeleton, the ECM, non-membrane bound organelles, and collagen.[16] Thus, gene ontology analyses of biological processes, biochemical pathways, and cellular components are highly consistent with cell replication and growth of the tissue in the proliferative phase, ECM remodeling that occurs with this growth, and steroid hormone action and subsequent signaling to effect these processes.

Laser capture microdissection (LCM) has proven to be an excellent adjunct in analyzing cell-specific gene expression. Yanaihara et al[27] studied mid-proliferative endometrial epithelium and stromal cell gene expression using this technique and subsequent cDNA microarray analysis. Of 1200 genes analyzed, 14 were highly expressed in epithelium and 12 in the stroma. Epithelium-enriched genes included WAP 4-disulfide core domain 2 (WGDC2, a protease inhibitor), HOX-1,-5, matrix metalloproteinase 7 (MMP-7; matrilysin), proenkephalin A, ID2, CDC28, glutathione-S-transferase-2, HSP27kD, tuberin, retinoic acid-BP2, and cyclin A_1 and B_1. Stromal-enriched genes included decorin, discoidin domain receptor family 2, PDGF-Rα, membrane channels/transporters, MMP-11 (stromelysin), TIMP-1, granzyme A, integrinβ_1, peripheral myelin protein-22, putative c-Myc-responsive gene, thymosin, and ribosomal protein-S19. In particular, decorin expression was validated in stromal fibroblasts and was found to be regulated by E_2 in this cell type in vitro.[27] Decorin may play a role in stromal matrix assembly and cell proliferation, perhaps involving the transforming growth factor β (TGFβ) family. Interestingly, many of these genes demonstrate the same cell-specific enrichment in the secretory phase of the cycle (see below), suggesting that they may be constitutively expressed in particular cell types in the endometrium. Also, while relatively few genes were differentially expressed in epithelium and stroma in proliferative endometrium in this study, genome-wide analysis (beyond the 1200 genes analyzed) would probably yield additional cell-specific candidates in this phase of the cycle.

With regard to E_2-regulated genes, insight derives from specific genes up-regulated in the proliferative phase. In particular, members of the insulin-like growth factor (IGF), epidermal growth factor (EGF), and vascular endothelial growth factor (VEGF) families and select members of their signaling cascades are up-regulated in proliferative endometrium,[16] suggesting that these pathways are primary mediators of E_2's proliferative effects in this tissue. Additional insight derives from a study in which gene expression in late PE (LPE, peak E_2) was compared to menstrual endometrium (very low E_2 levels) and E_2-treated endometrial explants, using the same Affymetrix platform.[23] Interestingly, LPE was less responsive to E_2 with regard to genes regulated, compared to menstrual endometrium. "Genes up-regulated in LPE vs menstrual endometrium included oviductal glycoprotein-1, connexin-37, olfactomedin-1, and secreted frizzled related protein 4 (SFRP-4), an inhibitor of the Wnt signaling pathway. Down-regulated genes included MMPs-1, -3, and -10, IL-1β, IL-8, IL-11, inhibin $β_A$, SOX4, and trefoil factor (important in perimenstrual repair of the endometrium)".[16] It should be noted that much tissue breakdown is ongoing in menstrual endometrium, accompanied by inflammation and hypoxia, and initiation of tissue repair. Thus, down-regulation of MMPs, inflammatory cytokines, and trefoil factor in LPE may reflect their high expression in menstrual endometrium, and these may or may not be directly regulated by E_2. Some of these genes regulated in LPE, however, are involved in cellular proliferation and tissue remodeling and may be direct or indirect mediators of E_2 action in this tissue. Mouse models of estrogen receptor (ER) deletions provide important additional insight into E_2-regulated genes and specific ERs associated with these responses (see 'Cycle- and steroid hormone-dependent gene expression in rodent uterus' section below).

Endometrial endothelial cells express ERβ,[28] and the transcriptome of E_2-treated human endometrial endothelial cells surprisingly reveals a lack of up-regulation of classical angiogenic factors, including VEGF, its receptors, FGF2, neuropilins or angiopoietins.[28] In contrast, classical E_2-regulated genes were observed – e.g. ERBB3, EGFR, SOD2. Interestingly, soluble factors from human proliferative phase endometrium promote angiogenesis in vitro, significantly affecting the endothelial transcriptome (e.g. vimentin, IL-1RtI, VE cadherin, GSTP-1, tissue factor inhibitor 2, and a variety of MMPs, among other genes).[29] The data suggest that there are probably paracine modulators that affect angiogenesis during the proliferative phase of the cycle. Additional research on this important part of endometrial development is needed for an understanding of endometrial vascular development and abnormal bleeding in women, a common and prevalent clinical condition.

The early secretory phase

In contrast to the proliferative phase in which the endometrium is stimulated by high levels of circulating E_2, after ovulation in the early secretory phase the endometrium is the target of low, but rising, circulating levels of progesterone (and E_2). During the first 36–48 hours after ovulation endometrial morphology is similar to the late proliferative phase.[11,12,25] Thereafter, the effects of progesterone become evident, and histological hallmarks of ovulation and progesterone action in ESE are cessation of cellular mitoses and synthesis and accumulation of glycogen in the basal region of the glands (subnuclear glycogen 'vacuoles' and 'palisading' of nuclei).[25,26] At the ultrastructural level, ovulation is heralded by an increase in mitochondrial size and an increased number of cristae (in response to an increased demand for energy for glycogen metabolism).[25,26] On days 19 and 20, few vacuoles remain, and the glycoprotein-rich supranuclear cytoplasmic products begin to be expelled by apocrine secretion into the glandular lumen. There is one study[16] that has compared global gene expression in ESE (cycle days [CD] 16–19) with that in late PE. Kinetic analysis of all genes regulated across the menstrual cycle revealed a cluster of genes highly expressed in ESE and with low expression in the remainder of the cycle. "This cluster is characterized by remarkably different biological processes, compared to the proliferative phase, and includes genes governing metabolism and biosynthesis of cholesterol, amino acids, organic acids, acetyl CoA and lipids, fatty acids, steroids, and prostaglandins, and also genes for transport of ions, peptides, and carboxylic acids. The cellular components involved are cell membranes, microsomes, peroxisomes, and mitochondria".[16] Furthermore, gene ontology analysis of up-regulated genes in ESE vs PE pair-wise comparisons demonstrates up-regulation of a variety of metabolic processes (enzymes for biosynthesis and transporters of precursors), as well as negative regulation of cell proliferation.[16] Thus, the molecular events derived from the clustering analysis and the pair-wise comparison support robust glycogen synthesis along with high energy demands, a concomitant increase in mitochondrial size and number of cristae, and a marked inhibition of cellular mitosis, consistent with the early secretory phase histological and electron microscopy observations.

With regard to specific genes and gene families (Table 14.1), the most highly up-regulated genes in the transition from proliferative to early secretory endometrium are those limiting estradiol availability within the endometrium (17β-hydroxysteroid dehydrogenase [17β-HSD] Type 2 converts $E_2 \rightarrow E_1$) and those encoding secretory proteins (secretoglobins and osteopontin (secreted phosphoprotein)). Up-regulation of 17β-HSD-2 in human ESE vs PE is consistent with results from Mustonen et al[30] and supports the beginning of curtailment of direct E_2 action in this phase, as a prelude to more pronounced curtailment of E_2 action in the mid-secretory phase in which ERs are down-regulated in the stroma and nearly completely absent in the epithelium.[31-34] Transporters for amino acids, peptides, and ions are highly up-regulated in ESE vs PE, as are enzymes involved in collagen metabolism, a variety of cytochrome P_{450} proteins (important in electron transport and energy pathways), and regulators of blood coagulation. Major inhibitors of the Wnt signaling, Dkk-1 and SFRP-1, are regulated, with Dkk-1 being increased six-fold, and SFRP-1 down-regulated.[16] MUC-1, an epithelial product, is an antibacterial agent that protects from microorganisms and their degradative enzymes and hydrates and lubricates cell surfaces.[35] It is only up-regulated in ESE (not in subsequent stages of secretory endometrium), as is aquaporin 3, important in water transport. Also, genes involved in lipid metabolism, phospholipase activity, and eicosanoid/prostaglandin metabolism are highly up-regulated. The metallothioneins are first noted to increase in the cycle in the early secretory phase, as are arginase 2, phospholipase C, keratin 8, IL-1R type I, IL-15, and monamine oxidase,[16] which are commonly attributed to being mid-secretory endometrial products.[5] The metallothioneins are important for protection from free radicals and detoxification. Evidence of EGF signaling is apparent, as is an antiapoptotic marker (FOXO1A). Most of these genes are known to be progesterone-regulated or subsequently have been determined to be progesterone-regulated.[5,6] Thus, the effect of progesterone in this part of the cycle extends beyond inhibition of E_2-stimulated cellular mitosis to regulation of specific genes, including osteopontin and MUC-1 in the epithelium and Dkk-1, FOXO1A, and IL-15 in stromal fibroblasts. Dkk-1 is a progesterone-regulated gene in endometrial stromal cells,[36] and IL-15 is progesterone-regulated and is important as a chemoattractant

and stimulator of natural killer (NK) cell replication.[37,38] FOXO1A is an important mediator of progesterone action and participates in progesterone signaling (Chapter 24).

Table 14.1 Highly up-regulated genes in early-secretory epithelium vs proliferative epithelium – the beginning of the response to progesterone

- 17β-HSD, Type 2 (27.1)
- Secreted proteins:
  - secretoglobins
    family 1D, member 2 (23.2)
    family 2A, members 1 (5.5) and 2 (4.4)
  - osteopontin (secreted phosphoprotein (2.8))
- Transporters:
  - amino acids [cysteine, SLC3A1 (21.6)]
  - peptides (12.1)
  - ions (9–12.1)
  - water [aquaporin (6.0)]
- Proteases:
  - ADAMTS8 (16.3), calpain 6 (16.1)
  - MMP-26 (4.0), MME (enkephalin, 3.8)
- FAIM [Fas apoptosis inhibitor molecule (13.8)]
- Electron transport (6.9–13.6):
  - cyp 26A1, 4B1, B5
- CD36 [collagen receptor 1(13.6)]
- Blood coagulation:
  - IL-20 receptor (11.8)
  - tissue factor pathway inhibitor 2 (8.1)
- Phospholipase C-like 1 (10.4)
- LRP4 (9.6)
- Dkk-1 (6.4)
- Nebulette (6.3)
- ALDH 1A3 (5.9), 3B2 (4.0)
- Prostaglandin metabolism/synthesis (3.1–4.8):
  - hydroxyprostaglandin dehydrogenase
  - PG-endoperoxide synthase
  - PG D-2 synthase
  - PG H-2 D-isomerase
- MUC-1 (3.8)
- Metallothionieins (2.4–3.7)1G, 1F, 1X, IL, 1E
- Monoamine oxidase (3.4)
- Toll-like receptor 5 (3.3)
- GABA-receptor π subunit (3.2)
- Interferon γ receptor1 (3.2)
- Thrombin receptor (3.1)
- Arginase 2 (3.0)
- Phospholipase (3.0)
- Folate receptor (3.1)
- Keratin 8 (3.1)
- IL-1R, type 1 (2.8)
- Apo D(2.3), L2 (2.3)
- EGF R pthwy15 (2.7)
- EGF-R pthwy EPS8 (2.1)
- PTHR-2 (2.1)
- FOXO1A (2.1)
- IL-15 (2.10)

Reproduced with permission from Talbi et al.[16]

"Gene ontology biological processes that are down-regulated in early secretory vs proliferative endometrium include cell motility, communication, and adhesion, Wnt receptor signaling, and the I-κB kinase/NF-κB cascade.[16] Also, strikingly, although not unexpectedly, genes involved in cell cycle regulation and cellular mitosis are highly represented among the down-regulated processes in this phase of the cycle. With regard to specific genes, the most highly down-regulated genes in the early secretory phase are MMP-11 (stromelysin), tissue plasminogen activator (tPA, PLAT) and ADAM-12, as well retinoic acid, IGF and TGFβ family members (TGFβ1, inhibin βA, BMP-1 and -7), and angiogenic factors (FGF1), HGF and FGF receptor (FGFR1,2,3), among others. The ECM reveals down-regulation of several members of the collagen family, laminin, dermatopontin, and tenascin-C".[16] Thus, genes and gene families regulated in ESE inhibit cellular mitosis, are involved in ECM homeostasis, and participate in the shift to increased cellular metabolism in this phase of the cycle, probably to prepare for embryonic implantation in the mid-secretory phase (see next section). These studies on gene expression profiling and gene ontology analysis provide important information on the biochemical participants, pathways, and processes underlying known histological observations in ESE. There is increasing interest in the early secretory phase because it is the 'prereceptive phase' (i.e. preceding the phase of receptivity to embryonic implantation (see 'The window of implantation' section below)). In addition, advancement of the endometrium in assisted reproductive treatment cycles accompanied by ovulation induction is observed first in ESE (see 'Gonadotropin-stimulated cycles' section below), and the early secretory phase appears to be the most informative about progesterone resistance in the disorder of endometriosis (see 'The endometrial transcriptome in women with endometriosis' section below).

The window of implantation

The endometrium is receptive to embryonic implantation only during a proscribed period of time, i.e. during 'the window of implantation', spanning 6–10 days after the luteinizing hormone (LH) surge, during the mid-secretory phase (cycle days 20–24) (see Figure 14.1) (and see Chapter 22). Histologically, by cycle day 20, few glycogen vacuoles remain in the glands, the nuclei are near the basal portion of the epithelial cells, and glycoprotein-rich products are largely expelled into the glandular lumen. The peak of glandular secretion coincides with implantation of the blastocyst.[25,26] Beginning on day 20, and subsequently, changes in the stroma are prominent, compared to in the glands prior to this day, and changes include increased capillary permeability, stromal edema, stromal fibroblast and endothelial cell mitoses, and coiling of the spiral arterioles.[11,26] Maximal capillary permeability and stromal edema occur on day 22 and are prerequisites for predecidual transformation of stromal fibroblasts, which begins first subepithelially and in the perivascular region by day 24, along with stromal mitoses.[11,26] On CD 24–25, there is a marked increase in lymphocyte infiltration. It is in this setting that the blastocyst attaches to the luminal epithelium, progresses through this cell layer, and begins the early events of trophoblast invasion into the endometrial stroma. The molecular dialogues between the epithelium and the blastocyst and the trophoblast and the stromal fibroblasts, vascular endothelium, and immune cells in the endometrium probably reflect a multiplicity of molecular and cellular interactions.[10,39] Several groups have investigated the transcriptome of human and non-human primate endometrium during this important phase of the menstrual cycle[15–24,40] (Figure 14.2 and below), which is the most widely studied endometrial cycle stage using global gene expression profiling. Kao et al,[17] Ace and Okulicz,[21] and Borthwick et al[19] investigated gene expression in the implantation window (peak progesterone) and compared the late proliferative phase (peak estradiol), whereas Carson et al,[18] Riesewijk et al,[20] Mirkin et al,[24,40] and Horcajadas et al[22,41] compared the implantation window (i.e. the 'receptive phase') to the prereceptive phase (i.e. the early secretory phase). Interestingly, while all of these groups used the Affymetrix platform for analysis, relatively few genes are in common (see below). Also, there is no information on the endometrial transcriptome in the presence of an embryo at this time of the cycle, where cross-talk between the embryo and endometrium may significantly affect each other, although studies in the mouse have given insight into this early process of implantation (see 'Cycle- and steroid hormone-dependent gene expression in rodent uterus' section). In the section below, the transcriptomes of human and non-human primate endometrium during the mid-secretory phase in the non-pregnant state are presented, which give valuable insight into the molecular events awaiting and perhaps participating in nidation of the blastocyst.

Up-regulated genes

Gene ontology analysis reveals that biological processes associated with up-regulated genes and gene families in MSE vs ESE include cellular differentiation, cell–cell communications, cell adhesion, suppression of cell

Table 14.2 Most highly up-regulated genes in mid-secretory vs early-secretory endometrium

- CXCL14 (61.2)
- Secreted proteins:
  - [a,b]glycodelin (43.6)
  - cysteine-rich secretory protein (CRSIP) 3 (10.8)
  - gastrin (6.5)
  - [a,c]osteopontin (4.9)
  - [b]secretoglobin, family 2A, member 2 (4.8)
  - [a]IGFBP-1 (5.2), IGFBP-3 (2.5)
- [a]Glutathione peroxidase 3 (40.2)
- [a]Solute carriers (glutamate, peptides) (22.8, 13.1)
- [a]Endothelin receptor B (12.7)
- [a]Transmemberane 4 superfamily member 2 (12.3)
- [a,b]Cartilage oligomeric matrix protein (11.7)
- Dipeptidyl peptidase 4/CD 26 (11.2)
- Complement components [DAF[a,c] (10.9), C4BPA (8.6), C4B (3.7), C3 (3.8)]
- [a]SOD2 (9.8)
- [a]Defensin, beta 1 (9.4)
- [a]MAO A (8.63)
- [a]Transcobalamin 1 (8.4)
- [a]Ceruloplasmin (7.)
- [a]RAR responder 1[c] (7.6)
- MUC 16 (7.4)
- [a]Laminin beta 3 [6.6, alpha 5 (2.5)]
- Serine protease inhibitor [SERPING1, 5.4]
- [a]Clusterin (5.3)
- [a,c]Versican [chondroitin sulfate proteoglycan (5.3)]
- [a,b]Dkk-1 (5.1)
- [a,c]Annexin A4 (4.9)
- Arginase 2 (4.85)
- [a]Retinol-binding protein 4 (4.84)
- [b]GABA receptor (4.7)
- [b]Protein tyrosine phosphatase receptor (4.6)
- Heparinase (4.6)
- [a]Keratin 7 (4.6)
- [a]Stanniocalcin 1 (4.2)
- [a,b]Thrombomodulin (4.2)
- Claudin 10 (4.1), claudin 4[a,b] (3.9)
- [a]Ephrin A1 (3.9)
- [a,b,c]IL-15 (3.9)
- [a,b]Apo D (3.8), Apo E (2.1)
- LIF (3.8)
- G0S2 (3.8)
- [a]ID4 [inhibitor of DNA binding (3.7)]
- [a]Granzyme A, B (3.6)
- [c]IL6ST (3.6)
- THBS2 (3.5); THBS1 (1.8)
- Metallothioneins 1G (3.4), [c]1H (3.0), [c]1E (3.0), 1F (2.8), 1L (2.6), 1X (2.6), 2A (2.5)
- [a]Cathepsin W (3.4)
- [a]Phospholipase A2
- [b]E-cadherin (2.9)
- TIMP-3 (2.8), TIMP-1 (2.0)
- [a]Endothelial cell growth factor (2.6)
- N-acetylglucosamine 6-O-sulfotransferase (2.5)
- [a]Integrin α_3
- Aquaporin 3 (2.3)
- Growth factors/effectors:
  - FOXO1A (2.3)
  - TGFB2 (2.1)
  - FGFR2 (2.1)
  - [a]inhibin beta B
  - Wnt 5B (2.0)
  - HGF (2.0)
  - VEGF (2.0)
- STAR (2.0)
- [a]GAS1 2.1
- TLR4 (1.7)

Reproduced with permission from Talbi et al.[16]
[a]Riesewijk et al,[20] [b]Carson et al,[18] and [c]Mirkin et al.[24]

proliferation, regulation of proteolysis, metabolism, growth factor and cytokine binding and signaling, and immune and inflammatory responses.[16] Striking up-regulation of genes encoding secreted proteins, cytokines, and genes involved in detoxification mechanisms are observed. Table 14.2 lists the most highly up-regulated genes in MSE vs ESE from the study by Talbi et al,[16] and has reference to genes found in common with other groups comparing these phases of the cycle.

Immune genes. CXCL14 is the most-highly up-regulated gene (61-fold) in MSE vs ESE.[16,22] It is also known as breast and kidney-expressed chemokine (BRAK) and is chemotactic for monocytes.[42] The cell type in endometrium in which CXCL14 is expressed and its function in this tissue are not known. However, it may attract the blastocyst to the endometrium or guide the trophoblast in the early invasive phase of implantation. Additionally, it may function to attract lymphocytes to the tissue or have other functions, and additional studies are needed to determine the role of this chemokine in the implantation window. Another highly up-regulated gene that peaks in MSE vs ESE is leukemia inhibitory factor (LIF),[16,41] a cytokine that is critical to embryo attachment and stromal decidualization in the mouse.[43,44] In humans, there is increasing evidence that it is important in successful implantation,[45] because some women with infertility and recurrent miscarriage have low levels of LIF in MSE,[46,47] and others have point mutations in the coding region of the LIF gene,[45] compared to normal, fertile women. Other immune genes regulated in the implantation window compared to the prereceptive phase are listed in Table 14.3. Overall, there is a striking up-regulation of genes involved in activation of the innate immune response, including members of the complement family (e.g. DAF), antimicrobial peptides, and Toll-like receptor expression.[16] These genes peak in MSE and drop in their expression after the implantation window (see below). Chemotaxis of monocytes, T cells, and NK cells by candidate genes CXCL14, granulysin, and IL-15, as well as up-regulation of carbohydrate sulfotransferase 2, and suppression of NK- and T-cell activation are observed in MSE vs ESE. Also, IL-15, a progesterone-regulated gene product of the stromal fibroblast (see above), plays a major role in secretory endometrium in the recruitment of peripheral blood CD16-NK cells in this phase of the cycle.[48] Many of the genes in Tables 14.2 and 14.3 were observed by Carson et al,[18] Riesewijk et al,[20] and Mirkin et al,[24] and, overall, the gene expression profiles are consistent with a marked increase in lymphocytes into the tissue in the implantation window observed histologically.[11,49]

Table 14.3   Immune genes peaking in mid-secretory endometrium vs early-secretory endometrium

1. **Complement-related**
   Decay accelerating factor
   Adispin
   Complement component 1
   Complement component 2
   Complement component 3
   Complement component 4 binding protein

2. **Activation of innate immunity**
   Toll-like receptor 3 (ligand for DS RNA)
   Toll-like receptor 4 (ligand for lipopolysaccharide)

   Antimicrobial
   Granulysin
   Defensin, β1
   Indoleamine-pyrrole 2,3 dioxygenase

3. **Suppression of T-cell proliferation (+/− activation) and/or NK cell cytotoxicity**
   Indoleamine-pyrrole 2,3 dioxygenase (IDO)
   Glycodelin

4. **Cytokines and receptors**
   IL-1 receptor, type I
   IL-6 receptor
   IL-15 (NK-cell proliferation and chemotaxis)
   IL-15 receptor α

5. **Involved in chemotaxis/lymphocyte migration**
   IL-15
   Granulysin
   Carbohydrate (N-acetylglucosamine-6-O) sulfotransferase 2 (migration of lymphocytes on endothelial venule ligands)

6. **Other**
   CD58 (LFA3)
   Interferon-induced protein 35
   Interferon regulatory factor 2
   Leukemia inhibitory factor (induces macrophage differentiation)

Reproduced with permission from Talbi et al.[16]

A focused study on the transcriptome of cytokine and cytokine-related genes expressed in receptive vs prereceptive endometrium[50] is in agreement with many of the genes observed in the studies described above. For example, up-regulation of glycodelin, osteopontin, TIMP-3, IGF-II, decorin, integrin α_3, and IL-1R, and down-regulation of IL-15 receptor and ephrin A2 were observed.

Secretory proteins.   A hallmark of the mid-secretory phase is secretion of glycoproteins into the glandular lumen.[11,26] The microarray approach[15-24] has enabled identification of some of these, including cysteine-rich secretory protein (CRISP) 3, secretoglobin family 2A member 2, glycodelin, osteopontin, and IGFBP-1 (see Table 14.2). While these are believed to be important

in embryonic attachment, immune suppression, and regulation of trophoblast migration, other functions, yet to be determined, may exist for these proteinaceous secretions in this time of the cycle.

Antioxidants/detoxification.   Glutathione peroxidase-3 (GPX-3) and metallothioneins (MT) 1G, 1H, 1E, 1F, 1L, 1X, and 2A are among the most highly up-regulated genes[16] (see Table 14.2). This is consistent with prior observations[20,24] (and in MSE vs PE[17,19,51]). GPX-3 is an antioxidant, and metallothioneins protect cells from unstable reactive radicals and heavy metals.[52] Up-regulation of these genes (and their gene products) may protect the implanting embryo from free radicals and heavy metal exposure. GPXs are selenium-dependent, and women with selenium deficiency have a higher rate of infertility and miscarriage, compared to normal women.[53] Whether abnormalities in GPX and MT expression (e.g. with an inadequate response to progesterone) result in a clinical phenotype remains to be determined.

Other.   Up-regulated genes also included apolipoproteins, phospholipase A_2, N-acetylglucosamine 6-O-sulfotransferase (for glycoprotein synthesis), members of the TGFb-signaling pathway, the Wnt signaling pathway (e.g. Dikkopf-1, a Wnt inhibitor), claudin-4 (also known as the CPE receptor), water and ion transporters, transcription factors, apoptosis family members, and others (see Giudice[5] for review).

Down-regulated genes

Talbi et al[16] found that the most highly down-regulated genes in MSE vs ESE include secreted frizzled related protein (SFRP), olfactomedin 1, the progesterone receptor (PR), PR membrane component 1, ERα, MUC-1, 17β-HSD-2, and MMP-11. Some of these genes were not detected in earlier MSE vs ESE microarray studies, probably due to different platforms, possibly different complements of cell types in samples, and different data analysis algorithms[5] (see below). Other down-regulated genes included intestinal trefoil factor, tenascin C, matrilysin (MMP-7), frizzled-related protein (FRP-HE, a Wnt inhibitor), Indian hedgehog receptor, and RAG2. Validation of multiple up- and down-regulated genes was conducted in all cases and confirmed differential expression.[5]

Progesterone-regulated genes

Analysis of genes expressed in various phases of the menstrual cycle and the presence of progesterone response elements (PREs) in their promoters (when known), as well as analysis of data on PR knockout mice and the use

Table 14.4 Candidate progesterone-regulated genes in human endometrium[16]

Up		Down	
ESE vs PE and MSE vs PE			
• Secretoglobin	• Aldehyde dehydrogenase I	• MMP-11	• proenkephalin
• Osteopontin	• MUC-1	• MMP-7	• CXCL12
• Aquaporin 3	• Metallothionein IG	• SFRP1	• SOX 4
• LRP4	• MAO	• Wnt 5A	• TGFb1
• Dkk-1	• GABA receptor π subunit	• Tenascin C	• MSX2
		• N-cadherin	• Sema 2 AE
MSE vs ES and MSE vs PE			
• Glycodelin (PAEP)	• Annexin A4	• CRISP2	
• Gastrin	• Arginase 2	• SFRP1	
• Osteopontin	• GABA receptor π subunit	• Olfactomedin 1	
• Secretoglobins	• Claudin 4	• MX2	
• Glutathione peroxidase	• IL-15	• Osteoblast specific factor	
• Solute carrier (glutamate)	• Apo D	• NDRG3	
• Monocarboxylic acid carrier	• Apo E	• Progesterone receptor membrane	
• Transmembrane 4 superfamily member	• G0S2	component 1	
• COMP	• Metallothioneins IG, IE, 2A,1! F	• Oviductal glycoprotein	
• MAO-A	• N-acetylglucosamine-6-	• MMP-11	
• Transcobalamin	O-sulfotransferase	• PR	
• Kdd-1	• Aquaporin 3	• ERα	

Reproduced with permission from Talbi et al.[16]

of PR antagonists in mice, and using human endometrial explants, all give insight into genes that are candidates for regulation by progesterone. While not all progesterone-regulated genes have PREs, and progesterone can have non-PR-mediated and non-genomic effects on gene expression,[54] the list of progesterone-regulated genes is growing, and some of this information is presented below. Additional information is found in Chapters 4 and 14. Of interest are genes in MSE (peak progesterone [and E_2]) vs PE (peak E_2, low progesterone) from *all* studies in humans and non-human primates[17,19,21] that are in *common* with those regulated in ESE vs PE[16] and MSE vs ESE.[16,18,20,24] The result of this comparison is shown in Table 14.4. These genes are likely to be regulated by progesterone, either directly or indirectly. Validation of such regulatory mechanisms awaits further investigation. By querying databases, electronic identification of PREs (and EREs) has been acheived in the promoters of many genes regulated (up or down) by Borthwick et al,[19] Mirkin et al,[24] and Talbi et al,[16] and support some of these conclusions, as do studies using antiprogestins[55] (and Chapter 4) and PR knockout of progesterone-regulated genes in mouse uterus/endometrium[56] (and Chapter 14). Mining databases affords an important tool to investigate candidate response elements and provides guidance toward searching for, e.g. steroid hormone-regulated genes in endometrium and other tissues.

The use of an antiprogestin on mid-secretory endometrial explant cultures has revealed insight into progesterone-regulated genes. Catalano et al[57] treated samples with E_2 and progesterone with and without RU-486 and analyzed the transcriptome using cDNAarrays containing approximately 1000 sequence-verified clones. Regulated genes included those involved in angiogenesis, apoptosis, cell signaling, ECM remodeling, and cell cycle regulation. The data demonstrated that two important signaling pathways in endometrium – namely, the JAK/STAT and the JNK pathways – are altered by RU-486, suggesting these may be involved in progesterone signaling and perhaps receptivity to embryonic implantation.

The effects of medroxyprogesterone acetate (MPA) on the endometrial endothelial cell transcriptome[28] reveal up-regulation of thrombin-activatable fibrinolysis inhibitor, creatine kinase, inositol polyphosphatas phosphatase-like 1, SOD2, protein-glutamine-γ-glutamyl transferase, placental alkaline phosphate-like gene, and uroporphyrinogen decarboxylase, and down-regulation of enterokinase, estrogen sulfotransferase, and lecithin retinol acyltransferase. The clinical significance of these effects is not clear at this time.

While progesterone can account for many of the genes that are up- or down-regulated in secretory phase endometrium, "differences between MSE and

ESE gene expression profiles may also reflect the loss of ERα during this transition. Inhibition of gene expression by estradiol (as occurs in T47D breast cancer cells[58]), and loss of this inhibition with the down-regulation of ERα in MSE, is an alternative explanation for some of the genes that appear during this time in the cycle".[16] In the setting of an inadequate endometrial response to progesterone, e.g. in luteal phase deficiency or endometriosis, effective loss of ERα may not occur, thus leading (for example) to some of the differences in gene expression.[59,60] In addition, while ERα expression in the epithelium is undetectable in MSE, ERα persists, albeit at low levels, in the stroma, and ERβ is expressed in the vascular endothelium.[28] Estrogen receptors act as dimers, and it is possible that some hetero/homodimers may not bind ligand, resulting in the equivalent of a dominant negative regulation of gene expression by these receptors[61] and perhaps differences between MSE and ESE gene expression profiles in normal women and those with inadequate production or response to progesterone.

Genes in common

Despite these studies having used similar platforms, the number of genes in common is surprisingly low. "For example, of the 75 genes up-regulated in MSE vs ESE in the study by Riesewijk et al,[20] 41 are identical to up-regulated genes in the study by Talbi et al,[16] and of the 56 down-regulated genes, 11 were the same. In the study by Carson et al,[18] of the 74 genes encoding cell surface components, ECM components, growth factors, and cytokines in MSE vs ESE, only 11 were in common, and of the 76 down-regulated genes, only 1 was in common with Talbi et al.[16] Also, of the 49 up-regulated genes in MSE vs ESE in the study by Mirkin et al,[24] 14 are similarly regulated, and of the 58 that were down-regulated, only 3 are common to Talbi et al.[16] These differences are probably the result of using different chip versions, hybridization conditions, scanners, and statistical programs for data analyses, subject-to-subject variability, where endometrium samples were obtained (fundus, lower uterine segment), different complements of cellular components in individual samples, and precisely the time in the cycle when samples were obtained".[5] For example, Rieswijk et al[20] obtained paired endometrial samples from the same subjects at 2 and 7 days after the LH surge, whereas most other studies analyzed non-paired samples that span groups of days in a particular phase. Also, one study pooled samples in a particular phase prior to hybridization of the RNA to the oligonucleotide chips (Borthwick et al[19]), whereas most others hybridized RNA from individual samples and performed statistical analyses on the data generated from each sample in a given stage and between stages.[4,5] Detailed comparative analyses of these data and reviews of these studies have recently been summarized by Horcajadas et al,[6,22] Sherwin et al,[62] Ponnampalam et al,[63] and Giudice.[5]

Non-human primate endometrium

Differential display-RT-PCR (DD-RT-PCR) was also used by Ace and Okulicz[64] and rhesus monkey endometrium from a simulated model of the proliferative phase and inadequate (low progesterone) and adequate (high progesterone) secretory phase, using silastic implants.[64] They sequenced several fragments and determined progesterone-dependent genes, including down-regulation of ser/thr protein phosphatase A, oxobutanoate dehydrogenase E1b-β, and up-regulation of six fragments homologous to uncharacterized ESTs, sequence site tags, and cosmid clones. In a subsequent study, also using DD-RT-PCR and endometrial samples from the window of implantation vs in a low progesterone environment, the same group[65] identified one fragment with high homology to secretory leukocyte protease inhibitor (antileukoprotease), an endometrial neutrophil elastase inhibitor with antibacterial and anti-inflammatory properties, and syncytin, a fusogenic membrane glycoprotein that induces formation of giant syncitia and may be important in decidual and placental development. In a subsequent study by this group, genes expressed on CD21–23 were compared to genes expressed on CD13, using oligonucleotide microarrays.[21] Several regulated genes were common with those regulated in human endometrium, including uteroglobin, metallothionein IG, and secretory leukocyte protease inhibitor, among the 39 up-regulated genes. TGFβ₁, stromelysin 3, proenkephalin, collagen type VII alpha 1, secreted frizzled-related protein 4, PR membrane component 1, CXCL12, and biglycan were among the 69 down-regulated genes. These studies underscore the validity of using the non-human primate model to investigate comparable processes in human endometrium and provide an insight into steroid hormone action on primate endometrium in general.

The transcriptome of cynomolgus monkey endometrium in the equivalent of the window of implantation vs the equivalent of the proliferative phase (in a model of ovariectomy and hormonal supplementation) was investigated by Allan and colleagues[66] using differential mRNA display and reverse Northern analysis. While numerous genes were differentially expressed, four were identified and further analyzed in human endometrium by in-situ hybridization. Iodothyronine deiodinase mRNA was found to be expressed in all stages of the menstrual cycle, primarily in stromal cells. Fibulin 1 was expressed in glandular epithelia during the menstrual phase and then in the stroma during the secretory phase. Osteopontin was expressed at high levels in glandular epithelium and isolated stromal cells (perhaps immune cells) in menstrual endometrium, and in the secretory phase expression was confined to a subpopulation of epithelial cells. Cathepsin H was expressed in menstrual and proliferative endometrium. These data raise interesting questions about, for example, the role of thyroid hormone, as well as fibulin 1, cathepsin H, and osteopontin, in the endometrium.

Other global approaches

Another technique used to investigate differences in gene expression between secretory and proliferative phase endometrium is subtractive cDNA hybridization, an early, large-scale profiling method in which cDNA libraries derived from two tissues, cell lines, or primary cell cultures are compared, using an excess of one library. Following denaturation and hybridization, cDNAs common to both tissues anneal, and the 'subtracted' unique cDNAs remain single stranded. Vaisse et al[67] used this approach and found that glycodelin is a specific product of secretory phase endometrium, confirming earlier work of Seppala and colleagues.[68] Also using this technique, Higushi et al[69] found marked up-regulation of tissue inhibitor of metalloproteinase-3 (TIMP-3) in secretory, compared to proliferative, phase endometrium. This is believed to be important later in the cycle and in early pregnancy to control matrix degradation (see next section) and to inhibit MMPs secreted by invading trophoblasts, respectively.

Martin et al[70] pursued differential display and cDNA microarray analyses of two human endometrial cell lines with 'receptive' phenotypes and endometrial biopsies from subjects (paired samples) on LH+7 vs LH+2. They found, for example, in the paired samples, up-regulation of glycodelin, MAC25, osteopontin, and IL-1RtI, and down-regulation of IL-15R and IFN-γRII. In low-receptivity cell lines, high expression of GM-CSF, TGFG-b, NFκBp65, and IGF-I were observed, and in high receptivity, G_1/S-cyclin D_1, GADD45, and MEKK3 were highly expressed. The use of cell lines to define receptivity is a novel approach and can minimize patient-to-patient variability observed in many studies.

Cell-specific gene expression

Laser capture microdissection of glands and stroma in mid-secretory endometrium in humans and non-human primates reveals several genes that are cell-specific.[71,72] Interestingly, in human endometrium, several epithelial and stromal enriched genes determined by cDNA analysis are the same as in the proliferative phase,[27] suggesting biomarkers for these cell types. In non-human primate (rhesus monkey) endometrium, LCM in mid-secretory phase specimens from the funtionalis and basalis, followed by DD-RT-PCR, revealed high expression of the leukotriene B_4 receptor in functionalis, high expression of an unknown gene only in the stroma of the functionalis, and a gene with 98% homology with an uncharacterized bacterial artificial chromosome clone sequence was expressed only in the glandular epithelium of the basalis.[72]

Gonadotropin-stimulated cycles

The endometrium during controlled ovarian hyperstimulation in assisted reproductive technology (ART) cycles has been noted to be advanced histologically by several days[73–75] and to have markedly reduced pinopodes.[76] While histological advancement is evident and ER and PR expression in glands and stroma are markedly decreased, as is Ki67 expression (a reflection of proliferative index), as early as the day of and 2 days after oocyte retrieval,[74] the transcriptome of the endometrium during gonadotropin-stimulated cycles has focused on the mid-secretory phase.[41,77] In the study by Mirkin et al,[77] endometrium was analyzed by global gene expression profiling from subjects in natural cycles (on day LH+8) and undergoing stimulated cycles (day human chorionic gonadotropin [hCG]+9) (recombinant follicle-stimulating hormone [FSH], gonadotropin-releasing hormone [GnRH] antagonist, with or without micronized progesterone luteal support, or down-regulation with GnRH agonist, and recombinant FSH and micronized progesterone for luteal support). They found that ER and PR in natural cycles on day 21 were fully expressed, whereas with rFSH and GnRH analogue, low expression was observed in both glands and stroma. Also, pinopodes were absent, and serum E_2 was nearly 10 times higher in stimulated cycles, with progesterone being similar on the day of egg retrieval; however, serum E_2 and progesterone levels on the day of endometrial biopsy were both about 10-fold higher than in natural cycles, with no differences in cycles with antagonist

Table 14.5 Effects on the endometrium by controlled ovarian hyperstimulation (COH) regimens in assisted reproductive technologies (ART)

COMP* (58.6)	Hyaluronan-binding protein 2 (6.7)	PGER2 (3.9)
Dipeptidylpeptidase 4* (CD26) (54.4)	Aldehyde oxidase 1* (6.2)	Gastrin* (3.6)
Thrombomodulin (24.28)	Amine oxidase* (6.0)	Small inducible cytokine subfamily E1 (3.6)
LIF* (23.02)	Transmembrane 4 superfamily member 3* (5.8)	CD36 (thrombospondin receptor) (3.6)
Mucin 16* (13.6)	Short-chaindehydrogenase/ reductase (5.8)	Thromboplastin(tissue factor) (3.5)
Cytochrome P450, family 3A5 (12.9)	Laminin beta 3* (5.6)	Sialyltransferase 1 (3.4)
GTX3* (12.5)	Dual specificity phosphatase 6 (5.7)	Alpha 2 adrenergic R (3.4)
IGFBP-1* (12.0)	RAR responder 1 (5.4)	Epithelial upregulated in carcinoma (3.3)
CFTR/MRP family (11.12)	Aldehyde oxidase (5.3)	Solute carrier family 22, member 5 (3.3)
Solute carrier family 15/member 1* (10.6); family 1, member 1 (8.2); family 22/5 (3.3)	Prominin 1 (5.0)	MMP-11 (stromelysin) (3.2)
Clusterin* (complement lysis inhibitor) (10.0)	G0/G1 switch (4.9)	E74-like factor 3 (ets, epithelial) (3.2)
Glycodelin* (PAEP; PP-14) (9.8)	Tetraspan 1 (4.7)	EGF-containing extracellular matrix (3.2)
Calponin 1 (9.3)	Vanin 1 (4.7)	Killer cell lectin-like R C1 (3.2)
Duffy blood group*(9.2)	IGFBP-3* (4.7)	Endothelin receptor B* (3.2)
CXCL1 4* (8.9)	Aquaporin 3* (4.6)	Fibroblast activation protein alpha (3.1)
Transcobalamin I* (vitB12 binding) (7.8)	FXYD domain containing ion transport regulator (4.6)	Monoamine oxidase A* (3.0)
Myosin heavy polypeptdie 11 (7.7)	CXCL12 (4.4)	Plastin 1 (3.0)
IL6 ST* (gp130, oncostatin M receptor) (7.4)	MMP-7 (4.2)	Complement component 4 binding protein alpha* (3.0)
Lipcalin (7.35)	Cadherin (4.1)	Thrombospondin 2* (3.0)
Stratifin (7.04)	Leiomodin (4.1)	Acetyl-CoA dehydrogenase (3.0)
CXCR4 (6.83)	Tropomodulin 1 (4.1)	
	PPAR-gamma coactivator 1 (4.01)	

ªMost highly down-regulated genes (hCG + 7 vs LH + 7): (*=highly up-regulated in MSE vs ESE[16]).
Reproduced with permission from Horcajadas et al.[41]

or agonist. Using statistical analysis of microarrays, in stimulated cycles vs natural cycles, there was a small variation in gene expression, with 18 genes/ESTs (expressed sequence tags) changing 1.55–3.0 fold. In cycles with antagonist and agonist, there were significant changes in 13 genes/ESTs, ranging between 1.42- and 2.10-fold, including, for example, IGFBP-5, and procollagen-lysine. This minimal response may be due to the days analyzed (LH+8 vs hCG+9).

In another study by Horcajadas et al,[41] endometrium from oocyte donors was obtained in each donor's natural cycle on day LH+7 and in the same donor's treatment cycle with GnRH agonist + human menopausal gonadotropin (hMG) + highly purified FSH (FSH HP), without exogenous luteal support on day hCG+7. By principal component analysis, LH+7 samples clustered together, as did hCG+7. More than 200 genes were differentially expressed with >three-fold change in hCG+7 vs LH+7. The most impressive observation was the most highly down-regulated genes (Table 14.5). Genes that were highly up-regulated in the window of implantation vs the prereceptive phase in the study by Talbi et al,[16] such as LIF, GTX2, IGFBP-1, glycodelin, CXCL14,

and aquaporin 3, gastrin, and MAO, thought to be important in endometrial development and implantation, were down-regulated in treatment cycles. These data underscore abnormal endometrial development in gonadotropin-stimulated cycles. Given that pregnancy rates in ART cycles range between 20 and 40% in women under the age of 40 years old (CDC 2004[78]), the question remains whether those women who do become pregnant happen to have normal maturation or does a 'healthy embryo' rescue an out-of-phase endometrium? Also, it is of great interest to investigate the prereceptive phase (ESE) in stimulated cycles, as this may respond to antiprogestins (of short duration) to alleviate accelerated maturation of the endometrium. Most valuable would be predictors of successful pregnancy from the perspective of endometrial biomarkers – the holy grail for infertility programs and patients, alike.

The late-secretory phase

The transition from the mid-secretory to late-secretory phase (CD 25–28), in the absence of embryonic implantation, is characterized by decreasing levels of progesterone locally and preparation for tissue desquamation and menstruation. While on CD 24–25, there is a marked infiltration of lymphocytes, by CD 26–28 there is a marked influx of extravasated polymorphonuclear leukocytes (PMNs).[11,12,25,26] Furthermore, by CD 27 most of the stroma in the functionalis layer appears as a solid sheet of predecidualized cells. Accordingly, gene expression profiling from three groups[15,16,79] reveals changes in genes involved in the ECM, the cytoskeleton, cell viability, vasoconstriction, smooth muscle contraction, hemostasis, and transition in the immune response to include an inflammatory response.

Immune profile

Data from Talbi et al[16] and Critchley et al[79] demonstrate that there is a major shift from an innate immune response in MSE to an inflammatory response in the LSE, consistent with histological observations of an influx of extravasated PMNs. For example, in LSE vs MSE, there is up-regulation of Fc receptors, MHC molecules, NK molecules, and T-cell molecules. By up-regulating Fc receptors, monocytes/granulocytes can readily respond to antibodies, and by expressing MHC-II molecules antigen-presenting cells become more effective. Interleukin (IL)-1, a proinflammatory cytokine, induces T-cell activation and, IL-1β and tumor necrosis factor α (TNFα), secreted by stromal leukocytes, stimulate release of matrix-degrading enzymes that proteolyze the vascular basement membrane and connective tissue of the endometrial functionalis, thus facilitating tissue shedding.[80,81] Withdrawal of progesterone up-regulates inflammatory mediators, including IL-1β, CXCL8 (IL-8), CCL2 (MCP-1),[82,83] and cyclooxygenase 2 (COX-2), with subsequent prostaglandin biosynthesis. In addition, genes involved in cellular apoptosis are up-regulated in LSE. Thus, the tissue is prepared for uterine smooth muscle contraction and vasospasm, promoted by elevated prostaglandin concentrations (PGE$_2$ and PGF$_{2\alpha}$)[84] whose synthases are elevated in this phase of the cycle. The microarray data are consistent with histological observations, and interestingly, an inflammatory environment, along with up-regulation of matrix-degrading enzymes and cellular apoptosis, probably would not be a receptive environment for embryonic implantation. Of interest is the immune profile in LSE in a conception cycle and the cross-talk between the implanting conceptus and the maternal decidua in the context of immune regulation – would, for example, the profile transition from innate immunity to a proinflammatory state?

Extracellular matrix degradation

Progesterone is known to inhibit stromal-derived proteases, including uPA, MMP-1, and MMP-3.[85] The global gene expression profiling of LSE vs MSE demonstrates striking up-regulation of metalloproteinases (MMPs and ADAMs), serine proteases [uPA (PLAU) and tPA (PLAT)], and their inhibitors. This is consistent with declining tissue progesterone levels and concomitant dysinhibition of expression of these genes. Progesterone also inhibits leukocyte transit into the endometrium,[86] controlled by stromal fibroblasts that retain PR in the secretory phase. Urokinase (uPA, PLAU) is up-regulated in LSE compared to MSE and is available to activate TGFβ1. It is regulated by tissue factor, which is also progesterone-dependent and activates plasminogen, which can activate MMPs. Thus, uPA probably plays a major role in preparing the tissue for desquamation. TGFβ family members also play a role in tissue breakdown. In particular, endometrial bleeding-associated factor (EBAF or Lefty A) is one of the most highly up-regulated genes in LSE vs MSE.[16] It stimulates production of proMMP-3 and -7 and is inhibited by progesterone.[87] Importantly, while these genes are up-regulated in LSE, tissue breakdown does not occur immediately. Also, these events should be carefully regulated, in magnitude and time, for menses to occur at an appropriate threshold of gene activation, to control hemorrhage and to permit subsequent repair of the tissue for the next cycle. In clinical disorders associated with endometrial bleeding at unexpected times[88] (Chapter 46), for example, it is possible that the endometrium has already undergone significant biochemical changes by the time clinical symptoms of spotting or bleeding occur. Indeed, Critchley and colleagues[79] analyzed global gene profiling in LSE and MSE in women with menstrual complaints (heavy menstrual bleeding and pelvic pain). Their data demonstrate heterogeneity among samples, as observed by others, and propose potential markers of endometrial bleeding/dysfunction, including lysyl oxidase (LOX) and protease activated receptor (PAR)-1, involved in wound healing and regulation of thrombin function, respectively.

In summary, events that occur across the menstrual cycle are shown schematically in Figure 14.4A. These have been deduced from the endometrial transcriptomes reported in the previous sections.

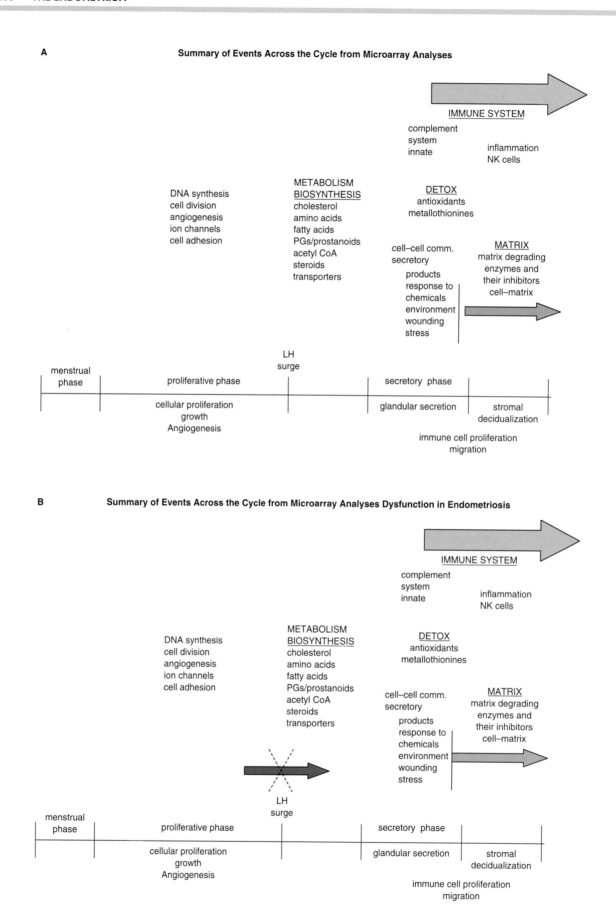

Figure 14.4 Summary of events occurring across the menstrual cycle, deduced from microarray analyses (see text). **(A)** Normally cycling women. **(B)** Women with endometriosis and progesterone resistance. (Reproduced with permission from reference 5.)

Cycle- and steroid hormone-dependent gene expression in rodent uterus

The mouse affords an excellent model for investigating cycle-dependent and estrogen- and progesterone-regulated gene expression in the uterus. This model permits hormonally well-defined environments and genetic manipulation of steroid hormone responsiveness that are more easily accomplished, compared to studies in humans for ethical and logistical reasons. The response to E_2 occurs as early and late events. Early responses include increased RNA transcription, hyperemia, and water imbibition, 2 and 6 hours after E_2 administration, and late responses include waves of DNA synthesis and epithelial mitoses, 10–16 hours after E_2 administration. The response to progesterone includes increased vascular permeability and stromal edema. Since progesterone-regulated genes in the mouse (using the PRKO and PR antagonist RU-486-treated animals) have been investigated primarily in the context of pregnancy, the progesterone-regulated uterine transcriptome in the mouse is discussed in the 'Lessons from selective progesterone receptor modulators in the mouse' section below (and in Chapter 14). Herein are reviewed changes in gene expression during the estrus cycle, in response to E_2 and selective ER modulators, as well as in the setting of genetic deletions of ERα and ERβ that provide understanding of steroid hormone gene regulation in this tissue.

The estrus cycle

Global gene expression profiling during the estrus cycle in the mouse was investigated by Tan et al.[89] Using cDNA arrays with 8192 probes, they compared gene expression in whole uteri obtained in CD-1 mature virgin mice during estrus (peak E_2 in the circulation) with diestrus (slightly increased basal levels of estradiol and high progesterone). There were 51 significantly up-regulated and down-regulated genes (greater than two-fold change, $p < 0.05$), with the most highly up-regulated genes being in the categories of structural protein (small proline-rich protein 2A), genes involved in protein turnover (a-1 protease inhibitors 5 and 1, several members of the cathepsin family), oncogenes, immune-related genes (complement component C3, factor B, factor h, lactransferrin), and interestingly, 17β-HSD type 2, which is progesterone-dependent in human endometrium (see above). Up-regulation of complement component C3, factor B, and factor H, and 24p3 suggests that E_2 is an important modulator of mucosal immunity. Down-regulated genes were involved in cytoskeleton and structural proteins, DNA binding, regulation of the cell cycle, and other categories.[89]

ERKO mice

To gain further insight into estrogen-regulated genes in mouse uterus, Watanabe et al[90] ovariectomized (OVX) ERKO and wild-type C57/BL6 mice at 8 weeks of age, and after 2 weeks, the mice were injected with 17β-E_2. A time course was conducted at 0, 1, 2, 6, 12, 24, and 48 hours, and total RNA from uteri were hybridized to mouse U74A high-density oligonucleotide microarrays. Kinetic analysis revealed that maximum changes in gene expression occurred between 6 and 12 hours after E_2 treatment. Temporal analysis of genes regulated between 1 and 6 hours of E_2 revealed six cluster patterns. Three clusters of induced genes were grouped into immediate early response genes (peaking at 2 hours; e.g. c-fos, c-jun, early growth response 1); continuously increasing during the 6-hour treatment; and marked increased expression only at 6 hours. Three repressed clusters included repressed between 1 and 2 hours; repressed at 1 hour and thereafter; and repressed between 2 and 6 hours. Interestingly, there was a large number of intermediate early genes, including HB-EGF. In the early–late genes, genes related to RNA processing were highly represented. With regard to down-regulated genes, cyclin G_2 was repressed, as was caspase-12. These genes are important in arresting cell cycle progression and in evoking apoptosis, respectively, which may allow rapid protein synthesis and secretion. The leptin receptor was down-regulated and is involved in fatty acid, cholesterol, and, thus, sterol biosynthesis. Some classically E_2-regulated genes, e.g. complement C3, EGF, MUC-1, lactoferrin, and PR, were not found to be regulated during the 6-hour time course after E_2 administration, consistent with their known activation at 12 hours or longer after E_2 administration. Analysis of genes up-regulated by E_2 in wild type vs ERKO mice revealed that most genes affected by E_2 in wild-type mice were not affected in the α-ERKO mice, demonstrating that E_2 effects on uterine gene expression are mainly mediated via ERα at the transcriptional level, consistent with αERKO mice having severe uterine defects.[91]

Hewitt and colleagues[92] (and see Chapter 13) investigated ER-dependent early and late global genomic responses (8700 probes) to E_2 in mouse uterus. Wild-type, αERKO and βERKO mice were ovariectomized and treated with E_2 for 2 hours (early response) and 24 hours (late response). Clusters of genes were regulated uniquely in the two response times or at both times. Both early and late responses in the βERKO mice were indistinguishable from the wild-type mice, whereas the

Table 14.6 E$_2$-regulated genes in mouse uterus

Short- and long-term estrogen-regulated genes in mouse uterus (hours after E)

	0.5	2	6	12	24
Known estrogen-regulated genes:					
c-Fos	2.07	3.77			
Lactoferrin					4.56
Sox4		0.47			0.51
Cyr61		4.35	2.15		
IGF signaling:					
IGF-1			4.3	3.2	2.2
IGFBP3			0.35	0.25	0.28
IGFBP5					2
RAMP3		5.56	10	5	2.7
Cell cyle:					
p21	1.8	2.8	2.4	2.9	
CyclinG				2.3	
MAD2		4.3	2.7		1.97
Stratifin					2.2
G$_1$ to S phase transition1				2.5	
cdc2					1.73
Chromatin:					
H2A histone fmz			2.9	3.16	2.08
H1 histone fm2			0.55		
HDAC5			0.44	0.55	
Apoptosis:					
BAD				2.7	2.03
Iκbα	1.8				
AKT-1		1.95	2.1	2	
Wnt signaling:					
Axin2 (Wnt signaling inhibitor)		1.7			
Expressed sequence AW227548 (fz-1)		0.5			
Case in kinase 1, α1		2.03			
ras Homolog gene family, member u (Wnt-1 responsive)		1.8			
Redox:					
Thioredoxin2	1.3		2.11	2.16	1.7
Thioredoxin reductase	1.3				2.15
Thioredoin-interacting protein	0.4		0.34		0.33
Keratinization:					
Small proline-rich protein 1A (cornifin)					3.6
Small proline-rich protein 2A (cornifin)				2.2	5.5
Stratifin					2.2
Transglutaminase2					2
Keratin complex 1, acidic, gene 13			2.6	2.4	1.77
Keratin complex 1, acidic gene 19					2.68
Keratin complex 2, basic gene 6a					2.25
Keratoepithelin			0.37	0.25	0.22

Reproduced with permission from Hewitt et al.[92]

αERKO mice demonstrated little response in gene expression to E$_2$, supporting a major role for ERα in the genomic response to E$_2$ in mouse uterus. Early and late E$_2$-regulated genes are shown in Table 14.6 and include c-fos, lactoferrin, SOX4, Cyr 61, members of the IGF family, cell cycle and chromatin regulators, and genes involved in apoptosis, Wnt signaling, oxidation/reduction reactions, and keratinization. Clearly, some of these are involved in DNA synthesis and cell division, and some have other functions. In a subsequent study by these same investigators,[93] they used a genomics approach to assess cross-talk between ERα and IGF and EGF signaling in the mouse uterus. They found that most of the E_2 response in wild type also occurred after IGF or EGF treatment, and some genes were uniquely regulated by E_2. Also, while E_2 did not induce gene expression changes in αERKO mice, the response to IGF and EGF was almost identical to that of the wild type, suggesting that ERα and IGF/EGF signaling have a point of convergence of similarly regulated genes.

The transcriptome of androgen response of the mouse uterus was investigated by Nantermet and colleagues.[94] Treatment of wild-type mice with E_2 or dihydrotestosterone (DHT) and subsequent analysis of genes using oligonucletoide arrays revealed that 491 genes were differentially expressed after E_2 treatment, including regulators of tissue remodeling, metabolism, and gene transcription. DHT regulated 164 specific genes, 86% of which were also regulated by E_2, including IGF-I and epithelial secretory genes such as uterocalin. In the αERKO mouse, DHT does not apparently activate ERα directly, because DHT induction of IGF-I was blocked by an androgen receptor (AR) antagonist and multiple genes regulated directly by ERα were not induced by DHT. Thus, the authors concluded that the gene expression profile in response to DHT is overlapping but distinct from the estrogen response.

Cell-specific estradiol gene regulation

Analysis of E_2-regulated genes was investigated by Hong et al[95] in a study involving treatment of OVX mice with E_2 for 6 and 12 hours, and cDNA microarray and LCM. They found that the most extensive regulation was observed at 12 hours and included up-regulation of cell cycle-, immune-, signal transduction-, transcription-, enzyme-, structure-, and apoptosis-related genes, as well as others, and similar categories for down-regulated genes. Furthermore, specific genes were identified as epithelial in origin, including Psmb 5, Ramp3, Sprp2A, Eif2s2, IF-1, and with cystatin B in both glands and stroma.

Rat uterus and estradiol gene regulation

A study on 3000 genes in rat uterus after ovariectomy and subsequent estradiol treatment, using cDNA arrays, revealed the transcriptome regulated by estradiol, in addition to some that are known E_2 mediators.[96] In this study, gene expression was compared with controls on days 1, 4, and 7 after E_2 treatment. Known and novel genes up-regulated by E_2 included growth response protein, Ladinin 1, thymosin b-4,

a-fodrin, immediate early response 5, ezrin, fas-activated Ser-Thr kinase, complement component C3, Sydecan 1, CD 24, IGFBP-2, follistation-related protein precursor, complement component C3, and secreted frizzled related protein 2 (SFRP-2). Some of these are in agreement with the study by Watanabe et al[90] in the mouse (e.g. glutathione S-transferase, epoxide hydrolase, 3-HMGCoA synthase 2, and farnesyl pyrophosphate synthase). In the study by Naciff et al,[97] the transcriptome of the developing rat female reproductive system (uterus and ovaries) was investigated on gestational day 20 in response to E_2, bisphenol A, and genistein. Analysis of 7000 rat genes and over 1000 ESTs revealed that, in dose–response experiments, a common set of genes was significantly and reproductively modified in the same way by all three estrogenic activities, although some genes were uniquely regulated by each of the agents. The authors suggest that transplacental exposure to chemicals with estrogenic activity can change the transcriptome of E-sensitive tissues that could determine the estrogenicity of different compounds – an interesting model to assess effects of, for example endocrine-disrupting chemicals with uncertain estrogen-like activities.

THE ENDOMETRIAL TRANSCRIPTOME IN WOMEN WITH ENDOMETRIOSIS

Endometriosis is a benign gynecological disorder in which endometrial glands and stroma are located in extra-endometrial/uterine sites[98–100] (see Chapter 45). It is believed to result from retrograde menstruation and transplantation of sloughed (eutopic) endometrial cells and tissue fragments onto the pelvic peritoneum, resulting in ectopic endometrial implants that elicit an inflammatory response and neoangiogenesis. Endometriomas are composed of endometrial tissue that is encapsulated in the ovary. In addition to peritoneal disease and endometriomas, deep endometriosis (e.g. in the rectovaginal septum) is another form of endometriosis. Other causes of endometriosis include coelomic metaplasia and genetic, immune, and environmental triggers.[98–100] Clinically, endometriosis is associated with pelvic pain and infertility, with the latter believed to be due, in part, to abnormal gene expression in the window of implantation. Over the past several years, two types of global gene expression profiling studies have been conducted on this tissue in humans – transcriptome analysis of ectopic vs matched eutopic endometrium (whole tissue or specific cell types) and transcriptome analysis of eutopic endometrium (whole tissues or specific cell types) from women with disease vs without disease. These are discussed below.

Ectopic vs eutopic endometrium

Eyster et al[101] investigated 4133 genes expressed in ovarian endometriomas, compared to paired eutopic endometrium during the proliferative phase of the cycle. Eight genes were up-regulated in ovarian endometriomas compared to eutopic endometrium, including genes encoding structural proteins (β-actin, α_2-actin, vimentin) and immune-related genes (Ig-l light chain, Ig germline H chain G-E-A region g-2 constant region, MCH class IC, and complement component 1S subcomponent). The relatively low number of differentially expressed genes in the two types of tissue may reflect the limited probe set used. While the significance of the up-regulation of genes associated with structural proteins and immune functions is not certain, the latter may reflect participants in immune dysfunction contributing to the pathogenesis of the disorder, and the structural proteins may be important for anchoring lipid droplets for steroid hormone biosynthesis by endometriosis tissue.[101]

Two recent studies have investigated global gene expression in ectopic vs eutopic endometrium. Hu and colleagues[102] investigated samples from 15 subjects with either minimal/mild disease (revised American Fertility Society [rAFS] scores [1985] of stage I/II) and moderate to severe disease (rAFS scores for stage III/IV) during either the proliferative or secretory phase. Peritoneal lesions (not endometriomas) constituted the ectopic disease. Of 78 candidate genes identified from the subtractive cDNA libraries, 76 were investigated by real-time RT-PCR in the 30 paired samples. Despite heterogeneity of cycle stage and disease severity, several genes and gene families were identified in the subtractive cDNA libraries, including ECM/cell adhesion proteins, ribosomal proteins, transcriptional regulators (including JUN and EGR1), RNA processing, signaling intermediates, cell cycle regulators (CDK2), GDP/GTP-binding proteins, metabolism, and other functions (e.g. semaphorin 4D, IGFBP-5). Fourteen candidate genes consistently expressed in 15 pairs of samples included up-regulation of IGFBP-5, PIM2 oncogene, RPL41, prosaposin, fibulin 1, SIPL protein, and four unknown genes and down-regulation of DLX5, 11β-HSD2, and Ras homologue gene family member E (RHOE). Some of these genes are known to participate in E_2 action and have antiapoptotic actions, suggesting that they may play a role in the pathogenesis

of the disorder and may be diagnostic biomarkers of the disorder or candidate therapeutic targets.

Wu and colleagues[103] investigated epithelial cells (isolated by LCM) from eutopic endometrium and ectopic endometrium (endometrioma and peritoneal lesions) and subsequent analysis using cDNA microarrays with 9600 genes/ESTs. Multidimensional scaling analysis revealed that samples clustered by site (ovarian endometriosis vs non-ovarian disease) (Figure 14.5A). Hierarchical clustering revealed five groups of genes (clusters) and two groups of patients (ovarian and non-ovarian endometriomas), further underscoring that ovarian and peritoneal endometriosis have different complements of gene expression. Cluster analysis revealed that both types of endometriosis had lower expression levels of genes involved in cell adhesion, Wnt signaling, and induction of apoptosis, and higher expression of genes participating in acute-phase response, cell proliferation, cell cycle, and regulation of transport, and differences in expression of genes associated with glycoprotein function, response to oxidative stress, and G-protein-coupled receptor signaling compared to paired eutopic endometrium. This may represent a response to the proinflammatory environment in which the lesions exist. Gene ontology analysis revealed, among differentially expressed genes, molecular functions of heparin binding, structural molecule activity, glcyosaminoglycan binding, and antioxidant activity. Biological processes included primarily cell growth and maintenance, cellular processes, among others, and KEGG pathways involving glutathione metabolism. IL-8 was found to be up-regulated, and IL-15 and PDGF-RA were down-regulated, consistent with other studies.[59,104] Importantly, members of the MAPK pathway and pathways involving oxidative stress were found to be up-regulated in endometriosis lesions compared to normal endometrium, as also found in an earlier study on deep endometriosis by Matsazuki et al[104] (see below). In summary, this study by Wu et al[103] underscores the differences in gene expression in ovarian and peritoneal disease and some important pathways that have been implicated in the pathogenesis of endometriosis.[105] Furthermore, it offers promise for another classification system of endometriosis, based on epithelial gene clustering and expression profiles.

Other studies include a spotted cDNA microarray analysis by Arimoto et al,[106] in which expression profiles of ovarian endometriomas, compared to eutopic endometrium, were investigated. Fifteen genes were found to be commonly up-regulated regardless of cycle phase, and 42 and 40 were up-regulated only in

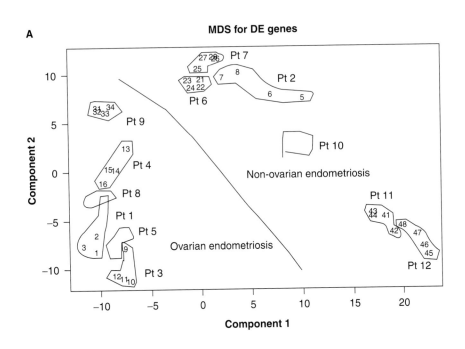

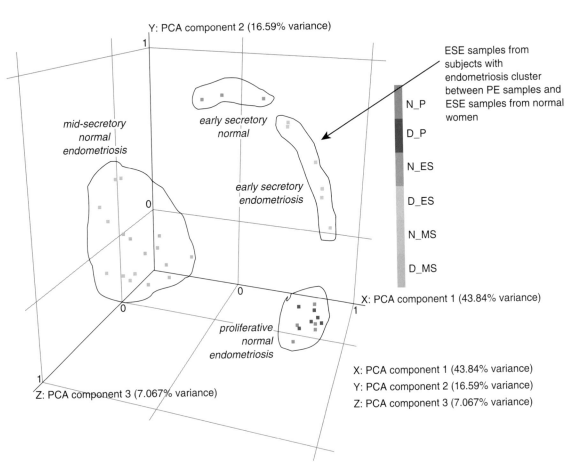

Figure 14.5   Multidimensional scaling (MDS) analysis of human endometriosis tissue. **(A)** Cluster by tissue type. Note that ovarian endometriomas cluster together, and non-ovarian endometriosis cluster separately. (Reproduction with permission from Wu et al).[103] **(B)**. Clustering or samples into cycle phase revealed by principal component analysis (see text). (Reproduction with permission from Burney et al.[60])

proliferative and secretory phases, respectively. Several genes were also found to be down-regulated uniquely in each phase or in both phases. In another study, genes involved in immunoreactions in endometriotic lesions were identified using cDNA chips.[107] Deep endometriosis (i.e. rectovaginal disease, compared to ovarian and peritoneal disease) has been characterized from a transcriptome perspective by Matsuzaki et al[104] using cDNA microarrays and LCM. They found that PDGF-RA, PKCb1, and JAK1 were up-regulated, and sprouty 2 and MAP kinase kinase 7 were down-regulated in endometriosis stromal cells, supporting a role for the RAS/RAF/ MAPK signaling pathway, perhaps through the PDGF-RA in the pathogenesis of the disorder. Furthermore, in endometriosis epithelial cells, COUP-TF2 and PGE2/ EP3, were down-regulated. Since these are putative negative regulators of aromatase, their down-regulation may contribute to the known estradiol synthesis that occurs in some endometriotic lesions (see Chapter 45). Three up-regulated genes were also identified that may be candidates that participate in the pathogenesis of the disorder: the tyrosine kinase receptor B (TRkB) in endometriosis epithelium and the serotonin transporter (5HTT) and the mu opioid receptor (MOR) in endometriosis stromal cells. The latter has been postulated to be involved in the proposed abnormal immune response observed in women with endometriosis.[104]

Endometrial stromal cells from eutopic endometrium and from endometriomas were evaluated for their response to IL-1β, an inflammatory cytokine produced by activated macrophages and central to monocyte chemotaxis and neoangiogenesis of endometriotic implants. Using a cDNA microarray approach, Taylor and colleagues[108] demonstrated altered expression of a cell cycle suppressor gene, Tob-1, in endometriotic stromal cells. Treatment with IL-1β of stromal cells isolated from endometriotic lesions and eutopic endometrium had differential responsiveness, with IL-1β down-regulating Tob-1 in endometriotic stromal cells and having minimal effect on normal stromal cells. Together, these results suggest that IL-1β promotes growth of endometriotic lesions through inhibition of Tob-1 and imply an association of IL-1β with an alteration of cell cycle gene expression in cells derived from endometriotic implants.[108]

Summary: thus, the data highly suggest that there is dysregulation in ectopic endometrium that involves genes that are members of the Ras, MAP kinase, and perhaps PI3 kinase signaling pathways. This is consistent with a mouse model of overexpression of k-ras and conditional Pten deletion in ovarian surface epithelium that resulted in endometriosis (and endometrioid ovarian carcinoma).[105]

Eutopic endometrium in women with vs without endometriosis

While ectopic and eutopic endometrium differ in their gene expression in subsets of endometriosis (e.g. peritoneal, deep lesions, and endometriomas), whether eutopic endometrium of women with endometriosis has equivalent responsiveness to steroid hormones and 'normalcy' of function, compared to women without disease, is an important question to resolve. Global transcriptome analysis has given insight into these issues, from the perspective of molecular mechanisms potentially acting in the pathogenesis of the disorder and for an opportunity to identify markers for the disease.

Taylor and colleagues[109] compared genes expressed in eutopic endometrium from women with endometriosis to those expressed in eutopic endometrium from women without disease, during the mid-proliferative phase of the cycle. Using differential display, they found up-regulation of a zinc-finger transcription factor coded by the early growth response (EGR)-1 gene in ectopic and eutopic endometrium of women with endometriosis compared to normal eutopic endometrium. EGR-1 is upregulated by E_2, IL-1β, IL-6, and TNFα (inflammatory cytokines) and may enhance angiogenesis via regulation of VEGF and its receptors. Many upstream regulators of EGR-1 are associated with endometriosis, and this gene has been proposed to play a central role in the pathogenesis of this disorder.[109]

Using high-density oligonucleotide microarrays, Kao et al[59] investigated genes differentially expressed in the implantation window in eutopic endometrium from women with minimal/mild endometriosis, compared to normal women. Of the 12 686 genes analyzed, 91 were significantly up-regulated and 115 genes were significantly down-regulated, greater than two-fold. Unsupervised clustering analysis revealed down-regulation of several known cell adhesion molecules, endometrial epithelial secreted proteins, and proteins not previously known to be associated with endometriosis, as well as up-regulated genes. Of note is the down-regulation of N-acetylglucosamine-6-O-sulfotransferase, glycodelin, IL-15, and Dikkopf-1, and up-regulation of semaphorin E. N-acetylglucosamine-6-O-sulfotransferase synthesizes a ligand for L-selectin which is important for blastocyst attachment to the endometrial epithelium.[110] Also, glycodelin and IL-15 are progesterone-regulated genes in the peri-implantation period that are believed to play a major role in immunomodulation of the implantation process. These data suggest that there is a relatively poor response to progesterone action in the endometrium during the implantation window in women with disease. Based on the findings in this study (and others[98]), dysfunctions in embryonic attachment, survival, and signaling are mechanisms postulated to be operational in eutopic endometrium of women with endometriosis that may contribute to infertility associated with this disorder.

Recently, Burney, Talbi, Giudice, and colleagues[100] have investigated the whole genome transcriptome of eutopic endometrium in late-proliferative, and early- and mid-secretory phases in women with moderate to severe disease (peritoneal lesions, no ovarian endometriomas), compared to women without disease. Marked dysregulation of gene expression in ESE in women with disease, compared to normal women, was found, with a fingerprint of persistence of cellular mitosis and minimal responsiveness of classically progesterone-regulated genes in ESE and in MSE. PCA revealed that ESE specimens from women with endometriosis collectively clustered closer to PE specimens than did the normal ESE specimens (Figure 14.5B), suggesting resistance to progesterone action on the molecular level in the transition from PE to ESE. Figure 14.4B shows the schematic of where resistance to progesterone is postulated to occur in eutopic endometrium in women with pelvic peritoneal disease. Furthermore, several genetic loci associated with endometriosis were identified among the dysregulated candidate genes. These data further support progesterone resistance as a common theme in endometrium of women with endometriosis, consistent with inadequate clinical response to progestins in women with this disorder.[98–100]

Cell-specific differences in gene expression, determined by LCM and cDNA microarray analysis in LPE, ESE, MSE, and LSE in women with deep endometriosis compared to women without disease, were recently reported by Matsuzaki et al.[111] They found up-regulation in LSE of RON, SOS, 14-3-3 protein eta, and uPAR in epithelial cells and KSR (a MAPK scaffold of the Ras pathway), and PI3K p85 regulatory subunit α in stromal cells. These genes are involved in two important signaling pathways – RAS/RAF/MAPK and PI3K. These results are strikingly similar to the abnormalities reported in ectopic lesions, suggesting a common dysregulation of signaling in eutopic and ectopic endometrium in women with endometriosis among pathways that participate in a variety of cellular functions, including cell cycle regulation and cell survival, with the ectopic lesions probably a more extreme phenotype.

THE ENDOMETRIAL TRANSCRIPTOME IN EARLY PREGNANCY

The decidua of early pregnancy

The decidua (the endometrium of pregnancy) is a unique tissue composed of primarily stromal fibroblasts and immune cells, as well as vascular components and epithelium. It is the tissue into which the extravillous trophoblast invades to reach the endometrial vessels for replacement as endovascular trophoblasts and establishing placental vasculature, in which the pregnancy is firmly anchored, and where immune tolerance of the conceptus proceeds.[112] Decidual fibroblasts are probably major regulators of these processes, as are resident and transient immune cells. Decidual cells have distinct phenotypes due to the action of progesterone on them and probably the result of paracrine interactions among cells within microenvironments in the decidua. The tissue is shed upon parturition, after which the endometrium begins the process of repair. This subsection presents the transcriptome of the decidua in early pregnancy in humans. Subsequent subsections present data on the transcriptome of decidualization of endometrial stromal fibroblasts in vitro in response to progesterone and analogues of cyclic AMP (cAMP). Included also are the transcriptomes of decidual cells in response to trophoblast-secreted products, and mouse implantation sites and inter-implantation sites. While the processes of implantation are unique in humans and rodents, there are some commonly regulated genes in the maternal endometrium that suggest broad categories of commonality of functions, including immune responses, ECM remodeling and signaling, and crosstalk between the conceptus and the decidua.

Chen and colleagues[113] investigated genes differentially expressed in early human pregnancy decidua and chorionic villi, obtained from first trimester abortus specimens (6–8 weeks' gestational age). Villi were separated from the decidua, and samples were processed for analysis on a 9600 cDNA microarray. Surprisingly, 641 genes were commonly expressed in the decidua and villi, underscoring potential redundancy of gene expression and processes in the floating villi and the decidua. The decidua was enriched in 49 genes, including CTGF, IGFBP-1, IGFBP-4, cathespin L, IL-1 type I receptor, the insulin receptor, and S-100 calcium-binding protein. These genes are also known to be expressed in the endometrium in response to progesterone from studies of human endometrial biopsies in the window of implantation[17,18] and also in decidualizing human endometrial stromal cells in response to progesterone and cAMP[114–116] (and see below). Chorionic villi were enriched in 75 genes, compared to decidua, including inhibin β_A, stromelysin-3, glycoprotein hormone α subunit, human GH-variant, LIF receptor, and other cell growth and cycle regulators, apoptosis-related factors, hormones, cytokines, ECM/cytoskeleton, stress-response factors, and signal transducers. This study gives an important insight into genes and processes occurring in decidua and in chorionic villi in early gestation. Additionally, the transcriptome reflecting interactions between the decidua and the invading trophoblast in the anchoring villous (compared to floating villi, as in the study by Chen et al[113]) has been investigated in in-vitro models and is described below.

Decidual natural killer cells

Natural killer cells constitute 50–90% of lymphocytes and about 30–50% of total cells in human uterine decidua in early pregnancy. Koopman and colleagues[117] investigated the transcriptome of the CD56[bright] uterine decidual NK cells (dNK) from early pregnancy, compared to CD56[dim] peripheral NK cells, using high-density oligonucleotide arrays containing about 10 000 probe sets. They found that 278 genes were significantly changed greater than three-fold, with the highest percentage represented by cell surface proteins, including lectin-like receptors NKG2E and Ly-49L, several NK Ig-like receptors, α^D, α^x, β_1, and β_5 integrin subunits, and several tetraspanins (CD9, CD151, CD53, CD63, and TSPAN-5), in addition to two secreted proteins, galectin-1 and glycodelin. The latter is a major product of cycling endometrial epithelium in the secretory phase (see 'The window of implantation' section), and the finding of its production in dNK cells was surprising. The data underscore a unique transcriptome of the dNK cell in early pregnancy decidua, and mining the significance of many of these genes in the process of implantation and pregnancy maintenance is an important area of research.

Decidualization of endometrial stromal fibroblasts

Decidualization (differentiation) of endometrial stromal fibroblasts is initiated by progesterone and, in humans, occurs independently of the presence of a conceptus, beginning in the mid–late secretory phase. It is essential for successful implantation and continues in conception cycles, accompanied by a distinct morphological appearance of the stromal fibroblasts and by a unique biosynthetic and secretory phenotype.[11,12,25,26] Decidualization in vitro can be achieved with progesterone, after estradiol priming, and also by cAMP and other ligands that activate the protein kinase A-dependent pathway (see Chapter 25), although the precise interactions of the pathways stimulated by these effectors remain to be determined. In vitro, achieving the secretory phenotype (measured by IGFBP-1 [a decidual 'marker'] secreted into the conditioned medium [CM]) in response to progesterone after E_2 priming takes about 7–10 days, whereas the response to cAMP in achieving equivalent levels of IGFBP-1 in the CM takes about 1–2 days. The early response to progesterone and subsequent molecular mechanisms underlying the process of decidualization are not completely understood, and several groups have investigated the transcriptome of human endometrial stromal fibroblasts in response to agents that are known to promote decidualization, with the goal of understanding the biological processes and biochemical pathways involved. These are described below.

The first study to address the transcriptome of stromal fibroblast decidualization was by Popovici et al,[114] in which the cells were treated for 10 days with progesterone and E_2 or for 48 hours with 8-Br-cAMP, compared to no treatment (non-decidualized controls), and subsequent analysis of RNA on cDNA microarrays containing 588 annotated genes. Up-regulation of the insulin and FSH receptors, some neurotransmitter receptors, neuromodulators, inhibin/activin β_A subunit, inhibin α, specific cytokines, growth factors, nuclear transcription factors, members of the cyclin family, and mediators of the cAMP signal transduction pathway were found, as were members of the angiotensin/renin family and the TNF-related apoptosis inducing ligand (TRAIL). Major contributions of this study were the discovery of new members of the TGFβ family up-regulated during decidualization, the expression of neuromodulators and neurotransmitter receptors, and many immune genes that had not been recognized in the process of decidualization of endometrial stromal fibroblasts.

Subsequently, Brar and colleagues[115] and Tierney and colleagues[116] reported the results of expanded transcriptomics studies. Brar et al,[115] using the Incyte human GEM-V microarray (6918 genes/ESTs), interrogated gene expression of human term decidual fibroblasts in response to combined treatment with progesterone, E_2, and 8Br-cAMP for 0, 2, 4, 6, 9, 12, and 15 days. Kinetic analysis revealed classification of the 121 up-regulated and 110 down-regulated and 51 biphasically regulated genes into five categories:

- cell and tissue function
- cell and tissue structure
- regulation of gene expression
- ESTs
- unknown function.

Temporal changes were observed in proteins involved in extracellular organization, cytoskeletal organization, and cell adhesion, transcription factors, members of the IGF family, early induction of genes involved in MAP kinase signaling, as well as others. Many genes were reprogrammed within specific functional groups and gene families with simultaneous induction and down-regulation of sets of genes with related functions, suggesting that reprogramming of gene expression within functional categories represents a fundamental aspect of cellular differentiation in general, and for the decidualizing pregnancy fibroblasts, in particular.

In the study by Tierney et al,[116] a kinetic analysis of gene expression was conducted, using stromal fibroblasts from cycling endometrium and treatment with 8Br-cAMP at 0, 2, 4, 6, 12, 24, and 48 hours. Of the nearly 6000 probe sets on the Affymetrix high-density oligonucleotide arrays, similar results of gene and gene family reprogramming during the decidualization process were observed. Most abundantly, up-regulated genes included neuropeptides, immune genes, IGF family members, cell cycle regulators, and genes involved in cholesterol trafficking, cell growth, and differentiation, hormone signaling, and signal transduction. Most abundantly, down-regulated genes included the activator of NF-kB, actin/troppomyosin/calmodulin-binding protein, cyclin B and E_2, IGFBP-5, and α1 type XVI collagen, and secreted frizzled related protein 1. Striking was the down-regulation of genes involved in G-protein signaling and up-regulation of genes involved in STAT pathway signaling, structural proteins, cellular differentiation, and secretory processes. The temporal analysis revealed that the early response to cAMP (0–6 hours) involves primarily cell cycle regulation; intermediate events (12–24 hours) involve genes regulating cellular differentiation, cell morphology, and the secretory phenotype; and late events (24–48 hours) had enrichment of genes mediating more specialized functions, including immunomodulation.

In another study, Okada et al[118] investigated gene expression in endometrial stromal fibroblasts from cycling endometrium treated for 3 days in 10% fetal calf serum containing progesterone. In this study, cDNA spotted arrays were used, containing nearly 1000 probes, and results similar to those of Brar et al[115] and Tierney et al[116] were observed (e.g. down-regulation of IGFBP-5 and changes in genes involved in cell differentiation and immunomodulation).

Animal studies in which homologous recombination and gene knockouts have resulted in defective decidualization and implantation phenotypes are valuable in identifying specific genes important in the decidualization process (see Lim et al,[19] for review): included in these are Hox A-10, Hox A-11, IL-11, and LIF. While decidualization in mice occurs in the presence of an embryo or can be induced mechanically or by inflammation (e.g. infusion of oil into the uterine cavity), participants in the decidualization process in mice may have commonalities with the process in humans. Indeed, the effector molecules listed above have important roles in decidualization in human endometrium (see Giudice,[5] for review).

Response of endometrial cells to trophoblast-secreted products

During the invasive phase of implantation, trophoblasts, decidual fibroblasts, and lymphocytes secrete products that probably contribute to regulation of trophoblast differentiation and migration and some of the phenotypes of other cells in situ. Global cross-talk between the trophoblast and the decidua has recently been investigated by Hess and colleagues,[120] in which human endometrial stromal fibroblasts were decidualized with progesterone and then treated with CM from human extravillous trophoblasts (TCM) or with control conditioned media (CCM) from non-decidualized stromal cells for 0, 3, and 12 hours. Samples were processed for transcriptome analysis on whole genome, high-density oligonucleotide arrays, containing 54 600 probe sets. Many genes (1374) were significantly up-regulated, and 3443 genes were significantly down-regulated after 12 hours of treating cells with products secreted by the TCM compared with CCM. The most highly up-regulated genes were the chemokines CXCL-1 (GRO1) and IL-8, CXCR4, and other immune related genes (SCYA8, PTX3, IL-6, and interferon-regulated and related genes), as well as TNFAIP6 and the matrix metalloproteinases MMP-1, MMP-10, and MMP-14. Gene ontology analysis and KEGG pathway analysis revealed cytokine/chemokine signaling pathways highly represented, including JAK/STAT, MAPK, and others. While the ligands in the TCM are not clearly defined, currently, the biochemical pathways and signaling pathways suggest the ligands may include IL-1 and interferon-like molecules. Indeed, analysis of the transcriptome of genes regulated by IL-1β in human endometrial stromal fibroblasts confirms marked up-regulation of CXCL-1 and IL-8.[121] The most highly down-regulated genes included growth factors, e.g. IGF-I, FGF-1, TGFβ$_1$ and angiopoietin-1, and genes involved in Wnt signaling (Wnt4, FZD2). In-situ expression of some proteins corresponding to the observed regulated genes was validated by immunohistochemistry of human placental bed specimens. Thus, there is a significant induction of proinflammatory cytokines and chemokines, as well as angiogenic/static factors in decidualized endometrial stromal fibroblasts in response to trophoblast-secreted products, suggesting that the trophoblast acts to alter the local immune environment of the decidua to facilitate the process of implantation and assure an enriched cytokine/chemokine environment, while limiting mitotic activity of the stromal cells during the early invasive phase of implantation. In a study by Popovici et al using co-cultured human first trimester trophoblasts and decidualized endometrial stromal fibroblasts,[122] strikingly similar results were obtained, with marked up-regulation of chemokines and angiogenic factors in the stromal fibroblasts. These complementary study designs with similar outcomes underscore the reliability of the data.

The transcriptome of human endometrial stromal fibroblasts co-cultured with BeWo cells, a choriocarcinoma cell line, was investigated by Cowan, Hines, and colleagues,[123] using DD-PCR. Several genes were identified to be up- and down-regulated and the complement of differentially regulated genes was a function of the degree of stromal fibroblast decidualization prior to co-culture and the duration of co-culture. Soares pregnant uterus gene was up-regulated in cells co-cultured with BeWo cells for 4 hours, and has been identified during endometrial stromal fibroblast decidualization.[116] The significance of this is not clear, although it may be that trophoblast enhances interactions with the stromal compartment as it invades through it.

Mouse implantation sites and inter-implantation sites

Implantation in the mouse occurs on day 4 (d4), where d0 = day of the vaginal plug. The uterine transcriptome just before (d3.5) and after (d5.0) implantation was investigated by Yoshioka et al,[124] using oligonucleotide microarrays containing 6500 probe sets: 192 genes were up-regulated and 207 were down-regulated as a result of the pre- to post-implantation transition. Since decidualization is prominent on d5, most of the enriched genes are probably decidual rather than implantation-specific. Also, some of the genes may be myometrial in origin, as whole uterine RNA was used. Nevertheless, several genes were subsequently found to agree with those of Cheon et al[55] on PR-regulated genes (see below).

The transcriptomes of mouse implantation and inter-implantation sites were investigated by Reese et al,[125] using oligonucleotide microarrays having 6500 probe sets. In addition, they investigated uterine gene expression in progesterone-treated, delayed implanting mice vs those in which delayed implantation is terminated by E$_2$ administration. The implantation sites, compared to the inter-implantation sites, contained 36 up-regulated genes and 27 down-regulated genes, and in delayed implantation, 128 genes were up-regulated and 101 were down-regulated. While a combined analysis revealed specific up-regulation of 27 genes both at the implantation site and during uterine activation, representing a broad diversity of molecular functions, the majority of genes that were decreased in the combined analysis were related to the immune response of the host. These data underscore the important role of the immune system in regulating the environment for an implanting blastocyst.

Lessons from selective progesterone receptor modulators in the mouse

Progesterone regulation of gene expression in the mouse has been investigated in the context of pregnancy in RU-486-treated animals. It should be noted that homologous recombination and gene deletion of the PR in the mouse[56] revealed that the females are sterile. Thus, delineation of the progesterone-regulated transcriptome using this model has not been possible, and the use of PR antagonists, such as RU-486, has been more informative. Cheon et al[55] investigated the uterine transcriptome regulated by progesterone acting through the PR, by administering a PR antagonist, RU-486, on d3 of pregnancy and collecting uteri on d4 and subsequently flushing out the embryos. Of over 6500 genes/ESTs interrogated, 78 genes were down-regulated in the RU-486-treated mice, compared to vehicle controls, and 70 genes were up-regulated, using a two-fold threshold. Immunohistochemical validation revealed that subsets of progesterone-regulated genes identified by the microarray analysis had distinct cell type-specific expression patterns, and that the spatial–temporal expression of these genes mimicked the expression of PR in the uterus during pregnancy, supporting their regulation by progesterone. Several of the down-regulated genes correspond to those observed by Yoshioka et al[124] including amphiregulin, fisp 12 (a member of the CTGF family), epidermal-12/15-lipoxygenase, follistatin, Rho B, and laminin-2-α2 chain. Of particular interest are genes, for example, involved in metabolism, such as lipoxygenases. Also, of interest are other metabolic enzymes likely to be important in the known increased oxygen consumption in uterine tissues and glucose regulation that occur on d4 and in suppressing FSH during pregnancy (follistatin). Several genes were also in agreement with the study by Reese et al,[125] in which the embryos were in the implantation sites during the analysis, and a different experimental paradigm was used.

Genes in common

That several genes and gene families are up- and down-regulated in early implantation (compared to pre-implantation or at inter-implantation sites) and are also regulated by progesterone, validates this approach of investigating the transcriptome of progesterone-regulated genes in the murine model. Also, the data provide important insight into mechanisms involved in implantation, especially since several genes are common to the window of implantation in humans.[17–20] This observation supports conservation of some mechanisms across species, and also the uniqueness of the implantation process that is species-specific.

SUMMARY AND EYE TO THE FUTURE

Transcriptomics is well suited to the endometrium, a tissue that dynamically changes in response to steroid hormones and mediators. Discovery-driven approaches have provided insights into biological processes and biochemical pathways, in general, and this is particularly true throughout the menstrual cycle in health and disease in human and non-human primate endometrium. Hypothesis-driven science is complementary to discovery-driven science,[126] and it is anticipated that more hypotheses will be generated based on insights gained from the discovery approach. Furthermore, development of candidate genes as diagnostic biomarkers and therapeutic targets is still in its infancy but offers

great opportunity for the future and would benefit from elucidation of at least some part of the endometrial proteome.[127] Functions of the multitude of components of the resulting proteome are indeed challenges for the future, as the complexities of the proteome are probably orders of magnitude greater than the transcriptome. Other 'omics', including, for example, the glycome and metabolome, are additional players in the equation of cellular function and dysfunction and remain an important part of investigation and translation of the biology of this important tissue.

ACKNOWLEDGMENTS

Supported (in part) by the NIH Specialized Cooperative Centers Program in Reproductive Research (U54-HD 31398) (LCG).

The authors wish to acknowledge members of the Giudice laboratory who have contributed over the years to an understanding of the biology and the transcriptome of human endometrium, and also would like to recognize Alexander Theologis for his help with the references. Also, Dr Giudice would like to dedicate this chapter to the memory of her PhD advisor, John G Pierce PhD who was an outstanding mentor, biochemist, and humanist. He demonstrated the highest standards of integrity in his quest for discovery and held his students to task. Dr Pierce passed away in 2006, and his memory will live on in his contributions to the science of glycoprotein hormone biology and biochemistry, and in the hearts of his students and colleagues for many years to come.

REFERENCES

1. Velculescu VE, Zhang L, Zhou W et al. Characterization of yeast transcriptome. Cell 1997; 88: 243–51.
2. Carter D. Cellular transcriptomics – the next phase of endocrine expression profiling. Trends Endocrinol Metab 2006; 17: 192–8.
3. Subramanian A, Tamayo P, Mootha VK et al. Gene set enrichment analysis: a knowledge-based approach for interpreting genome-wide expression profiles. Proc Natl Acad Sci USA 2005; 102: 15545–50.
4. Giudice, LC. Elucidating endometrial function in the post-genomic era. Hum Reprod Update 2003; 9: 223–35.
5. Giudice LC. Application of functional genomics to primate endometrium: insights into biological processes. Reprod Biol Endocrinol 2006; 9(4 Suppl 1): S4.
6. Horcajadas JA, Pellicer A, Simon C. Wide genomic analysis of human endometrial receptivity: new times, new opportunities. Human Reprod Update 2007; 13: 77–86.
7. Romero R, Tromp G. High-dimensional biology in obstetrics and gynecology: functional genomics in microarray studies. Am J Obstet Gynecol 2006; 195: 360–3.

8. Tarca AL, Romero R, Draghici S. Analysis of microarray experiments of gene expression profiling. Am J Obstet Gynecol 2006; 195: 373–88.

9. Ward K. Microarray technology in obstetrics and gynecology: a guide for clinicians. Am J Obstet Gynecol 2006; 195: 364–72.

10. Hess A, Nayak N, Giudice LC. Oviduct and endometrium: cyclic changes in the primate oviduct and endometrium. In: Knobil E, Neill JD, eds. The Physiology of Reproduction, 3rd edn. St Louis: Elsevier; 2006: 337–81.

11. Noyes RW, Hertig AT, Rock J. Dating the endometrial biopsy. Fertil Steril 1950; 1: 3–17.

12. Noyes RW, Hertig AT, Rock J. Dating the endometrial biopsy. Am J Obstet Gynecol 1975; 122: 262–3.

13. Coutifaris C, Myers ER, Guzick DS et al. Histological dating of timed endometrial biopsy tissue is not related to fertility status. Fertil Steril 2004; 82: 1264–72.

14. Murray MJ, Meyer WR, Zaino RJ et al. A critical analysis of the accuracy, reproducibility, and clinical utility of histologic endometrial dating in fertile women. Fertil Steril 2004; 81: 1333–43.

15. Ponnampalam AP, Weston GC, Trajstman AC et al. Molecular classification of human endometrial cycle stages by transcriptional profiling. Mol Hum Reprod 2004; 10: 879–93.

16. Talbi S, Hamilton AE, Vo KC et al. Molecular phenotyping of human endometrium distinguishes menstrual cycle phases and underlying biological processes in normo-ovulatory women. Endocrinology 2006; 147: 1097–121.

17. Kao LC, Tulac S, Lobo S et al. Global gene profiling in human endometrium during the window of implantation. Endocrinology 2002; 143: 2119–38.

18. Carson DD, Lagow E, Thathiah A et al. Changes in gene expression during the early to mid-luteal (receptive phase) transition in human endometrium detected by high-density microarray screening. Mol Hum Reprod 2002; 8: 871–9.

19. Borthwick JM, Charnock-Jones DS, Tom BD et al. Determination of the transcript profile of human endometrium. Mol Hum Reprod 2003; 9: 19–33.

20. Riesewijk A, Martín J, van Os R et al. Gene expression profiling of human endometrial receptivity on days LH+2 versus LH+7 by microarray technology. Mol Hum Reprod 2003; 9: 253–64.

21. Ace CI, Okulicz WC. Microarray profiling of progesterone-regulated endometrial genes during the rhesus monkey secretory phase. Reprod Biol Endocrinol 2004; 2: 54–62.

22. Horcajadas JA, Riesewijk A, Martín J et al. Global gene expression profiling of human endometrial receptivity. J Reprod Immunol 2004; 63: 41–9.

23. Punyadeera C, Dassen H, Klomp J et al. Oestrogen-modulated gene expression in the human endometrium. Cell Mol Life Sci 2005; 62: 239–50.

24. Mirkin S, Arslan M, Churikov D et al. In search of candidate genes critically expressed in the human endometrium during the window of implantation. Hum Reprod 2005; 20: 2104–17.

25. Ferenczy A, Bergeron C. Histology of the human endometrium: from birth to senescence. Ann NY Acad Sci 1991; 622: 6–27.

26. Giudice LC, Ferenczy A. The endometrial cycle: morphologic and biochemical events. In: Adashi EY, Rock JA, Rosenwaks Z, eds, Reproductive Endocrinology, Surgery, and Technology. New York: Raven Press, 1995; 1: 171–94.

27. Yanaihara A, Otsuka Y, Iwasaki S et al. Differences in gene expression in the proliferative human endometrium. Fertil Steril 2005; 83: 1206–15.

28. Krikun G, Schatz F, Taylor R et al. Endometrial endothelial cell steroid receptor expression and steroid effects on gene expression. J Clin Endocrinol Metab 2005; 90: 1812–18.

29. Print C, Valtola R, Evans A et al. Soluble factors from human endometrium promote angiogenesis and regulate the endothelial cell transcriptome. Hum Reprod 2004; 19: 2356–66.

30. Mustonen MV, Isomaa VV, Vaskivuo T et al. Human 17beta-hydroxysteroid dehydrogenase type 2 messenger ribonucleic acid expression and localization in term placenta and in endometrium during the menstrual cycle. J Clin Endocrinol Metab 1998; 83: 1319–24.

31. Lessey BA, Killam AP, Metzger DA et al. Immunohistochemical analysis of human uterine estrogen and progesterone receptors throughout the menstrual cycle. J Clin Endocrinol Metab 1988; 67: 334–40.

32. Bergqvist A, Ferno M. Oestrogen and progesterone receptors in endometriotic tissue and endometrium: comparison of different cycle phases and ages. Hum Reprod 1993; 8: 2211–27.

33. Mote PA, Balleine RL, McGowan EM, Clarke CL. Heterogeneity of progesterone receptors A and B expression in human endometrial glands and stroma. Hum Reprod 2000; 15(Suppl 3): 48–56.

34. Mylonas I, Jeschke U, Shabani N et al. Immunohistochemical analysis of estrogen receptor alpha, estrogen receptor beta and progesterone receptor in normal human endometrium. Acta Histochem 2004; 106: 245–52.

35. Brayman M, Thathiah A, Carson DD. MUC1: a multifunctional cell surface component of reproductive tissue epithelia. Reprod Biol Endocrinol 2004; 2: 4.

36. Tulac S, Overgaard MT, Hamilton AE et al. Dikkopf-1, an inhibitor of Wnt signaling, is regulated by progesterone in human endometrial stromal cells. J Clin Endocrinol Metab 2006; 91: 1453–61.

37. Dunn CL, Critchley HO, Kelly RW. IL-15 regulation in human endometrial stromal cells. J Clin Endocrinol Metab 2002; 87: 1898–901.

38. Okada H, Nakajima T, Sanezumi M et al. Progesterone enhances interleukin-15 production in human endometrial stromal cells in vitro. J Clin Endocrinol Metab 2000; 85: 4765–70.

39. Giudice LC. Microarray expression profiling reveals candidate genes for human uterine receptivity. Am J Pharmacogenomics 2004; 4: 299–312.

40. Schmmidt A, Groth P, Haendler B et al. Gene expression during the implantation window: microarray analysis of human endometrial samples. Ernst Schering Res Found Workshop 2005; 52: 139–57.

41. Horcajadas JA, Riesewijk A, Polman J et al. Effect of controlled ovarian hyperstimulation in IVF on endometrial gene expression profiles. Mol Hum Reprod 2005; 11: 195–205.

42. Muller WA. New mechanisms and pathways for monocyte recruitment. J Exp Med 2001; 194: F47–51.

43. Bhatt H, Brunet LJ, Stewart CL. Uterine expression of leukemia inhibitory factor coincides with the onset of blastocyst implantation. Proc Natl Acad Sci USA 1991; 88: 11408–12.

44. Stewart CL, Kaspar P, Brunet LJ et al. Blastocyst implantation depends on maternal expression of leukaemia inhibitory factor. Nature 1992; 359: 76–9.

45. Kondera-Anasz Z, Sikora J, Mielczarek-Palacz A. Leukemia inhibitory factor: an important regulator of endometrial function. Am J Reprod Immunol 2004; 52: 97–105.

46. Hambartsoumian E. Endometrial leukemia inhibitory factor (LIF) as a possible cause of unexplained infertility and multiple failures of implantation. Am J Reprod Immunol 1998; 39: 137–43.

47. Tsai HD, Chang CC, Hsieh YY, Lo HY. Leukemia inhibitory factor expression in different endometrial locations between fertile and infertile women throughout different menstrual phases. J Assist Reprod Genet 2000; 17: 415–18.

48. Kitaya K, Yamaguchi T, Honjo H. Central role of interleukin-15 in postovulatory recruitment of peripheral blood CD16(−) natural killer cells into human endometrium. J Clin Endocrinol Metab 2005; 90: 2932–40.

49. Booker SS, Jayanetti C, Karalak S et al. The effect of progesterone on the accumulation of leukocytes in the human endometrium. Am J Obstet Gynecol 1994; 171: 139–42.

50. Domínguez F, Avila S, Cervero A et al. A combined approach for gene discovery identifies insulin-like growth factor-binding protein-related protein 1 as a new gene implicated in human endometrial receptivity. J Clin Endocrinol Metab 2003; 88: 1849–87.

51. Ioachim EE, Kitsiou E, Carassavoglou C et al. Immuno-histochemical localization of metallothionein in endometrial lesions. J Pathol 2000; 191: 269–73.

52. Sies H. Strategies of antioxidant defense. Eur J Biochem 1993; 215: 213–19.

53. Kingsley PD, Whitin JC, Cohen HJ, Palis J. Developmental expression of extracellular glutathione peroxidase suggests antioxidant roles in deciduum, visceral yolk sac, and skin. Mol Reprod Dev 1998; 49: 343–55.

54. Leonhardt SA, Boonyaratanakornkit V, Edwards DP. Progesterone receptor transcription and non-transcription signaling mechanisms. Steroids 2003; 68: 761–70.

55. Cheon YP, Li Q, Xu X et al. A genomic approach to identify novel progesterone receptor regulated pathways in the uterus during implantation. Mol Endocrinol 2002; 16: 2853–71.

56. Lydon JP, DeMayo FJ, Conneely OM, O'Malley BW. Reproductive phenotypes of the progesterone receptor null mutant mouse. J Steroid Biochem Mol Biol 1996; 56: 67–77.

57. Catalano RD, Yanaihara A, Evans AL et al. The effect of RU486 on the gene expression profile in an endometrial explant model. Mol Hum Reprod 2003; 9: 465–73.

58. Pahl PM, Horwitz MA, Horwitz KB, Horwitz LD. Desferri-exochelin induces death by apoptosis in human breast cancer cells but does not kill normal breast cells. Breast Cancer Res Treat 2001; 69: 69–79.

59. Kao LC, Germeyer A, Tulac S et al. Expression profiling of endometrium from women with endometriosis reveals candidate genes for disease-based implantation failure and infertility. Endocrinology 2003; 144: 2870–81.

60. Burney RO, Talbi S, Hamilton AE et al. Gene expression analysis of endometrium reveals progesterone resistance and candidate genetic loci in women with endometriosis. Endocrinology 2007; 148: 3814–26.

61. Ogawa S, Inoue S, Watanabe T et al. Molecular cloning and characterization of human estrogen receptor β: a potential inhibitor of estrogen action in human. Nucleic Acids Res 1998; 6: 3505–12.

62. Sherwin R, Catalano R, Sharkey A. Large scale gene expression studies of the endometrium: what have we learnt? Reproduction 2006; 132: 1–10.

63. Ponnampalam AP, Weston GC, Susil B, Rogers PAW. Molecular profiling of human endometrium during the menstrual cycle. Austr NZ J Obstet Gynecol 2006; 46: 154–8.

64. Ace CI, Okulicz WC. Identification of progesterone-dependent messenger ribonucleic acid regulatory patterns in the rhesus monkey endometrium by differential-display reverse transcription-polymerase chain reaction. Biol Reprod 1999; 60: 1029–35.

65. Okulicz WC, Ace CI. Temporal regulation of gene expression during the expected window of receptivity in the rhesus monkey endometrium. Biol Reprod 2003; 69: 1593–9.

66. Allan G, Campen C, Hodgen G et al. Identification of genes with differential regulation in primate endometrium during the proliferative and secretory phases of the cycle. Endocr Res 2003; 29: 53–65.

67. Vaisse C, Atger M, Potier B, Milgrom E. Human placental protein 14 gene: sequence and characterization of a short duplication. DNA Cell Biol 1990; 9: 401–13.

68. Seppala M, Taylor RN, Koistinen H et al. Glycodelin: a major lipocalin protein of the reproductive axis with diverse actions in cell recognition and differentiation. Endocrine Rev 2002; 23: 401–30.

69. Higushi T, Kanzaki H, Nakayama H et al. Induction of tissue inhibitor of metalloproteinase 3 gene during in vitro decidualization of human endometrial stromal cells. Endocrinology 1995; 136: 4973–81.

70. Martín J, Domínguez F, Ávila S et al. Human endometrial receptivity: gene regulation. J Reprod Immunol 2002; 55: 131–9.

71. Yanaihara A, Otsuka Y, Iwasaki S et al. Comparison in gene expression of secretory human endometrium using laser microdissection. Reprod Biol Endocrinol 2004; 2: 66–72.

72. Torres MST, Ace CI, Okulicz WC. Assessment and application of laser microdissection for analysis of gene expression in the rhesus monkey endometrium. Biol Reprod 2002; 67: 1067–72.

73. Ubaldi F, Bourgain C, Tournaye H et al. Endometrial evaluation by aspiration biopsy on the day of oocyte retrieval in the embryo transfer cycles in patients with serum progesterone rise during the follicular phase. Fertil Steril 1997; 67: 521–6.

74. Bourgain C, Ubaldi F, Tavaniotou A et al. Endometrial hormone receptors and proliferation index in the periovulatory phase of stimulated embryo transfer cycles in comparison with natural cycles and relation to clinical pregnancy outcome. Fertil Steril 2002; 78: 237–44.

75. Devroey P, Bourgain C, Macklon NS, Fauser BC. Reproductive biology and IVF: ovarian stimulation and endometrial receptivity. Trends Endocrinol Metab 2004; 15: 84–90.

76. Nikas G, Develioglu OH, JP Toner, HW Jones Jr. Endometrial pinopodes indicate a shift in the window of receptivity in IVF cycles. Human Reprod 1999; 14: 787–92.

77. Mirkin S, Nikas G, Hsiu JG et al. Gene expression profiles and structural/functional features of the peri-implantation endometrium in natural and gonadotropin-stimulated cycles. J Clin Endocrinol Metab 2004; 89: 5742–52.

78. CDC 2004. http://www.cdc.gov/ART/ART2004/index.html

79. Critchley HOD, Robertson KA, Forster T et al. Gene expression profiling of mid to late secretory phase endometrial biopsies from women with menstrual complaint. Am J Obstet Gynecol 2006; 195: 406.e1–16.

80. Salamonsen LA. Matrix metalloproteinases and their tissue inhibitors in endocrinology. Trends Endocrinol Metab 1996; 7: 28–34.

81. Salamonsen LA, Woolley DE. Menstruation: induction by matrix metalloproteinases and inflammatory cells. J Reprod Immunol 1999; 44: 1–27.

82. Jones RL, Kelly RW, Critchley HO. Chemokine and cyclooxygenase-2 expression in human endometrium coincides with leukocyte accumulation. Hum Reprod 1997; 12: 1300–6.

83. Critchley HO, Kelly RW, Brenner RM, Baird DT. The endocrinology of menstruation – a role for the immune system. Clin Endocrinol (Oxf) 2001; 55: 701–10.

84. Pickles VR. Prostaglandins in the human endometrium. Int J Fertil 1967; 12: 335–8.

85. Schatz F, Krikun G, Runic R et al. Implications of decidualization-associated protease expression in implantation and menstruation. Semin Reprod Endocrinol 1999; 17: 3–12.

86. Booker SS, Jayanetti C, Karalak S et al. The effect of progesterone on the accumulation of leukocytes in the human endometrium. Am J Obstet Gynecol 1994; 171: 139–42.

87. Cornet PB, Picquet C, Lemoine P et al. Regulation and function of LEFTY-A/EBAF in the human endometrium. mRNA expression during the menstrual cycle, control by progesterone, and effect on matrix metalloprotenases. J Biol Chem 2002; 277: 42496–504.

88. Livingstone M, Fraser IS. Mechanisms of abnormal uterine bleeding. Hum Reprod Update 2002; 8: 60–7.

89. Tan YF, Li FX, Piao YS, Sun XY, Wang YL. Global gene profiling analysis of mouse uterus during the oestrous cycle. Reproduction 2003; 126: 171–82.

90. Watanabe H, Suzuki A, Kobayashi M et al. Analysis of temporal changes in the expression of estrogen-regulated genes in the uterus. J Mol Endocrinol 2003; 30: 347–58.

91. Lubahn DB, Moyer JS, Golding TS et al. Alteration of reproductive function but not prenatal sexual development after insertional disruption of the mouse estrogen receptor gene. Proc Natal Acad Sci USA 1993; 90: 11162–6.

92. Hewitt SC, Deroo BJ, Hansen K et al. Estrogen receptor-dependent genomic responses in the uterus mirror the biphasic physiological response to estrogen. Mol Endocrinol 2003; 17: 2070–83.

93. Hewitt SC, Collins J, Grissom S et al. Global uterine genomics in vivo: microarray evaluation of the estrogen receptor α-growth factor cross-talk mechanism. Mol Endocrinol 2005; 19: 657–68.

94. Nantermet PV, Masarachia P, Gentile MA et al. Androgenic induction of growth and differentiation in the rodent uterus involves the modulation of estrogen-regulated genetic pathways. Endocrinology 2005; 146: 564–78.

95. Hong SH, Nah HY, Lee JY et al. Analysis of estrogen-regulated genes in mouse uterus using cDNA microarray and laser capture microdissection. J Endocrinol 2004; 181: 157–67.

96. Wu X, Pang ST, Sahlin L et al. Gene expression profiling of the effects of castration and estrogen treatment in the rat uterus. Biol Reprod 2003; 69: 1308–17.

97. Naciff JM, Jump ML, Torontali SM et al. Gene expression profile induced by 17α-ethynyl estradiol, bisphenol A, and genistein in the developing female reproductive system of the rat. Toxicol Sci 2002; 68: 184–99.

98. Giudice LC, Kao LC. Endometriosis. Lancet Semin 2004; 364: 1789–99.

99. Swiersz LA, Giudice LC. Endometriosis. In: De Groot's Endocrinology, 5th edn. Philadelphia, PA: WB Saunders, 2005; Chapter 155: 2939–48.

100. Burney R, Giudice LC. Pathogenesis of endometriosis. In: Nezhat CR, ed. Operative Gynecologic Laparoscopy: Principles and Techniques. Cambridge, UK: Cambridge Press, 2006.

101. Eyster KM, Boles AL, Brannian JD, Hansen KA. DNA microarray analysis of gene expression markers of endometriosis. Fertil Steril 2002; 77: 38–42.

102. Hu WP, Tay SK, Zhao Y. Endometriosis-specific genes identified by real-time reverse transcription-polymerase chain reaction expression profiling of endometriosis versus autologous uterine endometrium. J Clin Endocrinol Metab 2006; 91: 228–38.

103. Wu Y, Kajdacsy-Balla A, Strawn E et al. Transcriptional characterization of differences between eutopic and ectopic endometrium. Endocrinology 2006; 147: 232–46.

104. Matsuzaki S, Canis M, Vaurs-Barrière C et al. DNA microarray analysis of gene expression profiles in deep endometriosis using laser capture microdissection. Mol Hum Reprod 2004; 10: 719–28.

105. Dinulescu DM, Ince TA, Quade BJ et al. Role of K-ras and Pten in the development of mouse models of endometriosis and endometrioid cancer. Nat Med 2005; 1: 63–70.

106. Arimoto T, Katagiri T, Oda K et al. Genome-wide cDNA microarray analysis of gene-expression profiles involved in ovarian endometriosis. Int J Oncol 2003; 22: 551–60.

107. Konno R, Yamada-Okabe H, Fujiwara H et al. Role of immunoreactions and mast cells in the pathogenesis of human endometriosis – morphologic study and gene expression analysis. Hum Cell 2003; 15: 141–9.

108. Lebovic DI, Baldocchi RA, Mueller MD, Taylor RN. Altered expression of a cell-cycle suppressor gene, Tob-1, in endometriotic cells by cDNA array analyses. Fertil Steril 2002; 78: 849–54.

109. Taylor RN, Lundeen SG, Giudice LC. Emerging role of genomics in endometriosis research. Fertil Steril 2002; 78: 694–8.

110. Genbacev OD, Prakobphol A, Foulk RA et al. Trophoblast L-selectin-mediated adhesion at the maternal–fetal interface. Science 2003; 299: 405–8.

111. Matsuzaki S, Canis M, Vaurs-Barrière C et al. DNA microarray analysis of gene expression in eutopic endometrium from patients with deep endometriosis using laser capture microdissection. Fertil Steril 2005; 84: 1180–90.

112. Lathi RA, Fisher SJ, Giudice LC. Implantation and placental physiology in early human pregnancy: the role of the maternal decidua and the trophoblast. In: De Groot's Endocrinology, 5th edn. Philadelphia, PA: WB Saunders, 2005; Chapter 181: 3341–51.

113. Chen HW, Chen JJW, Tzeng CR et al. Global analysis of differentially expressed genes in early gestational decidua and chorionic villi using a 9600 human cDNA microarray. Mol Hum Reprod 2002; 8: 475–84.

114. Popovici RM, Kao LC, Giudice LC. Discovery of new inducible genes in in vitro decidualized human endometrial stromal cells using microarray technology. Endocrinology 2000; 141: 3510–13.

115. Brar AK, Handwerger S, Kessler CA, Aronow BJ. Gene induction and categorical reprogramming during in vitro human endometrial fibroblast decidualization. Physiol Genomics 2001; 7: 135–48.

116. Tierney EP, Tulac S, Huang STJ, Giudice LC. Activation of the protein kinase A pathway in human endometrial stromal cells reveals sequential categorical gene regulation. Physiol Genomics 2003; 16: 47–66.

117. Koopman LA, Kopcow HD, Rybalov B et al. Human decidual natural killer cells are a unique NK cell subset with immunomodulatory potential. J Exp Med 2003; 198: 1201–12.

118. Okada H, Nakajima T, Yoshimura T et al. Microarray analysis of genes controlled by progesterone in human endometrial stromal cells in vitro. Gynecol Endocrinol 2003; 17: 271–80.

119. Lim H, Song H, Paria BC et al. Molecules in blastocyst implantation: uterine and embryonic perspectives. Vitamins Hormones 2002; 94: 43–76.

120. Hess AP, Dosiou CD, Hamilton AE et al. Decidual stromal cell response to paracrine signals from the trophoblast: amplification of immune and angiogenic modulators. Biol Reprod 2007; 76: 102–17.

121. Rossi M, Sharkey AM, Vigano P et al. Identification of genes regulated by interleukin-1β in human endometrial stromal cells. Reproduction 2005; 130: 721–9.

122. Popovici RM, Betzler NK, Krause MS et al. Gene expression profiling of human endometrial–trophoblast interaction in a coculture model. Endocrinology 2006; 147: 5662–75.

123. Cowan BD, Hines RS, Brackin MN, Case ST. Temporal and cell-specific gene expression by human endometrium after co-culture with trophoblast. Am J Obstet Gynecol 1999; 180: 806–14.

124. Yoshioka KI, Matsuda F, Takakura K et al. Determination of genes involved in the process of implantation: application of GeneChip to scan 6500 genes. Biochem Biophys Res Commun 2000; 272: 531–8.

125. Reese J, Das SK, Paria BC et al. Global gene expression analysis to identify molecular markers of uterine receptivity and embryo implantation. J Biol Chem 2001; 276: 44137–45.

126. Kell DB, Oliver SG. Here is the evidence, now what is the hypothesis? The complementary roles of inductive and hypothesis-driven science in the post-genomic era. BioEssays 2003; 26: 99–105.

127. LaBaer J, Carr SA. The marriage of proteomics and biomarkers. J Proteome Res 2005; 4: 1043–109.

15 Paracrine mediators of endometrial growth and differentiation

Robert M Bigsby and Kathleen E Bethin

Synopsis

Background

- Ovarian hormones regulate cell proliferation, cell differentiation, vascular development, and lymphoid cell infiltration into the endometrium in preparation for the arrival and eventual implantation of the developing embryo.
- Animal studies have demonstrated the existence of a temporal window of uterine receptivity to which the developing embryo must be synchronized to allow for attachment, implantation, and formation of the placenta.
- These processes result from a combination of the direct action of ovarian steroids and indirectly through induction of elaborated factors that affect neighboring cells and tissues, i.e. through juxtacrine or paracrine pathways.

Basic Science

- Paracrine mediation by stromal factors is important in hormonally induced changes in the endometrial epithelium and, reciprocally, an epithelial-to-stromal route also plays a role in hormone action.
- Experiments in genetically altered mice have shown that the uterine epithelial proliferative response to estradiol is partially dependent on stromal ERα.
- Similarly, the epithelial cell response to estradiol is blocked by progesterone only when the underlying stroma expresses PR; the PR status of the epithelium is irrelevant.
- Certain epithelial responses to hormones require expression of the cognate receptor in both the stroma and epithelium. The proteins lactoferrin and complement C3 are markers of estrogen-induced differentiation of mouse uterine epithelium which require ERα in both the stroma and epithelium.
- Likewise, progesterone inhibition of estrogen-induced gene expression in the epithelium requires both the stromal cell PR and the epithelial cell PR.
- Cell culture studies support the notion that hormonal regulation of human endometrial epithelial cells also requires paracrine factors derived from underlying stromal cells.
- The postnatal development of undifferentiatied uterine mesenchyme into endometrial stromal and myometrial layers in mouse requires the presence of epithelium.
- Detrimental effects of diethylstilbestrol (DES) on the development of the uterus are at least in part mediated by disruption of a paracrine pathway occurring in the epithelium-to-mesenchyme direction.
- In adult rats and mice, signals emanating from the epithelium are required for stromal decidualization.
- There is also evidence that systemic factors induced by estrogen may affect uterine cells even in the absence of uterine ERα.
- The paracrine mediators of these various effects are largely unknown, although IHH, IGF, EGF, FGF, prolactin, CG, LH, CRH, prostaglandin, GnRH, Wnt, VEGF, and TGFβ family ligands are implicated.

Clinical

- There are two components to luteal phase deficiency (LPD), the production of steroids by the ovary and the response of the endometrium to steroidal stimulation. It may be that inadequate production of hormonally regulated paracrine factors plays a role in LPD.

- PGE$_2$ synthesis and binding sites are increased in the uterus of women affected by menorrhagia, and cyclooxygenase (COX) inhibitors reduce menstrual blood loss.
- Estrogen receptor and aromatase activity are both high in endometriotic tissue. Paracrine actions of prostaglandins are implicated in the condition.
- COX inhibitors have also been successful in treating dysmenorrhea.
- Endometrial cancers exhibit either decreased expression or mutation of TGFβ receptor type II, suggesting that a lack of its growth inhibitory influence may play a role in endometrial carcinogenesis.

INTRODUCTION

Hormonal regulation of endometrial growth and differentiation

Human endometrium undergoes cyclic, hormonally driven changes in tissue morphology and functional differentiation.[1,2] Following menstruation, estrogen drives proliferation of the remaining epithelium and underlying stroma to regenerate the full thickness of the mature endometrium. Predominance of progesterone during the ovarian luteal phase pushes the epithelial cells towards a secretory phenotype and increases the complexity of the glandular structures within the endometrium. During the mid- to late-luteal phase, the subepithelial stromal cells undergo a round of proliferation and begin differentiation towards a decidualized phenotype. In addition, while under the influence of progesterone and estrogen, uterine spiral arteries grow, increasing in both length and tortuosity. Ovarian hormones also regulate infiltration of lymphoid cells into the endometrial stroma, particularly in the subepithelial, decidualizing region. All of this growth, differentiation, and tissue patterning takes place in preparation for the arrival and eventual implantation of the developing embryo. The secretory epithelial cells provide nutrients and stimuli that are required for maturation of the embryo. Proteins elaborated by the uterine epithelium activate the embryo to initiate attachment and implantation. The decidualized stromal cells participate in the formation of the maternal placenta and they secrete proteins that regulate the implantation reaction of the invading trophoblasts.

Animal studies have amply documented the existence of a temporal window of uterine receptivity to which the developing embryo must be synchronized to allow for attachment, implantation, and formation of the placenta.[3] The importance of embryo–uterine synchrony in early pregnancy in humans was shown to be crucial in a recent study of 189 human conceptions.[4] Embryo implantation, as determined by the appearance of human chorionic gonadotropin (hCG) in maternal urine, occurred 6–12 days after ovulation; the risk of early pregnancy loss increased dramatically when implantation occurred after day 10, rising to 52–82% in subjects with implantations on days 11–12. Such observations indicate that implantation occurring outside the window of uterine receptivity produces an imperfect pregnancy that is not maintained. This need for synchrony between embryo and uterus may serve as a mechanism whereby impaired embryos are eliminated.

Studies in animals and humans indicate that the processes of endometrial growth and maturation and of embryo implantation are regulated by ovarian steroids through both direct cellular action and indirectly through induction of elaborated factors that affect neighboring cells and tissues, i.e. through juxtacrine or paracrine pathways. This chapter focuses on growth and differentiation of endometrial tissues as regulated by paracrine mediators elaborated in response to ovarian hormone stimulation. A discussion of the molecules involved in cell–cell communications that regulate embryo attachment and implantation is covered in other chapters, and is not discussed herein.

Rodent models of hormonal regulation

Although they exhibit a greatly compressed ovarian cycle relative to humans, rodents have served as valuable animal models for the study of endometrial growth and differentiation. Intense study of the mouse uterus in particular has led to descriptions of hormonally regulated peptide growth factors, cell adhesion molecules, and small molecules, such as prostaglandins and nitric oxide, known to be involved in cell–cell interactions. An emerging theme that has developed from these correlative studies is the recapitulation in adulthood of tissue interactions occurring during organongenesis, but under the regulation of cyclic hormonal cues (see Chapter 1). Mouse models provide the experimental means of testing the importance of single or multiple paracrine factors in regulation of endometrial physiology. The information gained from rodent studies has been applied to investigations of human endometrial physiology, using both correlative studies to examine hormonal regulation of paracrine mediator expression and cell culture systems to test the hypothesized regulatory action of these molecules. We review investigations that led to the original paradigm of paracrine mediation in hormonally induced changes in the endometrial epithelium and examine evidence that the reciprocal paracrine pathway, an epithelial-to-stromal route, also plays a role in hormone action. In addition, we examine recent information regarding the likely mediators of these paracrine effects and how unregulated expression of these paracrine factors may play a role in endometrial pathologies.

Growth of the uterus in the ovariectomized or the immature (prepubertal) rodent has served as the standard bioassay for estrogens since the early part of the last century.[5] When a single dose of estradiol is administered to an ovariectomized adult mouse there is a dramatic proliferative response in the luminal epithelium and only a small increase in stromal cell proliferation.[6] When estradiol is administered to the immature animal, both the epithelium and the stroma respond.[7] Pretreatment of ovariectomized adult animals with progesterone 24 hours before estradiol inhibits the epithelial response to estradiol; the extent of inhibition to the epithelial response is dependent on the dose of progesterone, with a complete inhibition at doses of ≥ 20 mg/kg and approximately 50% inhibition at 10 mg/kg.[8] If the animal is pretreated with progesterone for at least 48 hours, there is a dramatic stromal cell response to a single dose of estradiol.[9] These effects mimic the physiological changes in the uterus of the normally cycling and early pregnant, ovary intact animal.[10,11] During proestrous–estrous, when estrogen levels are at the highest, the endometrium is in a growth stage; during diestrous, as estradiol secretion decreases and luteal progesterone secretion increases, cell proliferation wanes. At approximately day 4.5 of pregnancy there is surge in estrogen secretion that induces a round of proliferation in the epithelium and underlying stroma.[10,12,13] Thus, cellular proliferation and differentiation in the rodent uterus are regulated by changes in ovarian steroid secretion and these effects are analogous to those observed in the human endometrium in response to the ovarian cycle (Figure 15.1).

The stromal cell proliferative response to prenidatory estrogen is believed to be required for decidual differentiation of the stroma in rodents.[13,14] In humans there is also a round of cell proliferation that occurs in the subepithelial stroma during the mid–late luteal phase, prior to the time of embryo implantation, and these cells are referred to as predecidual.[2] The complete decidual reaction involving extensive proliferation and differentiation of the stroma requires stimuli from the attaching embryo.[3]

In rodents, the decidualization reaction in the stroma can be induced by experimentally injuring the luminal

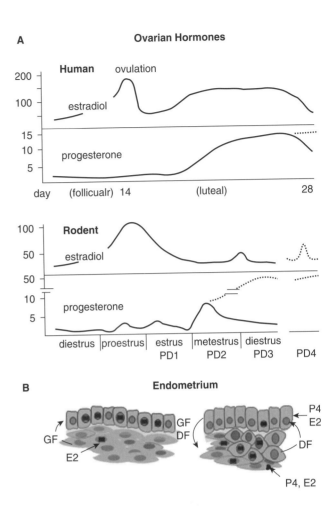

Figure 15.1 Comparison of human and rodent ovarian cycles and the endometrial responses to ovarian hormones. (A) Ovarian hormones: although the ovarian cycle in rodents is compressed relative to that of humans (4–5 days vs 28 days), the growth and differentiation effects of the hormones are very similar. Estrogen secreted during the follicular phase of the human cycle and during proestrous in rodents induces cell proliferation in the endometrium, most markedly in the epithelial compartment. In the mid–late luteal phase in humans, the presence of both progesterone and estradiol stimulates differentiation of the secretory phenotype in the epithelium and proliferation of the subepithelial stroma. In rodents, the corpus luteum is maintained by pituitary prolactin secreted in response to stimulation of the cervix by penile intromission, whether or not fertilization occurs, and thus there is increasing secretion of progesterone in early pregnancy or in a pseudopregnant state. Also, on pregnancy day 4 (PD4) in rodents there is a prenidatory surge in estrogen secretion, which stimulates proliferation of subepithelial stromal cells. The stromal cells that proliferate in response to the progesterone/estradiol hormonal milieu differentiate into large rounded cells with well-demarcated cell membranes; these are the predecidual cells. (B) Endometrium: the effects of estradiol (E_2) and progesterone (P_4) are mediated both directly through gene regulation in the responding cells and indirectly through induction of growth factors (GF) and differentiation factors (DF) that act in reciprocal paracrine fashions across tissues. Ovarian hormone patterns: units are pg/ml estradiol and ng/ml progesterone; dotted lines indicate hormone levels during early pregnancy/psuedopregnancy. (Modified from References 11 and 202–206).

epithelium through mechanical means or by intraluminal instillation of oil.[6,13,15–18] The decidual cell reaction has been studied in rodents that are made pseudopregnant by cervical stimulation at estrous or have been ovariectomized and maintained on a regimen of progesterone and estrogen. In these models, induction of trauma to the uterine epithelium causes a dramatic growth of the endometrial stroma. The trauma may be induced by crushing the uterus with a pair of clamps, passing a suture thread transversely through the uterine tissues, scratching the luminal epithelium with a bent needle, or instillation of a small volume of saline or paraffin oil into the lumen of the uterus. The enlarged uterine stroma that results during artificially induced decidualization is filled with large round cells and is referred to as a deciduoma. It should be noted that both progesterone and estrogen are required for the decidual cell reaction when saline or paraffin oil instillation is used as the stimulus; when excess trauma is used, such as occurs from crushing, or scratching the epithelium, priming with progesterone alone is sufficient.[6] Excess trauma probably explains how a decidual cell reaction was induced in estrogen receptor-alpha knockout (ERαKO) mice maintained on progesterone;[19,20] the uterus of the hormone-treated ERαKO mouse is only one-fifth the size of the uterus in hormone-treated, wild-type animals and it is therefore likely that insertion of a needle or catheter would induce extensive damage to the luminal epithelium.[21]

The rodent has also served as a model of hormonally induced uterine pathologies.[22] Although the study of non-human primate species is valuable for experimental reproductive endocrinology, it is not merely rhetorical to ask whether the mouse or a primate serves as a better model for biological activity in the human endometrium. Studies in primates did not predict the teratogenic and carcinogenic effects of diethylstilbestrol (DES) in the developing human reproductive tract, while the mouse exhibits numerous developmental effects that are analogous to those found in the human.[23,24]

PARACRINE MEDIATION OF HORMONE ACTION

Epithelial cell responses

Hormonal regulation of development and tissue maintenance in reproductive organ parenchyma is mediated by mesenchymal/stromal factors that direct epithelial cell proliferation and differentiation. From his early studies utilizing tissue recombinants grown in syngeneic mouse hosts, Gerald Cunha[25] showed that hormonal

regulation of tissue morphogenesis in the male reproductive accessory organs depended on mesenchymal–epithelial interactions. Cunha and colleagues went on to further demonstrate that development, differentiation, and neoplastic dysregulation of the male reproductive tract epithelia are all governed by an androgen responsive mesenchyme.[26,27] Those pioneering studies were facilitated by use of tissues derived from mice that carried a genetic mutation in the androgen receptor gene (Tfm). Before the availability of ERαKO mice, the neonatal mouse uterus provided a natural experimental model to test the role of stromal cell estrogen receptor (ER) in regulation of uterine epithelial cell proliferation. The uterus of the mouse is relatively undifferentiated at birth, consisting of a simple tube of cuboidal epithelial cells surrounded by a loose mesenchyme. During the first 5–6 days after birth the epithelium remains devoid of ER while the mesenchyme is ER-positive.[28,29] Taking advantage of this situation, we showed that estradiol could induce cellular proliferation in the ER-negative epithelium.[28] In similar experiments, Yamashita et al used a strain of mouse in which development of the epithelial ER expression occurred 2–3 days earlier but was patchy, i.e. the epithelium contained both ER-positive and ER-negative cells; the underlying mesenchyme was ER-positive.[30] In these animals, estradiol induced cellular proliferation in both the ER-positive and ER-negative epithelial cells but induction of the estrogen-sensitive gene marker, lactoferrin, occurred only in the ER-positive cells. These observations in neonatal mice suggest that estrogen exerts its action in uterine epithelium both indirectly through the ER of stromal cells or adjacent epithelial cells to induce cell proliferation and directly through the epithelial cell's own ER to induce specific gene expression.

With the advent of the ERαKO mouse, the role of the stromal ERα as the regulator of uterine and vaginal epithelial cell proliferation was definitively demonstrated using tissue recombinant experiments. Cooke et al used the Cunha technique of tissue separation and recombination starting with neonatal uteri of wild-type (WT) and ERαKO mice,[31] as depicted in Figure 15.2A. In this experimental set-up, uterine epithelium and mesenchyme of neonatal mice (WT and ERαKO) are separated as intact pieces of tissues; the remaining mesenchyme is slit longitudinally and placed on an agar plate. Epithelial sheets are placed on top of the mesenchyme and the recombined tissues are incubated overnight to allow them to attach to each other. All four possible combinations of epithelium and mesenchyme, ERαKO and WT, are constructed. The tissue recombinants are then grafted under the kidney capsule of either a syngeneic host

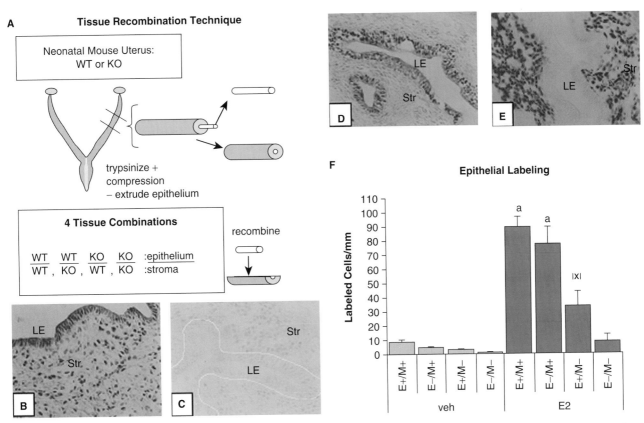

Figure 15.2 Demonstration of stromal mediation of estrogen-induced epithelial cell proliferation. (**A**) Uterine pieces from neonatal wild-type (WT) and ERαKO (KO) mice were subjected to trypsin digestion and gently compressed to extrude the intact tube of epithelium, as described in Bigsby et al.[207] The remaining sheath of mesenchyme was cut open longitudinally and a piece of epithelium was recombined with the mesenchyme in culture. The four possible tissue combinations were made and these were grafted under the kidney capsules of athymic mice. After 5 weeks the hosts were ovariectomized and 3 weeks later they were treated with vehicle (veh) or 4 μg/kg estradiol (E$_2$) and then ^{3}H-thymidine. The tissue recombinants produced pieces of fully formed uterus, with luminal and glandular epithelia, stroma, and myometrium. (**B–E**) Tissue ERα status was determined by immunohistochemistry. Luminal epithelium (LE) and stroma (Str) were both ERα-positive in WT/WT recombinants (**B**) or both ERα-negative in the KO/KO recombinants (**C**); the heterotypic recombinants WT/KO and KO/WT (**D** and **E**, respectively) produced ERα-positive or ERα-negative tissues as predicted. (**F**) Cell proliferation was assessed by thymidine autoradiography. The uterine epithelium (E) and mesenchyme (M) are designated as ERa-positive (+) or ERα-negative (−). ERα-negative epithelium fully responded to estradiol (E$_2$) when the underlying stroma was ERα-positive; there was a partial response in the ERα-positive epithelium growing on an ERα-negative stroma. Values are means ± SEM. a, $p<0.001$ or b, $p<0.01$ vs vehicle (veh) controls; d, $p<0.01$ E+/M− vs E−/M+ or E+/M+ recombinants. (Modified from Bigsby et al.[8])

or an athymic mouse. After a short growth period (4 weeks), the hosts are ovariectomized and then challenged with hormonal treatments 2 weeks later. Using this technique, it was found that the epithelial response to estradiol was entirely dependent on stromal ERα; epithelial cells proliferated when grown on ERα-positive mesenchyme, regardless of their own ERα status. In the course of examining the role of tissue interactions in combined progesterone + estrogen treatment, we performed similar studies, but we found that estradiol induced a partial response in ERα-positive epithelium grown on ERα-negative stroma[8] (Figure 15.2F). A major difference in experimental protocols between the two studies was that the tissue grafts in our study were allowed to mature longer before

hormonal challenge; this was required so that estradiol alone did not stimulate stromal cell proliferation, as it does in the immature rodent model.[7] It may be that the additional maturation allowed differentiation of an epithelial mechanism involved in estrogen-induced proliferation. The observation that ERα-positive epithelium is capable of responding partially in the absence of stromal ERα suggests that the role of the stroma may be facilitative, rather than directive in the mature tissues. Regardless of this fine point of interpretation, these experiments clearly indicate that estrogen induces important tissue interactions occurring in the stroma-to-epithelium direction.

Since estrogen stimulates uterine epithelial cell proliferation through elaboration of a stromal growth factor, then it might be expected that progesterone would inhibit this effect by a mechanism dependent upon stromal cell progesterone receptor (PR). Indeed, when tissue recombinants were prepared from wild-type and PR knockout (PRKO) tissues, the epithelial cell response to estradiol was blocked only when the underlying stroma expressed PR; the PR status of the epithelium was irrelevant.[32]

Some epithelial responses to hormones require expression of the cognate receptor in both the stroma and epithelium. The proteins lactoferrin and complement C3 serve as markers of estrogen-induced differentiation of the uterine epithelium in the mouse. Cooke and coworkers showed that estrogen induction of lactoferrin and complement C3 expression in the uterine epithelium require ERα in both the stroma and epithelium.[33] Likewise, progesterone inhibition of estrogen-induced gene expression in the epithelium requires both the stromal cell PR and the epithelial cell PR.[34]

Human endometrial cells in co-culture have been used to determine the requirement for stromal factor(s) in the epithelial response to estradiol or progesterone. Estradiol does not induce proliferation of human endometrial epithelial cells grown alone but when they are co-cultured with stromal cells estradiol is effective.[35] Epithelial cell telomerase activity is increased in the human endometrium during the proliferative phase. Estradiol failed to increase telomerase in epithelial cells cultured alone but the epithelial cells did respond when they were co-cultured with stromal cells.[36] Progesterone induces epithelial expression of 17β-hydroxysteroid dehydrogenase (17β-HSD), the enzyme that converts estradiol to the less potent estrogen, estrone. Ishikawa cells, an endometrial cancer cell line, express 17β-HSD under progesterone stimulation only when co-cultured with primary cultures of human endometrial stromal cells.[37] Similarly, progesterone inhibits expression of stromelysins in human endometrial epithlelial cells only when co-cultured with stromal cells.[38] These cell culture studies support the notion that hormonal regulation of human endometrial epithelial cells requires paracrine factors derived from the underlying stromal cells; however, the question remains of whether the stromal factors play a passive, facilitative role or act as directive regulators of epithelial physiology.

Stromal cell responses

Just as in development of other organs, it is likely that hormonal regulation of uterine physiology relies on reciprocal tissue interactions, i.e. while the stroma regulates

epithelial responses to hormonal stimulation, stromal responses to hormones may depend in part on the action of the overlying epithelium. As indicated above, the mouse uterus is undeveloped at the time of birth. The loose, unstructured mesenchyme will develop into the endometrial stroma and two layers of smooth muscle, the inner circular layer and the longitudinal outer layer. Full development of the three mesenchymal tissues occurs over the course of the first 10 days after birth.[39] By growing separated mesenchyme, with or without accompanying epithelium in syngeneic host mice, it was shown that development and organization of myometrium required the presence of the epithelium.[40] Although not tested in this study, it is well established that this differentiation process is not dependent on estrogen or ERα.[21] Nonetheless, abnormal exposure to the potent estrogen DES during the postnatal developmental period partially disrupts smooth muscle morphogenesis in the uterus.[41] DES induces a number of developmental abnormalities in the female reproductive tract, many of which are also seen in animals lacking the homeobox genes Hoxa10 and Hoxa11, or those that are null for the epithelially expressed secreted signaling molecule Wnt7a.[42] Neonatal DES treatment blocks Wnt7a expression during a critical developmental period; this effect and subsequent developmental changes require ERα.[43] Thus, although female reproductive tract development proceeds in the absence of estrogen signaling, it is sensitive to perturbations induced by inappropriate exposure to estrogen. Moreover, the detrimental effects of DES are at least in part mediated by disruption of a paracrine pathway occurring in the epithelium-to-mesenchyme direction.

The observation that it is only the subepithelial stromal cells that proliferate in the late secretory phase in humans[2] suggests that the stromal decidual cell response requires factor(s) from the overlying epithelium. In the rat model, the decidual cell reaction is absent in the stroma of a uterine horn in which the epithelium has been ablated; in fact, when the epithelium is partially ablated, the stromal response only occurs in the region of intact epithelium.[44,45] Thus, it is clear that signals emanating from the epithelium are required for the stromal decidualization reaction, but the nature of the signals is unknown.

We have examined the role of the epithelium in hormonal regulation of predecidual stromal cell proliferation induced by estrogen in the progesterone-primed uterus. Using a variation of the tissue recombination studies described above we found that uterine stromal cell proliferation requires the overlying epithelium.[46] Vaginal and uterine epithelia of the neonatal rodent is plastic until it becomes 'determined' approximately 10 days

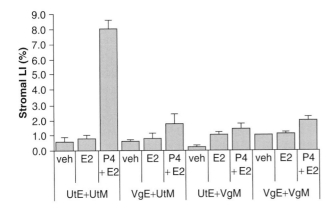

Figure 15.3 Endometrial stromal cell proliferation requires uterine epithelium. Uterine (UtE) and vaginal (VgE) epithelia were collected from 10- to 15-day-old mice and recombined with mesenchyme from uterus (UtM) or vagina (VgM) from neonatal rats. The recombinants were grown under the renal capsules of athymic mice. After 5 weeks the hosts were ovariectomized and 3 weeks later they were treated with three daily injections of vehicle (veh), two injections of vehicle followed by 5 μg/kg estradiol on the third day (E_2), or two injections of 40 mg/kg progesterone followed by progesterone + estradiol on the third day ($P_4 + E_2$). At 16 hours after the last treatment each host was injected with ^{3}H-thymidine and killed 1 hour later. Cell proliferation was assessed by thymidine autoradiography and expressed as labeling index (LI). Values are mean ± SEM; *, $p < 0.01$ vs vehicle control. (Modified from Bigsby et al.[46])

after birth: i.e. before postnatal day 10 its morphological development depends on the underlying mesenchyme and this can be changed experimentally by heterotypic tissue recombinations. Hence, neonatal uterine epithelium can be directed to become vaginal epithelium when grown on vaginal mesenchyme, and vice versa. When older, developmentally determined epithelium is transferred to the heterotypic mesenchyme, it does not change its morphological character. We made tissue recombinants using uterine or vaginal epithelium (UtE and VgE, respectively) from 10- to 15-day-old rats grown on neonatal uterine or vaginal mesenchyme (UtM and VgM, respectively). The four possible tissue recombinants were made and grown in athymic mice; after 4 weeks the hosts were ovariectomized and 3 weeks later they were treated with progesterone for 2 days followed by progesterone + estradiol on the third day. This regimen induces stromal cell proliferation in the host uterus and in the UtE+UtM recombinants, but not in the other tissue combinations (Figure 15.3). These observations indicate that uterine epithelium is required for the stromal cell response to estrogen after progesterone priming. Whether the epithelium performs a directive or a permissive role awaits further study.

Recently, we attempted to answer the question of whether epithelial cell ERα was required for estrogen-induced stromal cell proliferation using tissue recombinants made from neonatal wild-type and ERαKO mice.[8] Surprisingly, even the recombinants made from all ERα-negative tissues responded to estrogen after progesterone priming. Since the grafts were grown in athymic mice, which are wild type for ERα, the results suggested that estradiol induced a systemic factor in the host mouse, which in turn stimulated the progesterone-primed uterine tissue grafts. Indeed when ERαKO mouse uterus was grown in progesterone-primed ERαKO mice there was no stromal cell response to estradiol but when ERαKO uterus was grown in progesterone-primed wild-type mice, estradiol did induce stromal cell proliferation (Figure 15.4). Thus, it appears that uterine ERα is not required in either the epithelium or the stroma, but rather in other tissues to produce a systemic mediator of estradiol action. Preliminary evidence suggests that pituitary prolactin may mediate the effect of estradiol in the progesterone-primed uterus (RM Bigsby, unpublished observations). On the other hand, the stroma of wild-type uterus grown in progesterone-primed ERαKO mice did respond to estradiol stimulation. Since wild-type uterus does not require the systemic mediator, it may be that ERα-positive, progesterone-primed uterine tissues are capable of producing a paracrine factor, such as placental lactogen, that mediates the effect of estradiol. Although these tissue graft studies were performed in host mice that were ovariectomized, their uteri were left intact, leaving open the possibility that the systemic mediator of estradiol action may have been derived from ERα-positive uterine tissues. These studies also point out a technical problem with tissue grafting studies designed to discern the mechanisms through which estradiol controls stromal cell proliferation: i.e. tissue recombinants or mutant uterine tissues must be grown in ERα-negative hosts to remove the potential for a systemic factor inducing the estrogen response in progesterone-primed hosts. The issue of tissue-specific expression of ERα in regulation of the stromal cell response to hormones awaits additional investigation.

HORMONALLY REGULATED PARACRINE FACTORS IN THE ENDOMETRIUM

Observations described above clearly indicate that estrogen and progesterone regulate proliferation and differentiation of the endometrial tissues through paracrine mechanisms, and that these occur in both

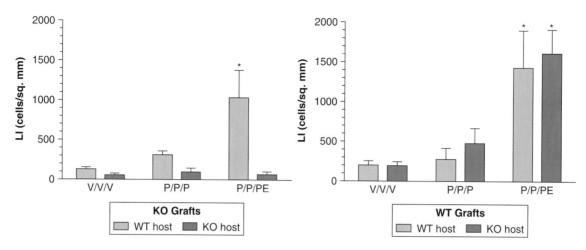

Figure 15.4 ERα-dependent systemic mediation of endometrial stromal cell proliferation. Pieces of whole uterus from neonatal wild-type (WT) or ERαKO (KO) mice were grown under the kidney capsules of WT or KO hosts. After 5 weeks the hosts were ovariectomized and 3 weeks later they were treated with three daily injections of vehicle (V/V/V), 10 mg/kg progesterone (P/P/P), or two injections of progesterone followed by progesterone plus 4 µg/kg estradiol on the third day (P/P/PE). At 20 hours after the last treatment, each host was injected with ³H-thymidine and killed 1 hour later. Cell proliferation was assessed by thymidine autoradiography and expressed as labeling index (LI). Values are mean ± SEM; *, $p < 0.01$ vs vehicle control. (Modified from Bigsby et al.[8])

directions, stroma-to-epithelium and epithelium-to-stroma (see Figure 15.1). Numerous growth factors have been shown to be hormonally responsive in uterine tissues (Table 15.1). However, there have been few definitive data pointing to any particular factor(s) as crucial to hormonally regulated paracrine action in the endometrium. Many of the observations made to date are purely correlative: i.e. expression patterns of growth factors have been correlated to hormonal fluctuations or experimental manipulations. Such observations are helpful in pointing the way to further, mechanistic examination of the role of particular putative growth-promoting factors.

The biggest impediments to defining the paracrine mediators of hormone action in the uterus, or any other organ, are redundancy among growth factors and their receptors and complex interactions among growth factor pathways.[47] Experimental results can be confounded by:

- receptor–ligand promiscuity within a family of growth factors and their cognate receptors
- receptor–ligand promiscuity through phylogenetically unrelated partners
- receptor/co-receptor promiscuity in which different receptors share a non-ligand binding receptor partner
- receptor/downstream mediator promiscuity in which common intracellular pathways are activated by numerous, unrelated receptors.

The EGF and Wnt families of growth factors and their receptors provide examples. As indicated in Table 15.1,

several members of the epidermal growth factor (EGF) family (transforming growth factor α [TGFα], heparin-binding EGF [HB-EGF], amphiregulin, epiregulin, NDF-1, and β-cellulin) are all expressed in the uterus and are regulated by hormones. Likewise, three of the four related tyrosine kinase receptor proteins, erbB1–4, have been identified in the uterus. Any one member of the EGF family may compensate for the experimental deletion of another member; thus it is difficult to interpret negative results from the use of knockout mice. Indeed, triple knockout mice lacking EGF, amphiregulin, and TGFα are fertile, suggesting a compensatory function of other members of the EGF family of ligands in reproduction.[48] In addition, EGF receptor (EGF-R) triggers numerous downstream signaling pathways, including RAS/RAF/MEK/MAPK, PLCγ/Ca²⁺, PKC, and STATs.[49] As indicated above, Wnt proteins may behave as growth factors in the uterus. Wnt signaling can occur through the canonical pathway mediated by the frizzled family of receptors inducing stabilization of β-catenin, or it may work through an unrelated receptor, RYK.[47] The angiogenic factor, vascular endothelial growth factor (VEGF), is produced in several splice variants and these interact differentially with the two VEGF receptors (VEGF-R1 and -R2, also known as Flt-1 and Flk-2); in addition, one isoform of VEGF (VEGF165) binds to neuropilin proteins (Npn-1 and -2), which are transmembrane proteins unrelated to VEGF-R (see Pavelock et al[50] and references therein). The interaction between VEGF165 and Npn-2 enhances the binding of VEGF165 to VEGF-R. Redundancy within pathways and cross-talk

Table 15.1 Growth factors and receptors expressed under hormonal regulation

Growth factor	Tissue expression	Hormonal regulation	References
IGF-1 and binding proteins			
IGF-1	Epithelium (m, r, h), stroma (m, r, h)	$\uparrow$ E$_2$, $\uparrow$ P$_4$ + E$_2$	52, 179, 180
IGFBP-1	Decid. stroma (h)	$\uparrow$ P$_4$ (+ GFs)	180
EGF family and receptors			
EGF	Epithelium (m, h)	$\uparrow$ E$_2$	61–63, 181
TGFα	Epithelium	$\uparrow$ P$_4$	181, 182
Amphiregulin	Epithelium	$\uparrow$ P$_4$	183
Epiregulin, ß-cellulin, NDF-1	Epithelium, subepithelial stroma (m)	$\uparrow$ P$_4$ + E$_2$	3
HB-EGF	Epithelium (m, h), stroma (m, h)	$\uparrow$ E$_2$, P$_4$ + E$_2$ $\uparrow$ E$_2$, P$_4$	3, 74, 184
EGF receptors (erbB1)	Epithelium (rab), stroma (m, h, rab)	$\uparrow$ E$_2$	63, 65, 71, 185
erbB2	Epithelium (m), decid. stroma (m)	$\uparrow$ E$_2$	65
erbB3	Epithelium (h)	=	67
erbB4	Epithelium (h), stroma (h)	$\uparrow$ fol ph, $\downarrow$ lut ph	67
TGF-ß family			
TGFß$_{1-3}$	Epithelium (stroma) (m)	$\uparrow$ E$_2$	186–189
TGFß$_4$	Stroma (h)	$\uparrow$ lut ph	190
Activin	Epithelium (h), decid. stroma (h)	$\uparrow$ fol ph; $\uparrow$lut ph	95
TGFß receptor types I, II, III	Epithelium (m), stroma (m, h)	$\downarrow$ E$_2$, P$_4$	189, 191, 129
Activin receptors	Stroma (h), endothelium (h)	$\uparrow$ lut ph	97
FGF family			
FGF-2	Perivascular stroma (h)	$\uparrow$ lut ph	85
FGF-7	Stroma (m, rh, h)	$\uparrow$ P$_4$	88, 90
FGF-9	Stroma (h)	$\uparrow$ fol ph; $\uparrow$ E$_2$	84
FGF-R	Epithelium, stroma (rh, h)	$\uparrow$ E$_2$	84, 89
Angiogenic factors			
VEGF	Epithelium, stroma (m, r, h)	$\uparrow$ E$_2$; $\uparrow$ E$_2$ + P$_4$	193–195
VEGF-R (1 and 2)	Endothelium (m, r)	$\uparrow$ E$_2$; $\uparrow$E$_2$ + P$_4$	50, 194
Neuropilin-1 and -2	Endothelium, gland, epithelium (h)	$\uparrow$ P$_4$, $\downarrow$ E$_2$	50, 194
Prokineticin-1 and -2 (PK-1 and PK-2)	Epithelium, stroma (h)	$\uparrow$ lut ph; $\uparrow$ P$_4$ (cult)	80
PK receptor 1 and 2	Epithelium, endothelium (h)	=	80
Chemokines			
IL-1a	Epithelium (m)	$\uparrow$ P$_4$	100
CXCR1, -2	Epithelium, stroma (h)	$\uparrow$ lut ph	196
CCR5	Epithelium, stroma (h)	$\uparrow$ lut ph	196
Prostaglandins			
COX-1	Epithelium (m, rh, h)	$\uparrow$ lut ph (rh, h) $\uparrow$ early pseudopreg (m)	142 144
COX-2	Epithelium, subepithelial stroma (m)	$\uparrow$ P$_4$ + E$_2$ + blastocyst	197
PGE$_2$	Epithelium (m, rh, h)	$\uparrow$ P$_4$ + E$_2$	137, 144, 198
PGF$_{2\alpha}$	Epithelium, stroma (m, r, h)	$\uparrow$ E$_2$	147, 198
PGE receptors (EP2, 3, 4)	Epithelium, stroma (m, r, h)	$\uparrow$ P$_4$ + E$_2$	137, 142, 143, 199
PGF$_{2\alpha}$ receptor (FP)	Stroma, myometrium (m)	$\uparrow$ fol ph (h); $\uparrow$ pseudopreg (m)	137, 142
Others			
PDGF	Epithelium (m), stroma (m, h)	$\uparrow$ E$_2$ (m); = (h)	63, 200
PDGFß receptor	Epithelium (h), stroma (m, h)	$\uparrow$ fol ph, $\downarrow$ lut ph; $\uparrow$ E$_2$ (m)	63, 200
CRF	Epithelium, stroma (h)	$\uparrow$ P$_4$ (cult)	134
CRF receptor type 1	Stroma (h)	=	134
Prl	Stroma (m), decid stroma (h)	$\uparrow$ P$_4$	118
PrlR	Epithelium, stroma (m, r, h)	=	119, 121, 122
Wnt-2, -3, 4, 5a, 7	Epithelium (m, h), stroma (m, h)	$\uparrow\downarrow$ E$_2$, P$_4$, tissue-dependent	42, 201
Fz-2, -6	Epithelium (m, h), stroma (m, h)	=	53, 54
LIF	Epithelium (m, h)	$\uparrow$ P$_4$ + E$_2$	10
Calcitonin	Epithelium (r, h)	$\uparrow$ P$_4$; $\downarrow$ E$_2$; $\uparrow$ lut ph	10

$\uparrow\downarrow$ = increased, decreased or not changed by estradiol (E$_2$) or progesterone (P$_4$), by hormones plus growth factors (+GF), or during follicular phase (fol ph) or luteal phase (lut ph); h, human; m, mouse; r, rat; rab, rabbit; rh, rhesus macaque; decid., decidualized; psuedopreg, pseudopregnant; cult, culture.

between pathways increases the complexity of biological responses, making it very difficult to dissect the molecular mechanisms involved in paracrine mediation of hormone action. Nonetheless, progress has been achieved through the use of genetically modified mice and cell culture systems. We will focus additional detail on experimental evidence, pro or con, concerning the role of several growth factors in regulation of endometrial cell proliferation and differentiation.

Peptide growth factors

Although correlative studies showing that estradiol increases uterine insulin-like growth factor I (IGF-I) expression suggested that it may act as a paracrine mediator of steroid action,[51,52] examination of estrogen responsiveness in IGF-I knockout mouse tissue or wild-type tissue grafted to wild-type or IGF-I knockout hosts indicates that systemic IGF-I is more important for estrogen action than local production of the growth factor at the tissue level.[53] Furthermore, targeted overexpression of IGF-I under the direction of the smooth muscle cell actin promoter induced elongation of the mouse uterine horns but did not induce epithelial hyperplasia or any other growth effect that would be associated with an excessive uterotropic effect.[54] Thus, it does not appear that IGF-I behaves as a local mediator of estrogen-induced cell proliferation in the mouse endometrium. However, co-culture studies of human endometrial cells suggest that stromal cell IGF-I is required for estradiol induction of epithelial cell proliferation. Proliferation of epithelial cells is stimulated by estradiol when stromal cells are included in the culture system; the effect of estradiol can be blocked by addition of an antibody against IGF-I, suggesting that it is the stromal cell factor that mediates the effect.[35] However, it cannot be ruled out that the effect of IGF-I is merely permissive and that systemic IGF-I would not be as effective in vivo.

Wnt genes, the vertebrate homolog to *Drosophila wingless*, encode secreted proteins known to regulate tissue growth and differentiation. Wnt signaling acts through the frizzled gene family of transmembrane receptor proteins; activation of the receptor leads to stabilization of cellular β-catenin, allowing it to localize in the nucleus and participate in specific transcriptional events.[55] Of the 16 known members of the Wnt gene family, three have been identified in the murine uterus, Wnt4, Wnt5a, and Wnt7a.[56,57] In the adult uterus, Wnt7a is expressed only within the luminal epithelium; Wnt4 and Wnt5a are both expressed in

the epithelium and the subepithelial stroma but the patterns of tissue expression vary according to the estrous cycle.[56] During estrogen dominance, Wnt4 is expressed in both the epithelial and stromal compartments but when progesterone predominates it is expressed mainly in the subepithelial stroma. On the other hand, Wnt5a is expressed almost exclusively in the subepithelial stroma during estrogen dominance but is expressed in both epithelium and stroma once estrogen wanes during estrous through diestrous. The Wnt receptor protein frizzled-2 (Fz-2) is expressed only in the epithelium.[57] In the ovariectomized mouse, Wnt4, Wnt5a, and Fz-2 are increased in the uterus within 6 hours of estradiol treatment and inhibition of Wnt signaling by artificial expression of the Wnt antagonist SFRP-2 blocks estradiol-induced epithelial cell proliferation.[57] Thus, it might appear that Wnt proteins may act as local mediators of estradiol-induced cell proliferation in the uterus. However, estradiol-induced Wnt signaling is not blocked by the potent estrogen antagonist ICI182,780 and estradiol induces Wnt proteins in both wild-type and ERαKO mice.[57,58] Since estrogen-induced cell proliferation does not occur in ERαKO mice[59] and is blocked by ICI182,780 in wild-type animals,[60] it may be concluded that the Wnt/Fz/β-catenin pathway is a required component of estrogen-induced growth but by itself is not sufficient to induce growth of the uterus.

The EGF family of growth factors may be involved in the paracrine (stromal-to-epithelial) or juxtacrine (epithelial-to-epithelial) mediation of estrogen-induced epithelial cell proliferation. Estradiol induces EGF expression in uterine epithelial cells.[61–63] In endocrine ablated mice, an antibody against EGF partially blocked the effect of estradiol on epithelial DNA synthesis and administration of EGF induced DNA synthesis in the epithelium to the same extent as estradiol.[61] The observation that uterine epithelium derived from EGF-R knockout mice did respond to estradiol suggests that another member of the erbB family of receptors might mediate the effect of estradiol.[64] EGF-R (erbB1) is not expressed in the uterine epithelium; erbB2 is expressed and it is up-regulated by estradiol.[65] Although erbB2 is a member of the family of EGF receptors, it does not include a ligand-binding domain, but rather it acts as a dimerization partner of other erbB transmembrane proteins.[66] ErbB3 and erbB4 are expressed in human uterine epithelium[67] but mouse uterine epithelium expresses only erbB3.[68] These observations indicate that estrogen regulation of members of the EGF family of growth factors and/or the corresponding family of receptor proteins plays a role in the epithelial proliferative response.

EGF and the related growth factor HB-EGF are also candidates for an epithelium-to-stroma paracrine effect of estradiol. When human endometrial stromal cells are grown in isolation of epithelial cells, progesterone increases cell proliferation only in the presence of either EGF, platelet-derived growth factor (PDGF), or basic fibroblast growth factor (bFGF); estradiol, administered alone or in combination with progesterone or growth factors, was ineffective.[69,70] In the murine uterus, estradiol induces EGF expression in the epithelium but not other tissues,[62] and EGF-R was detected only in the stroma and myometrium, not the epithelium.[71] When EGF-R knockout (EGFR-KO) uterus was grown in athymic mice, estradiol-induced stromal cell proliferation was impaired.[64] It should be pointed out that the tissue grafts behaved as immature uterus in that estradiol-stimulated stromal cell proliferation in wild-type tissues without progesterone priming, a situation that can be overcome by growing the grafts for a longer period before hormone challenge tests are performed.[8] Thus, it may be that EGF-R mediates estradiol action in the stroma of the immature uterus, but whether that holds true for the progesterone-primed, mature uterus has not been determined. HB-EGF also increases proliferation of cultured human endometrial stromal cells and this effect is enhanced by TNFα.[72] HB-EGF exists in both a transmembrane form and a soluble form, either of which stimulates human stromal cells in culture.[72,73] HB-EGF expression is increased in human stromal cells by either estradiol or progesterone stimulation but expression in the epithelium requires both hormones; furthermore, HB-EGF induces expression of epithelial biomarkers normally expressed during the window of implantation.[74]

Interactions between EGF-R and ERα pathways play important roles in estrogen-induced growth of the uterus. EGF induces DNA synthesis in the uterus of ovariectomized wild-type mice but not ERαKO mice, indicating that ERα is required for the growth-promoting effect of EGF.[75] It was suggested that activation of EGF-R leads to modification of ERα and associated coactivators through phosphorylation events, thereby increasing transcription of ERα-responsive genes. However, using gene arrays, Hewitt and coworkers found that growth factors (EGF or IGF-I) stimulated gene expression to the same extent in both wild-type and ERαKO mice: i.e. there was no additional set of genes activated by the growth factor when ERα was present.[76] Furthermore, most of the genes stimulated by estradiol in the wild-type mouse were also stimulated by the growth factors. Therefore, it is more likely that estradiol stimulates synthesis and activation of growth factors through ERα-mediated events, and these growth factors, along with activated ERα, regulate genes required for the growth response in the uterus. Although both estradiol and progesterone increase EGF-R transcript levels in the ovariectomized mouse uterus, activity of EGF-R is up-regulated only by estradiol, indicating that estradiol is required for EGF action in the uterus.[71] In addition, recent evidence suggests that a portion of cellular ERα resides in the cell membrane and this receptor interacts with G-protein-coupled receptors to stimulate a cascade of events leading to activation of pro-HB-EGF through matrix metalloproteases (MMPs).[77] Alternatively, estradiol may interact directly with the G-protein-coupled receptor GPR30 to activate EGF-R through this metalloprotease-mediated growth factor activation pathway.[78,79] Thus, estradiol-induced growth of the uterus may involve a complex interwoven array of pathways regulated by nuclear receptors and membrane-bound receptors, including membrane-bound ERα and GPR30.

A newly identified family of small protein growth factors, prokineticins, has been found in the human endometrium and was shown to be regulated by progesterone.[80] These proteins are known to be proangiogenic and it was suggested that this was their function in the uterus;[80] however, their activity has been shown to be more pleiotropic,[81] acting as a mitogen in bone marrow[82] and increasing secretion of VEGF by steroidogenic cells of the corpus luteum.[83] Since prokineticins and their G-protein-coupled receptors are expressed in both the stroma and epithelium of the uterus,[80] they warrant further investigation as potential paracrine mediators of hormone action.

Members of the fibroblast growth factor (FGF) family of growth factors are expressed in the uterus and may act as both paracrine and autocrine mediators of hormone action. FGF-9 is expressed in the human endometrial stroma and is highest in the late proliferative phase; receptors for FGF are expressed in the stroma (FGFR2IIIc, FGFR3IIIc, FGFR3IIIb) and the epithelium (FGF2IIIb, FGFR3IIIb).[84] FGF-9 expression is increased in cultured stromal cells by treatment with estradiol and estradiol-induced proliferation of stromal cells is blocked by an anti-FGF-9 antibody.[84] FGF-2 is believed to be involved in angiogenesis; it, and its receptor, are expressed in tissue surrounding blood vessels in the human endometrium, particularly during the early secretory phase.[85] FGF-7 and FGF-10 are expressed in the developing and adult ovine uterus, and their receptors are expressed mainly in the luminal and developing glandular epithelia.[86,87] In rhesus macaques, progesterone stimulates FGF-7 expression in endometrial stromal cells.[88] Likewise, in human endometrium FGF-7 expression is progesterone dependent while expression of its receptor is sensitive to estradiol.[89] In the mouse, FGF-7 is expressed in the uterine stroma and treatment of neonatal animals with FGF-7 stimulates proliferation of uterine and vaginal epithelia.[90] Application of FGF-7, either systemically or directly in the rhesus uterus, decreased apoptosis in glandular epithelium but did not stimulate cell proliferation.[91] Further research is required to define the responses of human endometrial cells to members of the FGF family.

Transforming growth factor β (TGFβ) is expressed in both the stroma and epithelium of the human endometrium; in cultured cells it inhibits epithelial cell proliferation, whereas it stimulates stromal cells.[92] Stromelysins, a family of matrix metalloproteases, are expressed in the human endometrium during the proliferative phase; progesterone suppression of stromelysins in the endometrial epithelium requires a stromal paracrine factor, most likely TGFβ.[93] These observations suggest that TGFβ secreted by stromal cells in response to progesterone may mediate inhibition of both cell proliferation and MMP expression in the epithelium.

The activin/inhibin/follistatin system plays a role in endometrial maturation and may be involved in a paracrine pathway in the epithelium-to-stroma direction that induces stromal cell proliferation and decidual differentiation.[94] Activin is a member of the TGFβ family of growth factors. Follistatin is a secreted activin-binding protein. In the non-pregnant uterus, the epithelium is the predominant source of activin A. Activin A is expressed by the epithelium during the proliferative phase and then in both the epithelium and stroma during the secretory phase; it appears that progestins up-regulate activin A expression in both epithelium and stroma.[95,96] Activin receptors (Ia, Ib, IIa, IIb) are expressed in the stroma and endothelium and are maximally expressed during early secretory phase and early pregnancy.[97] Activin A promotes decidualization of cultured stromal cells[98] and this can be inhibited by follistatin.[99] As differentiation progresses, the decidualized stromal cells secrete activin A.[94] Thus, activin is a candidate for an epithelial paracrine regulator of stromal cell proliferation and differentiation during the mid–late secretory phase. Extension of the decidual differentiation deeper into the stroma may be a juxtacrine effect of activin A secreted by cells that have already become decidualized.

The endometrial epithelial cells of both mouse and human secrete interleukin 1α (IL-1α) and it may regulate differentiated function of stromal cells. Tenascin C is an extracellular glycoprotein that is expressed by subepithelial stroma during the peri-implantation period. Tenascin C was induced in cultured mouse endometrial stromal cells when IL-1α and prostaglandins PGE_2 and $PGF_{2\alpha}$ were applied; furthermore, in co-culture of epithelial and stromal cells, progesterone-induced tenascin C expression in the stromal cells was blocked by an antibody against IL-1α.[100] In human stromal cells, IL-1α induced expression of MMP-1.[101,102] The roles of IL-1α and other cytokines are discussed further in other chapters of this book.

Recently it has been shown that progesterone induces expression of IHH in the murine uterine epithelium[103] and that hormonally induced stromal cell proliferation is absent in the uterus that has an *Ihh*-deficient epithelium.[104] These observations suggest that IHH is the epithelial factor required for the stromal response to progesterone plus estrogen. However, progesterone administered alone induces expression of IHH in the uterus[103,105] but it does not induce stromal cell proliferation.[8,106,107] Therefore the lack of a stromal response to progesterone plus estrogen in mice with an *Ihh*-deficient epithelium indicates that IHH may be required, but is not by itself sufficient to stimulate the stroma.

Pituitary prolactin (Prl) and uterine lactogen play critical roles in reproduction. In rodents, uterine lactogen is responsible for maintaining a functional corpus luteum (CL) during pregnancy.[14] As they differentiate into the decidual type cell under hormonal regulation, human endometrial stromal cells produce Prl,[108] but hCG, not Prl, is the utero/placental hormone that supports the CL in humans.[14] The uterus produces several other Prl-like proteins as well.[109–116] It has been suggested that Prl plays a paracrine role, mediating the stromally directed differentiation of the overlying epithelium.[117] Samples from luteal phase-deficient endometria produce less Prl than histologically matched control endometria, suggesting a key role for this paracrine factor.[118] Prl receptors (PrlR) are present in the stromal and epithelial cells of human endometrium.[119,120] Although PrlR is present in the rat uterus in fully decidualized stroma only,[121] it is present in the mouse uterine epithelium, myometrium, and undecidualized stromal cells.[122,123] Mice devoid of the Prl receptor (PrlR-KO) exhibit a failure of embryo implantation. This effect could be due to a lack of

Prl support of the corpus luteum, but it is only partially overcome by progesterone supplementation,[124] supporting the notion that Prl might have a direct effect on the uterus and is required for its full function. Prl has been shown to regulate expression of genes in the mouse uterine epithelium, undifferentiated stroma, and decidual stroma.[125–127] Prl and uterine lactogen bind to PrlR in uterine epithelial cells and stimulate gland development in the neonatal ovine uterus.[128,129] Prl enhances the progesterone response in the uterine epithelium of rabbits, most likely by augmenting the action of progesterone at the transcriptional level.[130–132] Human myometrial cells also produce Prl and leiomyoma cell proliferation is stimulated by Prl.[133] In the progesterone-primed mouse uterus, Prl can stimulate cell proliferation in the uterine stroma to a similar extent as induced by estradiol (RM Bigsby, unpublished observations). It is apparent that the role of Prl, or uterine lactogens, in the uterine response to estrogen warrants further investigation.

The hypothalamic hormones, corticotropin-releasing factor (CRF), and gonadotropin-releasing hormone (GnRH), have been identified in the uterus and these too may participate in the paracrine regulation of the endometrium. CRF is expressed by the epithelium and stroma, increasing as the cycle progresses from proliferative through the secretory phase; CRF-type 1 receptor is expressed only in the stroma.[134] Like activin, CRF decidualizes cultured stromal cells. GnRH is also expressed in the endometrium and it has been shown to up-regulate the expression of proteases in decidualized stromal cells.[135]

Prostaglandins

Prostaglandins are important endocrine and paracrine/autocrine regulators of female reproduction.[136] They are involved in menstruation, implantation, and parturition. They also appear to be important in pathological conditions, including endometrial carcinomas, menorrhagia, and dysmenorrhea.[137] Prostaglandin endoperoxide H synthases (PGHS 1 and 2), also known as cyclooxygenases 1 and 2 (COX-1 and COX-2), catalyze the first committed step in prostaglandin synthesis. In the endometrium, the two main prostaglandins are PGE_2 and $PGF_{2\alpha}$. There are four transmembrane, G-protein-coupled receptors for PGE_2: EP1, EP2, EP3, or EP4. $PGF_{2\alpha}$ exerts its effects through its own unique G-protein-coupled receptor, the FP receptor. Also, PGE_2 may be bound by EP receptors in the nucleus or by nuclear peroxisome proliferator-activated receptors

and thereby directly regulate transcription. Uterine $PGF_{2\alpha}$ is known to be very important for induction of luteolysis but its role in the endometrium is poorly understood.

Both COX-1 and COX-2 are expressed in the mouse endometrium. Prostaglandins produced from both COX-1 and COX-2 are important in reproduction.[138–140] COX-2 knockout mice are infertile because of a defect in implantation and decidualization.[140,141] COX-1 knockout mice are fertile but have abnormal parturition.[138,139] COX-1-deficient mice do not have any known defects in implantation, most likely because there is compensation from COX-2.[140] Interestingly, in some genetic backgrounds, COX-1 compensation can rescue the infertility phenotype in the COX-2 knockout mouse. In normal mouse pregnancy during preimplantation (days 1–4), COX-1 is expressed in the luminal and glandular endometrial cells, peaking on day 4 and decreasing after attachment of the blastocyst.[141] COX-1 expression increases again in the secondary decidual zone on days 7 and 8. COX-1 dramatically increases in the decidua between days 14.5 and 15.5, accounting for most of the $PGF_{2\alpha}$ produced by the uterus.[139] This rise in COX-1 and $PGF_{2\alpha}$ is critical for luteolysis and normally timed parturition in the mouse. During implantation, COX-2 is expressed in the luminal endometrium and underlying stromal cells at the antimesometrial pole surrounding the blastocyst and during the attachment reaction and then switching expression to the mesometrial pole on day 6.[140] In the ovariectomized mouse, treatment with progesterone and estradiol induce COX-1 but do not affect COX-2 expression in the uterine epithelium.

During preparation of the mouse endometrium for blastocyst implantation, expression of prostaglandin receptors is also regulated. EP1 mRNA is present throughout the uterus during the first 5 days of murine pregnancy.[142] After implantation on day 6, EP1 is primarily expressed in the decidua. EP3 is also present throughout the uterus on days 1 and 2 of pregnancy, but localizes to the circular layer of the myometrium and the mesometrial pole of the stroma on days 3 and 4 of pregnancy. EP4 demonstrates distinct expression in the luminal epithelium and stroma on days 3 and 4 that continues until after implantation; this pattern of expression is mimicked in ovariectomized mice treated with combined progesterone plus estradiol.[142,143] By days 6–8, EP4 is seen in primary and secondary decidual cells only. FP expression is very low in the stromal cells and circular myometrium on day 1 of pregnancy and gradually increases in the myometrium until day 4 and then declines until it is undetectable on days 6–8.

The prostaglandins are logical candidates for the mediators that orchestrate the changes that occur during the menstrual cycle. Immunohistochemistry localizes COX-1 expression to the luminal and glandular epithelium of the endometrium in the mouse, rhesus monkey, baboon, mink, and human.[144] In the rhesus monkey, cytosolic PGE_2 synthase along with COX-1 are maximally expressed in the luminal and glandular epithelia on days 16–20 of the menstrual cycle. This suggests that COX-1 is responsible for PGE_2 production in the rhesus endometrium. PGE_2 synthesis is maximal during the proliferative phase of the menstrual cycle and is found in the epithelial and perivascular cells of the endometrium.[136] In women, COX-2 is also found in the perivascular cells of the endometrium. However, there is controversy whether COX-2 is highly expressed in the epithelial cells and maximal in the proliferative phase[136] or highly expressed in the glandular cells and maximal in the late secretory phase[145] of the menstrual cycle. This controversy may be a result of the older studies using an antibody that recognizes both COX-1 and COX-2. In the rhesus monkey COX-2 localizes to the epithelial and stromal cells of the endometrium.[144] Timing of maximal $PGF_{2\alpha}$ synthesis is controversial.[136,146,147] Human endometrial cells isolated during the proliferative phase secrete more $PGF_{2\alpha}$ and PGE_2 than cells isolated during the secretory phase.[148] However, uterine flushings obtained during the menstrual cycle show that $PGF_{2\alpha}$ levels are significantly higher during the mid secretory phase than the proliferative phase of the cycle.[147] Expression and signaling of the receptors EP4 and FP are also maximal during the mid–late proliferative phase of the menstrual cycle.[136] EP4 is primarily expressed in glandular and vascular endometrium and FP is primarily expressed in the glandular epithelium. The location and expression patterns are consistent with the notion that prostaglandins may have a role in epithelial–epithelial or epithelial–perivascular cell interactions. The prostaglandins also regulate vascular tone. PGE_2 and PGI_2 vasodilate while $PGF_{2\alpha}$ and thromboxane A_2 (TXA_2) vasoconstrict the endometrial blood vessels. Endometrial prostaglandins also bind myometrial receptors to influence contractions in a paracrine manner. Similar to their effects on vascular smooth muscle, PGE_2 and PGI_2 inhibit myometrial contractions while $PGF_{2\alpha}$ stimulates contractions.

There is a significant hormonal influence on prostaglandin production. Estrogen stimulates the synthesis of $PGF_{2\alpha}$ in the endometrium and the withdrawal of progesterone during luteolysis enhances synthesis.[146] Progesterone also stimulates the conversion of PGE_2 and $PGF_{2\alpha}$ to inactive forms by prostaglandin dehydrogenase. Similarly, when antiprogestin is administered, there is decrease in prostaglandin dehydrogenase activity and an increase in menstrual bleeding. Administration of an antiprogestin during the luteal phase significantly decreased glandular COX-1 and luminal COX-2 protein but luminal COX-1 and perivascular COX-2 were unaffected.[149] In vitro, stromal cells grown in the presence of a progesterone antagonist show a dose-related increase in $PGF_{2\alpha}$ production.

Endometrial prostaglandin synthesis may also be regulated by pituitary luteinizing hormone (LH). LH receptors (LHR) have been found in the endometrium of cows, pigs, mice, baboons, sheep, and humans.[150] In the cow, endometrial LHR is highest during the proliferative phase. Activation of the bovine endometrial LHR increases expression of COX-2 and production of $PGF_{2\alpha}$. In endometrial cells obtained from non-pregnant women, administration of LH resulted in up-regulation of COX-2 and an increase in PGE_2.

The prostaglandin transporter (PGT), first cloned in the rat in 1995, is thought to play a role in regulating local prostaglandin levels by transporting prostaglandins across the cell membrane and enhancing metabolism of the prostaglandins.[151] The prostaglandin transporter carries newly synthesized PGE_2 and $PGF_{2\alpha}$ as well as PGD_2 and thromboxane B_2 (TXB_2) out of the cell. In the endometrium, PGT is expressed in both epithelial and stromal cells. In women, PGT expression varies throughout the menstrual cycle. Expression is lowest during the mid–late secretory phase while COX-2 expression increases during the late secretory phase. This may account for the increase in prostaglandins released from the endometrium during the middle and late secretory phases of the menstrual cycle.

PARACRINE MEDIATORS IN ENDOMETRIAL PATHOLOGY

Benign disease

Luteal phase deficiency (LPD) is described as inadequate progesterone stimulation of the endometrium due to insufficient development and/or hormonal responsiveness of the corpus luteum.[152–155] It has been linked to recurrent spontaneous abortion and unexplained infertility. In addition, LPD may be a frequent confounding factor in the success of in-vitro fertilization (IVF) procedures due to administration of excess GnRH.[156] LPD can be diagnosed through immunohistological examination of endometrial biopsies to determine whether there is an appropriate expression of biomarker proteins that are associated with maturation of the tissues that define the window of receptivity.[157] Thus, there are two components to LPD: the production of steroids by the ovary and the response of the endometrium to steroidal stimulation. Since expression of key players in uterine receptivity is under the control of paracrine mediators of progesterone and estrogen action,[157,158] it may be that inadequate production of these paracrine factors plays a role in LPD; this aspect of the problem requires investigation. However, the clinical relevance of the diagnosis of LPD is controversial because treatment with hormone regimens used in cases of unexplained infertility are usually successful in overcoming LPD, whether or not it has been identified through biopsy examination and extensive immunohistological characterization of marker proteins.[159]

Other benign diseases involving the endometrium are regulated by known paracrine mediators. The COX enzymes and prostaglandins play a significant role in uterine pathophysiology.[137] Menorrhagia, a condition of excess menstrual blood loss, affects 10–30% of women of reproductive age. Although the etiology of menorrhagia is unclear, it is evident that PGE_2 synthesis and binding sites are increased in the uterus of affected women. The increased bleeding may be related to increased vasodilatory factors, including nitric oxide and PGI_2. Consistent with a role for prostaglandins in menorrhagia, COX inhibitors do reduce menstrual blood loss.

Endometriosis is a condition in which endometrial glands and stroma grow outside of the uterus on peritoneal mesothelium, but the etiology is still unclear. It is an estrogen-dependent condition characterized by pelvic pain, infertility, and abnormal uterine bleeding.[137] Estrogen receptor and aromatase activity, which are absent in normal endometrium, are both highly expressed in endometriotic tissue. This results in a local increase in estrogen, which stimulates PGE_2 synthesis, inducing transcription of COX-2. Immunohistochemical analysis has confirmed an increased expression of COX-2 in the endometriotic endometrium.[137] Elevated prostaglandins have been found in the peritoneum of women with endometriosis, which may act in a paracrine manner to potentiate the dysfunction of endometriosis.

Primary dysmenorrhea is characterized by premenstrual tension and painful menstrual cramps. There is much evidence that women with dysmenorrhea have higher amounts of PGE_2 and $PGF_{2\alpha}$ in their menstrual fluid than women with painless periods.[137] Endometrial explants from women with dysmenorrhea produce more $PGF_{2\alpha}$ in response to arachidonic acid than from explants isolated from women with painless periods. COX inhibitors have been successful in treating dysmenorrhea and, more recently, selective COX-2 inhibitors appear to be even more efficacious.

Cancer

Recent literature has highlighted the importance of interactions between epithelial cancer cells and their surrounding stroma.[160] Those growth factors, which are regulated by estradiol in normal tissues, are candidates for paracrine or autocrine regulation of cancer cell growth. Although it is not hormonally regulated, endometrial stromal cell hepatocyte growth factor (HGF) may enhance growth of endometrial cancer cells. The stromal cells isolated from endometrial tumors express six-fold the amount of HGF compared to normal endometrial stromal cells and this may be due to signaling from the cancer cells via bFGF.[161] The angiogenic factors VEGF and FGF-1 and FGF-2 are up-regulated by estrogens and down-regulated by progestin in endometrial cancer cells.[162,163] Stromal TGFβ normally inhibits uterine epithelial cell proliferation; endometrial cancers exhibited either decreased expression or mutation of TGFβ receptor type II, suggesting that a lack of the growth inhibitory pathway plays a role in endometrial cancer.[164] Alternatively, endometrial cancers can express high levels of activin A, which reduces the growth inhibitory effects of $TGF\beta_1$.[165]

Paracrine regulation of secreted proteases may be involved in the spread of endometrial cancer and endometriotic lesions. Endometrial stromal cells secrete MMP-2, which is in turn translocated to the surface of endometrial cancer cells; proteolytic activity of the MMP-2 localized to the cell's outer surface allows the cancer cells to invade extracellular matrix.[166] In addition, systemic progesterone and local retinoic acid decrease MMP-3 expression and increase tissue inhibitor of metalloproteinase 1 (TIMP-1) expression by decidualized stromal cells, and these effects depend on $TGF\beta_2$.[167,168] Dysregulation of the paracrine effects of retinoic acid and $TGF\beta_2$ may be involved in establishment of endometriotic lesions.[167,168]

COX-1 and/or COX-2 may be up-regulated in endometrial cancers.[137] This coincides with increased synthesis of PGE_2 and increased expression and signaling of the EP receptors in endometrial carcinomas. Increased expression and signaling of the FP receptor has also been demonstrated in endometrial adenocarcinomas.[137] PGE_2 secreted by endometrial cancer cells induces COX-2 expression in normal endometrial stromal cells, thereby increasing stromal cell PGE_2 synthesis.[171] This paracrine action may enhance the ability of the stroma to support growth of the endometrial tumor. However, the exact role that the prostanoids play in tumorigenesis is unclear and a clearly beneficial effect of COX inhibitors has not been demonstrated in endometrial cancers.

As indicated above, IGF-I has been implicated as a paracrine stimulator of uterine epithelial cell proliferation. IGF-I was found to be secreted by several endometrial cancer cell lines and behaved as an autocrine stimulator of cell proliferation.[169] The action of IGF-I is attenuated by its binding protein, IGFBP-1, which is also found in the endometrium. Tamoxifen, which behaves as an ER agonist in the endometrium, increases IGF-I receptor activation in Ishikawa cells and this is mediated by a decrease in IGFBP-3, thereby increasing availability of IGF peptides.[170] The observation that IGFBP-1 is absent in preneoplastic conditions suggests that unopposed IGF-I may be involved in development of endometrial cancer.[172] However, two case-control studies suggest that IGF-I and IGFBP-1 have a limited effect on endometrial cancer risk.[173,174] Together, these observations suggest that the IGF-I system may be important to progression of endometrial cancer but it is not involved in its initial development.

The EGF-like protein amphiregulin was implicated as an autocrine growth factor in endometrial cancer by comparing gene expression profiles of endometrial cancer cells during treatment with estradiol, the partial ER agonist tamoxifen, or the full antiestrogen ICI182780.[175] Additional members of this family of growth factors, TGFα and β-cellulin and their receptor proteins, are also increased in endometrial cancers.[67,162] Amplification of the non-ligand-binding member of the receptor proteins, erbB2, is seen in approximately 20% of endometrial cancers and this is related to a poor prognosis.[176–178]

SUMMARY

Cellular proliferation in the endometrium is controlled by estrogen and progesterone in large part through paracrine mediators. Induction of cellular differentiation, such as the secretory phenotype in the epithelium and the decidualized phenotype in the stroma, requires both a direct action of steroid hormones and indirect action through paracrine factors. Numerous growth factors and their receptors have been shown to be under hormonal control in the endometrium, but a role as paracrine mediators of estrogen and progesterone action has been demonstrated for only a few. Many of the growth factors and their receptors belong to families of proteins that share function, making it difficult to define their roles through genetic deletion because of compensatory action of undeleted members of the same family. Additionally, growth factor receptors share intracellular signaling partners and the complexity of regulation is increased by cross-talk among these, including between steroid receptors and growth factor pathways. Nonetheless, clear roles for members of the EGF family of growth factors, the FGF family of growth factors, the TGFβ family, and the IGF-I/IGFBP system have been demonstrated in control of normal endometrial physiology. In addition, prostaglandins are likely candidates as paracrine regulators of endometrial function and, as discussed in other chapters, they are involved in embryo–uterine interactions as well. Dysregulation of paracrine pathways has been implicated to play a role in benign and malignant pathologies of endometrial tissues. Continued investigation of peptide and nonpeptide growth factors is warranted to fully define their roles in mediating or modifying hormonal action in the endometrium.

ACKNOWLEDGMENTS

The data derived from the authors' laboratory were gathered under the support of grants from NIH, HD23244 and HD37025.

REFERENCES

1. Markee JE. Physiology of reproduction. Annu Rev Physiol 1951; 13: 367–96.
2. Noyes RW, Hertig AT, Rock J. Dating the endometrial biopsy. Fertil Steril 1950; 1: 3–25.
3. Carson DD, Bagchi I, Dey SK et al. Embryo implantation. Dev Biol 2000; 223: 217–37.
4. Wilcox AJ, Baird DD, Weinberg CR. Time of implantation of the conceptus and loss of pregnancy. N Engl J Med 1999; 340: 1796–9.
5. Dorfman RI. Standard methods adopted by official organizations. In: Dorfman RI, ed. Methods in Hormone Research II. New York: Academic Press, 1962: 707–29.
6. Finn CA. Oestrogen and the decidual cell reaction of implantation in mice. J Endocrinol 1965; 32: 223–9.
7. Quarmby VE, Korach KS. The influence of 17β-estradiol on patterns of cell division in the uterus. Endocrinology 1984; 114: 694–702.

8. Bigsby RM, Caperell-Grant A, Berry N, Nephew K, Lubahn D. Estrogen induces a systemic growth factor through an estrogen receptor-alpha-dependent mechanism. Biol Reprod 2004; 70: 178–83.

9. Martin L, Finn CA, Trinder G. DNA synthesis in the endometrium of progesterone-treated mice. J Endocrinol 1973; 56: 303–7.

10. Yoshinaga K. Hormonal interplay in the establishment of pregnancy. Int Rev Physiol 1977; 13: 201–23.

11. Walmer DK, Wrona MA, Hughes CL, Nelson KG. Lactoferrin expression in the mouse reproductive tract during the natural estrous cycle: correlation with circulating estradiol and progesterone. Endocrinology 1992; 131: 1458–66.

12. Finn CA, Martin L. Hormone secretion during early pregnancy in the mouse. J Endocrinol 1969; 45: 57–65.

13. Finn CA, Pope M, Milligan SR. Control of uterine stromal mitosis in relation to uterine sensitivity and decidualization in mice. J Reprod Fertil 1995; 103: 153–8.

14. Weitlauf HM. Biology of implantation. In: Knobil E, Neill JD, eds. The Physiology of Reproduction, 2nd edn New York: Raven Press, 1994: 391–440.

15. Rothchild I, Meyer RK, Spielman MA. A quantitative study of oestrogen–progesterone interaction in the formation of placentomata in the castrate rat. Am J Physiol 1940; 128: 213–24.

16. Greenwald GS. Formation of deciduomata in the lactating mouse. J Endocrinol 1958; 17: 24–8.

17. Finn CA, Martin L. Endocrine control of the timing of endometrial sensitivity to a decidual stimulus. Biol Reprod 1972; 7: 82–6.

18. Rothchild I, Meyer RK. Studies of the pretrauma factors necessary for placentoma formation in the rat. Physiol Zool 1942; 15: 216–23.

19. Paria BC, Tan J, Lubahn DB, Dey SK, Das SK. Uterine decidual response occurs in estrogen receptor-alpha-deficient mice. Endocrinology 1999; 140: 2704–10.

20. Kurita T, Kj L, Saunders PT et al. Regulation of progesterone receptors and decidualization in uterine stroma of the estrogen receptor-alpha knockout mouse. Biol Reprod 2001; 64: 272–83.

21. Curtis HS, Goulding EH, Eddy EM et al. Studies using the estrogen receptor alpha knockout uterus demonstrate that implantation but not decidualization-associated signaling is estrogen dependent. Biol Reprod 2002; 67: 1268–77.

22. Hertz R. A review of the evidence linking estrogen and cancer in animals. Pediatrics 1978; 62: 1138–42.

23. Hertz R. The estrogen problem: retrospect and prospect. In: McLachlan JA, ed. Estrogen in the Environment II. New York: Elsevier, 1985: 1–14.

24. Newbold R. Cellular and molecular effects of developmental exposure to diethylstilbestrol: implications for other environmental estrogens. Environ Health Perspect 1995; 103(Suppl 7): 83–7.

25. Cunha GR, Chung LW, Shannon JM, Reese BA. Stromal–epithelial interactions in sex differentiation. Biol Reprod 1980; 22: 19–42.

26. Cunha GR, Cooke PS, Kurita T. Role of stromal–epithelial interactions in hormonal responses. Arch Histol Cytol 2004; 67: 417–34.

27. Cunha GR, Ricke W, Thomson A et al. Hormonal, cellular, and molecular regulation of normal and neoplastic prostatic development. J Steroid Biochem Mol Biol 2004; 92: 221–36.

28. Bigsby RM, Cunha GR. Estrogen stimulation of deoxyribonucleic acid synthesis in uterine epithelial cells which lack estrogen receptors. Endocrinology 1986; 119: 390–6.

29. Bigsby RM, Aixin L, Luo K, Cunha GR. Strain differences in the ontogeny of estrogen receptors in murine uterine epithelium. Endocrinology 1990; 126: 2592–6.

30. Yamashita S, Newbold RR, McLachlan JA, Korach KS. The role of the estrogen receptor in uterine epithelial proliferation and cytodifferentiation in neonatal mice. Endocrinology 1990; 127: 2456–63.

31. Cooke PS, Buchanan DL, Young P et al. Stromal estrogen receptors mediate mitogenic effects of estradiol on uterine epithelium. Proc Natl Acad Sci USA 1997; 94: 6535–40.

32. Kurita T, Young P, Brody JR et al. Stromal progesterone receptors mediate the inhibitory effects of progesterone on estrogen-induced uterine epithelial cell deoxyribonucleic acid synthesis. Endocrinology 1998; 139: 4708–13.

33. Buchanan DL, Setiawan T, Lubahn DB et al. Tissue compartment-specific estrogen receptor-alpha participation in the mouse uterine epithelial secretory response. Endocrinology 1999; 140: 484–91.

34. Kurita T, Lee KJ, Cooke PS et al. Paracrine regulation of epithelial progesterone receptor and lactoferrin by progesterone in the mouse uterus. Biol Reprod 2000; 62: 831–8.

35. Pierro E, Minici F, Alesiani O, et al. Stromal–epithelial interactions modulate estrogen responsiveness in normal human endometrium. Biol Reprod 2001; 64: 831–8.

36. Oshita T, Nagai N, Mukai K et al. Telomerase activation in endometrial epithelial cells by paracrine effectors from stromal cells in primary cultured human endometrium. Int J Mol Med 2004; 13: 425–30.

37. Yang S, Fang Z, Gurates B et al. Stromal PRs mediate induction of 17beta-hydroxysteroid dehydrogenase type 2 expression in human endometrial epithelium: a paracrine mechanism for inactivation of E2. Mol Endocrinol 2001; 15: 2093–105.

38. Osteen KG, Rodgers WH, Gaire M et al. Stromal–epithelial interaction mediates steroidal regulation of metalloproteinase expression in human endometrium. Proc Natl Acad Sci USA 1994; 91: 10129–33.

39. Brody JR, Cunha GR. Histologic, morphometric, and immunocytochemical analysis of myometrial development in rats and mice: I. Normal development. Am J Anat 1989; 186: 1–20.

40. Cunha GR, Young P, Brody JR. Role of uterine epithelium in the development of myometrial smooth muscle cells. Biol Reprod 1989; 40: 861–71.

41. Brody JR, Cunha GR. Histologic, morphometric, and immunocytochemical analysis of myometrial development in rats and mice: II. Effects of DES on development. Am J Anat 1989; 186: 21–42.

42. Kitajewski J, Sassoon D. The emergence of molecular gynecology: homeobox and Wnt genes in the female reproductive tract. Bioessays 2000; 22: 902–10.

43. Couse JF, Korach KS. Estrogen receptor-alpha mediates the detrimental effects of neonatal diethylstilbestrol (DES) exposure in the murine reproductive tract. Toxicology 2004; 205: 55–63.

44. Lejeune B, Leroy F. Role of the uterine epithelium in inducing the decidual cell reaction. Prog Reprod Biol 1980; 7: 92–101.

45. Lejeune B, Van HJ, Leroy F. Transmitter role of the luminal uterine epithelium in the induction of decidualization in rats. J Reprod Fertil 1981; 61: 235–40.

46. Bigsby RM, Aixin L, Everett L. Stromal–epithelial interactions regulating cell proliferation in the uterus. In: Magness RR, Naftolin F, eds. Local Systems in Reproduction. New York: Raven Press, 1993: 171.

47. Ben-Shlomo I. Sharing of unrelated receptors and ligands by cognate partners: possible implications for ovarian and endometrial physiology. Reprod Biomed Online 2005; 11: 259–69.

48. Luetteke NC, Qiu TH, Fenton SE et al. Targeted inactivation of the EGF and amphiregulin genes reveals distinct roles for

EGF receptor ligands in mouse mammary gland development. Development 1999; 126: 2739–50.

49. Wells A. EGF receptor. Int J Biochem Cell Biol 1999; 31: 637–43.

50. Pavelock K, Braas K, Ouafik L, Osol G, May V. Differential expression and regulation of the vascular endothelial growth factor receptors neuropilin-1 and neuropilin-2 in rat uterus. Endocrinology 2001; 142: 613–22.

51. Ghahary A, Chakrabarti S, Murphy LJ. Localization of the sites of synthesis and action of insulin-like growth factor-I in the rat uterus. Mol Endocrinol 1990; 4: 191–5.

52. Kapur S, Tamada H, Dey SK, Andrews GK. Expression of insulin-like growth factor-I (IGF-I) and its receptor in the peri-implantation mouse uterus, and cell-specific regulation of IGF-I gene expression by estradiol and progesterone. Biol Reprod 1992; 46: 208–19.

53. Sato T, Wang G, Hardy MP et al. Role of systemic and local IGF-I in the effects of estrogen on growth and epithelial proliferation of mouse uterus. Endocrinology 2002; 143: 2673–9.

54. Wang J, Niu W, Nikiforov Y et al. Targeted overexpression of IGF-I evokes distinct patterns of organ remodeling in smooth muscle cell tissue beds of transgenic mice. J Clin Invest 1997; 100: 1425–39.

55. Polakis P. Wnt signaling and cancer. Genes Dev 2000; 14: 1837–51.

56. Miller C, Pavlova A, Sassoon DA. Differential expression patterns of Wnt genes in the murine female reproductive tract during development and the estrous cycle. Mech Dev 1998; 76: 91–9.

57. Hou X, Tan Y, Li M, Dey SK, Das SK. Canonical Wnt signaling is critical to estrogen-mediated uterine growth. Mol Endocrinol 2004; 18: 3035–49.

58. Das SK, Tan J, Raja S et al. Estrogen targets genes involved in protein processing, calcium homeostasis, and Wnt signaling in the mouse uterus independent of estrogen receptor-alpha and -beta. J Biol Chem 2000; 275: 28834–42.

59. Couse JF, Curtis SW, Washburn TF et al. Analysis of transcription and estrogen insensitivity in the female mouse after targeted disruption of the estrogen receptor gene. Mol Endocrinol 1995; 9: 1441–54.

60. Geum D, Sun W, Paik SK, Lee CC, Kim K. Estrogen-induced cyclin D_1 and D_3 gene expressions during mouse uterine cell proliferation in vivo: differential induction mechanism of cyclin D_1 and D_3. Mol Reprod Dev 1997; 46: 450–8.

61. Nelson KG, Takahashi T, Bossert NL, Walmer DK, McLachlan JA. Epidermal growth factor replaces estrogen in the stimulation of female genital-tract growth and differentiation. Proc Natl Acad Sci USA 1991; 88: 21–5.

62. Huet-Hudson YM, Chakraborty C, De SK et al. Estrogen regulates the synthesis of epidermal growth factor in mouse uterine epithelial cells. Mol Endocrinol 1990; 4: 510–23.

63. Chegini N, Rossi MJ, Masterson BJ. Platelet-derived growth factor (PDGF), epidermal growth factor (EGF), and EGF and PDGF beta-receptors in human endometrial tissue: localization and in vitro action. Endocrinology 1992; 130: 2373–85.

64. Hom YK, Young P, Wiesen JF et al. Uterine and vaginal organ growth requires epidermal growth factor receptor signaling from stroma. Endocrinology 1998; 139: 913–21.

65. Lim H, Dey SK, Das SK. Differential expression of the erbB2 gene in the periimplantation mouse uterus: potential mediator of signaling by epidermal growth factor-like growth factors. Endocrinology 1997; 138: 1328–37.

66. Tzahar E, Waterman H, Chen X et al. A hierarchical network of interreceptor interactions determines signal transduction by Neu differentiation factor/neuregulin and epidermal growth factor. Mol Cell Biol 1996; 16: 5276–87.

67. Srinivasan R, Benton E, McCormick F et al. Expression of the c-erbB-3/HER-3 and c-erbB-4/HER-4 growth factor

receptors and their ligands, neuregulin-1 alpha, neuregulin-1 beta, and betacellulin, in normal endometrium and endometrial cancer. Clin Cancer Res 1999; 5: 2877–83.

68. Lim H, Das SK, Dey SK. erbB genes in the mouse uterus: cell-specific signaling by epidermal growth factor (EGF) family of growth factors during implantation. Dev Biol 1998; 204: 97–110.

69. Irwin JC, Utian WH, Eckert RL. Sex steroids and growth factors differentially regulate the growth and differentiation of cultured human endometrial stromal cells. Endocrinology 1991; 129: 2385–92.

70. Chegini N, Rossi MJ, Masterson BJ. Platelet-derived growth factor (PDGF), epidermal growth factor (EGF), and EGF and PDGF ß-receptors in human endometrial tissue: localization and in vitro action. Endocrinology 1992; 130: 2373–85.

71. Das SK, Tsukamura H, Paria BC et al. Differential expression of epidermal growth factor receptor (EGF-R) gene and regulation of EGF-R bioactivity by progesterone and estrogen in the adult mouse uterus. Endocrinology 1994; 134: 971–81.

72. Chobotova K, Muchmore ME, Carver J et al. The mitogenic potential of heparin-binding epidermal growth factor in the human endometrium is mediated by the epidermal growth factor receptor and is modulated by tumor necrosis factor-alpha. J Clin Endocrinol Metab 2002; 87: 5769–77.

73. Chobotova K, Karpovich N, Carver J et al. Heparin-binding epidermal growth factor and its receptors mediate decidualization and potentiate survival of human endometrial stromal cells. J Clin Endocrinol Metab 2005; 90: 913–19.

74. Lessey BA, Gui Y, Apparao KB et al. Regulated expression of heparin-binding EGF-like growth factor (HB-EGF) in the human endometrium: a potential paracrine role during implantation. Mol Reprod Dev 2002; 62: 446–55.

75. Curtis SW, Washburn T, Sewall C et al. Physiological coupling of growth factor and steroid receptor signaling pathways: estrogen receptor knockout mice lack estrogen-like response to epidermal growth factor. Proc Natl Acad Sci USA 1996; 93: 12626–30.

76. Hewitt SC, Collins J, Grissom S et al. Global uterine genomics in vivo: microarray evaluation of the estrogen receptor alpha-growth factor cross-talk mechanism. Mol Endocrinol 2005; 19: 657–68.

77. Levin ER. Bidirectional signaling between the estrogen receptor and the epidermal growth factor receptor. Mol Endocrinol 2003; 17: 309–17.

78. Filardo EJ. Epidermal growth factor receptor (EGFR) transactivation by estrogen via the G-protein-coupled receptor, GPR30: a novel signaling pathway with potential significance for breast cancer. J Steroid Biochem Mol Biol 2002; 80: 231–8.

79. Vivacqua A, Bonofiglio D, Recchia AG et al. The G protein-coupled receptor GPR30 mediates the proliferative effects induced by 17beta-estradiol and hydroxytamoxifen in endometrial cancer cells. Mol Endocrinol 2006; 20: 631–46.

80. Battersby S, Critchley HO, Morgan K et al. Expression and regulation of the prokineticins (endocrine gland-derived vascular endothelial growth factor and Bv8) and their receptors in the human endometrium across the menstrual cycle. J Clin Endocrinol Metab 2004; 89: 2463–9.

81. Kaser A, Winklmayr M, Lepperdinger G, Kreil G. The AVIT protein family. Secreted cysteine-rich vertebrate proteins with diverse functions. EMBO Rep 2003; 4: 469–73.

82. LeCouter J, Zlot C, Tejada M et al. Bv8 and endocrine gland-derived vascular endothelial growth factor stimulate hematopoiesis and hematopoietic cell mobilization. Proc Natl Acad Sci USA 2004; 101: 16813–18.

83. Kisliouk T, Podlovni H, Spanel-Borowski K et al. Prokineticins (endocrine gland-derived vascular endothelial growth factor

and BV8) in the bovine ovary: expression and role as mitogens and survival factors for corpus luteum-derived endothelial cells. Endocrinology 2005; 146: 3950–8.

84. Tsai SJ, Wu MH, Chen HM et al. Fibroblast growth factor-9 is an endometrial stromal growth factor. Endocrinology 2002; 143: 2715–21.

85. Moller B, Rasmussen C, Lindblom B, Olovsson M. Expression of the angiogenic growth factors VEGF, FGF-2, EGF and their receptors in normal human endometrium during the menstrual cycle. Mol Hum Reprod 2001; 7: 65–72.

86. Taylor KM, Chen C, Gray CA et al. Expression of messenger ribonucleic acids for fibroblast growth factors 7 and 10, hepatocyte growth factor, and insulin-like growth factors and their receptors in the neonatal ovine uterus. Biol Reprod 2001; 64: 1236–46.

87. Chen C, Spencer TE, Bazer FW. Fibroblast growth factor-10: a stromal mediator of epithelial function in the ovine uterus. Biol Reprod 2000; 63: 959–66.

88. Koji T, Chedid M, Rubin JS et al. Progesterone-dependent expression of keratinocyte growth factor mRNA in stromal cells of the primate endometrium: keratinocyte growth factor as a progestomedin. J Cell Biol 1994; 125: 393–401.

89. Siegfried S, Pekonen F, Nyman T, Ammala M. Expression of mRNA for keratinocyte growth factor and its receptor in human endometrium. Acta Obstet Gynecol Scand 1995; 74: 410–14.

90. Hom YK, Young P, Thomson AA, Cunha GR. Keratinocyte growth factor injected into female mouse neonates stimulates uterine and vaginal epithelial growth. Endocrinology 1998; 139: 3772–9.

91. Slayden OD, Rubin JS, Lacey DL, Brenner RM. Effects of keratinocyte growth factor in the endometrium of rhesus macaques during the luteal–follicular transition. J Clin Endocrinol Metab 2000; 85: 275–85.

92. Marshburn PB, Arici AM, Casey ML. Expression of transforming growth factor-beta 1 messenger ribonucleic acid and the modulation of deoxyribonucleic acid synthesis by transforming growth factor-beta 1 in human endometrial cells. Am J Obstet Gynecol 1994; 170: 1152–8.

93 Bruner KL, Rodgers WH, Gold LI et al. Transforming growth factor beta mediates the progesterone suppression of an epithelial metalloproteinase by adjacent stroma in the human endometrium. Proc Natl Acad Sci USA 1995; 92: 7362–6.

94. Salamonsen LA, Dimitriadis E, Jones RL, Nie G. Complex regulation of decidualization: a role for cytokines and proteases – a review. Placenta 2003; 24(Suppl A): S76–85.

95. Jones RL, Salamonsen LA, Critchley HO et al. Inhibin and activin subunits are differentially expressed in endometrial cells and leukocytes during the menstrual cycle, in early pregnancy and in women using progestin-only contraception. Mol Hum Reprod 2000; 6: 1107–17.

96. Mylonas I, Jeschke U, Wiest I et al. Inhibin/activin subunits alpha, beta-A and beta-B are differentially expressed in normal human endometrium throughout the menstrual cycle. Histochem Cell Biol 2004; 122: 461–71.

97. Jones RL, Salamonsen LA, Zhao YC et al. Expression of activin receptors, follistatin and betaglycan by human endometrial stromal cells; consistent with a role for activins during decidualization. Mol Hum Reprod 2002; 8: 363–74.

98. Jones RL, Salamonsen LA, Findlay JK. Activin A promotes human endometrial stromal cell decidualization in vitro. J Clin Endocrinol Metab 2002; 87: 4001–4.

99. Tierney EP, Giudice LC. Role of activin A as a mediator of in vitro endometrial stromal cell decidualization via the cyclic adenosine monophosphate pathway. Fertil Steril 2004; 81(Suppl 1): 899–903.

100. Noda N, Minoura H, Nishiura R et al. Expression of tenascin-C in stromal cells of the murine uterus during early pregnancy:

induction by interleukin-1 alpha, prostaglandin E(2), and prostaglandin F(2 alpha). Biol Reprod 2000; 63: 1713–20.

101. Singer CF, Marbaix E, Kokorine I et al. Paracrine stimulation of interstitial collagenase (MMP-1) in the human endometrium by interleukin 1alpha and its dual block by ovarian steroids. Proc Natl Acad Sci USA 1997; 94: 10341–5.

102. Singer CF, Marbaix E, Kokorine I et al. The matrix metalloproteinase-1 (MMP-1) expression in the human endometrium is inversely regulated by interleukin-1 alpha and sex steroids. Ceska Gynekol 2000; 65: 211–15.

103. Takamoto N, Zhau B, Tsai SY et al. Identification of Indian hedgehog as a progesterone-responsive gene in the murine uterus. Mol Endocrinol 2002; 16: 2338–48.

104. Lee K, Jeong J, Kwak I et al. Indian hedgehog is a major mediator of progesterone signaling in the mouse uterus. Nat Genet 2006; 38: 1204–9.

105. Khatua A, Wang X, Ding T et al. Indian hedgehog, but not histidine decarboxylase or amphiregulin, is a progesterone-regulated uterine gene in hamsters. Endocrinology 2006; 147: 4079–92.

106. Martin L, Finn CA, Hormonal regulation of cell division in epithelial and connective tissues of the mouse uterus. J Endocrinol 1968; 41: 363–71.

107. Bigsby RM, Cunha GR. Progesterone and dexamethasone inhibition of uterine epithelial proliferation in two models of estrogen-independent growth. Am J Obstet Gynecol 1988; 158: 646–50.

108. Maslar IA, Riddick DH. Prolactin production by human endometrium during the normal menstrual cycle. Am J Obstet Gynecol 1979; 135: 751–4.

109. Croze F, Kennedy TG, Schroedter IC, Friesen HG. Expression of rat prolactin-like protein B in deciduoma of pseudopregnant rat and in decidua during early pregnancy. Endocrinology 1990; 127: 2665–72.

110. Patel OV, Yamada O, Kizaki K et al. Temporospatial expression of placental lactogen and prolactin-related protein-1 genes in the bovine placenta and uterus during pregnancy. Mol Reprod Dev 2004; 69: 146–52.

111. Ain R, Tash JS, Soares MJ. Prolactin-like protein-A is a functional modulator of natural killer cells at the maternal–fetal interface. Mol Cell Endocrinol 2003; 204: 65–74.

112. Sahgal N, Knipp GT, Liu B et al. Identification of two new nonclassical members of the rat prolactin family. J Mol Endocrinol 2000; 24: 95–108.

113. Muller H, Ishimura R, Orwig KE et al. Homologues for prolactin-like proteins A and B are present in the mouse. Biol Reprod 1998; 58: 45–51.

114. Cohick CB, Xu L, Soares MJ. Prolactin-like protein-B: heterologous expression and characterization of placental and decidual species. J Endocrinol 1997; 152: 291–302.

115. Dai G, Liu B, Szpirer C et al. Prolactin-like protein-C variant: complementary deoxyribonucleic acid, unique six exon gene structure, and trophoblast cell-specific expression. Endocrinology 1996; 137: 5009–19.

116. Jayatilak PG, Gibori G. Ontogeny of prolactin receptors in rat decidual tissue: binding by a locally produced prolactin-like hormone. J Endocrinol 1986; 110: 115–21.

117. Jabbour HN, Critchley HO. Potential roles of decidual prolactin in early pregnancy. Reproduction 2001; 121: 197–205.

118. Daly DC, Maslar IA, Rosenberg SM, Tohan N, Riddick DH. Prolactin production by luteal phase defect endometrium. Am J Obstet Gynecol 1981; 140: 587–91.

119. Jones RL, Critchley HO, Brooks J, Jabbour HN, McNeilly AS. Localization and temporal expression of prolactin receptor in human endometrium. J Clin Endocrinol Metab 1998; 83: 258–62.

120. Jabbour HN, Critchley HO, Boddy SC. Expression of functional prolactin receptors in nonpregnant human endometrium: janus

kinase-2, signal transducer and activator of transcription-1 (STAT1), and STAT5 proteins are phosphorylated after stimulation with prolactin. J Clin Endocrinol Metab 1998; 83: 2545–53.

121. Gu Y, Srivastava RK, Clarke DL, Linzer DI, Gibori G. The decidual prolactin receptor and its regulation by decidua-derived factors. Endocrinology 1996; 137: 4878–85.

122. Yamashita M, Matsuda M, Mori T. In situ detection of prolactin receptor mRNA and apoptotic cell death in mouse uterine tissues with adenomyosis. In Vivo 1999; 13: 57–60.

123. Reese J, Binart N, Brown N et al. Implantation and decidualization defects in prolactin receptor (PRLR)-deficient mice are mediated by ovarian but not uterine PRLR. Endocrinology 2000; 141: 1872–81.

124. Binart N, Helloco C, Ormandy CJ et al. Rescue of preimplantatory egg development and embryo implantation in prolactin receptor-deficient mice after progesterone administration. Endocrinology 2000; 141: 2691–7.

125. Deb S, Tessier C, Prigent-Tessier A et al. The expression of interleukin-6 (IL-6), IL-6 receptor, and gp130-kilodalton glycoprotein in the rat decidua and a decidual cell line: regulation by 17beta-estradiol and prolactin. Endocrinology 1999; 140: 4442–50.

126. Baran N, Kelly PA, Binart N. Characterization of a prolactin-regulated gene in reproductive tissues using the prolactin receptor knockout mouse model. Biol Reprod 2002; 66: 1210–18.

127. Baran N, Kelly PA, Binart N. Decysin, a new member of the metalloproteinase family, is regulated by prolactin and steroids during mouse pregnancy. Biol Reprod 2003; 68: 1787–92.

128. Carpenter KD, Gray CA, Noel S et al. Prolactin regulation of neonatal ovine uterine gland morphogenesis. Endocrinology 2003; 144: 110–20.

129. Noel S, Herman A, Johnson GA et al. Ovine placental lactogen specifically binds to endometrial glands of the ovine uterus. Biol Reprod 2003; 68: 772–80.

130. Chilton BS, Daniel JCJ. Differences in the rabbit uterine response to progesterone as influenced by growth hormone or prolactin. J Reprod Fertil 1987; 79: 581–7.

131. Hewetson A, Chilton BS. Novel elements in the uteroglobin promoter are a functional target for prolactin signaling. Mol Cell Endocrinol 1997; 136: 1–6.

132. Mansharamani M, Chilton BS. Prolactin augments progesterone-dependent expression of a nuclear P-type ATPase that associates with the RING domain of RUSH transcription factors in the endometrium. Ann NY Acad Sci 2000; 923: 321–4.

133. Nowak RA, Mora S, Diehl T, Rhoades AR, Stewart EA. Prolactin is an autocrine or paracrine growth factor for human myometrial and leiomyoma cells. Gynecol Obstet Invest 1999; 48: 127–32.

134. Florio P, Rossi M, Sigurdardottir M et al. Paracrine regulation of endometrial function: interaction between progesterone and corticotropin-releasing factor (CRF) and activin A. Steroids 2003; 68: 801–7.

135. Harrison GS, Wierman ME, Nett TM, Glode LM. Gonadotropin-releasing hormone and its receptor in normal and malignant cells. Endocr Relat Cancer 2004; 11: 725–48.

136. Sales KJ, Jabbour HN. Cyclooxygenase enzymes and prostaglandins in reproductive tract physiology and pathology. Prostaglandins Other Lipid Mediat 2003; 71: 97–117.

137. Jabbour HN, Sales KJ. Prostaglandin receptor signalling and function in human endometrial pathology. Trends Endocrinol Metab 2004; 15: 398–404.

138. Gross G, Imamura T, Muglia LJ. Gene knockout mice in the study of parturition. J Soc Gynecol Investig 2000; 7: 88–95.

139. Muglia LJ. Genetic analysis of fetal development and parturition control in the mouse. Pediatr Res 2000; 47: 437–43.

140. Tranguch S, Daikoku T, Guo Y, Wang H, Dey SK. Molecular complexity in establishing uterine receptivity and implantation. Cell Mol Life Sci 2005; 62: 1964–73.

141. Wang H, Dey SK. Lipid signaling in embryo implantation. Prostaglandins Other Lipid Mediat 2005; 77: 84–102.

142. Yang ZM, Das SK, Wang J et al. Potential sites of prostaglandin actions in the periimplantation mouse uterus: differential expression and regulation of prostaglandin receptor genes. Biol Reprod 1997; 56: 368–79.

143. Katsuyama M, Sugimoto Y, Morimoto K et al. Distinct cellular localization of the messenger ribonucleic acid for prostaglandin E receptor subtypes in the mouse uterus during pseudopregnancy. Endocrinology 1997; 138: 344–50.

144. Sun T, Li SJ, Diao HL et al. Cyclooxygenases and prostaglandin E synthases in the endometrium of the rhesus monkey during the menstrual cycle. Reproduction 2004; 127: 465–73.

145. Jones RL, Kelly RW, Critchley HO. Chemokine and cyclooxygenase-2 expression in human endometrium coincides with leukocyte accumulation. Hum Reprod 1997; 12: 1300–6.

146. Baird DT, Cameron ST, Critchley HO et al. Prostaglandins and menstruation. Eur J Obstet Gynecol Reprod Biol 1996; 70: 15–17.

147. Poyser NL. The control of prostaglandin production by the endometrium in relation to luteolysis and menstruation. Prostaglandins Leukot Essent Fatty Acids 1995; 53: 147–95.

148. Smith SK, Kelly RW. The release of PGF_{2alpha} and PGE_2 from separated cells of human endometrium and decidua. Prostaglandins Leukot Essent Fatty Acids 1988; 33: 91–6.

149. Marions L, Danielsson KG. Expression of cyclo-oxygenase in human endometrium during the implantation period. Mol Hum Reprod 1999; 5: 961–5.

150. Fields MJ, Shemesh M. Extragonadal luteinizing hormone receptors in the reproductive tract of domestic animals. Biol Reprod 2004; 71: 1412–18.

151. Kang J, Chapdelaine P, Parent J et al. Expression of human prostaglandin transporter in the human endometrium across the menstrual cycle. J Clin Endocrinol Metab 2005; 90: 2308–13.

152. Ross GT, Hillier SG. Luteal maturation and luteal phase defect. Clin Obstet Gynaecol 1978; 5: 391–409.

153. Balasch J, Vanrell JA. Corpus luteum insufficiency and fertility: a matter of controversy. Hum Reprod 1987; 2: 557–67.

154. Ginsburg KA. Luteal phase defect. Etiology, diagnosis, and management. Endocrinol Metab Clin North Am 1992; 21: 85–104.

155. Wuttke W, Pitzel L, Seidlova-Wuttke D, Hinney B. LH pulses and the corpus luteum: the luteal phase deficiency (LPD). Vitam Horm 2001; 63: 131–58.

156. Tavaniotou A, Albano C, Smitz J, Devroey P. Impact of ovarian stimulation on corpus luteum function and embryonic implantation. J Reprod Immunol 2002; 55: 123–30.

157. Lessey BA. Adhesion molecules and implantation. J Reprod Immunol 2002; 55: 101–12.

158. Lessey BA. Two pathways of progesterone action in the human endometrium: implications for implantation and contraception. Steroids 2003; 68: 809–15.

159. Bukulmez O, Arici A. Luteal phase defect: myth or reality. Obstet Gynecol Clin North Am 2004; 31: 727–44.

160. Bhowmick NA, Moses HL. Tumor–stroma interactions. Curr Opin Genet Dev 2005; 15: 97–101.

161. Yoshida S, Harada T, Iwabe T et al. Induction of hepatocyte growth factor in stromal cells by tumor-derived basic fibroblast growth factor enhances growth and invasion of endometrial cancer. J Clin Endocrinol Metab 2002; 87: 2376–83.

162. Fujimoto J, Hori M, Ichigo S, Tamaya T. Antiestrogenic compounds inhibit estrogen-induced expression of fibroblast growth factor family (FGF-1, 2, and 4) mRNA in well-differentiated

endometrial cancer cells. Eur J Gynaecol Oncol 1997; 18: 497–501.

163. Hyder SM, Chiappetta C, Stancel GM. Triphenylethylene antiestrogens induce uterine vascular endothelial growth factor expression via their partial estrogen agonist activity. Cancer Lett 1997; 120: 165–71.

164. Sakaguchi J, Kyo S, Kanaya T et al. Aberrant expression and mutations of TGF-beta receptor type II gene in endometrial cancer. Gynecol Oncol 2005; 98: 427–33.

165. Tanaka T, Toujima S, Umesaki N. Activin A inhibits growth-inhibitory signals by TGF-beta1 in differentiated human endometrial adenocarcinoma cells. Oncol Rep 2004; 11: 875–9.

166. Park DW, Ryu HS, Choi DS et al. Localization of matrix metalloproteinases on endometrial cancer cell invasion in vitro. Gynecol Oncol 2001; 82: 442–9.

167. Osteen KG, Bruner-Tran KL, Ong D, Eisenberg E. Paracrine mediators of endometrial matrix metalloproteinase expression: potential targets for progestin-based treatment of endometriosis. Ann NY Acad Sci 2002; 955: 139–46.

168. Henriet P, Cornet PB, Lemoine P et al. Circulating ovarian steroids and endometrial matrix metalloproteinases (MMPs). Ann NY Acad Sci 2002; 955: 119–38.

169. Tamura M, Sebastian S, Yang S et al. Up-regulation of cyclooxygenase-2 expression and prostaglandin synthesis in endometrial stromal cells by malignant endometrial epithelial cells. A paracrine effect mediated by prostaglandin E_2 and nuclear factor-kappa B. J Biol Chem 2002; 277: 26208–16.

170. Reynolds RK, Hu C, Baker VV. Transforming growth factor-alpha and insulin-like growth factor-I, but not epidermal growth factor, elicit autocrine stimulation of mitogenesis in endometrial cancer cell lines. Gynecol Oncol 1998; 70: 202–9.

171. Kleinman D, Karas M, Danilenko M et al. Stimulation of endometrial cancer cell growth by tamoxifen is associated with increased insulin-like growth factor (IGF)-I induced tyrosine phosphorylation and reduction in IGF binding proteins. Endocrinology 1996; 137: 1089–95.

172. Rutanen EM. Insulin-like growth factors in endometrial function. Gynecol Endocrinol 1998; 12: 399–406.

173. Lacey JVJ, Potischman N, Madigan MP et al. Insulin-like growth factors, insulin-like growth factor-binding proteins, and endometrial cancer in postmenopausal women: results from a U.S. case-control study. Cancer Epidemiol Biomarkers Prev 2004; 13: 607–12.

174. Augustin LS, Dal Maso L, Franceschi S et al. Association between components of the insulin-like growth factor system and endometrial cancer risk. Oncology 2004; 67: 54–9.

175. Gielen SC, Burger CW, Kuhne LC et al. Analysis of estrogen agonism and antagonism of tamoxifen, raloxifene, and ICI182780 in endometrial cancer cells: a putative role for the epidermal growth factor receptor ligand amphiregulin. J Soc Gynecol Investig 2005; 12: e55–67.

176. Berchuck A, Rodriguez G, Kinney RB et al. Overexpression of HER-2/neu in endometrial cancer is associated with advanced stage disease. Am J Obstet Gynecol 1991; 164: 15–21.

177. Bigsby RM, Li AX, Bomalaski J et al. Immunohistochemical study of HER-2/neu, epidermal growth factor receptor, and steroid receptor expression in normal and malignant endometrium. Obstet Gynecol 1992; 79: 95–100.

178. Saffari B, Jones LA, el-Naggar A et al. Amplification and overexpression of HER-2/neu (c-erbB2) in endometrial cancers: correlation with overall survival. Cancer Res 1995; 55: 5693–8.

179. Croze F, Kennedy TG, Schroedter IC et al. Expression of insulin-like growth factor-I and insulin-like growth factor-binding protein-1 in the rat uterus during decidualization. Endocrinology 1990; 127: 1995–2000.

180. Giudice LC, Mark SP, Irwin JC. Paracrine actions of insulin-like growth factors and IGF binding protein-1 in non-pregnant

human endometrium and at the decidual–trophoblast interface. J Reprod Immunol 1998; 39: 133–48.

181. Tamada H, Das SK, Andrews GK, Dey SK. Cell-type-specific expression of transforming growth factor-alpha in the mouse uterus during the peri-implantation period. Biol Reprod 1991; 45: 365–72.

182. Paria BC, Das SK, Huet-Hudson YM, Dey SK. Distribution of transforming growth factor alpha precursors in the mouse uterus during the periimplantation period and after steroid hormone treatments. Biol Reprod 1994; 50: 481–91.

183. Das SK, Chakraborty I, Paria BC et al. Amphiregulin is an implantation-specific and progesterone-regulated gene in the mouse uterus. Mol Endocrinol 1995; 9: 691–705.

184. Lee DS, Yanagimoto Ueta Y, Xuan X et al. Expression patterns of the implantation-associated genes in the uterus during the estrous cycle in mice. J Reprod Dev 2005; 51: 787–98.

185. Klonisch T, Wolf P, Hombach-Klonisch S et al. Epidermal growth factor-like ligands and erbB genes in the peri-implantation rabbit uterus and blastocyst. Biol Reprod 2001; 64: 1835–44.

186. Das SK, Flanders KC, Andrews GK, Dey SK. Expression of transforming growth factor-beta isoforms (β_2 and β_3) in the mouse uterus analysis of the periimplantation period and effects of ovarian steroids. Endocrinology 1992; 130: 3459–66.

187. Takahashi T, Eitzman B, Bossert NL et al. Transforming growth factors β_1, β_2, and β_3 messenger RNA and protein expression in mouse uterus and vagina during estrogen-induced growth: a comparison to other estrogen-regulated genes. Cell Growth Diff 1994; 5: 919–35.

188. Tamada H, McMaster MT, Flanders KC et al. Cell type-specific expression of transforming growth factor-beta 1 in the mouse uterus during the periimplantation period. Mol Endocrinol 1990; 4: 965–72.

189. Wada K, Nomura S, Morii E et al. Changes in levels of mRNAs of transforming growth factor (TGF)-beta1, -beta2, -beta3, TGF-beta type II receptor and sulfated glycoprotein-2 during apoptosis of mouse uterine epithelium. J Steroid Biochem Mol Biol 1996; 59: 367–75.

190. Tabibzadeh S, Lessey B, Satyaswaroop PG. Temporal and site-specific expression of transforming growth factor-beta4 in human endometrium. Mol Hum Reprod 1998; 4: 595–602.

191. Chegini N, Zhao Y, Williams RS, Flanders KC. Human uterine tissue throughout the menstrual cycle expresses transforming growth factor-beta 1 (TGF beta 1), TGF beta 2, TGF beta 3, and TGF beta type II receptor messenger ribonucleic acid and protein and contains [^{125}I]TGF beta 1-binding sites. Endocrinology 1994; 135: 439–49.

192. Dumont N, O'Connor-McCourt MD, Philip A. Transforming growth factor-beta receptors on human endometrial cells: identification of the type I, II, and III receptors and glycosylphosphatidylinositol anchored TGF-beta binding proteins. Mol Cell Endocrinol 1995; 111: 57–66.

193. Hyder SM, Huang JC, Nawaz Z et al. Regulation of vascular endothelial growth factor expression by estrogens and progestins. Environ Health Perspect 2000; 108(Suppl 5): 785–90.

194. Halder JB, Zhao X, Soker S et al. Differential expression of VEGF isoforms and VEGF(164)-specific receptor neuropilin-1 in the mouse uterus suggests a role for VEGF(164) in vascular permeability and angiogenesis during implantation. Genesis 2000; 26: 213–24.

195. Ancelin M, Buteau-Lozano H, Meduri G et al. A dynamic shift of VEGF isoforms with a transient and selective progesterone-induced expression of VEGF189 regulates angiogenesis and vascular permeability in human uterus. Proc Natl Acad Sci USA 2002; 99: 6023–8.

196. Mulayim N, Palter SF, Kayisli UA et al. Chemokine receptor expression in human endometrium. Biol Reprod 2003; 68: 1491–5.

197. Chakraborty I, Das SK, Wang J, Dey SK. Developmental expression of the cyclo-oxygenase-1 and cyclo-oxygenase-2 genes in the peri-implantation mouse uterus and their differential regulation by the blastocyst and ovarian steroids. J Mol Endocrinol 1996; 16: 107–22.

198. Tawfik OW, Huet YM, Malathy PV et al. Release of prostaglandins and leukotrienes from the rat uterus is an early estrogenic response. Prostaglandins 1987; 34: 805–15.

199. Papay KD, Kennedy TG. Characterization of temporal and cell-specific changes in transcripts for prostaglandin E(2) receptors in pseudopregnant rat endometrium. Biol Reprod 2000; 62: 1515–25.

200. Gray K, Eitzman B, Raszmann K et al. Coordinate regulation by diethylstilbestrol of the platelet-derived growth factor-A (PDGF-A) and -B chains and the PDGF receptor alpha- and beta-subunits in the mouse uterus and vagina: potential mediators of estrogen action. Endocrinology 1995; 136: 2325–40.

201. Tulac S, Nayak NR, Kao LC et al. Identification, characterization, and regulation of the canonical Wnt signaling pathway in human endometrium. J Clin Endocrinol Metab 2003; 88: 3860–6.

202. Yoshinaga K, Hawkins RA, Stocker JF. Estrogen secretion by the rat ovary in vivo during the estrous cycle and pregnancy. Endocrinology 1969; 85: 103–12.

203. Park OK, Ramirez VD. Circulating blood progesterone is pulsatile throughout the rat oestrous cycle. Acta Endocrinol (Copenh) 1987; 116: 121–8.

204. Virgo BB, Bellward GD. Serum progesterone levels in the pregnant and postpartum laboratory mouse. Endocrinology 1974; 95: 1486–90.

205. Thorneycroft IH, Mishell DRJ, Stone SC, Kharma KM, Nakamura RM. The relation of serum 17-hydroxyprogesterone and estradiol-17-beta levels during the human menstrual cycle. Am J Obstet Gynecol 1971; 111: 947–51.

206. Ross GT, Cargille CM, Lipsett MB et al. Pituitary and gonadal hormones in women during spontaneous and induced ovulatory cycles. Recent Prog Horm Res 1970; 26: 1–62.

207. Bigsby RM, Cooke PS, Cunha GR. A simple efficient method for separating murine uterine epithelial and mesenchymal cells. Am J Physiol 1986; 251: E630–6.

16   A comparative view of prostaglandin action in the uterus

Flavia L Lopes, Joëlle Desmarais, and Bruce D Murphy

INTRODUCTION: COMPARATIVE MODELS OF ENDOMETRIAL FUNCTION

Viviparity is a defining characteristic of the eutherian or placental mammals. Evolution of this trait required extensive modification of the ovary,[1] as well as the uterus and the fetal membranes, which underwent modifications resulting in the establishment of the placenta.[2] The mammalian evolutionary pressure toward placental formation resulted in significant variation among the mechanisms of implantation, embryo invasion, and placentation.[3] The simplest mechanism, resulting in the least intimate maternal–fetal interaction, is known as epitheliochorial placentation. It comprises apposition and attachment of the embryonic chorion to the endometrial epithelium and is exemplified by the placentation in the pig, with variations in other hoofed mammals. In equids, for example, there is invasion of the specialized trophoblast cells of the chorionic girdle to form the endometrial cups.[4] In ruminants, specialized binucleate trophoblast cells invade the epitheliochorial interface and fuse with the endometrial epithelium.[4] A closer association of mother and fetus occurs in the endotheliochorial placental subtype, where the trophoblast erodes or bypasses the endometrial epithelium to associate directly with the maternal capillaries.[5] This placentation is found in species and groups as diverse as the mustelids, pinnepeds, shrews, squirrels, and elephants.[3] The most intimate of interactions, hemochorial placentation, is present when the trophoblast is in contact with maternal blood, following erosion of both the endometrial epithelium and the vascular endothelium. Versions of this subtype are found in primates, rodents, bats, and rabbits, among others.[3] Comparative morphological investigations across mammalian taxa have provided some surprises. The presence of trophoblast invasion, erosion of maternal epithelium, and endotheliochorial placentation in insectivores, believed to be the most primitive mammals, suggests that the least invasive subtype, epitheliochorial placentation, is a secondary specialization.[3] Moreover, there are variations in invasiveness of trophoblast

between closely related species (e.g. lemurs display the epitheliochorial mode, while hemochorial placentation is present in all other primates[6]). This diversity is indicative of convergent evolution of placental forms, and the frequency of the hemochorial subtype across diverse taxa argues for evolutionary pressure toward formation of this maternal–fetal interaction.[3]

The heterogeneity of processes by which successful viviparity was achieved in placental mammals suggests that there is parallel heterogeneity in the signaling mechanisms that regulate endometrial function and implantation. Although the comparative evidence is incomplete, it seems that function is characterized more by commonality than heterogeneity of mechanisms. Given this convergence, comparative analysis can provide insight relevant not only to understanding the endometrial events of early gestation, but also to evolution of the systems that regulate these events. In this chapter, we have attempted to take a comparative approach to examination of prostaglandin modulation of endometrial function, embryo implantation, and the early placentation. While there is a plethora of evidence linking prostaglandins to mammalian parturition, discussion of this phenomenon is out of the scope of this chapter. The reader is directed to informative recent reviews on the topic.[7-9]

PROSTAGLANDIN SYNTHESIS

Prostaglandins are bioactive lipid compounds in the eicosanoid family, derived from the essential fatty acid arachidonic acid. They were first identified more than 65 years ago by von Euler from semen and the prostate, and their chemical structures were elucidated by Bergström, Samuelsson, and van Dorp (for review, see Simmons et al[10]). Prostaglandins have widespread effects on cell and organ function and are essential regulators of reproductive processes, including ovulation, implantation, parturition, and cyclic endometrial changes. Figure 16.1 provides a simplified scheme of the synthesis of three categories of biologically active eicosanoids. More detailed information on the

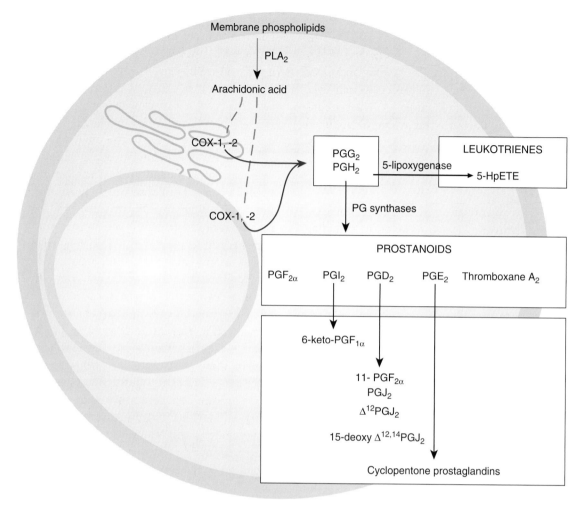

Figure 16.1   The cascade of prostaglandin synthesis. The parent molecule of prostaglandins is arachidonic acid, derived from membrane phospholipids cleaved by the enzyme phospholipase A_2 (PLA$_2$). The cyclooxygenase enzymes (COX) in the endoplasmic reticulum and nuclear membranes convert arachidonic acid to prostaglandin H_2 (PGH$_2$), which is then acted upon by other enzymes to produce the leukotrienes and prostanoids. The products with biological activity in the endometrium and placenta – e.g. prostaglandin E_2 (PGE$_2$) – are included in the diagram.

formation of these compounds can be found in any of a number of recent reviews of prostaglandin synthetic pathways.[10,11]

As can be seen from Figure 16.1, the parent molecule of the eicosanoids, arachidonic acid, is most commonly found in an esterified form in phospholipids of the membrane.[12] In order for it to become available for further formation of prostanoids, it must be cleaved from the membrane, achieved principally by phospholipase A_2 (PLA$_2$), in one of its two forms, cytosolic PLA$_2$ and the non-pancreatic, type II secretory PLA$_2$.[13] Following cleavage, the free arachidonate migrates to the luminal surface of the endoplasmic reticulum or to the nuclear membrane, where it enters the prostanoid formation cascade.[14] The first stages of prostaglandin formation require the cyclooxygenases (COX-1 and COX-2, also known as prostaglandin H_2 synthases) located on the endoplasmic reticulum or nuclear

membranes. These enzymes diooxygenate arachidonic acid to form the endoperoxide-containing prostaglandin G_2 (PGG$_2$), which then undergoes hydroperoxyl reduction to give rise to prostaglandin H_2 (PGH$_2$). This reaction is catalyzed by COX-1 and COX-2.[10] PGH$_2$ can then be converted by the specific synthases (prostaglandin and thromboxane synthases) to its biologically active products. These include the prostanoids (prostaglandin and thromboxanes) and the leukotrienes. The latter contain an oxane ring instead of the cyclopentane ring and are formed by action of the nuclear membrane enzyme 5-lipoxygenase on PGH$_2$. They are synthesized primarily in mast cells, leukocytes, macrophages, and other inflammatory cells.[15]

Several prostaglandins are formed from the PGH$_2$ precursor by the action of specific synthases and isomerases (see Figure 16.1). These include five primarily active forms – PGE$_2$, PGD$_2$, PGI$_2$, PGF$_{2\alpha}$, and thromboxane A_2.[16] Further modifications ensue to form other biologically active compounds, PGE_2 is converted to cyclopentone prostaglandins and PGD_2 to the J series of prostaglandins. The prostaglandins G, H, I, and thromboxane are unstable and have half-lives as brief as 30 seconds to a few minutes.[17] The remaining prostaglandins, while more stable, are metabolized and inactivated in a single passage through the lungs, which renders the local production of prostanoids a requirement for their prolonged action (for review, see Narumiya et al[18]).

Across mammalian tissues, an array of biological functions are provoked by prostanoids, including contraction and relaxation of smooth muscles, modulation of neurotransmitter release, fever responses, sleep induction, secretion of gastrointestinal enzymes, as well as regulation of gastrointestinal tract motility, transport of water and ions to the kidney, apoptosis, cell differentiation, immune responses, platelet aggregation, and vascular permeability and vasculogenesis. In the uterine context, prostaglandins modulate endometrial cyclicity, embryo implantation, placental formation and function, and parturition. The present discussion focuses on cyclicity and on the early events of gestation. The best-known prostanoid effects on the early embryo, endometrium, and on the establishment of gestation are mediated by prostaglandins of the E, F, D, I, and J series.

SIGNALING PATHWAYS FOR PROSTAGLANDIN ACTION IN THE ENDOMETRIUM

Receptor diversity and intracellular mechanisms

The variety of actions elicited by prostanoids are controlled by their temporally and spatially regulated synthesis, which is in turn regulated by expression of the synthetic enzymes and the availability of substrate. The heterogeneity and complexity of responses also results from diversity and specificity of membrane and nuclear receptors for prostaglandins. The membrane receptors are in the family of the G-protein-coupled rhodopsin-type receptors that consist of an extracellular ligand-binding domain, seven transmembrane domains, and an intracellular signaling component.[19] Although each prostanoid binds with high affinity to one or more receptors, there is some cross-reactivity amongst the ligands.[18] Nine different receptors, coded by separate genes, have been identified to date (Figure 16.2): the eponymous DP, IP, FP, TP, EP receptors, and the newly discovered CRTH2 (also known as DP_2) receptor that

displays equal affinity for PGD and thromboxane.[20,21] Four subtypes of the EP class of receptors are known, termed EP1 through EP4, each coded by a separate gene.[21] Intracellular pathways elicited by each receptor can also vary, and many can activate more than one receptor and signaling system (see Figure 16.2). The FP receptor activates the phospholipase C (PLC) pathway via the G protein Gq.[22] The IP receptor stimulates adenylate cyclase following ligand binding; however, activation of PLC and consequent elevation of Ca^{2+} levels have also been observed.[23] Ligand binding to the prostanoid receptor DP increases cyclic adenosine monophosphate (cAMP) and activates the protein kinase A (PKA) pathway.[24] The splice variants α and β of the thromboxane receptor, TP, both induce a PLC-dependent response through Gq and a PKA-related response through Gs.[25] They differ in their cAMP-related responses, as the α isoform inhibits while the β isoform increases cAMP synthesis.[21] The diverse actions of prostaglandin E_2 in target tissues result from the EP subtypes that activate different intracellular mechanisms. EP1 activation elevates Ca^{2+} concentrations[26] via activation of the PLC pathway.[23] Two of the subtypes, EP2 and EP4, are known mediators of cAMP signaling through Gs, thereby inducing responses via the PKA pathway.[21] Recent information suggests that these receptors can also signal through the Wnt/β-catenin pathway.[27] The receptor EP3 has eight splice variant isoforms, and, although its major signaling pathway involves inhibition of adenylate cyclase through Gi, activation of some isoforms increases cAMP levels.[28] At least one isoform can activate the PLC pathway.[29]

PPAR-activated pathways

Recently, the importance of another class of receptors in reproductive events has been demonstrated. These are the peroxisome proliferator-activated receptors (PPARs), members of the nuclear receptor family. Two PPARs bind prostaglandin ligands with consequence of modulation of physiological events in the embryo and uterus. PPARδ is activated by prostaglandin I_2,[30] while PPARγ is the receptor for the naturally occurring prostaglandin D and J series ligands.[31] Binding of ligands to PPARs engenders formation of heterodimers with the retinoic acid X receptor (RXR), most commonly with the RXRα isoform[32] (see Figure 16.2). The consequence of association of ligand-activated PPAR with RXR is the interaction with specific DNA sequences and enhancement or inhibition of transcription of target genes.[32] There are numerous candidates for targets of PPAR regulation in the endometrial and gestational context.

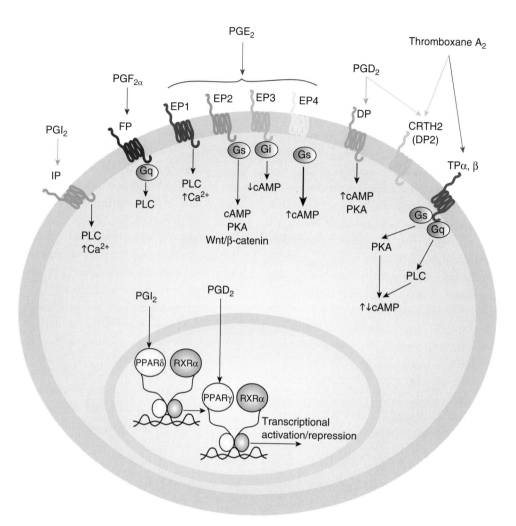

Figure 16.2 Prostaglandins induce a variety of effects in the uterus through membrane and nuclear receptors. Although the nine membrane receptors (e.g. IP, EP1) bind their eponymous ligands with high affinity, there is cross-reactivity, whereby a prostaglandin can bind to another receptor with lower affinity. The intracellular pathways known to be activated by each receptor subtype (e.g. protein kinase A) are found below the receptor (see text for further explanation). The nuclear peripheral peroxisome proliferator-activated receptors (PPARs) bind prostaglandins of the I series and metabolites of PGD_2. Binding induces heterodimerization with another nuclear receptor, the retinoic acid X receptor α isoform (RXRα) and the complex directly modulates target gene expression.

PROSTAGLANDIN REGULATION OF ENDOMETRIAL CYCLICITY

The cyclic ovarian events of follicle maturation, ovulation, formation and regression of the corpus luteum and consequent ovarian estrogen and progestin secretion provide dynamic regulation of endometrial differentiation, structure, and function. These events are discussed in depth in other chapters within this book. They comprise modification of the luminal and glandular epithelium, as well as stromal changes, including proliferation of and secretion by both cell types. In primates, decidualization, a terminal differentiation state of stromal cells with subsequent loss of approximately one-third of the endometrium by menstruation, is likewise under steroidal control.[33] Cyclic

variation in localization of prostaglandin synthetic enzymes and prostaglandin receptors implies a contribution of prostaglandins to cyclic changes in both the epithelium and stroma of the endometrium. Cyclic expression of both COX isozymes is present in both the stroma and epithelium of the endometrium of the rat,[34] baboon,[35] rhesus monkey,[36] cow,[37] and sheep.[38] EP family receptor transcript abundance is up-regulated in the rat endometrial stroma and glandular epithelium in response to progestin treatment,[39] and PGI and IP receptor expression are present in both the proliferative and secretory phases of the human endometrial cycle.[40]

There is evidence beyond the guilt by association for prostaglandin modulation of cyclic events in the endometrium. The principal control of the proliferative phase is exerted by ovarian estrogens, and estrogen has been shown to increase COX-2 expression in the endometrial epithelium and uterine glands.[41] Prostaglandin $F_{2\alpha}$ synthesis and FP receptor expression in human endometrial epithelial cells is greatest during the proliferative phase of the cycle, and $PGF_{2\alpha}$ has been shown to induce proliferation in human uterine cell lines.[22] Moreover, there is evidence for PGE induction of endometrial proliferation.[22,42] Most available information suggests that the I and J prostaglandins are not involved in this process, as their usual action is to attenuate the cell cycle.[43,44] The temporal and spatial pattern of expression of their synthetic enzymes and receptors[40] indicates that they are involved in the termination of endometrial proliferation.

Following ovulation, the endometrium undergoes extensive change associated with the dominant effects of progesterone of luteal provenance. Endometrial stromal cells in primates begin a progressive and terminal differentiation process known as decidualization, accompanied by marked development of the endometrial glands. Decidualization also takes place in the rodent uterus under progestin dominance, but only when provoked. Under biological conditions, it is the embryo that induces decidualization, but it can also be produced experimentally by mild mechanical trauma. During decidualization in both primates and rodents, stromal cells take on a polygonal shape and stromal vascular permeability increases. The essential role of prostaglandins in decidualization, particularly the PGEs, was proposed by TG Kennedy some years ago,[45] and is strongly supported by experimental evidence using cyclooxygenase inhibition and prostaglandin replacement.[46] Furthermore, decidual stimuli induce rapid expression of COX-2 but not COX-1 genes, and the null mutation of the COX-2 gene prevents both embryo and experimentally induced decidualization.[16] There is a current view, supported by results in the COX-2 knockout mouse, that PGI, acting through PPARδ, is the prostanoid that regulates decidualization.[47] Alternatively, there is evidence arguing for PGE_2 mediation of the decidual reaction in the rat.[48] The expression profile of a wide array of genes changes during the decidualization process in human endometrium[49] and at least three genes appear specifically up-regulated in the rat stroma.[50,51] The cellular mechanisms by which prostaglandin regulate the process of decidualization are not clearly understood at present.

Uterine $PGF_{2\alpha}$ plays a special role in regulating ovarian cyclicity, in that it induces regression of the corpus luteum in non-pregnant animals of several species. In ruminants, $PGF_{2\alpha}$ first reduces progesterone receptors and progesterone sensitivity in the uterus, and then acts to obliterate the luteal source of progesterone by means of multiple mechanisms.[52] The ruminant conceptus synthesizes a cytokine, interferon-τ, that modulates prostaglandin synthetic patterns to prevent $PGF_{2\alpha}$ synthesis and its luteolytic consequences.[52] This interesting phenomenon is the subject of Chapter 17, and thus will not be discussed further herein.

If conception does not occur in most mammals, the corpus luteum regresses, attenuating the progesterone support to the uterus. The consequence is endometrial regression. In many primates, luteal regression engenders menstruation, resulting in loss of approximately one-third of the endometrium. Common exceptions to the pattern of cyclic endometrial regression are found, usually in species in which ovulation is induced by copulation, such as carnivores and rabbits. In these species, the corpus luteum persists whether a conceptus is present or not, as does the secretory phase of the endometrium, resulting in a state of pseudopregnancy. Regression results from progesterone withdrawal, usually at the end of the normal gestational interval.

Prostaglandins modulate endometrial regression in non-primate mammals. Recent in-vitro studies indicate that $PGF_{2\alpha}$ directly modifies uterine stromal cell function, principally by altering genes associated with extracellular matrix turnover.[53] $PGF_{2\alpha}$ generation, induced by progesterone withdrawal, also appears to play a role in primate menstruation.[54] The downstream genes regulated by $PGF_{2\alpha}$ include the array of extracellular matrix proteins whose expression is dramatically altered during the extensive menstrual tissue remodeling of the endometrium.[55] Increased expression of PGI and its receptor in the endometrium during menstruation implicates this prostanoid in the process,[40] but the mechanisms and targets remain unexplored.

ESSENTIAL ROLE OF PROSTAGLANDINS IN IMPLANTATION

The regulated form of cyclooxygenase, COX-2, mediates embryo implantation

The landmark studies in the 1970s in which the cyclooxygenase inhibitor indomethacin was shown to delay the appearance of vascular permeability at the site of embryo attachment in the rat first linked prostaglandin synthesis to the process of implantation.[45] Early immunolocalization studies of COX enzymes demonstrated intense localization in early differentiating stromal cells adjacent to the luminal epithelium on day 5 after mating at the implantation site in the rat, and in the implanting blastocyst between days 5 and 7.[56] As the identity of the COX isoforms became known and specific antibodies against the regulated form, COX-2, became available, detailed analysis, beginning with the mouse,[57] showed its mRNA and protein to be highly expressed at implantation sites, in contrast to the constitutive form, COX-1 (Figure 16.3A). This proved true for the baboon, where COX-1 mRNA and protein were absent in implantation sites, while COX-2 expression was localized specifically to the decidualizing cells of the uterus.[35] Two studies confirmed a role for COX-2 in carnivore implantation. In a study in the western spotted skunk, *Spilogale gracilis*, expression of this enzyme was first observed in the uterus and trophoblast prior to blastocyst attachment and remained for the first 5–6 days of trophoblast invasion.[58] In the mink, *Mustela vison*, another carnivore presenting embryonic diapause, expression of COX-2 mRNA and protein was strongest in the uterus at early stages of implantation, again focused at the sites of embryo invasion.[59]

As noted above, prostaglandins participate in the decidual reaction, a necessary precursor to embryo invasion in rodents. In other species, such as the ferret *Mustela putorius* that have no decidual cells, indomethacin interferes with implantation.[60] This indicates that the nidatory events can be uncoupled from decidualization.

Specific inhibition of COX-2 and null mutation of the COX-2 enzyme impaired implantation in the mouse, supporting its essential role in the nidation process.[61] Further studies in which wild-type blastocysts were transplanted to the uteri of COX-2 knockout mice indicated delays in decidualization, without substantial effect on implantation,[62] suggesting that COX-1 can function in backup of COX-2. Support for this view comes from studies where COX-1 and COX-2 knockout mice were treated with the inhibitors of the alternative isoform, resulting in complete abrogation of the decidual response and implantation.[63] Reduction in COX-2 expression, induced by interdiction of extracellular lysophosphatidic acid (LPA) signaling through the LPA3 receptor subtype, disrupted implantation and embryo spacing.[64] As LPA3 activation induces COX-2 expression, these findings have been interpreted as further evidence for a specific role of COX-2 in implantation.[65]

Downstream prostaglandins in implantation

It is not surprising that elements and events up- and downstream of cyclooxygenase synthesis of prostaglandin precursors have effects on embryo implantation. Targeted disruption of the cytosolic form of phospholipase A_2, $PLA_{2\alpha}$ that mobilizes arachidonic acid from the membrane, defers implantation and disrupts embryo spacing in mice.[66] Strong evidence for a role for PGE synthase products comes from observation of temporal and spatial co-expression of this enzyme with COX-2 at hamster implantation sites[67] (see Figure 16.3B). In mice, the mRNA and protein for PGE synthase localize in the implantation site at the subluminal stroma surrounding the implanting blastocyst.[68,69] In bovine endometrial cells, the expression of PGE synthase correlates with the pattern of COX-2 expression during embryo implantation.[70] Nonetheless, null mutations, including a knockout of prostaglandin E synthase-1 that reduces prostaglandin E_2 abundance in tissues by a remarkable 80%[71] and knockout of the EP2 receptor,[72] did not prevent implantation. The lack of response is most likely due to redundancy in the system, as indicated by the occurrence of at least four cytosolic enzymes with PGE synthase activity,[73] and the presence of four isoforms of the EP receptors.[18] In support of this view, and, as noted above, PGE_2 administration rescues the decidual response that accompanies implantation in rats treated with indomethacin.[48] The capacity of the PGI analogue to rescue both blastocyst attachment and decidualization in the COX-2 knockout mouse strongly indicates its regulatory role.[47] Null mutation of the membrane PGI receptor did not affect implantation in mice, pointing to PPARδ as transducer of the PGI signal.[74]

Target genes in implantation

Information about the specific target genes for the prostaglandin signals and the patterns of gene expression modulated by prostaglandins in the implantation process is fragmentary. There is no shortage of candidates: differential expression studies comparing the pre- and postimplantation uteri in the mouse[75] and rat[50,51,76] have revealed a number of genes that are potentially up- or down-regulated during the temporal window of implantation. Likewise, comparison of the dormant and activated mouse embryos provided numerous candidate genes in the trophoblast with differential expression patterns associated with peri-implantation changes.[77] Among the classes of genes that one would expect to be regulated in implantation are those related to the extracellular matrix and cell adhesion. The protein products of these genes direct not only the attachment of the trophoblast to the endometrial epithelium but also the remodeling of the stroma during decidualization. An intriguing candidate is the adhesion molecule

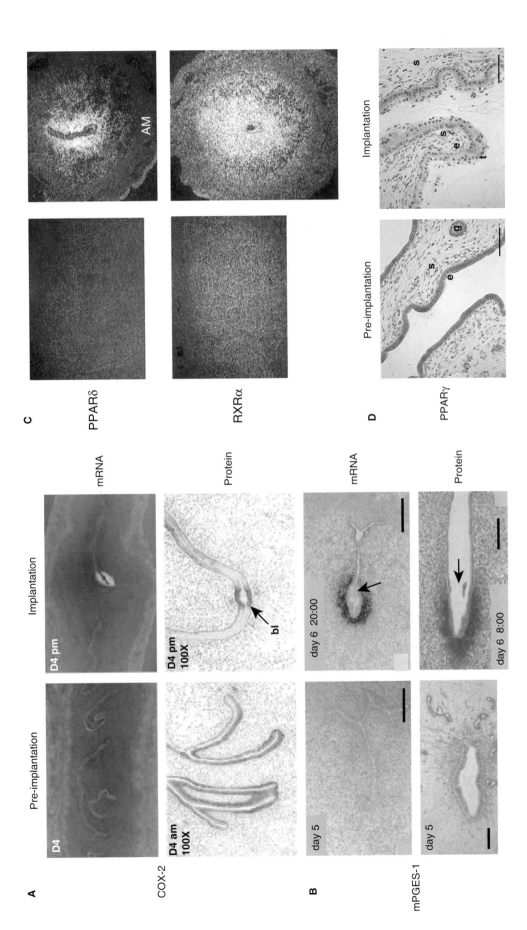

Figure 16.3 Expression of prostaglandin synthetic enzymes in rodents is temporally and spatially associated with early embryo implantation in the mouse and hamster. (A) Localization of COX-2 mRNA by in-situ hybridization and COX-2 protein on the morning prior to and on the evening of implantation in the mouse. (Reproduced from Wang et al,[67] with permission.) (B) Localization of the prostaglandin E synthase (PGES-1) signal, mRNA by in-situ hybridization and protein by immunohistochemistry on the morning and evening of the day of implantation (day 5 postcoitum) in the golden hamster. (Reproduced from Cong et al,[122] with permission.) (C) In situ hybridization reveals that PPARδ and RxR transcripts are co-expressed at the site and time of embryo implantation in the mouse (taken from Lim and Dey[74] with permission). (D) Immunohistochemical localization of PPARγ in the uterus of the non-pregnant (left) and pregnant pig (right). The bars at the bottom of each panel represent 8 μm and e g s, and t mark the endometrial epithelium, endometrial gland, endometrial stroma, and trophoblast, respectively. (Reproduced from Lord et al,[85] with permission).

L-selectin, which is highly expressed by the human uterus during the window of receptivity for trophoblast attachment to the uterus.[78] Although there is no demonstration of direct regulation of L-selectin by prostaglandins in the uterus, there is extensive information to indicate that a similar process in other tissues, L-selectin-based adhesion in leukocyte extravasation, requires local prostaglandin synthesis.[79] Negative regulation, preventing attachment, may be achieved by PGI_2, as this prostanoid reduces adhesion in capillary endothelial cells by direct effects on expression of L-selectin.[80] Molecules of the integrin family function not only in adhesion, but also in cell–cell signaling. The 15 or so integrin family members are regulated both spatially and temporally through the reproductive cycle, and are believed to play key roles in embryo implantation, regulating both the opening and closing of the window of endometrial receptivity.[81] One of these integrins, $a_v\beta_1$, is present on the human endometrial epithelial surface only during the window of attachment.[81] While no information appears available on uterine regulation of this heterodimer, its expression is associated with cell–cell adhesion and it is forcefully induced by PGE_2 in hepatocarcinoma cells.[82] This patchwork of evidence provides support for the view that prostaglandins, perhaps most predominantly PGE_2, regulate the adhesion and decidualization processes via effects on extracellular matrix protein expression.

PROSTAGLANDINS IN ESTABLISHMENT OF THE PLACENTA

Prostaglandins modulate invasion of the endometrium and early placental formation

As noted in the Introduction, some placental types involve limited or no invasion of the trophoblast into the maternal epithelium, while others invade and induce degeneration of the maternal epithelium, stroma, and vascular investments. In all cases, the establishment of pregnancy causes extensive tissue remodeling on both maternal and fetal sides of the placenta. Prostaglandins participate in and regulate the invasion process, and they induce the expression of an array of genes necessary for placental function.

All pregnancies fail in COX-2 knockout mice treated with COX-1 inhibitors and in COX-1 gene disrupted mice treated with COX-2 inhibitors during the implantation or early postimplantation phase.[63] This argues strongly for a requirement for prostaglandins in

trophoblast invasion and placental formation. Indeed, both the invading embryo and the endometrial stroma appear capable of prostaglandin synthesis in invasive placentas, as indicated by strong COX-2 expression.[59] As noted above and in Figure 16.3B, temporal investigation of PGE synthase in the hamster uterus demonstrates a rapid spread of expression of this enzyme across the stromal cells following implantation.[69] The activated preimplantation mink embryo produces E series prostaglandins,[83] indicating the functionality of the embryonic synthetic enzymes in the epitheliochorial context.

Prostaglandin receptors and placental formation

Membrane receptors for PGE and other prostaglandins have been characterized during invasion and uterine remodeling in the cow placenta, and are found in abundance on both maternal and fetal elements of the placenta. In mice, the individual EP receptors are redundant, as gestation continues following null mutations of each, although parturition is disrupted when the FP receptor is knocked out.[84] Multiple knockouts will be required to establish the PGE receptor requirement for invasion and placental establishment.

The story differs for the nuclear prostaglandin receptors, which appear essential to placental formation. Expression studies demonstrate that PPARδ is expressed following embryo attachment in the pig in both the trophoblast and the endometrial endothelium, with less prominent staining in the stroma.[85] In the mouse, PPARδ is expressed primarily in the stroma about the implanting embryo, spreading toward the myometrium as gestation progresses[86] (Figure 16.3C). In-situ hybridization revealed PPARδ transcripts to be present in stroma at implantation sites in the mink uterus during placental formation (J Desmarais and BD Murphy, unpublished work). PPARδ co-localizes with PGD synthase in human placenta, providing a local source of ligand.[87] PPARδ appears to participate in placental formation, as more than 90% of fertilized embryos from homozygous null mutation pregnancies are lost within a few days of implantation, due to lack of appropriate interaction between the trophoblast and the maternal deciduum.[88]

PPARγ is likewise indispensable to gestation in the mouse, as null mutation is embryo lethal, due to failure of trophoblast differentiation, placental formation, and vasculogenesis.[89] Expression studies suggest that PPARγ signaling is important to trophoblast function. PPARγ is weakly expressed in the porcine trophoblast and adjacent epithelium at attachment, but pronounced protein concentrations are present in both tissues some 10 days following attachment[85] (Figure 16.3D). In mink, an intense signal for PPARγ mRNA was found in the trophoblast soon after embryo attachment and in the invasive trophoblast in stroma within 72 hours of implantation.[90] The rat trophoblast also expresses PPARγ in a progressively stronger manner as the placenta develops and differentiates.[91] The same authors showed that 15-deoxy-$\Delta^{12,14}$-prostaglandin J$_2$ (15d-PGJ$_2$), a naturally occurring PPARγ ligand, localizes to the rat placenta, providing indication that the receptor is functional. Indeed, treatment of pregnant rats with PPARγ agonists increases the number of embryos that survive to term.[91] There is evidence for PPARγ signaling in primate fetal membrane development, as it induces both human cytotrophoblast differentiation[92] and reduces its invasiveness.[93]

Prostaglandin target genes in early placental formation

Compared to cyclic uterine variation and implantation, more information is available on prostaglandin regulation of early placentation. There is good evidence that prostaglandins drive extracellular matrix remodeling, via expression and activity of matrix-degrading enzymes, the matrix metalloproteinases (MMPs) and their inhibitors, the tissue inhibitors of MMPs (TIMPs). Among the MMPs whose expression correlates with invasion and placental formation in humans[94] and a number of other species, are MMP-2 and MMP-9. They are also known as gelatinases A and B, and they act to degrade the collagen of the extracellular matrix.[95] In-vitro studies of MMP-9 in human trophoblast cells[96] and MMP-2 in invasive pancreatic cancer cells[97] indicate the capability of PGE$_2$ to induce expression of these proteases. Infusion of rats with PGE$_2$ during early placental formation caused several-fold increases in the abundance of MMP-2 and MMP-9 proteins in the placenta.[98] This intervention, while pharmacological, indicates a potential role for PGE$_2$ in regulation of these remodeling enzymes.

As noted above, activation of PPARγ attenuates trophoblast invasion.[93] This presumably occurs by more than one mechanism and, therefore, by modulation of expression of a large array of target genes. Recent studies of myeloid cancer cell lines demonstrate that both the naturally occurring 15d-PGJ$_2$ ligand and the

PPARγ synthetic agonist, troglitazone, inhibit both the expression of MMP-2 and MMP-9 and their proteolytic activities.[99] No similar information is yet available in trophoblast or trophoblast cell lines. An interesting new finding is that null mutation of PPARγ results in loss of expression of the adhesion molecule Muc-1 on the trophoblast, impairing the union between trophoblast cells and inhibiting association with maternal vascular sinus in the mouse.[100] PPARγ also inhibits cell proliferation and promotes terminal differentiation in many cell types, a phenomenon best known in adipose tissue.[101] PPARγ expression is feeble in mouse trophoblast stem cells in vitro, but is strongly up-regulated with their differentiation from the pluripotent state.[100]

Cell cycle inhibition by PPARγ activation has not been studied in trophoblast cells, but information in other cell types suggests that this abrogation is visited on multiple targets. In colon cancer cells, PPARγ activation up-regulates the tumor suppressor p27^{kip1}, thereby blocking G$_1$/S transition.[102] Primary culture of hepatocytes provided confirmation of induction of p27^{kip1} but not other cell cycle suppressors induced by both 15d-PGJ$_2$ and pharmacological PPARγ agonists.[103] In immortalized cells of lymphocyte[104] and keratinocyte[43] lines, 15d-PGJ$_2$ inhibits the G$_1$S transition. Further investigation of the multiple roles of PPARγ in inhibition of proliferation and induction of differentiation should shed light on its role in placentation.

The deregulation of uterine and trophoblast vasculogenesis observed in mice bearing inactivating disruption of the COX-2 gene[105] provides insight into several potential target genes for prostanoids in placental formation. Endometrial and placental angiogenesis are treated more extensively elsewhere within this book, while the focus herein is the prostaglandin regulation of angiogenic factors. Vascular endothelial growth factor (VEGF) has been shown to be essential to the formation of the mouse placenta, as inactivation of a single allele in the mouse is embryo lethal.[106] VEGF is expressed by both trophoblast and endometrium during early placental formation in species from a number of mammalian species, including the mouse,[107] pig,[108] cow,[109] mink,[110,111] (Figure 16.4A), and primates.[112] Two receptors bind VEGF and initiate transduction of its signal by means of tyrosine kinase mechanisms: VEGFR1 (or Flt-1) and VEGFR2 (or KDR).[107] In the human placenta, they appear differentially expressed, with the former found in trophoblast and endometrium, while the latter appears restricted to decidual cells.[113] This distribution is not universal, as expression of both receptors was found in trophoblast, endometrial epithelium, and endometrial stroma of the cow[109] and mink.[110] VEGFR1, while expressed in trophoblast, endometrial epithelium, and stroma of the mouse, was found to be dispensable in the trophoblast.[114]

Down-regulation of COX-2 has been employed experimentally to interdict angiogenesis in a variety of tumors, providing evidence for prostaglandin regulation of VEGF and its receptors.[115] Prostaglandins of the E series are potent up-regulators of VEGF expression in human smooth muscle cells,[116] osteoblasts,[117] mast cells,[118] and in other tissues, including endometrial adenocarcinoma cells.[119] Promoter assays revealed that PGE, acting through EP2 and EP4, transactivates the mink VEGF promoter in a mink endometrial stromal cell line[83] (Figure 16.4B), providing a model for embryonic and endometrial paracrine regulation of VEGF expression during early gestation. As noted above, the PPARγ null mutation results in a failure to establish placental vasculature, with serious consequences on trophoblast angiogenesis,[89] leading to the hypothesis that PPARγ activation may be an important signaling mechanism in placental angiogenesis. While there appears to be no direct evidence to demonstrate that PPARγ ligands induce VEGF expression in the trophoblast or endometrium, there are numerous examples in extrauterine tissues. Among others, there are studies showing that 15d-PGJ₂ induces VEGF expression in tumor cell lines[120] and the synthetic PPARγ ligands ciglitazone and pioglitazone produce similar VEGF expression in osteoblasts. Yasuda et al[121] reported that administration of another PPARγ ligand, troglitazone, to pregnant rats, reduced rat fetal mortality by half, an effect they attributed to induction of differentiation of the trophoblast. It remains possible that enhanced survival induced by this PPARγ agonist resulted, entirely or in part, from PPARγ-mediated induction of placental vasculogenesis. In overview, the case for prostaglandin regulation of VEGF in the placenta through membrane and nuclear receptors is strong.

SUMMARY, CONCLUSIONS, AND PERSPECTIVES

Prostaglandins, derived from arachidonic acid under the rate-limiting regulation of COX enzyme isoforms, are synthesized nearly ubiquitously in mammalian tissues. Downstream metabolites of the parent molecule interact with specific membrane and nuclear receptors, thereby activating multiple intracellular

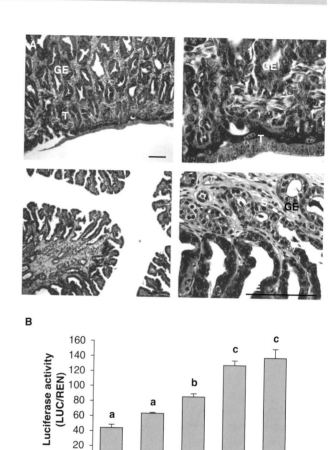

Figure 16.4 (A) Angiogenesis accompanies implantation in the mink uterus and there is immunohistochemical evidence for the expression of vascular endothelial growth factor (VEGF) in uterine surface epithelium (E) and glandular epithelium (GE) at the site of attachment on the day following implantation. (Reproduced from Lopes et al,[111] with permission.) Tissue labeled T is the trophoblast. (B) Dose-dependent activation of the mink VEGF gene promoter by PGE₂ in a transient transfection assay of a mink endometrial cell line demonstrating that this prostanoid regulates expression of VEGF in the uterus. (Reproduced from Lopes et al,[83] with permission.)

signaling pathways. Experimental evidence, accumulated over more than 35 years, has confirmed a role for prostaglandins as endocrine, paracrine, and autocrine mediators of reproductive processes in mammals. In the endometrium, they are necessary for regulation of steroid-driven cyclic modifications in the epithelium and stroma, for implantation, and for formation of a functional placenta (Figure 16.5). The localization of the rate-limiting enzymes and, consequently, their prostaglandin products, near their site of action indicates that effects on the endometrium and trophoblast are primarily local. Prostaglandin-induced effects common to endometrial cyclicity, implantation,

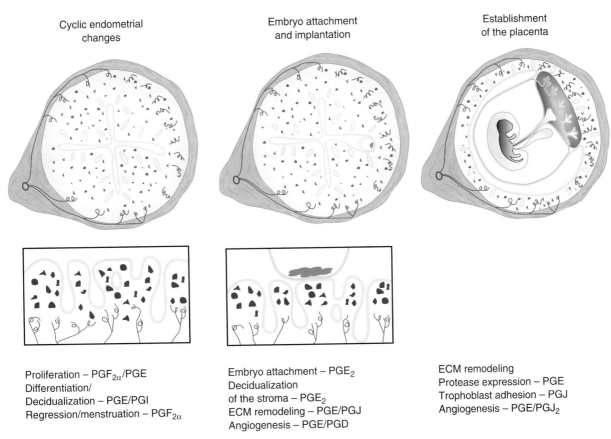

Cyclic endometrial
changes

Embryo attachment
and implantation

Establishment
of the placenta

Proliferation – PGF$_{2\alpha}$/PGE
Differentiation/
Decidualization – PGE/PGI
Regression/menstruation – PGF$_{2\alpha}$

Embryo attachment – PGE$_2$
Decidualization
of the stroma – PGE$_2$
ECM remodeling – PGE/PGJ
Angiogenesis – PGE/PGD

ECM remodeling
Protease expression – PGE
Trophoblast adhesion – PGJ
Angiogenesis – PGE/PGJ$_2$

Figure 16.5   Major prostaglandin products and their roles in cycling, implantation, and early placental formation. Depicted are representations of cross-sections of endometrium displaying decidualization, implantation, and placental formation. The principal known roles of prostaglandins in these processes are listed below each uterine depiction.

and placental formation include induction of cell differentiation, epithelial cell degradation, and remodeling of stromal cells and vascular elements (see Figure 16.5). Cell cycle regulatory factors, extracellular matrix proteins, and angiogenic elements are common targets of prostaglandins in many tissues and there is good evidence that these elements are local targets for paracrine prostaglandin signaling in the endometrium.

A common theme in the text of this chapter is the fragmentary understanding of the sequence of prostaglandin synthesis in reproductive events, as well as in the specific prostaglandins produced and the multiple target genes that they must regulate, directly and indirectly. It is more than likely that the ovary and the embryo, along with the reticuloendothelial system interact to control the complex pattern of prostaglandin expression that modulates cycling endometrial changes, embryo attachment and implantation, and placental formation. While clues can be divined from regulation in other tissues, uterine-specific regulation remains in the realm of mystery. Many null mutation studies of mice result in embryo

lethality, due to faulty establishment of the placenta a few days after implantation. The regulatory function of prostaglandins in the genes whose absence is marked by gestational failure merits further investigation.

ACKNOWLEDGMENTS

The original work from the laboratory of BD Murphy described herein was funded by generous support in the form of a Discovery Grant from the Natural Sciences and Engineering Research Council of Canada. The authors thank Dr DD Massion for valuable discussion and perspectives, and K Boisvert for aid with the figures.

REFERENCES

1. Rothchild I. The yolkless egg and the evolution of eutherian viviparity. Biol Reprod 2003; 68: 337–57.
2. Mess A, Carter AM. Evolutionary transformations of fetal membrane characters in Eutheria with special reference to Afrotheria. J Exp Zoolog B Mol Dev Evol 2006; 306: 140–63.

3. Carter AM, Enders AC. Comparative aspects of trophoblast development and placentation. Reprod Biol Endocrinol 2004; 2: 46.

4. Luckett WP. Uses and limitations of mammalian fetal membranes and placenta for phylogenetic reconstruction. J Exp Zool 1993; 266: 514–27.

5. Isakova GK, Skvortsova TE. [Mechanisms and frequency of nuclear divisions in trophoblast and decidua cells during postimplantation embryogenesis in the mouse]. Ontogenez 2003; 34: 472–7.

6. Carter AM. J. P. Hill on placentation in primates. Placenta 1999; 20: 513–17.

7. Mohan AR, Loudon JA, Bennett PR. Molecular and biochemical mechanisms of preterm labour. Semin Fetal Neonatal Med 2004; 9: 437–44.

8. Brown AG, Leite RS, Strauss JF 3rd. Mechanisms underlying "functional" progesterone withdrawal at parturition. Ann NY Acad Sci 2004; 1034: 36–49.

9. Myatt L, Lye SJ. Expression, localization and function of prostaglandin receptors in myometrium. Prostaglandins Leukot Essent Fatty Acids 2004; 70: 137–48.

10. Simmons DL, Botting RM, Hla T. Cyclooxygenase isozymes: the biology of prostaglandin synthesis and inhibition. Pharmacol Rev 2004; 56: 387–437.

11. Ruan KH. Advance in understanding the biosynthesis of prostacyclin and thromboxane A_2 in the endoplasmic reticulum membrane via the cyclooxygenase pathway. Mini Rev Med Chem 2004; 4: 639–47.

12. Irvine RF. How is the level of free arachidonic acid controlled in mammalian cells? Biochem J 1982; 204: 3–16.

13. Dennis EA. Diversity of group types, regulation, and function of phospholipase A_2. J Biol Chem 1994; 269: 13057–60.

14. Morita I, Schindler M, Regier MK et al. Different intracellular locations for prostaglandin endoperoxide H synthase-1 and -2. J Biol Chem 1995; 270: 10902–8.

15. Jones SM, Luo M, Peters-Golden M, Brock TG. Identification of two novel nuclear import sequences on the 5-lipoxygenase protein. J Biol Chem 2003; 278: 10257–63.

16. Wang H, Dey SK. Lipid signaling in embryo implantation. Prostaglandins Other Lipid Mediat 2005; 77: 84–102.

17. El Tahir KE, Williams KI, Betteridge DJ. Differences in the stability of prostacyclin in human, rabbit and rat plasma. Prostaglandins Leukot Med 1983; 10: 109–14.

18. Narumiya S, Sugimoto Y, Ushikubi F. Prostanoid receptors: structures, properties, and functions. Physiol Rev 1999; 79: 1193–226.

19. Foord SM, Bonner TI, Neubig RR et al. International Union of Pharmacology. XLVI. G protein-coupled receptor list. Pharmacol Rev 2005; 57: 279–88.

20. Hata AN, Lybrand TP, Breyer RM. Identification of determinants of ligand binding affinity and selectivity in the prostaglandin D_2 receptor CRTH2. J Biol Chem 2005; 280: 32442–51.

21. Hata AN, Breyer RM. Pharmacology and signaling of prostaglandin receptors: multiple roles in inflammation and immune modulation. Pharmacol Ther 2004; 103: 147–66.

22. Milne SA, Jabbour HN. Prostaglandin (PG) $F_{(2alpha)}$ receptor expression and signaling in human endometrium: role of $PGF_{(2alpha)}$ in epithelial cell proliferation. J Clin Endocrinol Metab 2003; 88: 1825–32.

23. Nasrallah R, Hebert RL. Prostacyclin signaling in the kidney: implications for health and disease. Am J Physiol Renal Physiol 2005; 289: F235–46.

24. Herlong JL, Scott TR. Positioning prostanoids of the D and J series in the immunopathogenic scheme. Immunol Lett 2006; 102: 121–31.

25. Hirata T, Ushikubi F, Kakizuka A et al. Two thromboxane A_2 receptor isoforms in human platelets. Opposite coupling to adenylyl cyclase with different sensitivity to Arg60 to Leu mutation. J Clin Invest 1996; 97: 949–56.

26. Watabe A, Sugimoto Y, Honda A et al. Cloning and expression of cDNA for a mouse EP1 subtype of prostaglandin E receptor. J Biol Chem 1993; 268: 20175–8.

27. Lee EO, Shin YJ, Chong YH. Mechanisms involved in prostaglandin E_2-mediated neuroprotection against TNF-alpha: possible involvement of multiple signal transduction and beta-catenin/T-cell factor. J Neuroimmunol 2004; 155: 21–31.

28. Hull MA, Ko SC, Hawcroft G. Prostaglandin EP receptors: targets for treatment and prevention of colorectal cancer? Mol Cancer Ther 2004; 3: 1031–9.

29. Ito Y, Murai Y, Ishibashi H et al. The prostaglandin E series modulates high-voltage-activated calcium channels probably through the EP3 receptor in rat paratracheal ganglia. Neuropharmacology 2000; 39: 181–90.

30. Lim H, Dey SK. A novel pathway of prostacyclin signaling – hanging out with nuclear receptors. Endocrinology 2002; 143: 3207–10.

31. Bos CL, Richel DJ, Ritsema T et al. Prostanoids and prostanoid receptors in signal transduction. Int J Biochem Cell Biol 2004; 36: 1187–205.

32. Tan NS, Michalik L, Desvergne B, Wahli W. Multiple expression control mechanisms of peroxisome proliferator-activated receptors and their target genes. J Steroid Biochem Mol Biol 2005; 93: 99–105.

33. Brenner RM, Slayden OD. Steroid receptors in blood vessels of the rhesus macaque endometrium: a review. Arch Histol Cytol 2004; 67: 411–16.

34. Fang L, Chatterjee S, Dong YL et al. Immunohistochemical localization of constitutive and inducible cyclo-oxygenases in rat uterus during the oestrous cycle and pregnancy. Histochem J 1998; 30: 383–91.

35. Kim JJ, Wang J, Bambra C et al. Expression of cyclooxygenase-1 and -2 in the baboon endometrium during the menstrual cycle and pregnancy. Endocrinology 1999; 140: 2672–8.

36. Sun T, Li SJ, Diao HL et al. Cyclooxygenases and prostaglandin E synthases in the endometrium of the rhesus monkey during the menstrual cycle. Reproduction 2004; 127: 465–73.

37. Arosh JA, Parent J, Chapdelaine P et al. Expression of cyclooxygenases 1 and 2 and prostaglandin E synthase in bovine endometrial tissue during the estrous cycle. Biol Reprod 2002; 67: 161–9.

38. Charpigny G, Reinaud P, Creminon C, Tamby JP. Correlation of increased concentration of ovine endometrial cyclooxygenase 2 with the increase in PGE_2 and PGD_2 in the late luteal phase. J Reprod Fertil 1999; 117: 315–24.

39. Papay KD, Kennedy TG. Characterization of temporal and cell-specific changes in transcripts for prostaglandin E_2 receptors in pseudopregnant rat endometrium. Biol Reprod 2000; 62: 1515–25.

40. Battersby S, Critchley HO, de Brum-Fernandes AJ, Jabbour HN. Temporal expression and signaling of prostacyclin receptor in the human endometrium across the menstrual cycle. Reproduction 2004; 127: 79–86.

41. Hertrampf T, Schmidt S, Laudenbach-Leschowsky U et al. Tissue-specific modulation of cyclooxygenase-2 (Cox-2) expression in the uterus and the v. cava by estrogens and phytoestrogens. Mol Cell Endocrinol 2005; 243: 51–7.

42. Sales KJ, Jabbour HN. Cyclooxygenase enzymes and prostaglandins in pathology of the endometrium. Reproduction 2003; 126: 559–67.

43. Matsuzaki Y, Koyama M, Hitomi T et al. 15-deoxy-$\Delta^{12,14}$-prostaglandin J_2 activates the expression of p15INK4b gene, a cyclin-dependent kinase inhibitor. Int J Oncol 2005; 27: 497–503.

44. Stewart SA, Kothapalli D, Yung Y, Assoian RK. Antimitogenesis linked to regulation of Skp2 gene expression. J Biol Chem 2004; 279: 29109–13.

45. Kennedy TG. Evidence for a role for prostaglandins in the initiation of blastocyst implantation in the rat. Biol Reprod 1977; 16: 286–91.

46. Kennedy TG. Prostaglandins and uterine sensitization for the decidual cell reaction. Ann NY Acad Sci 1986; 476: 43–8.

47. Lim H, Gupta RA, Ma WG et al. Cyclo-oxygenase-2-derived prostacyclin mediates embryo implantation in the mouse via PPARδ. Genes Dev 1999; 13: 1561–74.

48. Kennedy TG, Barbe GJ, Ross HE, Shaw TJ. Is prostaglandin E_2 (PGE_2) or prostaglandin I_2 (PGI_2) the physiological mediator of decidualization in rats? Biol Reprod 2000; 62: 344.

49. Mirkin S, Arslan M, Churikov D et al. In search of candidate genes critically expressed in the human endometrium during the window of implantation. Hum Reprod 2005; 20: 2104–17.

50. Simmons DG, Kennedy TG. Induction of glucose-regulated protein 78 in rat uterine glandular epithelium during uterine sensitization for the decidual cell reaction. Biol Reprod 2000; 62: 1168–76.

51. Simmons DG, Kennedy TG. Uterine sensitization-associated gene-1: a novel gene induced within the rat endometrium at the time of uterine receptivity/sensitization for the decidual cell reaction. Biol Reprod 2002; 67: 1638–45.

52. Spencer TE, Burghardt RC, Johnson GA, Bazer FW. Conceptus signals for establishment and maintenance of pregnancy. Anim Reprod Sci 2004; 82–83: 537–50.

53. Callegari EA, Ferguson-Gottschall S, Gibori G. PGF_{2alpha} induced differential expression of genes involved in turnover of extracellular matrix in rat decidual cells. Reprod Biol Endocrinol 2005; 3: 3.

54. Sugino N, Karube-Harada A, Taketani T et al. Withdrawal of ovarian steroids stimulates prostaglandin F_{2alpha} production through nuclear factor-kappaB activation via oxygen radicals in human endometrial stromal cells: potential relevance to menstruation. J Reprod Dev 2004; 50: 215–25.

55. Schatz F, Krikun G, Runic R et al. Implications of decidualization-associated protease expression in implantation and menstruation. Semin Reprod Endocrinol 1999; 17: 3–12.

56. Parr MB, Parr EL, Munaretto K et al. Immunohistochemical localization of prostaglandin synthase in the rat uterus and embryo during the peri-implantation period. Biol Reprod 1988; 38: 333–43.

57. Chakraborty I, Das SK, Wang J, Dey SK. Developmental expression of the cyclo-oxygenase-1 and cyclo-oxygenase-2 genes in the peri-implantation mouse uterus and their differential regulation by the blastocyst and ovarian steroids. J Mol Endocrinol 1996; 16: 107–22.

58. Das SK, Wang J, Dey SK, Mead RA. Spatiotemporal expression of cyclooxygenase 1 and cyclooxygenase 2 during delayed implantation and the periimplantation period in the Western spotted skunk. Biol Reprod 1999; 60: 893–9.

59. Song JH, Sirois J, Houde A, Murphy BD. Cloning, developmental expression, and immunohistochemistry of cyclooxygenase 2 in the endometrium during embryo implantation and gestation in the mink (*Mustela vison*). Endocrinology 1998; 139: 3629–36.

60. Mead RA, Bremner S, Murphy BD. Changes in endometrial vascular permeability during the periimplantation period in the ferret (*Mustela putorius*). J Reprod Fertil 1988; 82: 293–8.

61. Lim H, Paria BC, Das SK et al. Multiple female reproductive failures in cyclooxygenase 2-deficient mice. Cell 1997; 91: 197–208.

62. Cheng JG, Stewart CL. Loss of cyclooxygenase-2 retards decidual growth but does not inhibit embryo implantation or development to term. Biol Reprod 2003; 68: 401–4.

63. Reese J, Zhao X, Ma WG et al. Comparative analysis of pharmacologic and/or genetic disruption of cyclooxygenase-1 and cyclooxygenase-2 function in female reproduction in mice. Endocrinology 2001; 142: 3198–206.

64. Ye X, Hama K, Contos JJ et al. LPA3-mediated lysophosphatidic acid signaling in embryo implantation and spacing. Nature 2005; 435: 104–8.

65. Shah BH, Catt KJ. Roles of LPA3 and COX-2 in implantation. Trends Endocrinol Metab 2005; 16: 397–9.

66. Song H, Lim H, Paria BC et al. Cytosolic phospholipase A_{2alpha} is crucial [correction of A_{2alpha} deficiency is crucial] for 'on-time' embryo implantation that directs subsequent development. Development 2002; 129: 2879–89.

67. Wang X, Su Y, Deb K, Raposo M et al. Prostaglandin E_2 is a product of induced prostaglandin-endoperoxide synthase 2 and microsomal-type prostaglandin E synthase at the implantation site of the hamster. J Biol Chem 2004; 279: 30579–87.

68. Ni H, Sun T, Ma XH, Yang ZM. Expression and regulation of cytosolic prostaglandin E synthase in mouse uterus during the peri-implantation period. Biol Reprod 2003; 68: 744–50.

69. Ni H, Sun T, Ding NZ et al. Differential expression of microsomal prostaglandin E synthase at implantation sites and in decidual cells of mouse uterus. Biol Reprod 2002; 67: 351–8.

70. Parent J, Chapdelaine P, Sirois J, Fortier MA. Expression of microsomal prostaglandin E synthase in bovine endometrium: coexpression with cyclooxygenase type 2 and regulation by interferon-tau. Endocrinology 2002; 143: 2936–43.

71. Uematsu S, Matsumoto M, Takeda K, Akira S. Lipopolysaccharide-dependent prostaglandin E_2 production is regulated by the glutathione-dependent prostaglandin E^2 synthase gene induced by the Toll-like receptor 4/MyD88/NF-IL6 pathway. J Immunol 2002; 168: 5811–16.

72. Matsumoto H, Ma W, Smalley W et al. Diversification of cyclooxygenase-2-derived prostaglandins in ovulation and implantation. Biol Reprod 2001; 64: 1557–65.

73. Trebino CE, Stock JL, Gibbons CP et al. Impaired inflammatory and pain responses in mice lacking an inducible prostaglandin E synthase. Proc Natl Acad Sci USA 2003; 100: 9044–9.

74. Lim H, Dey SK. PPAR delta functions as a prostacyclin receptor in blastocyst implantation. Trends Endocrinol Metab 2000; 11: 137–42.

75. Reese J, Das SK, Paria BC et al. Global gene expression analysis to identify molecular markers of uterine receptivity and embryo implantation. J Biol Chem 2001; 276: 44137–45.

76. Simmons DG, Kennedy TG. Rat endometrial Vdup1 expression: changes related to sensitization for the decidual cell reaction and hormonal control. Reproduction 2004; 127: 475–82.

77. Hamatani T, Daikoku T, Wang H et al. Global gene expression analysis identifies molecular pathways distinguishing blastocyst dormancy and activation. Proc Natl Acad Sci USA 2004; 101: 10326–31.

78. Genbacev OD, Prakobphol A, Foulk RA et al. Trophoblast L-selectin-mediated adhesion at the maternal–fetal interface. Science 2003; 299: 405–8.

79. Gomez-Gaviro MV, Gonzalez-Alvaro I, Dominguez-Jimenez C et al. Structure–function relationship and role of tumor necrosis factor-alpha-converting enzyme in the down-regulation of L-selectin by non-steroidal anti-inflammatory drugs. J Biol Chem 2002; 277: 38212–21.

80. Zardi EM, Zardi DM, Cacciapaglia F et al. Endothelial dysfunction and activation as an expression of disease: role of prostacyclin analogs. Int Immunopharmacol 2005; 5: 437–59.

81. Reddy KV, Mangale SS. Integrin receptors: the dynamic modulators of endometrial function. Tissue Cell 2003; 35: 260–73.

82. Mayoral R, Fernandez-Martinez A, Bosca L, Martin-Sanz P. Prostaglandin E_2 promotes migration and adhesion in hepatocellular carcinoma cells. Carcinogenesis 2005; 26: 753–61.

83. Lopes FL, Desmarais J, Ledoux S et al. Transcriptional regulation of uterine vascular endothelial growth factor during early gestation in the carnivore model, *Mustela vison*. J Biol Chem 2006; 281: 24602–11.

84. Ushikubi F, Sugimoto Y, Ichikawa A, Narumiya S. Roles of prostanoids revealed from studies using mice lacking specific prostanoid receptors. Jpn J Pharmacol 2000; 83: 279–85.

85. Lord E, Murphy BD, Ledoux S et al. Modulation of peroxisome proliferator-activated receptor delta and gamma transcripts in swine endometrial tissue during early gestation. Reproduction 2006; 131: 929–42.

86. Ding NZ, Teng CB, Ma H et al. Peroxisome proliferator-activated receptor delta expression and regulation in mouse uterus during embryo implantation and decidualization. Mol Reprod Dev 2003; 66: 218–24.

87. Jowsey IR, Murdock PR, Moore GB et al. Prostaglandin D_2 synthase enzymes and PPARγ are co-expressed in mouse 3T3-L1 adipocytes and human tissues. Prostaglandins Other Lipid Mediat 2003; 70: 267–84.

88. Barak Y, Liao D, He W et al. Effects of peroxisome proliferator-activated receptor delta on placentation, adiposity, and colorectal cancer. Proc Natl Acad Sci USA 2002; 99: 303–8.

89. Barak Y, Nelson MC, Ong ES et al. PPARγ is required for placental, cardiac, and adipose tissue development. Mol Cell 1999; 4: 585–95.

90. Desmarais J, Lopes FL, Zhang H et al. The mink trophoblast expresses proliferator-activated receptor gamma during the initial steps of embryo implantation and cytotrophoblast differentiation. Biol Reprod 2005; Special Issue: 211.

91. Asami-Miyagishi R, Iseki S, Usui M et al. Expression and function of PPARγ in rat placental development. Biochem Biophys Res Commun 2004; 315: 497–501.

92. Tarrade A, Schoonjans K, Guibourdenche J et al. PPARγ/RXRα heterodimers are involved in human CG β synthesis and human trophoblast differentiation. Endocrinology 2001; 142: 4504–14.

93. Fournier T, Pavan L, Tarrade A et al. The role of PPAR-γ/RXR-α heterodimers in the regulation of human trophoblast invasion. Ann NY Acad Sci 2002; 973: 26–30.

94. Staun-Ram E, Goldman S, Gabarin D, Shalev E. Expression and importance of matrix metalloproteinase 2 and 9 (MMP-2 and -9) in human trophoblast invasion. Reprod Biol Endocrinol 2004; 2: 59.

95. Bischof P, Meisser A, Campana A. Biochemistry and molecular biology of trophoblast invasion. Ann NY Acad Sci 2001; 943: 157–62.

96. Oger S, Mehats C, Dallot E, Cabrol D, Leroy MJ. Evidence for a role of phosphodiesterase 4 in lipopolysaccharide-stimulated prostaglandin E_2 production and matrix metalloproteinase-9 activity in human amniochorionic membranes. J Immunol 2005; 174: 8082–9.

97. Ito H, Duxbury M, Benoit E et al. Prostaglandin E_2 enhances pancreatic cancer invasiveness through an Ets-1-dependent induction of matrix metalloproteinase-2. Cancer Res 2004; 64: 7439–46.

98. Lyons CA, Beharry KD, Nishihara KC et al. Regulation of matrix metalloproteinases (type IV collagenases) and their inhibitors in the virgin, timed pregnant, and postpartum rat uterus and cervix by prostaglandin E_2-cyclic adenosine monophosphate. Am J Obstet Gynecol 2002; 187: 202–8.

99. Liu J, Lu H, Huang R et al. Peroxisome proliferator activated receptor-gamma ligands induced cell growth inhibition and its influence on matrix metalloproteinase activity in human myeloid leukemia cells. Cancer Chemother Pharmacol 2005; 56: 400–8.

100. Shalom-Barak T, Nicholas JM, Wang Y et al. Peroxisome proliferator-activated receptor gamma controls Muc1 transcription in trophoblasts. Mol Cell Biol 2004; 24: 10661–9.

101. Cinti S. The adipose organ. Prostaglandins Leukot Essent Fatty Acids 2005; 73: 9–15.

102. Chen F, Harrison LE. Ciglitazone-induced cellular antiproliferation increases p27kip1 protein levels through both increased transcriptional activity and inhibition of proteasome degradation. Cell Signal 2005; 17: 809–16.

103. Cheng J, Nakamura H, Imanishi H et al. Peroxisome proliferator-activated receptor gamma ligands, 15-deoxy-$\Delta^{12,14}$-prostaglandin J_2, and ciglitazone, induce growth inhibition and cell cycle arrest in hepatic oval cells. Biochem Biophys Res Commun 2004; 322: 458–64.

104. Munoz U, de Las Cuevas N, Bartolome F et al. The cyclopentenone 15-deoxy-$\Delta^{12,14}$-prostaglandin J_2 inhibits G_1/S transition and retinoblastoma protein phosphorylation in immortalized lymphocytes from Alzheimer's disease patients. Exp Neurol 2005; 195: 508–17.

105. Matsumoto H, Ma WG, Daikoku T et al. Cyclooxygenase-2 differentially directs uterine angiogenesis during implantation in mice. J Biol Chem 2002; 277: 29260–7.

106. Carmeliet P, Collen D. Molecular analysis of blood vessel formation and disease. Am J Physiol 1997; 273: H2091–104.

107. Cheung CY. Vascular endothelial growth factor: possible role in fetal development and placental function. J Soc Gynecol Investig 1997; 4: 169–77.

108. Winther H, Ahmed A, Dantzer V. Immunohistochemical localization of vascular endothelial growth factor (VEGF) and its two specific receptors, Flt-1 and KDR, in the porcine placenta and non-pregnant uterus. Placenta 1999; 20: 35–43.

109. Pfarrer CD, Ruziwa SD, Winther H et al. Localization of vascular endothelial growth factor (VEGF) and its receptors VEGFR-1 and VEGFR-2 in bovine placentomes from implantation until term. Placenta 2006; 27: 889–98.

110. Winther H, Dantzer V. Co-localization of vascular endothelial growth factor and its two receptors flt-1 and kdr in the mink placenta. Placenta 2001; 22: 457–65.

111. Lopes FL, Desmarais J, Gevry NY et al. Expression of vascular endothelial growth factor isoforms and receptors Flt-1 and KDR during the peri-implantation period in the mink, *Mustela vison*. Biol Reprod 2003; 68: 1926–33.

112. Wang H, Li Q, Lin H et al. Expression of vascular endothelial growth factor and its receptors in the rhesus monkey (*Macaca mulatta*) endometrium and placenta during early pregnancy. Mol Reprod Dev 2003; 65: 123–31.

113. Clark DE, Smith SK, Sharkey AM, Charnock-Jones DS. Localization of VEGF and expression of its receptors flt and KDR in human placenta throughout pregnancy. Hum Reprod 1996; 11: 1090–8.

114. Hirashima M, Lu Y, Byers L, Rossant J. Trophoblast expression of fms-like tyrosine kinase 1 is not required for the establishment of the maternal–fetal interface in the mouse placenta. Proc Natl Acad Sci USA 2003; 100: 15637–42.

115. Gately S, Li WW. Multiple roles of COX-2 in tumor angiogenesis: a target for antiangiogenic therapy. Semin Oncol 2004; 31: 2–11.

116. Bradbury D, Clarke D, Seedhouse C et al. Vascular endothelial growth factor induction by prostaglandin E_2 in human airway smooth muscle cells is mediated by E prostanoid EP2/EP4 receptors and SP-1 transcription factor binding sites. J Biol Chem 2005; 280: 29993–30000.

117. Kanno Y, Tokuda H, Nakajima K et al. Involvement of SAPK/JNK in prostaglandin E_1-induced VEGF synthesis in osteoblast-like cells. Mol Cell Endocrinol 2004; 220: 89–95.

118. Abdel-Majid RM, Marshall JS. Prostaglandin E_2 induces degranulation-independent production of vascular endothelial growth factor by human mast cells. J Immunol 2004; 172: 1227–36.

119. Sales KJ, List T, Boddy SC et al. A novel angiogenic role for prostaglandin F_{2alpha}–FP receptor interaction in human endometrial adenocarcinomas. Cancer Res 2005; 65: 7707–16.

120. Haslmayer P, Thalhammer T, Jager W et al. The peroxisome proliferator-activated receptor gamma ligand 15-deoxy-$\Delta^{12,14}$-prostaglandin J_2 induces vascular endothelial growth factor in the hormone-independent prostate cancer cell line PC3 and the urinary bladder carcinoma cell line 5637. Int J Oncol 2002; 21: 915–20.

121. Yasuda E, Tokuda H, Ishisaki A et al. PPAR-γ ligands up-regulate basic fibroblast growth factor-induced VEGF release through amplifying SAPK/JNK activation in osteoblasts. Biochem Biophys Res Commun 2005; 328: 137–43.

122. Cong J, Diao HL, Zhao YC et al. Differential expression and regulation of cylooxygenases, prostaglandin E synthases and prostacyclin synthase in rat uterus during the peri-implantation period. Reproduction 2006; 131: 139–51.

17 Maternal recognition of pregnancy

Fuller W Bazer, Thomas E Spencer, Troy L Ott, and Greg A Johnson

Synopsis

Background

- During pregnancy, signals are transmitted from the conceptus to the ovary or to the uterus.
- These signals prevent regression of the corpus luteum (CL), ensuring continuing production of progesterone, which supports uterine function.
- In the absence of a conceptus, the corpus luteum regresses.
- Prostaglandin $F_{2\alpha}$ (PGF) is the signal for regression of the corpus luteum in most, if not all, mammals.

Basic Science

- The life span of the corpus luteum is controlled differently in different species.
- In most non-primate mammals, the endometrium secretes PGF in pulsatile patterns. PGF, in turn, acts on the corpus luteum, inducing luteolysis.
- Accordingly, in these species, hysterectomy extends CL life span to the corresponding gestation period.
- Pregnancy recognition signals are paracrine hormones from the trophoblast that modify endometrial production or secretion of PGF, and thus prevent luteolysis.
- These hormones may also affect gene expression in CL and immune cells, as well as exerting other effects on the endometrium.
- Antiluteolytic signals from trophectoderm include estrogen in pigs and interferon τ (IFNτ) in ruminants.
- Estrogen from the pig conceptus induces release of secretions, termed histotroph, from endometrial epithelium. Histiotroph supports conceptus development.
- In rodents, the anterior pituitary, decidua, and placenta produce luteotropic hormones such as prolactin and placental lactogens.
- In dogs and cats, the inherent life span of the CL is similar to the length of gestation; therefore, there appears to be no need for a pregnancy recognition signal at implantation.
- Pregnancy recognition signals can be luteotropic, luteal protective, or antiluteolytic in different species.
- At the time of implantation, progesterone receptors (PGR) are lost from epithelial cells in all species. Progesterone effects on endometrium are then mediated by its binding to PGR in stromal cells, which respond by targeting paracrine mediators such as hepatocyte growth factor (HGF), fibroblast growth factor 7 (FGF7), and FGF10 to epithelial cells.

Clinical

- In women, luteolysis is independent of the uterus.
- Chorionic gonadotropin (CG) produced by trophoblasts acts directly on the CL to abrogate the intraovarian luteolytic action of PGF.
- Pregnancy recognition in the baboon involves independent interactions between the conceptus and uterus and the conceptus and ovary. The same may well apply in humans, where CG receptors are present in endometrial cells.

- CG expression by trophectoderm appears to be limited to humans and non-human primates.
- During the peri-implantation period of pregnancy, interferon-stimulated genes such as chemokines appear in endometrium of humans as well as in many other species, suggesting that this may be a clinically relevant signaling pathway.

INTRODUCTION

Maternal recognition of pregnancy requires signaling between the conceptus (embryo and its associated membranes) and the maternal system for maintenance of the corpus luteum (CL). Progesterone, produced by the CL, is required for regulation of endometrial functions that support early embryonic development, implantation, placentation, and fetal/placental development.[1,2] Pregnancy recognition signals can be luteotropic, luteal protective, or antiluteolytic. Luteotropic signals include chorionic gonadotropin (CG), produced by human and primate conceptuses, which acts directly on CL via luteinizing hormone/chorionic gonadotropin receptor (LHCGR) to insure CL maintenance. The ovarian cycle of primates is independent of the uterus, as regression of the CL results from intraovarian effects of prostaglandins, oxytocin, or other undefined luteolytic agents. Therefore, it follows that CG acts directly on the CL to abrogate the intraovarian luteolytic mechanism.[3] Luteolytic agents induce structural and functional demise of the CL. Prostaglandin $F_{2\alpha}$ (PGF) is the luteolytic signal in most, if not all, mammals. Luteal protective signals, e.g. PGE_2 (PGE), may antagonize luteolytic effects of PGF.[4,5]

The ovarian cycle of most subprimate mammals is uterine-dependent, since endometrial epithelia of cyclic females secrete PGF in pulsatile patterns that act on the CL to induce luteolysis. In these species, hysterectomy extends CL life span for a period characteristic of the gestational period for that species. Therefore, pregnancy recognition signals are paracrine hormones from the trophectoderm that modify endometrial production or secretion of PGF to prevent luteolysis. These hormones may also affect gene expression in CL[6] and in circulating immune cells[7] in sheep and cattle,[8] but the functional significance of these effects has not been determined. Antiluteolytic signals from trophectoderm include estrogen in pigs and interferon τ (IFNτ) in ruminants. In rodents, lactogenic hormones from the anterior pituitary, decidua, and placenta are luteotropic although uterine-derived PGF induces luteolysis in pseudopregnant rodents. In dogs and cats, the inherent life span of their CL is similar to the length of gestation; therefore, there is no apparent need for a pregnancy recognition signal during the peri-implantation period.

ENDOCRINE REQUIREMENTS FOR LUTEOLYSIS AND PREGNANCY RECOGNITION

Primates

General

The menstrual cycle in humans averages 28 days from the beginning of menses in one cycle (day 0) to onset of menses in the subsequent cycle. Ovulation occurs in response to a luteinizing hormone (LH) surge on about day 14, and CL regression results from intraovarian effects of PGF,[9] oxytocin,[10] or other unidentified hormones. Although luteolysis is independent of the uterus, temporal and spatial changes in endometrial steroid receptors are associated with day of the menstrual cycle and pregnancy.[11,12] Estrogen receptor α (ESR1) expression is greatest in lumenal (LE) and glandular (GE) epithelia and stromal cells on days 10–14 and declines to low levels on days 22–28 just prior to onset of menses. Progesterone receptors (PGRs) are also highest in LE and GE on days 10–14 and decline to low levels on days 15–21. In stromal cells they do not change appreciably between days 10 and 21, but thereafter decrease. During pregnancy, PGRs are abundant in decidualized uterine stroma[13] to allow progesterone responsiveness for establishment and maintenance of pregnancy. However, ESR1 are undetectable in LE, GE, and stroma of endometria of pregnant baboons from as early as day 18 postovulation.[14] Thus, uterine stroma maintain abundant PGRs, which are required for conceptus development, implantation, decidualization, placentation, and successful fetal/placental development to term.

Pregnancy recognition

Primates utilize a luteotropic mechanism for pregnancy recognition signaling. Chorionic gonadotropin (CG) secreted by trophectoderm of primate conceptuses, beginning at implantation, acts directly on the CL to insure maintenance of structure and function.[15] The β subunit of CG (CGβ) confers biological and immunological specificity to CG and is detectable at the 6–8 cell stage of development of human embryos and its secretion increases in association with implantation and trophoblast outgrowth. In humans, implantation begins on days 7–9 of pregnancy and CG is detectable in peripheral blood between days 9 and 12 of gestation; a similar sequence of events occurs in other primates.[3] Luteolysis and termination of pregnancy is elicited by either passive (within 6 days) or active immunization (within 4 weeks) of marmoset monkeys against CG at 3–5 weeks of pregnancy. Although CG is the primary luteotropic signal in primates, gonadotropin-releasing hormone 1 (GnRH1), activin, interleukin (IL)-6, IL-1, colony-stimulating factor 1 (CSF1), γ-aminobutyric acid, retinoic acid, and dehydroepiandrosterone stimulate CG production by trophectoderm. Prostaglandins other than PGF, relaxin, and/or lactogenic hormones can also stimulate progesterone production by luteal cells and transforming growth factor β₁ (TFGβ₁), dopamine, inhibin, and progesterone inhibit CG production by trophectoderm.[3] Pregnancy recognition in primates may involve independent interactions between the conceptus and uterus and/or conceptus and ovary.

Uterine receptivity to implantation in baboons includes three phases.[16] Phase I is regulated by estrogen and progesterone between days 8 and 10 postovulation when (1) columnar epithelia contain microvilli, stromal cell proliferation increases, and ESR1 and PGR are lost from endometrial epithelia; (2) expression of mucin glycoprotein 1 (MUC1) decreases; and (3) expression of smooth muscle myosin (MYH11) and pinopods on LE and GE increase. Phase II of uterine receptivity to implantation is induced by CG, but is dependent on the actions of progesterone via PGR in stroma that include (1) plaque formation by LE that express abundant cytokeratin and proliferating cell nuclear antigen (PCNA); (2) increased expression of glycodelin by GE; (3) expression of α smooth muscle actin (ACTA2) and integrins by stroma that bind extracellular matrix (ECM) molecules critical to signal transduction; (4) transformation of GE to express pinopod structures; (5) differentiation of stroma to decidual cells; (6) inhibition of stromal apoptosis, perhaps through induction of NOTCH1; and (7) induction of stromal cell proteins. Phase III of the peri-implantation period of receptivity involves increased permeability of subepithelial capillaries surrounding the blastocyst, as

well as hypertrophy of GE, stroma decidualization, and increased secretion of ECM proteins. Known CG-induced genes include insulin-like growth factor binding protein-1 (IGFBP1), glycodelin, vascular endothelial growth factor (VEGF), leukemia-inhibiting factor (LIF), and matrix metalloproteinase-9 (MMP-9).[17,18]

In addition, the 'window of implantation' in humans is associated with both increases and decreases in expression of genes in the endometrium (see Chapters 13, 14, 18, and 21). The up-regulated genes include secreted phosphoprotein-1, apolipoprotein phospholipase A₂, PGE₂ receptor, glucuronyltransferase, glycodelin, mammaglobin, Dickkopf-1, IGFBPs, members of the TGFβ superfamily, monoamine oxidase, γ-aminobutyric acid receptor subunit, metallothioneins, enterotoxin 1 receptor, and potassium ion channel.[19]

Chorionic gonadotropin may act via multiple LHCGR, but the 4.5 kb form is most abundant. In the ovary, CG-induced signal transduction is primarily through activation of the heterotrimeric G-proteins, leading to an increase in cAMP, activation of protein kinase A, increases in intracellular calcium via activation of inositol triphosphate/phospholipase A₂ pathway, and possibly activation of protein kinase C via diacylglycerol. However, in human endometrial cell lines, CG does not activate cAMP and protein kinase A; rather, it induces phosphorylation of the extracellular signal-regulated kinase (ERK1/2) in a protein kinase A-independent manner.[16] This ERK1/2 pathway leads to CG-induced increases in prostaglandin synthase 2 (PTGS₂) expression and PGE₂ production.

Luteinizing hormone also binds to receptors in uteri of pig, rat, rabbit, human, mouse, and cow, where it inhibits myometrial contractions, increases cAMP and inositol phosphates, decreases gap junctions, promotes differentiation of endometrial stroma, increases expression of PTGS2, decreases vascular resistance, and increases uterine blood flow.[20] However, CG expression by trophectoderm appears to be limited to humans and non-human primates.

Ruminants

Estrous cycle

Sheep, cattle, and goats have estrous cycles of about 17, 21, and 20 days, respectively. An ovulatory surge of LH occurs at onset of estrus when the female accepts the male for mating and ovulation occurs about 30 hours later. With maturation of the CL, concentrations of progesterone in peripheral blood peak at mid-diestrus and luteolysis results from pulsatile release of PGF from endometrial LE and superficial GE (sGE) during late diestrus and proestrus. Three ovarian hormones are primarily responsible for endometrial secretion of luteolytic pulses of PGF: progesterone, estrogen, and oxytocin. Progesterone acts on endometrial epithelia to increase phospholipid stores (arachidonic acid source) and PTGS2 activity for conversion of arachidonic acid to PGF.[21] Oxytocin secreted by the CL and posterior pituitary binds oxytocin receptors (OXTRs), expressed by endometrial epithelia as PGR disappear and ESR1 increase, to stimulate pulsatile secretion of PGF and luteolysis. McCracken et al[22] proposed that progesterone binds PGR to inhibit synthesis of OXTR by ovine endometrial epithelia for 10–12 days, a period referred to as the progesterone-block. Afterwards, endometrial OXTRs increase as progesterone down-regulates PGR after about day 12 of the cycle to end the progesterone-block. With the decrease in endometrial PGR, an increase in OXTR is enhanced by estradiol,[23] allowing oxytocin to stimulate endometrial production of luteolytic pulses of PGF. Indeed, treatment of ewes[24] or goats[25] with an OXTR antagonist, passive or active immunization of ewes against oxytocin,[26,27] or continuous infusion of oxytocin to down-regulate OXTR[28] prevents or delays luteolysis. These results indicate central roles for estradiol and oxytocin in the PGF-induced luteolytic mechanism of ruminants.[26,29]

Pregnancy recognition signaling

The antiluteolytic signal for maternal recognition of pregnancy in ruminants is IFNτ.[1,2] Secretion of IFNτ by trophectoderm is limited to the peri-implantation period (days 11–20) when it exerts paracrine antiluteolytic effects on the endometrium to abrogate the luteolytic mechanism by blocking transcription of ESR1 (Figure 17.1). This precludes estrogen-induced expression of OXTR. In every studied mammal, estrogen is a key regulator of OXTR gene expression and, in sheep, administration of estrogen increases OXTR in the endometrium.[30–32] Administration of estrogen on either day 11 or day 12 postestrus induces structural and functional luteolysis in cyclic ewes, with the following temporal events:

- increase ESR1 mRNA and protein in endometrial epithelia between 12 and 24 hours
- a moderate increase in endometrial OXTR expression between 12 and 36 hours
- abundant OXTR expression between 36 and 48 hours

- a decline in concentrations of progesterone in plasma after 36 hours
- a decrease in CL weight by 48 hours.[30]

Similar temporal and spatial changes in ESR1 and OXTR gene expression occur in endometria of cyclic ewes between days 12 and 16 postestrus.[33]

Garrett et al[34] reported that administration of progesterone early in the estrous cycle of recipient cows advanced luteolysis. However, progesterone also changed uterine receptivity for transfer of older asynchronous embryos by accelerating conceptus development and the onset of IFNτ secretion to prevent luteolysis. These results indicate that progesterone-induced alterations in endometrial secretions accelerate conceptus development and advance the time that the conceptus secretes IFNτ for pregnancy recognition signaling.

Deletion and mutation analyses revealed that induction of ovine OXTR promoter activity by ligand-activated ESR1 depended on GC-rich SP1 binding sites at −104 and −64 in the minimal promoter, and basal activity of this promoter was also regulated by the same GC-rich SP1 elements adjacent to the transcriptional start site of the OXTR gene.[32] The SP1 transcription factor is constitutively expressed in most endometrial cell types from cyclic and pregnant ewes, but is most abundant in LE and sGE. Thus, the primary determinant of OXTR gene regulation in ovine endometrial epithelia is expression of the ESR1 gene. Therefore, antiluteolytic effects of IFNτ are to silence ESR1 gene transcription, which precludes ESR1 stimulation of OXTR gene transcription and, therefore, oxytocin-induced release of luteolytic pulses of PGF by uterine epithelia. The IFN family includes type I and type II IFNs.[35] Type I IFNs include IFNA (13 different subtypes), IFNB, IFND, IFNE, IFNK, IFNT, and IFNW. However, there is only one type II IFN, IFNG. IFNA, IFNB, IFNE, IFNK, and IFNW exist in humans, whereas IFND and IFNT are unique to pigs and ruminants, respectively.[35,36] IFNT and human type I IFNs share many biological activities, including inducing or increasing expression of interferon stimulated genes (ISGs) in endometria and human cell lines that influence endometrial differentiation and conceptus implantation.[37–40] During the peri-implantation period of pregnancy, there is induction or increases in ISGs in endometria of humans, baboons, domestic animals, and laboratory animals.[41–48] Thus, expression of ISGs is a common feature of endometria during the peri-implantation period when pregnancy recognition signaling and implantation is occurring. Available evidence[49] indicates that ISGs, such as chemokine

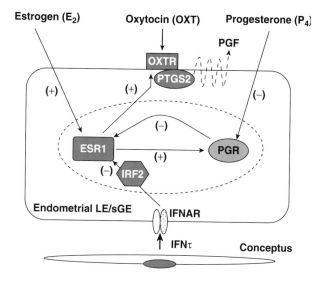

Figure 17.1 Hormonal regulation of the endometrial luteolytic mechanism and antiluteolytic effects of the conceptus on the endometrium in the ovine uterus. During estrus and metestrus, oxytocin receptors are present on the uterine lumenal epithelium and superficial ductal glandular epithelium (LE/sGE) because estrogen levels are high and increase expression of ESR1 and OXTR. The PGR is present, but low systemic levels of progesterone result in insufficient numbers of activated PGRs to suppress ESR1 and OXTR synthesis. During early diestrus, endometrial ESR1 and estrogen are low, but progesterone levels begin to increase with formation of the CL. Progesterone acts through the PGR to suppress ESR1 and OXTR synthesis for 8–10 days. Continuous exposure of the endometrium to progesterone eventually down-regulates PGR gene expression in the endometrial luminal epithelium by days 11–12 of the estrous cycle. The loss of PGR terminates the progesterone block to ESR1 and OXTR formation. Thus, ESR1 appears on days 11 and 12 postestrus, which is closely followed by OXTR on days 13 and 14. The increase in OXTR expression is facilitated by increasing secretion of estrogen by ovarian follicles. In both cyclic and pregnant sheep, oxytocin is released from the posterior pituitary and corpus luteum beginning on day 9. In cyclic sheep, OXT binds to OXTR on the endometrial epithelium and increases release of luteolytic pulses of PGF to regress the CL through a PTGS-dependent pathway. In pregnant sheep, IFNτ is synthesized and secreted by the elongating conceptus beginning on day 10 of pregnancy. IFN binds to type I IFN receptors (IFNAR) on the endometrial LE and inhibits transcription of the ESR1 gene through a signaling pathway involving IRF2. These antiluteolytic actions of IFNτ on the ESR1 gene prevent OXTR formation, thereby maintaining the CL and progesterone production. E$_2$, estrogen; ESR1, estrogen receptor; IFNAR, type I IFN receptor; IFNτ, interferon τ; IRF2, interferon regulatory factor 2; OXT, oxytocin; OXTR, oxytocin receptor; P$_4$, progesterone; PGF, prostaglandin F$_{2\alpha}$, PGR, progesterone receptor; PTGS2, prostaglandin-endoperoxide synthase 2 (prostaglandin G/H synthase and cyclooxygenase).

(C-X-C motif) ligand 10 (CXCL10), in sheep and goats, regulate conceptus implantation directly by affecting the conceptus or indirectly by affecting endometrial receptivity to implantation in ruminants.

Interferon τ signaling

The classical cell signaling pathway activated by type I IFNs is the JAK–STAT pathway. All type I IFNs bind a common receptor composed of two subunits, IFNAR1 and IFNAR2, which are associated with the Janus activated kinases (JAKs), tyrosine kinase 2 (Tyk2) and JAK1, respectively.[50] In sheep, both IFNAR1 and IFNAR2 are expressed in endometrial LE, GE, and stroma.[51] In the human uterus, IFNAR1 and IFNAR2 are expressed predominantly in uterine stroma and GE.[52] Activation of JAKs associated with type I IFN receptors results in tyrosine phosphorylation of STAT2 and STAT1 and then formation of a heterotrimeric STAT1–STAT2–ISGF3G complex known as ISGF3 (ISG factor 3). The ISGF3 translocates to the nucleus, binds IFN-stimulated response elements (ISREs) in DNA, and initiates transcription of target genes. Similar to type II IFNG, type I IFNs induce formation of STAT1–STAT1 homodimers (γ-activated factor or GAF) that translocate to the nucleus and bind GAS (γ-activated site) elements present in the promoter of certain ISGs. One of the GAS-regulated genes is interferon regulatory factor-1 (IRF1) that, in turn, activates ISREs of many ISGs to amplify effects of IFNs.[53]

Type I and type II IFNs can also regulate gene expression and cellular responses through STAT1-independent pathways.[50] One such pathway is the p38 MAPK pathway for signal transduction affecting biological processes such as inflammation, cell cycle, cell death, development, cell differentiation, senescence, and tumorigenesis.[54] The p38MAPK is phosphorylated and activated in a type I IFN-dependent manner in several IFN-sensitive cell lines.[55,56] Inhibition of p38MAPK activity can block expression of a number of ISGs regulated by ISREs.[55] There are no results on IFNτ activation of the p38MAPK pathway in uterine endometria. However, induction of PTGS2 by IFNτ in bovine myometrial cells does require activation of the p38MAPK pathway.[57] Thus, IFNτ activation of p38MAPK may be a signaling pathway that stimulates transcription of certain genes in STAT1-negative endometrial LE and human U3A (STAT1 null) cells.

Interferon-stimulated genes

Interferon τ activates the JAK–STAT–IRF signaling pathway in ovine endometrial stroma and GE as well as in human 2fTGH cells.[38,58,59] Candidate gene analyses and transcriptional profiling have identified a number of IFNτ-stimulated genes in endometria of ruminants (Table 17.1 and Figure 17.2). Although the JAK–STAT–IRF pathway is active in ovine endometrial stroma and GE, most ISGs are not induced or increased by IFNτ in LE and sGE.[60] This is because IRF2, a potent transcriptional repressor of ISGs, is expressed specifically in LE and sGE and represses transcriptional activity of ISRE- and IRFE-containing promoters.[60] Thus, IRF2 in LE and sGE restricts IFNT-induced ISGs to stroma and GE of the ovine uterus. In fact, all components of the ISGF3 transcription factor complex (STAT1, STAT2, and ISGF3G) are ISGs. Therefore, IFNT must utilize a non-classical STAT1-independent cell signaling pathway to regulate expression of genes in endometrial LE.[59,60] Using transcriptional profiling of human U3A (STAT1 null) cells and ovine endometrium treated with IFNT, IFNT-stimulated genes discovered in the endometrial LE and sGE include CTSL, LGALS15, and WNT7A.[59,61,62]

Cathepsins (CTS) are peptidases that can degrade extracellular matrix, catabolize intracellular proteins, and process prohormones, as well as regulate uterine receptivity for implantation and trophoblast invasion in a number of mammals.[63,64] In the ovine uterus, CTSL (cathepsin L) is the most abundant CTS and it is expressed only in LE and sGE of cyclic and pregnant ewes.[62] CTSL protein is also detected in conceptus trophectoderm and pro-CTSL is present in uterine flushings from ewes between days 12 and 16 of pregnancy. Cathepsin L is a novel progesterone-induced and IFNτ-stimulated gene in LE and sGE of ewes.

Galectin-15 (LGALS15; also known as ovgal11) was originally identified in ovine intestinal epithelium as being induced in response to infection by the nematode parasite *Haemonchus contortus*,[65] and it is one of the most abundant genes expressed in endometria of day 14 pregnant ewes.[40,61] The LGALS15 mRNA is detected after day 10 of pregnancy in ovine endometrial LE and sGE,[61] where its expression is induced by progesterone and stimulated by IFNτ. The LGALS15 has a nucleocytoplasmic distribution within LE and sGE, with most near and on the apical surface, and it is secreted into the uterine lumen.[66,67] Galectins bind β-galactosides and functionally cross-link glycoprotein and glycolipid receptors on the surface of cells to initiate biological responses that include cell proliferation, differentiation, motility, adhesion, and apoptosis.[67–69] A proposed extracellular role of LGALS15 is to functionally bind and cross-link β-galactosides on glycoproteins and glycolipids to allow heterophilic cell

adhesion molecules bridging conceptus trophectoderm and LE to stimulate biological responses within the trophoblast, such as migration, proliferation, and differentiation, which are critical for successful conceptus implantation.[61,70]

WNT7A is another novel IFNτ-stimulated gene expressed in ovine endometrial LE and sGE.[40] The WNT family (19 genes in human) includes many highly conserved and secreted glycoproteins that regulate cell and tissue growth and differentiation during embryonic development and play a central role in coordinating uterine–conceptus interactions required for implantation in mice,[71–74] and perhaps humans.[19,75] The canonical WNT (Wnt/β-catenin) signaling pathway plays a central role in coordinating interactions between blastocyst and uterus required for implantation in mice.[71–74]

CXCL10, also known as IFNG-inducible protein 10 kDa, is a member of the C-X-C chemokine family that regulates multiple aspects of inflammatory and immune responses primarily through chemotactic activity toward subsets of leukocytes.[76,77] CXCL10 preferentially targets natural killer cells and activates Th1 cells[78,79] through the C-X-C chemokine receptor 3 (CXCR3). Nagoaka et al[80] identified CXCL10 as a gene induced by IFNτ in the ovine uterus. CXCL10 mRNA was localized to monocytes in the subepithelial stroma of pregnant, but not cyclic uteri. In a chemotaxis assay, migration of peripheral blood mononuclear cells was stimulated by the addition of IFNτ, and the effect was significantly reduced by neutralization with an anti-CXCL10 antibody. In the ovine uterus, CXCL10 expression is also increased in the subepithelial stroma of the endometrium and is found in uterine flushings of early pregnant ewes.[80] Indeed, CXCR3 was localized to trophoblast cells and recombinant CXCL10 was shown to stimulate migration of trophoblast cells and promote their adhesion to fibronectin, as well as increase expression of integrins $α_5$, $α_V$, and $β_3$ subunit mRNAs in trophoblast cells. These findings suggest that endometrial CXCL10 regulates establishment of apical interactions between trophectoderm and uterine epithelia during early pregnancy and affects recruitment and/or distribution of immune cells in the pregnancy uterus.

The MX proteins belong to the mechanochemical enzyme superfamily typified by the dynamins. Dynamin superfamily members are subdivided into classical dynamins and dynamin-related proteins, including MX proteins.[81] Dynamins are involved in cellular processes such as intracellular vesicle trafficking,[82] clathrin-mediated endocytosis,[83] and cytokinesis.[84] Of the dynamin-related proteins, only MX proteins are

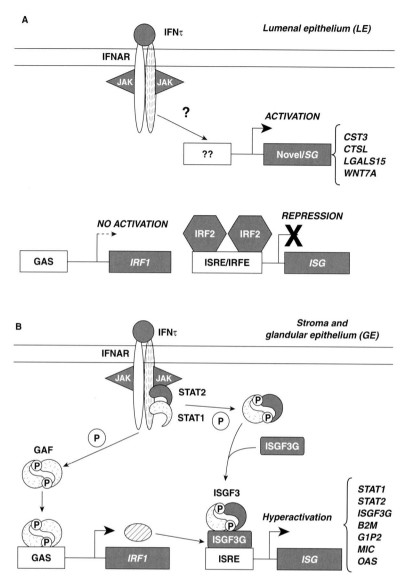

Figure 17.2 Current working hypothesis on IFNτ signaling in the endometrium of the ovine uterus. IFNτ produced in large amounts by the developing conceptus, binds to IFNAR present on cells of the ovine endometrium. In cells of the stroma and middle to deep glandular epithelium (**B**), IFNτ-mediated association of the IFNAR subunits facilitates the cross-phosphorylation and activation of JAK, which in turn phosphorylates the receptor and creates a docking site for STAT2. STAT2 is then phosphorylated, thus creating a docking site for STAT1, which is then phosphorylated. STAT1 and STAT2 are then released from the receptor and can form two transcription factor complexes. ISGF3, formed by association of the STAT1–2 heterodimer with ISG3G in the cytoplasm, translocates to the nucleus, and transactivates genes containing an ISRE(s), such as *STAT1, STAT2, ISGF3G, BMG, G1P2, MHC*, and *OAS*. GAF is formed by STAT1 homodimers, which translocates to the nucleus and transactivates genes containing a GAS element(s), such as *IRF1*. IRF1 can also bind and transactivate ISRE-containing genes as well an IRFE-containing genes. The simultaneous induction of *STAT2* and *ISGF3G* by IFNτ appears to shift transcription factor formation from GAF towards predominantly ISGF3. Therefore, IFNτ activation of the JAK–STAT signal transduction pathway allows for constant formation of ISGF3 and GAF transcription factor complexes and hyperactivation of ISG expression. In the luminal (LE) and superficial glandular epithelia (sGE), IFNτ is prevented from activating ISGs by IRF2 (**A**). IRF2, a potent and stable repressor present in the nucleus, increases during early pregnancy in the LE and sGE. The continual presence of IRF2 inhibits ISRE- and IRFE-containing target genes (*STAT1, STAT2, ISGF3G, BMG, G1P2, MHC, OAS*) through direct ISRE and IRFE binding and coactivator repulsion. Furthermore, critical factors in the JAK–STAT pathway (STAT1, STAT2, and ISGF3G) are not present, resulting in no ISGF3 or IRF1 transcription factors necessary to stimulate ISGs. However, IFNτ does activate an unknown signaling pathway that results in induction of *WNT7A* and stimulation of *CST3, CTSL*, and *LGALS15*, specifically in the endometrial LE and sGE. B2M, β₂-microglobulin; CST3, cystatin C; CTSL, cathepsin L; G1P2, interferon, α-inducible protein (clone IFI-15K); GAF, γ-activated factor; GAS, γ activation sequence; IFNAR, type I IFN receptor; IFNτ interferon tau; IRF1, interferon regulatory factor 1; IRF2, interferon regulatory factor 2; IRFE, IRF response element; ISGF3G, interferon-stimulated transcription factor 3, γ 48 kDa; ISRE, IFN-stimulated response element; JAK, janus activated kinase; LGALS15, galectin-15; MIC, MHC class I polypeptide-related sequence; OAS, 2′,5′-oligoadenylate synthetases; STAT1, signal transducer and activator of transcription 1, 91 kDa; STAT2, signal transducer and activator of transcription 2, 113 kDa; WNT7A, wingless-type MMTV integration site family, member 7A.

Table 17.1 Interferon τ-regulated genes identified in uteri of sheep and cattle

Gene symbol	Gene name	Alias/previous symbol	regulation[1]	Citation (Reference number)
APG4B	ATG4 autophagy related 4 homolog B (S. cerevisiae)	Apg4B, KIAA0943, DKFZp586D1822, AUTL1	I	Gray et al, 2006 (40)
B2M	β_2-2-microglobulin		I	Vallet et al, 1991; Choi et al, 2003; Chen et al, 2006 (218;39;217)
CIR	Complement component 1, r subcomponent		I	Chen et al, 2006 (217)
CISH	Cytokine inducible SH2-containing protein	CIS, G18, CIS-1, SOCS	I	Sandra et al, 2005 (220)
COL3A1	Collagen, type III, alpha 1 (Ehlers–Danlos syndrome type IV, autosomal dominant)	EDS4A	D	Gray et al, 2006 (40)
COL16A1	Collagen, type XVI, alpha 1		I	Chen et al, 2006 (217)
COL4A3BP	collagen, type IV, alpha 3 (Goodpasture antigen) binding protein	GPBP, STARD11, CERT	I	Gray et al, 2006 (40)
CST3	cystatin C (amyloid angiopathy and cerebral hemorrhage)		I	Song et al, 2006 (221)
CTSL	cathepsin L	FLJ31037	I	Song et al, 2005 (62)
CXCL10	chemokine (C-X-C motif) ligand 10	IFI10, IP-10, crg-2, mob-1, C7, gIP-10	I	Nagaoka et al, 2003; Nagaoka et al, 2003 (49;80)
DDX58	DEAD (Asp-Glu-Ala-Asp) box polypeptide 58	RIG-I, FLJ13599, DKFZp434J1111	I	Song, Spencer, and Bazer, unpublished results
DNPEP	aspartyl aminopeptidase	DAP, ASPEP	I	Gray et al, 2006 (40)
EIF3S6	eukaryotic translation initiation factor 3, subunit 6 48 kDa	eIF3-p48, eIF3e	I	Chen et al, 2006 (217)
ESR1	estrogen receptor 1 (estrogen receptor α)	NR3A1, Era	R	Spencer et al, 1995; Fleming et al, 2001 (33;31)
FAM14B	family with sequence similarity 14, member B	ISG12c	I	Gray et al, 2006 (40)
FXYD4	FXYD domain containing ion transport regulator 4	CHIF	I, NE	Gray et al, 2006 (40)
GBP2	guanylate binding protein 2, interferon-inducible		I	Kim et al, 2003; Chen et al, 2006 (59;217)
GRP	gastrin-releasing peptide		I	Gray et al, 2006 (40)
HIF1A	hypoxia-inducible factor 1, alpha subunit (basic helix-loop-helix transcription factor)	MOP1, HIF-1alpha, PASD8	I, D	Gray et al, 2006; Chen et al, 2006
HLA-A	major histocompatibility complex, class I, A		I	Chen et al, 2006 (217)
IEF SSP 5111	interferon gamma induced 1-5111 protein precursor		I	Chen et al, 2006 (217)
IFI6	interferon, alpha-inducible protein 6	G1P3, IFI616, FAM14C, 6-16, IFI-6-16	I	Gray et al, 2006; Chen et al, 2006 (40;217)
IFI16	interferon, gamma-inducible protein 16	IFNGIP1, PYHIN2	I	Chen et al, 2006 (217)
IFI27	interferon, alpha-inducible protein 27		I	Kim et al, 2003 (59)
IFIH1	interferon induced with helicase C domain 1	MDA-5, Hlcd, MDA5	I	Song et al, 2007 (222)
IFIT1	interferon-induced protein with tetratricopeptide repeats 1	GARG-16, G10P1, IFI56, IFNAI1	I	Kim et al, 2003 (59)
IFITM1	interferon-induced transmembrane protein 1 (9-27)	9-27, CD225, IFI17, LEU13	I	Pru et al, 2001; Chen et al, 2006 (223;217)
IFITM3	interferon-induced transmembrane protein 3 (1-8U)	1-8U	I	Pru et al, 2001; Gray et al, 2005 (223;217)
IFI35	interferon-induced protein 35	IFP35	I	Chen et al, 2006 (217)
IFNAR1	interferon (alpha, beta and omega) receptor 1	IFNAR, IFRC	NE	Chen et al, 2006 (217)
IFNAR2	interferon (alpha, beta and omega) receptor 2	IFNABR		Chen et al, 2006 (217)
IGF2	insulin-like growth factor 2		D	Chen et al, 2006 (217)
IRF1	interferon regulatory factor 1		I	Choi et al, 2003; Stewart et al, 2003; Chen et al, 2006 (39;219;217)
IRF2	interferon regulatory factor 2		I	Choi et al, 2003; Chen et al, 2006 (39;217)
ISG15	interferon, alpha-inducible protein (clone IFI-15K)	UCRP, ISG17	I	Austin et al, 1996; Hansen et al, 1997; Chen et al, 2006 (226;227;217)
ISGF3G	interferon-stimulated gene factor 3, gamma 48 kDa	IRF9, p48	I	Perry et al, 1999; Choi et al, 2001; Stewart et al, 2001; Chen et al, 2006 (225;39;219;217)
KERA	keratocan	CNA2, SLRR2B	I	Gray et al, 2006 (40)
LGALS15	galectin-15	ovgal11	I	Gray et al, 2004; Gray et al, 2006 (61;40)

Table 17.1   (Continued)

Gene symbol	Gene name	Aliases	Effect[a]	References
LUM	Lumican	SLRR2D	D	Gray et al, 2006 (40)
MAGED4	Melanoma antigen family D, 4	MAGE1, MGC3210, KIAA1859, MAGE-E1	I	Gray et al, 2006 (40)
MAP3K10	Mitogen-activated protein kinase kinase kinase 10	MLK2, MST	I	Chen et al, 2006 (217)
MIC	MHC class I polypeptide		I	Todd et al, 1998; Choi et al, 2003; Chen et al, 2006 (229;39;217)
MX1	Myxovirus (influenza virus) resistance 1, interferon-inducible protein p78 (mouse)	IFI-78K, MxA	I	Ott et al, 1998; Hicks et al, 2003; Chen et al, 2006 (91;87;217)
MX2	Myxovirus (influenza virus) resistance 2 (mouse)		I	Ott et al, 1998; Hicks et al, 2003; Chen et al, 2006 (91;87;217)
MYH9	Myosin, heavy polypeptide 9, non-muscle	DFNA17	I	Gray et al, 2006 (40)
NMI	N-myc (and STAT) interactor		I	Song, Spencer, and Bazer, unpublished results
OAS1	2',5'-oligoadenylate synthetase 1, 40/46 kDa	OIAS1, IFI-4	I	Short et al, 1991; Mirando et al, 1991; Schmitt et al, 1993; Johnson et al, 2001; Chen et al, 2006 (228;230;231;224;217)
OAS2	2'-5'-oligoadenylate synthetase 2, 69/71 kDa		I	Johnson et al, 2001; Chen et al, 2006 (224;217)
OAS3	2'-5'-oligoadenylate synthetase 3, 100 kDa		I	Johnson et al, 2001 (224)
PBP1	Scaffold protein Pbp1		I	Chen et al, 2006 (217)
PHGDH	phosphoglycerate dehydrogenase	SERA, PGDH, PDG	I	Chen et al, 2006 (217)
PHLDA1	pleckstrin homology-like domain, family A, member 1	TDAG51, DT1P1B11	I	Chen et al, 2006 (217)
PLSCR1	phospholipid scramblase 1	MMTRA1B	I	Song, Spencer, and Bazer, unpublished results
POLR3B	polymerase (RNA) III (DNA directed) polypeptide B	RPC2, FLJ10388	I	Gray et al, 2006 (40)
PPP5C	protein phosphatase 5, catalytic subunit	PPP5, PP5	I	Chen et al, 2006 (217)
PRKRA	protein kinase, interferon-inducible double-stranded RNA-dependent activator	PACT, RAX	I	Chen et al, 2006 (217)
PRLR	prolactin receptor		I	Martin et al, 2004 (233)
PTGS2	prostaglandin-endoperoxide synthase 2 (prostaglandin G/H synthase and cyclooxygenase 2)	COX2	I, D, NE	Doualla-Bell and Koromilas, 2001; Kim et al, 2003; Chen et al, 2006 (57;59;217)
PTMA	prothymosin, alpha (gene sequence 28)	TMSA	D	Gray et al, 2006 (40)
PUM1	pumilio homolog 1 (Drosophila)	PUMH1, KIAA0099	D	Gray et al, 2006 (40)
RBBP4	retinoblastoma binding protein 4	RbAp48, NURF55	I	Chen et al, 2006 (217)
RPL9	ribosomal protein L9		D	Gray et al, 2006 (40)
RSAD2	radical S-adenosyl methionine domain containing 2	cig5, viperin, vig1, 2510004L01Rik	I	Gray et al, 2006; Song et al, 2007 (40;222)
SEPP1	selenoprotein P, plasma, 1	Sep	I	Gray et al, 2006 (40)
SOCS1	suppressor of cytokine signaling 1	SOCS-1, SSI-1, JAB, TIP3, Cish1	I	Sandra et al, 2005 (220)
SOCS2	suppressor of cytokine signaling 2	STAT12, SSI2, SOCS-2, SSI-2, CIS2, Cish2	I	Sandra et al, 2005 (220)
SOCS3	suppressor of cytokine signaling 3	SSI-3, CIS3, SOCS-3, Cish3	I	Sandra et al, 2005 (220)
SPARC	secreted protein, acidic, cysteine-rich (osteonectin)	ON	D	Gray et al, 2006 (40)
STAT1	signal transducer and activator of transcription 1, 91 kDa	STAT91	I	Perry et al, 1999; Choi et al, 2001; Chen et al, 2006 (225;39;219;217)
STAT2	signal transducer and activator of transcription 2, 113 kDa	STAT113	I	Perry et al, 1999; Choi et al, 2001; Chen et al, 2006 (225;39;219;217)
TAGLN	transgelin	SM22, WS3-10, TAGLN1	I	Gray et al, 2006 (40)
UBE1L	Ubiquitin-activating enzyme E1-like	D8	I	Rempel et al, 2005 (232)
VIM	Vimentin		D	Gray et al, 2006 (40)
WNT7A	Wingless-type MMTV integration site family, member 7A		I	Kim et al, 2003 (59)

[a] Effect of interferon on gene expression in endometrium. D, decreased; I, increased; R, repressed; NE, no effect.

known to function in viral resistance.[81] In general, animals express one to three MX proteins that are products of different genes. The MX proteins are large GTPases containing three distinct domains: a GTPase (N-terminal) domain, a central interactive domain, and a GTPase effector (C-terminal) domain.[85] The GTPase domains of MX proteins include a highly conserved tripartite GTP-binding motif and GTPase activity at the N-terminus.[86] MX1 is expressed in endometria of cattle, sheep, pigs, and horses.[87] Of these species, MX1 expression is not regulated during the peri-implantation period in the mare,[87] which is consistent with the fact that horse conceptuses do not produce a type I IFN during pregnancy recognition signaling.[88]

Of the classical ISGs studied in the ovine endometrium, only MX1 expression remains in the LE and sGE during early pregnancy.[89] Expression of other ISGs (e.g. β_2-microglobulin B2MG, G1P2, MHCI, STAT1, STAT2, IRF1, ISGF3G, and OAS) is restricted to GE and stroma due to elevated expression of IRF2, a repressor of transcription, in LE and sGE.[60] Expression of MX1 mRNA is greater in the pregnant uterine horn of unilaterally pregnant ewes on day 13 due to a paracrine effect of IFNT.[90,91] However, MX1 expression also increases in CL following intrauterine injection of IFNT[92] and in peripheral blood mononuclear cells of early pregnant ewes[7] and cattle.[8] Interestingly, cyclic ewes express MX1 mRNA in endometrial LE and sGE, when both endometrial PGR and circulating progesterone concentrations are maximal.[91] This pattern of expression also occurs for other endometrial ISGs such as MHC class I and β2MG.[39] Endometrial expression of MX1 is greatest during periods of maximal IFNτ production by sheep (days 12–17) and cattle (days 15–21) conceptuses.[89] However, MX1 expression remains strong at day 25 of pregnancy in LE and sGE due to either the presence of immunoreactive IFNτ around day 25 of pregnancy or the long half-life of MX1 protein, which is detectable for 2 weeks following a single exposure of humans to IFNA.[91] The role(s) of MX proteins in pregnancy are not known, but they may regulate secretion by endometrial epithelia.[93]

Servomechanism regulating endometrial gland morphogenesis and function

Maintenance of pregnancy in sheep requires reciprocal communication between the conceptus and endometrium during implantation and synepithelio-chorial placentation which begins on days 15–16, but is not completed until days 50–60 of pregnancy.[94] During this period, the uterus grows and remodels substantially to accommodate conceptus development and growth during the latter two-thirds of pregnancy. In addition to placentomal development in the caruncular areas of the endometrium and changes in uterine vascularity, the intercaruncular endometrial glands grow substantially in length (four-fold) and width (10-fold) and undergo additional side-branching.[95] During gestation, endometrial gland hyperplasia occurs between days 15 and 50, followed by hypertrophy to increase surface area, which allows for maximal production of histotroph by GE after day 60 of gestation.[96]

The pregnant ovine uterus is exposed sequentially to estrogen, progesterone, IFNτ, placental lactogen or chorionic somatomammotropin hormone 1 (CSH1), and placental growth hormone (GH1), which initiate and maintain endometrial gland morphogenesis and differentiated secretory function (Figure 17.3). The placentas of a number of species, including rodents, humans, non-human primates, and sheep, secrete hormones structurally related to pituitary growth hormone and prolactin that are termed placental lactogens or chorionic somatomammotropic hormones.[97,98] Ovine CSH1 is produced by binucleate cells of conceptus trophectoderm beginning on days 15–16 of pregnancy, which is coordinated with induction of serine (or cysteine) peptidase inhibitors (SERPIN), also known as uterine milk proteins or UTMPs, by GE.[96,99] Ovine uterine SERPINs and secreted phosphoprotein 1 (SPP1; also known as osteopontin) are excellent markers for endometrial GE differentiation and secretory capacity during pregnancy. In maternal serum, CSH1 is detectable by day 50 and peaks between days 120 and 130 of gestation.[97] A homodimer of the prolactin receptor (PRLR), as well as a heterodimer of PRLR and GHR, transduce signals by ovine CSH1.[98] In the ovine uterus, PRLR gene expression is unique to GE.[100] Temporal changes in circulating levels of CSH1 are correlated with endometrial gland hyperplasia and hypertrophy and increased production of SERPINs and SPP1 during pregnancy. The ovine placenta also expresses GH1 between days 35 and 70 of gestation,[101] which is correlated with onset of GE hypertrophy and maximal increases in SERPIN and SPP1 production by GE. The sequential exposure of the pregnant ovine endometrium to estrogen, progesterone, IFNτ, CSH1, and GH constitutes a 'servomechanism' that activates and maintains endometrial remodeling, secretory function, and uterine growth during gestation. Chronic treatment of ovariectomized ewes with progesterone induces expression of SERPINs and SPP1 by GE. However, intrauterine infusions of CSH1 or GH1

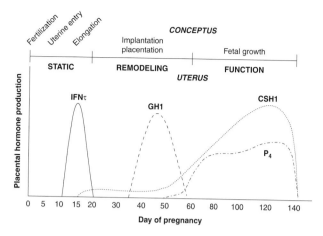

Figure 17.3 Placental hormone production during gestation in sheep and relation to development of the conceptus and uterus. CSH1, chorionic somatomammotropin hormone 1 (placental lactogen); GH1, growth hormone 1; IFNτ, interferon τ; P₄, progesterone.

further increase expression of SERPINs and SPP1 by GE of progesterone-treated ewes, but only when ewes receive intrauterine infusions of IFNτ between days 11 and 21. Indeed, Martin et al[102] reported that IFNτ increases expression of PRLR by GE in the ovine uterus. These results indicate that members of the lactogenic and somatogenic hormone family play key roles in stimulating endometrial gland morphogenesis and differentiated functions during pregnancy to facilitate conceptus growth and development; however, effects of those hormones require that the uterus first be exposed to IFNτ, the pregnancy recognition signal.

Swine

Luteolysis

In pigs, luteolysis occurs during late diestrus after the uterine endometrium has been continually exposed to progesterone stimulation for 10–12 days, causing loss of PGR from the endometrial epithelia. The ability of progesterone to down-regulate its own receptor within the endometrial epithelia is the foundation for the classical McCracken model for luteolysis in sheep.[22] The endocrine requirements for luteolysis in pigs are not as fully delineated as for ruminants.[103,104] However, uterine PGF is the luteolysin in pigs and CL regression occurs in response to pulsatile release of PGF into the uterine venous drainage beginning on days 15–16 of the estrous cycle[105] and hysterectomy extends CL life span to about 120 days.[103] Indeed, the CLs of pigs are refractory to PGF-induced luteolysis between days 1

and 13 of the estrous cycle, when they have few PGF receptors, and only respond to luteolyic effects of PGF when the CL expresses abundant receptors for PGF[105,106] from about day 14 of the estrous cycle. Unlike ruminants, pig CLs contain little oxytocin to be released and bind OXTR expressed by endometrial epithelia to stimulate pulsatile secretion of PGF.[107–109] Instead, the endometrium is a source of oxytocin that influences luteolysis.[110] Exogenous oxytocin decreases the interestrous interval when administered to pigs between days 10 and 16 of the estrous cycle, but not when administered to ovary-intact hysterectomized pigs.[103] The endometrium of pigs contains OXTR,[111] concentrations of oxytocin increase in the peripheral circulation of pigs during luteolysis,[112] oxytocin stimulates both inositol phosphate turnover[113] and secretion of PGF[112,114] from pig endometrial epithelial cells, and the effects of oxytocin on uterine secretion of PGF are reduced in pregnant and pseudopregnant compared to cyclic pigs.[103,112] Prostaglandins are important in pregnant pigs as inhibition of prostaglandin synthesis results in pregnancy failure.[115] Conceptuses and endometrium both secrete prostaglandins,[116,117] and conceptus expression of the PTGS2 gene increases immediately following trophoblast elongation and continues during conceptus attachment to endometrial LE.[104,118] Induction of PTGS2 expression promotes PGE synthesis[119] and endometrial secretion of PGE increases during the peri-implantation period in pigs.[120] PGE may stabilize extracellular matrix, inflammation and immune functions.[104] Inappropriate early expression of epithelial PTGS2 on day 10 of pregnancy correlates with embryonic loss in pigs.[121]

Estrogens

Estrogens, produced by pig conceptuses between days 11 and 12 of gestation, are the initial signal for pregnancy recognition in pigs.[1,115] This is reinforced by a second period of estrogen production by pig conceptuses between days 15 and 25–30 of pregnancy[122,123] and both periods of estrogen secretion by pig conceptuses are critical to establishment and maintenance of pregnancy in pigs. Administration of exogenous estradiol to gilts on days 11–15 of the estrous cycle results in CL maintenance for a period equivalent to or slightly longer than for pregnancy, a condition defined as pseudopregnancy. However, a single injection of estradiol on either day 9.5, 11, 12.5, 14, 15.5, or 14–16 extends CL life span by only 30 days, while administration of estradiol on day 11 and days 14–16 extends interestrous intervals to more than 60 days.[123]

*Endocrine–exocrine theory of
pregnancy recognition signaling*

The theory of maternal recognition of pregnancy in pigs[122–124] is based on evidence that:

1. The uterine endometrium secretes luteolytic PGF.
2. Pig conceptuses secrete estrogens which are antiluteolytic.
3. PGF is secreted in an endocrine direction (i.e. toward the uterine vasculature) in cyclic gilts to induce luteolysis.
4. Secretion of PGF in pregnant gilts is exocrine (i.e. into the uterine lumen), where it is sequestered to exert its biological effects in utero and/or be metabolized to prevent luteolysis (Figure 17.4).

Secretion of PGF by the uterus is not inhibited during pregnancy, pseudopregnancy, or the estrous cycle. Rather, there is a transition from endocrine to exocrine secretion of PGF between days 10 and 12 of pregnancy that is coincident with initiation of estrogen secretion by elongating pig conceptuses. Estrogen induces a transient release of calcium into the uterine lumen within 12 hours and an increase in endometrial expression of PRLR. Mean concentrations, peak frequency, and peak amplitude of PGF in utero–ovarian vein plasma are lower in pregnant and pseudopregnant pigs than in cyclic pigs. However, uterine flushings from pseudopregnant and pregnant pigs have significantly higher amounts of PGF than those from cyclic pigs. The switch in direction of endometrial secretion of PGF from endocrine to exocrine can be induced in an in-vitro perfusion chamber using endometria from estrogen-treated pigs exposed in vitro to the calcium ionophore A23187 (induces calcium flux across epithelial membranes) or PRL.[122] Therefore, it is hypothesized that estrogen induces endometrial PRLR in pigs, and that PRL acts on the endometrium to induce calcium cycling across the epithelia to facilitate exocrine secretion of PGF into the uterine lumen.[122]

There are reports that PGF from the uterus is taken up by the mesometrium and returned to the uterus in arterial blood by a countercurrent system within the broad ligament of the pig uterus.[125] Estrogen also increases the ratio of PGE to PGF[126,127] and maintains LHCGR in both CL and uterus.[128,129] Thus, PGE$_2$ may 'protect' CL from luteolytic effects of PGF and estrogens may have a luteotropic effect on pig CL.[130]

Uterine–conceptus interactions

Estrogen and progesterone play important roles in uterine–conceptus interactions in pigs to prepare the

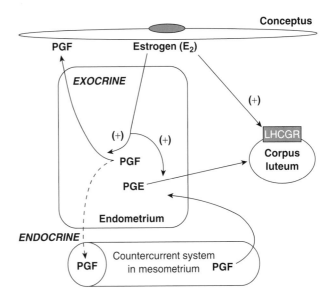

Figure 17.4 The inhibition of luteolysis in pigs. Estrogens produced by the conceptus alter the direction of PGF secretion from an endocrine to an exocrine direction (uterine lumen). Additionally, PGF of uterine origin is taken up by the mesometrium and transferred into the uterus in arterial blood by a countercurrent system operating in the broad ligament of the uterus. Estrogen also increases PGE secretion by the pig uterus, which is hypothesized to protect the corpus luteum from the luteolytic actions of PGF. Estrogen also maintains LHCGR in the corpus luteum and has a direct luteotropic effect. (Modified from Ziecik and coworkers.[129]) E$_2$, estrogen; LHCGR, luteinizing hormone/choriogonadotropin receptor; PGE, prostaglandin E$_2$; PGF, prostaglandin F$_{2\alpha}$.

uterus for implantation and to enhance maintenance of a successful pregnancy by increasing secretory activity of endometrial epithelia.[104,123,131,132] Conceptus estrogens induce a cascade of events mediated initially by activation of the kallikrein–kininogen–kinin system that cleaves an inter-α-trypsin inhibitor, a member of the Kunitz-type protease inhibitor superfamily, which is associated with conceptus elongation and adhesion.[123] Conceptus estrogens also increase expression of several genes in the pig endometrium that include retinol-binding protein, spermidine/spermine N1-acetyltransferase, integrin β$_5$, F-actin capping protein α$_1$ subunit, CD24a antigen, ubiquitin B precursor, and SPP1.[104] In pregnant and pseudopregnant pigs, SPP1 expression is induced by estrogen in endometrial LE; however, expression of SPP1 in LE is only in close proximity to conceptus trophectoderm on day 15 of pregnancy, suggesting a local effect of conceptus estrogens. In contrast, intramuscular injections of estrogen to induce pseudopregnancy results in uniform, albeit moderate, expression of SPP1 across the entire LE at day 15 after onset of estrus.[133] It is not known whether estrogen acts directly on LE to induce SPP1, or whether it acts indirectly through another uterine factor(s). A direct effect is possible since the promoter regions of rat and mouse SPP1 genes have response elements that are activated by ESR1, and the pig SPP1 promoter has an SP1 binding sequence, an AP1 site, and pig endometrial LE expresses both ESR1 and SPP1.[133] The exquisite restriction of SPP1 to LE near the conceptus is probably due to sulfatase activity of trophectoderm. During pregnancy, the pig endometrium rapidly converts estradiol to the biologically inactive estrone sulfate.[134] However, pig trophectoderm has sulfatase activity that restores the biological activity of estrone to allow it to exert localized effects that include induction of SPP1 expression. It is hypothesized that SPP1 protein at the apical surface of LE and interface with trophectoderm cross-links with itself and with other molecules to establish adhesion and implantation, as well as signal transduction, cell migration, tissue remodeling, and immune cell migration at implantation sites.[133] In support of this hypothesis, Burghardt et al[135] reported significant changes in expression of cell adhesion molecules and integrins during the peri-implantation period in swine. In particular, MUC1 is present at the apical surface of endometrial LE in the prereceptive stage of pregnancy, perhaps to block attachment of blastocyts while they are undergoing intrauterine migration and spacing. Then, during the receptive stage for implantation, MUC1 decreases coincidentally with increases in expression of α_4, α_5, α_v, β_1, and β_3 integrins (potential receptors for SPP1) at the site of contact between trophectoderm and uterine LE.

Pig conceptus estrogens also induce synchronous release of endometrial epithelial secretions, termed histotroph, which support conceptus development. A comparison of the composition of uterine flushings from pregnant and cyclic pigs between days 6 and 16 after the onset of estrus indicated that total protein increases significantly regardless of pregnancy status and that temporal changes in individual proteins differ due to pregnancy status. Pig histotroph of pregnancy is composed of a complex array of substances, including PGF, glucose for nutrition,[136] uteroferrin for iron transport and regulation of hematopoiesis,[137] retinol-binding protein,[138] and SPP1 for implantation and placentation.[133,140] There are also significant effects of day of pregnancy on total recoverable sodium and potassium, and total recoverable calcium is affected by both day and pregnancy status (Figure 17.5). In pregnant pigs, total recoverable calcium increases on day 11 and returns to basal levels by day 14; however, in cyclic gilts,

recoverable calcium increases in uterine flushings on day 11, but does not return to basal values by day 16. In the absence of the decrease in calcium by day 14, there is no transport of glucose into the uterine lumen (see Figure 17.5). Increases in uterine secretions and transport of glucose are more coordinated in pregnant pigs and this is probably favorable to survival and continued development of conceptuses. Recently, the phosphorylated form of mammalian target of rapamycin (mTOR) – a nutrient-sensing cell signaling pathway that stimulates migration, hypertrophy, and hyperplasia of trophectoderm cells – was immunolocalized to conceptus trophectoderm.[102] It is hypothesized that glucose, leucine, arginine, glutamine, and SPP1 act coordinately to activate mTOR within the conceptus to stimulate its development during the peri-implantation period (H Gao, FW Bazer, G Wu, and GA Johnson, unpublished results).

Estrogens secreted by pig conceptuses between days 10 and 15 of pregnancy are essential for both establishment of pregnancy and for increasing the presence of selected components of histotroph in the uterine lumen from day 11.[104] Placental estrogens act on endometrial epithelia in a paracrine manner to increase expression of specific growth factors, including insulin-like growth factor 1 (IGF1) and fibroblast growth factor-7 (FGF7), and perhaps SPP1, that act on trophectoderm to stimulate cell proliferation, conceptus attachment, and development of the conceptus.[140,141]

FGF7 is a paracrine mediator of epithelial growth and differentiation.[142] In all organs studied before the pig uterus, FGF7 was found to be expressed only in mesenchymal cells. Expression of FGF7 in the porcine uterus is particularly abundant in LE between days 12 and 15 of the estrous cycle and pregnancy, but expression shifts to GE and is maintained in the GE from day 30 until the end of the 114-day period of gestation.[143] The FGF7 protein is present in uterine flushings and FGFR2, the receptor for FGF7, is expressed by both endometrial epithelia and conceptus trophectoderm. Treatment of endometrial explants from day 9 cyclic gilts with estradiol-17β increased FGF7 expression, while treatment of porcine trophectoderm cells with recombinant rat FGF7 increased proliferation and expression of urokinase-type plasminogen activator and IFND, markers for trophectoderm cell differentiation.[144] These results indicate that estrogen, the pregnancy recognition signal from pig conceptuses, increases uterine epithelial expression of FGF7, which, in turn, stimulates proliferation and differentiation of trophectoderm in pigs which have a true epitheliochorial placenta.

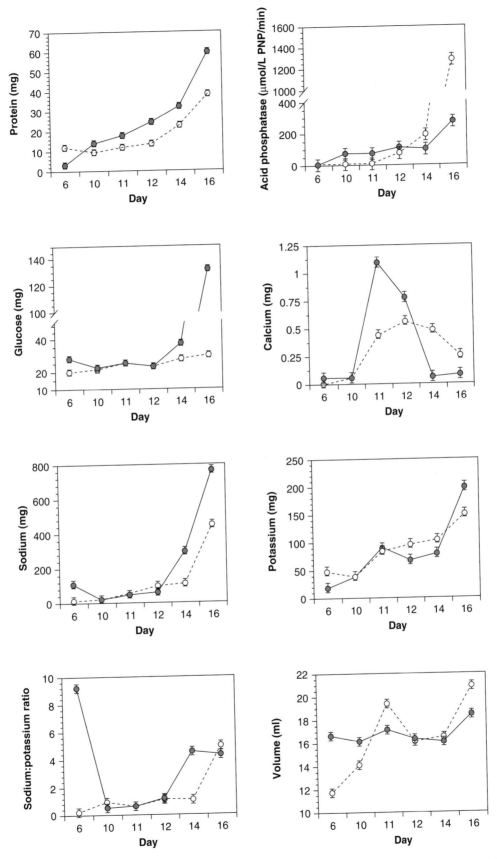

Figure 17.5 The composition of uterine flushings differs between cyclic (○) and pregnant (•) gilts. Effects of pregnancy are most notable on temporal changes in calcium between days 10 and 16, accumulation of glucose, accumulation of sodium, and changes in total recoverable protein (see text for additional details).

In addition to estrogen, the elongating pig conceptus secretes a wide array of growth factors and cytokines, including interleukin-1β (IL1β), PGE, IFND, IFNG, and transforming growth factors β₁, β₂, and β₃ that may influence implantation and pregnancy recognition signaling.[141] Indeed, it is hypothesized that conceptus estrogens modulate uterine responses to IL1β and activation of nuclear factor-κB (NFκB) during the inflammatory-like remodeling of the pig uterus during the peri-implantation period.[104] Interestingly, intrauterine infusion of IL1β at the time of implantation in non-pregnant baboons synergizes with CG to mimic early endometrial events associated with the presence of a conceptus.[18]

Trophoblast interferons

Peri-implantation pig conceptus trophectoderm produces both type I and type II IFNs, although their physiological role(s) in pregnancy recognition is only now emerging. The major species (75% of antiviral activity in pig conceptus secretory proteins) is IFNG and the other (25%) is a novel type I interferon, IFND.[145,146] There is no evidence that either IFNG or IFND are antiluteolytic or have any effect on interestrous interval or temporal changes in concentrations of progesterone in plasma.[122,146] However, paracrine effects for IFNG and IFND are suggested by localization of IFNAR1 and IFNGR2 receptors on endometrial epithelial cells[146] and evidence for induction of ISGs that may represent one aspect of complex temporal and spatial events affecting conceptus development throughout the peri-implantation period.[88,147]

Attachment of blastocysts to LE requires transitional labilization and remodeling of polarity of uterine LE in response to the synchronous exchange of signals between conceptus trophectoderm and endometrial cells.[148] Porcine trophoblast IFNG and/or IFND may stimulate remodeling and/or depolarization of uterine LE as a prerequisite for implantation and establishment of a functional placenta.[149] On day 15 of pregnancy, immunoreactive IFNG is detectable in cell clusters unevenly localized along the endometrial LE of the pig uterus. On day 15 of pregnancy, de-novo appearance of tight junction protein-1 (TJP1) can be detected at the basal side of LE, suggesting significant changes to polarity of endometrial epithelia in response to pig conceptus interferons. IFNG is a specific and potent inducer of major histocompatibility complex (MHC) II antigens[150] and, in endometrial stroma of pigs, MHC class II molecules are abundant only in uteri from day 15 pregnant pigs. These MHC class II antigens are localized to vascular elements beneath the LE. As in the ovine uterus during pregnancy, LE of pregnant porcine uteri is negative for MHC II antigens, suggesting that these cells are not responsive to IFNG. In addition, ISGs expressed by pig endometrial cells include G1P2, MX1, ISG15/17, IRF1, STAT1, and STAT2 that increase in the endometrial stroma of pigs between days 14 and 18 of pregnancy[88] (M Joyce and GA Johnson, unpublished results).

Horses

Estrous cycle

Mares are seasonally polyestrous from late winter through late fall in the Northern Hemisphere[151] with 21–22 day estrous cycles. Estrus lasts 3–7 days and ovulation occurs 24–48 hours before the end of behavioral estrus in response to a protracted LH surge over a period of up to 10 days. Progesterone production begins about 24 hours after ovulation, with maximal secretion between days 6 and 18–20 after onset of estrus when concentrations are 4–8 ng/ml before declining in response to PGF-induced luteolysis.[152]

Luteolysis

Uterine function in the mare is probably controlled by sequential exposure of the endometrium to the ovarian steroids, estrogen and progesterone, acting through their cognate nuclear receptors. Temporal and spatial expression of these receptors in the endometrium is similar to that for the ewe.[33,153] Endometrial expression of ESR1 and PGR mRNA and protein is greatest on day 0 and then declines to low levels by day 14 after ovulation when their patterns of expression diverge between cyclic and pregnant mares.[153] In cyclic mares, expression of both ESR1 and PGR increase by day 17 and reach maximal levels on day 20 after ovulation, whereas neither ESR1 nor PGR expression change between days 14 and 20 of pregnancy.[153] This divergence in the pattern of steroid receptor expression occurs around the time of onset of luteolysis in the mare, i.e. days 14–17 after ovulation. During this time endometria of cyclic mares release luteolytic PGF, but neither the pattern of release nor the endocrine regulation of uterine production of PGF are well-defined. Concentrations of PGF in uterine venous plasma and uterine flushings increase and concentrations of progesterone in plasma decrease between days 14 and 16 when luteolysis occurs. The amount of PGF bound by luteal receptors is maximal on day 14 of the estrous cycle and day 18 of pregnancy; however, the CL is responsive to luteolytic effects of PGF from day 5 after ovulation. Cervical stimulation induces the

Ferguson reflex, resulting in release of oxytocin from the posterior pituitary that stimulates uterine secretion of luteolytic PGF.[154] Administration of exogenous oxytocin also stimulates uterine secretion of PGF in cyclic mares.[155] The relationship between oxytocin and uterine PGF production in cyclic mares was also demonstrated by Sharp et al,[156] who reported that pregnancy status had no effect on Ferguson reflex-induced release of oxytocin in response to endometrial biopsy procedure; however, biopsy-induced release of oxytocin resulted in PGF production in cyclic, but not pregnant, mares. There is a report that PTGS2 is high in endometria of cyclic, but not pregnant, mares on day 15 after ovulation.[157] However, a more likely explanation is that uterine OXTRs are significantly lower in pregnant than cyclic mares.[156] There is no evidence that CL of mares produce oxytocin, but, as for pigs, high levels of oxytocin are present in uterine flushings and endometria from mares.[158,159] Therefore, oxytocin-induced PGF release appears to be a critical component of the luteolytic mechanism in mares that must be blocked to establish pregnancy.

Pregnancy recognition

In mares, pregnancy recognition may begin with early cleavage stage embryos that are transported from the oviduct into the uterine lumen while unfertilized oocytes remain 'locked' in the oviduct.[160] Cleavage stage embryos transported into the uterine lumen develop to large spherical blastocysts that hatch from the zona pellucida, but remain encased in a capsule that allows spherical expansion, but not elongation. The blastocysts migrate between uterine horns 12–15 times daily between days 7 and 17 of pregnancy in response to uterine contractions, and this is critical for pregnancy recognition. Intrauterine migration allows required physical contact between the conceptus and uterine endometrium for the equine conceptus to expose the entire uterus to an antiluteolytic factor(s) that inhibits uterine production of luteolytic PGF.[161] Equine conceptuses confined to the tip of one uterine horn fail to block luteolysis.[162] Around day 17 of pregnancy, intrauterine migration of the conceptus stops due to an increase in myometrial tone and fixation of the conceptus at the base of one uterine horn.[153] Pregnant mares have little PGF in uterine fluids, low concentrations of PGF in uterine venous plasma, and no episodic pattern of release of 15-keto-13,14-dihydro-prostaglandin $F_{2\alpha}$ (PGFM) into peripheral plasma. Furthermore, endometrial production of PGF in response to cervical stimulation and exogenous oxytocin is markedly reduced or absent in pregnant mares.[156]

Similar to the pig, equine conceptuses produce significant amounts of estradiol-17β and 17α-hydroxyprogesterone during the period of pregnancy recognition.[154,155] However, there is no clear evidence that estrogen is the antiluteolytic hormone in mares,[152] and the role of 17α-hydroxyprogesterone has not been determined. The fact that ESR1 and PGR are absent from LE and expressed at low levels in GE and stroma in the mare, as for ruminants, may explain the inability of exogenous estrogen to extend luteal life span in mares as it does in pigs.[122] Equine conceptuses also secrete low molecular weight molecules with apparent PGF-inhibitory activity between days 12 and 14 of pregnancy and they could play a role in pregnancy recognition.[161] In addition, several conceptus' secretory proteins without known functions have been identified.[163,164] However, as noted by Allen et al,[152] pregnancy recognition signaling in the mare remains a mystery.

Rats and mice

Estrous cycle

Laboratory rats and mice have estrous cycles of 4–5 days that are under photoperiodic control. Each phase of the estrous cycle can be defined by cytology of vaginal smears:[165] proestrus lasts 12–14 hours, estrus 25–27 hours, metestrus 6–8 hours, and diestrus 55–57 hours. In rats, mice, and hamsters, the CL secrete progestins for approximately 2 days, do not become fully functional, and regress during diestrus due to apoptosis, degeneration of the blood supply, leukocytic infiltration, and increased activity of 20α-hydroxysteroid dehydrogenase (HSD20A).[165] Although PGF is luteolytic in rodents, its mechanism of action is not well understood.[166] The CL of cyclic rodents secrete small amounts of progesterone, which is metabolized by HSD20A in the CL to 20α-hydroxyprogesterone, which does not support pregnancy or the uterine decidual reaction.[167] Thus, cyclic rodents lack a true luteal phase and have recurrent estrous cycles of short duration to ensure numerous opportunities for mating and establishment of pregnancy.

Maternal recognition of pregnancy

Gestation in rats and mice lasts 20–22 days, and functional CLs are required through day 17.[168] Although the placenta/decidua does not produce sufficient progesterone to supplant that from the CL, both of these tissues express isoforms of 3β-hydroxysteroid dehydrogenase (HSD3B) and trophoblast giant cells produce progesterone for at least a portion of early gestation in mice.[169] The locally produced progesterone may regulate immune cell function at the fetal–maternal interface.

Following mating, a nidatory surge of estrogen on day 4 is responsible for rendering the endometrium 'receptive' to blastocyst implantation (see[170]). This estrogen induces a rapid, but transient increase in expression of LIF in endometrial epithelia and stroma.[170] LIF –/– mice support pregnancy to the blastocyst stage, but the blastocysts are unable to undergo implantation due to failure to progress beyond attachment to the LE. Two homeobox genes, Hmx3 and HOXA11, are postulated to regulate the estrogen-induced increase in endometrial LIF expression.[170] Leukemia inhibitory factor receptor (LIF) acts on the uterine LE via the LIFR in association with IL6ST (IL-6 signal transducer) to activate the JAK–STAT signal transduction pathway. Activation of this pathway induces STAT3 phosphorylation, which, among other effects, increases interleukin-11 (IL-11) expression, which is thought to influence secondary decidualization and formation of trophoblast giant cells.[170,171] Furthermore, blastocyts express LIFR and LIF enhances blastocyst development; however, LIF –/– embryos can progress through the blastocyst stage of development.[170]

Establishment and maintenance of pregnancy in mice and rats requires two separate endocrine events.[166] First, mating or cervical stimulation induces nocturnal and diurnal surges of PRL from the maternal pituitary which are necessary for formation and maintenance of active CL and progesterone secretion[172] by increasing luteal cell receptors for LH[173] and inhibiting HSD20A activity.[174] This extends luteal function until days 10–12 of pregnancy or pseudopregnancy.[175] The HSD20A activity increases at the end of pseudopregnancy[176] when maternal surges of PRL cease around day 10 after mating.[177,178] Support for CL function then shifts from maternal PRL, to placental lactogen-I (CSH1).[175,178] By approximately day 12 of gestation, CSH1 expression decreases and placental lactogen-II (CSH2) expression increases and dominates until the end of gestation. Just prior to parturition, there is an increase in both maternal and fetal PRL production.[178] Serum concentrations of progesterone are similar for pseudopregnant and early pregnant rats through day 11 after mating and then increase two-fold between days 12 and 20 of pregnancy in rats.[179]

Prostaglandins are critical players in pregnancy recognition/implantation signaling in mice and rats. Expression of PTGS1 is low in LE and GE around the time of blastocyst attachment, but PTGS2 expression increases in LE and stroma adjacent to sites of blastocyst attachment.[180] Furthermore, homozygous mutants of cytoplasmic phospholipase A_2 (PLA2) experience delayed implantation, impaired spacing and development of conceptuses, and reduced fertility,[180] further emphasizing a role for prostanoids in implantation in mice and rats.

The second endocrine event required for pregnancy in rodents is implantation and development of placentas and deciduae that produce luteotropic PRL-like hormones which stimulate mammary gland development and production of progesterone and relaxin by CL during the middle and late stages of pregnancy.[178,181,182] Members of this diverse gene family exhibit different temporal–spatial patterns of expression in uteri and placentas of rodents.

Decidual PRL-like proteins

Implantation in rats and mice involves progesterone-dependent transformation of stromal cells into two unique populations of decidual cells.[183] The deciduae encase the developing blastocysts and provide a cellular microenvironment that supports and limits invasion and differentiation of trophoblast-derived cells and this requires both progesterone and activating signals for the implanting blastocysts.[178] The initial site of decidualization forms the antimesometrial decidua or decidua capsularis, which contains large polyploid cells that secrete numerous hormones, including follistatin, activin, TGFβ, and at least four members of the PRL family – PRL-like protein B (PLPB), decidual PRL-like protein (dPRP), PLPJ, and PRL.[178] Subsequent decidualization of mesometrial stroma results in formation of the mesometrial decidua or decidua basalis, comprised of fibroblast-like and binucleate cells that secrete α_2-macroglobulin and numerous growth factors.[184] The antimesometrial decidua produces primarily PRL-like hormones that stimulate luteal production of progesterone and reduce the ability of follicles to aromatize androgens to estradiol.[183] The dPRP is expressed only by antimesometrial decidual cells and PLP-B is expressed by both placentae and deciduae.[185] Decidual PRP binds PRL receptors on luteal cells to suppress HSD20A, and binds receptors in the mesometrial decidua to increase expression of α_2-macroglobulin. Thus, dPRP acts on both the ovary and the decidua.

Placental lactogens

At least 26 different PRL-related genes have been identified in mice, whereas only one GH1 gene is present[178] (see Chapter 22). Members of this gene family are synthesized as a single peptide of approximately

30 amino acids that is targeted for secretion.[178] They share general structural similarities, including conservation of cysteine positioning, a variety of post-translational glycosylation patterns, and a conformation that includes a four-helix bundle motif.[178]

Members of the CSH1 family are expressed in cell-, positional-, and temporal-specific patterns: mid pregnancy (CSH1) and late pregnancy (CSH2).[178,185] The CSH1 is expressed by mural trophoblast giant cells of implanting blastocysts and later by specific compartments of the choriovitelline and chorioallantoic placenta, is developmentally regulated by implantation and formation of trophoblast giant cells between days 4 and 5, while termination of CSH1 expression is coordinated with loss of the choriovitelline placenta around days 12–13 of gestation. On days 13 and 14 of gestation, the choriovitelline placenta degenerates, CSH1 expression ends, and CHS2 expression by trophoblast giant cells of the chorioallantoic placenta begins. CSH2 is expressed initially in trophoblast giant cells of the junctional zone and then by trophoblast giant cells of the labyrinth zone during late gestation.[178] Expression of PLPA, PLPC, and PLIv increases in cells of the chorioallantoic placental junctional zone just after mid gestation, with expression confined to spongiotrophoblast cells and some trophoblast giant cells of the junctional zone during the latter half of gestation. Although PLPB expression is restricted to spongiotrophoblast cells, its temporal expression is similar to that for PLPA, PLPC, and PLIv.[185] Glycogen cells and syncytial cells of rodent placentas do not express placental PRL family genes.[178]

Because rat placental PRL-like hormones display structural and functional similarity to PRL and diurnal surges of PRL cease when secretion of CSHs start, CSHs are postulated to functionally replace pituitary PRL. Like PRL, CSH1 and CSH2 bind PRL receptors and activate the JAK–STAT signal transduction pathway,[184] resulting in STAT5 and phosphotidylinositol 3-kinase/Akt activation. In contrast, PLPA, PLPB, and PLPC do not bind PRL receptors, and their activities are largely unknown. The likely roles of CSHs are (1) maintenance of progesterone and relaxin secretion by CL during pregnancy; (2) development of the mammary gland epithelium during pregnancy; and (3) control of maternal metabolic functions.[167]

Cats

Estrous cycle

Cats are seasonally polyestrous, induced ovulators with onset of cyclicity occurring as early as 4 months and as late as 21 months of age, depending on breed, photoperiod, and level of nutrition.[186,187] In the Northern Hemisphere, cats exhibit anestrus between October and January, but cats in the tropics are sexually active year round. In the absence of mating, estrus lasts an average of 7 days followed by an interestrous period of 10 days characterized by low estrogen levels and non-receptivity to mating. Rapid growth of ovarian follicles and increased secretion of estradiol occurs over the 2–3-day period prior to estrus.[186] At estrus the ovaries contain an average of five preovulatory follicles and an average of 4.3 ova are ovulated in response to mating. Mating induces a neuroendocrine reflex and a pulse of GnRH from the hypothalamus that induces an ovulatory surge of LH, which peaks at 20 minutes and returns to basal levels by 60 minutes post coitum.[188] Although some cats ovulate in the absence of cervical stimulation, amplitude and duration of the LH surge increases with number of copulations.[189,190] Multiple matings on successive days of estrus ensure ovulation in all queens, but less than 50% of estrus queens ovulate after a single copulation.[191]

Luteolysis

Feline CL are resistant to exogenous PGF at all stages of gestation; however, production of PGF by fetal–placental tissues and endometrium increases during the last half of pregnancy, plateaus around day 45, and increases rapidly just before parturition.[187] Administration of high levels of PGF after day 40 of pregnancy will induce abortion, but the mechanism is not known.[187] In addition, administration of the progesterone receptor antagonist aglepristone induces abortion after day 25 of gestation.[192]

Pregnancy recognition

In queens, ovulation occurs 25–50 hours postcoitum or 24–36 hours after the LH peak, with frequent matings reducing the time to ovulation. Fertilization occurs in the oviduct up to 48 hours after ovulation, embryos enter the uterus at the blastocyst stage 4–6 days postovulation, blastocysts undergo hatching on day 11, and implantation begins on days 12–13. Cats have an endotheliochorial placenta with zonary villous distribution (see Chapter 32). Following mating, CLs form and concentrations of progesterone in plasma increase from day 3 to maximal levels between days 10 and 40 of pregnancy or days 13 and 30 of pseudopregnancy. Cats that ovulate experience pseudopregnancy, which lasts about 40 days, while pregnancy averages 63–65 days. Therefore, there is no apparent requirement for a pregnancy recognition signal from cat conceptuses during the peri-implantation period. The placenta is not a significant source of progesterone. Ovariectomy on day 45 results in a rapid decline in plasma progesterone and abortion 6–9 days postsurgery.[193] Secretion of PRL increases throughout the last trimester of gestation and is considered an important luteotropin in late gestation.[187] In fact, PRL antagonists are effective abortifacients during the latter half of gestation of cats.[194]

The feline placenta produces substantial amounts of relaxin, while CL, uterus, and fetus also express detectable levels.[195] After implantation on days 13–14, relaxin is first detected in maternal serum on about day 20, peak values are between days 30 and 35 and then they decline gradually until parturition, and become undetectable within 24 hours after parturition.[195,196] The villous trophoblast cells of the labyrinth zone appear to be the sole source of feline placental relaxin.[195] The combination of relaxin and progesterone may maintain uterine quiescence and facilitate parturition.[197]

In addition to relaxin, other proteins are expressed by the feline uteroplacental tissues, including CSPL,[198] IGFBP1,[199] TGFα, EGF, and EGFR,[200] alkaline phosphatase and plasma membrane calcium-ATPase,[201] retinol-binding protein, α-fetoprotein, albumin, and transferrin,[202] and immunoreactive pregnancy-associated glycoprotein-2.[203] However, there are no known roles for these proteins in the establishment or maintenance of pregnancy in cats.

Dog

Estrous cycle

The dog is classified as monestrus and ovulates once or twice per year after reaching puberty at 7–12 months of age.[204] Ovarian follicles secrete estradiol and inhibin at the end of anestrus to induce an increase in LH and a slight reduction in follicle-stimulating hormone (FSH) just prior to proestrus. Ovarian inhibin suppresses FSH secretion during proestrus as estrogens increase. Proestrus lasts about 7 days, when there is a bloody vaginal discharge and increased size and turgidity of the vagina. The LH surge occurs near the onset of estrus. It results in a decrease in estrogen and an increase in progesterone in plasma, and an increase in sexual receptivity of bitches to males for mating. The LH surge lasts 2–3 days and is accompanied by an increase in plasma FSH, which peaks shortly after the LH surge and returns to basal levels in 1–2 days. In the

non-pregnant bitch, luteolysis is protracted: it begins around day 30 when progesterone secretion decreases gradually at the end of the luteal phase to below 1 ng/ml and remains low for weeks or months before the next ovarian follicular phase is initiated.[205] Hysterectomy does not prolong the life span of CL, which suggests that luteolysis in the bitch is not dependent on a uterine luteolysin.[198]

Pregnancy recognition

Ovulation occurs 48 hours after the LH surge to release oocytes at the germinal vesicle stage which achieve metaphase II in the isthmus of the oviduct.[187] They remain fertilizable for 2–3 days by spermatozoa, which are reported to be viable in the female reproductive tract for 6–7 days. Fertilization takes place approximately 4 days after the LH surge, embryos enter the uterus as morulae or blastocysts on days 9–10, and implantation occurs 16–18 days after the LH surge.[204] The length of the luteal phase in non-pregnant and pregnant bitches is similar; therefore, there is no apparent need for a pregnancy recognition signal to extend the life span of the CL. Concentrations of progesterone in plasma increase between days 10 and 40 after the LH surge and then decline gradually to term (days 64–66).[204] Concentrations of circulating estrogens increase during the second half of gestation and are thought to stimulate development of the mammary glands. Concentrations of PRL also increase from days 30–40 of gestation to peak values 24–48 hours prior to parturition. Prolactin appears to be luteotropic in bitches because suppression of prolactin secretion with a dopamine agonist decreases progesterone production early in pregnancy and results in luteolysis after about day 30.[205] Prolactin may regulate length of anestrus by affecting gonadotropin secretion or ovarian responsiveness to gonadotropins.[204,206] Relaxin, perhaps the only pregnancy-specific hormone in dogs, peaks during the last trimester of gestation and remains detectable for 1–2 months after parturition.[207] It is produced by both the ovary and the pregnant uterus. At the end of pregnancy there is rapid luteolysis due to inadequate gonadotropin support.[208]

SUMMARY

Pregnancy recognition signaling in primates having a uterine-independent ovarian cycle involves direct luteotropic effects of CG from conceptus trophectoderm on the CL. However, most subprimate species have a uterine-dependent ovarian cycle with life span of the CL controlled by PGF released from the uterus. Therefore, conceptuses of subprimate mammals must produce antiluteolytic factors such as IFNτ, estrogens, and/or lactogenic hormones or even luteotropic hormones such as prolactin and placental lactogens. Another strategy, used by the bitch and queen, is to have the life span of the CL equivalent to that required for full gestation to avoid the need for a pregnancy recognition signal, but perhaps require a signal such as prolactin to sustain CL function during the latter stages of pregnancy.

Interferon-stimulated genes are a common feature of the peri-implantation period of pregnancy recognition in humans, baboons, domestic animals, and laboratory animals. The ISGs expressed in defined temporal and spatial (cell-specific) patterns by endometrial cells may directly influence conceptus development and implantation or act indirectly by affecting endometrial receptivity to implantation and, in turn, pregnancy recognition and establishment of pregnancy.

Temporal and spatial changes in expression of ESR1 and PGR occur in uterine cells during the period of pregnancy recognition and implantation. Loss of expression of PGR by uterine epithelia is a hallmark of pregnancy in all mammalian species studied to date. During transition to the luteal phase and during the peri-implantation period in primates,[209] pigs,[210,211] sheep,[212] monkeys,[12] baboons,[14] and skunk,[213] LE and GE have no or few ESR1 and PGR, but ESR1 and PGR are abundant in stromal cells. Therefore, progesterone, the hormone of pregnancy, must mediate its effects on epithelial cells by inducing PGR-positive stromal and/or myometrial cells to secrete paracrine growth factors that regulate uterine epithelial cell proliferation and differentiated functions.[209,214] Stromal cells produce cytokines and growth factors which stimulate proliferation, differentiation, and secretions of epithelial cells,[143,214,215] as well as maintenance of polarity and unique functional characteristics of uterine epithelia required for conceptus development, pregnancy recognition signaling, and implantation.[216] Three growth factors known to be expressed by stromal cells are fibroblast growth factors FGF7 and FGF10, and hepatocyte growth factor (HGF), which act via their respective receptors expressed on epithelial cells (Figure 17.6). These three growth factors are secreted by stromal cells that express ESR1 and PGR in response to progestins and/or estrogens and are, therefore, known as progestamedins and estromedins. Thus, sex steroids probably mediate their effects on

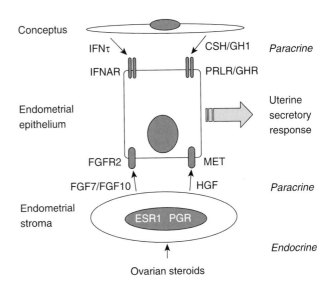

Figure 17.6 Ovarian steroid hormone regulation of endometrial function and uterine response to placental hormones during pregnancy. During early pregnancy, continuous exposure of the endometrium to progesterone down-regulates progesterone receptor in the endometrial epithelia. Indeed, the endometrial epithelia in the ovine uterus are negative for ESR1 and PGR during most of gestation. Therefore, the endocrine effects of ovarian steroids on endometrial function are promulgated by paracrine-acting growth factors produced by the steroid receptor-positive stroma. These progestamedins and estromedins include stromal FGFs (FGF7/FGF10) and HGF that activate their receptors, FGFR2 and MET, expressed only on epithelia. Furthermore, stromal-derived growth factors may be permissive for the effects of placental hormones IFNτ CSH1, and GH1 to activate their receptors and cellular functions, including secretion of proteins needed for conceptus growth and placentation. CSH1, chorionic somatomammotropin hormone 1 (placental lactogen); ESR1, estrogen receptor α; FGF7, fibroblast growth factor 7 (keratinocyte growth factor); FGF10, fibroblast growth factor 10; FGFR2, fibroblast growth factor receptor 2 (keratinocyte growth factor receptor); GH1, growth hormone 1; GHR, growth hormone receptor; HGF, hepatocyte growth factor (hepapoietin A; scatter factor); MET, met proto-oncogene (hepatocyte growth factor receptor); IFNAR, type I interferon receptor; IFNτ interferon τ; PGR, progesterone receptor; PRLR, prolactin receptor.

uterine epithelia indirectly through regulation of secretion of progestamedins, estromedins, and perhaps andromedins by stromal cells. The outcome is regulation of epithelial cell proliferation and secretion to support establishment and maintenance of pregnancy.

ACKNOWLEDGMENTS

We thank former and current members of our laboratories who contributed so much to the research presented in this paper. Financial support for studies from our laboratories over the past 10 years has been from BARD Grant OEP 9604563 (FWB, TES); NIH Grants HD08501 (GAJ), HD32534 (FWB, TES), P20 RR15587 (TLO), and P30 ES09106 (FWB, TES, GAJ); and USDA CSREES NRI Grants 91-37203-6548 (FWB), 96-35203-3916 (TLO), 98-01983 (FWB), 2000-35203-9137 (FWB), 2001-02259 (TES), 2002-02398 (TLO), and 2005-01476 (TES).

REFERENCES

1. Spencer TE, Bazer FW. Conceptus signals for establishment and maintenance of pregnancy. Reprod Biol Endocrinol 2004; 2: 49.
2. Spencer TE, Johnson GA, Burghardt RC et al. Progesterone and placental hormone actions on the uterus: insights from domestic animals. Biol Reprod 2004: 71: 2–10.
3. Stouffer RL, Hearn JP. Endocrinology of the transition from menstrual cyclicity to establishment of pregnancy in primates. In Bazer FW, eds. Endocrinology of Pregnancy. New Jersey: Humana Press, 1998: 35–58.
4. Pratt BR, Butcher RL, Inskeep EK. Antiluteolytic effect of the conceptus and or PGE_2 -in ewes. J Anim Sci 1977; 46: 784–91.
5. Silvia WJ, Ottobre JS, Inskeep EK. Concentrations of prostaglandins E2, F2 α and 6-keto-prostaglandin F1 α in the utero-ovarian venous plasma of nonpregnant and early pregnant ewes. Biol Reprod 1984; 30: 936–44.
6. Spencer TE, Stagg AG, Ott TL et al. Differential effects of intrauterine and subcutaneous administration of recombinant ovine interferon tau on the endometrium of cyclic ewes. Biol Reprod 1999; 61: 464–70.
7. Yankey SJ, Hicks BA, Carnahan KG et al. Expression of the antiviral protein Mx in peripheral blood mononuclear cells of pregnant and bred, non-pregnant ewes. J Endocrinol 2001; 170: R7–11.
8. Gifford CA, Racicot K, Clark DS et al. Regulation of interferon stimulated genes in peripheral blood leukocytes in pregnant and bred, non-pregnant dairy cows. J Dairy Sci 2007; 90: 274–80.
9. Zelinski-Wooten MB, Stouffer RL. Intraluteal infusions of prostaglandins of the E, D, I, and A series prevents $PGFI_{2\alpha}$-induced, but not spontaneous luteal regression in rhesus monkeys. Biol Reprod 1990; 43: 507–16.
10. Khan-Dawood FS, Marut EL, Dawood MY. Oxytocin in the corpus luteum of the cynomolgus monkey (*Macaca fascicularis*). Endocrinology 1984; 15: 570–4.
11. Lessey BA, Killarn AP, Metzger DA et al. Immunohistochemical analysis of human uterine estrogen and progesterone receptors throughout the menstrual cycle. J Clin Endocrinol 1988; 67: 334–40.
12. Okulicz WC, Hild-Petito S, Chilton B. Expression of steroid hormone receptors in the pregnant uterus. In Bazer FW, eds. Endocrinology of Pregnancy. New Jersey: Humana Press, 1998: 177–98.
13. Clark CL. Cell-specific regulation of progesterone receptor in the female reproductive system. Mol Cell Endocrinol 1990; 70: C29–C33.
14. Hild-Petito S, Verhage HG, Fazleabas AT. Estrogen and progestin receptor localization during implantation and early pregnancy in the baboon (*Papio anubis*) uterus. Endocrinology 1992; 130: 2343–53.
15. Hearn JP, Webley GE, Gidley-Baird AA. Chorionic gonadotrophin and embryo-maternal recognition during the peri-implantation period in primates. J Reprod Fertil 1991; 92: 497–509.
16. Cameo P, Srisuparp S, Strakova Z et al. Chorionic gonadotropin and uterine dialogue in the primate. Reprod Biol Endocrinol 2004; 2: 50.
17. Licht P, Russu V, Wildt L. On the role of human chorionic gonadotropin (hCG) in the embryo-endometrial microenvironment: implications for differentiation and implantation. Semin Reprod Med 2001; 19; 37–47.
18. Strakova Z, Mavrogianis P, Meng X et al. In vivo infusion of interleukin-1beta and chorionic gonadotropin induces endometrial changes that mimic early pregnancy events in the baboon. Endocrinology 2005; 146: 4097–104.
19. Kao LC, Tulac S, Lobo S et al. Global gene profiling in human endometrium during the window of implantation. Endocrinology 2002; 143: 2119–38.
20. Rao CV. Novel concepts in neuroendocrine regulation of reproductive tract functions. In Bazer, FW, eds. Endocrinology of Pregnancy. New Jersey: Humana Press, 1998: 125–44.
21. Eggleston DL, Wilken C, Van Kirk EA et al. Progesterone induces expression of endometrial messenger RNA encoding for cyclooxygenase (sheep). Prostaglandins 1990; 39: 675–83.
22. McCracken JA, Schramm W, Okulicz WC. Hormone receptor control of pulsatile secretion of PGF2a from ovine uterus during luteolysis and its abrogation in early pregnancy. Anim Reprod Sci 1984; 7: 31–56.
23. Meyer HHD, Mittermeier T, Schams D. Dynamics of oxytocin, estrogen and progestin receptors in the bovine endometrium during the estrous cycle. Acta Endocrinologica 1986; 118: 96–104.
24. Jenkin G. The interaction between oxytocin and prostaglandin $F_{2\alpha}$ during luteal regression and early pregnancy in sheep. Reprod Fertil Develop 1992; 4: 321–8.
25. Homeida AM, Khalafalla AE. Effects of oxytocin-antagonist injections on luteal regression in the goat. Brit J Pharmacol 1987; 90: 281–4.
26. Schams D, Prokopp S, Barth D. The effect of active and passive immunization against oxytocin on ovarian cyclicity in ewes. Acta Endocrinol 1983; 103: 337–44.
27. Wathes DC, Ayad VJ, McGoff SA et al. Effect of active immunization against oxytocin on gonadotrophin secretion and the establishment of pregnancy in the ewe. J Reprod Fertil 1989; 86: 653–64.
28. Flint APF, Sheldrick EL. Continuous infusion of oxytocin prevents induction of oxytocin receptors and blocks luteal regression in cyclic ewes. J Reprod Fertil 1985; 75: 623–31.
29. Hazzard TM, Pinckard KL, Stormshak F. Impact of chronic treatment of ewes with estradiol-17_β or progesterone on oxytocin receptor gene transcription and ovarian oxytocin secretion. Biol Reprod 1998; 59: 105–10.
30. Hixon JE, Flint AP. Effects of a luteolytic dose of oestradiol benzoate on uterine oxytocin receptor concentrations, phosphoinositide turnover and prostaglandin F-2 alpha secretion in sheep. J Reprod Fertil 1987; 79: 457–67.
31. Fleming JGW, Bazer FW, Johnson GA et al. Cloning of the ovine estrogen receptor alpha gene and regulation by interferon tau. Endocrinology 2001; 142: 2879–87.
32. Fleming JGW, Spencer TE, Safe SH et al, Estrogen regulates transcription of the ovine oxytocin receptor gene through GC-rich SP1 promoter elements. Endocrinology 2006; 147: 899–911.
33. Spencer TE, Becker WC, George P et al. Ovine interferon-tau inhibits estrogen receptor up-regulation and estrogen-induced luteolysis in cyclic ewes. Endocrinology 1995; 136: 4932–44.

34. Garret JE, Geisert RD, Zavy MT et al. Evidence for maternal regulation of early conceptus growth and development in the bovine. J Reprod Fertil 1988; 84: 437–46.

35. Pestka S, Krause CD, Walter MR. Interferons, interferon-like cytokines, and their receptors. Immunol Rev 2004: 202: 8–32.

36. Roberts RM, Ezashi T, Rosenfeld CS et al. Evolution of the interferon tau genes and their promoters, and maternal–trophoblast interactions in control of their expression. Reprod Suppl 2003; 61: 239–51.

37. Hansen TR, Austin KJ, Perry DJ et al. Mechanism of action of interferon-tau in the uterus during early pregnancy. J Reprod Fertil 1999; 54: 329–39.

38. Stewart DM, Johnson GA, Vyhlidal CA et al. Interferon-tau activates multiple signal transducer and activator of transcription proteins and has complex effects on interferon-responsive gene transcription in ovine endometrial epithelial cells. Endocrinology 2001; 142: 98–107.

39. Choi Y, Johnson GA, Spencer TE et al. Pregnancy and interferon tau regulate MHC class I and beta-2-microglobulin expression in the ovine uterus. Biol Reprod 2003; 68: 1703–10.

40. Gray CA, Abbey CA, Beremand PD et al. Identification of endometrial genes regulated by early pregnancy, progesterone, and interferon tau in the ovine uterus. Biol Reprod 2006; 4: 383–94.

41. Li Q, Zhang M, Kumar S et al. Identification and implantation stage-specific expression of an interferon-alpha-regulated gene in human and rat endometrium. Endocrinology 2001; 142: 2390–2400.

42. Kumar S, Li Q, Dua A et al. Messenger ribonucleic acid encoding interferon-inducible guanylate binding protein 1 is induced in human endometrium within the putative window of implantation. J Clin Endocrinol Metab 2001; 86: 2420–7.

43. Horcajadas JA, Riesewtjk A, Dominguez F et al. Determinants of endometrial receptivity. Ann NY Acad Sci 2004; 1034: 166–75.

44. Bebington C, Bell SC, Doherty FJ et al. Localization of ubiquitin and ubiquitin cross-reactive protein in human and baboon endometrium and decidua during the menstrual cycle and early pregnancy. Biol Reprod 1999; 60: 920–8.

45. Carson DD, Lagow E, Thathiah A et al. Changes in gene expression during the early to mid-luteal (receptive phase) transition in human endometrium detected by high-density microarray screening. Mol Hum Reprod 2002; 8: 871–9.

46. Austin KJ, Bany BM, Belden EL et al. Interferon-stimulated gene-15 (Isg15) expression is up-regulated in the mouse uterus in response to the implanting conceptus. Endocrinology 2003; 144: 3107–13.

47. Chen D, Xu X, Zhu LJ et al. Cloning and uterus/oviduct-specific expression of a novel estrogen-regulated gene (ERG1). J Biol Chem 1999; 274: 32215–24.

48. Cheon YP, Xu X, Bagchi MK et al. Immune-responsive gene 1 is a novel target of progesterone receptor and plays a critical role during implantation in the mouse. Endocrinology 2003; 144: 5623–30.

49. Nagaoka K, Sakai A, Nojima H et al. A chemokine, interferon (IFN)-gamma-inducible protein 10 kDa, is stimulated by IFN-tau and recruits immune cells in the ovine endometrium. Biol Reprod 2003; 68: 1413–21.

50. Platanias LC. Mechanisms of type-I- and type-II-interferon-mediated signalling. Nature Rev Immunol 2005; 5: 375–86.

51. Rosenfeld CS, Han CS, Alexenko AP et al. Expression of interferon receptor subunits, IFNAR1 and IFNAR2, in the ovine uterus. Biol Reprod 2002; 67: 847–53.

52. Ozaki T, Takahashi K, Kanasaki H et al. Expression of the type I interferon receptor and the interferon-induced Mx protein in human endometrium during the menstrual cycle. Fertil Steril 2005; 83: 163–70.

53. Taniguchi T, Takaoka A. The interferon-[alpha]/[beta] system in antiviral responses: a multimodal machinery of gene regulation by the IRF family of transcription factors. Cur Opin in Immunol 2002; 14: 111–16.

54. Zarubin T, Han J. Activation and signaling of the p38 MAP kinase pathway. Cell Res 2005; 15: 11–18.

55. Uddin S, Majchrzak B, Woodson J et al. Activation of the p38 mitogen-activated protein kinase by type I interferons. J Biol Chem 1999; 274: 30127–31.

56. Goh KC, Haque SJ, Williams BR. p38 MAP kinase is required for STAT1 serine phosphorylation and transcriptional activation induced by interferons. Embo J 1999; 18: 5601–8.

57. Doualla-Bell F, Koromilas AE. Induction of PG G/H synthase-2 in bovine myometrial cells by interferon-tau requires the activation of the p38 MAPK pathway. Endocrinology 2001; 142: 5107–15.

58. Stewart DM, Choi Y, Johnson GA et al. Roles of Statl, Stat2, and interferon regulatory factor-9 (IRF-9) in interferon tau regulation of IRF-1. Biol Reprod 2002: 66: 393–400.

59. Kim S, Choi Y, Bazer FW et al. Identification of genes in the ovine endometrium regulated by interferon tau independent of signal transducer and activator of transcription 1. Endocrinology 2003; 144: 5203–14.

60. Choi Y, Johnson GA, Burghardt RC et al. Interferon regulatory factor-two restricts expression of interereon-stimulated genes to the endometrial stroma and glandular epithelium in the ovine uterus. Biol Reprod 2001: 65: 1038–49.

61. Gray CA, Adelson DL, Bazer FW et al. Discovery and characterization of an epithelial-specific galectin in the endometrium that forms crystals in the trophectoderm. Proc Natl Acad Sci USA 2004; 101: 7982–7.

62. Song G, Spencer TE, Bazer FW. Cathepsins in the ovine uterus: regulation by pregnancy, progesterone, and interferon tau. Endocrinology 2005; 146: 4825–33.

63. Salamonsen LA. Role of proteases in implantation. Rev Reprod 1999; 4: 11–22.

64. Curry TE, Jr., Osteen KG. The matrix rnetalloproteinase system: changes, regulation, and impact throughout the ovarian and uterine reproductive cycle. Endocrine Rev 2003; 24: 428–65.

65. Dunphy JL, Balic A, Barcham GJ et al. Isolation and characterization of a novel inducible mammalian galectin. J Biol Chem 2000; 275: 32106–113.

66. Kazemi M, Amann JF, Keisler DH et al. A progesterone-modulated, low-molecular-weight protein from the uterus of the sheep is associated with crystalline inclusion bodies in uterine epithelium and embryonic trophectoderm. Biol Reprod 1990; 43: 80–96.

67. Cooper DN. Galecfnomics: finding themes in complexity. Biochim Biophys Acta 2002: 1572: 209–31.

68. Yang RY, Liu FT. Galectins in cell growth and apoptosis. Cell Mol Life Sci 2003; 60: 267–76.

69. Liu FT, Rabinovich GA. Galectins as modulators of tumour progression. Nat Rev Cancer 2005: 5: 29–411.

70. Spencer TE, Johnson GA, Bazer FW et al. Implantation mechanisms: insights from the sheep. Reproduction 2004; 128: 657–68.

71. Mohamed OA, Dufort D, Clarke HJ. Expression and estradiol regulation of wnt genes in the mouse blastocyst identify a candidate pathway for embryo-maternal signaling at implantation. Biol Reprod 2004; 71: 417–24.

72. Dey SK, Lim H, Das SK et al. Molecular cues to implantation. Endocrine Rev 2004; 25: 341–73.

73. Hou X, Tan Y, Li M et al. Canonical Wnt signaling is critical to estrogen-mediated uterine growth. Mol Endocrinol 2004; 18: 3035–49.

74. Mohamed OA, Jonnaert M, Labelle-Dumais C et al. Uterine Wnt/beta-catenin signaling is required for implantation. Proc Nat Acad Sci USA 2005; 102: S579–84.

75. Tulac S, Nayak NR, Kao LC et al. Identification, characterization, and regulation of the canonical Wnt signaling pathway in human endometrium. J Clin Endocrinol Metab 2003; 88: 3860–6.

76. Luster A, Unkeless J, Ravetch J. Interferon transcriptionally regulates an early-response gene containing homology to platelet proteins. Nature 1985; 315: 672–6.

77. Huang D, Han Y, Rani MR et al. Chemokines and chemokine receptors in inflammation of the nervous system: manifold roles and exquisite regulation. Immunol Rev 2000; 177: 52–67.

78. Taub DD, Lloyd AR, Conlon K et al. Recombinant human interferon-inducible protein 10 is a chemoattractant for human monocytes and T lymphocytes and promotes T cell adhesion to endothelial cells. J Exp Med 1993: 177: 1809–14.

79. Farber JM. Mig and IP-10: CXC chemokines that target lymphocytes. J Leukoc Biol 1997: 61: 246–57.

80. Nagaoka K, Nojima H, Watanabe F et al. Regulation of blastocyst migration, apposition, and initial adhesion by a chemokine, interferon gamma-inducible protein 10 kDa (IP-10), during early gestation. J Biol Chem 2003; 278: 29048–56.

81. Praefcke GJ, McMahon HT. The dynamin superfamily: universal membrane tabulation and fission molecules? Nat Rev Mol Cell Biol 2004: 5: 133–47.

82. McNiven MA, Kim L, Krueger EW et al. Regulated interactions between dynamin and the actin-binding protein cortactin modulate cell shape. J Cell Biol 2000; 151: 187–98.

83. Shupliakov O, Low P, Grabs D et al. Synaptic vesicle endocytosis impaired by disruption of dynamin–SH3 domain interactions. Science 1997; 276: 259–63.

84. Thompson HM, Skop AR, Euteneuer U et al. The large GTPase dynamin associates with the spindle midzone and is required for cytokinesis. Curr Biol 2002; 12: 2111–7.

85. Haller O, Kochs G. Interferon-induced rnx proteins: dynamin-like GTPases with antiviral activity. Traffic 2002; 3: 710–7.

86. Danino D, Hinshaw JE. Dynamin family of mechanoenzymes. Curr Opin Cell Biol 2001; 13: 454–60.

87. Hicks BA, Yankey SJ, Carnahan KG et al. Expression of the uterine Mx protein in cyclic and pregnant cows, gilts, and mares. J Anim Sci 2003: 81: 1552–61.

88. Baker CB, Adams MH, McDowell KJ. Lack of expression of alpha or omega interferons by the horse conceptus. J Reprod Fertil Suppl 1991: 44: 439–43.

89. Johnson GA, Joyce MM, Yankey SJ et al. The interferon stimulated genes (ISG) 17 and Mx have different temporal and spatial expression in the ovine uterus suggesting more complex regulation of the Mx gene. J Endocrinol 2002; 147: R7–R11.

90. Charleston B, Stewart HJ. An interferon-induced Mx protein: cDNA sequence and high-level expression in the endometrium of pregnant sheep. Gene 1993; 137: 327–31.

91. Ott TL, Yin J, Wiley AA et al. Effects of the estrous cycle and early pregnancy on uterine expression of Mx protein in sheep (Ovis aries). Biol Reprod 1998; 59: 784–94.

92. Spencer TE, Gray A, Johnson GA et al. Effects of recombinant ovine interferon tau, placental lactogen, and growth hormone on the ovine uterus. Biol Reprod 1999; 61: 1409–18.

93. Toyokawa K, Leite F, Ott TL. The antiviral protein ovine Mxl regulates secretion in an ovine glandular epithelial cell line. Am J Reprod Immunol 2007; 57: 23–33.

94. Spencer TE, Gray A, Johnson GA et al. Effects of recombinant ovine interferon tau, placental lactogen, and growth hormone on the ovine uterus. Biol Reprod 1999; 61: 1409–18.

95. Wimsatt WA. New histological observations on the placenta of the sheep. Am J Anat 1950; 3: 391–457.

96. Stewart DM, Johnson GA, Gray CA et al. Prolactin receptor and uterine milk protein expression in the ovine uterus during the estrous cycle and early pregnancy. Biol Reprod 2000; 62: 1779–89.

97. Anthony RV, Pratt SL, Liang R et al. Placental–fetal hormonal interactions: impact on fetal growth. J Anim Sci 1995; 73: 1861–71.

98. Gertler A, Djiane J. Mechanism of ruminant placental lactogen action: molecular and in vivo studies. Mol Genet Metab 2002: 75: 189–201.

99. Ing NH, Roberts RM. The major progesterone-modulated proteins secreted into the sheep uterus are members of the serpin superfamily of serine protease inhibitors. J Biol Chem 1989; 264: 3372–9.

100. Noel S, Herman A, Johnson GA et al. Ovine placental lactogen specifically binds to endometrial glands of the ovine uterus. Biol Reprod 2003; 68: 772–80.

101. Lacroix MC, Jatnmes H, Kann G. Occurrence of a growth hormone-releasing hormone-like messenger ribonucleic acid and immunoreactive peptide in the sheep placenta. Reprod Fertil Dev 1996; 8: 449–56.

102. Martin PM, Sutherland AE, Van Winkle LJ. Amino acid transport regulates blastocyst implantation. Biol Reprod 2003; 69: 1101–8.

103. Mirando MA, Prince BC, Tysseling KA et al. A proposed role for oxytocin in regulation of endometrial prostaglandin $F_{2\alpha}$ secretion during luteolysis in swine. Adv Exp Biol Med 1995; 395: 421–33.

104. Geisert RD, Ross JW, Ashworth MD et al. Maternal recognition of pregnancy signal or endocrine disrupter: the two faces of oestrogen during establishment of pregnancy in the pig. In Kraeling R, Ashworth C, eds. Control of Pig Reproduction VII. Nottingham, UK: University Press, 2005: 131–45.

105. Bazer FW. Establishment of pregnancy in sheep and pigs. Reprod Fertil Develop 1989; 1: 237–42.

105. Moeljono MPE, Bazer FW, Thatcher WW. A study of prostaglandin $F_{2\alpha}$ as the luteolysin in swine: I. Effect of prostaglandin $F_{2\alpha}$ in hysterectomized gilts. Prostaglandins 1976; 11: 737–43.

106. Gadsby JE, Balapure AK, Britt JH et al. Prostaglandin F2a receptors on enzyme-dissociated pig luteal cells throughout the estrous cycle. Endocrinology 1990; 126: 787–95.

107. Pitzel L, Welp K, Holtz W. The content of oxytocin and vasopressin in the corpus luteum of the pig. Acta Endocrinologica 1984; 105(Suppl 264):140–1.

108. Einspanier R, Pitzel L, Wuttke W et al. Demonstration of mRNAs for oxytocin and prolactin in porcine granulosa and luteal cells. FEES Letters 1986; 204: 37–40.

109. Choy VJ, Watkins WB. Arginine vasopressin and oxytocin in the porcine corpus luteum. Neuropeptides 1988: 11: 119–23.

110. Trout WE, Smith GW, Gentry PC et al. Oxytocin secretion by the endometrium of the pig during maternal recognition of pregnancy. Biol Reprod 1995; 52(Suppl 1): 188.

111. Soloff MS, Swartz TL. Characterization of a proposed oxytocin receptor in the uterus of the rat and sow. J of Biol Chem 1974: 249: 1376–81.

112. Edgerton LA, Karninski MA, Silvia WJ. Changes in uterine secretion of prostaglandin $F_{2\alpha}$ in response to oxytocin during the estrous cycle, early pregnancy, and estrogen-induced pseudopregnancy in swine. Biol Reprod 1996: 55: 657–62.

113. Mirando MA, Leen MP, Beers S, Harney JP, Bazer FW. Endometrial inositol phosphate turnover in pigs is reduced during pregnancy and estradiol-induced pseudopregnancy. J Anim Sci 1990; 68: 4285–91.

114. Gross TS, Lacroix MC, Bazer FW et al. Prostaglandin secretion by perifused porcine endometrium: further evidence for

an endocrine versus exocrine secretion of prostaglandins. Prostaglandins 1988; 35: 327–41.

115. Geisert RD, Zavy MT, Moffatt RJ et al. Embryonic steroids and the establishment of pregnancy.

116. Geisert RD, Brookband JW, Roberts RM et al. Establishment of pregnancy in the pig: I. Interrelationships between preimplantation development of the pig blastocyst and uterine endometrial secretions. Bio Reprod 1982; 27: 925–39.

117. Guthrie HD, Lewis GS. Production of prostaglandin F2 and estrogen by embryonal membranes and endometrium and metabolism of prostaglandin F2 by embryonal membranes, endometrium and lung from gilts. Pom Anim Endocrinol 1986; 3: 185–98.

118. Wilson ME, Fahrenkrug SC, Smith T et al. Differential expression of cyclooxygenase-2 around the time of elongation in the pig conceptus. Anim Reprod Sci 2002; 71: 229–37.

119. Murakami M, Kudo I. Recent advances in molecular biology and physiology of the prostaglandin E2-biosynthetic pathway. Prog Lipid Res 2004; 43: 3–35.

120. Bazer FW, Marengo SR, Geisert RD et al. Exocrine versus endocrine secretion of prostaglandin F in the control of pregnancy in swine. Anim Reprod Sci 1984; 7: 115–32.

121. Ashworth MD, Ross JW, Hu J et al. Porcine endometrial prostaglandin synthase expression during the estrous cycle, early pregnancy, and following endocrine disruption of pregnancy. Biol Reprod 2006; 74: 1007–15.

122. Bazer FW. Mediators of maternal recognition of pregnancy in mammals. Proc Soc Exp Biol Med 1992; 199: 373–84.

123. Geisert RD, Yelich JV. Regulation of conceptus development and attachment in pigs. J Reprod Fertil Suppl 1997; 52: 133–49.

124. Bazer FW, Ott TL, Spencer TE. Endocrinology of the transition from recurring estrous cycles to establishment of pregnancy in subprimate mammals. In Bazer FW, eds. Endocrinology of Pregnancy. New Jersey: Humana Press, 1998: 1–34.

125. Krzymowski T, Stefanczyk-Krzymowska S. The oestrous cycle and early pregnancy – a new concept of local endocrine regulation. Vet J 2004: 168: 285–96.

126. Akinlosotu BA, Diehl JR, Gimenez T. Prostaglandin E2 counteracts the effects of PGF2 alpha in indomethacin treated cycling gilts. Prostatdandins 1988; 35: 81–93.

127. Davis DL, Blair RM. Studies of uterine secretions and products of primary cultures of endometrial cells in pigs. J Reprod Fertil Suppl 1993: 48: 143–55.

128. Garverick HA, Polge C, Flint AP. Oestradiol administration raises luteal LH receptor levels in intact and hysterectomized pigs. J Reprod Fertil 1982; 66: 371–7.

129. Ziecik AJ. Old, new and the newest concepts of inhibition of luteolysis during early pregnancy in pig. Domest Anim Endocrinol 2002: 23: 265–75.

130. Conley AJ, Ford SP. Direct luteotrophic effect of oestradiol-17 beta on pig corpora lutea. J Reprod Fertil 1989: 87: 125–31.

131. Flint APF, Saunders PTK, Zeicak AJ. Blastocyst–endometrial interactions and their significance in embryonic mortality. In Cole DJA, Foxcroft GR, eds. Control of Pig Reproduction. London: Butterworths, 1982: 253–75.

132. Bazer FW, First NL. Pregnancy and parturition. J Anim Sci 1983; 57 Suppl 2: 425–60.

133. White FJ, Ross JW, Joyce MM et al. Steroid regulation of cell specific secreted phosphoprotein 1 (osteopontin) expression in the pregnant porcine uterus. Biol Reprod 2005; 73: 1294–1301.

134. Flood PF. Steroid-metabolizing enzymes in the early pig conceptus and in the related endometrium. J Endocrinol 1974: 64: 413–4.

135. Burghardt RC, Bowen JA, Newton GR et al. Extracellular matrix and the implantation cascade in pigs. J Reprod Fertil Suppl 1997: 52: 151–64.

136. Young KH, Bazer FW. The role of prolactin in the establishment of pregnancy in the pig: effects on fetal survival and uterine secretory function. J Reprod Fertil 1989; 86: 713–22.

137. Bazer FW, Worthington-White D, Fliss MFV et al. Uteroferrin: A progesterone-induced hematopoietic growth factor of uterine origin. J Exp Hematol 1991; 19: 910–15.

138. Harney JP, Ali M, Vedeckis WV et al. Porcine conceptus and endometrial retinoid-binding proteins. Reprod Fertil Develop 1994; 6: 211–19.

139. Garlow JE, Ka H, Johnson GA et al. Analysis of osteopontin at the maternal–placental interface in pigs. Biol Reprod 2002; 66: 718–25.

140. Simmen RCM, Ko Y, Simmen FA. Insulin-like growth factors and blastocyst development. Theriogenology 1993; 39: 163–75.

141. Jaeger LA, Johnson GA, Ka H et al. Functional analysis of autocrine and paracrine signaling at the porcine uterine-conceptus interface. Reproduction (Suppl, Control of Pig Reproduction VI) 2001; 58: 191–207.

142. Rubin JS, Bottaro DP, Chedid M et al. Keratinocyte growth factor as a cytokine that mediates mesenchymal–epithelial interaction. Exec Skills 1995; 74: 191–214.

143. Ka H, Spencer TE, Johnson GA et al. Keratinocyte growth factor: Expression by endometrial epithelia of the porcine uterus. Biol Reprod 2000; 62: 1772–8.

144. Ka H, Jaeger LA, Johnson GA et al. Keratinocyte growth factor in up-regulated in the porcine uterine endometrium and functions in trophectoderm cell proliferation and differentiation. Endocrinology 2001; 142: 2303–10.

145. LaBonnardiere C, Martinat-Botte F, Terqui M et al. Production of two species of interferon by Large White and Meishan pig conceptuses during the peri-attachment period. J Reprod Fertil 1991; 91(2):496–8.

146. Lefevre F, Martinat-Botte' F, Locatelli A et al. Intrauterine infusion of high doses of pig trophoblast interferons has no antiluteolytic effect in cyclic gilts. Biol Reprod 1998; 58: 1026–31.

147. Cencic A, La Bonnardiere C. Trophoblastic interferon-gamma: current knowledge and possible role(s) in early pig pregnancy. Vet Res 2002; 33: 139–57.

148. Denker HW. Implantation: a cell biological paradox. J Exp Zool 1993; 266: 541–58.

149. Cencic A, Guillomot M, Koren S et al. Trophoblastic interferons: do they modulate uterine cellular markers at the time of conceptus attachment in the pig? Placenta 2003; 24: 862–9.

150. Young HA, Hardy KJ. Role of interferon-gamma in immune cell regulation. J Leukoc Biol 995; 58: 373–81.

151. Irvine, CHG. The nonpregnant rnare: A review of some current research and of the last 25 years of endocrinology. In Bazer FW, Sharp DC, eds. Equine Reproduction IV, Biology of Reproduction Monograph Series 1.1995: 343–60.

152. Allen WR. Fetomaternal interactions and influences during equine pregnancy. Reproduction 2001; 121: 513–27.

153. Hartt L, Carling SJ, Joyce MM et al. Temporal and spatial associations of oestrogen receptor alpha and progesterone receptor expression in the endometrium of pregnant and non-pregnant rnares. Reproduction 2005; 130:1–11.

154. Zavy MT, Vernon MW, Sharp DC et al. Endocrine aspects of early pregnancy in pony mares: a comparison of uterine luminal and peripheral plasma levels of steroids during the estrous cycle and early pregnancy. Endocrinology 1984; 115(l): 214–9.

155. Goff AK, Leduc S, Poitras P et al. Steroid synthesis by equine conceptuses between days 7 and 14 and endometrial steroid metabolism. Dom Anim Endocrinol 1993; 10: 229–36.

156. Sharp DC, Thatcher M-J, Salute ME et al. Relationship between endometrial oxytocin receptors and oxytocin-induced prostraglandin $F_{2\alpha}$ release during the oestrous cycle and early pregnancy in pony mares. J Reprod Fertil 1997; 109: 137–44.

157. Boerboom D, Brown KA, Vaillancourt D et al. Expression of key prostaglandin synthases in equine endometrium during late diestrus and early pregnancy. Biol Reprod 2004; 70: 391–9.

158. Behrendt-Adam CY, Adams MH, Simpson KS et al. Oxytocin-neurophysin I mRNA abundance in equine uterine endometrium. Dom Anim Endocrinol 1999; 16: 183–92.

159. Bae SE, Watson, ED. A light microscopic and ultrastructural study on the presence of and location of oxytocin in the equine endometrium. Theriogenology 2003; 60: 909–21.

160. Freeman DA, Woods GL, Vanderwall DK et al. Embryo-initiated oviductal transport in mares.

161. Sharp DC, McDowell KJ, Weithenauer J et al. The continuum of events leading to maternal recognition of pregnancy in mares. J Reprod Fertil 1989; 37(Suppl): 101–7.

162. McDowell KJ, Sharp DC, Peck LS et al. Effect of restricted conceptus mobility on maternal recognition of pregnancy in mares. Equine Vet J Suppl 1985; 3: 23–4.

163. Betteridge KJ. Comparative aspects of equine embryonic development. Anim Reprod Sci 2000; 60–61: 691–702.

164. Sharp DC. The early fetal life of the equine conceptus. Anim Reprod Sci 2000; 60–61: 679–89.

165. Freeman ME, Smith MS, Nazian SJ et al. Ovarian and hypothalamic control of the daily surges of prolactin secretion during pseudopregnancy. Endocrinology 1974; 94: 875–82.

166. Niswender GD, Nett TM. Corpus luteum and its control in infraprimate species, In Knobil E, Neill JD, eds. The Physiology of Reproduction. New York: Raven Press, 1994: 781–816.

167. Shiota K, Hirosawa M, Hattori N et al. Structural and functional aspects of placental lactogens (Pls) and ovarian 20α-hydroxysteroid dehydrogenase (20α-HSD) in the rat. Endocrine J 1994; 41(Suppl): S43–S56.

168. Heap RB, Perry, JS, Challis JRG. Hormonal maintenance of pregnancy. In Greep RO, Astwood EB, Geiger SR, eds. Handbook of Physiology, Section 7: Endocrinology, Vol. II, Part 2. Baltimore, MD: Williams and Wilkins Company, 1973: 217–60.

169. Peng L, Arensburg J, Orly J et al. The murine 3β-hydroxysteroid dehydrogenase (3β-HSD) gene/family. A postulated role for 3β-HSD VI during early pregnancy. Mol Cell Endocrinol 2002; 187: 213–21.

170. Kimber SJ. Leukaemia inhibitory factor in implantation in uterine biology. Reproduction 2005; 130: 131–45.

171. Robb L, Dimitriadis E, Li R et al. Leukemia inhibitory factor and interleukin-11: cytokines with key roles in implantation. J Reprod Immunol 2002; 57: 129–41.

172. Freeman ME. The neuroendocrine control of the ovarian cycle of the rat, In Knobil E, Neill JD, eds. The Physiology of Reproduction, Second Edition. New York: Raven Press, 1994: 613–58.

173. Richards JS, Williams JL. Luteal cell receptor content for prolactin (PRL) and luteinizing hormone (LH). Regulation by LH and PRL. Endocrinology 1976; 99: 1571–81.

174. Hashimoto I, Henricks DM, Anderson LL et al. Progesterone and pregn-4-en-20α-ol-3-one in ovarian venous blood during various reproductive states in the rat. Endocrinology 1968; 82: 333–41.

175. Niswender GD, Juengel JL, Silva PJ et al. Mechanisms controlling the function and life span of the corpus luteum. Physiol Rev 2000; 80: 11–29.

176. Matsuda J, Noda K, Shiota K et al. Participation of ovarian 20α-hydroxysteroid dehydrogenase in luteotrophic and luteolytic processes during rat pseudopregnancy. J Reprod Fertil 1990; 88: 467–78.

177. Smith MS, Neill JD. Termination at midpregnancy of the two daily surges of plasma prolactin initiated by mating in the rat. Endocrinology 1976; 98: 696–701.

178. Soares MJ. The prolactin and growth hormone families: Pregnancy-specific hormones/cytokines and the maternal–fetal interface. Reprod Biol Endocrinol 2004; 2: 51.

179. Pepe GJ, Rothchild I. A comparative study of serum progesterone levels in pregnancy and in various types of pseudo-pregnancy in the rat. Endocrinology 1974; 95: 275–9.

180. Tranguch S, Diakoku T, Guo Y et al. Molecular complexity in establishing uterine receptivity and implantation. Cell Mol Life Sci 2005; 62: 1964–73.

181. Soares MJ, Julian JA, Glasser SR. Trophoblast giant cell release of placental lactogens: temporal and regional characteristics. Develop Biol 1985; 107: 520–6.

182. Galosy SS, Talamantes F. Luteotropic actions of placental lactogens at midpregnancy in the mouse. Endocrinology 1995; 136: 3993–4003.

183. Gibori G. The decidual hormones and their role in pregnancy recognition. In Glasser SR et al, eds. Endocrinology of Embryo-Endometrium Interactions. New York: Plenum Press, 1994: 217–22.

184. Gu Y, Gibori G. Isolation, culture and characterization of the two cell subpopulations forming the rat decidua: differential gene expression for activin, follistatin, and decidual prolactin-related protein. Endocrinology 1995; 36: 2451–8.

185. Soares MJ, Faria TN, Hamlin GP et al. Trophoblast cell differentiation: expression of the placental prolactin family. In Soares MJ, Handwerger S, Talamantes FJ, eds. Trophoblast Cells: Pathways for Maternal–Embryonic Communication. New York: Springer-Verlag, 1993: 45–67.

186. Chaffaux ST. Reproduction of the cat and dog. In: Thibault C, Levasseur MC, Hunter RHF, eds. Reproduction in Mammals and Man. Paris: Ellipses, 1993: 695–713.

187. Tsutsui T, Stabenfeldt G. Biology of ovarian cycles, pregnancy and pseudopregnancy in the domestic cat. J Reprod Fertil Suppl 1993; 47: 29–35.

188. Johnson LM, Gay VL. Luteinizing hormone in the cat. II. Mating-induced secretion. Endocrinology 1981; 109(1): 247–52.

189. Lawler DF, Johnston SD, Hegstad RL et al. Ovulation without cervical stimulation in domestic cats. J Reprod Fertil Suppl 1993; 47: 57–61.

190. Gudermuth DF, Newton L, Daels P et al. Incidence of spontaneous ovulation in young, group-housed cats based on serum and faecal concentrations of progesterone. J Reprod Fertil Suppl 1997; 51: 177–184.

191. Wildt DE, Chan SYW, Seager SWJ et al. Ovarian activity, circulating hormones, and sexual behavior in the cat. I. Relationships during the coitus-induced luteal phase and the estrous period without mating. Biol Reprod 1981; 25: 15–28.

192. Georgiev P, Wehrend A. Mid-gestation pregnancy termination by the progesterone antagonist aglepristone in queens. Theriogenology 2006; 65: 1401–6.

193. Verstegen JP, Onclin K, Silva LDM et al. Regulation of progesterone during pregnancy in the cat: studies on the roles of corpora lutea, placenta and prolactin secretion. J Reprod Fertil Suppl 1993; 47: 165–73.

194. Eilts BE. Pregnancy termination in the bitch and queen. Clin Tech Small Anim Practice 2002; 17: 116–23.

195. Klonisch T, Hombach-Klonisch S, Froehlich C et al. Nucleic acid sequence of feline preprorelaxin and its localization with the feline placenta. Biol Reprod 1999; 60: 305–11.

196. Stewart DR, Stabenfeldt GH. Relaxin activity in the pregnant cat. Biol Reprod 1985; 32: 848–54.

197. Concannon PW, McCann JP, Temple M. Biology and endocrinology of ovulation, pregnancy and parturition in the dog. J Reprod Fertil Suppl 1989; 39: 3–25.

198. Li W, Jaffe RC, Verhage HG. Immunocytochemical localization and messenger ribonucleic acid levels of a progesterone-dependent endometrial secretory protein (Cathepsin L) in the pregnant cat uterus. Biol Reprod 1992; 47: 21–8.

199. Boomsma RA, Mavrogianis PA, Fazleabas, AT et al. Detection of insulin-like growth factor binding protein-1 in cat implantation sites. Biol Reprod 1994; 51: 392–9.

200. Boomsma RA, Mavrogianis PA, Verhage HG. Immunocyto-chemical localization of transforming growth factor alpha, epidermal growth factor, and epidermal growth factor receptor in the cat endometrium and placenta. Histochemic 1997; 29: 495–504.

201. Champion EE, Glazier JD, Greenwood SL et al. Localization of alkaline phosphatase and Ca²⁺-ATPase in the cat placenta. Placenta 2003; 24: 453–61.

202. Thatcher M-J, Shille VM, Fliss MF et al. Characterization of feline conceptus proteins during/pregnancy. Biol Reprod 1991; 44: 108–20.

203. Amiri BE, de Sousa NM, Mecif K et al. Double radial immuno-diffusion as a tool to identify pregnancy-associated glycopro-teins in ruminant and nonruminant placentae. Theriogenology 2003; 59: 1291–1301.

204. Concannon PW. Biology of gonadotrophin secretion in adult and prepubertal female dogs. J Reprod Fertil Suppl 1993; 47: 3–27.

205. Hoffman B, Busges F, Engel E et al. Regulation of corpus luteum-function in the bitch. Reprod Domestic Anim 2004; 39: 232–40.

206. Jeffcoate IA. Endocrinology of anoestrous bitches. J Reprod Fertil Suppl 1993; 47: 69–76.

207. Steinetz BG, Goldsmith LT, Hasan SH et al. Diurnal variation of serum progesterone, but not relaxin, prolactin, or estradiol-17 beta in the pregnant bitch. Endocrinology 1990; 127(3): 1057–63.

208. Hoffmann B, Schneider S. Secretion and release of luteinizing hormone during the luteal phase of the oestrous cycle in the dog. J Reprod Fertil Suppl 1993; 47: 85–91.

209. Brenner RM, West NB, McClellan MC. Estrogen and prog-estin receptors in the reproductive tract of male and female primates. Biol Reprod 1990; 42: 11–19.

210. Geisert RD, Brenner RM, Moffatt RJ et al. Changes in oestro-gen receptor protein, mRNA expression and localization in the endometrium of cyclic and pregnant gilts. Reprod Fertil Develop 1993; 5: 247–60.

211. Geisert, RD, Pratt T, Bazer FW et al. Immunocytochemical localization and changes in endometrial progestin receptor protein during the porcine oestrous cycle and early preg-nancy. Reprod Fertil Develop 1994; 6: 749–60.

212. Spencer TE, Bazer FW. Temporal and spatial alterations in uterine estrogen receptor and progesterone receptor gene expression during the estrous cycle and early pregnancy in the ewe. Biol Reprod 1995; 53: 1527–43.

213. Mead RA, Eroschenko VP. Changes in uterine estrogen and progesterone receptors during delayed implantation and early implantation in the spotted skunk. Biol Reprod 1995; 53: 827–33.

214. Cooke PS, Buchanan DL, Kurita T, Lubahn D, Cunha GR. Stromal–epithelial cell communication in the female repro-ductive tract. In: Bazer FW, eds. Endocrinology of Pregnancy. New Jersey: Humana Press, 1998; 491–506.

215. Cunha GR. Growth factors as mediators of androgen action during male urogenital development. Prostate Suppl 1996; 6: 22–5.

216. Cunha GR, Chung LWK, Shannon, JM et al. Hormone-induced morphogenesis and growth: role of mesenchymal–epithelial interactions. Recent Prog Hormone Res 1983; 39: 1662–70.

217. Chen Y, Green JA, Antoniu E et al. Effect of interferon-τ admin-istration on endometrium of nonpregnant ewes: a comparison with pregnant ewes. Endocrinology 2006; 147: 2127–37.

218. Vallet JL, Barker PJ, Lamming GE et al. A low molecular weight endometrial secretory protein which is increased by ovine trophoblast protein-1 is a beta 2–microglobulin-like protein. J Endocrinol 1991; 130: R1–4.

219. Stewart MD, Johnson GA, Bazer FW et al. Interferon-tau (IFNtau) regulation of IFN-stimulated gene expression in cell lines lacking specific IFN-signaling components. Endocrinology 2001; 142: 1786–94.

220. Sandra O, Bataillon I, Roux P et al. Suppressor of cytokine sig-nalling (SOCS) genes are expressed in the endonetrium and regulated by conceptus signals during early pregnancy in the ewe. J Mol Endocrinol 2005; 34: 637–44.

221. Song G, Bazer FW, Spencer TE. Pregnancy and interferon tau regulate RSAD2 and IFIH1 expression in the ovine uterus. Reproduction 2007; 133: 1–12.

222. Song G, Spencer TE, Bazer FW. Progesterone and interferon tau regulate cystatin C (CST3) in the endometrium. Endocrinology 2006; 147: 3478–83.

223. Pru JK, Austin KJ, Haas AL et al. Pregnancy and interferon-tau upregulate gene expression of members of the 1-8 family in the bovine uterus. Biol Reprod 2001; 65: 1471–80.

224. Johnson GA, Stewart MD, Gray CA et al. Effects of the estrous cycle, pregnancy, and interferon tau on 2′,5′-oligoad-enylate synthetase expression in the ovine uterus. Biol Reprod 2001; 64: 1392–9.

225. Perry DJ, Austin KJ, Hansen TR. Cloning of interferon-stimulated gene 17: the promoter and nuclear proteins that regulate transcription. Mol Endocrinol 1999; 13: 1197–206.

226. Austin KJ, Ward SK, Teixeira MG et al. Ubiquitin cross-reactive protein is released by the bovine uterus in response to inter-feron during early pregnancy. Biol Reprod 1996; 54: 600–6.

227. Hansen TR, Austin KJ, Johnson GA. Transient ubiquitin cross-reactive protein gene expression in the bovine endonetrium. Endocrinology 1997; 138: 5079–82.

228. Short EC Jr, Geisert RD, Helmer SD et al. Expression of antiviral activity and induction of 2′,5′-oligoadenylate syn-thetase by conceptus secretory proteins enriched in bovine trophoblast protein-1. Biol Reprod 1991; 44: 261–8.

229. Todd I, McElveen JE, Lamming GE. Ovine trophoblast inter-feron enhances MHC class I expression by sheep endometrial cells. J Reprod Immunol 1998; 37: 117–23.

230. Mirando MA, Short EC Jr, Geisert RD et al. Stimulation of 2′,5′-oligoadenylate synthetase activity in sheep endometrium during pregnancy, by intrauterine infusion of ovine trophoblast protein-1, and by intramuscular administration of recombinant bovine interferon-alpha I1. J Reprod Fertil 1991; 93: 599–607.

231. Schmitt RA, Geisert RD, Zavy MT et al. Uterine cellular changes in 2′,5′-oligoadenylate synthetase during the bovine estrous cycle and early pregnancy. Biol Reprod 1993; 48: 460–6.

232. Rempel LA, Francis BR, Austin KJ et al. Isolation and sequence of an interferon-tau-inducible, pregnancy- and bovine interferon-stimulated gene product 15 (ISG15)-spe-cific, bovine ubiquitin-activating E1-like (UBE1L) enzyme. Biol Reprod 2005; 72: 365–72.

233. Martin C, Pessemesse L, De La Llosa-Hermier MP et al. Interferon-tau upregulates prolactin receptor mRNA in the ovine endometrium during the peri-implantation period. Reproduction 2004; 128: 99–105.

18 Chorionic gonadotropin signaling at the maternal–fetal interface

J Robert A Sherwin, Andrew M Sharkey, and Asgerally T Fazleabas

INTRODUCTION

The establishment of pregnancy requires an interaction between the embryo, uterus, and corpus luteum (CL). These interactions prevent luteal regression by extending the functional life span of the CL.[1] Successful implantation requires a genetically normal embryo and a receptive uterine endometrium.[2] Uterine receptivity has been defined as the limited period of time when the uterine luminal epithelium is favorable to blastocyst implantation.[3] Estrogen and progesterone play a critical role in establishing the receptive phase. However, it is becoming increasingly evident from rodent studies that the embryo induces functional receptivity, which is required for successful nidation.[4]

Chorionic gonadotropin (CG) is the most important early, embryo-derived signal in the primate and plays a pivotal role in implantation. The presence of luteinizing hormone LH/CG receptors (LH/CG-R) and associated G proteins has been documented in the human endometrium.[5] In addition, human chorionic gonadotropin (hCG) and the α-subunit of hCG have been shown to induce decidualization of human stromal fibroblasts in vitro.[6,7] Chorionic gonadotropin is synthesized by the 6–8 cell stage, preimplantation human embryo[8] and orthologues of CG are secreted by other primates and also equids.[9] CG exerts autocrine regulation of trophoblast invasion[10–12] as well as paracrine control of the endometrial environment to support embryo attachment and implantation.[13]

MOLECULAR BASIS OF CHORIONIC GONADOTROPIN ACTIVITY

CG is a heterodimeric glycoprotein, formed by the non-covalent binding of CGα and CGβ subunits. It is a member of a family of glycoprotein hormones that include pituitary derived follicle-stimulating hormone (FSH), luteinizing hormone (LH), and thyroid-stimulating hormone (TSH). These hormones share a common α subunit, but each has a unique β subunit, which accounts for their receptor affinities. The common α subunit

is encoded by a single gene on chromosome 6q21, which is translated into a 92 amino acid protein with two N-linked oligosaccharides. A free α subunit is also synthesized by the attachment of additional carbohydrate moieties and this acts as a ligand in its own right.[7,14] The CGβ subunit is a 145 amino acid polypeptide with two N-linked oligosaccharides and four O-linked oligosaccharides. This subunit is encoded by a gene cluster located on chromosome 19q13.3, near to the LHβ gene. There are six CGβ genes and one CGβ pseudogene in the cluster. Interestingly, there is a 96% identity between the CGβ and LHβ gene sequences, which explains their similar biological properties. However, human CGβ is characterized by a unique carboxy terminus peptide that confers a longer half-life for the hormone in serum.[15]

LH/CG-R is a seven transmembrane, G-protein-coupled receptor.[16] This is encoded for by a gene located on chromosome 2p21, which is about 880 kb in size and consists of 10 introns and 11 exons.[17,18] The 11th exon encodes the entire carboxyl terminal half of the receptor, which includes the seven transmembrane helices and the three interconnecting extracellular and intracellular loops, as well as the cytoplasmic tail. The majority of the naturally occurring, functionally important mutations in LH/CG-R occur in this 11th exon.[19–22] The first 10 exons of the LH/CG-R gene encode the extracellular N-terminal exodomain, which contains a number of leucine-rich repeat motifs that are likely to be involved in protein–protein interactions. Binding of CG to its receptor on the cell surface generates signal transduction through the activation of the heterotrimeric G protein (composed of one of 15 Gα, 6 Gβ, and 12 Gγ subunits), which is located on the inner membrane surface of the cell.[23] Activation of the G protein is achieved by the exchange of guanosine diphosphate (GDP) for guanosine triphosphate (GTP) by guanine exchange factors (GEFs), which causes the dissociation of the heterotrimer and the release of Gα-GTP and Gβγ, which are then free to activate downstream effectors. The intrinsic GTP hydrolysis rate of the Gα subunit limits the duration of the signal and causes the receptor to toggle back to the inactive state. In mature gonadal tissues, the major downstream effector of LH/CG-R signaling is cyclic adenosine monophosphate (cAMP).[19] In these tissues the Gα subunit associated with the receptor is G$_s$. This stimulatory G protein activates adenylyl cyclase to convert adenosine triphosphate (ATP) to cAMP, which activates protein kinase A (PKA), an enzyme that in turn phosphorylates a large number of proteins, including transcription factors.[24] LH/CG-R can also activate phospholipase C (PLC), leading to an increase in intracellular calcium through the inositol triphosphate (IP$_3$)/phospholipase A$_2$ (PLA$_2$) pathway. A possible activation of protein kinase C (PKC) through diacylglycerol (DAG) has also been suggested.[25] The intracellular signaling pathways activated by CG binding to the cell surface receptor are tissue specific. This is mediated by the specific G proteins that are present within the cell type. In addition to the complexity that is conferred by the presence of varying combinations of G proteins, G-protein-independent pathways such as the β arrestins[26] act as signal transducers. Also, there is growing evidence to show that cytokine and LH/CG-R signaling pathways are integrated.[27] Therefore, the effects of CG are regulated at many different levels, giving varied tissue-specific actions and also the possibility of misregulation.

The intracellular signal transduction system utilized in endometrium differs from that used in the ovary. Experiments performed using a human endometrial epithelial cell line (HES) and baboon epithelial endometrial cells[28] have shown that CG does not activate the G$_s$/adenyl cyclase/cAMP/PKA pathway but it does cause a rapid phosphorylation of the extracellular signal-regulated kinase (ERK 1/2) in a PKA-independent manner. This novel signal transduction pathway is functional and leads to an increase in cyclooxygenase 2 (COX-2) and prostaglandin E$_2$ (PGE$_2$). These results may be explained by the existence of an alternate spliced isoform of the LH/CG-R or by the presence of a different isoform of adenylate cyclase, of which nine are currently known.[24] It is also possible that competition for overlapping effector sites with other G proteins occurs.[29]

Multiple mRNA transcripts for LH/CG-R have been detected in human gonadal tissues. In the human ovary, 8.0, 7.0, and 4.5 kb transcripts are seen, with the 4.5 kb transcript being predominant.[30] However, there are no data to support the presence of protein products of these splice variants. In the testis LH/CG-R is expressed in the Leydig cells, whereas in the ovary LH/CG-R expression occurs in the thecal cells, interstitial cells, differentiated granulosa cells, and the luteal cells.[19] Extragonadal CG/LH-R expression has been reported in reproductive (uterus, placenta, and decidua)[5] and several non-reproductive tissues.[31–34] Although much work has been done aiming to clarify LH/CG-R expression regulation and signal transduction in the endometrium, there are still many unanswered questions. The structural and functional properties of extragonadal LH/CG-R, especially in the endometrium, are still controversial.[35,36] It is not yet clear which of the different isoforms of the receptor are expressed in this tissue and if there are differential expression patterns during the course of gestation. It is interesting to note that individuals with loss or gain of function mutations of the LH/CG-R do not show overt clinical abnormalities of uterine function.[21,22] However, these receptors are functional based on in-vivo experiments in baboons[37] and in-vitro studies of human endometrial cell lines.[38] In endometrium, LH/CG-R-like immunoreactivity has been demonstrated in several species, including the pig,[38] rat,[39] rabbit,[40] baboon,[37,41] and humans.[5] Also, Licht et al have shown a cycle-dependent expression of full-length human LH/CG-R in endometrium.[42] In trophoblast there is a selective expression of different LH/CG-R isoforms during the course of trophoblast differentiation[43] and, interestingly, case reports exist of patients with adrenal LH/CG-R expression who developed Cushing's syndrome during pregnancy and subsequently during the menopause.[44,45] These data, combined, support the presence of functional extragonadal LH/CG-R expression.

Transgenic mice in which the LH/CG-R gene has been knocked out are infertile[46,47] as are women who are homozygous for loss of function mutations, who have primary amenorrhea, but normal primary and secondary sexual characteristics. The phenotype of female mice carrying null mutations for the LH/CG-R gene includes small ovaries and uterine hypoplasia with a reduction in endometrial gland number and a reduced height of the luminal epithelium and vascular space.[48] In these mice serum levels of estrogen and progesterone are reduced.[46,47] Treatment with exogenous estrogen and progesterone does not restore fertility,[49] and in this model only partial rescue of the uterine phenotype occurs, suggesting that LH and hCG control uterine functions directly as well as indirectly through increasing ovarian synthesis of steroid hormones.[48] In another mouse model, however, normal fertility was restored after orthoptic transplantation of ovaries from wild-type mice into LH/CG-R knockout mice.[50] Further conditional knockout studies are needed to address the role in embryo implantation of uterine LH/CG-R in this species. Inactivating mutations in men result in varying phenotypes, from pseudohermaphroditism to micropenis/hypospadias, depending upon the residual functioning of the LH/CG-R. This occurs as fetal Leydig cells are unable to synthesize testosterone in response to maternal CG and so normal male external genitalia do not develop. In mice this phenotype can be reversed with exogenous testosterone.[51] Activating LH/CG-R mutations in women appear to have no phenotype, which can probably be explained as prepubertal girls express only low levels of the receptor and the mutant receptors may still be subject to negative feedback. Transgenic mice that overexpress CG show varied reproductive phenotypes, including elevated serum estradiol, hemorrhagic and cystic ovaries with thickened theca and stromal compartments, as well as enlarged uteri.[52,53] Females that overexpress LH can be superovulated and mated. Pregnancy fails at mid gestation possibly due to estrogen toxicity.[53]

AUTOCRINE ACTIONS OF CHORIONIC GONADOTROPIN

CG and other peptides such as insulin-like growth factor II (IGF-II) have been shown to stimulate trophoblast invasion[11,12] and are known to autoregulate the synthesis of matrix metalloproteinases.[10] Also, a number of trophoblast products, including CG, can increase the formation of human placental syncytium through the differentiation of mononuclear cytotrophoblasts.[54–57] Culturing cytotrophoblast with the LH/CG-R receptor antisense oligonucleotides significantly decreases LH/CG-R protein levels and inhibits CG-induced trophoblast differentiation. Reduction of LH/CG-R function also inhibits epidermal growth factor (EGF), transforming growth factor α (TGFα), leukemia inhibitory factor (LIF), but not 8-bromo-cAMP, induced trophoblast differentiation, suggesting that CG is required for EGF, TGFα, and LIF, but not for the cAMP actions.[58]

PARACRINE ACTIONS OF CG

In a series of experiments we have examined the paracrine actions of CG in vivo using a baboon (*Papio anubis*) model.[37,59–61] Infusion of CG into the uterine cavity of cycling animals between day 6 and day 10 postovulation mimics normal blastocyst transit and results in profound morphological changes within the uterine epithelial and stromal compartments.[37] Epithelial plaque formation, which occurs in the uterine luminal epithelium as an early maternal response to pregnancy, was seen after intrauterine CG infusion. This response is characterized by hypertrophy of the surface epithelium, with intense cytokeratin staining and rounding up of gland cells to form acinar clusters.[62] These changes can be inhibited by a progesterone receptor antagonist[63] and require synergy between ovarian and endometrial responses to hCG, as epithelial plaque formation is not seen in ovariectomized animals.[37] In contrast, CG effects on glandular transformation and stromal cell differentiation are direct and independent of the ovary.[37] The primary effect of CG on stromal fibroblasts is the induction of α-smooth muscle actin (αSMA),[37] which may be as a consequence of stromal integrin binding to secreted extracellular matrix (ECM) proteins.[64] The interaction between integrins and the ECM induces changes in the actin cytoskeleton that are thought to be critical for signal transduction and transformation of glandular epithelium.[65] Additional studies utilizing this model investigated the possible in-vivo relationship between two embryonic factors, CG and interleukin 1β (IL-1β), in preparing the endometrium for the establishment of pregnancy.[61] These studies revealed two distinct patterns associated with the IL-1β effect. First, the presence of IL-1β specifically contributed to decidualization (as evidenced by insulin-like growth factor binding protein 1 [IGFBP-1] expression) and COX-1 protein regulation, which are functional changes associated with the presence of the conceptus during early pregnancy.[66,67] The effect of IL-1β on in-vivo decidualization was in agreement with previous in-vitro studies in both baboon and human stromal fibroblasts.[68] In addition, IL-1β decreases COX-1 protein in epithelial cells of baboons, which is comparable to observations during early pregnancy.[66] Secondly, IL-1β in this model does not influence changes in cytokine levels detected in uterine flushings, as hCG alone is capable of regulating their secretion.

In recent experiments we have further tested the hypothesis that the direct action of CG on primate endometrium induces gene expression changes that enhance endometrial receptivity and support embryo implantation.[69] Utilizing microarray analysis of endometrial transcript abundance followed by confirmation of transcript changes using real-time PCR (polymerase chain reaction), these studies provided direct evidence that CG acts on the uterine endometrium to modulate function. In addition to confirming changes in transcript levels, for some of the genes up-regulated by intrauterine CG infusion, we also showed concomitant changes, in intrauterine flushings, of protein abundance. Endometrial expression of leukemia inhibitory factor (LIF) is known to be essential for implantation in rodents.[70] Expression of LIF mRNA and protein was up-regulated in the baboon model, by the action of CG. Although it is not clear whether LIF plays an essential role in human implantation, there is strong evidence that LIF plays an important role in implantation in other primates, as intrauterine injection of anti-LIF antibodies, on day 8 of pregnancy in rhesus monkeys significantly reduces implantation rates.[71] The experiments in the baboon showed that endometrial expression of LIF and gp130, the signal transducing part of the LIF receptor, are up-regulated in response to hCG treatment. In human endometrium, both in experiments using an intrauterine microdialysis catheter[72] and following systemic treatment, using a luteotropic regimen,[73] LIF has also been shown to be up-regulated by CG. It therefore appears that in the baboon and human, CG from the preimplantation embryo is able to stimulate expression in the endometrium of molecules essential for embryo attachment and previously thought to be primarily regulated by steroids.

This series of experiments also showed that CG regulates the immune environment surrounding the implanting blastocyst. Endometrial expression of complement C3 and C4A/B is up-regulated by CG. C3 is integral to the activation of complement via the classical, alternative and lectin activation pathways,[74] with C4 being part of the classical activation pathway. The multiple actions of C3 allow it to promote phagocytosis, support local inflammatory responses to pathogens, and also to select appropriate antigens for the humoral response. In response to CG treatment, C3 becomes localized to the stromal compartment, which parallels the pattern of staining for the CG receptor in baboon endometrium.[41] Previous baboon studies have demonstrated increased glycodelin secretion in response to intrauterine hCG infusion.[60] The biological role of glycodelin, which is the most abundant secreted protein in early human pregnancy, is unclear, although in-vitro immunosuppressive activity has been demonstrated.[75] We have previously demonstrated that endometrial expression of stromal cell protein (SCP) is up-regulated by CG.[76] SCP induces the expression of recombinant activating gene (RAG 1 and 2) and also activates T cells.[77] Taken together, the up-regulation of complement C3, C4, glycodelin, and SCP suggests that CG may orchestrate the endometrial immune adaptation to pregnancy. We have also shown that CG acts to modify the oxidative stressors that surround the implanting embryo. Superoxide dismutase 2 (SOD2) was shown in our microarray analysis to be up-regulated in response to CG infusion. SOD scavenges superoxide radicals, and

mice lacking SOD have reduced fertility.[78] Our finding that hCG significantly increases the expression of SOD suggests that in preparation for implantation the embryo also regulates an adaptive, endometrial response to oxidative stress.

Thus, these studies have shown that CG acts directly on the endometrium to regulate genes known to be important during the actual process of embryo attachment, endometrial remodeling, antioxidant defense mechanisms, and the modulation of the immune response around the implanting blastocyst.

REGULATION OF STROMAL CELL APOPTOSIS AND DECIDUALIZATION

Apoptosis has been shown to be an important regulator of endometrial function. In human endometrium, apoptosis was first described in 1976 by Hopwood and Levison,[79] and it was later reported that the level of apoptosis increases from proliferative phase through the cycle and peaks at menses.[80] However, recent studies have indicated that treatment with hCG or progesterone at the mid secretory phase inhibits apoptosis in the late secretory phase, implying a role for embryonic signals in the inhibition of apoptosis.[81]

Apoptosis is regulated by various gene products, including cytokines, interleukins, and steroid hormones. In addition, the cytoskeleton may also play a role in the early stages of induction of apoptosis.[82] This is suggested by the finding that DNase I, an endonuclease shown to be responsible for nuclear fragmentation during apoptosis, is associated with full-length actin in live cells, and this association down-regulates its endonuclease activity.[83] More supporting evidence comes from recent work indicating that the disruption of the actin cytoskeleton by dissociating agents induces apoptosis in some cell types.[84] Differentiation of stromal fibroblasts into the secretory decidual phenotype is initially associated with changes in the cytoskeleton.[85] We previously reported that stromal fibroblasts express αSMA, a cytoskeletal protein in response to in-vivo stimulation by CG.[37] It has been suggested that this induction of αSMA occurs as a consequence of integrins on the stromal cell membrane binding to secreted ECM proteins.[64] The interaction between integrins and the ECM induces changes in the actin cytoskeleton that are thought to be critical for signal transduction.[86] After implantation, additional signals from the embryo initiate the process of decidualization at the interface between the maternal endometrium and the embryo.[61,65,87]

This differentiation process is associated with the down-regulation of αSMA and the up-regulation of IGFBP-1. Previous in-vivo studies demonstrated that hCG and progesterone inhibited endometrial apoptosis in the late secretory phase.[81] Our studies suggest that both CG and dibutyryl cyclic AMP (dbcAMP) can prevent endometrial stromal fibroblasts from undergoing apoptosis after cytoskeletal disruption in vitro. The initial change in the cytoskeletal architecture in response to CG, together with the induction of Notch-1, may be the early signal required to prevent the normal apoptotic cascade that is initiated toward the latter part of the menstrual cycle. In the presence of an embryo, decidualization is initiated, and this transformation requires the disruption or down-regulation of αSMA.[68,85,87] Thus, the increase in IGFBP-1 and prolactin in decidual cells, coupled with the down-regulation of the CG receptor,[41] compensates for the disruption of the cytoskeleton, and the loss of CG signaling thus prevents the decidual cells from undergoing apoptosis as pregnancy proceeds.

The specific expression of LH/CG-R in the stromal cells at the implantation site in early pregnancy is also correlated with the expression of αSMA[37,61] and COX-2.[66] The induction of αSMA in these stromal cells is directly regulated by CG[37] and appears to be a necessary prerequisite to inhibit stromal cell apoptosis[81,88] and enable decidualization to proceed.[65,85] In addition, the co-expression of both LH/CG-R and COX-2 in stromal cells at the implantation site during early pregnancy is in agreement with previous in-vitro studies that demonstrated a direct effect of CG on COX-2 gene expression and the induction of decidualization in human stromal cells cultured in vitro.[38] Thus, the induction of the LH/CG-R in stromal cells at the maternal–fetal interface may play an essential role in inducing changes that are critical for both the establishment of pregnancy and the initiation of decidualization in the primate. In addition to the induction of LH/CG-R in stromal cells at the implantation site, the most dramatic increase in staining for the LH/CG-R was evident around the spiral arteries. The observed increase in LH/CG-R positive staining around the spiral arteries in early pregnancy was also correlated with positive staining for both inducible nitric oxide synthase (iNOS) and endothelial nitric oxide synthase (eNOS),[89] supporting the hypothesis that CG may play a key regulatory role in angiogenesis and vascular development in the female reproductive tract.[90]

LH/CG-R are present in the endothelium and smooth muscle of uterine blood vessels and their expression is significantly increased in the intramyometrial segment.[91,92] Recent studies have revealed that CG has a direct angiogenic effect and that LH/CG-R expressing uterine endothelial cells responded to physiological doses of hCG, with increased capillary formation in vitro.[90] In addition to its direct effects on uterine endothelial cells, CG also regulates vascular endothelial growth factor (VEGF) gene expression in the ovary, as well as macrophages.[90,93] These data suggest a potential function for CG in uterine adaptation to early pregnancy and underline the importance of hCG as an as-yet unrecognized vasculo-angiogenic factor.

In contrast to the dramatic increase in stromal cells expressing the LH/CG-R in early pregnancy, decidualization results in a marked down-regulation of LH/CG-R expression both in vivo and in vitro.[41] Licht et al[42] also demonstrated that, at the time of implantation, the human endometrium expresses full-length LH/CG-R, but with the onset of decidualization, the expression pattern switches to truncated isoforms, as a result of alternate splicing. It is unclear what the physiological implications of this dramatic down-regulation are or if this decrease in LH/CG-R expression is a direct effect of decidualization or if it occurs in response to the modification of the cellular phenotype.

These studies highlight the importance of CG during the secretory phase of the cycle and in early gestation, when the secretion of this hormone is high. The direct effects of CG on the endometrium via its receptor are necessary to induce the expression of specific genes that are important in modulating the decidualization process, the immune system, cell survival, and the vascularization at the maternal–fetal interface. The dynamic and cell-specific changes in LH/CG-R expression during the menstrual cycle and the establishment of pregnancy strongly suggest that CG, as an early embryonic signal, plays a critical role in primates, in establishing a receptive endometrium that is conducive to maintaining pregnancy.

CLINICAL USES OF CHORIONIC GONADOTROPIN

Endometrial function

Although the concept that LH and CG have been shown to regulate endometrial function, the impact of extragonadal LH/CG-R signaling on the outcome of clinical treatments has not been extensively studied. Oocyte donation programs offer a model system to study the uterine response to CG, independent of

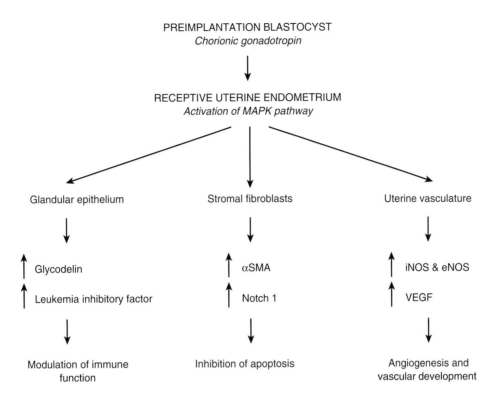

Figure 18.1 Diagrammatic illustration of the postulated actions of CG on epithelial and stromal cells and the uterine vasculature during the window of implantation. The major downstream signal transduction pathway in all cell types is the activation of the mitogen-activated protein kinase (MAPK) pathway by CG. The potential functions of the upregualted genes are highlighted. αSMA, α–smooth muscle actin; iNOS, inducible nitric oxide; e-NOS, and endothelial nitric oxide, VEGF, vascular endothelial growth factor.

ovarian function. Women receiving donated embryos undergo pituitary desensitization and down-regulation of both FSH and LH secretion, prior to direct stimulation of endometrial growth by exogenous estrogen and progesterone.[94] In such programs, high implantation and live birth rates can be achieved.[95] Interesting data have come from an oocyte donation study in which sibling oocytes were randomly allocated between two groups of recipients.[96] All women had undergone pituitary desensitization and endometrial preparation with exogenous steroids, but one group also received 5000 IU of hCG 5 days before embryo transfer. These women showed increased endometrial thickness at the time of embryo transfer and increased implantation rates compared to the placebo group. There was no difference in live birth rates between groups.

Conventional controlled ovarian hyperstimulation (COH) protocols often use urinary hCG as a substitute for the midcycle LH surge, which is essential for oocyte maturation and ovulation. Endometrial morphology,[97–100] steroid receptor expression,[101] and function[102] are all altered following COH and hCG treatment. Recently, global endometrial gene expression studies have compared endometrium from women undergoing natural menstrual cycles (LH+7) with that from women undergoing COH with hCG (CG+7).[73] More than 200 genes were shown to be differentially expressed by greater than three-fold between the two groups. The net effect of COH/hCG was to fail to up-regulate and down-regulate endometrial gene expression in a pattern consistent with the development of a receptive endometrium. Further studies are needed to establish whether endometrial function following COH/hCG can be improved and whether the global disregulation of endometrial gene expression that follows COH/hCG varies with time from hCG administration. Luteal phase support with hCG or progesterone after in-vitro fertilization (IVF) increases pregnancy rates.[103] Given the absence of full-length LH/CG-R in first timester decidua,[42] it is likely that hCG acts in this manner only to give luteotropic support.

Benign gynecological diseases

Leiomyomas, adenomyosis, and endometriotic implants have all been reported to express LH/CG-R.[104–107] A limited number of studies suggest that the invasion-promoting properties of CG[108] as well as its ability to increase angiogenesis[90] may promote myometrial invasion of endometrial glands in adenomyosis and increase the incidence of fibroids.[109] In contrast, treatment of women with endometriosis with CG resulted in a significant decrease in chronic pelvic pain associated with this disease.[110] Thus, it is evident that CG and its interaction with its extragonadal receptors in the reproductive tract may also influence the pathogenicity of benign gynecological diseases. However, further studies are required to fully understand the mechanisms by which CG influences these disease processes.

Preterm labor

Myometrial spiral arteries have been shown to express LH/CG-R, which are capable of binding CG.[92] CG was subsequently shown to reduce uterine vascular resistance and reduce abortion rates in women presenting with threatened miscarriages.[111] It has also been speculated that the use of CG as a tocolytic might improve pregnancy outcome later in gestation.[112] The possibility that CG can regulate progesterone receptors in the myometrium and may suppress myometrial contractivity provides a mechanism by which CG could be used to prevent preterm labor.[113]

CONCLUSIONS

In summary, the presence of LH/CG-R in the uterus and other extragonadal tissues indicates that CG mediates a multitude of functions in the reproductive tract. Within the intrauterine environment, CG, as an embryonic signal, activates a number of important genes in epithelial and stromal cells as well as the vasculature and so ensures that the endometrium is receptive to embryo implantation (Figure 18.1). In addition to the potential physiological role of CG in endometrial function, evidence is beginning to accumulate, that points to a potential therapeutic role for CG in benign gynecological diseases and preterm labor.

REFERENCES

1. Bazer FW, Ott TL, Spencer TE. In: Endocrinology of Pregnancy. Bazer FW (ed), Humana Press Inc, 1998: 1–34.
2. Yoshinaga K. Maternal and fetal endocrinology. In: Tulchinsky D, Little AB, eds. Maternal Fetal Endocrinology. Philadelphia: WB Saunders, 1994: 336–49.
3. Dey SK, Paria BC, Huet-Hudson YM. In: Dey SK, ed. Molecular and Cellular Aspects of Periimplantation Process. New York: Springer, 1995: 113–24.
4. Wang H, Dey SK. Roadmap to embryo implantation: clues from mouse models. Nat Rev Genet 2006; 7: 185–99.
5. Reshef ZM, Lei CV, Rao DD et al. The presence of gonadotropin receptors in nonpregnant human uterus, human placenta, fetal membranese and decidua. J Clin Endocrinol Metab 1990; 70: 421–30.
6. Rao CV. Tropic effects of LH and hCG on early pregnancy events in women's reproductive tract. Early Pregnancy 2001; 18–9.
7. Moy E, Kimzey LM, Nelson LM et al. Glycoprotein hormone alpha-subunit functions synergistically with progesterone to stimulate differentation of cultured human endometrial stromal cells to decidualized cells: a novel role for free alpha-subunit in reproduction. Endocrinology 1996; 137: 1332–9.
8. Fishel SB, Edwards RG, Evans CJ. Human chorionic gonadotropin secreted by preimplantation embryos cultured in vitro. Science 1984; 223: 816–18.
9. Leigh SE, Stewart F. Partial cDNA sequence for the donkey chorionic gonadotrophin-beta subunit suggests evolution from an ancestral LH-beta gene. J Mol Endocrinol 1990; 4: 143–50.
10. Bischof PE. Endocrine, paracrine and autocrine regulation of trophoblastic metalloproteinases. Early Pregnancy 2001; 5: 30–1.
11. Chakraborty C, Gleeson LM, McKinnon T et al. Regulation of human trophoblast migration and invasiveness. Can J Physiol Pharmacol 2002; 80: 116–24.
12. Hamilton GS, Lysiak JJ, Han VK et al. Autocrine–paracrine regulation of human trophoblast invasiveness by insulin-like growth factor (IGF)-II and IGF-binding protein (IGFBP)-1. Exp Cell Res 1998; 244: 147–56.
13. Cameo P, Srisuparp S, Strakova Z, Fazleabas AT. Chorionic gonadotropin and uterine dialogue in the primate. Reprod Biol Endocrinol 2004; 2: 50.
14. Nemansky M, Moy E, Lyons CD et al. Human endometrial stromal cells generate uncombined alpha-subunit from human chorionic gonadotropin, which can synergize with progesterone to induce decidualization. Clin Endocrinol Metab 1998; 83: 575–81.
15. Bousfield GR, Perry WM, Ward DN. Gonadotrophins: chemistry and biosynthesis. In: Knobil E, and Neill JD, eds. The Physiology of Reproduction. New York: Raven, 1994: 1749–92.
16. Dufau ML. The luteinizing hormone receptor. Annu Rev Physiol 1998; 60: 461–96.
17. Rousseau-Merck MF, Misrahi M, Atger M et al. Localization of the human luteinizing hormone/choriogonadotropin receptor gene (LHCGR) to chromosome 2p21. Cytogenet Cell Genet 1990; 54: 77–9.
18. Segaloff DL, Ascoli M. The lutropin/choriogonadotropin receptor … 4 years later. Endocr Rev 1993; 14: 324–47.
19. Ascoli M, Fanelli F, Segaloff DL. The lutropin/choriogonadotropin receptor, a 2002 perspective. Endocr Rev 2002; 23: 141–74.
20. Huhtaniemi IT, Themmen AP. Mutations in human gonadotropin and gonadotropin-receptor genes. Endocrine 2005; 26: 207–17.
21. Latronico AC, Segaloff DL. Naturally occurring mutations of the luteinizing-hormone receptor: lessons learned about reproductive physiology and G protein-coupled receptors. Am J Hum Genet 1999; 65: 949–58.
22. Themmen APN, Huhtaniemi IT. Mutations of gonadotropins and gonadotropin receptors: elucidating the physiology and pathophysiology of pituitary–gonadal function. Endocr Rev 2000; 21: 551–83.
23. Cabrera-Vera TM, Vanhauwe J, Thomas TO et al. Insights into G protein structure, function, and regulation. Endocr Rev 2003; 24: 765–81.
24. Daniel PB, Walker WH, Habener JF. Cyclic AMP signaling and gene regulation. Annu Rev Nutr 1998; 18: 353–83.

25. Ryu KS, Gilchrist RL, Koo Y et al. Gene, interaction, signal generation, signal divergence and signal transduction of the LH/CG receptor. Int J Gynaecol Obstet 1998; 60: S9–20.

26. Lefkowitz RJ, Shenoy SK. Transduction of receptor signals by beta-arrestins. Science 2005; 308: 512–17.

27. Shiraishi K, Ascoli M. Activation of the lutropin/choriogonadotropin receptor in MA-10 cells stimulates tyrosine kinase cascades that activate ras and the extracellular signal regulated kinases (ERK1/2). Endocrinology 2006; 147: 3419–27.

28. Srisuparp S, Strakova Z, Brudney A et al. Signal transduction pathways activated by chorionic gonadotropin in the primate endometrial epithelial cells. Biol Reprod 2003; 68: 457–64.

29. Antoni FA. Molecular diversity of cyclic AMP signalling. Front Neuroendocrinol 2000; 21: 103–32.

30. Nishimori K, Dunkel L, Hsueh AJ et al. Expression of luteinizing hormone and chorionic gonadotropin receptor messenger ribonucleic acid in human corpora lutea during menstrual cycle and pregnancy. J Clin Endocrinol Metab 1995; 80: 1444–8.

31. Pabon JE, Bird JS, Li X et al. Human skin contains luteinizing hormone/chorionic gonadotropin receptors. J Clin Endocrinol Metab 1996; 81: 2738–41.

32. Pabon JE, Li X, Lei ZM et al. Novel presence of luteinizing hormone/chorionic gonadotropin receptors in human adrenal glands. J Clin Endocrinol Metab 1996; 81: 2397–400.

33. Tao YX, Bao S, Ackermann DM et al. Expression of luteinizing hormone/human chorionic gonadotropin receptor gene in benign prostatic hyperplasia and in prostate carcinoma in humans. Biol Reprod 1997; 56: 67–72.

34. Thompson DA, Othman MI, Lei Z et al. Localization of receptors for luteinizing hormone/chorionic gonadotropin in neural retina. Life Sci 1998; 63: 1057–64.

35. Rao CV. No mRNAs for the LH/hCG receptor in human endometrium? Fertil Steril 1999; 72: 374–5.

36. Stewart EA. Gonadotropins and the uterus: is there a gonad-independent pathway? J Soc Gynecol Investig 2001; 8: 319–26.

37. Fazleabas AT, Donnelly KM, Srinivasan S et al. Modulation of the baboon (*Papio anubis*) uterine endometrium by chorionic gonadotrophin during the period of uterine receptivity. Proc Natl Acad Sci USA 1999; 96: 2543–8.

38. Zhou XL, Lei ZM, Rao CV. Treatment of human endometrial gland epithelial cells with chorionic gonadotropin/luteinizing hormone increases the expression of the cyclooxygenase-2 gene. J Clin Endocrinol Metab 1999; 84: 3364–77.

39. Bonnamy PJ, Benhaim A, Leymarie P. Uterine luteinizing hormone/human chorionic gonadotropin-binding sites in the early pregnant rat uterus: evidence for total occupancy in the periimplantation period. Endocrinology 1993; 132: 1240–6.

40. Jensen JD, Odell WD. Identification of LH/hCG receptors in rabbit uterus. Proc Soc Exp Biol Med 1988; 189: 28–30.

41. Cameo P, Szmidt M, Strakova Z et al. Decidualization regulates the expression of endometrial chorionic gonadotrophin receptor in the primate. Biol Reprod 2006; 75: 681–9.

42. Licht P, von Wolff M, Berkholz A et al. Evidence for cycle-dependent expression of full-length human chorionic gonadotropin/luteinizing hormone receptor mRNA in human endometrium and decidua. Fertil Steril 2003; 79 (Suppl 1): 718–23.

43. Licht P, Cao H, Zuo J et al. Lack of self-regulation of human chorionic gonadotropin biosynthesis in human choriocarcinoma cells. J Clin Endocrinol Metab 1994; 78: 1188–94.

44. Lacroix A, Hamet P, Boutin JM. Leuprolide acetate therapy in luteinizing hormone-dependent Cushing's syndrome. N Engl J Med 1999; 341: 1577–81.

45. Lacroix A, Ndiaye N, Tremblay J et al. Ectopic and abnormal hormone receptors in adrenal Cushing's syndrome. Endocr Rev 2001; 22: 75–110.

46. Lei Z, Mishra M, Zou S et al. Targeted disruption of luteinizing hormone/human chorionic gonadotropin receptor gene. Mol Endocrinol 2001; 15: 184–200.

47. Zhang FP, Poutanen, Wilbertz J et al. Normal prenatal but arrested postnatal sexual development of luteinizing hormone receptor knockout (LuRKO) mice. Mol Endocrinol 2001; 15: 172–83.

48. Lin DX, Lei ZM, Li X et al. Targeted disruption of LH receptor gene revealed the importance of uterine LH signaling. Mol Cell Endocrinol 2005; 234: 105–16.

49. Rao CV, Lei ZM. Consequences of targeted inactivation of LH receptors. Mol Cell Endocrinol 2002; 187: 57–67.

50. Pakarainen T, Zhang FP, Poutanen M et al. Fertility in luteinizing hormone receptor-knockout mice after wild-type ovary transplantation demonstrates redundancy of extragonadal luteinizing hormone action. J Clin Invest 2005; 115: 1862–8.

51. Yuan FP, Lin DX, RaoCV et al. Cryptorchidism in LhrKO animals and the effect of testosterone-replacement therapy Hum Reprod 2006; 21: 936–42.

52. Matzuk MM, DeMayo FJ, Hadsell LA et al. Overexpression of human chorionic gonadotropin causes multiple reproductive defects in transgenic mice. Biol Reprod 2003; 69: 338–46.

53. Nilson JH, Abbud RA, Keri RA et al. Chronic hypersecretion of luteinizing hormone in transgenic mice disrupts both ovarian and pituitary function, with some effects modified by the genetic background. Recent Prog Horm Res 2000; 55: 69–89.

54. Cronier L, Bastide B, Herve JC et al. Gap junctional communication during human trophoblast differentiation: influence of human chorionic gonadotropin. Endocrinology 1994; 135: 402–8.

55. Cronier L, Herve JC, Deleze J et al. Regulation of gap junctional communication during human trophoblast differentiation. Microsc Res Tech 1997; 38: 21–8.

56. Sawai K, Azuma C, Koyama M et al. Leukemia inhibitory factor (LIF) enhances trophoblast differentiation mediated by human chorionic gonadotropin (hCG). Biochem Biophys Res Commun 1995; 211: 137–43.

57. Shi QJ, Lei ZM, Rao CV et al. Novel role of human chorionic gonadotropin in differentiation of human cytotrophoblasts. Endocrinology 1993; 132: 1387–95.

58. Yang M, Lei ZM, Rao CV. The central role of human chorionic gonadotropin in the formation of human placental syncytium. Endocrinology 2003; 144: 1108–20.

59. Hild-Petito S, Donnelly KM, Miller JB et al. A baboon (*Papio anubis*) simulated-pregnant model: cell specific expression of insulin-like growth factor binding protein-1 (IGFBP-1), type I IGF receptor (IGF-I R) and retinol binding protein (RBP) in the uterus. Endocrine 1995; 3: 639–51.

60. Hausermann HM, Donnelly KM, Bell SC et al. Regulation of the glycosylated beta-lactoglobulin homolog, glycodelin [placental protein 14: (PP14)] in the baboon (*Papio anubis*) uterus. J Clin Endocrinol Metab 1998; 83: 1226–33.

61. Strakova Z, Mavrogianis P, Meng X et al. In vivo infusion of interleukin-1beta and chorionic gonadotropin induces endometrial changes that mimic early pregnancy events in the baboon. Endocrinology 2005; 146: 4097–104.

62. Tarara R, Enders AC, Hendrickx AG et al. Early implantation and embryonic development of the baboon: stages 5, 6 and 7. Anat Embryol 1987; 176: 267–75.

63. Banaszak S, Brudney A, Donnelly K et al. Modulation of the action of chorionic gonadotropin in the baboon (*Papio anubis*) uterus by a progesterone receptor antagonist (ZK 137.316). Biol Reprod 2000; 63: 820–5.

64. Fazleabas AT, Bell SC, Fleming S et al. Distribution of integrins and the extracellular matrix proteins in the baboon endometrium during the menstrual cycle and early pregnancy. Biol Reprod 1997; 56: 348–56.

65. Christensen S, Verhage HG, Nowak G et al. Smooth muscle myosin II and alpha smooth muscle actin expression in the baboon (*Papio anubis*) uterus is associated with glandular secretory activity and stromal cell transformation. Biol Reprod 1995; 53: 598–608.

66. Kim JJ, Wang J, Bambra C et al. Expression of cyclooxygenase-1 and -2 in the baboon endometrium during the menstrual cycle and pregnancy. Endocrinology 1999; 140: 2672–8.

67. Tarantino S, Verhage HG, Fazleabas AT. Regulation of insulin-like growth factor-binding proteins in the baboon (*Papio anubis*) uterus during early pregnancy. Endocrinology 1992; 130: 2354–62.

68. Strakova Z, Srisuparp S, Fazleabas AT. Interleukin 1β induces the expression of insulin-like growth factor binding protein-1 during decidualization in the primate. Endocrinology 2000; 141: 4664–70.

69. Sherwin JRA, Sharkey AM, Cameo P et al. Identification of novel genes regulated by chorionic gonadotrophin in the baboon endometrium during the implantation window. Endocrinology 2007; 148: 618–26.

70. Stewart CL, Kaspar P, Brunet LJ et al. Blastocyst implantation depends on maternal expression of leukaemia inhibitory factor. Nature 1992; 359: 76–9.

71. Yue ZP, Yang ZM, Wei P et al. Leukemia inhibitory factor, leukemia inhibitory factor receptor, and glycoprotein 130 in rhesus monkey uterus during menstrual cycle and early pregnancy. Biol Reprod 2000; 63: 508–12.

72. Licht P, Russu V, Lehmeyer S. Molecular aspects of direct LH/hCG effects on human endometrium – lessons from intrauterine microdialysis in the human female in vivo. Reprod Biol 2001; 1: 10–19.

73. Horcajadas JA, Riesewijk A, Polman J et al. Effect of controlled ovarian hyperstimulation in IVF on endometrial gene expression profiles. Mol Hum Reprod 2005; 11: 195–205.

74. Sahu A, Lambris JD. Structure and biology of complement protein C3, a connecting link between innate and acquired immunity. Immunol Rev 2001; 180: 35–48.

75. Bolton AE, Pockleym AG, Clough KJ et al. Identification of placental protein 14 as an immunosuppressive factor in human reproduction. Lancet 1987; 1: 593–5.

76. Lobo SC, Srisuparp S, Peng X et al. Uterine receptivity in the baboon: modulation by chorionic gonadotropin. Semin Reprod Med 2001; 19: 69–74.

77. Tagoh H, Kishi H, Muraguchi A. Molecular cloning and characterization of a novel stromal cell-derived cDNA encoding a protein that facilitates gene activation of recombination activating gene (RAG)-1 in human lymphoid progenitors. Biochem Biophys Res Commun 1996; 221: 744–9.

78. Ho YS, Gargano M, Cao J et al. Reduced fertility in female mice lacking copper-zinc superoxide dismutase. J Biol Chem 1998; 273: 7765–69.

79. Hopwood D, Levison DH. Atrophy and apoptosis in the cyclical human endometrium. J Pathol 1978; 119: 159–66.

80. Vaskivuo TE, Stenback F, Karhumaa P et al. Apoptosis and apoptosis-related proteins in human endometrium. Mol Cell Endocrinol 2000; 165: 75–83.

81. Lovely LP, Fazleabas AT, Fritz MA et al. Prevention of endometrial apoptosis: randomized prospective comparison of human chorionic gonadotropin versus progesterone treatment in the luteal phase. J Clin Endocrinol Metab 2005; 90(4): 2351–6.

82. Suria H, Chau LA, Negrou E et al. Cytoskeletal disruption induces T cell apoptosis by a caspase-3 mediated mechanism. Life Sci 1999; 65: 2697–707.

83. Kayalar C, Ord T, Testa MP et al. Cleavage of actin by interleukin 1β-converting enzyme to reverse DNase I inhibition. Proc Natl Acad Sci USA 1996; 93: 2234–8.

84. Kim SJ, Hwang SG, Kim IC et al. Actin cytoskeletal architecture regulates nitric oxide-induced apoptosis, de-differentitation and cyclooxygenase-2 expression in articular chondrocytes via mitogen-activated protein kinase and protein kinase C pathways. J Biol Chem 2003; 278: 42448–56.

85. Kim JJ, Jaffe RC, Fazleabas AT. Insulin-like growth factor binding protein-1 expression in baboon endometrial stromal cells: regulation by filamentous actin and requirement for de novo protein synthesis. Endocrinology 1999; 140: 997–1004.

86. Clark EA, Brugge JS. Integrins and signal transduction pathways: the road-taken. Science 1995; 268: 233–9.

87. Jasinska A, Han V, Fazleabas AT et al. Induction of insulin-like growth factor binding protein-1 expression in baboon endometrial stromal cells by cells of trophoblast origin. J Soc Gynecol Invest 2004; 11: 399–405.

88. Jasinska A, Strakova A, Szmidt M et al. Human chorionic gonadotrophin and decidualization in vitro inhibits cytochalasin-D induced apoptosis in cultured endometrial stromal fibroblasts. Endocrinology 2006; 147: 4112–21.

89. Chwalisz K, Garfield RE. Role of nitric oxide in implantation and menstruation. Hum Reprod Update 2000; 15: 96–111.

90. Zygmunt M, Herr F, Keller-Schoenwetter S et al. Characterization of human chorionic gonadotropin as a novel angiogenic factor. J Clin Endocrinol Metab 2002; 87: 5290–6.

91. Lei ZM, Reshef E, Rao V. The expression of human chorionic gonadotropin/luteinizing hormone receptors in human endometrial and myometrial blood vessels. J Clin Endocrinol Metab 1992; 75: 651–9.

92. Toth P, Li X, Rao CV et al. Expression of functional human chorionic gonadotropin/human luteinizing hormone receptor gene in human uterine arteries. J Clin Endocrinol Metab 1994; 79: 307–15.

93. Neulen J, Yan Z, Raczek S et al. Human chorionic gonadotropin-dependent expression of vascular endothelial growth factor/vascular permeability factor in human granulosa cells importance in ovarian hyperstimulation syndrome. J Clin Endocrinol Metab 1995; 80: 1967–71.

94. Devroey P, Pados G. Preparation of endometrium for egg donation. Hum Reprod Update 1998; 4: 856–61.

95. Klein J, Sauer MV. Oocyte donation. Best Pract Res Clin Obstet Gynaecol 2002; 16: 277–91.

96. Tesarik J, Hazout A, Mendoza C. Luteinizing hormone affects uterine receptivity independently of ovarian function. Reprod Biomed Online 2003; 1: 59–64.

97. Seif MW, Pearson JM, Ibrahim ZH et al. Endometrium in in-vitro fertilization cycles: morphological and functional differentiation in the implantation phase. Hum Reprod 1992; 7: 6–11.

98. Psychoys A. The implantation window: basic and clinical aspects. In: Perspectives on Assited Reproduction. Ares-Serono Symposium 4, 1994.

99. Kolb BA, Paulson RJ. The luteal phase of cycles utilizing controlled ovarian hypersimulation and the possible impact of this hypersimulation on embryo implantation. Am J Obstet Gynecol 1997; 176: 1262–7.

100. Kolibianakis EM, Bourgain C, Platteau P et al. Abnormal endometrial development occurs during the luteal phase of nonsupplemented donor cycles treated with recombinant follicle-stimulating hormone and gonadotropin-releasing hormone antagonists. Fertil Steril 2003; 80: 464–6.

101. Develioglu OH, Hsiu JG, Nikas G et al. Endometrial estrogen and progesterone receptor and pinopode expression in stimulated cycles of oocyte donors. Fertil Steril 1999; 71: 1040–7.

102. Paulson RJ, Sauer MV, Lobo RA. Embryo implantation after human in vitro fertilization: importance of endometrial receptivity. Fertil Steril 1990; 53: 870–4.

103. Daya S, Gunby J. Luteal phase support in assisted reproduction cycles. Cochrane Database Syst Rev 2004; (3): CD004830.

104. Stewart EA, Rein MS, Friedman AJ et al. Glycoprotein hormones and their common alpha-subunit stimulate prolactin production by explant cultures of human leiomyoma and myometrium. Am J Obstet Gynecol 1994; 170: 677–83.

105. Singh M, Zuo J, Li X et al. The decreased expression of functional human chorionic gonadotropin/luteinizing hormone receptor gene in human uterine leiomyomas. Biol Reprod 1995; 53: 591–7.

106. Lei ZM, Rao CV, Lincoln S et al. Increased expression of human chorionic gonadotropin/human luteinizing hormone receptors in adenomyosis. J Clin Endocrinol Metab 1993; 76: 763–8.

107. Lincoln S, Lei ZM, Rao CV et al. The expression of human chorionic gonadotropin/human luteinizing hormone receptors in ectopic human endometrial implants. J Clin Endocrinol Metab 1992; 75: 1140–4.

108. Lei ZM, Taylor DD, Gercel-Taylor C et al. Human chorionic gonadotropin promotes tumorigenesis of choriocarcinoma JAR cells. Trophoblast Res 1999; 13: 147–59.

109. Baird DD, Kesner JS, Dunson DB. Luteinizing hormone in premenopausal women may stimulate uterine leiomyomata development. J Soc Gynecol Invest 2006; 13: 130–5.

110. Huber AV, Huber JC, Kolbus A et al. Systemic HCG treatment in patients with endometriosis: a new perspective for a painful disease. Wien Klin Wochenschr 2004; 116: 839–43.

111. Toth P, Lukacs H, Gimes G et al. Clinical importance of vascular LH/hCG receptors. Reprod Biol 2001; 1: 5–11.

112. Kurtzman JT, Wilson H, Rao CV. A proposed role for hCG in clinical obstetrics. Semin Reprod Med 2001; 19: 63–8.

113. Ticconi C, Piccione E, Belmonte A et al. HCG – a new kid on the block in prematurity prevention. J Matern Fetal Neonatal Med 2006; 19: 687–92.

19 Embryo–endometrial signaling

Francisco Dominguez and Carlos Simón

Synopsis

Background

- As the preimplantation embryo moves through the fallopian tube and enters the uterus, signals pass between it and the maternal host tissues.
- After hatching, the blastocyst becomes apposed to the endometrial luminal epithelium. At this stage, local bidirectional signals are particularly important in the initiation of the cascade of adhesive interactions that mediates implantation.
- Maternal epithelial cells are hormonally activated to become receptive to embryonic stimuli.

Basic Science

- Lymphocyte–endothelial interactions at sites of inflammation occur by a coordinated series of adhesion mechanisms, beginning with a low-affinity carbohydrate-mediated interaction and progressing to higher-affinity integrin-mediated binding. It is likely that embryos attach via a comparable cascade.
- Uterine epithelial cells release chemokines, including RANTES, MIP-1α, MIP-1β, MCP-1, and IL-8, in response to ovarian steroids.
- Steroids also regulate chemokine receptors such as CXCR4, which is maximal in the inplantation phase.
- In-vitro evidence suggests that the blastocyst up-regulates maternal epithelial expression of the chemokine receptors CXCR1, CXCR4, and CCR5.
- Chemokines act on maternal leukocyte subsets, which in turn release proteases and other mediators that facilitate embryo invasion.
- They also probably act on the blastocyst, which (in humans) expresses receptors CCR2B and CCR5.
- The OB gene product leptin secreted by adipose tissue is tightly linked to food consumption, energy balance, and body weight.
- Leptin is involved in the regulation of reproductive function. Its receptor is encoded by the OB-R gene and belongs to the class I superfamily of cytokine receptors.
- There is evidence that leptin and its receptor are expressed both by the endometrium and the implanting blastocyst.
- ob/ob female mice (which lack functional leptin) and db/db mice (which lack functional leptin receptor) are characterized by obesity and sterility.
- In humans, one of the pathological consequences of obesity is infertility, indicating a link between adipose tissue and the reproductive system.

Clinical

- The prevalence of obesity has doubled in the past decade.
- High BMI has been associated with low IVF pregnancy rates, suggesting the involvement of endometrial receptivity and implantation in these conditions.

INTRODUCTION

Successful implantation requires a functionally normal embryo at the blastocyst stage and a receptive endometrium, while the communication between them is also vital. This embryonic–endometrial cross-communication, already described in rodents[1] and non-human primates,[2] is a highly regulated mechanism with the involvement of many systems at the paracrine and autocrine levels.

During apposition, the human blastocyst finds a location to attach, in a specific area of the maternal endometrium. In the adhesion phase, which occurs 6–7 days after ovulation, within the 'implantation window', direct contact occurs between the endometrial epithelium (EE) and the trophoectoderm (TE). Finally, in the invasion phase, the embryonic trophoblast breaches the basement membrane and invades the endometrial stroma up to the uterine vessels.

The EE is a monolayer of cuboidal cells that covers the interior of the uterus. As a reproductive tract mucosal barrier, EE must provide continuous protection against pathogens that gain access to the uterine cavity (see Chapter 33), while allowing embryonic implantation, a unique event crucial for the continuation of the species in mammals. Initial adhesion of the TE of the embryo to the EE plasma membrane is the prerequisite for implantation and placental development (see Chapter 19). EE is a specialized hormonally regulated cell population that must undergo cyclical morphological and biochemical changes to maintain an environment suitable for preimplantation embryonic development. Acting as a modulator, it translates and controls the impact of the embryo on the stromal and vascular compartments, and converts hormonal into embryonic signals.

In this chapter, we summarize the existing information concerning the embryo–endometrial cross-talk implicated in human implantation. We compare this process with the well-studied leukocyte transendothelial migration and select specific systems for further detailed study. We also present new strategies based on array technology that will clarify the fragmented information existing in the field.

COMPARATIVE MODEL: EMBRYONIC IMPLANTATION VS TRANSENDOTHELIAL MIGRATION

A parallelism between the different steps in human embryo–endometrial apposition/adhesion/invasion and leukocyte–endothelium rolling/adhesion/extravasation has been established in recent years.[3–5] Cascades of events that take place during both processes show similarities, although some details with respect to time scale, size of cells, identity of involved molecules, and others are obviously different.

During the apposition phase in implantation and leukocyte adhesion, the blastocyst/endometrium and leukocyte/endothelium dialogue relies on a first wave of soluble mediators, such as cytokines, chemokines, and other factors, produced and acting in a bidirectional fashion.[6,7] These molecules regulate the expression and functional activity of adhesion molecules such as L-selectin and integrins that mediate both processes.

The first step in the extravasation sequence in leukocytes corresponds to the interaction of selectins with their carbohydrate-based ligands.[8] This interaction, known as tethering, allows the leukocyte to roll on the endothelial cell wall. These selectin interactions are highly dynamic and short-lived, so they are able to slow down the leukocytes through transient contacts with the endothelial monolayer, facilitating their firm adhesion (Figure 19.1). Leukocytes express L-selectin, which is shed from their surface to allow the transmigration process to proceed. The L-selectin system is also critically involved in the embryonic apposition phase.[4] Carbohydrate ligands that bind L-selectin are localized on the luminal epithelium at the time of implantation, while the trophoectoderm expresses L-selectin strongly after hatching. Trophoblast lineages use L-selectin to bind to uterine epithelial oligosaccharide ligands, and, when L-selectin is blocked with specific antibodies, adhesion to the epithelium is impaired.[4]

Also exposed in the glycocalyx of human endometrial epithelial cells (EEC) are mucins such as mucin glycoprotein 1 (MUC1), which increases its expression from the proliferative to secretory phase in endometrial tissue[9] and is also regulated by the human blastocyst.[10] The possible substrate candidates for MUC1 binding include L-selectins,[9] or intercellular adhesion molecules; however, its function as an adhesion or antiadhesion molecule is still controversial.

During leukocyte rolling, chemokines induce the activation in situ of leukocyte integrins[11] and, in cooperation with integrin-dependent signals, the polarization of the cell.[12,13] Many authors have studied integrins in human implantation. A subset of epithelial endometrial integrin subunits may be relevant to the process of implantation based on spatiotemporal considerations. Therefore, the embryo could induce a favorable epithelial integrin pattern for its implantation. Integrin knockout studies reveal that, in β1–/– mice, embryos develop normally to the blastocyst stage but fail to implant.[14] However, no implantation-related phenotypes have been observed in other integrin knockouts.

In the diapedesis step, leukocytes have to squeeze into the endothelial cell-to-cell junctions. During this process, the permeability of the endothelial monolayer is not usually compromised. Leukocyte integrins interact with tight junction molecules such as junctional adhesion molecules (JAMs), establishing heterotypic connections that are replaced by JAM–JAM homotypic interactions once the leukocyte has traversed the monolayer, thus restoring the initial situation[15,16] (see Figure 19.1).

The size of the blastocyst prevents its migration between EEC; therefore, another strategy is needed. In

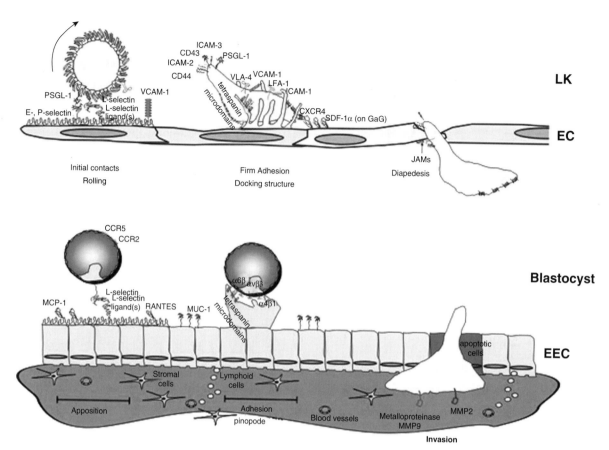

Figure 19.1 Comparison of the sequential adhesion steps involved in (**A**) leukocyte transendothelial migration and (**B**) embryonic implantation and their molecular players. LK, leukocyte; EC, embryonic cell; EEC, endometrial epithelial cells. (Reproduced from Domínguez et al,[3] with permission.)

humans and mice when the blastocyst adheres to the EEC monolayer, a paracrine apoptotic reaction is induced.[17,18] This embryo-induced apoptotic mechanism is triggered by direct contact between the blastocyst and the EEC, and is mediated at least in past by the Fas–Fas ligand system. To achieve successful invasion, trophoblasts must induce a repertoire of genes involved in the degradation of the extracellular matrix. Matrix metalloproteinase 9 (MMP-9) is closely associated with the invasive phenotype of trophoblasts.[19]

Comparison of these two processes point to aspects of similarity and divergence that open new fields of research for both immunologists and reproductive biologists.

CHEMOKINES IN IMPLANTATION

Chemokines (short for chemoattractant cytokines), a family of small polypeptides with molecular weight in the range 8–12 kDa, attract specific leukocyte subsets by binding to cell surface receptors (see Chapter 35). Two main subfamilies are distinguished by the arrangement of the first two of four (second and fourth) conserved cysteine residues near the amino terminus. CXC chemokines attract neutrophils and CC chemokines act upon monocytes, eosinophils, T lymphocytes, and natural killer (NK) cells. The other two subfamilies are CX3C (fractalkine or neurotactin) with three amino acids between the two cysteines and the C subfamily (also named lymphotactins),[20] with only a single cysteine near the N-terminal domain eliciting potent lymphocyte chemoattractant capacity but no action on monocytes. Chemokines act through cell surface G-protein-coupled receptors (GPCRs).[21] One receptor might bind one or more chemokines from the same subfamily and chemokines can bind several different receptors.[22] Consequently, the activity of chemokines is the outcome of a complex cascade that depends on the cell type, the ligand, the structure and configuration of the receptor, and the activation enzymes.

In reproductive biology, these molecules have been implicated in crucial processes such as ovulation, menstruation, embryo implantation, and parturition, and in pathological processes such as preterm delivery, HIV infection, endometriosis, and ovarian hyperstimulation syndrome[23,24] (see also Chapter 35). Chemokines produced by the endometrial epithelium and the human blastocyst are implicated in this molecular network. We know that different subsets of leukocytes are recruited into the endometrium during implantation. The regulation of the uterine tissue during this process is thought to be orchestrated by uterine epithelial cells, which release an array of chemokines in a precise temporal pattern driven mainly by ovarian steroids.[25] Chemokines act on a range of leukocyte subsets, which in turn release a number of proteases and other mediators that facilitate embryo invasion.[26]

Chemokine receptors belong to the superfamily of GPCRs. These receptors display seven sequences of 20–25 hydrophobic residues that form an α-helix and span the plasma membrane, an extracellular N-terminus, three extracellular loops, three intracellular domains, and an intracellular C-terminal tail. These receptors transmit information to the cell about the presence of chemokine gradients in the extracellular environment. They are named depending on the structure of their ligand (CXC or CC).

Chemokine expression has been found in EE cells, including regulated on activation, normal T-cell expressed and secreted (RANTES), macrophage inflammatory protein (MIP-1α, MIP-1β), and macrophage chemotactic protein (MCP-1).

Interleukin-8 (IL-8), a CXC chemokine with neutrophil chemotactic/activating and T-cell chemotactic activity, is produced by human endometrial stromal and glandular cells in culture. IL-8 is found in both the surface epithelium and glands throughout the menstrual cycle. It has been suggested that it might be implicated in the recruitment of neutrophils and lymphocytes into the endometrium.[27] After ovulation, the number of large granular lymphocytes increases in the uterus,[28] and this effect might be mediated by endometrial epithelial chemokines. There is a synergism between prostaglandin E (PGE) and IL-8 in the infiltration of neutrophils from the peripheral circulation.[29] Cyclooxygenase 2 (COX-2), IL-8, and MCP-1 also have similar modulators; IL-1β up-regulates MCP-1, IL-8, and COX-2 production and this induction can be inhibited by dexamethasone and progesterone, and endometrial explants in culture produce IL-8, which is inhibited by progesterone.[30] Estrogen has also been implicated in the control of endometrial leukocyte migration by regulating the production of granulocyte–macrophage colony-stimulating factor (GM-CSF) by endometrial epithelial cells.[31] In summary, progesterone and estrogen withdrawal initiates

a cascade of events, involving EE chemokine production (IL-8, MCP-1, and GM-CSF), which plays a role in inducing the premenstrual influx of leukocytes.

In rodents, on day 1 of pregnancy, there is a high density of leukocytes in the luminal epithelium, macrophages being the most predominant cell type. Granulocytes crawl across the epithelium into the lumen to phagocytose sperm debris, suggesting that semen may contain granulocyte-specific chemokines. On day 3 (when apposition occurs), macrophages decrease and are evenly distributed through the uterine tissue.[32] On day 5 (when adhesion occurs), they become more closely associated with the epithelium. All these findings suggest that there is a preimplantation surge of chemokines, including RANTES and MCP-1, as well as growth factors, including GM-CSF produced by the EE in response to ovarian steroids, that may contribute to the initiation of implantation.

Endometrial epithelial chemokines can be regulated also by the embryo. Examination of the embryonic regulation of IL-8 mRNA[33] and production and secretion in human endometrial epithelial cells demonstrates no effect of the human blastocyst on EE IL-8 production and secretion. However, 4–8 cell embryos inhibit IL-8 secretion by EEC, suggesting that endometrial IL-8 might be relevant for migration of the early preimplantation embryo. Interestingly, there is an up-regulation of IL-8 mRNA expression on EEC co-cultures with embryos compared to those without embryos.[33]

Our group has analyzed the mRNA expression of four chemokine receptors (CXCR4, CXCR1, CCR5, and CCR2) throughout the human menstrual cycle using quantitative fluorescence polymerase chain reaction (QF-PCR). CXCR1 and CCR5 receptors showed a progesterone-dependent pattern in the early secretory phase that continued into the mid secretory phase and was maximal in the late secretory phase. The CXCR4 (SDF-1 receptor) presented a more pronounced up-regulation in the mid luteal phase than in the early and late luteal phases. Therefore, this receptor, which is located in the endometrial epithelium, is specifically up-regulated during the implantation window.[34]

To study the in-vivo hormonal regulation of the four chemokine receptors, endometrial samples were analyzed by immunohistochemistry. On day 13, when patients were treated solely with estradiol, a very weak staining for CCR2B, CCR5, and CXCR4 was localized in the luminal and glandular epithelium and endothelial cells. During the prereceptive and receptive periods (days 18 and 21, respectively), an increase of staining intensity for the CXCR1 receptor was noted in the glandular compartment. The CCR5 receptor was also immunolocalized, mainly at the luminal epithelium but also in the stromal and perivascular cells, showing a slight increase compared to the non-receptive phase. The CCR2B receptor showed a moderate increase of staining on days 18 and 21 in the luminal epithelium, while no staining was observed in endothelial cells or stroma. The CXCR4 receptor showed the same staining as CCR5, mainly expressed in the epithelium on days 18 and 21. Endothelial and stromal cells were also positive.[34]

The embryonic impact on chemokine receptors CXCR1, CXCR4, CCR5, and CCR2B polarization in cultured EEC was investigated using our apposition model for human implantation. This model consists of culturing human blastocysts in a monolayer of EEC cells. When the blastocyst was absent, chemokine receptors CXCR1, CXCR4, and CCR5 were barely detectable in few cells of the EEC monolayer. However, when a human blastocyst was present, there was an increase in the number of stained cells for CXCR1, CXCR4, and CCR5, and these receptors were polarized in one of the cell poles of the endometrial epithelium. Immunolocalization and polarization changes in CCR2B receptor were not present in the EEC monolayer and this receptor was not regulated by the presence of the human blastocyst.[34]

Finally, we have detected immunoreactive CCR2B and CCR5 receptors in the human blastocyst. CCR2B staining was localized mainly at the inner cell mass, whereas CCR5 staining can be visualized across the trophoectoderm. In all cases ($n = 3$), CCR5 staining was more intense than that of the CCR2B receptor, while the zona pellucida was not stained in any case. Immunoreactive CXCR4 and CXCR1 were not detected in human blastocysts (Figure 19.2).[34]

Other clues about the relevance of the chemokines in the process of implantation come from the chemokine interferon-inducible protein 10 kDa (IP-10). IP-10 has been implicated in the regulation of blastocyst migration, apposition, and initial adhesion in ruminants.[35] More indirect evidence on the implication of chemokines in the attraction of the blastocyst comes from clinical trials, demonstrating that scar tissue (i.e. a persistent inflammatory focus) from previous cesarean section or endometrial surgery became an attractive implantation site.[36] Furthermore, some chemokines such as CX3CL1 (fractalkine), CCL14 (HCC-1), and CCL4 (MIP-1β) seem to promote human trophoblast migration at the feto–maternal interface.[37]

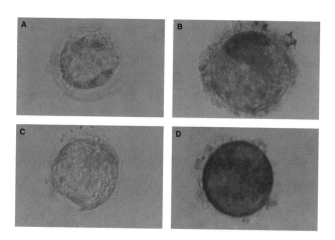

Figure 19.2 Inmunolocalization of chemokine receptors CCR2B and CCR5 in human blastocysts. (**A**) Negative control and (**B**) CCR2B. (**C**) Negative control and (**D**) CCR5. (Reproduced from Domínguez et al,[34] with permission.) (See also color plate section.)

RELEVANCE OF THE LEPTIN SYSTEM IN THE EMBRYO–ENDOMETRIAL DIALOGUE

Obesity is a condition that is reaching epidemic proportions in the United States. The prevalence of obesity has doubled in the past decade[38] and one of the pathological consequences is infertility, indicating a link between adipose tissue and the reproductive system.[39] Recently, high body mass index (BMI) has been associated with low in-vitro fertilization (IVF) pregnancy rates,[40] suggesting the involvement of endometrial receptivity and implantation in these conditions.

Leptin is a 16 kDa non-glycosylated polypeptide of 146 amino acids discovered in 1994 by Zhang et al.[41] It is the OB gene product, a small pleiotrophic peptide initially thought to be secreted by adipose tissue. Secretion is tightly linked to food consumption, energy balance, and body weight.[42] More recently, investigations have implicated leptin in the regulation of reproductive function.[39]

Leptin receptor is the product of the LEPR or OB-R gene and belongs to the class I superfamily of cytokine receptors. The full-length receptor has the signaling capabilities of an IL-6 type receptor.[43] In humans and rodents, two major leptin receptor isoforms (OB-R) are expressed. The short form (OB-RS) is detected in many organs and is considered to lack signaling capability,[44] as it has a truncated intracellular domain.[45] The long form (OB-RL), with a complete intracellular domain, predominates in the hypothalamus and anterior pituitary, and is also expressed in low amounts in peripheral tissues.[46]

OB-RL activation involves the signal transduction cascade of Janus activated kinases (JAKs) and signal transducers and activators of transcription (STATs). Leptin binding leads to receptor oligomerization and activation of the JAK–STAT pathway.[42]

An early observation indicated that ob/ob female mice (which lack functional leptin) and db/db mice (which lack functional leptin receptor) are characterized by obesity and sterility.[42] Fertility in the ob/ob animals can be restored by exogenous administration of leptin but not by food restriction, indicating that leptin per se is required for normal reproductive functioning.[47] Moreover, impaired reproductive function of ob/ob male mice is corrected only with leptin treatment.[48]

Similar findings in congenital leptin deficiency[49] and leptin mutation[50] have also been reported in humans; however, there are discrepancies in reports concerning normal reproduction in leptin-deficient patients with lipoatropic diabetes.[51] In keeping with its predominant role as a signal for starvation, leptin also seems to be important in mediating undernutrition-induced deficits in reproductive function. In starved mice, the lack of reproductive function coincides with the fall of plasma leptin level and several neuroendocrine changes. An exogenous leptin injection restores fertility in these mice.[52] In addition, leptin infusions restore ovulatory function in an animal model of starvation.

Human obesity is not characterized by leptin deficiency. It is possible that obesity is a state of leptin resistance, However, evidence for this hypothesis is limited, with only a few cases having been reported of splice-site mutation leading to a truncated form of the receptor with no signaling function.[53]

Although the leptin system clearly influences reproduction, whether leptin exerts its effect as an endocrine or paracrine mediator is yet to be resolved. A large body of data support the notion that the reproductive actions of leptin involve a direct effect on the brain, specifically the hypothalamus. Leptin receptor and actions of leptin have been described in the pituitary in both rodents and humans.[54] Expression of functional leptin receptors has also been detected in rodents[55] and humans[56] and follicular and serum leptin production seems to be influenced by the ovarian functional state. To the present date, the mechanism linking leptin, luteinizing hormone (LH), and estradiol levels has not been clearly established. Endocrine data from in-vitro fertilization patients suggest that leptin production may be influenced by the ovarian functional state.[57]

In recent years, components of the leptin system have been studied in human endometrium.[58–60] The long form of leptin receptor (OB-RL) mRNA is detectable by Northern blot analysis[59] and reverse transcriptase polymerase chain reaction (RT-PCR). Furthermore, OB-RL protein is detected by Western blot analyses[58,59] and in glandular and luminal epithelium[58] by immunohistochemistry.[60] In addition, OB-RL has been detected by RT-PCR and Western blotting in cultured human EEC.[58] Interestingly, OB-R mRNA expression peaks in the early secretory phase, as assayed by semiquantitative RT-PCR[59] and semiquantitative immunohistochemistry.[60]

Leptin secretion is regulated in EEC by the human embryo during the apposition phase. Using a co-culture model, leptin and leptin receptor mRNA and protein were identified in secretory endometrium and in EEC co-cultured with human embryos by RT-PCR and immunoblot, respectively.[61] Individual human blastocysts and EEC also secrete leptin. The concentration of immunoactive leptin secreted by competent blastocysts was significantly higher than that secreted by arrested blastocysts cultured alone.[58] In contrast, leptin secreted from co-cultures of arrested blastocysts with EEC was significantly higher than that secreted from co-cultures of competent blastocysts with EEC. These findings suggest that the endometrium is a target tissue for circulating leptin and, in addition, is a site of local production. Moreover, the leptin receptor is present throughout human early preimplantation development,[61] confirming similar data in the mouse.[62] Leptin expression is detected specifically at the blastocyst stage in humans (Figure 19.3). Expression of components of the leptin signaling system in the endometrium and regulation of leptin secretion by EEC due to the presence of the human embryo implicates the leptin system in the embryo–endometrial dialogue.

In the embryonic context, leptin and STAT3 proteins have been immunolocalized in a polarized manner in mouse and human oocytes and in preimplantation embryos.[44] Both molecules were found in preimplantation embryos, with differences in the allocation of blastomeres occurring after the first cell division (2–4 cell stage). A cell-borne concentration gradient of these proteins extended along the surface of the embryo at the morula stage. A potential role of these proteins in early development has been suggested by the fact that at the morula stage inner blastomeres contain little leptin/STAT3, while outer cells contain both leptin/STAT3-rich and -poor cells. In humans, this pattern has also been observed at the blastocyst stage.[61] Higher levels of leptin were present in conditioned media from

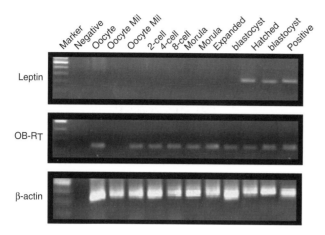

Leptin

OB-Rt

β-actin

Figure 19.3   Leptin and leptin receptor (OB-Rt) mRNA expression throughout human embryo development. (Reproduced from Cerveró et al,[61] with permission.)

single human blastocysts, suggesting that this molecule may be a marker of embryonic vitality. However, when competent blastocysts were co-cultured with EEC, leptin concentrations in conditioned media did not differ to those of EEC cultured alone. This finding suggests various possibilities: leptin secreted by a competent blastocyst may bind to EEC or the secretion of leptin is regulated in EEC and/or in the human blastocyst. In any case, all these findings strongly suggest that this molecule takes part in the embryonic–endometrial dialogue during the adhesion phase of human embryonic implantation.

FUTURE DIRECTIONS

DNA microarray technology[63–65] allows analysis of the gene expression profile in one biological sample in a single experiment (see Chapter 14). The action of progesterone on an estrogen-primed endometrium results in a particular gene expression profile which renders the endometrium receptive.[66,67] Several studies have analyzed, in a global way, the gene expression profile of the endometrium during the window of implantation (WOI) in comparison to other phases of the menstrual cycle.[68–70] These analyses have produced long lists of genes that are up- or down-regulated during this short period in which the endometrium is receptive. Some of the identified genes have known roles in human endometrial receptivity, such as PP-14[71] (glycodelin), osteopontin,[72] or insulin-like growth factor binding protein 3 (IGFBP-3),[73] but other genes were not previously known to be involved in endometrial receptivity. However, it is not clear from these studies which of the many genes altered during the WOI are functionally important for implantation. It is therefore important to analyze the gene expression profile of the endometrium

in non-fertile or subfertile conditions. Several groups have addressed this question by investigating mRNA expression in endometrium from women with endometriosis,[68] treated with RU486,[74] or under IVF protocols.[75,76] These approaches have generated indirect evidence of the regulation or dysregulation of the WOI genes in those non-physiological situations that produce a decrease in the embryonic implantation rate. Characterization of the effect of the blastocyst on gene expression in endometrial epithelial cells is a priority for current research[77] (Figure 19.4).

CONCLUSION

The endometrium is a hormonally regulated tissue that responds through paracrine pathways to the presence of the blastocyst. Transcriptomic and other biochemical changes are thought to be crucial for the acquisition of receptivity. Chemokines produced locally by the epithelium may act to recruit leukocytes and further induce a second wave of cytokines that, through binding to their specific receptors, regulate the expression of adhesion molecules essential for the adhesion of the blastocyst. Microarray studies will help decipher the gene products involved in this complex phenomenon.

REFERENCES

1. Shiotani M, Noda Y, Mori T. Embryo-dependent induction of uterine receptivity assessed by an in vitro model of implantation in mice. Biol Reprod 1993; 49: 794–801.
2. Cameo P, Srisuparp S, Strakova Z et al. Chorionic gonadotropin and uterine dialogue in the primate. Reprod Biol Endocrinol 2004; 2: 50.
3. Domínguez F, Yanez-Mo M, Sanchez-Madrid F et al. Embryonic implantation and leukocyte transendothelial migration: different processes with similar players? FASEB J 2005; 19(9): 1056–60.
4. Genbacev OD, Prakobphol A, Foulk RA et al. Trophoblast L-selectin-mediated adhesion at the maternal–fetal interface. Science 2003; 299(5605): 405–8.
5. Thie M, Denker HW. In vitro studies on endometrial adhesiveness for trophoblast: cellular dynamics in uterine epithelial cells. Cells Tissues Organs 2002; 172(3): 237–52.
6. Paria BC, Reese J, Das SK, Dey SK. Deciphering the cross-talk of implantation: advances and challenges. Science 2002; 296: 2185–8.
7. Moser B, Loetscher P. Lymphocyte traffic control by chemokines. Nat Immunol 2001; 2: 123–8.
8. Ley K, Kansas GS. Selectins in T-cell recruitment to non-lymphoid tissues and sites of inflammation. Nat Rev Immunol 2004; 4: 1–11.
9. Hey NA, Graham RA, Seif MW et al. The polymorphic epithelial mucin MUC1 in human endometrium is regulated with maximal expression in the implantation phase. J Clin Endocrinol Metab 1994; 78: 337–42.
10. Meseguer M, Aplin JD, Caballero-Campo P et al. Human endometrial mucin MUC1 is up-regulated by progesterone and down-regulated in vitro by the human blastocyst. Biol Reprod 2001; 64: 590–601.

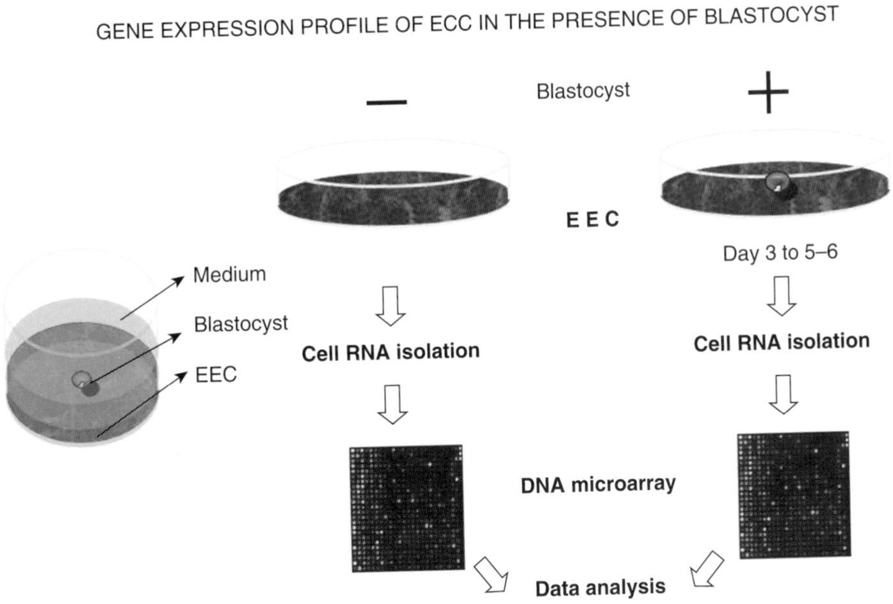

GENE EXPRESSION PROFILE OF ECC IN THE PRESENCE OF BLASTOCYST

Figure 19.4   Gene expression profile of endometrial epithelial cells (EEC) in the presence of a blastocyst. cDNA array experiments using EEC in culture in the presence or absence of a human blastocyst. RNA from both situations was extracted, labeled, and hybridized into the same arrays and differential expression data were obtained.

11. Vicente-Manzanares M, Sánchez-Madrid F. Role of the cytoskeleton during leukocyte responses. Nat Rev Immunol 2004; 4: 110–22.

12. Vicente-Manzanares M, Sancho D, Yáñez-Mó M, Sanchez-Madrid F. The leukocyte cytoskeleton in cell migration and immune interactions. Int Rev Cytol 2002; 216: 233–89.

13. Sanchez-Madrid F, del Pozo MA. Leukocyte polarization in cell migration and immune interactions. EMBO J 1999; 18: 501–11.

14. Fássler R, Meyer M. Consequences of lack of β_1 integrin gene expression in mice. Genes Dev 1995; 9: 1876–908.

15. Luscinskas FW, Ma S, Nusrat A et al. The role of endothelial cell lateral junctions during leukocyte trafficking. Immunol Rev 2002; 186: 57–67.

16. Vestweber D. Regulation of endothelial cell contacts during leukocyte extravasation. Curr Opin Cell Biol 2002; 14: 587–93.

17. Galan A, Herrer R, Remohi J et al. Embryonic regulation of endometrial epithelial apoptosis during human implantation. Hum Reprod 2000; 15(Suppl 6): 74–80.

18. Kamijo T, Rajabi MR, Mizunuma H et al. Biochemical evidence for autocrine/paracrine regulation of apoptosis in cultured uterine epithelial cells during mouse embryo implantation in vitro. Mol Hum Reprod 1998; 4: 990–8.

19. Bischof P, Meisser A, Campana A. Control of MMP-9 expression at the maternal–fetal interface. J Reprod Immunol 2002; 55: 3–10.

20. Kelner GS, Kennedy J, Bacon KB et al. Lymphotactin: a novel cytokine which represents a new class of chemokine. Science 1994; 266: 1395–9.

21. Vaddi K, Keller M, Newton RC. The Chemokine Fact Book. London: Academic Press, 1997.

22. Horuk R, Peiper SC. Chemokines: molecular double agents. Curr Biol 1996; 6: 1581–2.

23. Cocchi F, DeVico AL, Garzino-Demo A et al. Identification of RANTES, MIP-1 alpha, and MIP-1 beta as the major HIV-suppressive factors produced by CD8+ T cells. Science 1995; 270: 1811–15.

24. Simón C, Caballero-Campo P, García-Velasco JA, Pellicer A. Potential implications of chemokines in reproductive function: an attractive idea. J Reprod Immunol 1998; 38: 169–93.

25. Robertson SA, Mayrhofer G, Seamark RF. Ovarian steroid hormones regulate granulocyte–macrophage colony-stimulating factor synthesis by uterine epithelial cells in the mouse. Biol Reprod 1996; 54: 2183–96.

26. Dudley DJ, Trantman MS, Mitchel MD. Inflammatory mediators regulate interleukin-8 production by cultured gestational tissues: evidence for a cytokine network at the chorio–decidual interface. J Clin Endocrinol Metab 1993; 76: 404–10.

27. Arici A, Seli E, Senturk LM et al. Interleukin-8 in the human endometrium. J Clin Endocrinol Metab 1998; 83: 1783–7.

28. King A, Loke Y. Uterine large granular lymphocytes: a possible role in embryonic implantation. Am J Obstet Gynecol 1990; 162: 308–10.

29. Colditz, LG. Effects of exogenous prostaglandin E$_2$ and actinomycin D on plasma leakage induced by neutrophil-activating peptide-1/interleukin-8. Immunol Cell Biol 1990; 68: 397–403.

30. Kelly RW, Illingworth P, Baldie G et al. Progesterone control of one interleukin-8 production in endometrium and chorio-decidual cells underlines the role of the neutrophil in menstruation and parturition. Hum Reprod 1994; 9: 253–8.

31. Robertson SA, Mau VJ, Tremellen KP, Seamork RF. Role of high molecular weight seminal vesicle proteins in eliciting the uterine inflammatory response to semen in mice. J Reprod Fertil 1996; 107: 265–77.

32. De Choudhuri R, Wood GW. Determination of the number and distribution of macrophages, lymphocytes and granulocytes in the mouse uterus from mating through implantation. J Leukocyte Biol 1991; 50: 252–62.

33. Caballero-Campo P, Bernal A, Mercader A et al. Embryonic regulation of IL-8 production and secretion in human endometrial cells. J Soc Gynecol Invest 1998; 5(Suppl): 117A.

34. Domínguez F, Galan A, Martin JJ et al. Hormonal and embryonic regulation of chemokine receptors CXCR1, CXCR4, CCR5 and CCR2B in the human endometrium and the human blastocyst. Mol Hum Reprod 2003; 9: 189–98.

35. Nagaoka K, Nojima H, Watanabe F et al. Regulation of blastocyst migration, apposition, and initial adhesion by a chemokine, interferon gamma-inducible protein 10 kDa (IP-10), during early gestation. J Biol Chem 2003; 278: 29048–56.

36. Shufaro Y, Nadjari M. Implantation of a gestational sac in a cesarean section scar. Fertil Steril 2001; 75: 1217.

37. Hannan NJ, Jones RL, White CA, Salamonsen LA. The chemokines, CX3CL1, CCL14, and CCL4, promote human

trophoblast migration at the feto–maternal interface. Biol Reprod 2006; 74: 896–904.

38. Houseknecht KL, Baile CA, Matteri RL, Spurlock ME. The biology of leptin: a review. J Anim Sci 1998; 76: 1405–20.

39. Frisch RE. The right weight: body fat, menarche and ovulation. Ballieres Clin Obstet Gynaecol 1990; 4: 419–39.

40. Wang JX, Davies M, Norman RJ. Body mass and probability of pregnancy during assisted reproduction treatment: retrospective study. BMJ 2000; 321: 1320–1.

41. Zhang Y, Proenca R, Maffei M et al. Positional cloning of the mouse obese gene and its human homologue. Nature 1994; 372: 425–32.

42. Friedman JM, Halaas JL. Leptin and the regulation of body weight in mammals. Nature 1988; 395: 763–70.

43. Baumann H, Morella KK, White DW. The full-length leptin receptor has signaling capabilities of interleukin 6-type cytokine receptors. Proc Natl Acad Sci USA 1996; 93: 8374–8.

44. Wang Y, Kuropatwinski KK, White DW. Leptin receptor action in hepatic cells. J Biol Chem 1997; 272: 16216–23.

45. Campfield LA, Smith FJ, Burn P. The OB protein (leptin) pathway – a link between adipose tissue mass and central neural networks. Horm Metab Res 1996; 28: 619–32.

46. Finn PD, Cunningham MJ, Pau KY et al. The stimulatory effect of leptin on the neuroendocrine reproductive axis in the monkey. Endocrinology 1998; 139: 4652–62.

47. Barash IA, Cheung CC, Weigle DS. Leptin is a metabolic signal to the reproductive system. Endocrinology 1996; 137: 3144–7.

48. Mounzih K, Lu R, Chehab FF. Leptin treatment rescues the sterility of genetically obese ob/ob males. Endocrinology 1997; 138: 1190–3.

49. Montague CT, Farooqi IS, Whitehead JP. Congenital leptin deficiency is associated with severe early-onset obesity in humans. Nature 1997; 387: 903–8.

50. Strobel A, Issad T, Camoin L, Ozata M, Strasbery AD. A leptin missense mutation associated with hypogonadism and morbid obesity. Nat Genet 1998; 18: 213–15.

51. Andreelli F, Hanaire-Broutin H, Laville M et al. Normal reproductive function in leptin-deficient patients with lipoatropic diabetes. J Clin Endocrinol Metab 2000; 85: 715–19.

52. Ahima RS, Prabakaran D, Mantzoros C. Role of leptin in the neuroendocrine response to fasting. Nature 1996; 382: 250–2.

53. Clement K, Vaisse C, Lahlou N. A mutation in the human leptin receptor gene causes obesity and pituitary dysfunction. Nature 1998; 392: 398–401.

54. Shimon I, Yan X, Magoffin DA et al. Intact leptin receptor is selectively expressed in human fetal pituitary and pituitary adenomas and signals human fetal pituitary growth hormone secretion. J Clin Endocrinol Metab 1998; 83: 4059–64.

55. Zachow RJ, Magoffin DA. Direct intraovarian effects of leptin: impairment of the synergistic action of the insulin-like growth factor I on follicle-stimulating hormone-dependent estradiol-17β production by rat ovarian granulosa cells. Endocrinology 1997; 138: 847–50.

56. Karlsson C, Lindell K, Svensson E et al. Expression of functional leptin receptors in human ovary. J Clin Endocrinol Metab 1997; 82: 4144–8.

57. Bützow TL, Moilanen JM, Lehtovirta M. Serum and follicular fluid leptin during in vitro fertilization: relationship among leptin increase, body fat mass, and reduced ovarian response. J Clin Endocrinol Metab 1999; 84: 3135–9.

58. González RR, Caballero-Campo P, Jasper M et al. Leptin and leptin receptor are expressed in the human endometrium and

endometrial leptin secretion is regulated by the human blastocyst. J Clin Endocrinol Metabol 2000; 85: 4883–8.

59. Kitawaki J, Koshiba H, Ishihara H. Expression of leptin receptor in human endometrium and fluctuation during the menstrual cycle. J Clin Endocrinol Metabol 2000; 85: 1946–50.

60. Alfer J, Müller-Schöttle F, Classen-Linke I. The endometrium as a novel target for leptin: differences in fertility and subfertility. Mol Hum Reprod 2000; 6: 595–601.

61. Cerveo A, Horcajadas JA, Martín J et al. The leptin system during human endometrial receptivity and preimplantation development. J Clin Endocrinol Metab 2004; 89(5): 2442–51.

62. Kawamura K, Sato N, Fukuda J et al. Leptin promotes the development of mouse preimplantation embryos in vitro. Endocrinology 2002; 143: 1922–31.

63. Schena M, Shalon D, Davis RW et al. Quantitative monitoring of gene expression patterns with a complementary DNA microarray. Science 1995; 270: 467–70.

64. Stoughton RB. Applications of DNA microarrays in biology. Ann Rev Biochem 2005; 74: 53–82.

65. Mata J, Marguerat S, Bahler J. Post-transcriptional control of gene expression: a genome-wide perspective. Trend Biochem Sci 2005; 30: 506–14.

66. Giudice LC. Elucidating endometrial function in the postgenomic era. Hum Reprod Update 2003; 9: 223–35.

67. Salamonsen LA, Nie G, Findlay JK. Newly identified endometrial genes of importance for implantation. J Reprod Immunol 2002; 53(1–2): 215–25.

68. Kao LC, Germeyer A, Tulac S et al. Expression profiling of endometrium from women with endometriosis reveals candidate genes for disease-based implantation failure and infertility. Endocrinology 2003; 144: 2870–81.

69. Carson D, Lagow E, Thathiah A et al. Changes in gene expression during the early to mid-luteal (receptive phase) transition in human endometrium detected by high-density microarray screening. Mol Hum Reprod 2002; 8: 871–9.

70. Borthwick J, Charnock-Jones S, Tom B et al. Determination of the transcript profile of human endometrium. Mol Hum Reprod 2003; 9: 19–33.

71. Julkunen M, Koistenen R, Sjoberg J et al. Secretory endometrium synthesizes placental protein 14. Endocrinology 1986; 118: 1782–6.

72. Apparao KB, Murray MJ, Fritz MA et al. Osteopontin and its receptor alpha (v) beta (3) integrin are coexpressed in the human endometrium during the menstrual cycle but regulated differentially. J Clin Endocrinol Metab 2001; 86: 4991–5000.

73. Zhou J, Dsupin BA, Giudice L et al. Insulin-like growth factor system gene expression in human endometrium during the menstrual cycle. J Clin Endocrinol Metab 1994; 79: 1723–34.

74. Catalano RD, Yanaihara A, Evans AL et al. The effect of RU486 on the gene expression profile in an endometrial explant model. Mol Human Reprod 2003; 9: 465–73.

75. Horcajadas JA, Riesewijk A, Polman J et al. Effect of controlled ovarian hyperstimulation in IVF on endometrial gene expression profiles. Mol Hum Reprod 2005; 11: 195–205.

76. Simon C, Oberye J, Bellver J et al. Similar endometrial development in oocyte donors treated with either high- or standard-dose GnRH antagonist compared to treatment with a GnRH agonist or in natural cycles. Hum Reprod 2005; 20(12): 3318–27.

77. Horcajadas JA, Catalano R, Gadea B et al. The human embryo–endometrial dialogue: impact of a single blastocyst in the gene expression pattern of endometrial epithelial cells. Fertil Steril 2005; 84(Suppl 1): S60.

20 Endometrial receptivity

Bruce A Lessey and Stanley Glasser

Synopsis

Background

- The endometrium undergoes cyclic growth and differentiation in preparation for pregnancy.
- Synchronous events in the corpus luteum, endometrium, and embryo are critical to successful implantation.
- Estrogen is required for postmenstrual regeneration.
- Progesterone effects changes in the endometrium that are essential for successful implantation.
- Endometrial luminal epithelium acts as a barrier to implantation except under appropriate and defined hormonal conditions.
- While nidatory E_2 is critical for implantation in rodents, there are questions regarding whether estrogen is necessary at all during the receptive phase in humans.
- The window of implantation is the period during which the endometrium is receptive to an embryo that has developed to the hatched blastocyst stage.
- Trophoblast interacts with endometrial cells to mediate implantation.

Basic Science

- In the human, the embryo enters the uterine cavity at 72–96 hours after fertilization.
- Hatching of the embryo (escape from the zona pellucida) occurs by day 5 (about 110–120 hours after ovulation).
- Direct studies of human implantation sites suggest that embryos attach and implant a full week after ovulation.
- Observations in donor/recipient cycles suggest a window of implantation spanning cycle days 20–24.
- Correspondingly, in normal women, implantation appears to occur at peak serum progesterone concentration, around 7–10 days after ovulation.
- Pinopods are dome-like protrusions from the apical surface of luminal epithelial cells seen in the secretory phase. They may interact transiently with the embryo at implantation but appear not to be reliable markers of receptivity.
- Estrogen up-regulates expression in endometrium of the steroid receptors ERα and PR. At the time of implantation, both these receptors are lost from epithelial cells.
- Transcriptomics, proteomics, genetics, and other approaches have led to the identification of biomarkers with a high probability of being involved in implantation in humans. These include adhesion molecules such as integrins and cadherins, and the secreted glycoproteins osteopontin, glycodelin, and calcitonin.

Clinical

- The traditional method of dating endometrium uses a series of defined histological criteria.
- Prospective, randomized re-examination of these criteria in normal fertile women has shown that they do not provide the accuracy or precision necessary to correctly assign the endometrium to a given day or series of days.
- Variability is highest during the time of implantation.
- Endometrial biopsy combined with histological dating fails to discriminate between fertile and infertile couples, and is not recommended for the routine evaluation of infertile women.
- Much has been learned about dysfunction of the endometrium and its consequences for implantation through the study of its structure and function in women with infertility or recurrent pregnancy loss.

- Women who conceive and implant at LH+10 or later exhibit a high miscarriage rate, suggesting that certain types of infertility or pregnancy loss result from defects in uterine receptivity associated with aberrant synchrony between the embryo, endometrium, and ovary.
- Loss of epithelial ERα and PR in endometrium correlates closely with the establishment of receptivity. A delay in acquisition of receptivity is associated with a correctable delay in the down-regulation of epithelial PR.
- Normal down-regulation of ERα during mid-secretory phase does not occur in some women with infertility, including those with PCOS and endometriosis. Failure of ERα down-regulation leads to uterine receptivity defects, as suggested by the loss of integrin.
- Altered progestin responses seen in endometriosis may be explained by abnormal expression of aromatase, leading to increased local estrogen production.
- PCOS patients exhibit elevated androgen receptor (AR) in their endometrium. Here, overexpression of steroid receptor coactivators may help explain prolonged estrogenic activity and a poor progesterone response.
- Future treatment options may include stronger progestins, antiestrogens (to block the receptor), or aromatase inhibitors.

INTRODUCTION

There is increasing interest in the role of the endometrium in trophoblast attachment and invasion during implantation.[1,2] The endometrium represents a barrier to implantation except under appropriate and defined hormonal conditions. To understand the regulatory biology that governs uterine receptivity requires an appreciation not only of the many endometrial peptides, cytokines, and signaling molecules that are expressed during the reproductive cycle, but also of the eloquent interplay between the embryo and the endometrium. Synchrony between the corpus luteum, endometrium, and embryo appears to be a critical element of normal implantation. The developmental strategy of the blastocyst requires cooperation with the maternal tissues that is highly regulated and temporally coordinated. Because of this complexity, it is not surprising that these mechanisms sometimes fail, resulting in pregnancy loss or infertility. By understanding the role of the endometrium in defining receptivity for the embryo, we begin to understand how the process of implantation itself works.

The endometrium of many species, including humans, undergoes cyclic development in preparation for implantation and pregnancy. Historically, animal models were used to study implantation. The concept of a defined window of implantation, during which time the embryo and endometrium first interact, was suggested by Psychoyos,[3–6] McLaren,[7,8] and Finn and Martin.[9] Studies in primate models helped to refine these concepts further[10] and much has been learned from studies of comparative placentation.[11–19] More recently, modern molecular biology techniques have identified many of the genes that are expressed in the endometrium during the reproductive cycle in humans.[20–23] This approach has set the stage for a more complete understanding of the regulation of these highly coordinated events, leading to successful pregnancy and birth: endocrine, paracrine, autocrine, and juxtacrine mechanisms of cellular communication.

Based on the paradigm of receptor-mediated interactions at implantation,[24] much work has been published on cell adhesion and the role of extracellular matrix (ECM) and receptors for ECM as key participants in the functional role of the endometrium. Degradation of endometrial ECM by endometrial or embryo-derived proteases is also a critical element of the events surrounding both implantation and subsequent menstruation when embryos fail to implant (see Chapter 23). Finally, much has been learned about dysfunction of the endometrium and its consequences for implantation through the study of endometrial structure and function in women with infertility or recurrent pregnancy loss. The purpose of this chapter is to examine the processes that arise within the endometrium that shepherd interstitial implantation, while remaining cognizant of the many aspects that remain to be understood.

ENDOMETRIAL DEVELOPMENT AND THE TIMING OF IMPLANTATION

In eutherian mammals, embryo attachment is precisely timed within the reproductive cycle. Constraints on the maturation of the fertilized egg, the endometrial lining, and the need to signal that pregnancy has been established contribute to this limitation. Synchrony between the embryo, endometrium, and the corpus luteum appears essential to the success of the pregnancy. There is general agreement that the endometrium in women exhibits a defined period of receptivity towards embryo implantation.[25,26] In rodents, the luminal surface of the endometrium appears to be a barrier to implantation except during a narrow window of receptivity[27] and the endometrium is inhospitable towards the embryo except during this period, even though embryos can implant and survive in a variety of other places within the body.[28,29] Thus, the question is raised as to what extent receptivity is an integral part of the window of implantation.

One of the earliest human studies demonstrating when embryos attach during a normal menstrual cycle was undertaken by Hertig and colleagues 50 years ago.[30] These researchers examined luteal phase hysterectomy specimens obtained from women suspected of being pregnant. Of the hundreds of specimens studied, these investigators identified 34 embryos: 8 were free floating within the uteri of women prior to cycle days 19–20; the other 26 embryos had already undergone the attachment reaction and came from women who were beyond day 20 of their menstrual cycle. While these cycles were not timed with precision, this early study suggested that embryos attach and implant a full week after ovulation.

Navot and co-workers used donor/recipient cycles to study when implantation occurs in the human.[31, 32] Using extremely sensitive serum β human chorionic gonadotropin (βhCG) measurements in cryopreserved embryo transfer cycles, these investigators determined that successful pregnancy depended on the time of embryo transfer. In these studies, a window of implantation spanning cycle days 20–24 was suggested. Most recently, Wilcox and coworkers studied a normal population of women trying to conceive and measured the timing of pregnancy using sensitive urinary markers. In this study, the window of implantation appears to be expressed during peak serum progesterone concentrations, around 7–10 days after ovulation. Interestingly, Wilcox noted that women who conceived but implanted beyond this window (luteinizing hormone [LH] + 10 or later) exhibited a high miscarriage rate.[33] These data support the hypothesis that certain types of infertility or pregnancy loss result from defects in uterine receptivity, leading to a loss of synchrony between the embryo, endometrium, and ovary.

MECHANISMS OF IMPLANTATION

There does not appear to be a unified mechanism of implantation shared by all mammalian species.

The evolutionary dialogue between mother and fetus has generated many types of placentation and a corresponding diversity in mechanisms of implantation.[11,34] The human exhibits a particularly invasive phenotype, and similarities have been drawn between placental invasion and malignant metastasis.[34]

Endometrial receptivity in humans and other mammals depends on the ovarian cycle. Folliculogenesis and selection of the dominant follicle is accompanied by elevation in circulating estrogen, promoting growth and thickening and the development of new blood vessels. Progesterone transforms the proliferating endometrium into a secretory tissue capable of nurturing the embryo and facilitating attachment.

In the human and primates, the endometrium is made up of two layers: the upper 'functionalis' and the lower 'basalis' layer. Interesting differences in hormone regulation have been noted between these zones.[35] Epithelial cells of the functionalis layer undergo mitosis and cell division in response to estrogen during the proliferative phase, while stromal cells divide during the progesterone-dominant secretory phase.[35] Interestingly, epithelial cells from the basalis undergo cell division in response to progesterone, an effect opposite to that seen in the functionalis layer.[35] The luminal surface appears to be a site of distinct responsiveness to ovarian steroids, with the development of specialized protrusions known as pinopods peaking during the mid-secretory phase, and a less pronounced secretory activity than is seen in glandular epithelial cells[36,37] (see also Chapter 5).

UTERINE RECEPTIVITY AND IMPLANTATION

Development of the endometrium depends on the programmed secretion of ovarian estradiol (E_2) and progesterone (P). The peak of serum progesterone corresponds to the time that implantation normally occurs[33] between 7 and 10 days after ovulation. Following egg release, secretory changes occur in response to the sex steroids that prepare the endometrium for the blastocyst. Progesterone appears to be essential for successful implantation.[38] While nidatory E_2 is critical for implantation in rodents, there are questions regarding whether estrogen is necessary at all during the receptive phase of the menstrual cycle of humans.[39]

Assessment of endometrial receptivity has steadily progressed over the past 60 years. As shown in Figure 20.1, the traditional method of dating the endometrium using defined histological criteria was established in 1950.[40] Early use of this technique led to the description of luteal phase defect (LPD).[41]

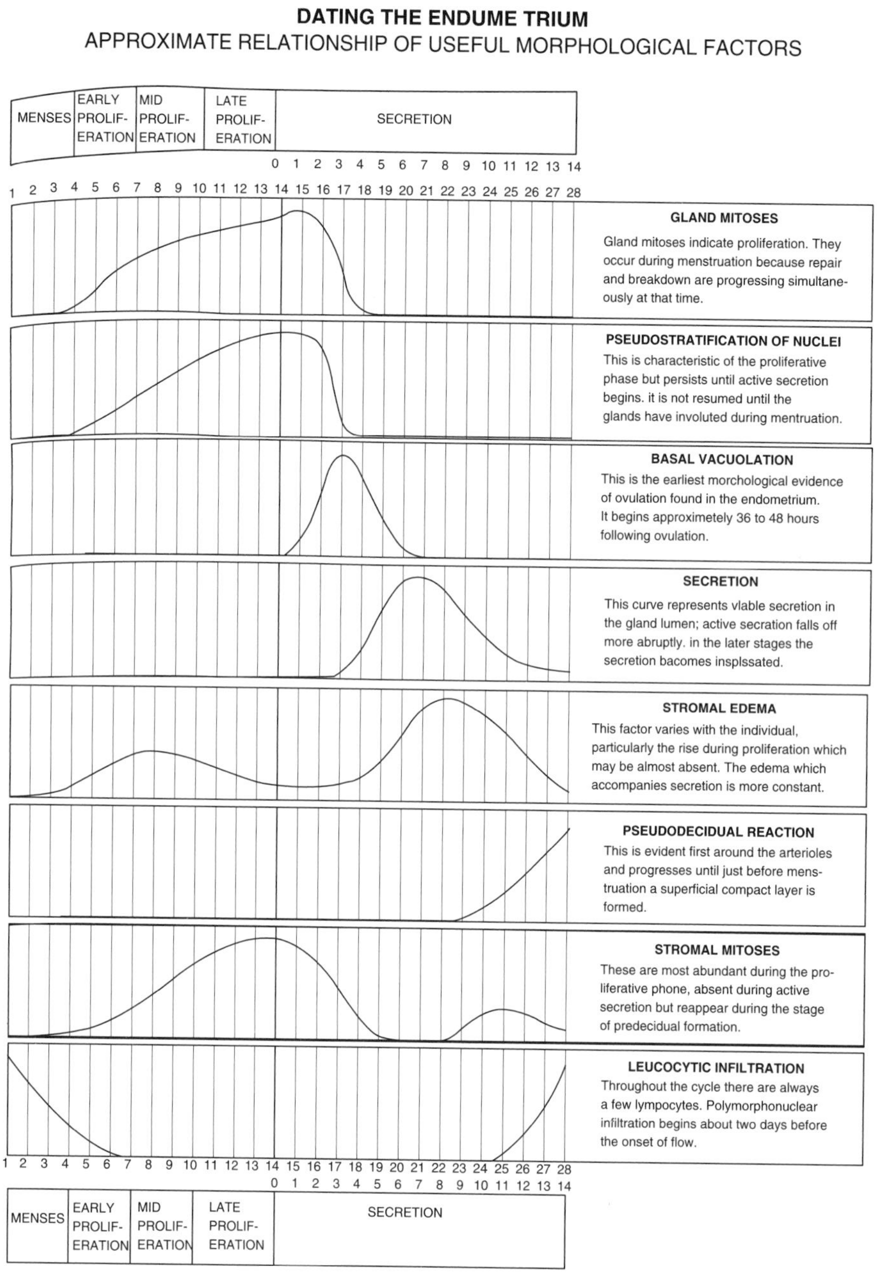

DATING THE ENDUME TRIUM
APPROXIMATE RELATIONSHIP OF USEFUL MORPHOLOGICAL FACTORS

| MENSES | EARLY PROLIF-ERATION | MID PROLIF-ERATION | LATE PROLIF-ERATION | SECRETION |

0 1 2 3 4 5 6 7 8 9 10 11 12 13 14

1 2 3 4 5 6 7 8 9 10 11 12 13 14 15 16 17 18 19 20 21 22 23 24 25 26 27 28

GLAND MITOSES

Gland mitoses indicate proliferation. They occur during menstruation because repair and breakdown are progressing simultaneously at that time.

PSEUDOSTRATIFICATION OF NUCLEI

This is characteristic of the proliferative phase but persists until active secretion begins. it is not resumed until the glands have involuted during mentruation.

BASAL VACUOLATION

This is the earliest morchological evidence of ovulation found in the endometrium. It begins approximetely 36 to 48 hours following ovulation.

SECRETION

This curve represents vlable secretion in the gland lumen; active secration falls off more abruptly. in the later stages the secretion bacomes insplssated.

STROMAL EDEMA

This factor varies with the individual, particularly the rise during proliferation which may be almost absent. The edema which accompanies secretion is more constant.

PSEUDODECIDUAL REACTION

This is evident first around the arterioles and progresses until just before menstruation a superficial compact layer is formed.

STROMAL MITOSES

These are most abundant during the proliferative phone, absent during active secretion but reappear during the stage of predecidual formation.

LEUCOCYTIC INFILTRATION

Throughout the cycle there are always a few lympocytes. Polymorphonuclear infiltration begins about two days before the onset of flow.

1 2 3 4 5 6 7 8 9 10 11 12 13 14 15 16 17 18 19 20 21 22 23 24 25 26 27 28

0 1 2 3 4 5 6 7 8 9 10 11 12 13 14

| MENSES | EARLY PROLIF-ERATION | MID PROLIF-ERATION | LATE PROLIF-ERATION | SECRETION |

Figure 20.1 Dating criteria for histological development established by Noyes et al.[40] (Reproduced with permission of the publisher, The American Fertility Society.)

This entity was commonly thought to occur in couples with infertility and recurrent pregnancy loss and to result from dyssynchronous development of the endometrium due to inadequate P or a lessened response to P.[42] The usefulness of histological dating has been repetitively challenged due to the high inter- and intra-observer variation, and the fact that the patients sampled in the original study all had infertility. A recent prospective, randomized study re-examined the dating criteria of Noyes et al in normal fertile women.[43] This study found that the criteria themselves were too variable to provide either the accuracy or precision to correctly assign the endometrium to a given day or series of days based on these criteria alone. Other studies found that variability was highest during the time of implantation, precisely when accuracy of timing may be most critical.[44] In addition, comparing fertile and infertile women, Coutifaris and colleagues found that the endometrial biopsy combined with histological dating did not discriminate between the two populations, and recommended against its use for the routine evaluation of infertile women.[45]

The proliferative phase (Figure 20.2A) of the endometrial cycle is characterized by epithelial proliferation, generalized growth of the endometrium, and an increase in expression of estrogen and progesterone receptors.[46–48] The secretory phase (Figure 20.2B) represents a period of conversion, from epithelial to stromal dominance. In response to progesterone, the early secretory phase endometrial glands are transformed in the direction of protein synthesis and secretion.[22] Both epithelial estrogen receptor (ER) and progesterone receptors (PR) decline during this transition, while stromal PR are maintained.[48,49] This transformation is accompanied by sequential and well-orchestrated expression of specific genes that may facilitate and/or limit the ability of the blastocyst and trophoblast to invade.[21,23] As the embryo invades into the endometrium, decidualization of the endometrial stroma occurs in response to rising levels of P and in response to the embryo, associated with rapid changes in stromal protein expression. Of note, these changes represent an epithelialization of the endometrial stroma, with expression of ECM components, cell surface receptors, and cellular proteins that in certain respects recapitulate the epithelial phenotype.[50,51]

The time of endometrial receptivity corresponds to entry of the blastocyst into the uterine cavity. When the embryo hatches out of the zona pellucida, it exposes elements on the outer trophoblast; these apical epithelial surfaces are probably involved in initial embryo–endometrial interactions.[52] Morrish et al point out that the embryo is genetically programmed and fully equipped to undergo development and invasion independent of endometrial input.[53] Attachment, however, must wait until the endometrium recognizes the trophoblast.

Implantation in the human can be viewed as a stepwise progression involving apposition, then attachment and adhesion, and then a species-specific, oriented interaction between trophoblast and endometrial epithelial cells. Implantation can be divided into distinct and separate stages, relating to the developmental progression of the nascent embryo and its interaction with maternal cells. The newly ovulated oocyte is transported through the Fallopian tube where fertilization may occur, defining stage I of implantation. Stage II is defined by the initiation of cell division by the embryo. At stage III, the ball of embryonic cells, now called a morula, enters the uterine cavity where further divisions result in formation of the blastocyst. In the human, the embryo enters the uterine cavity at 72–96 hours after fertilization.[54] Hatching of the embryo (escape from the zona pellucida) occurs by day 5 (about 110–120 hours after ovulation).[55]

Stage IV corresponds to the time of apposition. Apposition/adhesion is quickly followed by epithelial

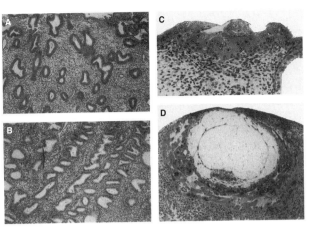

Figure 20.2 Photomicrographs of proliferative (**A**) and secretory (**B**) endometrium. Also shown are an early (**C**) implantation site during stage 5a of implantation. At this stage the maternal vasculature remains intact, but becomes surrounded by the expanding syncytium. By the later stage 5c (**D**), the embryo is fully below the luminal surface. A layer of cytotrophoblast which will soon bud to form villi surrounds the embryo and lacunae have formed as a result of maternal vascular invasion. (These examples of human implantation sites were generously provided and photographed from the Carnegie Collection by Dr Allen Enders and were used with his permission.)

penetration and invasion, signifying the beginning of stage V of implantation.[11] What triggers these orderly cells lining the blastocyst to begin to intrude through the surface epithelium is incompletely understood, but it is almost certain that endometrial receptors, enzymes, cytokines, chemokines, and other gene products are critical to this event (see Chapters 18 and 35). Despite the production of digestive enzymes by the embryo, this intrusive event does not appear to be a destructive one; rather it appears, in the mouse at least, that the syncytial trophoblasts send out processes that attach to lateral maternal epithelium surfaces, spreading the luminal epithelium apart and providing an avenue involving ECM components that facilitate entry of the embryo.[56,57] Pinopods may serve as a pseudolateral surface that allows the embryo to attach and intrude,[58] thus answering the paradox of how two epithelial apical surfaces might interact.[59]

The acquisition of specific proteins on the apical pole of the luminal surface of the endometrium and on the apex of the embryonic epithelium may be critical for processes that initiate normal placentation.[60–67] The nature of many of these biomarkers of uterine receptivity suggests that apposition and/or attachment are mediated by cell adhesion molecules (CAMs) and/or CAM/ECM interactions. Once the embryo has established an expanded 'trophoblastic plate', cytotrophoblast cells invade through the basement membrane into the underlying stroma and continue to proliferate[68] (Carnegie stage 5a embryo, Figure 20.2C).

Once embryo attachment and invasion have occurred, access to the vascularized maternal endometrium becomes a priority for the embryo. Its increase in size and metabolism quickly requires increasing quantities of nutrients, oxygen, and better management of cellular waste for survival. By Carnegie stage 5c, the embryo is fully below the luminal surface and is surrounded by a layer of cytotrophoblast which will soon bud to form villi (shown in Figure 20.2D). Development of the placenta and stage 5 ends approximately 11–12 days after ovulation, with the development of the primary villi (see Chapters 31b and 28, respectively, for further details of early implantation stages and placental development).

With further growth and time, cytotrophoblast cells begin to invade the maternal vasculature, becoming incorporated into the wall of maternal vasculature securing access to maternal resources. Fisher and colleagues suggest that cellular mimicry is an essential part of the deception that placental cells use to incorporate into the maternal vasculature, adopting a phenotype matching that of maternal endothelium.[69] Penetration of extravillous cytotrophoblast deeper into the endometrium represents a threat to the maternal endometrium that must be controlled. How the endometrium meets these challenges to be at once receptive and resistive to the invasive behavior of the newly formed placenta is the subject of other chapters of the book.

BIOMARKERS OF UTERINE RECEPTIVITY

Researchers and clinicians continue to search for the best biomarker of uterine receptivity. Biomarkers that predict functionality will be useful for the diagnosis and treatment of couples with infertility. Prediction of success in embryo transfer following in-vitro fertilization (IVF) would offer advantages to the clinician and patient as well as improving the efficiency of allocation of healthcare resources. Progress has been made in this direction.

Histological dating of the endometrium was first described in 1950 and was one of the first approaches to assessing uterine receptivity. As discussed above, these criteria are no longer thought to be discriminatory or useful by themselves for the assessment of infertile couples.[45] With the advent of electron microscopy and immunological and molecular techniques, the number of potential endometrial biomarkers has increased dramatically over the last 20 years.[70–73]

Progesterone is responsible for stimulating a host of endometrial proteins.[74,75] Discovery of new markers has been accelerated by the advent of DNA microarray analyses.[21–23] Some of the best-characterized endometrial biomarkers are shown in Figure 20.3, illustrated with their temporal pattern of maximal expression relative to the putative window of implantation. These and others are discussed below.

Pinopods

Since embryos first interact with the endometrial surface, structural changes on luminal epithelium have been a focus of much attention. Perhaps the best recognized structure associated with the receptive endometrium is the pinopod. These structural adaptations of the apical pole of the luminal surface epithelium were first described by Psychoyos and Mandon.[4] The name was given by Enders and Nelson[16] as 'drinking foot' based on the observation in rats that these projections took up ferritin from the uterine lumen. Best viewed by scanning electron microscopy, these projections have been suggested to function in the absorption of luminal fluid from the endometrial cavity.[70] Much of the value of pinopods was placed on the reported correlation between the timing of their appearance and the putative window of implantation.[76] Nikas and co-workers reported that pinopods are expressed for only 1–2 days and the appearance of these structures varies within the window of implantation.[77] It has further been suggested, as with other markers, that a delay in expression may predict poor reproductive outcome.[78] Ordi et al reported on the variability of pinopods between cycles and between patients.[79] Examination of prospectively collected, LH-timed biopsies indicates that pinopods peak during maximal progesterone secretion but their presence extends well beyond the narrow window of implantation.[37,80] It appears that these structures are a generalized phenomenon of the secretory phase that acquire a dome-like appearance in the late secretory phase.[36,37] The high variability in the temporal and perhaps spatial distribution of pinopods argues against their usefulness as specific biomarkers of a receptive endometrium.

Despite these questions, possible functional significance has been ascribed to the pinopod. In-vitro culture of blastocysts on human endometrium have shown interactions of the embryo with pinopod-like structures.[58] While pinopods are usually observed using scanning electron microscopy (Figure 20.4A), they can also be visualized in paraffin-embedded

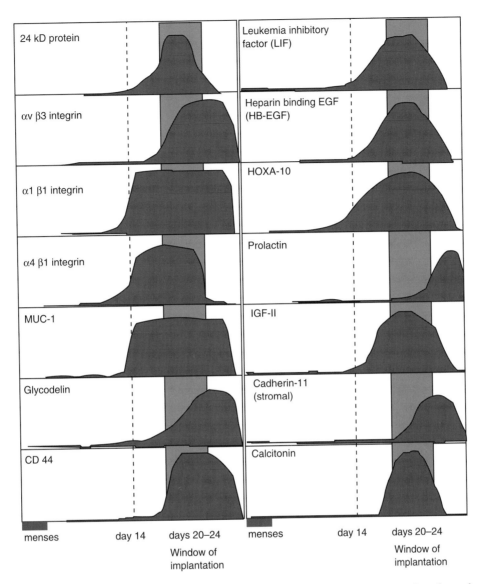

Figure 20.3 The temporal distribution of several endometrial peptides during the menstrual cycle with reference to the window of implantation (shaded bar, cycle days 20–24). The cycle-dependent nature of their expression makes each a potential marker of uterine receptivity. Except for prolactin and cadherin-11, all are expressed on the endometrial epithelium. IGF-II, insulin-like growth factor-II.

endometrial tissue. As shown, secretory phase epithelial proteins such as $\alpha_v\beta_3$ can be detected using immunohistochemistry, staining structures that seem to correspond to these dome-like structures[81] (Figure 20.4B). Other known luminal proteins such as osteopontin (Figure 20.4C) and the L-selectin ligand, as detected using MECA79 antibody (Figure 20.4D), also appear to be associated with these structures. Using novel scanning electron microscopy combined with immunohistochemical techniques, we previously reported that osteopontin specifically localized to pinopods, using silver-enhanced back-scatter.[82] As a privileged site of protein localization, pinopods may function to elevate the surface epithelium to facilitate

embryo–endometrial interaction.[58,83] Further study will be required to establish their true function.

Immunohistochemical biomarkers

Immunohistochemical assessment of the endometrial lining has identified a large number of endometrial proteins that exhibit cycle-dependent expression around the time of implantation.[21,71,84] The first such protein described was the 24 kDa heat shock protein, which is differentially expressed on glandular vs. luminal epithelium but is found on the luminal epithelium around the time of implantation.[85]

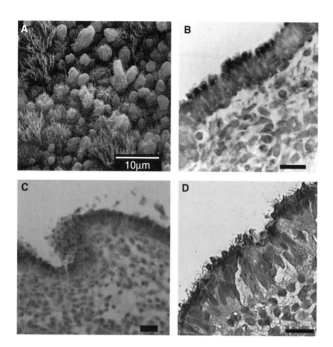

Figure 20.4 Scanning electron micrographs and photomicrographs showing pinopods on the mid-secretory endometrial surface. By scanning electron microscopy, classic pinopods can be seen (**A**). Using various specific antibodies to surface proteins, luminal pinopod-like structures can be visualized by high-powered microscopy for the $\alpha_v\beta_3$ integrin (**B**), osteopontin (**C**), and the ligand for L-selectin (**D**). Relative size is indicated by the bar, which is equal to 10 μm. (See also color plate section.)

Integrins are heterodimeric CAMs that serve as receptors for ECM or cell surface ligands and act as modulators of endometrial and embryonic function. They are perhaps the best characterized of the immunohistochemical markers of uterine receptivity.[86,87] There has been increasing interest in integrins in the reproductive tract, and accumulating data suggest their involvement in both fertilization and implantation.[20,88,89] The endometrium shows a combination of constitutive and cycle-dependent integrin expression.[90–95] Decidualized endometrial stromal cells also display alteration of integrins at the time of implantation.[51,96]

At least three integrins are temporally and spatially restricted, present on endometrial epithelium, and co-expressed only during the window of implantation, on cycle days 20–24 (Figure 20.5). The apical pole of the luminal epithelium contains $\alpha_v\beta_3$, one of the few integrins expressed on the apical surface.[97] This distribution suggests a role in initial embryo–endometrial interaction.

Integrins may interact with extracellular ligands; in the case of the $\alpha_v\beta_3$ integrin, the preferred ligand appear to be osteopontin.[98,99] Expression patterns are similar for both the receptor and ligand, but the regulatory stimuli for each appear to be distinct.[82]

Progesterone induces osteopontin, while the epidermal growth factor (EGF) family induce the β_3 integrin subunit. New insights on certain integrins include their participation in innate immunity. For example, the $\alpha_v\beta_3$ integrin, acting in concert with its ligand osteopontin, and decay-accelerating factor (DAF or factor H) are thought to limit complement activation.[100] Interestingly, complement regulatory proteins are up-regulated at the time of implantation, suggesting the importance of prevention of complement activation at this time.[101] Studies in animal models have demonstrated the essential nature of integrin function during implantation. In the mouse and rabbit, blockade of the $\alpha_v\beta_3$ integrin prevents implantation.[102,103]

Glycodelin, formerly known as PP14, is the major secretory glycoprotein of the glandular endometrium and is expressed during and after the window of implantation. It is also present in blood and may have a role in immune modulation, perhaps in preventing the fetal allograft from eliciting a maternal response.[104] Glycodelin can also block the interaction between sperm and zona pellucida, effectively preventing fertilization.[105] It has been examined as a marker of uterine receptivity, since expression is tied to the levels of progesterone and corpus luteum function.[106] Klentzeris and co-workers found reduced serum glycodelin levels in women with LPD compared to normal cycles,[107] but others have not found a good correlation between glycodelin levels and endometrial histology.[108] Its expression is reduced during the window of implantation in women with endometriosis, suggesting a trend toward progesterone insensitivity in eutopic endometrium in women with this disorder.[109]

Other CAMs have been examined in the endometrium at the time of implantation in either epithelial or stromal cells as possible participants in embryo/trophoblast interactions. These include the hyaluronic acid receptor CD44,[95,110,111] trophinin,[61] and cadherin-11.[112,113] CD44 is present in various isotypes[114] and is more strongly expressed in the secretory endometrium and deciduas. Trophinin is a novel CAM that has been well-described in the human[61,115] but is present in animal models as well.[116,117] It is expressed on the luminal surface in both rodents and humans and may mediate cell–cell interaction between epithelial cells from maternal and epithelial surfaces. Targeted disruption of the gene in mice suggests it is not involved in implantation in the murine model.[118] Cadherin-11 is an epithelial marker and is also expressed in decidua[113] and trophoblast, suggesting a role in endometrial–embryo interaction.[112]

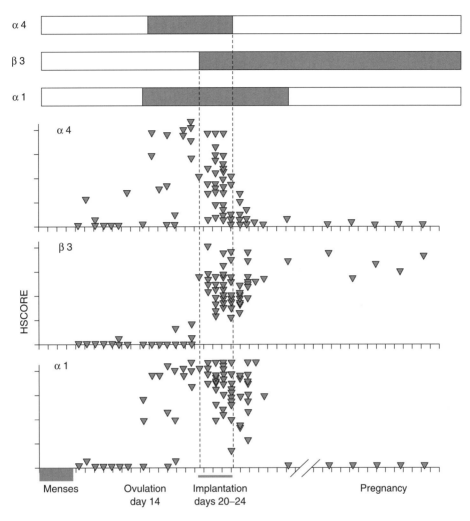

Figure 20.5   Relative intensity of staining for the epithelial α_4, β_3 and α_1 integrin subunits throughout the menstrual cycle and in early pregnancy. Immunohistochemical staining was assessed by a blinded observer using the semi-quantitative HSCORE (ranging from 0 to 4) , as described in the Materials and Methods section, and correlated to the estimate of histological dating based on pathological criteria or by LMP in patients undergoing therapeutic pregnancy termination. The negative staining (open bars) was shown for immunostaining of an HSCORE = 0.7, for each of the three integrin subunits. Positive staining for all three integrin subunits was seen only during a 4-day interval corresponding to cycle days 20–24, based on the histological dating criteria of Noyes et al.[40] This interval of integrin co-expression corresponds to the putative window of implantation. Of the three, only the $\alpha_v\beta_3$ integrin was seen in the epithelium of pregnant endometrium. (Reproduced from Lessey et al,[92] with permission from the publisher, The American Society for Reproductive Medicine.)

Adhesion systems in embryo–endometrial interaction are further discussed in Chapter 19.

Calcitonin is a hormone that is well known for its endocrine role in regulating calcium metabolism. Bagchi and co-workers first reported calcitonin expression in the endometrium of rats[119,120] and its expression is tightly confined to the window of implantation in humans.[121] It appears that this hormone is also a paracrine factor that communicates with the blastocyst to stimulate its activity and differentiation.[122] Other roles for calcitonin may include the regulation of cellular adhesion, providing a potential

mechanism to loosen lateral attachments in luminal epithelium at the time of implantation.[123]

REGULATION AND DYSREGULATION OF ENDOMETRIAL RECEPTIVITY

The discovery of a wide array of specific marker proteins has led to a renewed interest in the regulation of implantation. Furthermore, dysregulation of specific biomarkers may provide an insight into the underlying defects leading to implantation failure in the infertility clinic. Central to the action of steroid hormones in endometrium are the steroid hormone receptors, primarily ERα and the PR.[124] It has long been known that estrogen up-regulates both ERα and PR in the human[46,48,125] as well as in primates and other mammals,[126–128] while progesterone down-regulates both ERα and PR in epithelial cells during the secretory phase of the cycle.[129] Sustained expression is seen in endometrial stromal cells.[48,49,130,131] Interestingly, loss of epithelial ERα and PR correlates closely with the onset of uterine receptivity in humans as well as most other mammals.[132–134] A delay in the opening of the window of implantation is associated with a correctable delay in the down-regulation of epithelial PR.[135]

The normal down-regulation of ERα during the mid-secretory phase of the menstrual cycle does not occur in some women with infertility, including those with polycystic ovary syndrome (PCOS)[136] and endometriosis.[137] In turn, this leads to uterine receptivity defects, as suggested by the delay in the expression of the epithelial integrin $\alpha_v\beta_3$ in such patients.[137] Conversely, in most cases so far tested, loss of this integrin in infertile women is associated with failure of down-regulation of the estrogen receptor. Since this biomarker is negatively regulated by estrogen,[138] it follows that loss of ERα coincides with its onset of expression in the mid-secretory phase.

Causes of persistent endometrial ERα in mid-secretory phase might include inadequate circulating progesterone or loss of cellular sensitivity to progesterone. In either case, reduced expression of 17β-hydroxysteroid dehydrogenase would be predicted. This progestin-induced enzyme metabolizes estradiol to the less active estrone. Increased estrogenic activity might play a role as well, since estrogen up-regulates its own receptor. Precise causes of persistent ERα may vary with diagnosis and therefore treatment will need to be tailored. In endometriosis, for example, abnormal expression of aromatase could increase local estrogen production.[139] Abnormal progestin responses have been noted in women with endometriosis, including a reduction in 17β-hydroxysteroid dehydrogenase activity.[109,140–144] In addition to elevated ERα, PCOS patients exhibit elevated endometrial androgen receptors (AR). In the case of PCOS, overexpression of steroid receptor coactivators may also help explain the elevated estrogenicity coupled with a poor progesterone response.[136] Treatment in each instance might include administration of stronger progestins,[143] antiestrogens (to block the ERα)[137] or aromatase inhibitors.[145,146]

In summary, endometrial receptivity is determined by the coordinated influences of estrogen and progesterone. These steroids require receptors and their associated enzymes and regulators, and their actions induce a large cadre of other proteins, including CAMs, ECM, growth factors, and cytokines that contribute to the process of embryo attachment. Amongst biomarkers of uterine receptivity, there are several candidates that may help predict fertility while at the same time contributing to improved understanding of endocrine dysfunction. Provided with these clues, better treatment options for women with implantation failure are evolving, and targeted therapeutics are on the horizon.

REFERENCES

1. Bischof P, Aplin JD, Bentin-Ley U et al. Implantation of the human embryo: research lines and models. From the implantation research network 'Fruitful'. Gynecol Obstet Invest 2006; 62: 206–16.
2. Aplin JD, Kimber SJ. Trophoblast–uterine interactions at implantation. Reprod Biol Endocrinol 2004; 2: 48.
3. Psychoyos A. Hormonal control of ovoimplantation. Vitam Horm 1973; 31: 201–56.
4. Psychoyos A, Mandon P. [Study of the surface of the uterine epithelium by scanning electron microscopy.] C R Hebd Seances Acad Sci D 1971; 272: 2723–5. [in French]
5. Psychoyos A, Martel D. Embryo–endometrial interactions at implantation. J Reprod Fertil 1985; 41: 195.
6. Psychoyos A, Mori T, Tominaga T, Aono T, Hiroi M. The implantation window: basic and clinical aspects. Frontiers in Endocrinology. Tokyo: Ares-Serono Symposia, 1995 (vol 4).
7. McLaren A, Michie D. Studies on the transfer of fertilized mouse eggs to uterine foster-mothers. J Exp Biol 1954; 33: 394.
8. McLaren A, Segal SJ, Crozier R, Corfman PA, Condliffe PG. Blastocyst activation. The Regulation of Mammalian Reproduction. London: Thomas Springfield, 1973.
9. Finn CA. The implantation reaction. In: Wynn RM, ed. Biology of the Uterus. New York: Plenum Press, 1977.
10. Hodgen GD. Surrogate embryo transfer combined with estrogen–progesterone therapy in monkeys: implantation, gestation, and delivery without ovaries. JAMA 1983; 250: 2167–71.
11. Enders AC. Implantation (embryology). Encycloped Hum Biol 1991; 4: 423–30.
12. Enders AC. Transition from lacunar to villous stage of implantation in the macaque, including establishment of the trophoblastic shell. Acta Anat (Basel) 1995; 152: 151–69.
13. Enders AC, Glasser SR, Mulholland J, Psychoyos A. Contributions of comparative studies to understanding mechanisms of implantation. Endocrinology of Embryo–Endometrium Interactions. New York: Plenum Press, 1994.
14. Enders AC, Liu IK. Trophoblast–uterine interactions during equine chorionic girdle cell maturation, migration, and transformation. Am J Anat 1991; 192: 366–81.
15. Enders AC, Mead RA. Progression of trophoblast into the endometrium during implantation in the western spotted skunk. Anat Rec 1996; 244: 297–315.
16. Enders AC, Nelson DM. Pinocytotic activity of the uterus of the rat. Am J Anat 1973; 138: 277.
17. Enders AC, Schlafke S. Cytological aspects of trophoblast–uterine interactions in early implantation. Am J Anat 1969; 125: 1.
18. Enders AC, Schlafke S. Implantation in the ferret: epithelial penetration. Am J Anat 1979; 133: 291.
19. Enders AC, Schlafke S, Welsh AO. Trophoblastic and uterine luminal epithelial surfaces at the time of blastocyst adhesion in the rat. Am J Anat 1980; 159: 59–72.

20. Carson DD, Bagchi I, Dey SK et al. Embryo implantation. Dev Biol 2000; 223: 217–37.

21. Carson DD, Lagow E, Thathiah A et al. Changes in gene expression during the early to mid-luteal (receptive phase) transition in human endometrium detected by high-density microarray screening. Mol Hum Reprod 2002; 8: 871–9.

22. Talbi S, Hamilton AE, Vo KC et al. Molecular phenotyping of human endometrium distinguishes menstrual cycle phases and underlying biological processes in normo-ovulatory women. Endocrinology 2006; 147: 1097–121.

23. Kao LC, Tulac S, Lobo S et al. Global gene profiling in human endometrium during the window of implantation. Endocrinology 2002; 143: 2119.

24. Yoshinaga K, Yoshinaga K, Mori T. Receptor concept in implantation research. Development of Preimplantation Embryos and Their Environment. New York: Alan Liss, 1989.

25. Anderson TL, Hodgen GD. Uterine receptivity in the primate. Prog Clin Biol Res 1989; 294: 389–99.

26. Rogers PAW, Murphy CR, Yoshinaga K. Uterine receptivity for implantation: human studies. Blastocyst Implantation: Serono Symposia, USA, 1989.

27. Cowell TP. Implantation and development of mouse eggs transferred to the uterus of non-progestational mice. J Reprod Fertil 1969; 19: 239–45.

28. Fawcett DW. The development of mouse ova under the capsule of the kidney. Anat Rec 1950; 108: 71–91.

29. Kirby DR. The development of mouse blastocysts transplanted to the scrotal and cryptorchid testis. J Anat 1963; 97: 119–30.

30. Hertig AT, Rock J, Adams EC. A description of 34 human ova within the first 17 days of development. Am J Anat 1956; 98: 435–93.

31. Navot D, Bergh PA, Williams M et al. An insight into early reproductive processes through the in vivo model of ovum donation. J Clin Endocrinol Metab 1991; 72: 408–14.

32. Navot D, Scott RT, Droesch K et al. The window of embryo transfer and the efficiency of human conception in vitro. Fertil Steril 1991; 55: 114–18.

33. Wilcox AJ, Baird DD, Wenberg CR. Time of implantation of the conceptus and loss of pregnancy. N Engl J Med 1999; 340: 1796–9.

34. Murray MJ, Lessey BA. Embryo implantation and tumor metastasis: common pathways of invasion and angiogenesis. Semin Reprod Endocrinol 1999; 17: 275–90.

35. Slayden OD, Brenner RM. Hormonal regulation and localization of estrogen, progestin and androgen receptors in the endometrium of nonhuman primates: effects of progesterone receptor antagonists. Arch Histol Cytol 2004; 67: 393–409.

36. Murphy CR. Understanding the apical surface markers of uterine receptivity: pinopods -or uterodomes? Hum Reprod 2000; 15: 2451–4.

37. Usadi RS, Murray MJ, Bagnell RC et al. Temporal and morphologic characteristics of pinopod expression across the secretory phase of the endometrial cycle in normally cycling women with proven fertility. Fertil Steril 2003; 79: 970–4.

38. Baulieu EE. RU486: a compound that gets itself talked about. Hum Reprod 1994; (9 Suppl 1): 1–6.

39. De Ziegler D, Frydman R, Bouchard P. Contribution of estrogen to the morphology of "secretory" endometrium? Fertil Steril 1995; 63: 1135.

40. Noyes RW, Hertig AI, Rock J. Dating the endometrial biopsy. Fertil Steril 1950; 1: 3–25.

41. Jones GS. Some newer aspects of management of infertility. JAMA 1949; 141: 1123–9.

42. Fritz MA, Lessey BA. Defective luteal function. In: Fraser IS, Jansen RPS, Lobo RA, Whitehead MI, eds. Estrogens and Progestogens in Clinical Practice. London: Churchhill Livingstone, 1998 : 437–53.

43. Murray MJ, Meyer WR, Zaino RJ et al. A critical analysis of the accuracy, reproducibility, and clinical utility of histologic endometrial dating in fertile women. Fertil Steril 2004; 81: 1333–43.

44. Myers ER, Silva S, Barnhart K et al. Interobserver and intraobserver variability in the histological dating of the endometrium in fertile and infertile women. Fertil Steril 2004; 82: 1278–82.

45. Coutifaris C, Myers ER, Guzick DS et al. Histological dating of timed endometrial biopsy tissue is not related to fertility status. Fertil Steril 2004; 82: 1264–72.

46. Flickinger GL, Elsner C, Illington DV, Muechler EK, Mikhail G. Estrogen and progesterone receptors in the female genital tract of humans and monkeys. Ann NY Acad Sci 1977; 286: 180.

47. Elsner CW, Illingworth DV, De Groot K, Flickinger GL, Mikhail G. Cytosol and nuclear estrogen receptor in the genital tract of the rhesus monkey. J Steroid Biochem 1977; 8: 151–5.

48. Lessey BA, Killam AP, Metzger DA et al. Immunohistochemical analysis of human uterine estrogen and progesterone receptors throughout the menstrual cycle. J Clin Endocrinol Metab 1988; 67: 334–40.

49. Garcia E, Bouchard P, De Brux J et al. Use of immunocytochemistry of progesterone and estrogen receptors for endometrial dating. J Clin Endocrinol Metab 1988; 67: 80–7.

50. Aplin JD, Charlton AK, Ayad S. An immunohistochemical study of human endometrial extracellular matrix during the menstrual cycle and first trimester of pregnancy. Cell Tissue Res 1988; 253: 231–40.

51. Ruck P, Marzusch K, Kaiserling E et al. Distribution of cell adhesion molecules in decidua of early human pregnancy: an immunohistochemical study. Lab Invest 1994; 71: 94–101.

52. Aplin JD. The cell biology of human implantation. Placenta 1996; 17: 269–75.

53. Morrish DW, Dakour J, Li HS. Functional regulation of human trophoblast differentiation. J Reprod Immunol 1998; 39: 179–95.

54. Croxotto HB, Ortiz ME, Diaz S et al. Studies on the duration of egg transport by the human oviduct. II. Ovum location at various intervals following luteinizing hormone peak. Am J Obstet Gynecol 1978; 132: 629–34.

55. Buster J, Bustillo M, Rodi I et al. Biologic and morphologic development of donated human ova recovered by nonsurgical uterine lavage. Am J Obstet Gynecol 1985; 153: 211–17.

56. Klaffky EJ, Gonzales IM, Sutherland AE. Trophoblast cells exhibit differential responses to laminin isoforms. Dev Biol 2006; 292: 277–89.

57. Sutherland A. Mechanisms of implantation in the mouse: differentiation and functional importance of trophoblast giant cell behavior. Dev Biol 2003; 258: 241–51.

58. Bentin-Ley U, Sjögren A, Nilsson L et al. Presence of uterine pinopodes at the embryo–endometrial interface during human implantation in vitro. Hum Reprod 1999; 14: 515–20.

59. Denker HW. Implantation: a cell biological paradox. J Exp Zool 1993; 266: 541–58.

60. Campbell S, Swann HR, Seif MW, Kimber SJ, Aplin JD. Cell adhesion molecules on the oocyte and preimplantation human embryo. Hum Reprod 1995; 10: 1571–8.

61. Fukuda MN, Sato T, Nakayama J et al. Trophinin and tastin, a novel cell adhesion molecule complex with potential involvement in embryo implantation. Genes Dev 1995; 9: 1199–210.

62. Turpeenniemi-Hujanen T, Feinberg RF, Kauppila A, Puistola U. Extracellular matrix interactions in early human embryos: implications for normal implantation events. Fertil Steril 1995; 64: 132–8.

63. Aplin JD, Spanswick C, Behzad F, Kimber SJ, Vicovac L. Integrins β_5, β_3, α_v are apically distributed in endometrial epithelium. Mol Hum Reprod 1996; 2: 527–34.

64. Lessey BA, Ilesanmi AO, Lessey MA et al. Luminal and glandular endometrial epithelium express integrins differentially throughout the menstrual cycle: implications for implantation, contraception, and infertility. Am J Reprod Immunol 1996; 35: 195–204.

65. Raab G, Kover K, Paria BC et al. Mouse preimplantation blastocysts adhere to cells expressing the transmembrane form of heparin-binding EGF-like growth factor. Development 1996; 122: 637–45.

66. Yoo HJ, Barlow DH, Mardon HJ. Temporal and spatial regulation of expression of heparin-binding epidermal growth factor-like growth factor in the human endometrium: a possible role in blastocyst implantation. Dev Genet 1997; 21: 102–8.

67. Genbacev OD, Prakobphol A, Foulk RA et al. Trophoblast L-selectin-mediated adhesion at the maternal–fetal interface. Science 2003; 299: 405–8.

68. Chobotova K, Karpovich N, Carver J et al. Heparin-binding epidermal growth factor and its receptors mediate decidualization and potentiate survival of human endometrial stromal cells. J Clin Endocrinol Metab 2005; 90: 913–19.

69. Zhou Y, Fisher SJ, Janatpour M et al. Human cytotrophoblasts adopt a vascular phenotype as they differentiate. A strategy for successful endovascular invasion? J Clin Invest 1997; 99: 2139–51.

70. Anderson TL, Yoshinaga K. Biomolecular markers for the window of uterine receptivity. Blastocyst Implantation. Boston, MA: Adams Publishing Group, 1993 (vol. 1).

71. Ilesanmi AO, Hawkins DA, Lessey BA. Immunohistochemical markers of uterine receptivity in the human endometrium. Microsc Res Tech 1993; 25: 208–22.

72. Yaron Y, Botchan A, Amit A et al. Endometrial receptivity in the light of modern assisted reproductive technologies. Fertil Steril 1994; 62: 225–32.

73. Bulletti C, Flamigni C, de Ziegler D. Implantation markers and endometriosis. Reprod Biomed Online 2005; 11: 464–8.

74. Joshi SG. Progestin-regulated proteins of the human endometrium. Semin Reprod Endocrinol 1983; 1: 221–36.

75. Bell SC, Drife JO. Secretory proteins of the endometrium – potential markers for endometrial dysfunction. Baillière's Clin Obstet Gynaecol 1989; 3: 271–91.

76. Martel D, Frydman R, Sarantis L et al. Scanning electron microscopy of the uterine luminal epithelium as a marker of the implantation window. In: Yoshinaga K, ed. Blastocyst Implantation. Boston, MA: Adams Publishing Group, 1993: 225–30.

77. Nikas G, Drakakis P, Loutradis D et al. Uterine pinopodes as markers of the 'nidation window' in cycling women receiving exogenous oestradiol and progesterone. Hum Reprod 1995; 10: 1208–13.

78. Edwards RG. Physiological and molecular aspects of human implantation. Hum Reprod 1995; 10(Suppl)2: 1.

79. Ordi J, Creus M, Ferrer B et al. Midluteal endometrial biopsy and alphavbeta3 integrin expression in the evaluation of the endometrium in infertility: implications for fecundity. Int J Gynecol Pathol 2002; 21: 231–8.

80. Acosta AA, Elberger L, Borghi M et al. Endometrial dating and determination of the window of implantation in healthy fertile women. Fertil Steril 2000; 73: 788–98.

81. Apparao KB, Illera J, Beyler SA, et al. Regulated expression of Osteopontin in the peri-implantation rabbit uterus. Biol Reprod 2003; 68: 1484–90.

82. Lessey BA. Two pathways of progesterone action in the human endometrium: implications for implantation and contraception. Steroids 2003; 68: 809–15.

83. Bentin-Ley U, Horn T, Sjögren A et al. Ultrastructure of human blastocyst–endometrial interactions in vitro. J Reprod Fertil 2000; 120: 337–50.

84. Lindhard A, Bentin-Ley U, Ravn V et al. Biochemical evaluation of endometrial function at the time of implantation. Fertil Steril 2002; 78: 221–33.

85. Ciocca DR, Asch RS, Adams DJ, McGuire WL. Evidence for the modulation of a 24K protein in human endometrium during the menstrual cycle. J Clin Endocrinol Metab 1983; 57: 496–9.

86. Lessey BA. Endometrial integrins and the establishment of uterine receptivity. Hum Reprod 1998; 13(Suppl 3): 247–58.

87. Lessey BA. Endometrial receptivity and the window of implantation. Baillière's Clin Obst Gynaecol 2000; 14: 775.

88. Bronson RA, Fusi FM. Integrins and human reproduction. Mol Hum Reprod 1996; 2: 153–68.

89. Sueoka K, Shiokawa S, Miyazaki T et al. Integrins and reproductive physiology: expression and modulation in fertilization, embryogensis, and implantation. Fertil Steril 1997; 67: 799–811.

90. Lessey BA. Integrin cell adhesion molecules: immunohistochemical evaluation of endometrial integrin receptor subunits and extracellular matrix components in endometriosis. Am Fert Soc Ann Mtg 1992; O-19: S8.

91. Tabibzadeh S. Patterns of expression of integrin molecules in human endometrium throughout the menstrual cycle. Hum Reprod 1992; 7: 876–82.

92. Lessey BA, Castelbaum AJ, Buck CA et al. Further characterization of endometrial integrins during the menstrual cycle and in pregnancy. Fertil Steril 1994; 62: 497–506.

93. Lessey BA, Castelbaum AJ, Sawin SJ et al. Aberrant integrin expression in the endometrium of women with endometriosis. J Clin Endocrinol Metab 1994; 79: 643–9.

94. Meyer WR, Castelbaum AJ, Somkuti S et al. Hydrosalpinges adversely affect markers of endometrial receptivity. Hum Reprod 1997; 12: 1393–8.

95. Albers A, Thie M, Hohn HP, Denker HW. Differential expression and localization of integrins and CD44 in the membrane domains of human uterine epithelial cells during the menstrual cycle. Acta Anat (Basel) 1995; 153: 12–19.

96. Grosskinsky CM, Yowell CW, Sun J, Parise LV, Lessey BA. Modulation of integrin expression in endometrial stromal cells in vitro. J Clin Endocrinol Metab 1996; 81: 2047–54.

97. Lessey BA, Ilesanmi AO, Sun J et al. Luminal and glandular endometrial epithelium express integrins differentially throughout the menstrual cycle: implications for implantation, contraception, and infertility. Am J Reprod Immunol 1996; 35: 195–204.

98. Apparao KB, Murray MJ, Fritz MA et al. Osteopontin and its receptor alpha(v)beta(3) integrin are coexpressed in the human endometrium during the menstrual cycle but regulated differentially. J Clin Endocrinol Metab 2001; 86: 4991–5000.

99. von Wolff M, Strowitzki T, Becker V et al. Endometrial osteopontin, a ligand of β_3-integrin, is maximally expressed around the time of the "implantation" window. Fertil Steril 2001; 76: 775–81.

100. Jain A, Karadag A, Fohr B, Fisher LW, Fedarko NS. Three SIBLINGs (small integrin-binding ligand, N-linked glycoproteins) enhance factor H's cofactor activity enabling MCP-like cellular evasion of complement-mediated attack. J Biol Chem 2002; 277: 13700–8.

101. Hasty LA, Lambris JD, Lessey BA, Pruksananonda K, Lyttle CR. Hormonal regulation of complement components and receptors throughout the menstrual cycle. Am J Obstet Gynecol 1994; 170: 168–75.

102. Illera MJ, Cullinan E, Gui Y et al. Blockade of the alpha(v)beta(3) integrin adversely affects implantation in the mouse. Biol Reprod 2000; 62: 1285–90.

103. Illera MJ, Lorenzo PL, Gui YT A role for alpha(v)beta(3) integrin during implantation in the rabbit model. Biol Reprod 2003; 68: 766–71.

104. Clark GF, Oehninger S, Patankar MS et al. A role for glycoconjugates in human development: the human feto-embryonic defence system hypothesis. Hum Reprod 1996; 11: 467–73.

105. Oehninger S, Coddington CC, Hodgen GD, Seppala M. Factors affecting fertilization: endometrial placental protein

14 reduces the capacity of human spermatozoa to bind to the human zona pellucida. Fertil Steril 1995; 63: 377–83.

106. Stewart DR, Erikson MS, Erikson ME et al. The role of relaxin in glycodelin secretion. J Clin Endocrinol Metab 1997; 82: 839–46.

107. Klentzeris LD, Bulmer JN, Seppälä M et al. Placental protein 14 in cycles with normal and retarded endometrial differentiation. Hum Reprod 1994; 9: 394–8.

108. Batista MC, Cartledge TP, Nieman LK et al. Characterization of the normal progesterone and placental protein 14 responses to human chorionic gonadotropin stimulation in the luteal phase. Fertil Steril 1994; 61: 637–44.

109. Kao LC, Germeyer A, Tulac S et al. Expression profiling of endometrium from women with endometriosis reveals candidate genes for disease-based implantation failure and infertility. Endocrinology 2003; 144: 2870–81.

110. Yaegashi N, Fujita N, Yajima A, Nakamura M. Menstrual cycle dependent expression of CD44 in normal human endometrium. Hum Pathol 1995; 26: 862–5.

111. Saegusa M, Hashimura M, Okayasu I. CD44 expression in normal, hyperplastic, and malignant endometrium. J Pathol 1998; 184: 297–306.

112. MacCalman CD, Furth EE, Omigbodun A et al. Regulated expression of cadherin-11 in human epithelial cells: a role for cadherin-11 in trophoblast–endometrium interactions? Dev Dyn 1996; 206: 201–11.

113. Getsios S, Chen GTC, Stephenson MD et al. Regulated expression of cadherin-6 and cadherin-11 in the glandular epithelial and stromal cells of the human endometrium. Dev Dyn 1998; 211: 238–47.

114. Behzad F, Seif MW, Campbell S, Aplin JD. Expression of two isoforms of CD44 in human endometrium. Biol Reprod 1994; 51: 739–47.

115. Suzuki N, Nakayama J, Shih IM et al. Expression of trophinin, tastin, and bystin by trophoblast and endometrial cells in human placenta. Biol Reprod 1999; 60: 621–7.

116. Suzuki N, Nadano D, Paria BC et al. Trophinin expression in the mouse uterus coincides with implantation and is hormonally regulated but not induced by implanting blastocysts. Endocrinology 2000; 141: 4247–54.

117. Nakano S, Kishi H, Ogawa H et al. Trophinin is expressed in the porcine endometrium during the estrous cycle. J Reprod Dev 2003; 49: 127–34.

118. Nadano D, Sugihara K, Paria BC et al. Significant differences between mouse and human trophinins are revealed by their expression patterns and targeted disruption of mouse trophinin gene. Biol Reprod 2002; 66: 313–21.

119. Zhu LJ, Bagchi MK, Bagchi IC. Attenuation of calcitonin gene expression in pregnant rat uterus leads to a block in embryonic implantation. Endocrinology 1998; 139: 330–9.

120. Zhu LJ, Cullinan-Bove K, Polihronis M, Bagchi MK, Bagchi IC. Calcitonin is a progesterone-regulated marker that forecasts the receptive state of endometrium during implantation. Endocrinology 1998; 139: 3923–34.

121. Kumar S, Zhu LJ, Polihronis M et al. Progesterone induces calcitonin gene expression in human endometrium within the putative window of implantation. J Clin Endocrinol Metab 1998; 83: 4443–50.

122. Wang J, Rout UK, Bagchi IC, Armant DR. Expression of calcitonin receptors in mouse preimplantation embryos and their function in the regulation of blastocyst differentiation by calcitonin. Development 1998; 125: 4293–302.

123. Li Q, Wang J, Armant DR, Bagchi MK, Bagchi IC. Calcitonin down-regulates E-cadherin expression in rodent uterine epithelium during implantation. J Biol Chem 2002; 277: 46447–55.

124. Katzenellenbogen BS. Dynamics of steroid hormone receptor action. Ann Rev Physiol 1980; 42: 17–35.

125. Sanborn BM, Kuo KS, Held B. Estrogen and progesterone binding site concentrations in human endometrium and cervix throughout the menstrual cycle and in tissue from women taking oral contraceptives. J Steroid Biochem 1978; 9: 951.

126. Brenner RM, West NB, McClellan MC. Estrogen and progestin receptors in the reproductive tract of male and female primates. Biol Reprod 1990; 42: 11–19.

127. Lessey BA, Gorell TA. A cytoplasmic estradiol receptor in the immature beagle uterus. J Steroid Biochem Mol Biol 1980; 13: 211–17.

128. Lessey BA, Gorell TA. Analysis of the progesterone receptor in the beagle uterus and oviduct. J Steroid Biochem Mol Biol 1980; 13: 1173–80.

129. Savouret JF, Chauchereau A, Misrahi M et al. The progesterone receptor. Biological effects of progestins and antiprogestins. Hum Reprod 1994; 9(Suppl 1): 7–11.

130. Press MF, Nousek Goebl NA, Bur M, Greene GL. Estrogen receptor localization in the female genital tract. Am J Pathol 1986; 123: 280–92.

131. Press MF, Udove JA, Greene GL. Progesterone receptor distribution in the human endometrium. Analysis using monoclonal antibodies to the human progesterone receptor. Am J Pathol 1988; 131: 112–24.

132. Geisert RD, Pratt TN, Bazer FW, Mayes JS, Watson GH. Immunocytochemical localization and changes in endometrial progestin receptor protein during the porcine oestrous cycle and early pregnancy. Reprod Fertil Dev 1994; 6: 749–60.

133. Mead RA, Eroschenko VP. Changes in uterine estrogen and progesterone receptors during delayed implantation and early implantation in the spotted skunk. Biol Reprod 1995; 53: 827–33.

134. Tan J, Paria BC, Dey SK, Das SK. Differential uterine expression of estrogen and progesterone receptors correlates with uterine preparation for implantation and decidualization in the mouse. Endocrinology 1999; 140: 5310.

135. Lessey BA, Yeh I, Castelbaum AJ et al. Endometrial progesterone receptors and markers of uterine receptivity in the window of implantation. Fertil Steril 1996; 65: 477–83.

136. Gregory CW, Wilson EM, Apparao KB et al. Steroid receptor coactivator expression throughout the menstrual cycle in normal and abnormal endometrium. J Clin Endocrinol Metab 2002; 87: 2960–6.

137. Lessey BA, Palomino WA, Apparao KB, Young SL, Lininger RA. Estrogen receptor-alpha (ER-alpha) and defects in uterine receptivity in women. Reprod Biol Endocrinol 2006; Suppl 1: 59.

138. Somkuti SG, Yuan L, Fritz MA, Lessey BA. Epidermal growth factor and sex steroids dynamically regulate a marker of endometrial receptivity in Ishikawa cells. J Clin Endocrinol Metab 1997; 82: 2192–7.

139. Noble L, Simpson E, Johns A, Bulun S. Aromatase expression in endometriosis. J Clin Endocrinol Metab 1996; 81: 174–9.

140. Lessey BA, Metzger DA, Haney AF, McCarty KS Jr. Immunohistochemical analysis of estrogen and progesterone receptors in endometriosis: comparison with normal endometrium during the menstrual cycle and the effect of medical therapy. Fertil Steril 1989; 51: 409–15.

141. Sharpe-Timms KL. Endometrial anomalies in women with endometriosis. Ann NY Acad Sci 2001; 943: 131–47.

142. Igarashi TM, Bruner-Tran KL, Yeaman GR et al. Reduced expression of progesterone receptor-B in the endometrium of women with endometriosis and in cocultures of endometrial cells exposed to 2,3,7,8-tetrachlorodibenzo-p-dioxin. Fertil Steril 2005; 84: 67–74.

143. Bruner-Tran KL, Zhang Z, Eisenberg E, Winneker RC, Osteen KG. Down-regulation of endometrial matrix metalloproteinase-3 and -7 expression in vitro and therapeutic regression of experimental endometriosis in vivo

by a novel nonsteroidal progesterone receptor agonist, tanaproget. J Clin Endocrinol Metab 2006; 91: 1554–60.

144. Cheng YH, Imir A, Suzuki T et al. SP1 and SP3 mediate progesterone-dependent induction of the 17beta hydroxy-steroid dehydrogenase type 2 gene in human endometrium. Biol Reprod 2006; 75: 605–14.

145. Casper RF, Mitwally MF. Review: aromatase inhibitors for ovulation induction. J Clin Endocrinol Metab 2006; 91: 760–71.

146. Mitwally MF, Biljan MM, Casper RF. Pregnancy outcome after the use of an aromatase inhibitor for ovarian stimulation. Am J Obstet Gynecol 2005; 192: 381–6.

21 Connexins: indicators for hormonal and blastocyst-mediated endometrial differentiation

Ruth Grümmer and Elike Winterhager

Synopsis

Background

- Gap junctions are channels formed in the plasma membranes of adherent cells.
- They are formed by a family of 21 proteins in the human genome known as connexins.
- Each gap junction channel consists of a pair of hemichannels (connexons), which contain six connexins arranged around a water-filled pore.
- Gap junction-mediated communication is used in intercellular signaling.
- Cell–cell communication serves as a general control mechanism for coordinated tissue differentiation.
- Connexins are also thought to have channel-independent functions.
- Connexins are discussed as tumor suppressor genes.

Basic Science

- The main connexin (Cx) isoforms expressed in the rodent and human endometrium have been identified as Cx26 and Cx43.
- In the preimplantation period of pregnancy, cells in the endometrium of several animal species lack gap junctional communication due to suppression by maternal progesterone.
- Non-physiological concentrations of estradiol disturb this progesterone-mediated suppression in the receptive phase via the estrogen receptor ERα.
- Endometrial Cx26 expression can be used as a sensitive reporter of estrogenic action in bioassays.
- At implantation, the blastocyst induces Cx26 locally in the epithelial cells of the implantation chamber and Cx43 in the surrounding decidua in both rats and mice.
- This blastocyst-mediated up-regulation is independent of the receptor isoform ERα.
- IL-1β, catechol estrogen, and $PGF_{2\alpha}$ can be regarded as candidates involved in embryonic signaling.
- Cx26 may transmit apoptotic signals laterally through epithelial cells in the implantation chamber.

Clinical

- Gap junction proteins exhibit variations in expression in endometrium during the menstrual cycle.
- In endometriosis, the ectopic lesions reveal a connexin pattern different from healthy endometrium.
- Gap junctional communication is diminished in both endometrial hyperplasia and carcinoma.

INTRODUCTION

Implantation of a mammalian blastocyst into the endometrium is a complex process and requires a series of precisely synchronized physiological and cell biological events. Disruption of this synchrony in the differentiation process of the blastocyst and the uterine epithelium leads to failure of implantation. Although reproduction is critical to species survival, establishment of pregnancy is inefficient in humans. Here, 20% of spontaneous abortions during pregnancy are estimated to occur before pregnancy is detected clinically,[1] and the pregnancy rate in in-vitro fertilization (IVF) programs still remains as low as 20–30% in spite of the high rate of successful fertilization.[2] Although this inefficiency of the implantation process could in part be considered as a gatekeeper to support only healthy embryos for ongoing pregnancies, the molecular mechanisms of this impairment in the feto–maternal cross-talk need clarification.

In preparation for embryo implantation, the endometrium has to differentiate into a receptive state which allows adhesion and invasion of the trophoblast.[3,4] This endometrial differentiation is primarily coordinated by the ovarian hormones progesterone and estrogen that modulate uterine events in a spatiotemporal manner as a prerequisite for the endometrium to interact with blastocyst signals.[5,6] In recent years, several important signal cascades have been identified using gene targeting in mice and gene array approaches. However, the comprehensive cell biological mechanisms, regulation of genes, and signal cascades that are involved in the changes of the endometrial program on the one hand and in those induced by the implanting blastocyst on the other hand are only partly defined.[7] Identification of the genes needed for the different cell biological processes involved in the consecutive steps of the implantation reaction, such as apposition, adhesion, and invasion,[8] is indispensable to understanding blastocyst–endometrial cross-talk.

To gain more insight into the impact of the embryo on the maternal program, animal models – mostly rodents – have been used in recent years. Numerous molecules regulated by ovarian hormones preceding the implantation reaction have been identified, including cytokines, chemokines, and growth factors as well as factors involved in prostaglandin synthesis.[9,10]

As the first remarkable sign of a rodent blastocyst signal, an increasing vascular permeability at the site of blastocyst implantation has been described.[11] Signal cascades involved in the cross-talk between the blastocyst and the receptive uterus have been described in rodents.[7,12,13] In rabbit, blastocyst signals trigger local reprogramming of the uterine epithelium by induction of cell–cell communication.[14] Gap junction connexin genes are very sensitively regulated not only by blastocyst signals but also by ovarian hormones, providing the opportunity to separate these processes – hormonal regulation vs regulation by blastocyst signaling – from each other.[15–17]

In humans, many genes are regulated by ovarian steroids during the receptive phase.[18] To evaluate the changing gene pattern during preimplantation, in recent years microarray analyses comparing human endometrium of the late proliferative phase with that of the mid-luteal phase, representing the receptive phase, have been performed. Specific functions in the endometrium during implantation remain to be established for many of these genes.[19–22] Effects of the

embryo on the molecular events in the endometrium are difficult to investigate in humans. Using in-vitro co-cultures of human blastocysts and endometrial epithelial cells, regulation of endometrial expression of interleukin-8 and certain chemokine receptors has been demonstrated in the presence of a blastocyst,[23] and a role for MUC1, a mucin of the epithelial glycocalyx, has been proposed in blastocyst adhesion.[24]

In this chapter, we focus on the ovarian steroid regulation of connexin genes during the receptive phase in the endometrium of humans and rodents, and their induction in response to embryo implantation in the rodent endometrium. Furthermore, we add some more information for the role of gap junction connexins in human reproduction and their possible involvement in endometrial diseases.

GAP JUNCTIONS: STRUCTURE AND FUNCTION

Connexin proteins form intercellular channels in vertebrates as a simple pathway for rapid, direct communication between adjacent cells. Each gap junction channel consists of a pair of hemichannels (connexons), which contain six connexin proteins arranged around a water-filled pore (Figure 21.1). Up to the present, 21 members of the connexin gene family have been identified in the human and 20 in the mouse genome.[25,26] The capability for direct exchange of small molecules, ions, and second messengers between cells enables the channels to control and coordinate diverse physiological roles during embryonal development as well as in adult organisms. Consequently, mutations in the connexin proteins resulting in modulations of channel properties are associated with a large variety of diseases in humans and very specific pathologies in experimental animals.[27] The specific function of the connexins in development and organ functions has been evaluated by systemically knocking out the corresponding genes. The phenotypes resulting from the absence of specific connexin isoforms have been summarized.[26,27] Replacing one channel isoform by another (knock-ins) revealed that channel redundancy is incomplete. Each channel has unique functions but at least some capacities are shared because knock-ins are able to rescue partially the phenotype of the knockouts.[28,29]

The high diversity and specification of channel functions cannot only be explained by transfer of ions and second messengers but needs additional explanations. Recent publications suggested a channel-independent role for connexins in intracellular signaling by interacting

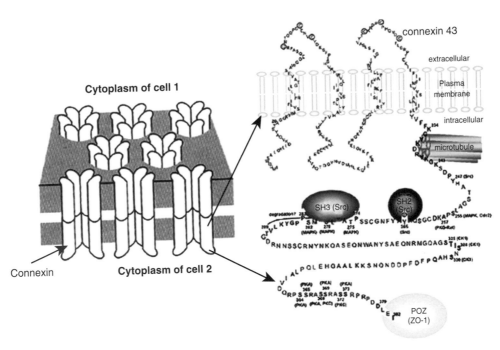

Figure 21.1 Gap junction structure and amino acid sequence of Cx43. Each gap junction channel consists of a pair of hemichannels (connexons), which contain six connexin proteins arranged around a water-filled pore. Each connexin reveals four transmembrane domains. The C-terminal region differs in length and amino acid sequence among the various connexin isoforms and may contain binding sites for interacting partners like ZO-1, α- and β-tubulin, and c-Src. (Modified from Giepmans.[93])

with other proteins. It could be demonstrated that, independent from gap junction channel formation, the connexin43 (Cx43) protein is able to effect growth control as well as influencing cellular functions like adhesion and migration.[30,31] The C-terminal region, which differs in length and amino acid sequence among the various connexin isoforms, plays an important role in signal transduction processes. Besides numerous phosphorylation sites for protein kinases,[32] several interacting partners are known that bind to the Cx43 tail, including ZO-1,[33] α- and β-tubulin, and c-Src[34,35] (see Figure 21.1). The group of Naus[36] as well as ours[37] gave evidence that Cx43 binds to the C-terminus of the growth regulator protein NOV (CCN3), thereby reducing proliferation and growth of tumor cells. Thus, there is a need for further investigation of gap junction proteins to discriminate between channel and other functions.

REGULATION OF ENDOMETRIAL CONNEXIN EXPRESSION DURING EARLY PREGNANCY IN THE RODENT

The main connexin isoforms expressed in the rodent endometrium have been identified as connexin26 (Cx26) and Cx43.[15,38] Transcripts of these two connexins can be found in high amounts in the endometrium of mice and rats (Figure 21.2). With regard to protein expression, immunohistochemical analyses demonstrated that in non-pregnant rats only the uterine epithelium of the estrous phase shows a weak immunoreaction to Cx26 antibodies, whereas the Cx43 protein is missing in cycling endometrium.[38] In pregnancy, the connexin expression pattern changes impressively. During the first 3 days of pregnancy, when rising progesterone levels influence endometrial differentiation to the receptive phase, both connexins – Cx26 in the uterine epithelium and Cx43 in the stromal compartment – are rapidly down-regulated and completely suppressed before implantation (see Figure 21.2).[16,38] A simultaneous up-regulation of other connexins, such as Cx30, 32, 37, 40, and 45, which could compensate for the missing communication properties, was not found during this phase. Thus, in the preimplantation period, cells in the endometrium lack direct junctional communication as already proven in an earlier study in the rabbit.[14] This phenomenon of a non-communicating epithelium is most unusual since nearly all tissues except for blood cells and skeletal muscle are connected by connexin channels. The phenomenon is mirrored in the down-regulation of Cx43 in the myometrial compartment during pregnancy to keep the smooth muscle cells in a quiescent state.[39]

Remarkably, with the beginning of the implantation reaction, a strong induction of gap junction connexins is

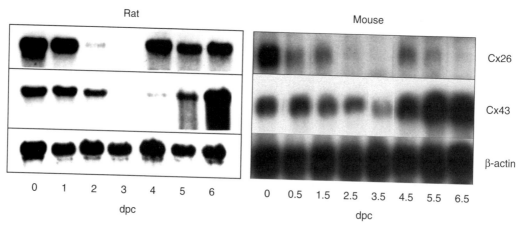

Figure 21.2 Northern blot of RNA from rat endometrium from day 1 to day 6 of pregnancy and from mice uteri during 0–6.5 dpc (days postcoitum). Transcription of Cx26 and Cx43 is significantly suppressed during the receptive phase in both species and is induced in the presence of the blastocysts. Whereas Cx26 expression in rats maintains after implantation due to its expression in the developing decidua, Cx26 transcripts in mice are not detectable anymore from 6.5 dpc onwards when the epithelium of the implantation chamber has vanished.

observed in the endometrium: however, it is exclusively in the epithelial cells of the implantation chamber. Transcripts for Cx26 are clearly expressed in both rat and mouse already on 4 dpc (days postcoitum) (see Figure 21.2), followed by a distinct expression of the Cx26 protein restricted to the luminal epithelium of the implantation chamber on 4.5 dpc in mice and on 5 dpc in rats (Figure 21.3a).[15,16] This seems to be a local effect due to the presence of a blastocyst, because this antigen is neither detected in the interblastocyst segments nor in pseudopregnant animals.[15,16,40] This local restriction of Cx26 induction has been confirmed by comparing mouse uterine tissue of implantation and interimplantation sites by microarray analysis, demonstrating an up-regulation of Cx26 only in the implantation sites.[41]

Concomitantly, with the decidualization of the stromal cells surrounding the implantation chamber,[42] intense staining for the Cx43 antigen is detectable in this primary decidual zone (Figure 21.3b) and increases and spreads out with ongoing decidualization in both rodent species.[15,16] A tremendous increase of gap junctional structures in the developing decidua has been already described in mice[43] and rats.[44] In the rat decidua, Cx26 is coexpressed with Cx43 restricted to the primary decidual zone. In contrast, in mice, although a similar pattern occurs during trophoblast invasion in the decidua with regard to Cx43 expression, Cx26 is not induced in decidual cells.[45,46]

These results raise the question of whether this precisely defined connexin expression pattern varies in animals with different modi of implantation. Another species with invasive placentation, the rabbit, shows a

similar connexin expression pattern, although there is no hormonally regulated estrous cycle and the invasion modus (fusion–implantation) is different from rodents with a replacement–invasion modus.[47] The uterine epithelium of the non-cycling non-pregnant rabbit, as well as of the preimplantation phase, lacks connexin expression and functional coupling. As in rodents, a strong expression of functional gap junction channels is induced by the blastocyst in the uterine epithelium of the implantation chamber as a response to embryo recognition as evidenced by tubal ligation experiments.[14] In contrast to rodents, however, another gap junction isoform, Cx32, connects the epithelial cells.[14] In species with non-invasive placentation like pigs and horses, such a gap junctional response in the epithelium is missing, which supports the hypothesis that induction of connexins is related to the invasion process. However, the phenomenon of a non-communicating uterine epithelium in early pregnancy is the same as in the invasive types of implantation.[48] In sheep, which also have non-invasive placentation, increasing amounts of stromal Cx43 and epithelial Cx26 were found in the endometrium during implantation;[49] thus, here the endometrial connexin response resembles more the invasive type of implantation.

In conclusion, there is substantial evidence that in numerous mammalian species a non-coupled uterine epithelium is a characteristic physiological status in the preimplantation phase, and in invasive types of implantation a local induction of connexin channels by the blastocyst seems to be required (Figure 21.3f). The different regulatory pathways involved are examined more closely in the following sections.

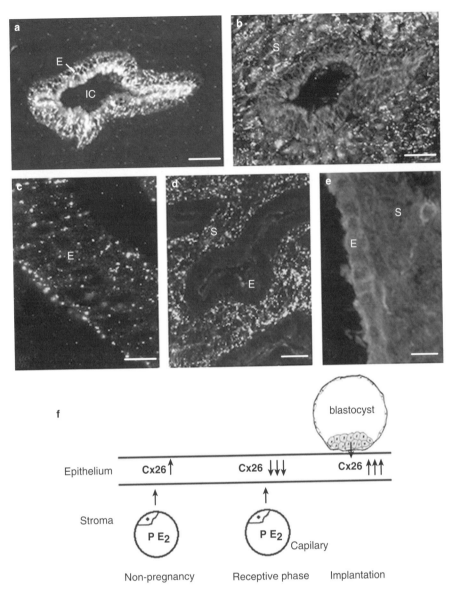

Figure 21.3 Immunohistochemical staining for Cx26 and Cx43 in the endometrium. During implantation in the rat, on 5 dpc, Cx26 proteins are locally restricted to the epithelium (E) of the implantation chamber (IC) (a), whereas Cx43 is expressed at the lateral borders of the stromal cells (S) surrounding the implantation chamber (b). In the cyclic human endometrium, Cx26 is expressed in the uterine epithelial cells of the proliferative phase (c); however, it is not detected in the late proliferative phase (e). Cx43 characterizes the stromal compartment throughout the menstrual cycle (d). The regulation of epithelial Cx26 expression during pre- and peri-implantation in rodents (f): P, progesterone; E_2, estradiol. The bars in a, b, d, and e = 40 μm; in c = 15 μm.

Hormonal regulation of connexin expression during preimplantation

Substantial literature indicates that, in target tissues, connexins are able to respond to a variety of hormones and stimuli at the transcriptional level, which closely relates to the functional status of the tissue. The most dramatic hormonal regulation of gap junctional communication is observed in the uterine myometrium. It is obvious that the missing cell–cell communication in the myometrium during pregnancy is to avoid muscular

contraction leading to premature labor. In normal pregnancies, the onset of labor is indicated by a tremendous increase in gap junctional communication, which leads to a coordinated electrical activity prior to parturition.[39,50] This myometrial Cx43 expression has been proven to be suppressed by progesterone[51] and elevated by estrogen.[52]

As described above, in the endometrial compartment down-regulation of connexins occurs during preimplantation. To prove that the suppression of connexins during the preimplantation phase in rats is under control of

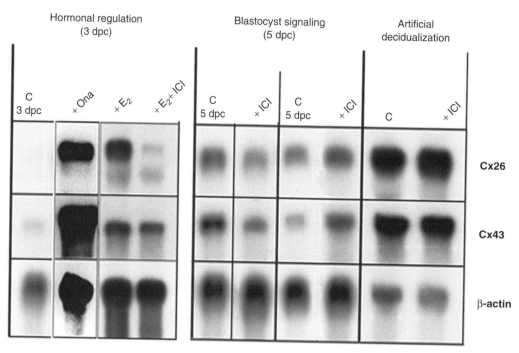

Figure 21.4 Northern blot of rat endometrial RNA probed for Cx26 and Cx43. During the receptive phase on 3 dpc, gene expression of Cx26 and Cx43 is suppressed in rat endometrium (C 3 dpc). This inhibition can be abolished by application of the antiprogestin onapristone (Ona) or by application of 1 μg estradiol (E$_2$) on day 1 and 2 pc. The Cx26 induction by estradiol was inhibited by simultaneous application of the antiestrogen ICI. Blots were hybridized to β-actin as a loading control. The induction of Cx26 and Cx43 by the blastocyst on 5 dpc (C 5dpc) is not inhibited by application of the antiestrogen (ICI) neither in normal nor in delayed implantation. Cx26, as well as Cx43, is strongly induced by a traumatic stimulus, leading to artificial decidualization (C). This induction is not inhibited by application of the antiestrogen (+ICI).

maternal progesterone, the antiprogestin onapristone (Schering AG, Berlin) was applied during the first 3 days of pregnancy. This treatment prevented the physiological suppression of connexin transcripts of both Cx26 and Cx43 on 3 dpc (Figure 21.4). Simultaneously, the corresponding Cx26 protein was expressed throughout the uterine epithelium and the Cx43 protein in the stromal compartment.[16] Furthermore, induction of Cx26 is dependent on estradiol. Supraphysiological estradiol concentrations during the receptive phase led to an induction of Cx26 in the uterine epithelium, overriding the suppressive effect of progesterone. Application of 1 μg estradiol on the first 2 days of pregnancy, which represents 10-fold the physiological amount during receptivity, induced a strong expression of Cx26 mRNA on 3 dpc, which was inhibited by simultaneous application of the antiestrogen ICI 182780 (see Figure 21.4), suggesting estrogen receptor (ER)-mediated regulation. The corresponding protein was localized at this time point to the membranes of the uterine epithelial cells but was not detected in rats which simultaneously had received the antiestrogen.[46] Basal Cx43 gene transcription was present during the receptive phase of pregnancy, revealing no significant regulation of either

transcript or protein expression by estradiol and/or antiestrogen treatment. Thus, these two gap junction genes react differently to estradiol, revealing that the Cx26 gene is much more responsive to estrogen.

The steroid hormone-regulated balance of connexin expression has been further analyzed in ovariectomized rats using different progesterone:estradiol ratios. A hormonal profile similar to pregnancy, with a high amount of progesterone in combination with low estradiol levels, was able to suppress transcripts of both connexins, Cx26 and Cx43, comparable to the situation during preimplantation. Again, Cx26 and Cx43 revealed a different sensitivity to the ratio of progesterone:estradiol, since with increasing estradiol levels Cx26 was reinduced despite high progesterone concentrations, whereas Cx43 mRNA levels remained suppressed.[17]

How sensitive is the response of these genes to estrogen? To test this, OVX rats which express low levels of Cx43 mRNA in the endometrium and no transcripts for Cx26 were treated with different concentrations of estradiol. We demonstrated that the Cx26 gene reacts more sensitively to estradiol compared with Cx43, i.e. at lower estradiol concentrations,[53] and as an early gene response already after 3 hours of estradiol injection, whereas Cx43 transcripts were not seen before 14 hours after injection of estradiol.[17]

Mice which reveal a similar spatiotemporal pattern of connexins were used to clarify the role of the different estrogen receptors. Experiments with mice deficient for ERα (ERαKO) or ERβ (ERβKO) revealed that induction of connexins is mediated in the endometrium via the ERα, but not the ERβ. ERα has been shown to be the most important form of ER in the uterus, whereas ERβ is weakly transcribed in the mouse uterus[54] and only faint staining for the protein is seen in the glandular epithelium and stromal cells of rats.[55,56] ERα-dependent induction of Cx26 is regulated at the transcriptional level, since addition of the transcription inhibitor actinomycin D prevents Cx26 gene induction in an organ culture model.[46]

In summary, the expression of Cx26 and Cx43 in the rat endometrium is sensitively and differentially regulated by the ovarian steroid hormones estradiol and progesterone. Transcription of the Cx26 gene is more sensitive to estrogen than Cx43, and only a hormonal milieu similar to that in early pregnancy is able to suppress transcription of both genes.[17]

Induction of connexin expression during embryo implantation

As described above, progesterone-mediated suppression of connexins can be abolished by elevated estrogen concentrations via an ER-mediated pathway, but also by an unknown signal from the implanting embryo. Blastocyst signaling is mediated by an ER-independent signal cascade since application of a pure antiestrogen to pregnant rats had no effect on epithelial Cx26 induction (see Figure 21.4).[46] In the progesterone-treated delayed implantation model, Cx26 transcripts are induced in the uterine epithelium solely by the presence of the blastocyst. In this experimental model, blastocysts remain closely apposed to the uterine luminal epithelium without initiation of decidualization. Related to the lack of a decidualization reaction in the stromal compartment, Cx43 up-regulation was not observed.[46] Also in delayed implantation, like in normal pregnancy, blastocyst-mediated Cx26 induction was not impaired by application of an antiestrogen, again confirming an ER-independent pathway.

It remained to be clarified if the tremendous increase in Cx43 mRNA and protein expression in the decidualizing stromal cells is hormone dependent and regulated via the ER or is induced by the implanting blastocyts. We demonstrated that artificially induced decidualization in pseudopregnant rats leads to an induction of Cx43 in deciduoma.[16] As in the case for the epithelial Cx26 response, the expression of Cx43 in the decidual cells is also not changed by application of an antiestrogen (see Figure 21.4), and also ERα-deficient mice decidualize and express high amounts of Cx43.[46] Both experiments demonstrate a Cx43 up-regulation concomitantly with the decidualization process independent from ER action.

While estradiol leads to an induction of Cx26 transcripts only in the uterine epithelium but not in the stromal cells, a traumatic stimulus as well as the implantation of the blastocyst cause a strong induction of Cx26 in addition to Cx43 in the developing rat decidua. Thus, induction of Cx26 in the stromal cells, in contrast to epithelial cells, seems to be regulated solely via the ER-independent signal pathway. The stromal cell response is primarily dependent on progesterone, while the luminal epithelium which controls the initiation of implantation is highly sensitive to estrogen.[57] Thus, estrogen is essential for epithelial proliferative and implantation responses but is dispensable for signaling leading to the decidual response.

Molecular signals guiding the interactions between the blastocyst and uterus to initiate the process of implantation still remain ill-defined. Different hormones, second messengers, growth factors, cytokines, transcription factors, and even mechanical manipulations have been suggested to act as embryonic signals[6,13,58,59] and could be involved in stimulating cell–cell communication in the endometrium. In addition, recent discoveries suggest a role for prostaglandins in the implantation process.[12,13]

Using an organ culture model, we demonstrated that ER-independent induction of Cx26 gene expression can be achieved by interleukin-1β (IL-1β), catechol estrogen, and prostaglandin $F_{2\alpha}$ (PGF$_{2\alpha}$),[46] factors that have been shown to be involved in the implantation process and may act as blastocyst-derived signals.[60,61]

Up to now we have not been able to demonstrate the physiological importance either the local induction of Cx26 or of Cx43 expression for decidualization, since Cx26 deletion causes lethality in mice at early gestation due to an impairment in glucose transport across the placental barrier,[62] and Cx43 gene deficiency results in fetal death directly after birth.[63] Appropriate tissue-specific knockouts for the two connexins in the uterine epithelium as well as in the decidua using the Cre-lox system are still missing. We hypothesize that in the case of the epithelial connexins the communication channels help to coordinate and restrict the local apoptotic process of the epithelium in response to the interacting blastocyst during the replacement implantation modus in rodents. In support of this idea, a correlation between

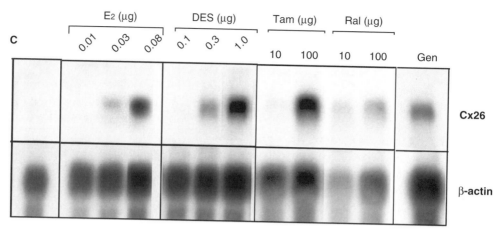

Figure 21.5   Northern blot evaluation of rat endometrial RNA 24 hours after injection of different compounds. Induction of Cx26 gene expression was observed from a concentration of 0.03 µg estradiol/rat and 0.3 µg diethylstilbestrol (DES)/rat, respectively, onwards. The SERM tamoxifen (Tam) showed a clear inductive effect on Cx26 at a concentration of 100 µg/rat, whereas raloxifene (Ral) only revealed a weak estrogenic action in regard to Cx26 induction at this concentration. Also, application of the phytoestrogen genistein (Gen, 2.5 mg/rat) exhibited an estrogenic effect on the endometrium in regard to the induction of Cx26 gene expression. Blots were hybridized to β-actin as a loading control.

cells expressing Cx26 and undergoing apoptosis has been observed.[64]

CX26 – A SENSITIVE INDICATOR FOR COMPOUNDS WITH ESTROGENIC ACTIVITY IN THE ENDOMETRIUM

Since the endometrium is one of the main target tissues for ovarian hormones, it reacts to estrogens as well as to compounds with estrogenic activity. Exposure to such possible endocrine disruptors has been associated with an increased incidence of tumorigenesis in hormone-dependent tissues such as testis, endometrium, and breast.[65–67] Thus, sensitive and reliable markers to screen different compounds for estrogenic activity in this target tissue are of interest. A remarkable diversity of naturally occurring and synthetic compounds have been shown to mimic the biological effects of estradiol. These include drugs for hormonal replacement therapy during menopause, selective estrogen receptor modulators (SERMs) like tamoxifen and raloxifene, which have been developed as antiestrogens for the therapy of breast cancer,[68,69] phytoestrogens from plant origin,[70] as well as pesticides and industrial chemicals.[71] Since identifying Cx26 as a very sensitive marker for estrogen action in rat endometrium, we have evaluated its value for determination of the estrogenic activity of these different compounds.

Cx26 gene expression in the rat endometrium can serve as a model for biological activity of estrogens since it is induced at an estradiol concentration as low as 0.03 µg/rat, and increases in a gene-dose-dependent

manner (Figure 21.5). The strong estrogen agonist diethylstilbestrol (DES) had to be applied at about 10-fold higher concentration to induce comparable levels of Cx26 transcript (see Figure 21.5). Expression of Cx26 protein after estrogen and DES treatment was detected 24 hours after application of the highest concentration of estrogen or DES, whereas Cx43 mRNA as well as protein was not regulated by these hormonal treatments.[53] The SERMs tamoxifen and raloxifene also induced Cx26 gene expression, but more than 100-fold higher concentrations were needed compared to DES. In comparison to tamoxifen, however, the same concentration of raloxifene acts only as a weak agonist on endometrial gene expression (see Figure 21.5).[53] The agonistic effect of tamoxifen on Cx26 induction supports observations that these compounds lead to an increased risk of development of endometrial cancer after long-time tamoxifen therapy,[72,73] whereas raloxifene, which also acts as an estrogen antagonist in breast tissue,[74] showed a much lower agonistic effect in the endometrium.

Interestingly, an increase in Cx26 transcription was also seen 24 hours after a single subcutaneous injection of 2.5 mg of the soy phytoestrogen genistein, which means that phytoestrogens are able to shift the endometrial gene program even at a relatively low dose (see Figure 21.5). It is known that phytoestrogens reveal multiple biological effects, including beneficial effects on osteoporosis, breast cancer, prostate cancer, and menopausal symptoms, and on the cardiovascular system,[75] but may also cause severe reproductive tract disorders including impaired fertility,[76] which could be explained by the estrogenic activity of phytoestrogens.

All these drug effects described above on endometrial Cx26 induction were mediated by the estrogen receptor, since they could be inhibited by simultaneous application of an antiestrogen.[53]

In conclusion, to obtain more comprehensive information about the estrogenic activity of natural and synthetic estrogens, the regulation of Cx26 in the rat endometrium is a reliable marker. In regard to DES, which reveals an even higher binding capacity to the ER than estradiol,[77] the physiological effect seems to be less than might have been expected from ER-binding assays. This confirms the observation of other groups that ER-binding assays do not allow conclusions in regard to the biological activity of estrogenic substances,[78,79] and that hormonal activity can only be evaluated in a biological model.

CONNEXINS IN THE HUMAN ENDOMETRIUM

Corresponding to the situation in rodents, Cx26 and Cx43 are the main connexin isoforms expressed in the human endometrium. Their expression seems to be hormonally regulated during the cycle. Three gap junction isoforms – Cx26, Cx43, and, to a lesser extent Cx32 – are detected, each with a distinct distribution and spatial and temporal regulation.[80] Cx26 was demonstrated to be expressed with increasing intensity in the uterine epithelial cells during the course of the proliferative phase (Figure 21.3c); however, it could hardly be detected in the secretory phase including the receptive window (Figure 21.3e). Cx43 characterizes the stromal compartment (Figure 21.3d) and, like Cx26, decreased during the secretory phase.[80] However, in the late secretory phase in some women, expression of Cx43 was observed in epithelial cells instead of Cx26 (unpublished results). This is in accordance with a report suggesting a slight increase in Cx43 mRNA in the mid secretory phase on day 21 and an increase in Cx43 protein in the late secretory phase on day 25; however, this study did not include histological localization.[81]

For Cx32, a constant weak expression could be observed at the basal portion of the epithelial cells,[80] whereas other studies demonstrated an increase in early secretory and a decrease in late secretory phase.[82] The basal immunolocalization of Cx32 is probably related to gap junctions of the basal cell projections mainly found in early to late proliferative phase which share numerous gap junctions with projections from adjacent cells.[83]

In conclusion, connexins are allocated to the different tissue compartments in the human endometrium and seem to be hormonally regulated in the course of the menstrual cycle. While species with short cycles like rats demonstrate a regulation of connexin expression mainly on the transcriptional level, in humans the protein pattern changes during the cyclic phases of the endometrium. Cell–cell communication could serve as a general control mechanism for coordinated tissue differentiation upon sex hormone stimulation.

CONNEXINS IN ENDOMETRIAL DISEASES

Loss of communication properties or the aberrant expression of connexins has long been considered as one important step in carcinogenesis.[84] Numerous studies have shown that growth of communication-deficient tumor cells in vitro and in vivo could be reduced if transfected with the appropriate connexin, suggesting a role of these proteins in tumor suppression.[85] Very convincing results were obtained from Cx32-deficient mice and a dominant-negative liver mutant of Cx32: neither shows an increase in incidence of spontaneous tumors but both have elevated susceptibility to chemical hepatocarcinogenesis.[86–88] However, the mechanisms by which the channels are involved in cell cycle control are not fully understood. As already described above, the growth regulatory protein NOV has been discovered to interact with the C-terminus of Cx43, thereby reducing the proliferation of glioma and choriocarcinoma cells.[36,37] In some tumor cell lines, proliferation is reduced after Cx43 transfections by a prolonged G_0/G_1 phase.[31,89]

Up to now, there have only been a few studies on connexin expression in endometrial hyperplasia and carcinoma. All of them support the idea that gap junctional transcript and protein expression, and as a consequence gap junctional communication, is down-regulated in both hyperplasia and carcinoma. Cx26, normally found to be expressed in uterine epithelium, is less expressed and aberrantly localized in hyperplasia and mostly missing in carcinomas. A similar reduction in expression was found for Cx32, whereas all samples of neoplasia as well as carcinoma showed only weak expression of Cx43.[90] Carcinoma cell lines representing different grades of endometrial cancer show a continuous decrease in Cx43 expression which could be paralleled to endometrial tumors of patients diagnosed for grade 1 to grade 3 endometrial cancer. The suppression of connexins in endometrial cancer is considered to be mediated via estrogen and the presence of ERα without the effect of progestins because it has been shown that estrogen treatment in endometrial carcinoma cells overexpressing ERα down-regulates gap junctional communication.[91]

In endometriosis, the benign uterine ectopic lesions reveal a connexin pattern different from healthy endometrium. Here the glandular epithelial cells exhibit mostly a strong Cx43 expression, whereas Cx26 expression was missing in half of the cohort investigated, and Cx32 was not detectable.[92] The aberrant expression of connexins in all those endometrial diseases indicates that connexins are a sensitive marker for the differentiation state and could be associated with the pathogenesis of endometriosis and endometrial cancer.

CONCLUSIONS

Transformation of the endometrium into the receptive phase is under the control of ovarian steroid hormones and, in addition, the endometrial program is modulated by embryonic signals at implantation. During these early stages of pregnancy, cell–cell communication via gap junction channels is precisely temporally and spatially regulated in the endometrium of different species in response to both ovarian hormones and embryonic signals. During endometrial receptivity, the complete suppression of connexin genes leads to a non-communicating epithelium in most species investigated. In addition, in species with invasive implantation, connexins are induced only in the epithelium of the implantation chamber due to embryo recognition. In rodents as well as in humans, these endometrial connexins could be identified as Cx26 in the epithelium and Cx43 in the stromal cells. Connexin gene expression in the rodent endometrium is regulated via two distinct signaling pathways during the different stages of early pregnancy. During preimplantation, transcription of connexins is hormonally regulated by steroid receptor-dependent pathways, whereas the Cx26 gene showed a more pronounced estrogen responsiveness compared to Cx43. Induction by blastocyst signaling prior to implantation is mediated by a signaling cascade independent of both estrogen receptors ERα and ERβ.

Thus, intercellular communication via gap junctions, which is involved in cell differentiation, seems to play an important role in preparing the uterus for embryo implantation as well as in controlling the implantation process of the trophoblast. In addition, modulation of epithelial Cx26 transcript expression could serve as a reliable indicator for compounds with estrogenic effects as well as for non-physiological changes in steroid hormone serum levels. Furthermore, a low expression of the different connexins is correlated with endometrial diseases such as endometrial hyperplasia, carcinoma, and endometriosis. The physiological role of this highly regulated expression pattern of endometrial connexins is not known yet. The restricted expression pattern of the cell–cell communication channels could be responsible for coordinating the local cell program at the implantation site and separating the fate of this cell population from the rest of the uterine tissue. Using connexins as marker genes will help to map endometrial signaling cascades induced by the embryo which are necessary for successful implantation.

REFERENCES

1. Wilcox AJ, Weinberg CR, O'Connor JF et al. Incidence of early loss of pregnancy. N Engl J Med 1988; 319(4): 189–94.
2. Barash A, Dekel N, Fieldust S et al. Local injury to the endometrium doubles the incidence of successful pregnancies in patients undergoing in vitro fertilization. Fertil Steril 2003; 79(6): 1317–22.
3. Schlafke S, Welsh AO, Enders AC. Penetration of the basal lamina of the uterine luminal epithelium during implantation in the rat. Anat Rec 1985; 212: 47–56.
4. Denker HW. Implantation: a cell biological paradox. J Exp Zool 1993; 266(6): 541–58.
5. Psychoyos A. Hormonal control of ovoimplantation. Vitam Horm 1973; 31: 201–56.
6. Carson DD, Bagchi I, Dey SK et al. Embryo implantation. Dev Biol 2000; 223(2): 217–37.
7. Dey SK, Lim H, Das SK et al. Molecular cues to implantation. Endocr Rev 2004; 25(3): 341–73.
8. Enders AC, Schlafke S. Cytological aspects of trophoblast–uterine interaction in early implantation. Am J Anat 1969; 125(1): 1–29.
9. Tranguch S, Daikoku T, Guo Y et al. Molecular complexity in establishing uterine receptivity and implantation. Cell Mol Life Sci 2005; 62(17): 1964–73.
10. Dimitriadis E, White CA, Jones RL et al. Cytokines, chemokines and growth factors in endometrium related to implantation. Hum Reprod Update 2005; 11(6): 613–30.
11. Psychoyos A, Bitton V. [Chronologic aspects of the anti-implantation effect of the presence of a thread in the uterus of the rat]. C R Seances Soc Biol Fil 1966; 160(2): 229–32. [in French]
12. Paria BC, Reese J, Das SK et al. Deciphering the cross-talk of implantation: advances and challenges. Science 2002; 296(5576): 2185–8.
13. Norwitz ER, Schust DJ, Fisher SJ. Implantation and the survival of early pregnancy. N Engl J Med 2001; 345(19): 1400–8.
14. Winterhager E, Brummer F, Dermietzel R et al. Gap junction formation in rabbit uterine epithelium in response to embryo recognition. Dev Biol 1988; 126(1): 203–11.
15. Winterhager E, Grummer R, Jahn E et al. Spatial and temporal expression of connexin26 and connexin43 in rat endometrium during trophoblast invasion. Dev Biol 1993; 157(2): 399–409.
16. Grümmer R, Chwalisz K, Mulholland J et al. Regulation of connexin26 and connexin43 expression in rat endometrium by ovarian steroid hormones. Biol Reprod 1994; 51(6): 1109–16.

17. Grümmer R, Traub O, Winterhager E. Gap junction connexin genes cx26 and cx43 are differentially regulated by ovarian steroid hormones in rat endometrium. Endocrinology 1999; 140(6): 2509–16.

18. Cavagna M, Mantese JC. Biomarkers of endometrial receptivity – a review. Placenta 2003; 24 (Suppl B): S39–47.

19. Carson DD, Lagow E, Thathiah A et al. Changes in gene expression during the early to mid-luteal (receptive phase) transition in human endometrium detected by high-density microarray screening. Mol Hum Reprod 2002; 8(9): 871–9.

20. Dominguez F, Remohi J, Pellicer A et al. Human endometrial receptivity: a genomic approach. Reprod Biomed Online 2003; 6(3): 332–8.

21. Kao LC, Tulac S, Lobo S et al. Global gene profiling in human endometrium during the window of implantation. Endocrinology 2002; 143(6): 2119–38.

22. Riesewijk A, Martin J, van Os R et al. Gene expression profiling of human endometrial receptivity on days LH+2 versus LH+7 by microarray technology. Mol Hum Reprod 2003; 9(5): 253–64.

23. Dominguez F, Pellicer A, Simon C. The chemokine connection: hormonal and embryonic regulation at the human maternal–embryonic interface – a review. Placenta 2003; 24(Suppl B): S48–55.

24. Aplin JD, Meseguer M, Simon C et al. MUC1, glycans and the cell-surface barrier to embryo implantation. Biochem Soc Trans 2001; 29(Pt 2): 153–6.

25. Willecke K, Eiberger J, Degen J et al. Structural and functional diversity of connexin genes in the mouse and human genome. Biol Chem 2002; 383(5): 725–37.

26. Söhl G, Willecke K. An update on connexin genes and their nomenclature in mouse and man. Cell Commun Adhes 2003; 10(4–6): 173–80.

27. Willecke K. Connexin and pannexin genes in the mouse and human genome. In: Winterhager E, ed. Gap Junctions in Development and Disease. Berlin: Springer, 2005: 1–12.

28. Plum A, Hallas G, Magin T et al. Unique and shared functions of different connexins in mice. Curr Biol 2000; 10(18): 1083–91.

29. Zheng-Fischhöfer Q, Ghanem A, Kim JS et al. Connexin31 cannot functionally replace connexin43 during cardiac morphogenesis in mice. J Cell Sci 2006; 119: 693–701.

30. Dang X, Doble BW, Kardami E. The carboxy-tail of connexin-43 localizes to the nucleus and inhibits cell growth. Mol Cell Biochem 2003; 242(1–2): 35–8.

31. Zhang YW, Nakayama K, Morita I. A novel route for connexin 43 to inhibit cell proliferation: negative regulation of S-phase kinase-associated protein (Skp 2). Cancer Res 2003; 63(7): 1623–30.

32. Lampe PD, Lau AF. Regulation of gap junctions by phosphorylation of connexins. Arch Biochem Biophys 2000; 384(2): 205–15.

33. Giepmans BN, Moolenaar WH. The gap junction protein connexin43 interacts with the second PDZ domain of the zona occludens-1 protein. Curr Biol 1998; 8(16): 931–4.

34. Giepmans BN, Hengeveld T, Postma FR et al. Interaction of c-Src with gap junction protein connexin-43. Role in the regulation of cell–cell communication. J Biol Chem 2001; 276(11): 8544–9.

35. Giepmans BN, Verlaan I, Moolenaar WH. Connexin-43 interactions with ZO-1 and alpha- and beta-tubulin. Cell Commun Adhes 2001; 8(4–6): 219–23.

36. Fu CT, Bechberger JF, Ozog MA et al. CCN3 (NOV) interacts with connexin43 in C6 glioma cells: possible mechanism of connexin-mediated growth suppression. J Biol Chem 2004; 279(35): 36943–50.

37. Gellhaus A, Dong X, Propson S et al. Connexin43 interacts with NOV: a possible mechanism for negative regulation of cell growth in choriocarcinoma cells. J Biol Chem 2004; 279(35): 36931–42.

38. Winterhager E, Stutenkemper R, Traub O et al. Expression of different connexin genes in rat uterus during decidualization and at term. Eur J Cell Biol 1991; 55(1): 133–42.

39. MacKenzie LW, Garfield RE. Hormonal control of gap junctions in the myometrium. Am J Physiol 1985; 248(3 Pt 1): C296–308.

40. Grümmer R, Winterhager E. Regulation of gap junction connexins in the endometrium during early pregnancy. Cell Tissue Res 1998; 293(2): 189–94.

41. Reese J, Das SK, Paria BC et al. Global gene expression analysis to identify molecular markers of uterine receptivity and embryo implantation. J Biol Chem 2001; 276(47): 44137–45.

42. Glasser SR. Biochemical and structural changes in uterine endometrial cell types following natural or artificial deciduogenic stimuli. In: Denker HW, Aplin JD, eds. Trophoblast Research 4: Trophoblast Invasion and Endometrial Receptivity. New York: Plenum Medical 1990: 377–416.

43. Finn CA, Lawn AM. Specialized junctions between decidual cells in the uterus of the pregnant mouse. J Ultrastruct Res 1967; 20(5): 321–7.

44. Kleinfeld RG, Morrow H, DeFeo VJ. Intercellular junctions between decidual cells in the growing deciduoma of the pseudopregnant rat uterus. Biol Reprod 1976; 15(5): 593–603.

45. Pauken CM, Lo CW. Nonoverlapping expression of Cx43 and Cx26 in the mouse placenta and decidua: a pattern of gap junction gene expression differing from that in the rat. Mol Reprod Dev 1995; 41(2): 195–203.

46. Grümmer R, Hewitt SW, Traub O et al. Different regulatory pathways of endometrial connexin expression: preimplantation hormonal-mediated pathway versus embryo implantation-initiated pathway. Biol Reprod 2004; 71(1): 273–81.

47. Enders AC, Schlafke S. Penetration of the uterine epithelium during implantation in the rabbit. Am J Anat 1971; 132(2): 219–30.

48. Day WE, Bowen JA, Barhoumi R et al. Endometrial connexin expression in the mare and pig: evidence for the suppression of cell–cell communication in uterine luminal epithelium. Anat Rec 1998; 251(3): 277–85.

49. Gabriel S, Winterhager E, Pfarrer C et al. Modulation of connexin expression in sheep endometrium in response to pregnancy. Placenta 2004; 25(4): 287–96.

50. Ou CW, Orsino A, Lye SJ. Expression of connexin-43 and connexin-26 in the rat myometrium during pregnancy and labor is differentially regulated by mechanical and hormonal signals. Endocrinology 1997; 138(12): 5398–407.

51. Chwalisz K, Fahrenholz F, Hackenberg M et al. The progesterone antagonist onapristone increases the effectiveness of oxytocin to produce delivery without changing the myometrial oxytocin receptor concentrations. Am J Obstet Gynecol 1991; 165(6 Pt 1): 1760–70.

52. Di WL, Lachelin GC, McGarrigle HH et al. Oestriol and oestradiol increase cell to cell communication and connexin43 protein expression in human myometrium. Mol Hum Reprod 2001; 7(7): 671–9.

53. Heikaus S, Winterhager E, Traub O, Grümmer R. Responsiveness of endometrial genes Connexin26, Connexin43, C3 and clusterin to primary estrogen, selective estrogen receptor modulators, phyto- and xenoestrogens. J Mol Endocrinol 2002; 29(2): 239–49.

54. Couse JF, Lindzey J, Grandien K et al. Tissue distribution and quantitative analysis of estrogen receptor-alpha (ERalpha) and estrogen receptor-beta (ERbeta) messenger ribonucleic acid in the wild-type and ERalpha-knockout mouse. Endocrinology 1997; 138(11): 4613–21.

55. Hiroi H, Inoue S, Watanabe T et al. Differential immunolocalization of estrogen receptor alpha and beta in rat ovary and uterus. J Mol Endocrinol 1999; 22(1): 37–44.

56. Shughrue PJ, Lane MV, Scrimo PJ et al. Comparative distribution of estrogen receptor-alpha (ER-alpha) and beta (ER-beta)

mRNA in the rat pituitary, gonad, and reproductive tract. Steroids 1998; 63(10): 498–504.

57. Curtis Hewitt S, Goulding EH, Eddy EM et al. Studies using the estrogen receptor alpha knockout uterus demonstrate that implantation but not decidualization-associated signaling is estrogen dependent. Biol Reprod 2002; 67(4): 1268–77.

58. Lim H, Song H, Paria BC et al. Molecules in blastocyst implantation: uterine and embryonic perspectives. Vitam Horm 2002; 64: 43–76.

59. Salamonsen LA, Dimitriadis E, Robb L. Cytokines in implantation. Semin Reprod Med 2000; 18(3): 299–310.

60. Simon C, Moreno C, Remohi J et al. Molecular interactions between embryo and uterus in the adhesion phase of human implantation. Hum Reprod 1998; 13(Suppl 3): 219–32; discussion 233–6.

61. Pakrasi PL, Dey SK. Blastocyst is the source of prostaglandins in the implantation site in the rabbit. Prostaglandins 1982; 24(1): 73–7.

62. Gabriel HD, Jung D, Butzler C et al. Transplacental uptake of glucose is decreased in embryonic lethal connexin26-deficient mice. J Cell Biol 1998; 140(6): 1453–61.

63. Reaume AG, de Sousa PA, Kulkarni S et al. Cardiac malformation in neonatal mice lacking connexin43. Science 1995; 267(5205): 1831–4.

64. Joswig A, Gabriel HD, Kibschull M et al. Apoptosis in uterine epithelium and decidua in response to implantation: evidence for two different pathways. Reprod Biol Endocrinol 2003; 1: 44.

65. Davis DL, Bradlow HL, Wolff M et al. Medical hypothesis: xenoestrogens as preventable causes of breast cancer. Environ Health Perspect 1993; 101(5): 372–7.

66. Cotton P. Environmental estrogenic agents area of concern. JAMA 1994; 271(6): 414, 416.

67. Safe S. Endocrine disruptors and human health: is there a problem. Toxicology 2004; 205(1–2): 3–10.

68. Nass SJ, Hahm HA, Davidson NE. Breast cancer biology blossoms in the clinic. Nat Med 1998; 4(7): 761–2.

69. Overmoyer BA. The breast cancer prevention trial (P-1 study). The role of tamoxifen in preventing breast cancer. Cleve Clin J Med 1999; 66(1): 33–40.

70. Beck V, Unterrieder E, Krenn L et al. Comparison of hormonal activity (estrogen, androgen and progestin) of standardized plant extracts for large scale use in hormone replacement therapy. J Steroid Biochem Mol Biol 2003; 84(2–3): 259–68.

71. Brevini TA, Zanetto SB, Cillo F. Effects of endocrine disruptors on developmental and reproductive functions. Curr Drug Targets Immune Endocr Metabol Disord 2005; 5(1): 1–10.

72. Burke C. Endometrial cancer and tamoxifen. Clin J Oncol Nurs 2005; 9(2): 247–9.

73. Assikis VJ, Jordan VC. Gynecologic effects of tamoxifen and the association with endometrial carcinoma. Int J Gynaecol Obstet 1995; 49(3): 241–57.

74. Burckhardt P. [Selective estrogen receptor modulators (SERM): new substances for hormone replacement therapy]. Schweiz Med Wochenschr 1999; 129(49): 1926–30. [in German]

75. Branca F, Lorenzetti S. Health effects of phytoestrogens. Forum Nutr 2005; 57: 100–11.

76. Jefferson WN, Padilla-Banks E, Newbold RR. Adverse effects on female development and reproduction in CD-1 mice following neonatal exposure to the phytoestrogen genistein at environmentally relevant doses. Biol Reprod 2005; 73(4): 798–806.

77. Kuiper GG, Carlsson B, Grandien K et al. Comparison of the ligand binding specificity and transcript tissue distribution of estrogen receptors alpha and beta. Endocrinology 1997; 138(3): 863–70.

78. Hopert AC, Beyer A, Frank K et al. Characterization of estrogenicity of phytoestrogens in an endometrial-derived experimental model. Environ Health Perspect 1998; 106(9): 581–6.

79. Strunck E, Stemmann N, Hopert A et al. Relative binding affinity does not predict biological response to xenoestrogens in rat endometrial adenocarcinoma cells. J Steroid Biochem Mol Biol 2000; 74(3): 73–81.

80. Jahn E, Classen-Linke I, Kusche M et al. Expression of gap junction connexins in the human endometrium throughout the menstrual cycle. Hum Reprod 1995; 10(10): 2666–70.

81. Granot I, Dekel N, Bechor E et al. Temporal analysis of connexin43 protein and gene expression throughout the menstrual cycle in human endometrium. Fertil Steril 2000; 73(2): 381–6.

82. Saito T, Oyamada M, Yamasaki H et al. Co-ordinated expression of connexins 26 and 32 in human endometrial glandular epithelium during the reproductive cycle and the influence of hormone replacement therapy. Int J Cancer 1997; 73(4): 479–85.

83. Roberts DK, Walker NJ, Lavia LA. Ultrastructural evidence of stromal/epithelial interactions in the human endometrial cycle. Am J Obstet Gynecol 1988; 158(4): 854–61.

84. Mesnil M. Connexins and cancer. Biol Cell 2002; 94(7–8): 493–500.

85. King TJ, Fukushima LH, Yasui Y et al. Inducible expression of the gap junction protein connexin43 decreases the neoplastic potential of HT-1080 human fibrosarcoma cells in vitro and in vivo. Mol Carcinog 2002; 35(1): 29–41.

86. Dagli ML, Yamasaki H, Krutovskikh V et al. Delayed liver regeneration and increased susceptibility to chemical hepatocarcinogenesis in transgenic mice expressing a dominant-negative mutant of connexin32 only in the liver. Carcinogenesis 2004; 25(4): 483–92.

87. Temme A, Buchmann A, Gabriel HD et al. High incidence of spontaneous and chemically induced liver tumors in mice deficient for connexin32. Curr Biol 1997; 7(9): 713–16.

88. Evert M, Ott T, Temme A et al. Morphology and morphometric investigation of hepatocellular preneoplastic lesions and neoplasms in connexin32-deficient mice. Carcinogenesis 2002; 23(5): 697–703.

89. Koffler L, Roshong S, Kyu Park I et al. Growth inhibition in G(1) and altered expression of cyclin D1 and p27(kip-1) after forced connexin expression in lung and liver carcinoma cells. J Cell Biochem 2000; 79(3): 347–54.

90. Saito T, Nishimura M, Kudo R et al. Suppressed gap junctional intercellular communication in carcinogenesis of endometrium. Int J Cancer 2001; 93(3): 317–23.

91. Saito T, Tanaka R, Wataba K et al. Overexpression of estrogen receptor-alpha gene suppresses gap junctional intercellular communication in endometrial carcinoma cells. Oncogene 2004; 23(5): 1109–16.

92. Regidor PA, Regidor M, Schindler AE et al. Aberrant expression pattern of gap junction connexins in endometriotic tissues. Mol Hum Reprod 1997; 3(5): 375–81.

93. Giepmans BN. Gap junctions and connexin-interacting proteins. Cardiovasc Res 2004; 62(2): 233–45.

22 Blastocyst implantation: the adhesion cascade

Susan J Kimber

Synopsis

Background

- At implantation, the outer trophectoderm cells attach the blastocyst to the apical surface of the endometrial luminal epithelium.
- In humans, this interaction is transient, the embryo rapidly migrating through the epithelium into the underlying stroma where trophoblast adheres to maternal cells and extracellular matrix.
- Numerous families of adhesion receptors mediate binding between trophectoderm and maternal cells. Multiple ligand–receptor pairs are likely to be needed for successful implantation.
- A useful paradigm for embryo attachment is the adhesion of neutrophils to activated vascular endothelium at sites of inflammation, which occurs in a cascade that begins with low-affinity carbohydrate-mediated interactions, progressing to more avid interactions involving other families of adhesion molecules including CAMs and integrins, and rapid transendothelial migration.

Basic Science

- Trophectoderm in mouse blastocysts must be activated by catechol estrogen to enable interaction with the luminal epithelium (LE). It then undergoes a type of epithelial–mesenchymal transition for invasion into the uterus.
- The estrogen- and progesterone-sensitized mouse LE is activated by binding of 17β-estradiol to its receptor, thus becoming directly or indirectly receptive to the activated blastocyst.
- Rat and mouse embryos can only undergo the implantation interaction with the LE during a period of less than 24 hours, known as the 'window of receptivity'.
- In humans, the receptive phase is about 4 days in length. An estrogen peak in the secretory phase may not be an absolute requirement for a receptive uterus, although progesterone is essential.
- It is believed that a complex spatiotemporally regulated cascade of interactions mediates the various stages of implantation.
- The embryo may initially undergo low-affinity carbohydrate-mediated interactions with the apical maternal epithelial glycocalyx. This is followed by higher-affinity interactions mediated by other types of receptor.
- Alterations in the occurrence and distribution of tight junctions and desmosomes coincident with the implantation period indicate that cell–cell interactions within the LE are modulated.
- Later, as the LE is breached, interaction occurs between trophoblast and the maternal subepithelial basal lamina and, later still, the stromal ECM.

Clinical

- Although candidate adhesion systems that may mediate implantation have been identified, the molecular signature of a receptive endometrium has not yet been decoded.

ABSTRACT

The sequence of cell adhesion events occurring during implantation of the mammalian embryo is described, concentrating on data from mouse and human. Changes occurring in the luminal endometrial epithelium prior to implantation are dissected. The analogy is explored between initial attachment of trophoblast to the uterine epithelium and that of neutrophils to the endothelial lining of blood vessels at sites of inflammation. The possible role of various carbohydrate ligands in initial attachment of the blastocyst is reviewed. The evidence for subsequent stabilization of cell adhesion via integrins is discussed. In spite of many years of research, the precise sequence of events during interaction of the embryo with the uterus is still not clearly understood.

INTRODUCTION

Reproduction in mammals is characterized by fertilization together with early embryonic development within the female reproductive tract, after which the conceptus implants in the wall of the uterus. This allows development of the placenta to supply the fetus with nutrients and oxygen and remove waste products. In spite of the variation between species in the detailed events of embryo implantation, there is considerable similarity in particular phases as for other developmental processes. Control of uterine differentiation by ovarian steroids is a common factor. Implantation requires an attachment phase in which the outer layer of the blastocyst, the trophectoderm (TE), interacts with the luminal epithelium (LE) of the uterus. Both human and murine implantation involve invasion of maternal tissues by trophoblast cells, although the extent of this invasion is greater in humans. The size and complexity of the mouse and human placentas are considerably different, reflecting the length of time the placenta is needed to support the fetus (19–20 days' gestation in the mouse and 42 weeks in humans). However, similarities in cell biology and architecture are also being recognized.[1] The erosion of maternal cell layers occurs in parallel in the formation of murine and human hemochorial placental.

We know little about the initial events of implantation in humans because even rare histological specimens are too late to be very informative. Intimate contact with the uterine wall takes place over a short period in the luteal phase of the menstrual cycle. Ethical considerations prevent observation, so much of our knowledge of how the embryo develops from a blastocyst in the uterine lumen, to a firmly embedded conceptus within the uterine wall, comes from animal models. A few studies have been carried out on human blastocyst attachment to luminal epithelium (LE) in vitro[2–4] or interaction with stroma[5] but few data have come from non-human primate implantation models in vitro. The human blastocyst proteome is being progressively mapped.[6–12] This will help us to predict whether factors implicated in implantation in other species could also be involved in humans.

Requirements for initial implantation

Successful implantation requires both that the uterus has undergone a specified sequence of differentiation controlled by ovarian steroids and that the blastocyst has reached a precise stage of activation.[13–15] The TE of the rodent blastocyst undergoes a stepwise maturation, leading to a state known as 'activated' (trophoblast),[15] including changes in metabolism[16] and development of the ability both to interact with LE[17] and undergo an epithelial–mesenchymal transition for invasion into the uterus.[18] For implantation to occur, both the blastocyst and the uterus must differentiate in synchrony so that they express, at the same time, the precise molecular repertoire required for adhesive interaction between TE/trophoblast and LE and subsequent penetration into the stroma.[15]

Rat and mouse embryos can only undergo the implantation interaction with the LE during a short period of less than 24 hours, known as the 'window of receptivity'.[19] This is determined by the sequential actions on the endometrium of progesterone from the corpus luteum, followed by a small peak of estrogen on day 4 of pregnancy, the nidatory estrogen. At the end of the receptive period the uterus becomes refractory and a transferred embryo cannot implant. Receptive sensitivity is thought to be at the level of the LE because the hormone-regulated restriction on attachment and invasion of the intact uterus is abolished if the epithelium is broken or absent[20,21] or when implantation occurs at ectopic sites. In women the period when the uterus is favorable for implantation appears to be longer, probably between days 19–20 and day 24 of a standard menstrual cycle.[22,23] Moreover, an estrogen peak in the secretory phase may not be an absolute requirement for a receptive uterus,[19,24] although progesterone is essential.

The mechanism by which a blastocyst is activated to become implantation competent was for a long time an enigma. It is now clear that there is a critical molecular dialogue that ensues between endometrium and blastocyst which determines the stepwise maturation of the blastocyst[17] as well as the establishment of molecular changes in LE required to permit trophoblast adhesion and subsequent implantation.[25,26] This dialogue includes soluble and membrane-bound signals which modulate cell surface receptors. A metabolite of estradiol, 4-hydroxyestradiol-17β (catechol estrogen), is required to activate the murine blastocyst while interaction of estradiol-17β (E_2) with its nuclear receptor is needed for uterine receptivity. When pregnant mice are ovariectomized before sufficient nidatory estrogen, early on the morning of day 4, embryos fail to implant. Blastocysts can be maintained in utero in a state of dormancy (known as delay of implantation) if the dams are given daily injections of progesterone (P_4). Such dormant embryos are implanted up to 16 hours after injection of E_2 to recipient females, but only up to 1 hour of recipient injection if transferred from culture.[27,28] This suggests rapid induction of a 'blastocyst activating factor' by E_2. Injection of an inhibitor of E_2 hydroxylation, 2-Fl-E_2, blocked implantation in these delayed animals,[29] while dormant blastocysts cultured with catecholestrogen (but not E_2) became activated and implanted after transfer to P_4 injected pseudopregnant females. Activation of blastocysts by catecholestrogen was unaffected by blocking estrogen receptor (ER) nuclear signaling, but prevented by inhibition of prostaglandin (PG) synthesis, adenyl cyclase, or protein kinase A (PKA). Assuming activation from dormancy mimics the normal signaling pathway associated with blastocyst acquisition of implantation competence, activation of the blastocyst may therefore occur by PG stimulating cAMP synthesis and is mediated by PKA.

Implantation comprises a number of steps by which TE undergoes a distinct series of interactions with the LE. The embryo must first contact the apical surface of the LE (apposition), facilitated by the closure of the uterine lumen,[30] which requires fluid absorption by the LE.[31] Following apposition, firmer attachment occurs, which may continue for weeks for instance in sheep, after which epithelial–trophoblast fusion occurs,[32,33] or be a transient event, as in the mouse and human. In the latter species, trophoblast penetrates the epithelium and into the stroma with formation of a hemochorial placenta. In mice TE cells squeeze between LE cells, developing desmosome-like membrane specializations with lateral and basal LE cell surfaces.[34] Passage through the underlying basement membrane is facilitated by decidual-cell-mediated breakdown of this structure in advance of trophoblast penetration.[35] Coordinately, cell death is initiated in the LE starting at the regions of initial contact with the embryos[36] and there is molecular evidence that the embryo initiates this in mouse and human.[37,38] Co-culture of embryos of cow, mouse, or human with endometrial epithelium from the same species[2,3] verify the species-specific nature of the interaction. Thus, human blastocysts exhibit intrusive-type epithelial penetration as for other primates,[39,40] while in the mouse, trophoblast intrudes between endometrial epithelial cells and then displaces them,[2,41] although the flattened epithelial cells' phenotype on plastic culture dishes prompts caution.[2] Primary (mural) trophoblast penetrates only a few cell diameters into the stroma in contrast to the extensive invasion of human cytotrophoblast. However, about a day later, trophoblast from the ectoplacental cone adjacent to the inner cell mass-derived embryo proper moves deeper into the stroma to form both giant cells and syncytiotrophoblast of the placenta.[19]

Changes in LE in preparation for implantation

Molecular and ultrastructural studies support the cyclic differentiation of LE during the reproductive cycle, which correlates with the pattern of hormonal changes.[15] A simple model to account for the restricted period of receptivity is for new adhesion molecules to be synthesized and expressed on the apical LE membrane, with counter receptors appearing on the tr phoblast, but new endometrial RNA or protein synthesis is not required,[42] arguing against de-novo expression in LE. Rather, adhesive components appear to be unmasked, modified, or relocated from basolateral aspects to the apical region of the cell. Apical epithelial surfaces are normally non-adhesive, yet during implantation, apical interaction between TE and LE occurs. This suggests that the transition of the prereceptive to receptive uterus requires fundamental changes in epithelial cell organization.[20,43,44] At the time of implantation, the apical–basal polarity of LE cells becomes less marked with appearance of laterobasal markers in the apical membrane.[20,45] The cells are flatter and have reduced microvilli, which are replaced by bulbous protrusions in many species.[46,47] Although morphometric analysis through the human menstrual cycle indicates little change in LE cell height or a number of other parameters, basement membrane thickness decreases.[48] There are also changes in apicolateral distribution of cell surface molecules; for instance, α_6 integrin distribution changes from basal to both lateral and basal during the secretory phase.[49] This implies alterations in LE cell–cell interactions at the time of implantation. In the mouse, estrogen-induced E-cadherin degradation leads to reduced lateral epithelial adhesion on day 4.5 of pregnancy[50] and previously lateral cadherins relocate to the apical LE surface at implantation in rats[51] or become more basal in rabbit LE.[20] Desmosomal proteins are down-regulated and redistributed along the lateral cell surfaces in murine LE[52] and the density of desmosomes similarly decreases in human LE at the expected time of implantation.[48] The distribution and complexity of tight junction particle networks also changes in the lateral membrane at this time, in several species including humans.[53,54] Indeed, this may reflect an opening up of the lateral epithelial junctions in anticipation of interaction with trophoblast. Additionally, specific gap junction connexins are expressed in implantation chamber epithelium[55] tightly regulated by ovarian steroids[56,57] (see Chapter 20). Furthermore, in the human uterine epithelial cell line RL95-2, epithelial reorganization may be triggered by trophoblast binding. Activation of Rho-GTPase, with associated reorganization of the actin cytoskeleton, takes place in response to trophoblast attachment.[43]

In mouse, the apical microvilli of LE cells, characteristic of regular simple epithelia, give way to bulbous endocytic pinopods as the uterus moves into the receptive period.[46,47] Pinopod formation has been shown to be stimulated by progesterone and inhibited by estrogen, and pinopods are absent in leukemia inhibitory factor (LIF)-null females at the expected implantation window, suggesting direct or indirect regulation by LIF.[58] The human equivalents of pinopods (uterodomes) are not pinocytotic[59] but have been associated with receptivity[60] and it has been suggested that they carry potential adhesion molecules.[3,61] The bulbous uterodomes appear between days 20 and 22 of the menstrual cycle, correlating with the beginning of the expected period for implantation.[3,60] Repeated biopsy of the endometrium suggests that uterodomes have a lifetime of less than 48 hours in women. Furthermore, in one study, all three human blastocysts co-cultured with endometrial epithelial cells were reported to attach where clusters of uterodomes were present.[3] So uterodomes may be important in the initial attachment of human embryos. Little is known about whether they carry qualitatively or quantitatively different molecules, but a recent study showed uterodomes are not associated with the antiadhesive factor mucin glycoprotein 1 (MUC-1)[62] (see below). It is possible that the failure of embryos to develop intimate association with the LE of LIF-null mice relates to the lack of pinopod formation by these cells,[58] suggesting similarity between rodents and humans. Hoxa-10 is also required for murine pinopod formation. After Hoxa-10-antisense treatment, embryos do not implant and these structures fail to appear on the luminal epithelium at the start of the period of receptivity.[63] Moreover, recent observations suggest that fine tuning of the attachment reaction may involve repulsion between ephrins expressed on the blastocyst and Eph A1 on the endometrial epithelium. The latter is decreased at the attachment site and inhibits blastocyst attachment in vitro.[64] Gathering together these observations, it becomes clear that postovulatory LE and receptive LE have very different cell surface phenotypes. A change in epithelial cell organization at the time of implantation and at the attachment site may be a general principle across the range of mammals, irrespective of differences in control mechanisms and subsequent trophoblast behavior.

Molecular basis of initial attachment

As adhesion between trophoblast and LE occurs, engagement of cell adhesion molecules leads to transduction of cytoplasmic signals that trigger the next steps in implantation. Since adhesion must be transient, the molecular environment must evolve rapidly to facilitate penetration of trophoblast through the LE and into the stroma. So what do we know about the molecules involved? Targeted gene deletion has led to the identification of surprisingly few genes with an implantation phenotype, perhaps because of compensatory capacity associated with the importance of implantation being successful. Therefore, our knowledge of the key molecules comes from less direct approaches.

ANALOGY WITH NEUTROPHIL–ENDOTHELIAL INTERACTION

The analogy has been made between interaction of leukocytes with endothelial cells at sites of inflammation and that of the blastocyst with LE at implantation.[26,65] However, the blastocyst moves through the luminal fluid under very gentle flow conditions, while neutrophils experience shear stress even in capillaries and venules. In damaged or infected tissues, neutrophils adhere to activated vascular endothelium. Initial adhesion is mediated by selectins, transmembrane proteins with terminal C-type, calcium-dependent lectin domains.[66] Under conditions of flow they induce the slowed rolling motion of leukocytes preceding attachment, by low-affinity, specific, carbohydrate binding. Although shear stress does not apply in the uterus, it is likely that trophoblast interaction with LE proceeds stepwise, starting with a 'tethering' step that leads to a sequence of further adhesive interactions.[65] Rolling leukocytes then adhere by low avidity interactions between β_2 integrins and immunoglobulin superfamily endothelial receptors. Binding-induced increase in avidity leads to firmer adhesion, which is followed by extravasation,[67] with morphological similarities to trophoblast penetration of LE. Unfortunately, current in-vitro models for TE–LE interactions cannot accurately reflect the changing time course of adhesive events, so the sequential nature of TE–LE interactions is still to be documented.

GLYCOSYLATION OF THE LUMINAL EPITHELIUM AND IMPLANTATION

In common with other epithelial surfaces, the LE contains an apical glycocalyx that allows diffusion of small molecules but inhibits adhesion.[68] Carbohydrate chains within this glycocalyx extend into the extracellular space for varying distances: in the case of mucins, by as much as 1 µm and well beyond the projection of proteins, suggesting that mucin oligosaccharide chains of the glycocalyx are the first point of contact for the embryo as it approaches the LE.[26] This is supported by the observation of a 0.2–0.7 µm space between LE and TE surfaces of blastocysts attached to cultured uterine strips,[69] although whether this occurs in vivo is not clear.

ROLE OF MUCINS IN REGULATING IMPLANTATION

LE acts as a barrier to microbial infection as well as maintaining tissue homeostasis. Thus, the balance between antiadhesive molecules such as mucins and adhesive molecules in generally is in favor of non-adhesion but this balance must change to allow blastocyst implantation. Large glycosylated mucins, such as Muc-1, have long-core proteins with multiple O-glycosylation sites carrying sialylated and sulfated carbohydrate chains that give the molecule a highly extended conformation able to project hundreds of nanometers from the membrane. This, together with their negative charge, is likely to prevent interaction between less extensive adhesion molecules on adjacent

cell surfaces.[68,70] Indeed Muc-1 has been shown to sterically block E-cadherin-based cell–cell interactions and Muc-1 and -4 to block integrin-based cell–matrix interactions.[71–73] In keeping with this idea, Muc-1 exhibits species-dependent steroidal and implantation-related regulation. In murine LE, Muc-1 integral membrane protein is down-regulated at implantation under the control of maternal steroids,[74] as similarly demonstrated in vitro for pigs.[33] Indeed, after injection of mice on day 3 of pregnancy with RU-486, Muc-1 increased six-fold,[75] nicely demonstrating its progesterone repression. In rabbits and primates, although it is *stimulated* by progesterone, it is still selectively reduced at implantation adjacent to the implanting rabbit blastocyst[76] and in baboon in LE but not glands.[77] Removal of its ectodomain by cleavage, as occurs in vitro,[78] might allow trans-binding between other adhesive molecules on TE and LE. Null mice are fertile despite suffering from reproductive tract infections.[79] In-vitro studies have illuminated the function of Muc-1 in several species. Murine blastocyst attachment to cultured polarized LE cells from Muc-1 null female mice was greater than for wild-type LE. Treatment of wild-type LE cells with O-sialoglycoprotein endopeptidase to remove mucins similarly increased embryo attachment compared to wild type but had no effect on Muc-1 null epithelium. However, after embryo transfer, the percentages of implanted fetuses in Muc-1 null, wild-type, or O-sialoglycoprotein endopeptidase-injected wild-type uteri were similar even when transfer took place the day before the normal day of implantation.[79] Thus, removal of Muc-1 alone does not control the opening of the implantation window in vivo, nor is reduction of Muc-1 sufficient to allow normal LE–TE attachment since it occurs on schedule in LIF-null females but implantation does not take place.[58] In rats, another mucin, Muc-4, is expressed in LE, under similar ovarian steroid control to murine Muc-1. It also disappears at the time of implantation.[80] So, Muc-4 may have a similar barrier function in preventing attachment in prereceptive LE of rats.

In women, during the receptive phase, MUC-1 is strongly expressed at the epithelial apical cell surface and in uterine secretions,[81] although the pattern of its glycosylation changes during the menstrual cycle.[82–84] It has been suggested to act as a selective barrier to prevent adhesion of substandard blastocysts to LE.[68,85] In this way, it might contribute to the recognized greater success of implantation in mice compared to humans, reflected in the higher frequency of pregnancy for mouse embryo transfer compared to human IVF replacement. In support of this idea, when human embryos are allowed to attach to endometrial epithelial cell monolayers, MUC-1 expression disappears from the area around the attached blastocyst, suggesting that the human embryo may play an active role in MUC-1 removal at implantation.[70] The mechanism by which Muc-1 is removed is not entirely clear. However, the disintegrin metalloproteinase ADAM9 accumulates at the site of blastocyst attachment in rabbits[86] and ADAM17/TACE, which is expressed in LE, has been shown to release Muc-1 ectodomain from cells in culture.[87] Moreover, tumor necrosis factor, known to be secreted by receptive endometrium and detected in media from human embryo culture, has been shown to induce loss of MUC1 from a human epithelial cell line in a metalloproteinase-dependent manner.[88] Interestingly, in patients with recurrent miscarriage, MUC-1 is less abundant, suggesting a reduction in the barrier, which might lead to implantation of embryos with reduced developmental potential.[89]

In women, carbohydrate structures such as keratan sulfate, associated with implantation success, are carried by MUC-1,[90,91] as are potential selectin ligands like sialyl Le-x and sialyl Le-y.[84] It is possible that special properties of human MUC-1 render it an initial adhesion molecule with carbohydrate groups functioning as tethering agents interacting with trophoblast sugar-binding molecules. At the same time it might sterically block interaction with other cell adhesion molecules (CAMs) on substandard blastocysts lacking lectin-type receptors. A specific epitope of MUC-1, although highly expressed in most proliferative phase endometrial epithelium, is drastically reduced in mid secretory phase[91,92] but restored by keratinase or neuraminidase treatment. This suggests that specific glycosylation occurs at the expected time of implantation to mask the epitope and reinforces the possibility that lectin-like trophoblast molecules may interact first with temporally regulated sialylated or sulfated sugars expressed on large mucins.

Fucosylated carbohydrates and ligands at implantation

Carbohydrate–lectin binding has been suggested to mediate initial weak attachment in parallel with the known leukocyte–endothelial interaction that occurs at inflammatory sites.[26,65,93] There is evidence for involvement of a number of carbohydrate ligands and some lectin-like molecules in initial embryo attachment.

The fucosylated H-type-1 antigen ($Fuc_{\alpha1-2}Gal_{\beta1-3}GlcNAc_{\beta1-}$) has been suggested as one possible initial attachment ligand and it is expressed in the LE in several species.[26,33,94] Expression on murine LE is estrogen-dependent and controlled by an α_{1-2} fucosyltransferase ($\alpha_{1-2}FT$).[95–98] In-vitro attachment of blastocysts to cultured LE is inhibited by an H-type-1 pentasaccharide, or a monoclonal antibody (mAb) that recognizes it.[99] The H-type-1 sugar is abundant on the apical LE cell surface up to day 4 of pregnancy[100] and so could interact with the trophoblast at attachment. Its disappearance between day 5 and day 6[100] may contribute to the refractory phase when implantation can no longer occur. Binding sites for H-type-1 are detected on abembryonic TE (which first contacts the LE in mice) of hatching blastocysts,[101,102] suggesting the presence of receptor(s) on the trophoblast. H-type-1 on LE may be unavailable to trophoblast receptors up to the normal time of implantation or the H-type-1 sugar present in luminal fluid may act as a competitive inhibitor in the preimplantation period.[103] In the absence of LIF, H-type-1 antigen is dramatically enhanced adjacent to the embryo on day 5 of pregnancy and not down-regulated by day 6 of pregnancy when the wild-type uterus shows no H-type-1 expression and has become refractory to implantation.[58] Since the embryo does not attach to the LE in the LIF-null uterus it is clear that the increase in H-type-1 is insufficient to drive embryo attachment to LE without other changes taking place. It is possible that it has a dual function: as a component of a barrier against embryo attachment or as an attachment molecule, depending on the molecular environment in the apical LE. It is clear that H-type-1 interaction is not essential to implantation, or its loss can be compensated, because implantation is normal in mice carrying a deletion of Fut2, the fucosyltransferase required for H-type-1 biosynthesis.[104] Furthermore, uterine injection of antibody to H-type-1 fails to block implantation.[105] From successful antibody inhibition in vivo, the possible involvement of the Le-y carbohydrate antigen ($Fuc_{\alpha1-2}Gal_{\beta1-4}[Fuc_{\alpha1-3}]GlcNAc_{\beta1-}$) in attachment has also been suggested.[105,106] This carbohydrate epitope is present on the blastocyst surface in mice[107,108] and on LE in both mice[100,105] and humans.[93,109] Since Le-y glycolipid has been demonstrated to bind H-type-1 and -2 chain glycolipids, Le-y on the blastocyst could interact with H-type-1 on apical LE. However, the Fut2 enzyme is again required to produce the ligand.

Selectins and galectins and other carbohydrate-binding receptors

The selectins are calcium-dependent carbohydrate-binding molecules with well-established roles in the initial interaction of leukocytes with endothelial cells at sites of inflammation and in lymphocyte homing.[67] Several selectin ligands are expressed by murine and human trophectoderm (see above)[7,12,110,111] and LE, where sialyl Le-x increases during the murine receptive period[112] and is modulated during the menstrual cycle.[84] L-selectin and E-selectin proteins are expressed on murine blastocysts but not earlier stages,[111] while human hatched blastocysts and invasive trophoblast express L-selectin[12] and bind to 6-sulfo sialyl Le-x beads. In sheep, the mucin GlyCAM-1, a ligand for L-selectin in lymph node endothelium, is expressed both by LE and trophectoderm during the initial interaction period.[113] In homozygotic mutant mice null for each of the three selectins, and in mice lacking two or all three selectins, embryonic development, implantation, and pregnancy appear normal.[114,115] Although gene deletion experiments may be misleading because of possible compensatory functions of other contributing molecules, there is no direct evidence that any of the selectins plays an essential role in implantation.

There is good evidence for expression of members of the carbohydrate-binding galectin family by the blastocyst. Galectins are calcium-independent animal lectins which share structural similarities and specificity for saccharides containing N-acetyl lactosamine repeats.[116] They are widely expressed and have been implicated in multiple functions. Galectin-1, -3, and -5 are expressed first by the murine blastocyst at hatching and both galectins -1 and -3 are present on the surface of implanting blastocyst TE but not ICM.[9,117–119] Since galectins-1 and -3 have some affinity for the H-type-1 epitope, either might act as a receptor for the H-type-1 antigen on the LE.[9] Galectins bind laminin[120] and can modulate its interaction with integrin $\alpha 7\beta 1$,[121] suggested to be involved in trophoblast invasion in mice.[18,122,123] However, gene deletion militates against a unique role of either galectin-1 or -3. In mice lacking functional genes for either or both of these galectins, reproduction is unaffected.[117,124,125] It is still possible that galectin-5 can compensate for loss of the galectins-1 and -3 or plays a role in its own right. Since several members of the galectin family are expressed by trophoblast at implantation, they may function interchangeably, thus safeguarding this critically important process. Interestingly, expression of galectin-9 increases in human endometrial epithelium during the mid and late secretory phase,[126] while galectin-15 is secreted by the endometrial glandular and luminal epithelium in sheep and absorbed onto the placental trophoblast.[127] So there are potential roles for endometrial galectins in materno–fetal/placental interactions at implantation in these species.[128] Galectin-3 has been found in decidua in the mouse and a potential ligand, cubilin, identified in yolk sac endoderm,[129] suggesting a role in maternal–fetal interactions in the early postimplantation embryo.

Other carbohydrate-binding molecules such as CD44 could potentially be involved in TE adhesion, although the evidence is circumstantial. CD44 consists of a family of alternatively spliced membrane glycoproteins that are involved in cell–cell and cell–matrix interactions. Unspecified isoforms are expressed both by preimplantation human embryos (but not first trimester trophoblast) and endometrial epithelium.[6,130] CD44 isoforms could form bridging ligands interacting with the abundant sialylated and sulfated carbohydrates on the apical surface of human and murine LE.[68,84,90] Other potential CD44 ligands are present both in endometrium and blastocyst,[68] osteopontin being arguably the most important.[130] However, ablation of CD44 does not appear to perturb fertility,[131] so again neither expression in the uterus nor embryo appears essential.

Heparan sulfate proteoglycan

Heparan sulfate proteoglycan (HSPG) exists in a variety of membrane-bound and extracellular matrix (ECM)-associated forms. The specificity of interactions is based on both tissue-specific core protein expression and complex differential modification of the characteristic repeat disaccharide (Glc–GlcNAc).[132] A basement membrane form of HSPG, perlecan, surrounds the blastocyst after hatching and expression of the mRNA and protein correlates with acquisition of attachment competence.[133,134] This suggests a possible role in implantation: HSPG is in the right position to act as a bridging ligand binding TE to LE and mouse embryos can attach to HSPG-binding proteins. Once again, gene deletion offers little help because perlecan-null embryos show no implantation phenotype, being indistinguishable from wild-type embryos until day 9.5, nearly mid gestation.[135] In the human it is not known if perlecan or other ECM-associated HSPG is expressed by hatched blastocysts. However, attachment of labeled JAR cells (human choriocarcinoma-derived trophoblast cell line) to RL95 monolayers (human endometrial adenocarcinoma line) occurs by an HSPG/heparin-dependent mechanism.[136] RL-95 cells are one of the few human endometrial epithelial cell lines which allow trophoblast adhesion at their apical surface.[43,44] An HSPG-binding protein, heparin/heparan sulfate proteoglycan interacting protein (HIP) cloned from RL-95 cells, is expressed by murine and human endometrial epithelium throughout the reproductive cycle.[137] Purified HIP supports attachment of JAR cells in an HS-dependent manner,[138] and since HIP also binds perlecan,[139] a

HIP–perlecan–HS interaction may occur at the TE–LE interface. HIP is also expressed preferentially at points of chorionic villus attachment and where cytotrophoblast invasion is initiated in first trimester placenta. However, enrichment on cytotrophoblast that has penetrated maternal blood vessel walls suggests a role in trophoblast invasion. This is supported by the effect of antibodies to HIP, which block invasion of JAR cells into Matrigel but not their attachment. Moreover, in pre-eclampsia, when infiltration of trophoblast through arterial walls is compromised, HIP expression is very low.[139] It is possible that different LE or TE HSPG-binding molecules function in attachment of human blastocysts from those in cytotrophoblast invasion. Furthermore, a truncated form of heparin-binding EGF-like growth factor (HB-EGF; see below) is induced in the LE by the embryo and could also interact with HSPG.[140] Importantly, findings from *Drosophila* and vertebrate development suggest that HSPGs have important roles in regulating growth factor morphogen signaling (e.g fibroblast growth factor [FGF], hedgehog, and wnt families).[141] Therefore, this may be an additional or alternative function at the maternal–fetal interface.

Heparin binding EGF-like growth factor

HB-EGF is a member of the epidermal growth factor (EGF) family. It binds to HSPG as well as the EGF receptor family members ErbB1 and ErbB4,[142] all three of which are expressed by the hatching murine blastocyst.[28,140] It is now clear that it has two functions in relation to the blastocyst: trophoblast maturation and LE–trophoblast interaction. Soluble HB-EGF accelerates murine trophoblast maturation to adhesion competence and promotes hatching and outgrowth.[143,144] Similarly, HB-EGF increases the percentage of human embryos reaching the blastocyst stage and promotes hatching.[145] HB-EGF triggered EGF-R phosphorylation in murine trophoblast,[143] suggesting that this is at least one signaling route to modifying trophoblast cell phenotype. Maturation of the murine trophectoderm induced by HB-EGF requires influx of extracellular calcium and activity of calmodulin and correlated with cell surface appearance of ErbB4.[144] Transactivation of ErbB4 or ErbB1 by lysophosphatidic acid induced accumulation of HB-EGF at the trophectoderm surface and accelerates trophoblast outgrowth.[146] Interestingly, the knockout strategy has implicated uterine LPA receptor 3 in regulation of later events in implantation,[147] but blastocysts lack LPA receptor 3 while expressing LPA receptors 1 and 2.[146]

HB-EGF expression is regulated by estrogen in murine endometrium and by progesterone in stroma.[148,149] In LE it mediates estrogenic effects on cell proliferation.[150] During early pregnancy, HB-EGF mRNA is absent from LE on days 2 and 3. However, 6–7 hours before the expected time of blastocyst attachment, a transmembrane form of HB-EGF is induced by the blastocyst on the apical LE surface of the implantation chamber.[143] Activated blastocysts can adhere to cells transfected with this form of HB-EGF by a mechanism which involves an EGF-R family member, probably ErbB4.[140] HB-EGF–blastocyst interaction is partially heparitinase-sensitive, suggesting involvement of HSPG. HB-EGF binding to EGF-R[151] is enhanced by HSPG, suggesting this may be the major function of trophectoderm HSPG. Alternatively HSPG may bind to transmembrane HBEGF on LE to form a component of the initial attachment mechanism. Other members of the EGF family are subsequently expressed in the LE.[152] ErbB4-null embryos die early in gestation, while the majority of HB-EGF null progeny die before weaning. Both these nulls develop heart problems.[153,154] However, surviving HB-EGF–/– adult females are fertile, and fertile erbB4 nulls can be produced after cardiomyocyte-specific rescue of the heart defect, so a unique role in murine implantation may be questionable.

Human endometrium shows menstrual cycle-dependent changes in HB-EGF mRNA. It increases in the secretory phase and is highest just prior to the opening of the implantation window, after which it declines. The protein is expressed in proliferative phase stroma, but at midsecretory phase (expected receptive phase) it is expressed at the apical surface of the LE.[155,156] HB-EGF protein expression was highest on endometrial epithelium when receptivity-associated uterodomes were well developed.[157] ErbB4 but not ErbB1 is expressed by human peri-implantation blastocysts and they adhere to cells or substrates carrying transmembrane HB-EGF,[155] suggesting that this molecule may function in adhesion of human blastocysts to LE, as in mice.

Signaling events at initial implantation

Interaction between the blastocyst and uterus (Figure 22.1) contributes to synchronization of their development and differentiation. Some of the proposed cell adhesive interactions between LE and TE may function mainly to initiate signaling cascades that induce further changes in blastocyst and uterine cell phenotypes. These signaling pathways drive the epithelial–mesenchymal

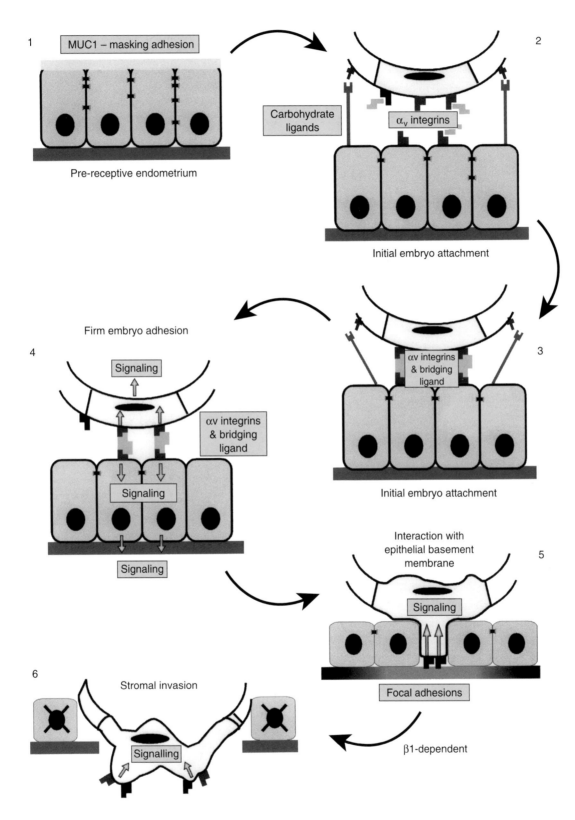

Figure 22.1 The series of interactions between the TE/trophoblast and LE and subjacent stroma. Potential roles of cell adhesion molecules at each stage are indicated. (1) Prereceptive endometrium: desmosomes distributed along lateral LE cell surfaces and non-adhesive apical cell surface. (2) Receptive endometrium and initial embryo attachment: reorganization of lateral LE adhesion complexes accompanies apical carbohydrate ligand engagement to tether blastocyst, α_v integrins now becoming available for binding. (3) Stabilization of initial attachment: α_v integrin-mediated adhesion involving bridging ligands shown but other ligand binding also probably functional. (4) Potential signaling through cell adhesion ligand–receptor interaction. (5) Penetration of LE and interaction with extracellular matrix via β_1 integrins (basement matrix degraded). (6) Invasion into stroma: continuing β_1 integrin activity and trophoblast signaling.

transition of the TE to form trophoblast and, in rodents, the differentiation or decidualization of uterine stroma.

The essential function of calcium signaling during implantation both in endometrium[158,159] and in trophoblast[17] is well established. Transcripts encoding the calcium-binding protein calbindin-d9k (CABP-d9k) are increased in the luminal epithelium at the interimplantation site.[159,160] Down-regulation of both calbindin-d9k and d28K occurs at the implantation site[159,160] or after blastocyst transfer,[161] suggesting precise spatial and temporal regulation of calcium-mediated signaling, or calcium availability. The importance of calbindin regulation of calcium transport for implantation is revealed by the prevention of implantation by use of antisense removal of calbindin d9k transcripts in a calbindin d28K null uterus.[159] This suggests that stimulation of calcium transport before implantation is needed for some implantation-related function in LE, but it is also possible that upsetting the normal calcium flux impaired the calcium-dependent activation of trophectoderm. The progesterone-regulated endometrial gland cell secretory product calcitonin[162] is important for implantation in rats, where reduction in implantation rates is observed when maternal expression is blocked using antisense oligonucleotide.[158] Calcitonin binds to a G-protein-coupled receptor on the preimplantation embryo, triggering an increase in intracellular calcium, activation of adenyl cyclase, and expression of the fibronectin receptor, integrin $\alpha_5\beta_1$,[163] a component of trophoblast activation which can interact with endometrial ligands.

Murine blastocyst signals lead to local induction of cyclooxygenase 2 (Cox-2) in the LE and stroma adjacent to the embryo.[164] Cox-2, a key enzyme in prostaglandin and prostacyclin synthesis, appears to be central to a number of the signaling pathways involved in early implantation events. It has profound regulatory effects through the mediation of prostaglandins and vascular endothelial growth factor (VEGF) on vascular permeability and angiogenesis.[165] COX-2 null females have multiple reproductive failure, including defects in ovulation, fertilization, and delayed decidualization with (in some strains) inability to support implantation[166] but in others normal pregnancy outcome.[167] These conflicting findings have been suggested to stem from differences in genetic makeup that drive altered levels of compensatory Cox-1 in the Cox-2 knockout.[168] In females lacking Cox-2, supplementing with a prostacyclin (PGI$_2$) analogue was much more effective than PGE$_2$ in restoring the decidual reaction and implantation.[169] This suggests that PGI$_2$ may be an important missing Cox-2 product in mice lacking this enzyme and responsible for the induction of uterine stromal changes required for implantation. Since PGI$_2$ has been shown to induce increased vascular permeability,[170] a key feature of the decidual reaction, this may be its prime target at implantation. PGI$_2$ may interact with the cellular machinery through activation of the nuclear peroxisome proliferator-activated receptor δ (PPARδ) receptor, rather than through its membrane receptor whose mRNA is very low in the uterus.[169] A PPARδ agonist was effective in restoring implantation in Cox-2 null females. Interestingly, in the absence of LIF, uteri cannot support implantation of an embryo[171,172] and Cox-2 transcript and protein expression is observed only in the LE at the implantation site without later expression in the stroma.[58,173] In women, prostaglandin levels rise in the luteal phase of the menstrual cycle and COX-2 protein increases in the glands in late luteal phase,[174] while in the mid luteal phase COX-2 protein was reported to be mainly in perivascular cells and LE.[175] LE but not perivascular expression was mifepristone-sensitive and therefore progesterone dependent.[175] Thus, LE COX-2 may also play a role in preparation of the human uterus for implantation.

CONTINUED INTERACTION WITH LE

Once the embryo is tethered, possibly by a low binding–strength link, other molecules probably establish firmer contact with LE in preparation for its penetration. Some of the best candidates are integrin cell adhesion molecules and their ligands[176,177] but the trophinin–tastin–bystin complex[178] has also been suggested.

Trophinin–tastin–bystin complex

Cell adhesion between a human trophoblast cell line and an endometrial adenocarcinoma cell line has been shown to occur through a unique intrinsic membrane protein, trophinin, but only when complexed to a cytoplasmic protein, tastin.[179] Trophinin and tastin do not bind directly to one another but both bind an intermediate protein bystin, also expressed by both cell lines.[180] Functional complex formation is facilitated by interaction of these molecules with cytokeratins 8 and 18, suggesting the assembly of a true functional adhesion complex. Trophinin appears to mediate calcium-dependent homophilic binding and its structure – with its 69 serine/threonine-rich decapeptide repeats – has been likened to a mucin.[68]

In mice, trophinin is specifically expressed by the blastocyst and uterus between 3.5 and 5.5 days post-coitum. Null mice have been produced by homologous recombination in embryonic stem (ES) cells and on a 129/SvJ background, but not some others, there is partial lethality. It appears that in the mouse trophinin is not essential for implantation.[181] However it is possible that it still plays some role, and maternal trophinin may persist from the oocyte and be used at the blastocyst stage.[179] Parallel endometrial expression of trophinin and tastin occurs in human: they are absent in proliferative phase but appear at days 16/17, in early secretory phase, at the apical endometrial epithelial surface. Then they disappear rapidly during the mid/late secretory period and when implantation should occur they are apparently absent from epithelium but present in uterine mucus. However, trophinin is present later at the uteroplacental interface at 6–7 weeks of human pregnancy.[179] Naturally, the implantation site in a conception cycle has not been examined, but it would be interesting to know if this adhesion complex is retained in LE specifically adjacent to the blastocyst. In the mouse, although trophinin is hormonally regulated in LE, the embryo does not induce expression.[182] Certainly, at the macaque implantation site, trophinin expression is observed at the apposed apical surfaces of trophoblast and LE and similarly on the apical surface of rhesus monkey blastocyst TE, predominantly at the embryonic pole which first contacts the LE in primates.

Integrins

A number of α and β integrin subunits are expressed continuously from the fertilized murine egg through to the peri- and postimplantation period, including α_5, α_{6B}, α_v, β_1, and β_3,[123] while other integrins are regulated in the embryo. In particular α_2, α_7, and α_{6A} mRNAs are detected from the fully expanded blastocyst stage and α_3, α_2, and α_1 can be detected as protein in trophoblast outgrowths in vitro.[17,123] Therefore several β_1 and α_v integrin heterodimers may be expressed at the time of blastocyst attachment (Table 22.1) and $\alpha_v\beta_3$, $\alpha_5\beta_1$, and $\alpha_6\beta_1$ are present at the cell surface.[123] Identified ligands for the different heterodimers are shown in Table 22.2. Of the blastocyst integrins, $\alpha_5\beta_1$ and $\alpha_6\beta_1$ integrins are not regulated and are expressed between inner cell mass (ICM) cells and adjacent to the blastocyst cavity, rather than the external TE surface[123] of early expanded blastocysts. This makes them unlikely candidates for adhesion to LE. However, as differentiation

of the TE continues in culture, $\alpha_5\beta_1$ does translocate to the apical surface of abembryonic TE, which first contacts the uterus and generates the primary trophoblast[163,183] and is fundamental to strong fibronectin adhesion.[184] Integrin translocation is regulated by ligation of the blastocyst calcitonin receptor and receptor-mediated Ca^{2+} signaling and is a prerequisite for attachment and outgrowth on fibronectin.[163,183] Furthermore, $\alpha_{IIb}\beta_3$ integrin, another fibronectin receptor, also regulates adhesion, only translocating to the TE surface on ligand binding.[184] This exemplifies the crucially important and complex signaling function of cell adhesion molecule engagement. In contrast, $\alpha_v\beta_3$ can be demonstrated on the external surface of TE and later, in vitro, in focal contacts of spreading trophoblast. It is therefore in a position to mediate initial adhesion and/or subsequent invasion. $\alpha_v\beta_3$ integrin interacts with fibronectin, vitronectin, tenascin, osteopontin, and thrombospondin and with a cryptic domain of laminin (see Table 22.2). All are found in the trophoblast adhesion/invasion pathway. Furthermore, function-blocking antibodies to $\alpha_v\beta_3$ in utero have been reported to reduce the number of implantation sites.[185] Thus, $\alpha_5\beta_1$, $\alpha_v\beta_3$, and $\alpha_{II}\beta_3$ integrins appear to act in concert to regulate at least fibronectin-based trophoblast adhesion.[184] Integrin cell surface expression and interactions contribute to the differentiation of the trophoblast in terms of resultant immediate signaling response and subsequent autocrine signaling.[17] Human preimplantation embryos have also been shown to express a number of integrin subunits, and at the blastocyst stage these include α_3, α_v, β_1, β_3, and β_5.[7,110] So far, there is little evidence for developmental regulation at the protein level. However, trophoblast $\alpha_v\beta_3$ integrin may be available for adhesion of human embryos to LE (as in the mouse), as may other integrins ($\alpha_3\beta_1$, $\alpha_6\beta_4$, $\alpha_v\beta_5$ and theoretically $\alpha_v\beta_1$).

A number of ligands for integrins are also expressed at or by the blastocyst stage. In the mouse these include fibronectin, laminin and entactin 1,[186] and type IV collagen,[187] but apart from laminin they are predominantly in the ICM and developing basement membrane of TE. In 8-cell+ bovine embryos, fibronectin, and in human morulae laminin, is expressed at the cell surface.[188,189] Osteopontin is expressed by human cytotrophoblast and mRNA levels are stimulated by progesterone.[190] Laminin, HSPG, and thrombospondin are detected around the external cell surface of the murine blastocyst.[191-193] Laminin and osteopontin might be anchored by $\alpha_v\beta_3$, while thrombospondin can interact with both $\alpha_v\beta_3$ and HSPG core protein.[194,195]

Table 22.1 Expression of adhesion molecules potentially involved in the trophoblast adhesion cascade

Cell adhesion molecule	Mouse blastocyst	Mouse luminal epithelium	Human/primate blastocyst	1st trimester trophoblast	Human endometrium
$\alpha_1\beta_1$				↑	+
$\alpha_2\beta_1$	+				+
$\alpha_3\beta_1$			+		
$\alpha_3\beta_3$					+
$\alpha_4\beta_1$					+
$\alpha_5\beta_1$	+			↑	+
$\alpha_6\beta_1$	+	+		+[r]	+?
$\alpha_6\beta_4$			+?	↓	
$\alpha_7\beta_1$	+				
$\alpha_v\beta_1$			+?	+?	+?
$\alpha_v\beta_3$	+	+	+	+	+
$\alpha_v\beta_5$		+	+		+?
$\alpha_{IIb}\beta_3$	+				
E-cadherin	+	+	+	+ → −	+
Cadherin-11				− → +	+
N-CAM	+				
P-selectin		+[u]			
L-selectin	+[u]		+		
Trophinin/tastin	+	+	+[p]		+
CD44			+		+
Perlecan	+	+			
HIP				+	+
Muc-1					+
HB-EGF		+[r]			+
Galectin-1	+		+		
Galectin-3	+				
Galectin-5	+				
Le-y	+	+			+
H-type-1		+			+
Laminin	+	+	+?		+
Thrombospondin	+				
Osteopontin				+	+

r, restricted expression; p, primate; ?, requires confirmation due to low numbers or weak staining or inferred integrin heterodimer; u, Stones and Kimber unpublished data; ↑, increasing expression on subset of cells; ↓, decreasing expression on subset of cells.

For references refer to text.

HSPG also has a number of other potential ligands on LE or trophoblast (above). Theoretically, any of these ECM molecules could act as a bridge, binding the TE to the luminal surface. However, fibronectin and vitronectin null mouse embryos implant normally,[196,197] suggesting no TE requirement and these molecules are probably not present on the apical LE. The best candidates for a bridging function are osteopontin, embryonic laminin, and HSPG. Osteopontin is expressed on ruminant endometrial epithelium[198] and by human endometrial epithelium, particularly apically and with highest levels in the secretory phase glands.[199]

If ECM components expressed by the embryo or LE are to act as bridging-type molecules, the LE surface must carry appropriate receptors. The ability of different human uterine epithelial cell lines to support embryo attachment has been correlated with the apical expression of normally basolateral cell adhesion molecules such as E-cadherin, but also α_6, β_1, and β_4

Table 22.2 Extracellular matrix ligands of β_1- and α_v-family integrins

$\alpha_1\beta_1$	COL	LM								PE	
$\alpha_2\beta_1\ \alpha_3\beta_1$	COL	LM									
$\alpha_4\beta_1\ \underline{\alpha_5\beta_1}$			FN								
$\alpha_6\beta_1\ \alpha_7\beta_1$		LM									
$\alpha_8\beta_1$			FN		VN		TN				
$\alpha_9\beta_1$							TN				
$\underline{\alpha_v\beta_1}$	COL		FN	FB	VN	vWF					
$\underline{\alpha_v\beta_3}$		LM	FN	FB	VN	vWF	TN	OST	TSP	PE	PEC
$\underline{\alpha_v\beta_5}$			FN	FB	VN						
$\underline{\alpha_v\beta_6}$			FN				TN				
$\alpha_v\beta_8$					VN						

COL, collagen; LM, laminin; FN, fibronectin; FB, fibrinogen; VN, vitronectin; vWF, Von Willebrand factor; TN, tenascin; OST, osteopontin; TSP, thrombospondin; PE, perlecan; platelet endothelial cell adhesion molecule – 1, PEC.
Integrins known to recognize the RGD motif found in most ligands are underlined.
Based on References 235–237.

integrins.[200] However, the reduction in proposed antiadhesive factors like Muc-1 may also contribute to the adhesivity of some of these cell lines.[85] A number of β_1 integrins – $\alpha_1\beta_1$, $\alpha_2\beta_1$, $\alpha_3\beta_3$, $\alpha_4\beta_1$, $\alpha_5\beta_1$, and $\alpha_6\beta_1$ – are expressed on human endometrial epithelial cells while $\alpha_1\beta_1$, $\alpha_4\beta_1$, and $\alpha_5\beta_1$ are also expressed by stromal cells: with the exception of $\alpha_1\beta_1$ and $\alpha_4\beta_1$, most show little menstrual cycle regulation[201,202] (reviewed in references 26 and 203). Expression of $\alpha_4\beta_1$ is highest in glandular epithilium (GE) between mid proliferative and mid secretory phase. However $\alpha_1\beta_1$ shows possible implantation phase-related changes: its expression is restricted to early and mid secretory phase in epithelium and in stroma is only expressed in the predecidual stage. α_v integrin protein is expressed in the endometrium[202,204] and a potential β subunit partner, β_5, is expressed by LE and stroma but not regulated at the protein level.[204] Higher levels of β_6 integrin protein in secretory phase LE have been reported.[205] Another partner, β_3, appears abruptly on the GE on day 19 of the menstrual cycle at the initiation of the window of receptivity for implantation, but slightly later on the LE.[206] $\alpha_v\beta_3$ integrin has many potential ligands (see Table 22.2). As well as those mentioned above, it binds vitronectin, which may be present on the trophoblast, but vitronectin-null mice show no apparent reproductive defect. Another ligand, oncofetal fibronectin, is expressed by human trophoblast.[207] Proposed bridging between trophoblast $\alpha_v\beta_3$ and luminal epithelial osteopontin seems unlikely in ruminants due to lack of appropriate trophoblast integrin expression.[208] Some indirect evidence of $\alpha_v\beta_3$ expression related to fertility comes from the absence of β_3 as well as α_1 and α_4 in menopausal endometrium.[209] β_3 integrin is also absent or expressed

late in infertility-related delayed endometrial differentiation[210] and lacking in endometriosis.[211] Most importantly for initial TE–LE interaction, $\alpha_v\beta_3$ is expressed apically in both mouse and human endometrial epithelium, as is another α_v partner β_5, which can also bind fibronectin and vitronectin.[204] Although none of α_v, β_3, and β_5 appear to be hormonally regulated in mouse LE,[204] their apical location would allow a role in strengthening the initial interaction between TE and LE. Temporally regulated interaction only during the receptive period might be accounted for if α_v heterodimers are masked[33] prior to the period of receptivity in mice. Recently, a teraspanin protein shown to regulate cell surface expression of proteins, including the integrins $\alpha_5\beta_1$ and $\alpha_6\beta_1$, has been implicated in implantation. Epithelial membrane protein 2 (EMP2) is expressed in mouse LE and becomes located in the apical membrane during the receptive period. RNAi for EMP2 in a number of human endometrial carcinoma cell lines reduced murine embryo attachment and RNAi inhibition of EMP2 in the uterus reduced implantation sites.[212]

LATER EVENTS IN ADHESION–INVASION

Laminin and collagen IV disappear from the LE basement membrane before trophoblast reaches the basal LE cell surface,[35] so they are unavailable for trophoblast interaction following penetration between the LE cells. However, decidualization leads to increased secretion by stromal cells of laminin, entactin, type 4 collagen, and HSPG (all trophoblast substrates). ECM is rearranged into a pericellular matrix layer around the cells in humans, or into patches in mice, and there is decreased production of fibronectin by mouse decidua.[213,214] These molecules are available for adhesion and migration of trophoblast late in the adhesion cascade but also as a source of bound growth factors[141,215] and induction of differentiation.[216] Evidence that these ECM components actually function in trophoblast interactions has come from adhesion and outgrowth of trophoblast on single two-dimensional (2D) extracellular matrix substrates, or invasion into three-dimensional (3D) matrix substrates in vitro. This has been considered to resemble the 3D invasion in utero, but care must be taken in interpreting observations on single substrates, and particularly in 2D systems. Cultured trophoblast may upregulate appropriate matrix receptors according to environment. Mouse trophoblast invades endometrial ECM[217] and human and primate blastocysts attach to and invade into Engelbreth-Holm-Swarm sarcoma (EHS) matrix.[218,219] Protease production, particularly of matrix metalloproteinases (MMPs), is an important moderator of invasion/outgrowth.[220] One of these, MMP-2, also binds $\alpha_v\beta_3$ to facilitate directed cell migration.[221] Antisense or antibodies to the tretraspanin protein CD9 enhances trophoblast outgrowth apparently at least partly by induction of MMP-2 through the PI3 kinase signaling pathway. Since CD9 is expressed during preimplantation development and by trophoblast (as well as peri-implantation LE) it may regulate trophoblast invasion by repressing MMP-2-induced ECM remodeling.[222]

Trophoblast is likely to be adaptable and capable of reacting to and migrating on a number of substrates. This responsiveness is exemplified by the reaction to fibronectin. Murine blastocysts bind by their abembryonic pole to the cell-binding fragment of fibronectin attached to microspheres and adhesion is inhibited by soluble fibronectin or antibodies to α_v, α_5, β_1, or β_3 integrin subunits. Interaction with fibronectin is required to induce translocation of integrin to the trophoblast cell surface, thereby achieving adhesion.[183,223]

As murine trophoblast outgrowth proceeds in vitro, α_1, α_{6A}, and α_7 integrin become trophoblast specific[123] and they are also expressed during invasion in utero, suggesting an integrin switch at this stage. In combination with β_1, these integrins form laminin and collagen receptors (see Table 22.2). Murine trophoblast spreads on both the P1' fragment of laminin via its RGD sequence and the E_8 fragment, independent of RGD and possibly via its IKVAV cell recognition domain known to bind trophoblast.[123,224] The P1' fragment, recognized by $\alpha_v\beta_3$, seemed to be cryptic in intact laminin and the E_8 fragment is thought to facilitate trophoblast invasion in vivo.[123] However, antibodies

against one E_8 receptor, $\alpha_6\beta_1$, failed to block outgrowth and in the absence of available antibodies against, $\alpha_7\beta_1$, the latter was predicted to be a major outgrowth receptor for mouse trophoblast on laminin, although α_7 null mice do not appear to have defective implantation.[225] Mice null for integrin α_1 also implant and develop normally, as do those null for α_v (a candidate for initial adhesion), although most die at mid gestation from placental failure.[226,227] Perhaps other α subunits may compensate for loss of α_1 or α_v integrins at implantation. Galactosyl transferase expressed on secondary ectoplacental cone trophoblast was reported to function in their migration on laminin in vitro,[228] suggesting that carbohydrate chains of laminin may influence later invasion of trophoblast. These experiments also suggest that secondary trophoblast uses multiple interaction mechanisms during invasion. Anti-β_1 integrin antibodies prevent mouse trophoblast adhesion and outgrowth on fibronectin[223] and adhesion of human cytotrophoblast to fibronectin or laminin.[229] Outgrowth of mouse trophoblast on human decidual cells is also inhibited by anti-β_1 treatment of decidual cells[230,231] and trophoblast invasion is reduced in β_1 −/− mouse embryos. The null trophoblast invades through LE but only poorly into decidua,[230,231] supporting a role on trophoblast at implantation. However, the major defect has been ascribed to failure in the β_1 −/− ICM because trophoblast outgrowth on fibronectin and vitronectin appeared normal. Lack of ICM signals to trophoblast may account for the limited invasion. However, β_1 −/− trophoblast did not outgrow on laminin (a likely substrate in vivo) and anti β_1 antibodies block trophoblast outgrowth on laminin. Thus, β_1 integrins may indeed be involved in invasion of the laminin-enriched decidua.

In the human the changing pattern of integrin subunits expressed by different populations of cytotrophoblast at different states of differentiation and invasion implies a complex sequence of interactions with different ECM molecules.[219,232] The phenomenon of evolving integrin expression during differentiation and invasion of the trophoblast, or integrin switching,[219] may reflect changes in available matrix in utero, but in-vitro evidence suggests that it is preprogrammed. In utero, α_6 integrin is restricted to cytotrophoblast stem cells and lost on invasion, while invasive differentiating cytotrophoblast upregulates $\alpha_5\beta_1$ and $\alpha_1\beta_1$. The same pattern of changing human cytotrophoblast integrin expression is seen on cells invading EHS matrix.[219] Antibody inhibition of $\alpha_1\beta_1$ interaction with laminin and collagen IV inhibited invasion, whereas antibody to $\alpha_6\beta_1$, the fibronectin receptor, accelerated invasion. This suggests the regulated counterbalancing of adhesive- and migration-promoting machinery in invasive cytotrophoblast, driven by integrin cell surface expression which controls the interactions between laminin/collagen and their receptors (adhesion) and fibronectin-integrin binding (migration). The lack of a normal cytotrophoblast integrin differentiation program in pregnancies with preeclampsia,[233] where infiltration of the arterial system and endovascular remodeling is restricted,[234] supports this idea.

CONCLUSION

A summary model for the adhesion cascade which drives implantation of the embryo is outlined in Figure 22.1. This is simplified to allow representation of a complex series of interactions. The major masking substances in the prereceptive uterus are depicted as mucins (Muc-1) associated with the apical LE surface. However, these could equally be other membrane-bound mucins or molecules secreted into the uterine fluid, which, by binding to the cell surface, mask blastocyst or LE receptors. Carbohydrate ligands on LE are shown as the initiators of attachment by their (low-avidity?) tethering function. HSPG on the TE might be involved in interacting with HB-EGF on the LE in this initial phase. Once tethered, the proximity of cell surface proteins facilitates firmer adhesion mediated by α_v family integrins probably interacting with ECM components at the trophoblast–LE interface. To fulfill their function as bridging molecules, ECM molecules will need at least two accessible (integrin?) binding sites, or they may bridge by forming complexes with other ECM components at the trophoblast–LE interface. Integrin $\alpha_v\beta_3$ is a prime candidate for a functional integrin receptor on both trophoblast and apical LE, especially in human. This is particularly because its ligands are found at this interface in mouse and human (laminin, osteopontin) and it shows appropriate cyclic regulation in human LE. The absence of an implantation phenotype in the α_v knockout embryo precludes a unique function. However, $\alpha_v\beta_5$ might interact with human trophoblast oncofetal fibronectin or vitronectin. The relaxation of polarity in the LE during the window of receptivity suggests that appropriate integrins and even ECM substrates become available on the *lateral* aspect of LE cells to act as substrates for trophoblast invasion. The clearance of laminin and type IV collagen from the LE basement membrane in mice allows direct interactions with stromal matrix components from the point that trophoblast leaves the lateral surface of LE. Finally, interaction with decidual matrix appears to be driven by β_1 integrins in human with the up-regulation of cytotrophoblast $\alpha_5\beta_1$ and $\alpha_1\beta_1$. Similarly, β_1 integrins

become important from an early stage in stromal invasion in mice, with modulation of MMP-induced ECM degradation an important regulator of invasion.

The search for molecules that mediate the initial stages of implantation has identified several strong candidates. However, the scarcity of implantation phenotypes observed after gene deletion of adhesion molecules, either individually or in families, emphasizes that in most cases different molecular mechanisms work in parallel to drive trophectoderm adhesion, and invasion, allowing compensation when one mechanism fails. Following initial TE–LE adhesion, the species differences in detailed cellular architecture of implantation and placentation indicate that various strategies have been evolutionarily successful in establishing a functional placenta. The lack of molecular systems that are specific to particular implantation functions suggests a relatively weak evolutionary drive to eliminate surplus mechanisms. This may help to account for the observed redundancy, which confers the added evolutionary benefit of securing implantation success in the presence of random mutations affecting the function of individual components.

ACKNOWLEDGMENTS

We thank Ian Illingworth for his assistance in producing Figure 22.1. Work from our laboratory was supported by the Wellcome Trust, John Pinto Foundation, and the BBSRC UK.

REFERENCES

1. Cross JC. Genetic insights into trophoblast differentiation and placental morphogenesis. Semin Cell Dev Biol 2000; 11: 105–13.
2. Lindenberg S, Hyttel P, Sjogren A et al. A comparative study of attachment of human, bovine and mouse blastocysts to uterine epithelial monolayer. Hum Reprod 1989; 4: 446–56.
3. Bentin-Ley U, Sjogren A, Nilsson L et al. Presence of uterine pinopodes at the embryo–endometrial interface during human implantation in vitro. Hum Reprod 1999; 14: 515–20.
4. Bentin-Ley U, Horn T, Sjogren A et al. Ultrastructure of human blastocyst–endometrial interactions in vitro. J Reprod Fertil 2000; 120: 337–50.
5. Carver J, Martin K, Spyropoulou I et al. An in vitro model for stromal invasion during implantation of the human blastocyst. Hum Reprod 2003; 18: 283–90.
6. Campbell S, Swann HR, Aplin JD et al. CD44 is expressed throughout pre-implantation human embryo development. Hum Reprod 1995; 10: 425–30.
7. Campbell S, Swann HR, Seif MW et al. Cell-adhesion molecules on the oocyte and preimplantation human embryo. Hum Reprod 1995; 10: 571–8.
8. Sharkey AM, Dellow K, Blayney M et al. Stage-specific expression of cytokine and receptor messenger ribonucleic

acids in human preimplantation embryos, Biol Reprod 1995; 53: 974–81.

9. Poirier F, Kimber S. Cell surface carbohydrates and lectins in early development. Mol Hum Reprod 1997; 3: 907–18.

10. Jurisicova A, Antenos M, Kapasi K et al. Variability in the expression of trophectodermal markers beta-human chorionic gonadotropin, human leukocyte antigen-G and pregnancy specific beta-1 glycoprotein by the human blastocyst. Hum Reprod 1999; 14: 1852–8.

11. Adjaye J, Huntriss J, Herwig R et al. Primary differentiation in the human blastocyst: comparative molecular portraits of inner cell mass and trophectoderm cells. Stem Cells 2005; 23: 1514–25.

12. Genbacev OD, Prakobphol A, Foulk RA et al. Trophoblast L-selectin-mediated adhesion at the maternal–fetal interface. Science 2003; 299: 405–8.

13. Denker HW. Implantation – a cell biological paradox. J Exp Zool 1993; 266: 541–58.

14. Dey SK, Lim H, Das SK et al. Molecular cues to implantation. Endocr Rev 2004; 25: 341–73.

15. Aplin JD, Kimber SJ. Trophoblast–uterine interactions at implantation. Reprod Biol Endocrinol 2004; 2: 48.

16. Leese HJ. Quiet please, do not disturb: a hypothesis of embryo metabolism and viability. Bioessays 2002; 24: 845–9.

17. Armant DR. Blastocysts don't go it alone. Extrinsic signals fine-tune the intrinsic developmental program of trophoblast cells. Dev Biol 2005; 280: 260–80.

18. Sutherland A. Mechanisms of implantation in the mouse: differentiation and functional importance of trophoblast giant cell behavior. Dev Biol 2003; 258: 241–51.

19. Psychoyos A. Hormonal control of ovoimplantation. Vitam Horm 1973; 31: 201–56.

20. Denker HW. Implantation: a cell biological paradox. J Exp Zool 1993; 266: 541–58.

21. Cowell TP. Implantation and the development of mouse eggs transferred to uterine foster mothers. J Reprod Fertil 1969; 19: 239–45.

22. Bergh PA, Navot D. The impact of embryonic development and endometrial maturity on the timing of implantation. Fertil Steril 1992; 58: 537–42.

23. Navot D, Bergh PA, Williams M et al. An insight into early reproductive processes through the in vivo model of ovum donation. J Clin Endocrinol Metab 1991; 72: 408–14.

24. de Ziegler D, Fanchin R, de Moustier B et al. The hormonal control of endometrial receptivity: estrogen (E2) and progesterone. J Reprod Immunol 1998; 39: 149–66.

25. Kimber SJ. Molecular interactions at the maternal–embryonic interface during the early phase of implantation. Semin Reprod Med 2000; 18: 237–53.

26. Kimber SJ, Spanswick C. Blastocyst implantation: the adhesion cascade. Semin Cell Dev Biol 2000; 11: 77–92.

27. Paria BC, Huet-Hudson YM, Dey SK. Blastocyst's state of activity determines the "window" of implantation in the receptive mouse uterus. Proc Natl Acad Sci USA 1993; 90: 10159–62.

28. Paria BC, Lim H, Das SK et al. Molecular signaling in uterine receptivity for implantation. Semin Cell Dev Biol 2000; 11: 67–76.

29. Paria BC, Lim H, Wang XN et al. Coordination of differential effects of primary estrogen and catecholestrogen on two distinct targets mediates embryo implantation in the mouse. Endocrinology 1998; 139: 5235–46.

30. Finn CA. The implantation reaction. In: Wynn RA, ed. Biology of the Uterus. New York: Plenum Press, 1977.

31. Enders AC, Nelson DM. Pinocytotic activity in the uterus of the rat. Am J Anat 1973; 138: 277–99.

32. Spencer TE, Johnson GA, Bazer FW, Burghardt RC. Implantation mechanisms: insights from the sheep. Reproduction 2004; 128: 657–68.

33. Bowen JA, Burghardt RC. Cellular mechanisms of implantation in domestic farm animals. Semin Cell Dev Biol 2000; 11: 93–104.

34. Schlafke S, Enders AC. Cellular basis of interaction between trophoblast and uterus at implantation. Biol Reprod 1975; 12: 41–65.

35. Blankenship TN, Given RL. Loss of laminin and type IV collagen in uterine luminal epithelial basement membranes during blastocyst implantation in the mouse. Anat Rec 1995; 243: 27–36.

36. Parr EL, Tung HN, Parr MB. Apoptosis as the mode of uterine epithelial cell death during embryo implantation in mice and rats. Biol Reprod 1987; 36: 211–25.

37. Kamijo T, Rajabi MR, Mizunuma H et al. Biochemical evidence for autocrine/paracrine regulation of apoptosis in cultured uterine epithelial cells during mouse embryo implantation in vitro. Mol Hum Reprod 1998; 4: 990–8.

38. Galan A, O'Connor JE, Valbuena D et al. The human blastocyst regulates endometrial epithelial apoptosis in embryonic adhesion. Biol Reprod 2000; 63: 430–9.

39. Enders AC, Hendrickx AG, Schlafke S. Implantation in the rhesus monkey: initial penetration of endometrium. Am J Anat 1983; 167: 275–98.

40. Smith CA, Moore HD, Hearn JP. The ultrastructure of early implantation in the marmoset monkey (Callithrix jacchus). Anat Embryol (Berl) 1987; 175: 399–410.

41. He ZY, Liu HC, Mele CA et al. Expression of 42 inhibin/activin subunits and their receptors and binding proteins in human preimplantation embryos. J Assist Reprod Genet 1999; 16: 73–80.

42. Finn CA, Bredl JC. Studies on the development of the implantation reaction in the mouse uterus: influence of actinomycin D. J Reprod Fertil 1973; 34: 247–53.

43. Heneweer C, Adelmann HG, Kruse LH et al. Human uterine epithelial RL95-2 cells reorganize their cytoplasmic architecture with respect to Rho protein and F–actin in response to trophoblast binding. Cells Tissues Organs 2003; 175: 1–8.

44. Thie M, Denker HW. In vitro studies on endometrial adhesiveness for trophoblast: cellular dynamics in uterine epithelial cells. Cells Tissues Organs 2002; 172: 237–52.

45. Thie M, Fuchs P, Denker HW. Epithelial cell polarity and embryo implantation in mammals. Int J Dev Biol 1996; 40: 389–93.

46. Murphy CR. Understanding the apical surface markers of uterine receptivity: pinopods or uterodomes? Hum Reprod 2000; 15: 2451–4.

47. Lopata A, Bentin-Ley U, Enders A. "Pinopodes" and implantation. Rev Endocr Metab Disord 2002; 3: 77–86.

48. Sarani SA, Ghaffari-Novin M, Warren MA et al. Morphological evidence for the 'implantation window' in human luminal endometrium. Hum Reprod 1999; 14: 3101–6.

49. Albers A, Thie M, Hohn HP, Denker HW. Differential expression and localization of integrins and CD44 in the membrane domains of human uterine epithelial cells during the menstrual cycle. Acta Anat (Basel) 1995; 153: 12–19.

50. Potter SW, Caza G, Morris JE. Estradiol induces E-cadherin degradation in mouse uterine epithelium during the etrous cycle and early pregnancy. J Cell Physiol 1996; 169: 1–14.

51. Hyland RA, Shaw TJ, Png FW, Murphy CR. Pan-cadherin concentrates apically in uterine epithelial cells during uterine closure in the rat. Acta Histochem 1998; 100: 75–81.

52. Illingworth IM, Kiszka I, Bagley S et al. Desmosomes are reduced in the mouse uterine luminal epithelium during the preimplantation period of pregnancy: a mechanism for facilitation of implantation. Biol Reprod 2000; 63: 1764–73.

53. Murphy CR, Rogers PA, Hosie MJ et al. Tight junctions of human uterine epithelial cells change during the menstrual cycle: a morphometric study. Acta Anat (Basel) 1992; 144: 36–8.

54. Winterhager E, Kuhnel W. Alterations in intercellular junctions of the uterine epithelium during the preimplantation phase in the rabbit. Cell Tissue Res 1982, 224: 517–26.

55. Winterhager E, Grummer R, Jahn E, Willecke K, Traub O. Spatial and temporal expression of connexin26 and connexin43 in rat endometrium during trophoblast invasion. Dev Biol 1993; 157: 399–409.

56. Grummer R, Hewitt SW, Traub O et al. Different regulatory pathways of endometrial connexin expression: preimplantation hormonal-mediated pathway versus embryo implantation-initiated pathway. Biol Reprod 2004; 71: 273–81.

57. Grummer R, Traub O, Winterhager E. Gap junction connexin genes cx26 and cx43 are differentially regulated by ovarian steroid hormones in rat endometrium. Endocrinology 1999; 140: 2509–16.

58. Fouladi-Nashta AA, Jones CJ, Nijjar N et al. Characterization of the uterine phenotype during the peri-implantation period for LIF-null, MF1 strain mice. Dev Biol 2005; 281: 1–21.

59. Adams SM, Gayer N, Hossie MJ et al. Human uterodomes (pinopods) do not display pinocytotic function. Hum Reprod 2002; 17: 1980–6.

60. Nikas G, Develioglu OH, Toner JP et al. Endometrial pinopodes indicate a shift in the window of receptivity in IVF cycles. Hum Reprod 1999; 14: 787–92.

61. Creus M, Ordi J, Fabregues F et al. alphavbeta3 integrin expression and pinopod formation in normal and out-of-phase endometria of fertile and infertile women. Hum Reprod 2002; 17: 2279–86.

62. Horne AW, Lalani EN, Margara RA et al. The expression pattern of MUC1 glycoforms and other biomarkers of endometrial receptivity in fertile and infertile women. Mol Reprod Dev 2005; 72: 216–29.

63. Bagot CN, Troy PJ, Taylor HS. Alteration of maternal Hoxa 10 expression by in vivo gene transfection affects implantation. Gene Ther 2000; 7: 1378–84.

64. Fujii H, Tatsumi K, Kosaka S, et al. Eph-ephrin A system regulates murine blastocyst attachment and spreading. Dev Dyn 2006; 235: 3250–8.

65. Kimber S, White S, Cooke A et al. The initiation of implantation. Parallels between attachment of the embryo and neutrophil–endothelial interaction. In: Mastrioianni LJ, ed. Gametes and Embryo Quality. Carnforth: Parthenon, 1994: 171–98.

66. Drickamer K, Taylor ME. Biology of animal lectins. Annu Rev Cell Biol 1993; 9: 237–64.

67. Simon SI, Green CE. Molecular mechanics and dynamics of leukocyte recruitment during inflammation. Annu Rev Biomed Eng 2005; 7: 151–85.

68. Aplin JD. Adhesion molecules and implantation. Rev Reprod 1997; 2: 84–93.

69. Shiotani M, Noda Y, Mori T. Embryo-dependent induction of uterine receptivity assessed by an in-vitro model of implantation in mice. Biol Reprod 1993; 49: 794–801.

70. Meseguer M, Pellicer A, Simon C. MUC1 and endometrial receptivity. Mol Hum Reprod 1998; 4: 1089–98.

71. Komatsu M, Carraway CA, Fregien NL et al. Reversible disruption of cell–matrix and cell–cell interactions by overexpression of sialomucin complex. J Biol Chem 1997; 272: 33245–54.

72. Wesseling J, van der Valk SW, Vos HL et al. Espisialin (MUC1) overexpression inhibits integrin-mediated cell adhesion to extracellular matrix components. J Cell Biol 1995; 129: 255–65.

73. Ligtenberg MJ, Buijs F, Vos HL et al. Suppression of cellular aggregation by high levels of episialin. Cancer Res 1992; 52: 2318–24.

74. Surveyor GA, Gendler SJ, Pemberton L et al. Expression and steroid hormonal control of Muc-1 in the mouse uterus. Endocrinology 1995; 136: 3639–47.

75. Cheon YP, Li Q, Xu X et al. A genomic approach to identify novel progesterone receptor regulated pathways in the uterus during implantation. Mol Endocrinol 2022; 16: 2853–71.

76. Hoffman LH, Olson GE, Carson DD et al. Progesterone and implanting blastocysts regulate Muc1 expression in rabbit uterine epithelium. Endocrinology 1998; 139: 266–271.

77. Hild-Petito S, Fazleabas AT, Julian J et al. Mucin (Muc-1) expression is differentially regulated in uterine luminal and glandular epithelia of the baboon (Papio anubis). Biol Reprod 1996; 54: 939–47.

78. Pimental RA, Julian J, Gendler SJ et al. Synthesis and intracellular trafficking of Muc-1 and mucins by polarized mouse uterine epithelial cells. J Biol Chem 1996; 271: 28128–37.

79. DeSouza MM, Surveyor GA, Price RE et al. MUC1/episialin: a critical barrier in the female reproductive tract. J Reprod Immunol 1999; 45: 127–58.

80. McNeer RR, Carraway CA, Fregien NL et al. Characterization of the expression and steroid hormone control of sialomucin complex in the rat uterus: implications for uterine receptivity. J Cell Physiol 1998; 176: 110–19.

81. Hey NA, Li TC, Devine PL et al. MUC1 in secretory phase endometrium: expression in precisely dated biopsies and flushings from normal and recurrent miscarriage patients. Hum Reprod 1995; 10: 2655–62.

82. Aplin JD. MUC-1 glycosylation in endometrium: possible roles of the apical glycocalyx at implantation. Hum Reprod 1999; 14(Suppl 2): 17–25.

83. Hey NA, Graham RA, Seif MW et al. The polymorphic epithelial mucin MUC1 in human endometrium is regulated with maximal expression in the implantation phase. J Clin Endocrinol Metab 1994; 78: 337–42.

84. Hey NA, Aplin JD. Sialyl-Lewis x and Sialyl-Lewis a are associated with MUC1 in human endometrium. Glycoconj J 1996; 13: 769–79.

85. Chervenak JL, Illsley NP. Episialin acts as an antiadhesive factor in an in vitro model of human endometrial–blastocyst attachment. Biol Reprod 2000; 63: 294–300.

86. Olson GE, Winfrey VP, Matrisian PE et al. Blastocyst-dependent upregulation of metalloproteinase/disintegrin MDC9 expression in rabbit endometrium. Cell Tissue Res 1998; 293: 489–98.

87. Thathiah A, Blobel CP, Carson DD. Tumor necrosis factor-alpha converting enzyme/ADAM 17 mediates MUC1 shedding. J Biol Chem 2003; 278: 3386–94.

88. Thathiah A, Brayman M, Dharmaraj N et al. Tumor necrosis factor alpha stimulates MUC1 synthesis and ectodomain release in a human uterine epithelial cell line. Endocrinology 2004; 145: 4192–203.

89. Aplin JD. The cell biology of human implantation. Placenta 1996; 17: 269–75.

90. Graham RA, Li TC, Cooke ID et al. Keratan sulphate as a secretory product of human endometrium: cyclic expression in normal women. Hum Reprod 1994; 9: 926–30.

91. Aplin JD, Hey NA, Graham RA. Human endometrial MUC1 carries keratan sulfate: characteristic glycoforms in the luminal epithelium at receptivity. Glycobiology 1998; 8: 269–76.

92. DeLoia JA, Krasnow JS, Brekosky J et al. Regional specialization of the cell membrane-associated, polymorphic mucin (MUC1) in human uterine epithelia. Hum Reprod 1998; 13: 2902–9.

93. Kimber S. Carbohydrates as low affinity agents involved in initial attachment of the mammalian embryo at implantation. In: Ward RHT, Smith SK, Donnai D, eds. Early Foetal Growth and Development. London: Royal College of Obstetricians and Gynaecologists, 1994: 75–102.

94. Kimber SJ, Illingworth IM, Glasser SR. Expression of carbohydrate antigens in the rat uterus during early pregnancy and after ovariectomy and steroid replacement. J Reprod Fertil 1995; 103: 75–87.

95. Kimber SJ, Lindenberg S. Hormonal control of a carbohydrate epitope involved in implantation in mice. J Reprod Fertil 1990; 89: 13–21.

96. White S, Kimber SJ. Changes in alpha (1–2)-fucosyltransferase activity in the murine endometrial epithelium during the estrous cycle, early pregnancy, and after ovariectomy and hormone replacement. Biol Reprod 1994; 50: 73–81.

97. Illingworth IM, Kimber SJ. Demonstration of oestrogenic control of H-type-1 carbohydrate antigen in the murine endometrial epithelium by use of ICI 182,780. J Reprod Fertil 1999; 117: 89–95.

98. Sidhu SS, Kimber SJ. Hormonal control of H-type alpha (1–2)fucosyltransferase messenger ribonucleic acid in the mouse uterus. Biol Reprod 1999; 60: 147–57.

99. Lindenberg S, Sundberg K, Kimber SJ et al. The milk oligosaccharide lacto-N-fucopentaose I, inhibits attachment of mouse blastocysts on endometrial monolayers. J Reprod Fertil 1988; 83: 149–58.

100. Kimber SJ, Lindenberg S, Lundblad A. Distribution of some Gal beta 1–3(4)GlcNAc related carbohydrate antigens on the mouse uterine epithelium in relation to the peri-implantational period. J Reprod Immunol 1988; 12: 297–313.

101. Lindenberg S, Kimber SJ, Kallin E. Carbohydrate binding properties of mouse embryos. J Reprod Fertil 1990; 89: 431–9.

102. Yamagata T, Yamazaki K. Implanting mouse embryo stain with a LNF-I bearing fluorescent probe at their mural trophectodermal side. Biochem Biophys Res Commun 1991; 181: 1004–9.

103. Kimber SJ, Waterhouse R, Lindenberg S. In vitro models for implantation. In: Bavister B, ed. Preimplantation Embryo Development. New York: Springer Verlag, 1993: 244–63.

104. Domino SE, Zhang L, Gillespie PJ et al. Deficiency of reproductive tract alpha(1,2)fucosylated glycans and normal fertility in mice with targeted deletions of the FUT1 or FUT2 alpha(1,2)fucosyltransferase locus. Mol Cell Biol 2001; 21: 8336–45.

105. Zhu ZM, Kojima N, Stroud MR et al. Monoclonal antibody directed to Le(y) oligosaccharide inhibits implantation in the mouse. Biol Reprod 1995; 52: 903–12.

106. Wang XQ, Zhu ZM, Fenderson BA et al. Effects of monoclonal antibody directed to Le(Y) on implantation in the mouse. Mol Hum Reprod 1998; 4: 295–300.

107. Fenderson BA, Holmes EH, Fukushi Y, Halfamori S. Coordinate expression of X and Y haptens during murine embryogenesis. Dev Biol 1986; 114: 12–21.

108. Kimber SJ. Glycoconjugates and cell surface interactions in pre- and peri-implantation mammalian embryonic development. Int Rev Cytol 1990; 120: 53–167.

109. Ravn V, Teglbjaerg CS, Mandel U et al. The distribution of type-2 chain histo-blood group antigens in normal cycling human endometrium. Cell Tissue Res 1992; 270: 425–33.

110. Bloor DJ, Metcalfe AD, Rutherford A et al. Expression of cell adhesion molecules during human preimplantation embryo development. Mol Hum Reprod 2002; 8: 237–45.

111. Stones RE. The expression of glycosyltransferases and their products in the murine uterus during early pregnancy. University of Manchester, 1999: 275.

112. Kimber SJ, Stones RE, Sidhu SS. Glycosylation changes during differentiation of the murine uterine epithelium. Biochem Soc Trans 2001; 29: 156–62.

113. Spencer TE, Bartol FF, Bazer FW et al. Identification and characterization of glycosylation-dependent cell adhesion molecule 1-like protein expression in the ovine uterus. Biol Reprod 1999; 60: 241–50.

114. Robinson SD, Frenette, PS, Rayburn H et al. Multiple, targeted deficiencies in selectins reveal a predominant role for P-selectin in leukocyte recruitment. Proc Natl Acad Sci USA 1999; 96: 11452–7.

115. Collins RG, Jung U, Ramirez M et al. Dermal and pulmonary inflammatory disease in E-selectin and P-selectin double-null mice is reduced in triple-selectin-null mice. Blood 2001; 98: 727–35.

116. Leffler H, Carlsson S, Hedlund M et al. Introduction to galectins. Glycoconj J 2004; 19: 433–40.

117. Colnot C, Fowlis D, Ripoche MA et al. Embryonic implantation in galectin 1/galectin 3 double mutant mice. Dev Dyn 1998; 211: 306–13.

118. Poirier F, Robertson EJ. Normal development of mice carrying a null mutation in the gene encoding the L14 S-type lectin. Development 1993; 119: 1229–36.

119. Poirier F, Timmons PM, Chan CT, Gunet JL, Rigby PW. Expression of the L14 lectin during mouse embryogenesis suggests multiple roles during pre- and post-implantation development. Development 1992; 115: 143–55.

120. Cooper DN, Massa SM, Barondes SH. Endogenous muscle lectin inhibits myoblast adhesion to laminin. J Cell Biol 1991; 115: 1437–48.

121. Gu M, Wang W, Song WK et al. Selective modulation of the interaction of alpha 7 beta 1 integrin with fibronectin and laminin by L-14 lectin during skeletal muscle differentiation. J Cell Sci 1994; 107 (Pt 1): 175–81.

122. Klaffky E, Williams R, Yao CC et al. Trophoblast-specific expression and function of the integrin alpha 7 subunit in the peri-implantation mouse embryo. Dev Biol 2001; 239: 161–75.

123. Sutherland AE, Calarco PG, Damsky CH. Developmental regulation of integrin expression at the time of implantation in the mouse embryo. Development 1993; 119: 1175–86.

124. Colnot C, Ripoche MA, Scaerou F et al. Galectins in mouse embryogenesis. Biochem Soc Trans 1996; 24: 141–6.

125. Sparrow CP, Leffler H, Barondes SH. Multiple soluble beta-galactoside-binding lectins from human lung. J Biol Chem 1987; 262: 7383–90.

126. Popovici RM, Krause MS, Germeyer A et al. Galectin-9: a new endometrial epithelial marker for the mid- and late-secretory and decidual phases in humans. J Clin Endocrinol Metab 2005; 90: 6170–6.

127. Gray CA, Adelson DL, Bazer FW et al. Discovery and characterization of an epithelial-specific galectin in the endometrium that forms crystals in the trophectoderm, Proc Natl Acad Sci USA 2004; 101: 7982–7.

128. Baldwin HS, Shen HM, Yan HC et al. Platelet endothelial-cell adhesion molecule-1 (Pecam-1 Cd31) – alternatively spliced, functionally distinct isoforms expressed during mammalian cardiovascular development. Development 1994; 120: 2539–53.

129. Crider-Pirkle S, Billingsley P, Faust C et al. Cubilin, a binding partner for galectin-3 in the murine utero-placental complex. J Biol Chem 2002; 277: 15904–12.

130. Behzad F, Seif MW, Campbell S et al. Expression of two isoforms of CD44 in human endometrium. Biol Reprod 1994; 51: 739–47.

131. Schmits R, Filmus J, Gerwin N et al. CD44 regulates hematopoietic progenitor distribution, granuloma formation, and tumorigenicity. Blood 1997; 90: 2217–33.

132. Perrimon N, Bernfield M. Specificities of heparan sulphate proteoglycans in developmental processes. Nature 2000; 404: 725–8.

133. Julian J, Das SK, Dey SK et al. Expression of heparin/heparan sulfate interacting protein-ribosomal protein L29 during the estrous cycle and early pregnancy in the mouse. Biol Reprod 2001; 64: 1165–75.

134. Sutherland AE, Sanderson RD, Mayes M et al. Expression of syndecan, a putative low affinity fibroblast growth factor receptor, in the early mouse embryo. Development 1991; 113: 339–51.

135. Costell M, Gustafsson E, Aszodi A et al. Perlecan maintains the integrity of cartilage and some basement membranes. J Cell Biol 1999; 147: 1109–22.

136. Rhode LH, Carson DD. Heparin-like glycosaminoglycans participate in binding of a human trophoblastic cell-line (Jar) to a human uterine epithelial-cell line (R195). J Cell Physiol 1993; 155: 185–96.

137. Rhode LH, Julian J, Babaknia A et al. Cell surface expression of HIP, a novel heparin/heparan sulface binding protein of human uterine epithelial cells and cell lines. J Biol Chem 1996; 271: 11824–30.

138. Liu S, Hoke D, Julian J et al. Heparin/heparan sulfate (HP/HS) interacting protein (HIP) supports cell attachment and selective, high affinity binding of HP/HS. J Biol Chem 1997; 272: 25856–62.

139. Rohde LH, Janatpore MJ, McMaster MT et al. Complementary expression of HIP, a cell-surface heparan sulfate binding protein, and perlecan at the human fetal–maternal interface. Biol Reprod 1998; 58: 1075–83.

140. Paria BC, Elenius K, Klagsbrun M et al. Heparin-binding EGF-like growth factor interacts with mouse blastocysts independently of ErbB1: a possible role for heparan sulfate proteoglycans and ErbB4 in blastocyst implantation. Development 1999; 126: 1997–2005.

141. Hacker U, Nybakken K, Perrimon N. Heparan sulphate proteoglycans: the sweet side of development. Nat Rev Mol Cell Biol 2005; 6: 530–41.

142. Raab G, Klagsbrun M. Heparin-binding EGF-like growth factor. Biochim Biophys Acta 1997; 1333: F179–99.

143. Das SK, Wang XN, Paria BC et al. Heparin-binding EGF-like growth factor gene is induced in the mouse uterus temporally by the blastocyst solely at the site of its apposition: a possible ligand for interaction with blastocyst EGF-receptor in implantation. Development 1994; 120: 1071–83.

144. Wang J, Mayernik L, Schultz JF, Armant DR. Acceleration of trophoblast differentiation by heparin-binding EGF-like growth factor is dependent on the stage-specific activation of calcium influx by ErbB receptors in developing mouse blastocysts. Development 2000; 127: 33–44.

145. Martin KL, Barlow DH, Sargent IL. Heparin-binding epidermal growth factor significantly improves human blastocyst development and hatching in serum-free medium. Hum Reprod 1998; 13: 1645–52.

146. Liu Z, Armant DR. Lysophosphatidic acid regulates murine blastocyst development by transactivation of receptors for heparin-binding EGF-like growth factor. Exp Cell Res 2004; 296: 317–26.

147. Ye X, Hama K, Contos JJ et al. LPA3-mediated lysophosphatidic acid signaling in embryo implantation and spacing. Nature 2005; 435: 104–8.

148. Zhang Z, Funk C, Roy D et al. Heparin-binding epidermal growth factor-like growth factor is differentially regulated by progesterone and estradiol in rat uterine epithelial and stromal cells. Endocrinology 1994; 134: 1089–94.

149. Wang XN, Das SK, Damm D et al. Differential regulation of heparin-binding epidermal growth factor-like growth factor in the adult ovariectomized mouse uterus by progesterone and estrogen. Endocrinology 1994; 135: 1264–71.

150. Zhang Z, Laping J, Glasser S et al. Mediators of estradiol-stimulated mitosis in the rat uterine luminal epithelium. Endocrinology 1998; 139: 961–6.

151. Higashiyama S, Abraham JA, Klagsbrun M. Heparin-binding EGF-like growth factor stimulation of smooth muscle cell migration: dependence on interactions with cell surface heparan sulfate. J Cell Biol 1993; 122: 933–40.

152. Das SK, Das N, Wang J et al. Expression of betacellulin and epiregulin genes in the mouse uterus temporally by the blastocyst soley at the site of its apposition is coincident with the "window" of implantation. Dev Biol 1997; 190: 178–90.

153. Jackson LF, Qiu TH, Sunnarborg SW et al. Defective valvulogenesis in HB-EGF and TACE-null mice is associated with aberrant BMP signaling. EMBO J 2003; 22: 2704–16.

154. Iwamoto R, Yamazaki S, Asakura M et al. Heparin-binding EGF-like growth factor and ErbB signaling is essential for heart function. Proc Natl Acad Sci USA 2003; 100: 3221–6.

155. Chobotova K, Spyropoulou I, Carver J et al. Heparin-binding epidermal growth factor and its receptor ErbB4 mediate implantation of the human blastocyst. Mech Dev 2002; 119: 137–44.

156. Yoo HJ, Barlow DH, Mardon HF. Temporal and spatial regulation of expression of heparin-binding epidermal growth factor-like growth factor in the human endometrium: a possible role in blastocyst implantation. Dev Genet 1997; 21: 102–8.

157. Stavreus-Evers A, Aghajanova L, Brismar H et al. Co-existence of heparin-binding epidermal growth factor-like growth factor and pinopodes in human endometrium at the time of implantation. Mol Hum Reprod 2002; 8: 765–9.

158. Zhu LJ, Bagchi MK, Bagchi IC. Attenuation of calcitonin gene expression in pregnant rat uterus leads to a block in embryonic implantation. Endocrinology 1998; 139: 330–9.

159. Luu KC, Nie GY, Salamonsen LA. Endometrial calbindins are critical for embryo implantation: evidence from in vivo use of morpholino antisense oligonucleotides. Proc Natl Acad Sci USA 2004; 101: 8028–33.

160. Nie GY, Li Y, Wang J et al. Complex regulation of calcium-binding protein D9k (calbindin-d(9k)) in the mouse uterus during early pregnancy and at the site of embryo implantation. Biol Reprod 2000; 62: 27–36.

161. Tatsumi K, Higuchi T, Fujiwara H et al. Expression of calcium binding protein D-9k messenger RNA in the mouse uterine endometrium during implantation. Mol Hum Reprod 1999; 5: 153–161.

162. Kumar S, Brudney A, Cheon P et al. Progesterone induces calcitonin expression in the baboon endometrium within the window of uterine receptivity. Biol Reprod 2003; 68: 1318–23.

163. Wang J, Rout UK, Bagchi IC et al. Expression of calcitonin receptors in mouse preimplantation embryos and their function in the regulation of blastocyst differentiation by calcitonin. Development 1998; 125: 4293–302.

164. Chakraborty I, Das SK, Wang J et al. Developmental expression of the cyclo-oxygenase-1 and cyclo-oxygenase-2 genes in the peri-implantation mouse uterus and their differential regulation by the blastocyst and ovarian steroids. J Mol Endocrinol 1996; 16: 107–22.

165. Matsumoto H, Ma WG, Daikoku T et al. Cyclooxygenase-2 differentially directs uterine angiogenesis during implantation in mice. J Biol Chem 2002; 277: 29260–7.

166. Lim H, Paria BC, Das SK et al. Multiple female reproductive failures in cyclooxygenase 2-deficient mice. Cell 1997; 91: 197–208.

167. Cheng JG, Stewart CL. Loss of cyclooxygenase-2 retards decidual growth but does not inhibit embryo implantation or development to term. Biol Reprod 2003; 68: 401–4.

168. Wang H, Ma WG, Tejada L et al. Rescue of female infertility from the loss of cyclooxygenase-2 by compensatory up-regulation of cyclooxygenase-1 is a function of genetic makeup. J Biol Chem 2004; 279: 10649–58.

169. Lim H, Gupta RA, Ma WG et al. Cyclo-oxygenase-2-derived prostacyclin mediates embryo implantation in the mouse via PPARdelta. Genes Dev 1999; 13: 1561–74.

170. Murohara T, Horowitz JR, Silver M et al. Vascular endothelial growth factor/vascular permeability factor enhances vascular permeability via nitric oxide and prostacyclin. Circulation 1998; 97: 99–107.

171. Stewart CL, Kaspar P, Brunet LJ et al. Blastocyst implantation depends on maternal expression of leukaemia inhibitory factor. Nature 1992; 359: 76–9.

172. Kimber SJ. Leukaemia inhibitory factor in implantation and uterine biology. Reproduction 2005; 130: 131–45.

173. Song H, Lim H, Das SK et al. Dysregulation of EGF family of growth factors and COX-2 in the uterus during the preattachment and attachment reactions of the blastocyst with the luminal epithelium correlates with implantation failure in LIF-deficient mice. Mol Endocrinol 2000; 14: 1147–61.

174. Jones RL, Kelly RW, Critchley HO. Chemokine and cyclooxy-genase-2 expression in human endometrium coincides with leukocyte accumulation. Hum Reprod 1997; 12: 1300–6.

175. Marions L, Danielsson KG. Expression of cyclo-oxygenase in human endometrium during the implantation period. Mol Hum Reprod 1999; 5: 961–5.

176. Yoshimura Y. Integrins: expression, modulation, and signaling in fertilization, embryogenesis and implanation. Keio J Med 1997; 46: 16–24.

177. Reddy K, Mangale SS. Integrin receptors: the dynamic modu-lators of endometrial function. Tissue Cell 2003; 35: 260–73.

178. Aoki R, Fukuda MN. Recent molecular approaches to eluci-date the mechanism of embryo implantation: trophinin, bystin, and tastin as molecules involved in the initial attach-ment of blastocysts to the uterus in humans. Semin Reprod Med 2002; 18: 265–71.

179. Fukuda MN, Nozawa S. Trophinin, tastin, and bystin: a com-plex mediating unique attachment between trophoblastic and endometrial epithelial cells at their respective apical cell membranes. Semin Reprod Endocrinol 1999; 17: 229–34.

180. Suzuki N, Zara J, Sato T et al. A cytoplasmic protein, bystin, interacts with trophinin, tastin, and cytokeratin and may be involved in trophinin-mediated cell adhesion between tro-phoblast and endometrial epithelial cells. Proc Natl Acad Sci USA 1998; 95: 5027–32.

181. Nadano D, Sugihara K, Paria BC et al. Significant differences between mouse and human trophinins are revealed by their expression patterns and targeted disruption of mouse trophinin gene. Biol Reprod 2002; 66: 313–21.

182. Suzuki N, Nadano D, Paria B et al. Trophinin expression in the mouse uterus coincides with implantation and is hormonally regulated but not reduced by implanting blastocysts. Endocrinology 2000; 141: 4247–54.

183. Schultz JF, Mayernik L, Rout UK et al. Intergrin trafficking reg-ulates adhesion to fibronectin during differentiation of mouse peri-implantation blastocysts. Dev Genet 1997; 21: 31–43.

184. Rout UK, Wang J, Paria BC et al. alpha 5 beta 1, alpha V beta 3 and the platelet-associated integrin alpha IIb beta 3 coordinately regulate adhesion and migration of differenti-ating mouse trophoblast cells. Dev Biol 2004; 268: 135–51.

185. Illera MJ, Cullinan E, Gui YT et al. Blockade of the alpha(v)beta(3) integrin adversely affects implantation in the mouse. Biol Reprod 2000; 62: 1285–90.

186. Dziadek M, Timpl R. Expression of nidogen and laminin in basement membranes during mouse embryogenesis and in teratocarcinoma cells. Dev Biol 1985; 111: 372–82.

187. Adamson ED, Ayers SE. The localization and synthesis of some collagen types in developing mouse embryos. Cell 1979; 16: 953–65.

188. Turpeenniem-Hujanen T, Feinberg RF, Kauppila A, Puistola U. Extracellular matrix interactions in early human embryos: implications for normal implantation events. Fertil Steril 1995; 64: 132–8.

189. Larson RC, Ignotz GG, Currie WB. Effect of fibronectin on early embryo development in cows. J Reprod Fertil 1992; 96: 289–97.

190. Omigbodun A, Ziolkiewicz P, Tessler C et al. Progesterone regulates osteopontin expression in human trophoblasts: a model of paracrine control in the placenta? Endocrinology 1997; 138: 4308–15.

191. Carson DD, Tang JP, Julian J. Heparan sulfate proteoglycan (perlecan) expression by mouse embryos during acquisition of attachment competence. Dev Biol 1993; 155: 97–106.

192. O'Shea KS, Liu LH, Kinnunen LH et al. Role of the extracel-lular matrix protein thrombospondin in the early development of the mouse embryo. J Cell Biol 1990; 111: 2713–23.

193. Dziadek M, Fujiwara S, Paulsson M et al. Immunological char-acterization of basement membrane types of heparan sulfate proteoglycan. EMBO J 1985; 4: 905–12.

194. Gao AG, Lindberg FB, Finn MB et al. Integrin-associated pro-tein is a receptor for the C-terminal domain of throm-bospondin. J Biol Chem 1996; 271: 21–4.

195. Hayashi K, Madri JA, Yurchenco PD. Endothelial cells inter-act with the core protein of basement membrane perlecan through beta1 and beta 3 integrins: an adhesion modulated by glycosaminoglycan. J Cell Biol 1992; 119: 945–59.

196. George EL, Georges-Labouesse EN, Patel-King RS et al. Defects in mesoderm, neural tube and vascular development in mouse embryos lacking fibronectin. Development 1993; 119: 1079–91.

197. Zheng X, Saunders TL, Camper SA et al. Vitronectin is not essential for normal mammalian development and fertility. Proc Natl Acad Sci USA 1995; 92: 12426–30.

198. Johnson GA, Burghardt RC, Bazer FW et al. Osteopontin: roles in implantation and placentation. Biol Reprod 2003; 69: 1458–71.

199. Von Wolff M, Strowitzki T, Becker V et al. Endometrial osteo-pontin, a ligand of beta(3)-integrin, is maximally expressed around the time of the "implantation window". Fertil Steril 2001; 76: 775–81.

200. Thie M, Harrachruprecht B, Sauer H et al. Cell-adhesion to the apical pole of epithelium – a function of cell polarity. Euro J Cell Biol 1995; 66: 180–91.

201. Lessey BA, Castelbaum AJ, Wolf L et al. Use of integrins to date the endometrium. Fertil Steril 2000; 73: 779–87.

202. Lessey BA, Ilesanmi AO, Lessey MA et al. Luminal and glan-dular endometrial epithelium express integrins differentially throughout the menstrual cycle: implications for implantation, contraception and infertility. Am J Reprod Immunol 1996; 35: 195–204.

203. Tabibzadeh S. Patterns of expression of integrin molecules in human endometrium throughout the menstrual cycle. Hum Reprod 1992; 7: 876–82.

204. Aplin JD, Spanswick C, Behzad F et al. Integrins beta 5, beta 3 and alpha v are apically distributed in endometrial epithe-lium. Mol Hum Reprod 1996; 2: 527–34.

205. Breuss JM, Gallow J, DeLisser HM et al. Expression of the beta 6 integrin subunit in development, neoplasia and tissue repair suggests a role in epithelial remodelling. J Cell Sci 1995; 108 (Pt 6): 2241–51.

206. Lessey BA, Castelbaum AJ, Buck CA et al. Further character-ization of endometrial integrins during the menstrual cycle and in pregnancy. Fertil Steril 1994; 62: 497–506.

207. Feinberg RF, Kliman HJ, Lockwood CJ. Is oncofetal fibronectin a trophoblast glue for human implantation? Am J Pathol 1991; 138: 537–43.

208. Kimmins S, Lim HC, MacLaren LA. Immunohistochemical localization of integrin alpha V and beta 3 and osteopontin suggests that they do not interact during embryo implanta-tion in ruminants. Reprod Biol Endocrinol 2004; 2: 19.

209. Lessey BA, Albelda S, Buck CA et al. Distribution of integrin cell adhesion molecules in endometrial cancer. Am J Pathol 1995; 146: 717–26.

210. Lessey BA, Castelbaum AJ, Sawin SW et al. Integrins as markers of uterine receptivity in women with primary unex-plained infertility. Fertil Steril 1995; 63: 535–42.

211. Lessey BA, Castelbaum AJ, Sawin SW et al. Aberrant integrin expression in the endometrium of women with endometrio-sis. J Clin Endocrinol Metab 1994; 79: 643–9.

212. Wadehra M, Dayal M, Mainigi M et al. Knockdown of the tetraspan protein epithelial membrane protein-2 inhibits implantation in the mouse. Dev Biol 2006; 292: 430–41.

213. Wewer UM, Damjanov A, Weiss J et al. Mouse endometrial stromal cells produce basement-membrane components. Differentiation 1986; 32: 49–58.

214. Church HJ, Vicovac LM, Williams JD et al. Laminins 2 and 4 are expressed by human decidual cells. Lab Invest 1996; 74: 21–32.

215. Ornitz DM. FGFs, heparan sulfate and FGFRs: complex interactions essential for development. Bioassays 2000; 22: 108–12.

216. Damsky CH, Moursi A, Zhou Y et al. The solid state environment orchestrates embryonic development and tissue remodelling. Kidney Int 1997; 51: 1427–33.

217. Armant DR, Kameda S. Mouse trophoblast cell invasion of extracellular matrix purified from endometrial tissue: a model for peri-implantation development. J Exp Zool 1994; 269: 146–56.

218. Librach CL, Werb Z, Fitzgerald ML et al. 92-kD type IV collagenase mediates invasion of human cytotrophoblasts. J Cell Biol 1991; 113: 437–49.

219. Damsky CH, Librach C, Lim KH et al. Integrin switching regulates normal trophoblast invasion. Development 1994; 120: 3657–66.

220. Salamonsen LA. Role of proteases in implantation. Rev Reprod 1999; 4: 11–22.

221. Brooks PC, Stromblad S, Sanders LC et al. Localization of matrix metalloproteinase MMP-2 to the surface of invasive cells by interaction with integrin alpha v beta 3. Cell 1996; 85: 683–93.

222. Liu WM, Cao YJ, Yang YJ et al. Tetraspanin CD9 regulates invasion during mouse embryo implantation. J Mol Endocrinol 2006; 36: 121–30.

223. Schultz JF, Armant DR. Beta 1- and beta 3-class integrins mediate fibronectin binding activity at the surface of developing mouse peri-implantation blastocysts. Regulation by ligand-induced mobilization of stored receptor. J Biol Chem 1995; 270: 11522–31.

224. Armant DR. Cell interactions with laminin and its proteolytic fragments during outgrowth of mouse primary trophoblast cells. Biol Reprod 1991; 45: 664–72.

225. Hynes RO. Targeted mutations in cell adhesion genes: what have we learned from them? Dev Biol 1996; 180: 402–12.

226. Bader BL, Rayburn H, Crowley D et al. Extensive vasculogenesis, angiogenesis, and organogenesis precede lethality in mice lacking all alpha v integrins. Cell 1998; 95: 507–19.

227. Gardner H, Kreidberg J, Koteliansky V et al. Deletion of integrin alpha 1 by homologous recombination permits normal murine development but gives rise to a specific deficit in cell adhesion. Dev Biol 1996; 175: 301–13.

228. Romagnano L, Babiarz B. The role of murine cell surface galactosyl transferase in trophoblast:laminin interactions in vitro. Dev Biol 1990; 141: 254–61.

229. Burrows TD, King A, Smith SK et al. Human trophoblast adhesion to matrix proteins: inhibition and signal transduction. Hum Reprod 1995; 10: 2489–500.

230. Stephens LE, Sutherland AE, Klimanskaya IV et al. Deletion of beta-1 integrins in mice results in inner cell mass failure and peri-implantation lethality. Genes Dev 1995; 9: 1883–95.

231. Brakebusch C, Hirsch E, Potocnik A et al. Genetic analysis of beta 1 integrin function: confirmed, new and revised roles for a crucial family of cell adhesion molecules. J Cell Sci 1997; 110 (Pt23): 2895–904.

232. Aplin JD. Expression of integrin alpha 6 beta 4 in human trophoblast and its loss from extravillous cells. Placenta 1993; 14: 203–15.

233. Zhou Y, Damsky CH, Chiu K et al. Preeclampsia is associated with abnormal expression of adhesion molecules by invasive cytotrophoblasts. J Clin Invest 1993; 91: 950–60.

234. Pijnenborg R, Vercruysse L, Verbist L et al. Interaction of interstitial trophoblast with placental bed capillaries and venules of normotensive and pre-eclamptic pregnancies. Placenta 1998; 19: 569–75.

235. Sugimori T, Griffith DL, Arnaout MA. Emerging paradigms of integrin ligand binding and activation. Kidney Int 1997; 51: 1454–62.

236. Plow EF, Haas TA, Zhang L et al. Ligand binding to integrins. J Biol Chem 2000; 275: 21785–8.

237. Humphries MJ. The molecular basis and specificity of integrin–ligand interactions. J Cell Sci 1990; 97 (Pt 4): 585–92.

23 The prolactin family: regulators of uterine biology

Michael J Soares, SM Khorshed Alam, Toshihiro Konno, and Rupasri Ain

Synopsis

Background

- In rats and mice, the uterus is bicornuate with a mesometrial vascular supply.
- The chorioallantoic placenta develops at the mesometrial pole.
- Above the basal decidua is a triangular area rich in blood vessels known as the metrial gland or the mesometrial lymphoid aggregate of pregnancy (MLAP).
- Uterine natural killer (uNK) cells are abundant in the metrial gland at mid gestation.
- The placenta comprises two anatomically distinct regions: the junctional zone, an endocrine and invasive tissue; and the labyrinth, which is the site of maternal–fetal exchange.
- Prolactin (PRL) is a polypeptide hormone with effects on reproduction, lactation, the brain, immune system, and metabolism in rodents, humans, and other mammals.
- Members of the PRL family are produced by the anterior pituitary, the decidua, and the placenta.

Basic Science

- In mid pregnancy in the rat a subpopulation of trophoblasts exits the junctional zone and infiltrates the metrial gland and its blood vessels. This coincides with the degeneration of the uNK cell population.
- In the mouse, trophoblast infiltration is restricted to the mesometrial decidua.
- A subset of mammals, including the rat, mouse, and cow have genes encoding numerous PRL family members, while other species, such as dogs and humans, have only a single orthologous member, PRL.
- The PRL family seems to have expanded in the mouse and rat to enable adaptations to environmental challenges during pregnancy. These challenges might have included nutrient availability, exposure to pathogens, or changes in atmospheric conditions or temperature.
- The anterior pituitary, uterine decidual cells, and various lineages of trophoblast cells all contribute to the production of these ligands.
- PRL and the placental lactogens (PLs) are PRL receptor agonists.
- They are critical to pregnancy and lactation through their actions on the corpus luteum and mammary gland.
- Human decidual PRL binds to heparin and probably accumulates in extracellular matrix at the maternal–fetal interface.
- Its targets in the uterus may include epithelial glands, angiogenesis, trophoblast development, and immune cells. In addition, it may target amniotic and possibly fetal tissues.
- The remaining members of the PRL family have a broad spectrum of targets, including but not limited to hematopoietic precursor cells and immune cells and cells of the vasculature. PLP-A produced by trophoblast binds receptors on uNK cells.
- Expression of decidual PRL family ligands is most abundant in antimesometrial decidua in the mouse and the rat.
- Gene ablation studies in the mouse have demonstrated that two family members, dPRP and PLP-A, are both dispensable under normal breeding conditions but their absence renders mice susceptible to hypoxia-induced pregnancy failure.

Clinical

- Insights into the mechanisms controlling pregnancy-dependent adaptations to physiological stressors may be useful in understanding the etiology of pregnancy-related diseases such as preeclampsia and intrauterine growth restriction.

INTRODUCTION

Pregnancy requires significant changes in the functioning of maternal tissues. Of primary importance is the redirection of resources and nutrients to the uterus, the site of embryonic development. Pregnancy is associated with two key uterine adaptations:

- the differentiation of uterine stromal cells, a process referred to as decidualization
- the modification of the uterine arterial vessels supplying the placenta.

The latter adaptation is directed, at least in part, by invasive trophoblast cells exiting the chorioallantoic placenta. Some of the functions of decidual cells and invasive trophoblast are mediated by their secretion of a family of hormones related to prolactin (PRL).

The purpose of this chapter is to provide a framework for understanding the biology of the PRL family in the context of uterine events contributing to the establishment and maintenance of pregnancy. The discussion focuses primarily on the rat and mouse and, where applicable, on other species for comparative purposes.

ORGANIZATION OF THE UTEROPLACENTAL COMPARTMENT

The uteroplacental compartments of the rat and mouse are similar and they share the same basic organizational plan of other species with hemochorial placentation.[1,2] Schematic representations of rat uteroplacental anatomy are presented in Figure 23.1.

The site where blood enters the uterus determines the orientation of the uteroplacenta. This region is referred to as the mesometrial compartment, and the opposite side is antimesometrial. The uterine mesometrial compartment is composed of stromal cells, blood vessels, immune/inflammatory cells, smooth muscle cells of the myometrium, and trophoblast cells. Cellular composition is dynamic. Following implantation, natural killer cells expand in number, and infiltrate the

mesometrial decidua, located adjacent to the developing chorioallantoic placenta. Decidual cells are derived from uterine stromal cells.[3,4] A triangular-shaped area rich in blood vessels is situated between the mesometrial decidua and the surface of the uterus and is referred to as the metrial gland.[5,6] A subpopulation of trophoblast giant cells represents the earliest extraembryonic invaders of the uterine mesometrial vasculature. While pregnancy progresses, placental and embryonic structures expand in size and the decidua regresses. The chorioallantoic placenta is established in the mesometrial compartment and consists of two functionally distinct regions:

- a junctional zone, an endocrine and invasive tissue, which is composed of trophoblast giant cells, spongiotrophoblast cells, glycogen cells, and the source of an invasive trophoblast cell population
- a labyrinth zone, which is the site of maternal–fetal exchange and the location of syncytial trophoblast, cytotrophoblast, and labyrinthine trophoblast giant cell lineages.

Accompanying the development of the chorioallantoic placenta, natural killer cells vacate the mesometrial decidua and infiltrate the metrial gland where they associate with the resident vasculature. Subsequently, the antimesometrial deciduum and mesometrial-associated natural killer cells degenerate. As natural killer cells vacate, the specialized population of invasive trophoblast cells exits the junctional zone of the chorioallantoic placenta, invades the mesometrial decidua, and associates with the vasculature[7] (Figure 23.2). In the mouse, trophoblast invasion is limited to the mesometrial decidua; in the rat, trophoblast cells penetrate through the mesometrial decidua and infiltrate the metrial gland.

THE PRL FAMILY

PRL is a hormone initially isolated from the mammalian anterior pituitary with effects on reproduction and lactation.[8,9] Subsequent analyses expanded the

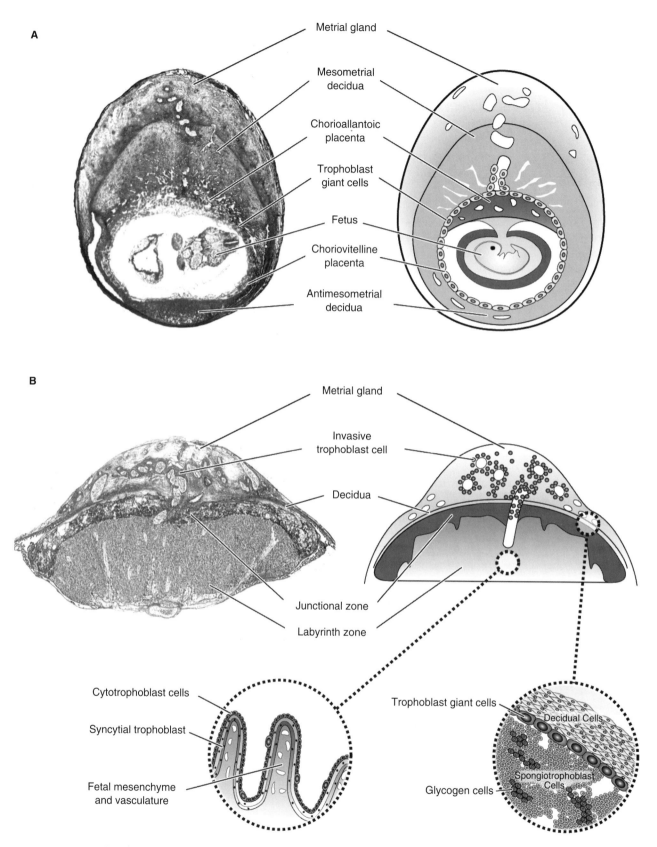

Figure 23.1 Mid and late gestation uteroplacental compartments. (**A**) Hematoxylin and eosin-stained tissue section of the mid gestation rat uteroplacental compartment (left, day 11 of gestation) and a corresponding schematic diagram (right). (**B**) Hematoxylin and eosin-stained tissue section of the late gestation rat uteroplacental compartment (left, day 18 of gestation) and a corresponding schematic diagram (right) with highlighted expanded views of the labyrinth and junctional zones (lower panels). (Reproduced in modified form from Ain et al,[103] with permission from Humana Press. See also color plate section.)

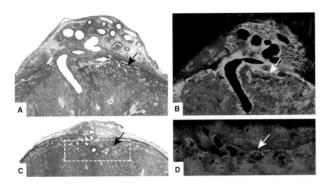

Figure 23.2   Identification of invasive trophoblast cells in the rat and mouse. Rat and mouse placentation sites were recovered at day 18 of gestation, and 10 μm sections prepared. Trophoblast cells were identified by cytokeratin immunostaining. (**A**) Hematoxylin and eosin staining of the rat placentation site. (**B**) Cytokeratin immunolocalization with the rat placentation site. (**C**) Hematoxylin and eosin staining of the mouse placentation site (the area shown in the box is present in **D**). (**D**) Cytokeratin immunolocalization within the mouse placentation site. All magnifications are at 100×. Arrows indicate the trophoblast giant cell boundary between the placenta and decidua. (Reproduced from Ain et al,[7] with permission from Academic Press. See also color plate section.)

range of biological actions for PRL to effects on the brain, immune system, and metabolism.[10] Concurrent with these efforts, it also became evident that the PRL locus was expanded in a subset of mammals, including the rat, mouse, and cow; however, PRL loci of other species, as exemplified by the dog and human, have only a single orthologous member, PRL.[11] The expanded PRL families, like other gene families, arose via gene duplication and have evolved to their present form by natural selection, resulting in both subfunctionalization and neofunctionalization.[12]

The rat genome contains at least 24 genes related to PRL, spanning approximately 1.7 megabases on chromosome 17.[13] Organization of the rat PRL family locus is similar to the 1-megabase mouse PRL family locus situated on chromosome 13, which includes at least 26 genes related to PRL.[14] Phylogenetic relationships of rat and mouse PRL families are presented in Figure 23.3. Each PRL family gene encodes for a secretory protein that has been linked to pregnancy.[11] All PRL family genes possess five conserved exons. A subset of PRL family genes clustered in the middle of the locus contains an additional exon(s) situated between exon-II and exon-III of the prototypical PRL 5-exon structure.[13,14] The anterior pituitary, uterine decidual cells, and various lineages of trophoblast cells all contribute to the production of these ligands. They are elaborated during gestation in specific temporal and spatial profiles.

Biological activities of PRL family ligands can be categorized as classical and non-classical.[11] Classical actions are mediated by ligand interactions with the PRL receptor and non-classical modes of actions utilize other signaling pathways. PRL and the placental lactogens (PLs) are PRL receptor agonists, and are critical to pregnancy and lactation through their actions on the corpus luteum and mammary gland.[11] The remaining members of the PRL family have a broad spectrum of targets, including but not limited to hematopoietic and immune cells and cells of the vasculature. Overviews of PRL family members associated with decidual tissue and those potentially impacting the uterine vasculature are provided below.

DECIDUAL PRL FAMILY

The seminal research leading to the discovery of uterine decidua as a source of PRL related ligands was directed towards elucidation of a decidual factor that promoted corpus luteum survival and function.[15–17] Such biological activities are classified as luteotropic actions and are hallmarks of PRL (see Chapter 17). These investigative efforts culminated in the identification of four PRL family ligands in the deciduum, including PRL-like protein-B (PLP-B), decidual PRL-related protein (dPRP), PLP-J, and PRL. The exact contribution of any of these decidual products to the luteotropic activities intrinsic to decidual tissue is unknown. A couple of generalizations are appropriate for the decidual PRL family ligands: i) expression is most abundant in antimesometrial decidua of pregnancy; and ii) expression is evident in deciduomal tissue of pseudopregnancy. The decidual PRL family ligands will be discussed in the order of their discovery.

PLP-B

Friesen and co-workers first identified PLP-B in the rat placenta[18] and subsequently demonstrated its expression in rat decidual tissue.[19] PLP-B is encoded by a 5-exon gene with significant homology to the prototypical PRL gene.[13,14] Temporally, decidual PLP-B production follows the growth, development, and regression of the antimesometrial deciduum.[19,20] After mid gestation, PLP-B expression shifts to spongiotrophoblast cells of the rat chorioallantoic placenta, where it is expressed at high levels until it declines during the final days of gestation.[18,20–22] The PLP-B protein is secreted as a glycoprotein by both decidua

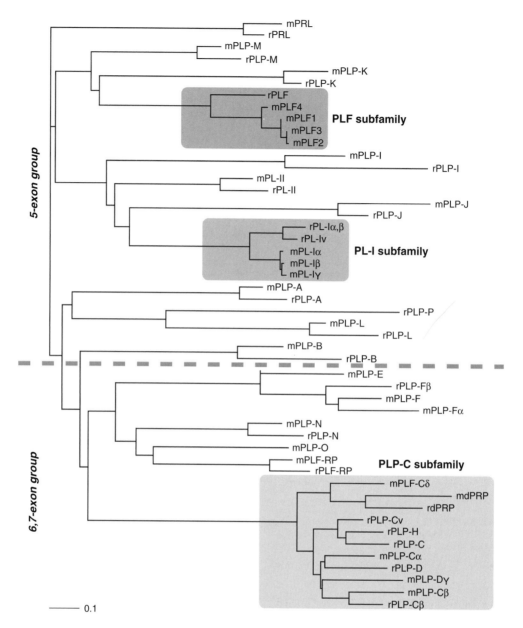

Figure 23.3   Phylogenetic analysis of the PRL family in the rat (*Rattus norvegicus*) and mouse (*Mus musculus*). Multiple amino acid sequence alignments and phylogenetic tree construction were performed using the CLUSTAL X and TREEVIEW software programs.[104,105] GenBank accession numbers for each member of the rat and mouse PRL family are provided in Table 23.1. The PRL families of the rat and mouse are largely orthologous. The rat and mouse expanded PRL families contain subsets of 5-exon and 6-exon members which can be further subdivided into subfamilies (e.g. PL, PLF, PLP-C). Although the rat and mouse PRL family loci are similar, each possesses some notable unique features (e.g. rat PLP-P, mouse PLP-O, mouse PLP-E, PLF, and some features of the PLP-C subfamily).

and placental tissues.[20] PLP-B exhibits similar structural features and expression profiles in the mouse.[23,24] There is some evidence that PLP-B expression is induced by tissue injury, at least in the placenta,[22] but there is little information on its biological activities. PLP-B does not effectively bind to PRL receptors, nor does it activate the PRL receptor signaling pathway;[20] thus, it is unlikely to be directly responsible for the luteotropic actions of decidual tissue.

dPRP

dPRP was discovered in an attempt to characterize the PLP-B protein from rat decidual tissue.[25] Once isolated, dPRP was found to be more closely related to another PRL family member, termed PLP-C, which facilitated its cloning and characterization.[25] dPRP is a member of the 6-exon cluster of genes,[26] centrally located within the rat and mouse PRL

Table 23.1   Rat and mouse PRL families

PRL family[a]	Rat GenBank Accession No.	Mouse GenBank Accession No.	References
PRL	NM_012629	NM_011164	82–84
PL-Iα	NM_017363	AF525162	13, 14, 85–87
PL-Iβ	DQ329283	NM_172155	13, 14
PL-Iγ	—	NM_172156	14
PLP-J	NM_031316	NM_013766	34–37
PL-II	NM_012535	M14647	87–89
PLP-I	NM_153736	AF525154	14, 36
PLP-B	M31155	NM_011166	23, 24, 61
dPRP	NM_022846	NM_010088	23, 25, 26
PLP-K	NM_138861	NM_025532	14, 36, 37
PLP-D	NM_022537	—	90
PLP-Cv	NM_020079	—	91
PLP-C	M76537	—	92
PLP-H	NM_021580	—	93
PL-Iv	NM_033233	—	94, 95
PLP-Cγ	—	NM_023741	14
PLP-Cβ	NM_134385	NM_023332	96
PLP-Cδ	—	NM_028477	14
PLP-Cα	—	NM_011167	97
PLP-N	NM_153738	NM_029355	14, 77
PLP-E	None	NM_008930	98, 99
PLP-F	None	NM_011168	98, 99
PLP-Fβ	AY741310	—	Unpublished[b]
PLP-Fα	NM_022530	—	56
PLP-O	—	NM_026206	14
PLF-RP	NM_053364	NM_011120	50, 56, 78
PLF1	—	NM_031191	49
PLF2	—	K03235	100
PLF3	—	NM_011954	101
PLF4	—	AF128884	102
PLP-M	NM_053791	NM_019991	78
PLF	DQ329281	—	13
PLP-A	NM_017036	NM_011165	61
PLP-L	NM_138527	NM_023746	36, 78
PLP-P	DQ329280	—	13

[a]Abbreviations: PRL, prolactin; PL, placental lactogen; PLP, prolactin-like protein; dPRP, decidual prolactin-related protein; PLF, proliferin; PLF-RP, proliferin-related protein.
[b]JK Ho-Chen, J Bustamante, MJ Soares, unpublished results.

family loci.[13,14] The temporal and tissue-specific expression profiles for dPRP are similar to PLP-B, except in magnitude.[25–29] Levels of dPRP production in uterine decidua and the chorioallantoic placenta are inversely related. dPRP expression is abundant in the uterine decidua and modest in the chorioallantoic placenta.[29] The dPRP protein is secreted as a glycoprotein but probably resides primarily in the decidual extracellular matrix where it binds with high affinity to heparin-containing molecules.[28,30] dPRP exhibits similar structural features and expression profiles in the mouse.[23,31]

The potential for dPRP as an activator of both classical and known non-classical mechanisms has been examined. dPRP failed to bind to PRL receptors and showed minimal ability to promote the proliferation of the PRL-dependent Nb2 lymphoma cell line.[28] Two members of the mouse PRL family, proliferin (PLF) and proliferin-related protein (PLF-RP), are known modulators of angiogenesis through non-classical mechanisms.[32] dPRP did not markedly influence the development of vascular structures, as evaluated through both in-vitro and in-vivo assays;[28] however, in-vivo analysis indicated that dPRP could facilitate heterologous tissue transplantation into athymic mice.[28] Additional experiments with dPRP fusion proteins implicated eosinophils as potential targets for dPRP action.[30] These findings suggested that dPRP could potentially contribute to decidual signals responsible for the establishment of pregnancy and prompted the creation and characterization of a dPRP null mouse.

dPRP null mice were made by replacing exons II–VI of the dPRP gene with an inframe enhanced green fluorescent protein gene and a neomycin resistance cassette.[33] Under standard animal husbandry conditions, some modest phenotypic changes were observed, including a decrease in decidual PLP-J expression, but none sufficient to impair the progression of pregnancy. A prominent phenotype was observed when pregnant dPRP null mice were exposed to a physiological stressor. Pregnancies were disrupted when dPRP null mice were exposed to hypoxia. In contrast, wild-type mice adapted to the hypoxic challenge and their pregnancies proceeded. These observations suggest that dPRP may participate in pregnancy-dependent adaptations to physiological stressors. The mechanism underlying dPRP's role in the adaptive response to hypoxia is unknown at present.

PLP-J

Two approaches were used to identify a third decidual mRNA related to PRL:

- screening a decidual cDNA library with a human PRL cDNA[34]
- inspection of expressed sequence tag (EST) databases for cDNAs with sequence similarity to members of the PRL family.[35–37]

One of the groups referred to the new gene as PLP-I, whereas the other three termed the new decidual transcript as PLP-J. We refer to the gene as PLP-J, since there is another trophoblast-derived PRL family member with the name PLP-I.[14,36] The PLP-J mRNA and protein are abundant within the antimesometrial decidua. It is curious that PLP-J is embedded between the PL-I genes and the PL-II gene within the PRL family locus[13,14] and structurally is also most closely related to the PLs. However, unlike the PLs, PLP-J does not interact with the PRL receptor (S Alam, MJ Soares, unpublished results). Similar to dPRP, PLP-J avidly binds to heparin-containing molecules (S Alam, MJ Soares, unpublished results). We view PLP-J as a potential autocrine/paracrine modulator of the establishment of pregnancy, and/or similar to dPRP, as a contributor to pregnancy-dependent adaptations to physiological stressors.

PRL

The PRL gene has also been shown to be expressed in rat and mouse decidual tissue.[38,39] The overall abundance of decidual PRL is less than for other members of the decidual PRL family. PRL transcripts in the decidua are most readily detected by reverse transcription-polymerase chain reaction (RT-PCR). PRL signals through the PRL receptor. In the early postimplantation uterus, the PRL receptor is primarily associated with undecidualized stromal cells in the antimesometrial border and a restricted population of mesometrial stromal cells associated with the developing chorioallantoic placenta.[40] As gestation advances, decidual cell expression of the PRL receptor increases and then declines as the antimesometrial decidua regresses.[41] Local production of PRL by decidual cells may contribute to decidual cell survival.[38,42] Trophoblast giant cells of the chorioallantoic placenta are situated at the decidual cell–placental interface and produce PL-I and PL-II, which are PRL receptor agonists, and probably also contribute to the modulation of uterine decidual cell function.[11]

PRL is a prominent product of the uterine decidua in primates, and has been best studied in the human.[43,44] Human decidual PRL binds to heparin,[45] a feature it shares with two rodent decidual PRL family members (dPRP and PLP-J), and thus probably accumulates in the decidual extracellular matrix. Targets for human decidual PRL include intrauterine (uterine gland development, angiogenesis, trophoblast cell development, and immune regulation), amniotic, and possibly fetal tissues.[46,47] The expansion of decidual PRL-related ligands in rodents might represent a subspecialization of biological activities ascribed to PRL in human decidua.

THE PLACENTAL PRL FAMILY AND THE UTERINE VASCULATURE

Establishment of an effective delivery system of nutrients and waste products between the mother and the fetus is imperative for a successful pregnancy.[48] Trophoblast cells contribute to the remodeling of the uterine vasculature, at least in part, through their secretion of hormones/cytokines, which influence cell types within the uterine mesometrial compartment. PRL family ligands are produced by trophoblast cells as they establish relationships with the uterine mesometrial vasculature.

PLF and PLF-RP

As indicated above, two members of the mouse placental PRL family (PLF and PLF-RP) modulate blood vessel development.[32] PLF was originally discovered as a growth factor regulated gene in serum-starved mouse fibroblasts[49] and PLF-RP was identified based on its structural relationships with PLF.[50] PLF is the product of at least four closely related genes in the mouse,[14] whereas in the rat there is only a single PLF gene.[13] PLFs and PLF-RP are products of the placenta.[50,51] Trophoblast giant cells contribute significantly to the initial invasion and remodeling of the uterine vasculature and are the source of PLFs.[52,53] PLF-RP expression differs in the mouse and rat. In the mouse, PLF-RP is a product of the spongiotrophoblast;[54,55] however, in the rat, PLF-RP is expressed at the leading edge of invasive trophoblast at mid gestation and then within the labyrinth zone during the last week of gestation.[56] Linzer and his colleagues have demonstrated that PLF is angiogenic and PLF-RP is antiangiogenic.[32] These two hormones/cytokines reciprocally influence blood vessel formation as demonstrated by both in-vitro and in-vivo analyses.[32,57–59] The biological activities of the rat PLF and PLF-RP orthologues have not been reported. Collectively, PLF and PLF-RP represent the major placental factors regulating angiogenesis in the mouse.[60]

PLP-A

PLP-A modulates the establishment of the hemochorial placenta. Rat PLP-A was first discovered as a by-product of the cDNA cloning of PL-II.[61] Subsequently, mouse orthologues were revealed and characterized from EST databases.[23,24] In the mouse, PLP-A is primarily a product of trophoblast giant cells,[24,62] whereas in the rat PLP-A is synthesized by trophoblast giant cells, spongiotrophoblast cells, and invasive trophoblast cells.[7,63] PLP-A is secreted as a glycoprotein hormone,[24,64,65] circulates in maternal blood as a high molecular mass complex,[66,67] and specifically interacts with uterine natural killer cells.[68,69] Uterine natural killer cells are the principal leukocytes of the uterus[70–72] and have been implicated in mediating uterine mesometrial inflammatory/immune responses[73] and vascular remodeling.[74] The latter effects on the uterine mesometrial vasculature facilitate nutrient flow to the placenta and fetus[74] and are proposed to be mediated by interferon γ (IFNγ).[75] PLP-A is an intermediary in trophoblast cell modulation of natural killer cells, including their production of IFNγ.[69,76]

The physiology of PLP-A has been further explored in PLP-A-deficient mice.[76] PLP-A null mice were made by replacing exons II–V of the PLP-A gene with a neomycin resistance cassette.[76] As was true for the dPRP gene, the PLP-A gene was also dispensable when mice were maintained under standard animal husbandry conditions. However, when pregnant PLP-A null mice were challenged by exposure to hypoxia, they were not able to adapt and their pregnancies terminated.[76] Pregnancies failed because of inadequate placentation (Figure 23.4). Exposure to maternal hypoxia disrupted trophoblast cells of the PLP-A-deficient chorioallantoic placenta from establishing connectivity with the uterine mesometrial vasculature. This is in contrast to pregnant mice expressing PLP-A, which successfully adapt to low oxygen and maintain their pregnancies. The potential involvement of natural killer cells in mediating PLP-A-regulated adaptations to maternal hypoxia is unknown.

PRL family and invasive trophoblast cells

During the last week of gestation, invasive trophoblast cells exit the chorioallantoic placenta and enter the mesometrial uterine compartment.[7] These invasive trophoblast cells possess a unique phenotype, which is distinguished by their elaboration of PRL family ligands. In the rat, invasive trophoblast cells express five members of the PRL family: PLP-A, PLP-L, PLP-M, PLP-N, and PLP-P.[7,13,77] The structure and function of PLP-A were discussed above. The remaining PRL-related proteins expressed in invasive trophoblast were first identified through searches for PRL-related sequences in rat EST and genomic databases.[13,36,37,77,78] Orthologues were identified from mouse EST and genomic databases,[14,37,78] except for PLP-P, which is unique to the rat.[13] Minimal characterization of the corresponding mRNAs and proteins has been performed beyond tissue expression profiles. In comparison to the junctional zone of the rat chorioallantoic placenta, PLP-A expression in invasive trophoblast cells is weak.[7] PLP-M and PLP-P are dually expressed in invasive trophoblast cells and in trophoblast cells situated within the chorioallantoic placenta,[7,13] whereas PLP-L and PLP-N expression is restricted to invasive trophoblast cells.[7] Rat invasive trophoblast cells expressing genes related to PRL penetrate throughout the uterine mesometrial compartment.[7] In contrast, mouse invasive trophoblast cells do not penetrate beyond the mesometrial decidual boundary and only prominently express two members of the PRL family (PLP-M and PLP-N).[7] Invasive trophoblasts can replace the endothelium of the uterine arterial vessels

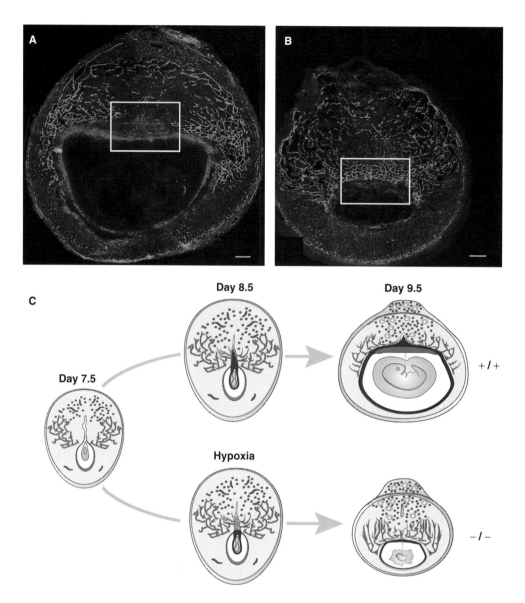

Figure 23.4 Defect in hemochorial placentation and trophoblast–vascular interactions in PLP-A null mutant mice exposed to hypoxia. Double immunohistochemical staining for trophoblast cells by using a cytokeratin-8-specific antibody (TROMA-1) and for endothelial cells by using an endoglin antibody within implantation sites of wild-type and PLP-A null mutant mice after 48 hours (**A** and **B**) of hypoxia starting on gestation day 7.5 (scale bars = 250 μm). (**C**) Cellular dynamics at implantation sites of wild-type and PLP-A null mutant mice exposed to hypoxia for 48 hours starting on gestation day 7.5. Note the lack of trophoblast expansion into the mesometrial chamber on days 8.5 and 9.5 of pregnancy in PLP-A null mutant mice after exposure to hypoxia. Also note the aberrant vasculature and underdeveloped placentas at the implantation sites on day 9.5 of pregnancy in PLP-A null mutant mice exposed to hypoxia. (Reproduced in modified form from Ain et al,[74] with permission from the National Academy of Sciences of the USA. See also color plate section.)

(endovascular) and accumulate around the vessels (interstitial), where their presence is associated with the disappearance of vascular smooth muscle.[7,79,80] These changes impact the permeability and distention properties of the vessels and alter their delivery of cellular and molecular components of maternal blood. A distant relative of the PRL family, growth hormone variant (also known as placental growth hormone), is a known autocrine/paracrine stimulator of invasiveness in human trophoblast.[81] Whether the different PRL family expression patterns in invasive trophoblast cells of the rat and mouse are responsible for the species difference in the depth of trophoblast invasion remains to be determined.

FINAL THOUGHTS

The PRL family is an intriguing example of the evolution of a set of genes directed towards the regulation of viviparity and species-specific reproductive success. At this juncture, we possess a modicum of knowledge on the evolution of the PRL family but we do have enough insights from the few mammalian species that have been studied to know that conservation is not the rule. The lack of species conservation would direct some scientists elsewhere. However, based on emerging gene targeting experimentation, this would be an unfortunate oversight.[33,76] Evolution of the PRL family and its various expansions did not occur in the laboratory setting. The PRL family expanded in the mouse and rat to ensure pregnancy-dependent adaptations to environmental challenges. These challenges might have included nutrient availability, exposure to pathogens, and temperature excesses. The ability to reproductively adapt to environmental challenges provides a selective advantage for a species, ensuring its survival.

The insights discussed in the preceding paragraph are based on the phenotypic analysis of mice with disruptions in two mouse PRL family genes, dPRP and PLP-A.[33,76] The physiological relevance of the remainder of the mouse PRL family locus is unknown. If the mouse PRL family locus was modified to resemble the human locus, consisting of only PRL, what would be the impact on pregnancy? The generation of new genes by gene duplication and natural selection results in a purification process, leading to subspecialization from the ancestral gene (subfunctionalization) or the development of new functions not previously attributed to the ancestral gene (neofunctionalization). Have rodent PRL family ligands undergone subfunctionalization and/or neofunctionalization? Are mouse PRL and human PRL functionally equivalent or have they undergone specialization? These questions can be addressed through chromosomal engineering and gene replacement experiments and will provide important information about the evolution of the PRL family locus.

Finally, it is important to emphasize that we gain insights about human pregnancy from studying rodent pregnancy and the rodent PRL family. Pregnancy is characterized by adaptive responses to physiological stressors. Appropriate adaptive responses result in successful progression of gestation and healthy offspring, whereas ineffective adaptations compromise pregnancy and the health of the fetus and newborn. Insights into the mechanisms controlling pregnancy-dependent adaptations to physiological stressors are essential to understanding the etiology of pregnancy-related diseases, such as preeclampsia and intrauterine growth restriction. The rodent PRL family provides a means for identification of key cellular and molecular participants in pregnancy-dependent adaptations.

ACKNOWLEDGMENTS

We would like to acknowledge current colleagues in our laboratory and also past trainees that made valuable contributions. This work was supported by grants from the National Institutes of Health (HD20676, HD039878, HD48861) and the Hall Family Foundation.

REFERENCES

1. Rossant J, Cross JC. Extraembryonic lineages. In: Rossant J, Tam PPL, eds. Mouse Development. New York: Academic Press, 2002: 155–80.
2. Georgiades P, Ferguson-Smith AC, Burton GJ. Comparative developmental anatomy of the murine and human definitive placentae. Placenta 2002; 23: 3–19.
3. DeFeo VJ. Decidualization. In: Wynn RM, ed. Cellular Biology of the Uterus. New York: Appleton-Century-Crofts, 1967: 191–290.
4. Bell SC. Decidualization: regional differentiation and associated function. Oxf Rev Reprod Biol 1983; 5: 220–71.
5. Selye H, McKeown T. Studies on the physiology of the maternal placenta in the rat. Proc R Soc Lond Biol 1935; 119: 1–31.
6. Peel S. Granulated metrial gland cells. Adv Anat Embryol Cell Biol 1989; 115: 1–112.
7. Ain R, Canham LN, Soares MJ. Gestational stage-dependent intrauterine trophoblast cell invasion in the rat and mouse: novel endocrine phenotype and regulation. Dev Biol 2003; 260: 176–90.
8. Nicoll CS. Ontogeny and evolution of prolactin's functions. Fed Proc 1980; 39: 2563–66.
9. Nicoll CS, Bern HA. On the actions of prolactin among the vertebrates: is there a common denominator? In: Wolstenholme GEW, Knight J, eds. Lactogenic Hormones. London: Churchill Livingstone, 1972: 99–337.
10. Goffin V, Binart N, Touraine P, Kelly PA. Prolactin: the new biology of an old hormone. Annu Rev Physiol 2002; 64: 47–67.
11. Soares MJ. The prolactin and growth hormone families: pregnancy-specific hormones/cytokines at the maternal–fetal interface. Reprod Biol Endocrinol 2004; 2: 51.
12. Francino MP. An adaptive radiation model for the origin of new gene functions. Nat Genet 2005; 37: 573–7.
13. Alam SMK, Ain R, Konno T et al. The rat prolactin gene family locus: species-specific gene family expansion. Mamm Genome 2006; 17: 858–77.
14. Wiemers DO, Shao L-J, Ain R et al. The mouse prolactin gene family locus. Endocrinology 2003; 144: 313–25.
15. Ershoff BH, Deuel HJ. Prolongation of pseudopregnancy by induction of deciduomata in the rat. Proc Soc Exp Biol Med 1943; 54: 167–218.
16. Gibori G, Rothchild I, Pepe GI et al. Luteotrophic action of decidual tissue in the rat. Endocrinology 1974; 95: 1113–18.
17. Rothchild I, Gibori G. The luteotrophic effect of decidual tissue: the stimulating effect of decidualization on serum progesterone level of pseudopregnant rats. Endocrinology 1975; 97: 838–42.
18. Duckworth ML, Peden LM, Friesen HG. A third prolactin-like protein expressed by the developing rat placenta: complementary deoxyribonucleic acid sequence and partial structure of the gene. Mol Endocrinol 1988; 2: 912–20.
19. Croze F, Kennedy TG, Schroedter IC, Friesen HG. Expression of rat prolactin-like protein-B in deciduoma of pseudopregnant rat and in decidua during early pregnancy. Endocrinology 1990; 127: 2665–72.
20. Cohick CB, Xu L, Soares MJ. Prolactin-like protein-B: heterologous expression and characterization of placental and decidual species. J Endocrinol 1997; 152: 291–302.

21. Duckworth ML, Schroedter IC, Friesen HG. Cellular localization of rat placental lactogen-II and rat prolactin-like proteins A and B by in situ hybridization. Placenta 1990; 11: 143–55.

22. Lu X-J, Deb S, Soares MJ. Spontaneous differentiation of trophoblast cells along the spongiotrophoblast pathway: expression of the placental prolactin gene family and modulation by retinoic acid. Dev Biol 1994; 163: 86–97.

23. Lin J, Poole J, Linzer DIH. Three new members of the mouse prolactin/growth hormone family are homologous to proteins expressed in the rat. Endocrinology 1997; 138: 5541–9.

24. Müller H, Ishimura R, Orwig KE et al. Homologues for prolactin-like protein-A and B are present in the mouse. Biol Reprod 1998; 58: 45–51.

25. Roby KF, Deb S, Gibori G et al. Decidual prolactin-related protein. Identification, molecular cloning, and characterization. J Biol Chem 1993; 268: 3136–42.

26. Orwig KE, Dai G, Rasmussen CA, Soares MJ. Decidual/trophoblast prolactin-related protein: characterization of gene structure and cell-specific expression. Endocrinology 1997; 138: 2491–500.

27. Gu Y, Soares MJ, Srivastava RK, Gibori G. Expression of decidual prolactin-related protein in the rat decidua. Endocrinology 1994; 135: 1422–7.

28. Rasmussen CA, Hashizume K, Orwig KE et al. Decidual prolactin-related protein: heterologous expression and characterization. Endocrinology 1996; 137: 5558–66.

29. Rasmussen CA, Orwig KE, Soares MJ. Dual expression of prolactin-related protein in decidua and trophoblast tissues during pregnancy in rats. Biol Reprod 1997; 56: 647–54.

30. Wang D, Ishimura R, Walia DS et al. Eosinophils are cellular targets of the novel uteroplacental heparin-binding cytokine, decidual/trophoblast prolactin-related protein. J Endocrinol 2000; 167: 15–29.

31. Orwig KE, Ishimura R, Müller H et al. Identification and characterization of a mouse homolog for decidual/trophoblast prolactin-related protein. Endocrinology 1997; 139: 5511–17.

32. Jackson D, Volpert OV, Bouck N, Linzer DIH. Stimulation and inhibition of angiogenesis by placental proliferin and proliferin-related protein. Science 1994; 266: 1581–4.

33. Alam SMK, Konno T, Dai G et al. A uterine decidual cell cytokine ensures pregnancy-dependent adaptations to hypoxia. Development 2007; 17: 858–77.

34. Hiraoka Y, Ogawa M, Sakai Y et al. PLP-I: a novel prolactin-like gene in rodents. Biochim Biophys Acta 1999; 1447: 291–7.

35. Toft DJ, Lizer DIH. Prolactin (PRL)-like protein J, a novel member of the PRL/growth hormone family, is exclusively expressed in maternal decidua. Endocrinology 1999; 140: 5095–101.

36. Ishibashi K, Imai M. Identification of four new members of the rat prolactin/growth hormone gene family. Biochem Biophys Res Commun 1999; 262: 575–8.

37. Dai G, Wang D, Liu B et al. Three novel paralogs of the rodent prolactin gene family. J Endocrinol 2000; 166: 63–75.

38. Prigent-Tessier A, Tessier C, Hirosawa-Takamori M et al. Rat decidual prolactin. Identification, molecular cloning, and characterization. J Biol Chem 1999; 274: 37982–9.

39. Kimura F, Takakura K, Takebayashi K et al. Messenger ribonucleic acid for the mouse decidual prolactin is present and induced during in vitro decidualization of endometrial stromal cells. Gynecol Endocrinol 2001; 15: 426–32.

40. Reese J, Binart N, Brown N et al. Implantation and decidualization defects in prolactin receptor (PRLR)-deficient mice are mediated by ovarian but not uterine PRLR. Endocrinology 2000; 141: 1872–81.

41. Gu Y, Srivastava RK, Clarke DL et al. The decidual prolactin receptor and its regulation by decidua-derived factors. Endocrinology 1996; 136: 4878–85.

42. Tessier C, Prigent-Tessier A, Ferguson-Gottschall S et al. PRL antiapoptotic effect in the rat decidua involves the PI3K/protein kinase B-mediated inhibition of caspase-3 activity. Endocrinology 2001; 142: 4086–94.

43. Handwerger S, Markoff E, Richards R. Regulation of the synthesis and release of decidual prolactin by placental and autocrine/paracrine factors. Placenta 1991; 12: 121–30.

44. Telgmann R, Gellersen B. Marker genes of decidualization: activation of the decidual prolactin gene. Hum Reprod Update 1998; 4: 472–9.

45. Khurana S, Kuns R, Ben-Jonathan N. Heparin-binding property of human prolactin: a novel aspect of prolactin biology. Endocrinology 1999; 140: 1026–9.

46. Jabbour HN, Critchley HO. Potential roles of decidual prolactin in early pregnancy. Reproduction 2001; 121: 197–205.

47. Handwerger S, Brar A. Human uteroplacental lactogens: physiology and molecular biology. In: Horseman ND, ed. Prolactin. Norwell, MA: Kluwer Academic Publishers, 2001: 169–87.

48. Enders AC, Welsh AO. Structural interactions of trophoblast and uterus during hemochorial placenta formation. J Exp Zool 1993; 266: 578–87.

49. Linzer DIH, Nathans D. Nucleotide sequence of a growth-related mRNA encoding a member of the prolactin-growth hormone family. Proc Natl Acad Sci USA 1984; 81: 4255–9.

50. Linzer DIH, Nathans D. A new member of the prolactin-growth hormone gene family expressed in mouse placenta. EMBO J 1985; 4: 1419–23.

51. Linzer DIH, Lee SJ, Ogren L et al. Identification of proliferin mRNA and protein in mouse placenta. Proc Natl Acad Sci USA 1985; 82: 4356–9.

52. Lee SJ, Talamantes F, Wilder E et al. Trophoblastic giant cells of the mouse placenta as the site of proliferin synthesis. Endocrinology 1988; 122: 1761–7.

53. Hemberger M, Nozaki T, Masutani M, Cross JC. Differential expression of angiogenic and vasodilatory factors by invasive trophoblast giant cells depending on depth of invasion. Dev Dyn 2003; 227: 185–91.

54. Colosi P, Swiergiel JJ, Wilder EL et al. Characterization of proliferin-related protein. Mol Endocrinol 1988; 2: 579–86.

55. Carney EW, Prideaux V, Lye SJ, Rossant J. Progressive expression of trophoblast-specific genes during formation of mouse trophoblast giant cells in vitro. Mol Reprod Dev 1993; 34: 357–68.

56. Sahgal N, Knipp GT, Liu B et al. Identification of two new nonclassical members of the rat prolactin family. J Mol Endocrinol 2000; 24: 95–108.

57. Volpert O, Jackson D, Bouck N, Linzer DIH. The insulin-like growth factor II/mannose 6-phosphate receptor is required for proliferin-induced angiogenesis. Endocrinology 1996; 137: 3871–6.

58. Bengtson NW, Linzer DIH. Inhibition of tumor growth by the antiangiogenic placental hormone, proliferin-related protein. Mol Endocrinol 2000; 14: 1934–43.

59. Toft DJ, Rosenberg SB, Bergers G et al. Reactivation of proliferin gene expression is associated with increased angiogenesis in a cell culture model of fibrosarcoma tumor progression. Proc Natl Acad Sci USA 2001; 98: 13055–9.

60. Linzer DIH. Placental angiogenic and anti-angiogenic factors. J NIH Res 1995; 7: 57–8.

61. Duckworth ML, Peden LM, Friesen HG. Isolation of a novel prolactin-like cDNA clone from developing rat placenta. J Biol Chem 1986; 61: 10879–84.

62. Ma GT, Linzer DIH. GATA-2 restricts prolactin-like protein A expression to secondary trophoblast giant cells in the mouse. Biol Reprod 2000; 63: 570–4.

63. Campbell WJ, Deb S, Kwok SC et al. Differential expression of placental lactogen-II and prolactin-like protein-A in the rat chorioallantoic placenta. Endocrinology 1989; 125: 1565–74.

64. Deb S, Youngblood T, Rawitch AB, Soares MJ. Placental pro-lactin-like protein A. Identification and characterization of two major glycoprotein species with antipeptide antibodies. J Biol Chem 1989; 264: 14348–53.

65. Manzella SM, Dharmesh SM, Cohick CB et al. Developmental regulation of a pregnancy-specific oligosaccharide structure, NeuAcα2,6GalNAcβ1,4GlcNAc, on select members of the rat placental prolactin family. J Biol Chem 1997; 272: 4775–82.

66. Deb S, Soares MJ. Characterization of placental prolactin-like protein-A in intracellular and extracellular compartments. Mol Cell Endocrinol 1990; 74: 163–72.

67. Deb S, Hamlin GP, Roby KF et al. Heterologous expression and characterization of prolactin-like protein-A. Identification of serum binding proteins. J Biol Chem 1993; 268: 3298–305.

68. Müller H, Liu B, Croy BA et al. Uterine natural killer cells are targets for a trophoblast cell-specific cytokine, prolactin-like protein A. Endocrinology 1999; 140: 2711–20.

69. Ain R, Tash JS, Soares MJ. Prolactin-like protein-A is a func-tional modulator of natural killer cells at the maternal–fetal interface. Mol Cell Endocrinol 2003; 204: 65–74.

70. Croy BA, Luross JA, Guimond M-J, Hunt JS. Uterine natural killer cells: insights into lineage relationships and functions from studies of pregnancies in mutant and transgenic mice. Nat Immun 1996; 15: 22–33.

71. Moffett-King A. Natural killer cells and pregnancy. Nat Rev Immunol 2002; 2: 656–63.

72. Dosiou C, Giudice LC. Natural killer cells in pregnancy and recurrent pregnancy loss: endocrine and immunologic per-spectives. Endocr Rev 2005; 26: 44–62.

73. Murphy SP, Fast LD, Hanna NN, Sharma S. Uterine NK cells mediate inflammation-induced fetal demise in IL-10-null mice. J Immunol 2005; 175: 4084–90.

74. Croy BA, Ashkar AA, Minhas K, Greenwood JD. Can murine uterine natural killer cells give insights into the pathogenesis of preeclampsia? J Soc Gynecol Invest 2000; 7: 12–20.

75. Ashkar AA, Croy BA. Functions of uterine natural killer cells are mediated by interferon gamma production during murine pregnancy. Semin Immunol 2001; 13: 235–41.

76. Ain R, Dai G, Dunmore JH et al. A prolactin family paralog regulates reproductive adaptations to a physiological stressor. Proc Natl Acad Sci USA 2004; 101: 16543–8.

77. Wiemers DO, Ain R, Ohboshi S, Soares MJ. Migratory tro-phoblast cells express a newly identified member of the pro-lactin gene family. J Endocrinol 2003; 179: 335–46.

78. Toft DJ, Linzer DIH. Identification of three prolactin-related hormones as markers of invasive trophoblasts in the rat. Biol Reprod 2000; 63: 519–25.

79. Vercruysse L, Caluwaerts S, Luyten C, Pijnenborg R. Interstitial trophoblast invasion in the decidua and mesome-trial triangle during the last third of pregnancy in the rat. Placenta 2006; 27: 22–33.

80. Caluwaerts S, Vercruysse L, Luyten C, Pijnenborg R. Endovas-cular trophoblast invasion and associated structural changes in uterine spiral arteries of the pregnant rat. Placenta 2005; 26: 574–84.

81. Lacroix MC, Guibourdenche J, Fournier T et al. Stimulation of human trophoblast invasion by placental growth hormone. Endocrinology 2005; 146: 2434–44.

82. Gubbins EJ, Maurer RA, Hartley JL, Donelson JE. Construction and analysis of recombinant DNAs containing a structural gene for rat prolactin. Nucleic Acids Res 1979; 6: 915–30.

83. Cooke NE, Coit D, Weiner RI et al. Structure of cloned DNA complementary to rat prolactin messenger RNA. J Biol Chem 1980; 255: 6502–10.

84. Linzer DI, Talamantes F. Nucleotide sequence of mouse pro-lactin and growth hormone mRNAs and expression of these mRNAs during pregnancy. J Biol Chem 1985; 260: 9574–9.

85. Robertson MC, Croze F, Schroedter IC, Friesen HG. Molecular cloning and expression of rat placental lactogen-I

86. Hirosawa M, Miura R, Min KS et al. A cDNA encoding a new member of the rat placental lactogen family, PL-I mosaic (PL-Im). Endocr J 1994; 41: 387–97.

87. Dai G, Imagawa W, Liu B et al. Rcho-1 trophoblast cell placental lactogens: complementary deoxyribonucleic acids, heterologous expression, and biological activities. Endocrin-ology 1996; 137: 5020–7.

88. Duckworth ML, Kirk KL, Friesen HG. Isolation and identifi-cation of a cDNA clone of rat placental lactogen II. J Biol Chem 1986; 261: 10871–8.

89. Jackson LL, Colosi P, Talamantes F, Linzer DIH. Molecular cloning of mouse placental lactogen cDNA. Proc Natl Acad Sci USA 1986; 83: 8496–500.

90. Iwatsuki K, Shinozaki M, Hattori N et al. Molecular cloning and characterization of a new member of the rat placental prolactin (PRL) family, PRL-like protein D (PLP-D). Endocrinology 1996; 137: 3849–55.

91. Dai G, Liu B, Szpirer C et al. Prolactin-like protein-C variant: complementary deoxyribonucleic acid, unique six exon gene structure, and trophoblast cell-specific expression. Endocrin-ology 1996; 137: 5009–19.

92. Deb S, Roby KF, Faria TN et al. Molecular cloning and char-acterization of prolactin-like protein C complementary deoxyribonucleic acid. J Biol Chem 1991; 266: 23027–32.

93. Iwatsuki K, Oda M, Sun W et al. Molecular cloning and charac-terization of a new member of the rat placental prolactin (PRL) family, PRL-like protein H. Endocrinology 1998; 139: 4976–83.

94. Robertson MC, Schroedter IC, Friesen HG. Molecular cloning and expression of rat placental lactogen-Iv, a variant of rPL-I present in late pregnant rat placenta. Endocrinology 1991; 129: 2746–56.

95. Cohick CB, Dai G, Xu L et al. Placental lactogen-I variant uti-lizes the prolactin receptor signaling pathway. Mol Cell Endocrinol 1996; 116: 49–58.

96. Hwang IT, Lee YH, Moon BC et al. Identification and characteri-zation of a new member of the placental prolactin-like protein-C (PLP-C) subfamily, PLP-Cβ. Endocrinology 2000; 141: 3343–52.

97. Dai G, Chapman BM, Liu B et al. A new member of the mouse prolactin (PRL)-like protein-C subfamily, PRL-like protein-C alpha: structure and expression. Endocrinology 1998; 139: 5157–63.

98. Lin J, Poole J, Linzer DIH. Two novel members of the prolactin/growth hormone family are expressed in the mouse placenta. Endocrinology 1997; 138: 5535–40.

99. Müller H, Orwig KE, Soares MJ. Identification of two new members of the mouse prolactin gene family. Biochim Biophys Acta 1998; 1396: 251–8.

100. Wilder EL, Linzer DIH. Expression of multiple proliferin genes in mouse cells. Mol Cell Biol 1986; 6: 3283–6.

101. Fassett JT, Nilsen-Hamilton M. Mrp3, a mitogen-regulated protein/proliferin gene expressed in wound healing and in hair follicles. Endocrinology 2001; 142: 2129–37.

102. Fassett JT, Hamilton RT, Nilsen-Hamilton M. Mrp4, a new mitogen-regulated protein/proliferin gene; unique in this gene family for its expression in the adult mouse tail and ear. Endocrinology 2000; 141: 1863–71.

103. Ain R, Konno T, Canham LN, Soares MJ. Phenotypic analysis of the placenta in the rat. In: Soares MJ, Hunt JS, eds. Placenta and Trophoblast: Methods and Protocols. Totowa, New Jersey: Humana Press, 2006; 1: 295–313.

104. Page RD. TreeView: an application to display phylogenetic trees on personal computers. Comput Appl Biosci 1996; 2: 357–8.

105. Thompson JD, Gibson TJ, Plewniak F et al. The CLUSTAL_X windows interface: flexible strategies for multiple sequence alignment aided by quality analysis tools. Nucleic Acids Res 1997; 25: 4876–82.

complementary deoxyribonucleic acid. Endocrinology 1990; 127: 702–10.

24　Endometrial extracellular matrix

John D Aplin

Synopsis

Background

- Extracellular matrix (ECM) is the connective tissue material found between cells.
- The three-dimensional interstitial matrix comprises mainly fibrillar collagens, which provide strength and shape, and proteoglycans, which bind water and provide resistance to compression.
- In addition, there is basement membrane, a sheet of ECM of specialized composition that separates epithelial cells from the underlying stroma. Basement membranes are also found in the walls of blood vessels.
- Muscle tissue, including vascular smooth muscle, also contains elastin, which forms highly cross-linked fibers with elastic properties.
- Secreted matrix metalloproteinases (MMPs) and serine proteases of the plasminogen activator family break down ECM in tissues.

Basic Science

- ECM production is required along with cell proliferation in the course of endometrial regeneration in the proliferative phase.
- ECM remodeling, comprising breakdown of existing components and deposition of new ones, occurs coincident with cyclic histological changes such as angiogenesis, stromal edema in midsecretory phase, and decidualization.
- Decidual ECM is important in providing a substrate for invading trophoblast during pregnancy.
- Trophoblast, a potent source of MMPs and plasminogen-related enzymes, remodels the walls of maternal spiral arteries during pregnancy, including transforming the ECM.
- ECM breakdown occurs at menstruation due to the up-regulation of numerous MMPs as progesterone levels decline.
- Finely tuned local MMP activity is important for normal placentation and decidualization.

Clinical

- A remarkable increase in numerous MMP family members occurs on steroid withdrawal from endometrium.
- Focal expression of matrix metalloproteinases may explain irregular dysfunctional endometrial bleeding.

INTRODUCTION

The function of the extracellular matrix (ECM) can be broadly divided into two. First, it acts as a structural framework for tissue. The structural demands on endometrium change with pregnancy, and after parturition there is a need to return the ECM to its non-pregnant state. The hormonally controlled compositional and biomechanical changes in endometrial ECM during the reproductive cycle are some of the most rapid and extensive seen in adult physiology.

The second major function of the ECM is that it interacts, via integrins and other receptors, with resident cell populations. These interactions mediate cell adhesion, survival, growth, migration, and differentiation.[1] Virtually all components of ECM participate in interactions with the cell surface. The details of the respective receptors and their downstream effects on cells lie beyond the scope of this chapter. The ECM also contains embedded cytokines and growth factors and harbors cryptic information that may be revealed by the action of extracellular enzymes, in turn altering the cell phenotype.[2]

The life cycle of a typical ECM component comprises gene expression and regulation, polypeptide biosynthesis, subunit association, post-translational

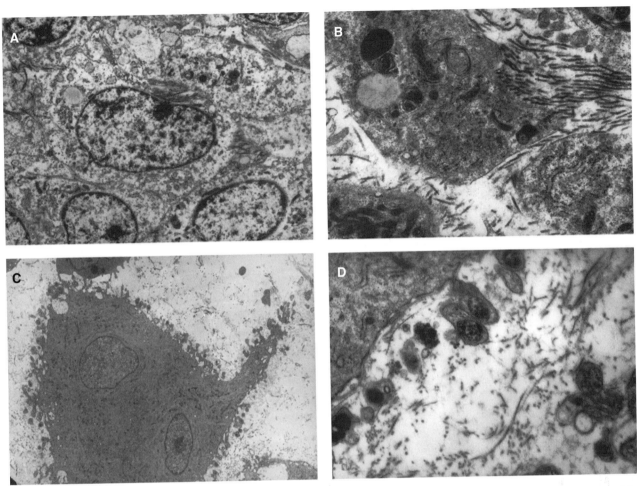

Figure 24.1   Ultrastructure of human endometrium and decidua showing extracellular matrix. (**A,B**) Early secretory phase stroma with uniform bundles of collagen fibrils in the narrow intercellular spaces. Microfibrils are seen in **B** closely associated with the larger collagen fibrils. Part of a gland cell is visible in the lower left corner of **B**. (**C,D**) First trimester decidua. The decidual cell shown in **C** is set in a sparsely fibrillar ECM. It has an associated bone marrow-derived cell (top). The decidual cell shows large numbers of typical peripheral processes (pedicels). At higher magnification (**D**) a basal lamina is associated with the plasma membrane, but does not surround the pedicels. (Reproduced from Aplin et al,[25] with permission.)

modification (especially glycosylation), secretion, further extracellular modification (especially conversion of procollagen to mature collagen), assembly into the ECM (a process that utilizes cell surface receptors, with the existing ECM as a template), restructuring by the local action of cells, then eventual breakdown by a combination of extracellular proteolysis, endocytosis, and further processing in lysosomes. Since this sequence occurs in a time frame that may vary from hours to years, it is important to note that neither spot measurements nor biosynthetic studies of mRNA or polypeptide can be extrapolated to indicate the composition of the ECM at the same time point. However, studies of the endometrial transcriptome provide important clues indicating that alterations in ECM and associated tissue components are central to differentiation, as discussed in Chapter 14. Most ECM components are relatively large in molecular mass, and many are modular: i.e. specific regions play different

(even independent) functional roles, e.g. in relation to cell binding, binding of other ECM components, or growth factors.

MORPHOLOGY OF ENDOMETRIAL ECM

Humans and other primates

In women, following menstrual shedding, the endometrium regenerates in the proliferative phase to produce a densely cellular stroma containing narrow tubular glands and small blood vessels. In addition to cellular proliferation, this requires the deposition of a scaffolding of ECM into the often narrow intercellular spaces. Early secretory stroma retains these features. Collagen is organized into bundles of uniform 30 nm fibrils that form an anastomosing network in the intercellular spaces (Figure 24.1A,B). Microfibrils are associated with the larger fibrils.

The mid secretory stroma shows histological changes that represent the earliest phase of the cascade of differentiative events leading to decidualization. Focal areas of edema appear in which the density of stromal cells is reduced. As a result, blood vessels in these areas are more obvious, although no overt vascular differentiation is yet evident. Other areas of the stroma are still densely populated with elongated mesenchymal cells. As in the other phases of the cycle, but now more obviously, the periglandular stroma contains a layer of flattened cells in close apposition to the epithelial basement membrane.

In the late secretory phase, these areas of edematous stroma become more extensive, although more densely cellular areas also persist. At this time, vascular differentiation occurs to produce prominent spiral arterioles surrounded by a cuff of enlarged stromal cells that resemble the decidual cells of pregnancy. There is a large infiltration by inflammatory cells on the day before menstruation occurs.

In fully differentiated decidua of late first trimester pregnancy (Figure 24.1C,D), the cells are greatly enlarged and, in many areas, intercellular spaces are prominent. A diversity of cellular morphology is found with large rounded cell profiles adjacent to elongated fibroblastic cells and cells with numerous complex filopodial extensions. The ECM is characterized by appearance of a discontinuous pericellular basement membrane (see Figure 24.1D),[3–5] also observed in other primates.[6] There is now a very significant population of bone marrow-derived cells amounting to some 40% of the total, and comprising large granular lymphocytes (LGLs), macrophages, and a few T cells. Close associations are often observed between these cells, which are discussed in Chapters 14, 33, 34, and 35, and resident decidual stromal cells or their basement membrane (see Figure 24.1C).

The intercellular spaces now contain banded collagen fibrils of widely varying diameter, oriented anisotropically and set amidst amorphous ground substance. Fibril bundles are lacking (see Figure 24.1C,D). The decidual collagen network therefore lacks many of the most notable features of ECM in the cycling endometrium, suggesting a radical reorganization, including both breakdown and de-novo deposition.

Rodents

Mouse estrous phase stroma contains banded collagen fibrils of approximately 50 nm diameter, and these are also observed on the second day of pregnancy.

Phagocytosis of the fibrils by stromal cells leads to a reduction in their abundance such that there are few fibrils by day 4. However, biosynthesis continues so that in subepithelial decidua the narrow intercellular spaces contain very large banded fibrils of up to 300 nm diameter as well as fine fibrillar and amorphous material. The large fibrils appear to arise by lateral association of smaller fibrils. Both synthesis and phagocytosis of fibrillar collagen by decidual cells continue into mid pregnancy.[7] In the rat, intercellular spaces are reduced during decidualization, particularly in the primary decidual zone, and the spaces contain a mixture of banded collagen fibrils and densely stained amorphous, probably basal laminal material. In contrast, the basal endometrium contains wider intercellular spaces with dense bundles of collagen fibrils. There is therefore considerable remodeling of the ECM in both species during decidualization, with regional variation in superficial and deeper locations, and variations between the mesometrial and antimesometrial stroma.[8,9]

MAJOR FIBRIL-FORMING COLLAGENS I, III, AND V AND SHORT-CHAIN COLLAGEN XIII

Humans

The major interstitial fibril-forming collagens I, III, and V[10] are all present in the undifferentiated stroma of human endometrium, based on light microscopic immunolabeling with specific antibodies and sodium dodecyl sulfate–polyacylamide gel electrophoresis (SDS-PAGE) of pepsinized tissue.[5,11,12] They are also associated with blood vessels.

As in many tissues, collagen I $[\alpha1(I)_2\alpha2(I)]$ is the most abundant species in proliferative and secretory phase endometrium as well as decidua. Collagen III $[\alpha1(III)_3]$ is present in all three phases, but becomes less abundant in relation to collagen I in first trimester decidual tissue. In contrast, the relative amount of collagen V increases during decidualization. There is conflicting evidence regarding the chain composition of collagen V in human endometrium, with evidence for the relatively unusual homotrimeric form $[\alpha1(V)_3]$[11] and other data indicating the more widespread form $[\alpha1(V)_2\alpha2(V)]$.[12] Collagen V epitopes in proliferative phase endometrium are masked, suggesting close interactions with other components of the ECM, possibly collagen I.[5] Examination of expression databases (see, for example Unigene at www.ncbi.nlm.nih.gov) suggests that another large fibril-forming collagen, type XI, may be present in both uterus and placenta. Prolyl hydroxylase, which is essential for collagen production, is present in stromal cells of both pregnant and non-pregnant endometrium.[11] In postmenopausal endometrium, collagen I is again predominant, with relatively little collagen III. However, after treatment with estrogen, the relative level of collagen III increases.[13] Other uterine collagen transcripts include types VIII, IX, XII, XIV, XV, XVI, XXI, XXIII, XXV, and XXVII (Unigene).

Biosynthetic studies confirm the continuing production of collagens I, III, and V in decidua.[14] During decidualization, unmasking of collagen V epitopes occurs, consistent with both an increase in abundance and reorganization of the fibril arrangement. Human decidual cells express mRNA encoding the short-chain collagen type XIII [α1(XIII)$_3$] and a complex pattern of alternative splicing has been documented that differs markedly from that observed in placental villous mesenchymal cells.[15] Decidual cells also express collagen XVIII/endostatin.[16]

Rodents

In the rat, the major endometrial collagen is type I, although its concentration declines during pregnancy in both implantation and non-implantation sites. Comparison of its abundance in implantation site and inter-site stroma on days 6, 7, and 8 – i.e. the time period during which the primary decidual zone expands and decidualization occurs in the mesometrial sector – indicates that the relative proportion of collagen I decreases.[17] Analysis of dissected tissue has confirmed that the overall collagen content (measured as hydroxyproline) of the mesometrial region declines by about half from day 6 to day 8 of pregnancy.[18] When localized immunochemically, collagen I is absent from the stroma surrounding the embryo on the evening of day 5 of pregnancy, and staining progressively decreases in the primary and secondary zones as decidualization progresses. On day 8 the primary decidual zone is negative for collagen I, while the secondary decidua, including the glycogen-rich (angiogenic) areas, are weakly reactive.[19] In contrast, non-decidualized stroma (including the mesometrial and antimesometrial basalis) continues to be collagen I-positive throughout.

In addition to collagen I, collagens III and V are present in the rat.[17,20,21] Collagen I is present in banded 30–35 nm fibrils while collagen III occurs in finer beaded 10–15 nm fibrils. Their concentrations decrease in implantation sites but not in inter-site stroma during this period. Collagen V contains two distinct polypeptides, suggesting the presence of α1(V)$_2$α2(V). Localization studies have confirmed that only low levels of these collagens are present in decidualized stroma. While synthesis of all three isoforms, as monitored by incorporation of [^{3}H]glycine, continues in decidual tissue on days 6–8, 3.5 times more label is incorporated into collagens I and III than into type V.

Another approach to studying collagen production is immunolocalization using antibodies directed to the propeptide sequences of procollagen chains. Proteolytic processing of procollagens is required for extracellular fibril formation and matrix assembly, so the method gives details of sites at which collagen production and maturation are occurring. Regions of tissue that contain mature ECM will not be stained if no procollagen production is occurring.

At day 8 of pregnancy, rat antimesometrial decidua lacks procollagen I. The superficial mesometrial area shows small areas of staining, but is mostly negative. The basal mesometrial decidua, however, shows evidence of strong procollagen I production.[21a] Procollagen III staining is much weaker in decidua, although it can be detected in the basalis and myometrium. At day 9.5, both mesometrial and basal decidua are procollagen I positive, while procollagen III again appears much weaker, although it is strongly expressed in a restricted area adjacent to the maternal central artery.

In the mouse, both total collagen (measured as hydroxyproline) and the relative abundance of collagen V increase significantly during decidualization (days 5–8), correlating with the appearance of unusually large banded collagen fibrils (see above). Biochemical analysis suggests the presence of the unusual isoforms [α1(V)$_3$].[22] Collagens I and III are also present throughout this period, and ultrastuctural evidence indicates that the large fibrils contain all three collagens, while thinner fibrils contain much less type V.[23]

MICROFIBRILS, COLLAGEN VI, AND FIBRILLIN

Microfibrils are found in human endometrial stroma where they are associated with bundles of larger banded collagen fibrils (see Figure 24.1). Microfibrils are also associated with elastic fibers in the walls of vessels. Type VI collagen and fibrillin are both microfibrillar glycoproteins of the ECM. Elastin itself, the major elastic fiber polypeptide, is present only in vessel walls, while fibrillin and collagen VI are present in stromal ECM as well as vessel walls.

Collagen VI occurs as a disulfide-linked heterotrimer of three α chains, α1(VI), α2(VI), and α3(VI).[24] The α1(VI) and α2(VI) chains have a molecular mass of 140 000 while α3(V) is larger with a molecular mass of

260 000 to 280 000. There is a relatively short (105 nm; 335 or 336 amino acids per subunit) central collagenous triple helical domain which contains several interruptions in the GXY repeat sequence. Several alternatively spliced variants of the α2(VI) and α3(VI) chains have been identified in endometrium.[25] The triple helix is flanked by large N- and C-terminal globular domains that constitute about two-thirds of the molecular mass. All three chains are glycosylated. Collagen VI monomers assemble intracellularly into dimers and then tetramers that are in turn secreted.

Collagen VI is found in endometrial stroma and myometrium.[5,26–29] In proliferative and early secretory phase endometrium, immunolocalization studies using subunit-specific antibodies have shown that it is present as a component of the intercellular collagenous network. In mid secretory phase, an alteration is apparent, with the appearance of areas of reduced immunoreactivity, and punctate staining in place of some of the continuous network. In late secretory phase, there remain areas of fibrillar reactivity, but areas devoid of immunoreactivity are also apparent. Blood vessel walls, however, remain immunoreactive. In decidua of first trimester the stroma lacks all three subunits of collagen VI, although immunoreactivity persists in arterial walls.

Similar observations have been made in rats and mice, with loss of collagen VI immunoreactivity from the stroma at the time of decidualization in both pregnant animals and deciduoma. In the undifferentiated basal endometrium, expression persists. In rat, precise correlations can be made between cell differentiation and matrix remodeling by comparing desmin, an established marker of decidualization, with collagen VI immunoreactivity. Collagen VI is removed from the stroma shortly after the onset of desmin expression.[5,26–29] This may reflect the different kinetics of two distinct regulatory processes, transcriptional activation of desmin being more rapid than proteolytic digestion of extracellular matrix.

To determine whether down-regulation is transcriptionally controlled, mRNA studies have been carried out in humans and mice. The mRNA coding for all three collagen VI chains is present in stromal cells throughout the non-pregnant cycle.[25,29,30] In decidua, by late first trimester, little mRNA is present in the differentiated stromal cells, but vascular cells contain mRNA for all three chains. Mouse decidual cells also down-regulate all three mRNA species.[26] These data suggest that regulation is occurring at two levels: transcriptional down-regulation is associated with decidualization of stromal cells, while in the human non-pregnant cycle the loss of collagen VI from stromal

ECM appears to be mediated by a non-transcriptional mechanism, perhaps a change in the balance between secretion and extracellular proteolysis.

Fibrillin is a large single-subunit glycoprotein (~350 kDa) that self-associates to form beaded microfibrils. It occurs as two distinct gene products, fibrillins 1 and 2. Fibrillin 1 is found in human endometrial stroma throughout the normal cycle and in decidua, where it is associated with the pericellular basement membrane as well as intercellular ECM.[31,32] It is absent from blood vessel walls and glands.

Microfibrils surround and interconnect bundles of the larger banded fibrils of the major collagen types I, III and V. In endometrium they encapsulate the major macrostructural elements, i.e. glands and blood vessels. Fibrillin 1 is associated with the stromal interface of basal laminae. It appears likely that both collagen VI and fibrillin 1 play a role in the integration and structural stabilization of tissue architecture, perhaps by cross-linking the major scaffolding elements. The contribution of these two distinct microfibrillar components to ECM function during stromal remodeling remains to be defined. It is possible that the regions of lower cell density and increased edema that become apparent in mid secretory phase stroma may be related to the focal loss of collagen VI. Loss of collagen VI during decidualization may help to provide an environment into which trophoblast infiltration may occur more readily.[33,34] In rats, it is also possible that the loss of collagen VI (and collagen I; see above) is required to allow close apposition of subluminal decidual cells. During the same events, however, fibrillin 1 levels increase.

OTHER GLYCOPROTEINS OF THE INTERSTITIAL ECM

Fibronectin, a homodimeric glycoprotein with well-established cell adhesion and migration-promoting properties, is abundant in both endometrial and decidual ECM in human and rat,[5,35,36] although there is evidence for an increase in production by human stromal cells as a result of progestin stimulation.[37] The extra domain A (EDA) domain-containing splice variant is present in human decidua but not extra domain B (EDB). Fibronectin in decidual tissue is associated with both the pericellular ECM and fibrillar matrix in the intercellular spaces.

Fibulin 1 is an ECM protein with cell-binding properties that is associated with elastic fibers in blood vessel walls and with basement membranes. It is present in both rat and human endometrial stroma;

expression is increased by estrogen in the former species, while in human, expression is highest in mid secretory phase and is progesterone-regulated.[38]

Tenascin C is a member of a gene family that also contains tenascins R, X, and W. It is a large disulfide-linked hexameric glycoprotein containing polypeptide splice variants (190–330 kDa) derived from one primary transcript. It is commonly associated with stromal cells surrounding proliferative or developing epithelia. Its functions are not well defined,[39] but it binds several integrins, ECM components such as heparin, fibronectin, and collagen, and can act as an inhibitor of cell adhesion to fibronectin. It is found in human proliferative phase subepithelial stroma,[40] persists into the early secretory phase in a thin area of stroma beneath the glandular epithelium, but is absent in the mid secretory phase.[41,42] There is a correlation between stromal tenascin and proliferating epithelial cells,[43] and stromal cells express tenascin C more strongly in the presence of carcinomatous epithelium.[44] Tenascin C is also associated with vascular smooth muscle, and is evident in the late secretory phase spiral arterial walls as they become muscularized.

In mouse, tenascin C is expressed weakly in estrous and early pregnancy stroma, and is very strongly up-regulated in the subepithelial stroma precisely beneath the site of embryo attachment on day 4.5–5.5 of pregnancy.[45] This appears to be the result of an epithelial signal, since stromal cells in oil-induced deciduomata also express tenascin. In-vitro experiments suggest that stromal tenascin C expression in the preimplantation period is under the indirect control of progesterone, mediated by interleukin-1α (IL-1α) secreted by epithelial cells and prostaglandins PGE_2 and $PGF_{2\alpha}$ secreted by the stromal cells themselves.[46] Tenascin C decreases epithelial cell adhesion to Matrigel in vitro, and up-regulates matrix metalloproteinase 3 (MMP-3),[47] results that suggest the possible involvement of stromal ECM in the loss of epithelial integrity that occurs immediately after blastocyst attachment in the mouse. Tenascin C has been studied in rat endometrium during the estrous cycle and pregnancy.[48] In cycling rats, the periglandular stroma is variably immunopositive, but the subluminal stroma is negative in proestrus, weakly positive in estrus, and intensely positive in diestrus. Subluminal tenascin is stimulated by progesterone (P) but not estrogen (E_2) or a combination of P and E_2 in ovariectomized rats. On day 6 of pregnancy the antimesometrial basement membrane zone surrounding the blastocyst and the surrounding superficial stroma are both intensely immunopositive. Tenascin expression extends throughout the primary and secondary decidua on days 7–9, but thereafter diminishes except in the walls of blood vessels and in myometrial smooth muscle.

Thrombospondin-1 (TSP-1) is a 420 kDa glycoprotein comprising three similar or identical disulfide-linked subunits. A second related product, TSP-2, has been reported. TSP-1 has been implicated in modulation of cell adhesion, as well as in promoting cell proliferation in synergy with growth factors. It is also known to inhibit angiogenesis. It is present in platelet α granules and expressed by endothelial and smooth muscle cells. In endometrium, TSP-1 is absent in the proliferative phase, but expressed in the stroma adjacent to glands in the secretory phase.[49] Blood vessel walls are also immunopositive in the secretory phase. Cultured stromal cells express TSP-1 in response to P, and this effect is inhibited by RU486. Expression is decreased by epidermal growth factor (EGF) but increased by interferon-γ.[50] When stromal cells are decidualized in vitro, expression increases. TSP-1 is produced in sufficient concentration to inhibit migration of endothelial cells in vitro, suggesting a role in inhibition of angiogenesis in late cycle. TSP-1 is found in the periglandular stroma in mouse endometrium and also in decidua and trophoblast giant cells. TSP-1 and TSP-2 have been reported in neoplastic endometrium.[51]

Dermatopontin is a small (22 kDa) ECM protein with a role in the control of collagen fibrillogenesis and the ability to bind to proteoglycans including decorin. In mouse, its expression is regulated by progesterone and switches from the uterine epithelium on days 2 and 3 of pregnancy to the stroma on days 4 and 5. After implantation, dermatopontin mRNA locates to the outer edge of the decidualized stroma.[52] These observations are consistent with a role in ECM remodeling that occurs as decidualization proceeds.

PROTEOGLYCANS AND GLYCOSAMINOGLYCANS (GAGS)

Proteoglycans (PGs) are important in the regulation of collagen fibrillogenesis. Chondroitin sulfate (CS), dermatan sulfate (DS), and heparan sulfate PGs are present in rat and mouse endometrial stroma.[53,54] The CS/DS proteoglycan versican, a member of the large aggregating chondroitin sulfate proteoglycan family (lecticans) is present in undifferentiated stroma and accumulates subepithelially as decidualization commences.[55] The family of small leucine-rich proteoglycans (SLRPs) has several members including decorin, lumican, fibromodulin, and biglycan. Decorin, which bears CS and DS chains, is present in human decidual ECM. It binds transforming growth factor β (TGFβ) and inhibits its action.[56] Decorin and lumican are present in mouse uterine stroma in early pregnancy prior to the onset of decidualization. Biglycan and lesser amounts of lumican are found in decidualized stroma.[57] Biglycan is associated with thick collagen fibrils in the mouse decidua while decorin is associated with the thinner ones that are more abundant in undecidualized tissue.[58] Correspondingly, biglycan mRNA is higher in the mouse IL-11Rα-null uterus than in controls 48 hours after a decidualizing stimulus;[59] IL-11Rα nulls show defective decidualization. In addition to their role in controlling ECM morphology, all these PGs are capable of influencing cell phenotype[60] but their functions in the uterus in this respect remain undefined. The cell surface proteoglycan syndecan 4 has been reported in mouse decidual cells.[61] The enzyme heparanase 1 has been shown to be stimulated by estrogen and to be present in late proliferative and secretory phase human endometrium.[62]

Biochemical analysis of whole decidual swellings from pregnant and pseudopregnant mice indicates that the overall abundance of hyaluronan (HA) increases on pregnancy days 5 and 6, decreasing on day 7.[54,63] Localization studies suggest that HA is present in undifferentiated mouse endometrial stroma and is lost from the antimesometrial stroma during decidualization, but expression continues in the region of maternal angiogenesis (glycogen-rich region) and in the basal mesometrial stroma.[64,65] Peaks of HA deposition occur in human endometrium in midproliferative and midsecretory phases, likely to be important in creating the transiently elevated tissue hydration observed in both these phases.[66]

BASEMENT MEMBRANE COMPONENTS

Humans and rodents

Endometrial glandular and luminal epithelium and blood vessels are surrounded by basement membranes. Fully differentiated human decidual cells are encapsulated in a pericellular basal lamina through which pedicels protrude (see Figure 24.1D).[3,5,67] The pedicels contain secretory granules probably involved in the release of basement membrane components.[4]

Heterogeneity occurs in the tissue; while most stromal cells produce basement membrane components to some degree,[5,40] not all of them complete the deposition of a continuous pericellular basal lamina. In rodents, basement membrane components are produced in the decidualizing stroma and are incorporated into amorphous or fine fibrillar ECM in the narrow intercellular spaces between subepithelial decidual cells. However, there is not continuous pericellular basement membrane as seen in primates.

The human decidual cell basement membrane contains laminins, collagen types IV, VII, and XVII, heparan sulfate proteoglycan/perlecan and BM-40/SPARC.[3–5,68–71] The basic structural framework of the basement membrane is provided by a polymeric lattice of collagen type IV.[72] Six different collagen IV α chain genes have been described, but the pattern of expression in uterine tissues has not been fully analyzed. $\alpha 1(IV)$ and $\alpha 2(IV)$ are strongly expressed in mouse decidua.[73]

Laminins are large heterotrimeric glycoproteins ($\alpha\beta\gamma$) associated with all basement membranes where they function in cell attachment, polarization, and differentiation and bind other matrix macromolecules including collagen IV, heparan sulfate proteoglycan and entactin/nidogen.[72] Molecules have a cross-shaped structure in which the long arm comprises a linear assembly of α-helical domains (about 600 residues) associated into a triple helix, while each short arm arises from the N-terminal region of a single subunit polypeptide. Chain association via the coiled coil heterotrimer is a constant feature, but the short arms are isoform-specific and of variable length. There are known to be at least 5α, 5β, and 2γ subunits, giving rise to at least 13 heterotrimeric isoforms.

Glandular and vascular basement membranes are strongly immunopositive in human proliferative phase endometrium, indicating that a laminin-containing basement membrane is deposited during reepithelialization, glandular growth, and angiogenesis following menstrual shedding. Further experiments with subunit-specific monoclonal antibodies have demonstrated that both the epithelial and vascular basement membranes contain subunits α_2, α_5, β_1, β_2 and γ_1. All persist in these locations throughout the cycle. The laminin α_1 chain is restricted to the epithelial basement membrane, being absent from endometrial blood vessels.[74]

Human decidual stromal cell laminin contains subunits α_2, α_4, β_1, β_2 and γ_1, along with small amounts of α_5. Laminin has been isolated from decidual tissue, confirming that laminins 2 ($\alpha_2\beta_1\gamma_1$) and 4 ($\alpha_2\beta_2\gamma_1$) are present (CP Chen, HJ Church, and JD Aplin, unpublished work). This is consistent with the observation that cells of mesenchymal as well as epithelial origin tend to produce the α_2 subunit.[75] However, decidual cells in culture switch to predominant production of laminin 10 ($\alpha_5\beta_1\gamma_1$), and increased α_5 expression has been reported in the decidua basalis.[76] Trophoblast produces several laminin isoforms, including those containing α_2 and α_5 chains.[77,78]

When non-pregnant endometrium was assayed for specific laminin subunits, punctate deposits of α_2 chain were detected in the perivascular stroma in late secretory phase, but not earlier in the cycle. This correlates with the appearance of decidual cells in these locations in late secretory phase and suggests that laminin α_2 chain expression may be specifically regulated by P in this tissue compartment.[70] In agreement with this, endometrium exposed to levonorgestrel exhibits well-developed decidual cells with laminin α_2-positive basement membranes.[79]

Laminin 2/4 mediates efficient trophoblast attachment and spreading (HJ Church and JD Aplin, unpublished work). It is interesting to speculate that it may play a role in interstitial or intravascular trophoblast migration and/or migration of bone marrow-derived cells that can sometimes be observed attached to the pericellular basal lamina (see Figure 24.1C). It is also possible that the decidual basement membrane plays a role in the structural organization and integration of the decidual extracellular matrix, which is required to support the developing conceptus, to expand as the fetoplacental compartment grows, and to be permeable to macromolecules such as prolactin secreted by decidual cells and destined for the fetal compartment.

Laminin expression has also been reported in rodent decidua. Polyclonal antibodies to laminin 1 ($\alpha_1\beta_1\gamma_1$) show pericellular deposits in decidualized stroma as well as in vascular and epithelial basement membranes. Furthermore, cultured stromal cells produce laminin.[80] Comparisons have been made in mice of the levels of mRNA encoding laminin β_1 and γ_1 chains (previously known as β_1 and β_2, respectively). The latter is strongly expressed in all areas of decidua, but expression of the former is restricted to the primary decidual zone on day 6 of pregnancy.[73] By day 8 there is little β_1 expression in the superficial decidua, while γ_1 expression remains strong in all areas. This suggests that other β subunits are utilized, perhaps β_2 as seen in humans.[70] The α_1 subunit (previously known as A) is largely absent from decidual stroma, consistent with other data suggesting it is confined to epithelial cells. This suggests that other α chains may be utilized, perhaps α_2 as in human.[70] Laminin 1 promotes mouse blastocyst attachment and outgrowth of trophoblast.[81] The laminin α_5 null mouse suffers pregnancy failure as the result of abnormalities of placental vascularization.[82]

The glycoprotein nidogen, also known as entactin, performs an important function in basement membrane, linking laminin via the short arm of the γ_1 subunit to the collagen IV network. In its own right it supports cell adhesion and migration and outgrowth of trophoblast from mouse blastocysts in vitro.[83] Nidogen has been immunolocalized to mouse decidual cells.[84] Its mRNA has been shown to be expressed in mouse decidua from up to day 10, after which it is confined to endothelial cells lining maternal blood spaces within the basal decidua. Nidogen mRNA is detectable on days 8 and 9 not only in the decidua but also the endometrial basalis.[73,85] Cultured mouse stromal cells produce nidogen.[80]

MMPS AND ADAMS

Overview

The matrix metalloproteinases (MMPs) are a family of at least 23 zinc-dependent endopeptidases (Table 24.1).[86] They belong to the metzincin superfamily of metalloproteinases, which also includes astacins and ADAM (a protein with a disintegrin and metalloprotease domain) and ADAM-TS (an ADAM with a thrombospondin-like motif) proteases.[87,88] ADAMs have a major role as cell surface sheddases, but also cleave ECM components.

MMPs are secreted as proenzymes containing an N-terminal propeptide, requiring proteolytic activation. Six members of the family (membrane-type MMPs, MT-MMPs) are anchored to the cell surface via a C-terminal membrane-spanning domain, although secreted splice variants also exist. Two other members are GPI-anchored. Each MMP acts on a range of substrates in the ECM, and substrate repertoires vary. One MMP may activate another; thus, for example, MMP-2 (gelatinase A) activates proMMP-9 and MMP-7 (Matrilysin) activates proMMP-1. It is noteworthy that MMP action on ECM components can reveal cryptic cell-binding sites, as, for example, in the action of MMP-2 on laminin 5 or MMP-1 on collagen 1. MMP-2 is targeted to the cell surface by binding to integrin $\alpha_v\beta_3$. The MMPs are inhibited in vitro by tissue inhibitors of metalloproteinases (TIMPs 1–4). Thus, ECM remodeling is controlled by the production, targeting, activation, and inhibition of MMPs. The protein basigin (EMMPRIN, CD147), which is required for normal fertility in mice,[89] is expressed in both human luminal epithelium and secretory phase stroma[90] and activates MMPs. MMP action releases cryptic information from the ECM by cleaving large insoluble ECM components and ECM-associated molecules, liberating bioactive fragments and growth factors that subsequently act on cells.[2] Particularly relevant examples are the release of peptides with either angiogenic or antiangiogenic activity.[2] These are likely to be important in postmenstrual regeneration.

MMPs 1–3, 7, 9, 10, 11, 13–16, 19, and 26 are all expressed in endometrium,[91] and there is a striking

Table 24.1   The matrix metalloproteinases and their substrates

Enzyme		Substrate
Gelatinases		Denatured collagens, native collagens IV, V, VII, X, elastin, FN
MMP-2	Gelatinase A	Also proMMP-9
MMP-9	Gelatinase B	
Collagenases		Collagens I, II, III, VII, VIII, X
MMP-1		
MMP-8		
MMP-13		Also proMMP-9
Stromelysins		Proteoglycan core protein, FN, LN, elastin, collagens IV, V, IX, X
MMP-3	Stromelysin 1	Also proMMP-2, proMMP-7, proMMP-9
MMP-10	Stromelysin 2	Also proMMP-1, proMMP-8, proMMP-8, proMMP-9
MMP-11	Stromelysin 3	
Matrilysins		
MMP-7	Matrilysin 1	FN, LN, collagen IV, proteoglycan core protein, proMMP-1
MMP-26	Matrilysin 2	
Membrane-MMPs		FN, TN, nidogen, collagens I, III, aggrecan, perlecan, proMMP-2, proTNF
MMP-14	MT1-MMP	
MMP-15	MT2-MMP	Also laminin
MMP-16	MT3-MMP	
MMP-17	MT4-MMP	GPI anchored
MMP-24	MT5-MMP	
MMP-25	MT6-MMP	GPI anchored
Others		
MMP-12	Macrophage elastase	Elastin and other substrates
MMP-19		
MMP-20	Enamelysin	
MMP-23	CA-MMP	Transmembrane
MMP-28	Epilysin	

up-regulation of several members of the family at menstruation, extending into early proliferative phase. Transcriptomic analysis indicates that several other family members are present (see Unigene at www.ncbi.nlm.nih.gov). Useful immunolocalization data can be obtained at the Human Protein Atlas (http://www.proteinatlas.org/). ADAMs 8, 9, 10, 12, 15, and 19 have been reported in mouse or monkey endometrium.[92,93] Endothelial MT-MMPs may be important in angiogenesis during endometrial regeneration.[94]

TIMPs 1–3 are present in endometrium and the enzyme:inhibitor ratio increases at menstruation.[95,96] Inhibition of MMP action can inhibit steroidally triggered menstruation in an explant culture model,[97] suggesting a role for MMPs in tissue breakdown. Similarly, in densely cultured human endometrial stromal cells, up-regulation of MMP leads to cell detachment, apparently due to degradation of the associated ECM.[98]

When endometrial tissue fragments were put into the peritoneal cavity of nude mice to simulate retrograde menstruation in women, the establishment of endometriotic implants was suppressed by inhibiting MMP action.[99] All the above findings indicate the importance of MMP-mediated matrix remodeling in endometrial pathophysiology. As a result it has been suggested that focally dysregulated MMP activity may explain irregular uterine bleeding.[100,101]

However, conflicting results have been obtained in a mouse model of menstruation.[50,102] Here decidualization was induced by mechanical trauma in females sensitized with estrogen followed by progesterone. Withdrawal of progesterone led to shedding of the decidua within 24 hours. Re-epithelialization had occurred by 36 hours with MMP-3 and MMP-7 localizing near the epithelium. The endometrium had largely regenerated by 48 hours. MMP-9 and MMP-7 colocalized with leukocyte subsets, particularly neutrophils, whereas MMP-13 was detected extracellularly. When the MMP inhibitors doxycycline and batimistat were introduced, both effectively reduced MMP activity, but there was no significant effect on endometrial breakdown or repair. This could be interpreted as an indication that elevated widespread MMP activity in endometrium is not required for breakdown or repair. However, microenvironments close to the cell surface may be protected from diffusible inhibitors and it would be rash to exclude the possibility that local MMP activity may be critically important.

It is likely that MMP action plays an important role at the maternal–fetal interface in pregnancy. Trophoblast produces MMPs 1, 2, 7, 9, 11, 12, and 14.[103–105] Trophoblast is involved in remodeling uterine spiral arterial ECM to allow increased blood to flow to the placenta, either by direct ECM breakdown or by stimulating resident cells.[105] Stromal TIMPs 1–3 increase at decidualization, both in humans[96] and mice. TIMP-3 is bound to heparan and chondroitin sulfates in the ECM.[106] Intrauterine inhibition of MMP action gives rise to disturbances in decidualization and implantation in the mouse and baboon,[107,108] although without a full block to either process. Collagenases (MMPs 1, 8, 13) catalyze cleavage of fibrillar collagens at a few specific sites, leading to denaturation and, in turn, degradation by gelatinases. A targeted mutation introduced into the mouse α1(I) chain rendered type I collagen resistant to collagenase cleavage.[109] This did not have any major effect on pregnancy, but postpartum remodeling of the uterus was severely impaired, with persistence of collagenous nodules in the uterine wall.

A case has been presented based on expression studies that MMP and TIMP activity may be important in postnatal uterine morphogenesis.[110]

Localization and regulation of specific MMPs

MMP-1 is present in human and rhesus monkey endometrium during the menstrual and early proliferative phases.[111–113] Expression is confined to groups of stromal cells in the functionalis and correlates with foci of overt tissue lysis. The same cells also produce MMP-2 and MMP-3 as well as laminin; since laminin is a marker for early decidual change, the latter observation implicates the decidual-like cells observed in superficial and perivascular regions of late secretory phase tissue in menstrual breakdown. After decline of P, MMP-1 mRNA peaks, and then appears to decrease more rapidly than is the case for stromal MMP-2 and MMP-11. Thus, by 5 days after P withdrawal from a spayed rhesus monkey, MMP-1 mRNA has dropped to baseline values.[113] MMP-1 is also released by ovine stromal cells.[114] In cultured human stromal cells, MMP-1 production (and similarly MMP-3 and MMP-9, but not MMP-2) is stimulated by both IL-1α and tumor necrosis factor-α (TNFα);[115] these data may hint at the mechanisms that lead to localized and focal MMP production in vitro.

MMP-7 (matrilysin) expression is confined to the epithelial cell compartment in human[116,117] and rhesus endometrium.[113] Evidence from in-situ hybridization, Northern blotting, and immunohistochemistry shows it is abundant in proliferative and menstrual epithelium but is not seen in early or mid secretory phases. In artificial cycles induced in spayed macaques, P withdrawal leads after 2 days to an increase in epithelial MMP-7 mRNA and the level remains high for 8–10 days of estrogen (E$_2$) administration.[113] Immunolocalization shows regional specificity: initially, the strongest signal is in the glandular epithelium (GE) and its associated secretions in the residual functionalis, with much lower levels in the basalis and the (shedding) upper functionalis. Later in the proliferative phase, expression shifts to the deeper glands. Similar observations are made after withdrawal of both E$_2$ and P, and these results may suggest that paracrine interactions with stroma vary at different levels of the tissue, thus controlling the remodeling process. MMP-7 binds in an active form to the epithelial cell surface.[118] MMP-7 appears to participate in postmenstrual ECM remodeling by epithelium, with early activity in the functionalis and a later phase in the basalis. MMP-7 activates proMMP-1, suggesting a possible role for epithelial mesenchymal interaction in the control of perimenstrual ECM remodeling.

These observations are consistent with suppression of MMP-7 transcription by P, but the effect is stromally mediated; P stimulates stromal cells to produce TGFβ, and this in turn suppresses production of MMP-7 by the epithelium in a P-independent step.[119,120] Antibody to TGFβ inhibits the paracrine effect, up-regulating MMP-7.

Another TGFβ family member, LEFTY-A, has been demonstrated to be involved in the regulation of MMP activity. The abundance of LEFTY-A increases steeply in the menstrual phase, and similarly if ovarian steroids are withdrawn from proliferative phase explant cultures. Addition of recombinant LEFTY-A to proliferative phase explants stimulates increases in MMP-3, MMP-7, and MMP-9, and this increase is inhibited by ovarian steroids.[121,122]

Expression of MMP-2 (gelatinase A), and MMP-11 (stromelysin 3) is consistently detected in human and rhesus menstrual and proliferative endometrium[117] and shows a pattern of mRNA up-regulation after P withdrawal in rhesus that resembles that observed with MMP-7.[113] One important difference, however, is that MMP-2 and MMP-11 are expressed exclusively in the stromal compartment of the tissue. At menstruation in the rhesus the shedding stroma is intensely reactive with anti-MMP-2 antibody; by day 10 of E$_2$ this had died away. In spayed animals, the initial pattern of reactivity is the same, but MMP-2 persists up to 14 days in the absence of E$_2$. It is seen in the cytoplasm of stromal cells and, in addition, very strongly in the walls of spiral arteries. P inhibits MMP-2 secretion in a human tissue explant model and this effect can be antagonized by RU486.[123] P withdrawal from cultured human stromal cells induces up-regulation of MMP-2.[98] Similarly, the production of MMP-8 is mostly by endometrial stromal cells and its level is elevated at menstruation or steroid withdrawal.[124]

MMP-3 (stromelysin 1), which, in addition to degrading ECM, activates MMP-9 (see Table 24.1) is expressed in human endometrial stromal cells at menstruation.[124] It is transiently, focally, and more weakly present in the stroma in mid proliferative and mid secretory phases, stages at which local stromal edema is observed. In rhesus monkey endometrium, it is up-regulated after menstruation; 2 days after P withdrawal, expression is intense in the upper (fragmenting) stromal functionalis, especially around glands and spiral arteries. Three days later, expression is more restricted, being mainly seen in groups of stromal cells immediately beneath the luminal epithelium, but also in a widely dispersed population of single cells that were not identified but were probably bone marrow-derived. MMP-3 is also present in sheep endometrium,[125] an indication that its function in the uterus is not solely to aid interstitial placentation, nor specifically in relation to ECM breakdown at menstruation.

MMP-3 is transcriptionally suppressed in cultured human stromal cells by the progestins medroxyprogesterone acetate (MPA) or R5020, and more so by E_2 and MPA in combination.[126,127] The same can be observed in cultured decidual cells. Inflammatory cytokines, including IL-1α, can stimulate MMP-3 (and MMP-7) expression, but this effect is opposed by P, indicating a mechanism by which ECM integrity is preserved during pregnancy.[128] This pathway appears to involve endogenous retinoic acid.[129] When human stromal cells were co-cultured with first trimester cytotrophoblast, there was also inhibition of MMP-3 production. Separation of the two cell types by a polycarbonate membrane such that no heterotypic contact was possible caused the inhibition to become substantially weaker, suggesting the need for close interactions.[126]

Transcripts for MMP-10 (stromelysin 2) are present in stromal cells in human late secretory and menstrual phase endometrium, while MMP-11 (stromelysin 3) is also found in the proliferative phase.[117] In the spayed rhesus monkey model, similar findings have been reported, with P withdrawal leading to up-regulation of both MMP-10 and MMP-11. The former mRNA species returned to baseline by 5 days after withdrawal, while the latter species persisted longer into the proliferative phase.[113]

The MMP-9/gelatinase B transcript is detected in menstrual phase cells, especially stromal foci.[121]

Cultured stromal cells produce MMP-9 as a 180 kDa homodimer and production is stimulated by phorbol myristate acetate, 1L-1α, and TNFα,[115] as well as by P withdrawal.[95,123] MMP-9 is also associated with populations of eosinophils, neutrophils, mast cells, and macrophages in the tissue at menstruation;[130] these cells may release regulators of MMP production as well as proenzyme activator.

MMP-9 has been detected in other phases of the cycle, with immunolocalization in the GE in late proliferative phase and just after ovulation, and reactivity in epithelial secretions in the peri-implantation phase.[130] In endometrial carcinoma, there is an increase in epithelial expression of MMP-9.[131]

In mouse, a postcoital neutrophil influx into the endometrium is associated with rising levels of MMP-9, and in-situ zymography has been used to show co-distribution of gelatinase activity and neutrophils. MMP-9 gene expression by resident cells remains unchanged and neutropenic mice do not show the increase. Furthermore, removing the seminal vesicles from male mice abolishes the effect. Thus, infiltrating cells attracted from the uterine serosa by components in ejaculate may be responsible for ECM remodeling that occurs in the days prior to implantation.[132]

MMP-9 is produced by trophoblast at the early maternal–placental interface in both the mouse[133] and human.[134,135] Expression of TIMP-3 by adjacent decidual cells is likely to regulate trophoblast-mediated proteolysis. As MMP-9 expression by trophoblast giant cells declines after day 9.5 of pregnancy in the mouse, decidual TIMP-3 expression also diminishes.[136]

Collagen VI is resistant to cleavage by MMPs, including collagenases and stromelysins. However, it is susceptible to breakdown by certain serine proteases, including mast cell chymase and tryptase and neutrophil elastase and cathepsin G. The population of mast cells in endometrium remains fairly constant during the menstrual cycle;[137] however, there is a good correlation between mast cell activation (protease secretion) and the onset of extracellular breakdown of collagen VI in the mid secretory phase.[137] Mast cells have been implicated in decidualization in rodents. Breakdown of collagen VI may be mediated at least in part by mast cells.

Localization studies of several ADAMs in the mouse suggest a predominant epithelial rather than stromal expression.[93] For example, ADAM-9 (also known as MDC-9 or meltrin gamma) has been localized to the rabbit uterine epithelium at the implantation site[138] where it is up-regulated by the adjacent blastocyst, suggesting a role in implantation. However, mice that lack ADAM-9 expression are viable and fertile.[139] ADAM-19 is present in macaque epithelium at implantation and later in pregnancy it appears in stroma and strongly in trophoblast.[92]

CONCLUSION

During the menstrual cycle and pregnancy in humans, the endometrium undergoes one of the most radical and rapid changes of ECM seen in normal adult physiology. This is likely to be a cooperative adaptation to interstitial implantation, with its requirement for initially rapid access of the conceptus to maternal stroma and vessels followed by a more prolonged period of placental growth, trophoblast infiltration, and vascular remodeling. There is a complex interplay of ECM production, deposition, and degradation, the course of which is fundamentally different in non-pregnant cycles and pregnancy. In the absence of a conceptus, some of the early events in pregnancy ECM remodeling (loss of collagen VI, production of basement membrane components by perivascular decidual-like cells) are evident, but declining progesterone levels and an influx of inflammatory cells lead to a large up-regulation of MMPs, the activities of which contribute importantly to tissue breakdown at menstruation. In pregnancy, maternal MMP activities are suppressed. Trophoblast and decidua cooperate at the tissue interface to produce an ECM that stabilizes placental anchorage. The local activity of trophoblast-derived MMPs is important in infiltration and vascular remodeling. Rodents also remodel the ECM at decidualization, and, as in the human, there is an interplay between trophoblast-derived MMP action and regulation by maternal TIMP. Experimental manipulation of ECM composition and breakdown in mice has begun to demonstrate the importance of these events in pregnancy outcome.

REFERENCES

1. Streuli C. Extracellular matrix remodelling and cellular differentiation. Curr Opin Cell Biol 1999; 11: 634–40.
2. Mott JD, Werb Z. Regulation of matrix biology by matrix metalloproteinases. Curr Opin Cell Biol 2004; 16: 558–64.
3. Wewer UM, Faber M, Liotta LA, Albrechtsen R. Immunochemical and ultrastructural assessment of the nature of the pericellular basement membrane of human decidual cells. Lab Invest 1985; 53: 624–33.
4. Kisalus LL, Herr JC. Immunocytochemical localization of heparan sulfate proteoglycan in human decidual cell secretory bodies and placental fibrinoid. Biol Reprod 1988; 39: 419–30.
5. Aplin JD, Charlton AK, Ayad S. An immunohistochemical study of human endometrial extracellular matrix during the menstrual cycle and first trimester of pregnancy. Cell Tissue Res 1988; 253: 231–40.
6. Enders AC. Current topic: structural responses of the primate endometrium to implantation. Placenta 1991; 12: 309–25.
7. Abrahamsohn PA, Zorn TM. Implantation and decidualization in rodents. J Exp Zool 1993; 266: 603–28.
8. O'Shea JD, Kleinfeld RG, Morrow HA. Ultrastructure of decidualization in the pseudopregnant rat. Am J Anat 1983; 166: 271–98.
9. Parr MB, Tung HN, Parr EL. The ultrastructure of the rat primary decidual zone. Am J Anat 1986; 176: 423–36.
10. Canty EG, Kadler KE. Procollagen trafficking, processing and fibrillogenesis. J Cell Sci 2005; 118: 1341–53.
11. Iwahashi M, Muragaki Y, Ooshima A et al. Alterations in distribution and composition of the extracellular matrix during decidualization of the human endometrium. J Reprod Fertil 1996; 108: 147–55.
12. Kisalus LL, Herr JC, Little CD. Immunolocalization of extracellular matrix proteins and collagen synthesis in first-trimester human decidua. Anat Rec 1987; 218: 402–15.
13. Iwahashi M, Ooshima A, Nakano R. Effects of oestrogen on the extracellular matrix in the endometrium of postmenopausal women. J Clin Pathol 1997; 50: 755–9.
14. Kisalus LL, Nunley WC, Herr JC. Protein synthesis and secretion in human decidua of early pregnancy. Biol Reprod 1987; 36: 785–98.
15. Juvonen M, Pihlajaniemi T, Autio-Harmainen H. Location and alternative splicing of type XIII collagen RNA in the early human placenta. Lab Invest 1993; 69: 541–51.
16. Pollheimer J, Bauer S, Huber A et al. Expression pattern of collagen XVIII and its cleavage product, the angiogenesis inhibitor endostatin, at the fetal–maternal interface. Placenta 2004; 25: 770–9.
17. Hurst PR, Gibbs RD, Clark DE, Myers DB. Temporal changes to uterine collagen types I, III and V in relation to early pregnancy in the rat. Reprod Fertil Dev 1994; 6: 669–77.
18. Clark DE, Hurst PR, Myers DB, Spears GF. Collagen concentrations in dissected tissue compartments of rat uterus on days 6, 7 and 8 of pregnancy. J Reprod Fertil 1992; 94: 169–75.
19. Clark DE, Hurst PR, McLennan IS, Myers DB. Immunolocalization of collagen type I and laminin in the uterus on days 5 to 8 of embryo implantation in the rat. Anat Rec 1993; 237: 8–20.
20. Karkavelas G, Kefalides NA, Amenta PS, Martinez-Hernandez A. Comparative ultrastructural localization of collagen types III, IV, VI and laminin in rat uterus and kidney. J Ultrastruct Mol Struct Res 1988; 100: 137–55.
21. Hurst PR, Palmay RD, Myers DB. Localization and synthesis of collagen types III and V during remodelling and decidualization in rat uterus. Reprod Fertil Dev 1997; 9: 403–9.
21a. Kitaoka M, Iyama K, Yashioka H et al. Immunohistochemical localisation of procollagen types I and III during placentation in pregnant rats by type-specific procollagen antibodies. J Histochem Cytochem 1994; 42: 1453–61.
22. Teodoro WR, Witzel SS, Velosa AP et al. Increase of interstitial collagen in the mouse endometrium during decidualization. Connect Tissue Res 2003; 44: 96–103.
23. Spiess K, Zorn TM. Collagen types I, III, and V constitute the thick collagen fibrils of the mouse decidua. Microsc Res Tech 2007; 70: 18–25.
24. Ball S, Bella J, Kielty C, Shuttleworth A. Structural basis of type VI collagen dimer formation. J Biol Chem 2003; 278: 15326–32.
25. Aplin JD, Mylona Y, Kielty CM et al. Collagen VI and laminin as markers of decidualisation in human endometrial stroma. In: Dey SK, ed. Molecular and Cellular Aspects of Peri-implantation Processes. New York: Springer-Verlag, 1995: 331–51.
26. Dziadek M, Darling P, Zhang RZ et al. Expression of collagen alpha 1(VI), alpha 2(VI), and alpha 3(VI) chains in the pregnant mouse uterus. Biol Reprod 1995; 52: 885–94.
27. Dziadek M, Darling P, Bakker M et al. Deposition of collagen VI in the extracellular matrix during mouse embryogenesis

correlates with expression of the alpha 3(VI) subunit gene. Exp Cell Res 1996; 226: 302–15.

28. Mulholland J, Aplin JD, Ayad S et al. Loss of collagen type VI from rat endometrial stroma during decidualization. Biol Reprod 1992; 46: 1136–43.

29. Mylona P, Kielty CM, Hoyland JA, Aplin JD. Expression of type VI collagen mRNAs in human endometrium during the menstrual cycle and first trimester of pregnancy. J Reprod Fertil 1995; 103: 159–67.

30. Aplin JD. Molecular and Cellular Aspects of Peri-implantation Processes, Boston, Massachusetts, 15–18 July 1994. Placenta 1995; 16: 109–11.

31. Fleming S, Bell SC. Localization of fibrillin-1 in human endometrium and decidua during the menstrual cycle and pregnancy. Hum Reprod 1997; 12: 2051–6.

32. Jacobson SL, Kimberly D, Thornburg K, Maslen C. Localization of fibrillin-1 in the human term placenta. J Soc Gynecol Invest 1995; 2: 686–90.

33. Aplin JD. Implantation, trophoblast differentiation and haemochorial placentation: mechanistic evidence in vivo and in vitro. J Cell Sci 1991; 99(Pt 4): 681–92.

34. Aplin JD, Glasser SR. The interaction of trophoblast with endometrial stroma. In: Glasser SR, Mulholland J, Psychoyos A, eds. Endocrinology of Embryo–Endometrial Interactions. New York: Plenum Press, 1994: 327–41.

35. Glasser SR, Lampelo S, Munir MI, Julian J. Expression of desmin, laminin and fibronectin during in situ differentiation (decidualization) of rat uterine stromal cells. Differentiation 1987; 35: 132–42.

36. Rider V, Carlone DL, Witrock D et al. Uterine fibronectin mRNA content and localization are modulated during implantation. Dev Dyn 1992; 195: 1–14.

37. Zhu HH, Huang JR, Mazela J et al. Progestin stimulates the biosynthesis of fibronectin and accumulation of fibronectin mRNA in human endometrial stromal cells. Hum Reprod 1992; 7: 141–6.

38. Haendler B, Yamanouchi H, Lessey BA et al. Cycle-dependent endometrial expression and hormonal regulation of the fibulin-1 gene. Mol Reprod Dev 2004; 68: 279–87.

39. Hsia HC, Schwarzbauer JE. Meet the tenascins: multifunctional and mysterious. J Biol Chem 2005; 280: 26641–4.

40. Harrington DJ, Lessey BA, Rai V et al. Tenascin is differentially expressed in endometrium and endometriosis. J Pathol 1999; 187: 242–8.

41. Vollmer G, Siegal GP, Chiquet-Ehrismann R et al. Tenascin expression in the human endometrium and in endometrial adenocarcinomas. Lab Invest 1990; 62: 725–30.

42. Yamanaka M, Taga M, Minaguchi H. Immunohistological localization of tenascin in the human endometrium. Gynecol Obstet Invest 1996; 41: 247–52.

43. Taguchi M, Kubota T, Aso T. Immunohistochemical localization of tenascin and ki-67 nuclear antigen in human endometrium throughout the normal menstrual cycle. J Med Dent Sci 1999; 46: 7–12.

44. Sedele M, Karaveli S, Pestereli HE et al. Tenascin expression in normal, hyperplastic, and neoplastic endometrium. Int J Gynecol Pathol 2002; 21: 161–6.

45. Julian J, Chiquet-Ehrismann R, Erickson HP, Carson DD. Tenascin is induced at implantation sites in the mouse uterus and interferes with epithelial cell adhesion. Development 1994; 120: 661–71.

46. Noda N, Minoura H, Nishiura R et al. Expression of tenascin-C in stromal cells of the murine uterus during early pregnancy: induction by interleukin-1 alpha, prostaglandin E(2), and prostaglandin F(2 alpha). Biol Reprod 2000; 63: 1713–20.

47. Nishiura R, Noda N, Minoura H et al. Expression of matrix metalloproteinase-3 in mouse endometrial stromal cells during early pregnancy: regulation by interleukin-1alpha and tenascin-C. Gynecol Endocrinol 2005; 21: 111–18.

48. Michie HJ, Head JR. Tenascin in pregnant and non-pregnant rat uterus: unique spatio-temporal expression during decidualization. Biol Reprod 1994; 50: 1277–86.

49. Iruela-Arispe ML, Porter P, Bornstein P, Sage EH. Thrombospondin-1, an inhibitor of angiogenesis, is regulated by progesterone in the human endometrium. J Clin Invest 1996; 97: 403–12.

50. Kawano Y, Nakamura S, Nasu K et al. Expression and regulation of thrombospondin-1 by human endometrial stromal cells. Fertil Steril 2005; 83: 1056–9.

51. Seki N, Kodama J, Hashimoto I et al. Thrombospondin-1 and -2 messenger RNA expression in normal and neoplastic endometrial tissues: correlation with angiogenesis and prognosis. Int J Oncol 2001; 19: 305–10.

51a. Corless CL, Mendoza A, Collins T, Lawler J. Colocalization of thrombospondin and syndecan during mouse development. Dev Dynam 1992; 193: 346–58.

52. Kim HS, Cheon YP. Spatio-temporal expression and regulation of dermatopontin in the early pregnant mouse uterus. Mol Cells 2006; 22: 262–8.

53. Cidadao AJ, Thorsteinsdottir S, David-Ferreira JF. Immunocytochemical study of tissue distribution and hormonal control of chondroitin-, dermatan- and keratan sulfates from rodent uterus. Eur J Cell Biol 1990; 52: 105–16.

54. Zorn TM, Pinhal MA, Nader HB et al. Biosynthesis of glycosaminoglycans in the endometrium during the initial stages of pregnancy of the mouse. Cell Mol Biol (Noisy-le-grand) 1995; 41: 97–106.

55. San Martin S, Soto-Suazo M, Zorn TM. Distribution of versican and hyaluronan in the mouse uterus during decidualization. Braz J Med Biol Res 2003; 36: 1067–71.

56. Lysiak JJ, Hunt J, Pringle GA, Lala PK. Localization of transforming growth factor beta and its natural inhibitor decorin in the human placenta and decidua throughout gestation. Placenta 1995; 16: 221–31.

57. San Martin S, Soto-Suazo M, De Oliveira SF et al. Small leucine-rich proteoglycans (SLRPs) in uterine tissues during pregnancy in mice. Reproduction 2003; 125: 585–95.

58. San Martin S, Zorn TM. The small proteoglycan biglycan is associated with thick collagen fibrils in the mouse decidua. Cell Mol Biol (Noisy-le-grand) 2003; 49: 673–8.

59. White CA, Robb L, Salamonsen LA. Uterine extracellular matrix components are altered during defective decidualization in interleukin-11 receptor alpha deficient mice. Reprod Biol Endocrinol 2004; 2: 76.

60. Kinsella MG, Bressler SL, Wight TN. The regulated synthesis of versican, decorin, and biglycan: extracellular matrix proteoglycans that influence cellular phenotype. Crit Rev Eukaryot Gene Expr 2004; 14: 203–34.

61. San Martin S, Soto-Suazo M, Zorn TM. Perlecan and syndecan-4 in uterine tissues during the early pregnancy in mice. Am J Reprod Immunol 2004; 52: 53–9.

62. Xu X, Ding J, Rao G et al. Estradiol induces heparanase-1 expression and heparan sulphate proteoglycan degradation in human endometrium. Hum Reprod 2007; 22: 927–37.

63. Carson DD, Dutt A, Tang JP. Glycoconjugate synthesis during early pregnancy: hyaluronate synthesis and function. Dev Biol 1987; 120: 228–35.

64. Brown JJ, Papaioannou VE. Distribution of hyaluronan in the mouse endometrium during the periimplantation period of pregnancy. Differentiation 1992; 52: 61–8.

65. Fenderson BA, Stamenkovic I, Aruffo A. Localization of hyaluronan in mouse embryos during implantation, gastrulation and organogenesis. Differentiation 1993; 54: 85–98.

66. Salamonsen LA, Shuster S, Stern R. Distribution of hyaluronan in human endometrium across the menstrual cycle. Implications for implantation and menstruation. Cell Tissue Res 2001; 306: 335–40.

67. Wynn RM. Ultrastructural development of the human decidua. Am J Obstet Gynecol 1974; 118: 652–70.

68. Faber M, Wewer UM, Berthelsen JG et al. Laminin production by human endometrial stromal cells relates to the cyclic and pathologic state of the endometrium. Am J Pathol 1986; 124: 384–91.

69. Wewer UM, Albrechtsen R, Fisher LW et al. Osteonectin/SPARC/BM-40 in human decidua and carcinoma, tissues characterized by de novo formation of basement membrane. Am J Pathol 1988; 132: 345–55.

70. Church HJ, Vicovac LM, Williams JD et al. Laminins 2 and 4 are expressed by human decidual cells. Lab Invest 1996; 74: 21–32.

71. Maatta M, Salo S, Tasanen K et al. Distribution of basement membrane anchoring molecules in normal and transformed endometrium: altered expression of laminin gamma2 chain and collagen type XVII in endometrial adenocarcinomas. J Mol Histol 2004; 35: 715–22.

72. Timpl R, Brown JC. Supramolecular assembly of basement membranes. Bioessays 1996; 18: 123–32.

73. Farrar JD, Carson DD. Differential temporal and spatial expression of mRNA encoding extracellular matrix components in decidua during the peri-implantation period. Biol Reprod 1992; 46: 1095–108.

74. Virtanen I, Gullberg D, Rissanen J et al. Laminin alpha 1-chain shows a restricted distribution in epithelial basement membranes of fetal and adult human tissues. Exp Cell Res 2000; 257: 298–309.

75. Vuolteenaho R, Nissinen M, Sainio K et al. Human laminin M chain (merosin): complete primary structure, chromosomal assignment, and expression of the M and A chain in human fetal tissues. J Cell Biol 1994; 124: 381–94.

76. Korhonen M, Virtanen I. The distribution of laminins and fibronectins is modulated during extravillous trophoblastic cell differentiation and decidual cell response to invasion in the human placenta. J Histochem Cytochem 1997; 45: 569–81.

77. Leivo I, Engvall E. Merosin, a protein specific for basement membranes of Schwann cells, striated muscle, and trophoblast, is expressed late in nerve and muscle development. Proc Natl Acad Sci USA 1988; 85: 1544–8.

78. Church HJ, Richards A, Aplin JD. Laminins in decidua, placenta and choriocarcinoma cells. Trophoblast Res 1997; 10: 143–62.

79. Kohnen G, Campbell S, Irvine GA et al. Endothelin receptor expression in human decidua. Mol Hum Reprod 1998; 4: 185–93.

80. Wewer UM, Damjanov A, Weiss J et al. Mouse endometrial stromal cells produce basement-membrane components. Differentiation 1986; 32: 49–58.

81. Armant DR. Cell interactions with laminin and its proteolytic fragments during outgrowth of mouse primary trophoblast cells. Biol Reprod 1991; 45: 664–72.

82. Miner JH, Cunningham J, Sanes JR. Roles for laminin in embryogenesis: exencephaly, syndactyly, and placentopathy in mice lacking the laminin alpha5 chain. J Cell Biol 1998; 143: 1713–23.

83. Yelian FD, Edgeworth NA, Dong LJ et al. Recombinant entactin promotes mouse primary trophoblast cell adhesion and migration through the Arg-Gly-Asp (RGD) recognition sequence. J Cell Biol 1993; 121: 923–9.

84. Wu TC, Wan YJ, Chung AE, Damjanov I. Immunohistochemical localization of entactin and laminin in mouse embryos and fetuses. Dev Biol 1983; 100: 496–505.

85. Thomas T, Dziadek M. Expression of laminin and nidogen genes during the postimplantation development of the mouse placenta. Biol Reprod 1993; 49: 1251–9.

86. Visse R, Nagase H. Matrix metalloproteinases and tissue inhibitors of metalloproteinases: structure, function, and biochemistry. Circ Res 2003; 92: 827–39.

87. Sternlicht MD, Werb Z. How matrix metalloproteinases regulate cell behavior. Annu Rev Cell Dev Biol 2001; 17: 463–516.

88. White JM: ADAMs: modulators of cell–cell and cell–matrix interactions. Curr Opin Cell Biol 2003; 15: 598–606.

89. Xiao LJ, Chang H, Ding NZ et al. Basigin expression and hormonal regulation in mouse uterus during the peri-implantation period. Mol Reprod Dev 2002; 63: 47–54.

90. Braundmeier AG, Fazleabas AT, Lessey BA et al. Extracellular matrix metalloproteinase inducer regulates metalloproteinases in human uterine endometrium. J Clin Endocrinol Metab 2006; 91: 2358–65.

91. Goffin F, Munaut C, Frankenne F et al. Expression pattern of metalloproteinases and tissue inhibitors of matrix-metalloproteinases in cycling human endometrium. Biol Reprod 2003; 69: 976–84.

92. Wang HX, Zhao YG, Wang HM et al. Expression of adamalysin 19/ADAM19 in the endometrium and placenta of rhesus monkey (Macaca mulatta) during early pregnancy. Mol Hum Reprod 2005; 11: 429–35.

93. Kim J, Kim H, Lee SJ et al. Abundance of ADAM-8, -9, -10, -12, -15 and -17 and ADAMTS-1 in mouse uterus during the oestrous cycle. Reprod Fertil Dev 2005; 17: 543–55.

94. Plaisier M, Kapiteijn K, Koolwijk P et al. Involvement of membrane-type matrix metalloproteinases (MT-MMPs) in capillary tube formation by human endometrial microvascular endothelial cells: role of MT3–MMP. J Clin Endocrinol Metab 2004; 89: 5828–36.

95. Salamonsen LA, Butt AR, Hammond FR et al. Production of endometrial matrix metalloproteinases, but not their tissue inhibitors, is modulated by progesterone withdrawal in an in vitro model for menstruation. J Clin Endocrinol Metab 1997; 82: 1409–15.

96. Zhang J, Salamonsen LA. Tissue inhibitor of metalloproteinases (TIMP)-1, -2 and -3 in human endometrium during the menstrual cycle. Mol Hum Reprod 1997; 3: 735–41.

97. Marbaix E, Kokorine I, Moulin P et al. Menstrual breakdown of human endometrium can be mimicked in vitro and is selectively and reversibly blocked by inhibitors of matrix metalloproteinases. Proc Natl Acad Sci USA 1996; 93: 9120–5.

98. Irwin JC, Kirk D, Gwatkin RB et al. Human endometrial matrix metalloproteinase-2, a putative menstrual proteinase. Hormonal regulation in cultured stromal cells and messenger RNA expression during the menstrual cycle. J Clin Invest 1996; 97: 438–47.

99. Bruner KL, Matrisian LM, Rodgers WH et al. Suppression of matrix metalloproteinases inhibits establishment of ectopic lesions by human endometrium in nude mice. J Clin Invest 1997; 99: 2851–7.

100. Vincent AJ, Salamonsen LA. The role of matrix metalloproteinases and leukocytes in abnormal uterine bleeding associated with progestin-only contraceptives. Hum Reprod 2000; 15(Suppl 3): 135–43.

101. Galant C, Berliere M, Dubois D et al. Focal expression and final activity of matrix metalloproteinases may explain irregular dysfunctional endometrial bleeding. Am J Pathol 2004; 165: 83–94.

102. Kaitu'u TJ, Shen J, Zhang J et al. Matrix metalloproteinases in endometrial breakdown and repair: functional significance in a mouse model. Biol Reprod 2005; 73: 672–80.

103. Huppertz B, Kertschanska S, Demir AY et al. Immunohistochemistry of matrix metalloproteinases (MMP), their substrates, and their inhibitors (TIMP) during trophoblast invasion in the human placenta. Cell Tissue Res 1998; 291: 133–48.

104. Teesalu T, Masson R, Basset P et al. Expression of matrix metalloproteinases during murine chorioallantoic placenta maturation. Dev Dyn 1999; 214: 248–58.

105. Harris LK, Aplin JD. Arterial remodelling during pregnancy. Reprod Sci 2008; in press.

106. Yu WH, Yu S, Meng Q et al. TIMP-3 binds to sulfated gly-cosaminoglycans of the extracellular matrix. J Biol Chem 2000; 275: 31226–32.

107. Alexander CM, Hansell EJ, Behrendtsen O et al. Expression and function of matrix metalloproteinases and their inhibitors at the maternal–embryonic boundary during mouse embryo implantation. Development 1996; 122: 1723–36.

108. Strakova Z, Szmidt M, Srisuparp S, Fazleabas AT. Inhibition of matrix metalloproteinases prevents the synthesis of insulin-like growth factor binding protein-1 during decidualization in the baboon. Endocrinology 2003; 144: 5339–46.

109. Liu X, Wu H, Byrne M et al. A targeted mutation at the known collagenase cleavage site in mouse type I collagen impairs tissue remodeling. J Cell Biol 1995; 130: 227–37.

110. Hu J, Zhang X, Nothnick WB, Spencer TE. Matrix metallo-proteinases and their tissue inhibitors in the developing neonatal mouse uterus. Biol Reprod 2004; 71: 1598–604.

111. Marbaix E, Kokorine I, Henriet P et al. The expression of interstitial collagenase in human endometrium is controlled by progesterone and by oestradiol and is related to menstrua-tion. Biochem J 1995; 305(Pt 3): 1027–30.

112. Kokorine I, Marbaix E, Henriet P et al. Focal cellular origin and regulation of interstitial collagenase (matrix metallopro-teinase-1) are related to menstrual breakdown in the human endometrium. J Cell Sci 1996; 109(Pt 8): 2151–60.

113. Rudolph-Owen LA, Slayden OD, Matrisian LM, Brenner RM. Matrix metalloproteinase expression in Macaca mulatta endometrium: evidence for zone-specific regulatory tissue gradients. Biol Reprod 1998; 59: 1349–59.

114. Salamonsen LA, Nagase H, Suzuki R, Woolley DE. Production of matrix metalloproteinase 1 (interstitial collage-nase) and matrix metalloproteinase 2 (gelatinase A: 72 kDa gelatinase) by ovine endometrial cells in vitro: different regu-lation and preferential expression by stromal fibroblasts. J Reprod Fertil 1993; 98: 583–9.

115. Rawdanowicz TJ, Hampton AL, Nagase H et al. Matrix met-alloproteinase production by cultured human endometrial stromal cells: identification of interstitial collagenase, gelati-nase-A, gelatinase-B, and stromelysin-1 and their differential regulation by interleukin-1 alpha and tumor necrosis factor-alpha. J Clin Endocrinol Metab 1994; 79: 530–6.

116. Rodgers WH, Osteen KG, Matrisian LM et al. Expression and localization of matrilysin, a matrix metalloproteinase, in human endometrium during the reproductive cycle. Am J Obstet Gynecol 1993; 168: 253–60.

117. Rodgers WH, Matrisian LM, Giudice LC et al. Patterns of matrix metalloproteinase expression in cycling endometrium imply differential functions and regulation by steroid hor-mones. J Clin Invest 1994; 94: 946–53.

118. Berton A, Selvais C, Lemoine P et al. Binding of matrilysin-1 to human epithelial cells promotes its activity. Cell Mol Life Sci 2007; 64: 610–20.

119. Bruner KL, Rodgers WH, Gold LI et al. Transforming growth factor beta mediates the progesterone suppression of an epithelial metalloproteinase by adjacent stroma in the human endometrium. Proc Natl Acad Sci USA 1995; 92: 7362–6.

120. Osteen KG, Rodgers WH, Gaire M et al. Stromal–epithelial interaction mediates steroidal regulation of metalloproteinase expression in human endometrium. Proc Natl Acad Sci USA 1994; 91: 10129–33.

121. Cornet PB, Galant C, Eeckhout Y et al. Regulation of matrix metalloproteinase-9/gelatinase B expression and activation by ovarian steroids and LEFTY-A/endometrial bleeding-associated factor in the human endometrium. J Clin Endocrinol Metab 2005; 90: 1001–11.

122. Cornet PB, Picquet C, Lemoine P et al. Regulation and function of LEFTY-A/EBAF in the human endometrium. mRNA expression during the menstrual cycle, control by progesterone,

and effect on matrix metalloproteinases . J Biol Chem 2002; 277: 42496–504.

123. Marbaix E, Donnez J, Courtoy PJ, Eeckhout Y. Progesterone regulates the activity of collagenase and related gelatinases A and B in human endometrial explants. Proc Natl Acad Sci USA 1992; 89: 11789–93.

124. Vassilev V, Pretto CM, Cornet PB et al. Response of matrix metalloproteinases and tissue inhibitors of metalloproteinases messenger ribonucleic acids to ovarian steroids in human endometrial explants mimics their gene- and phase-specific differential control in vivo. J Clin Endocrinol Metab 2005; 90: 5848–57.

125. Salamonsen LA, Nagase H, Woolley DE. Production of matrix metalloproteinase 3 (stromelysin) by cultured ovine endometrial cells. J Cell Sci 1991; 100(Pt 2): 381–5.

126. Bellingard V, Hedon B, Capony F et al. Identification of prometalloproteinase-3 as a major protein secreted by human endometrial fibroblasts and inhibited by coculture with tro-phoblast cells. Biol Reprod 1996; 55: 604–12.

127. Schatz F, Papp C, Toth-Pal E, Lockwood CJ. Ovarian steroid-modulated stromelysin-1 expression in human endometrial stromal and decidual cells. J Clin Endocrinol Metab 1994; 78: 1467–72.

128. Keller NR, Sierra-Rivera E, Eisenberg E, Osteen KG. Progesterone exposure prevents matrix metalloproteinase-3 (MMP-3) stimulation by interleukin-1alpha in human endome-trial stromal cells. J Clin Endocrinol Metab 2000; 85: 1611–19.

129. Osteen KG, Igarashi TM, Bruner-Tran KL. Progesterone action in the human endometrium: induction of a unique tis-sue environment which limits matrix metalloproteinase (MMP) expression. Front Biosci 2003; 8: d78–86.

130. Jeziorska M, Nagase H, Salamonsen LA, Woolley DE. Immunolocalization of the matrix metalloproteinases gelati-nase B and stromelysin 1 in human endometrium throughout the menstrual cycle. J Reprod Fertil 1996; 107: 43–51.

131. Soini Y, Alarakkola E, Autio-Harmainen H. Expression of mes-senger RNAs for metalloproteinases 2 and 9, type IV collagen, and laminin in nonneoplastic and neoplastic endometrium. Hum Pathol 1997; 28: 220–6.

132. Daimon E, Wada Y. Role of neutrophils in matrix metallopro-teinase activity in the preimplantation mouse uterus. Biol Reprod 2005; 73: 163–71.

133. Behrendtsen O, Alexander CM, Werb Z. Metalloproteinases mediate extracellular matrix degradation by cells from mouse blastocyst outgrowths. Development 1992; 114: 447–56.

134. Librach CL, Werb Z, Fitzgerald ML et al. 92-kD type IV collagenase mediates invasion of human cytotrophoblasts. J Cell Biol 1991; 113: 437–49.

135. Polette M, Nawrocki B, Pintiaux A et al. Expression of gelati-nases A and B and their tissue inhibitors by cells of early and term human placenta and gestational endometrium. Lab Invest 1994; 71: 838–46.

136. Leco KJ, Edwards DR, Schultz GA. Tissue inhibitor of metalloproteinases-3 is the major metalloproteinase inhibitor in the decidualizing murine uterus. Mol Reprod Dev 1996; 45: 458–65.

137. Jeziorska M, Salamonsen LA, Woolley DE. Mast cell and eosinophil distribution and activation in human endometrium throughout the menstrual cycle. Biol Reprod 1995; 53: 312–20.

138. Olson GE, Winfrey VP, Matrisian PE et al. Blastocyst-dependent upregulation of metalloproteinase/disintegrin MDC9 expres-sion in rabbit endometrium. Cell Tissue Res 1998; 293: 489–98.

139. Weskamp G, Cai H, Brodie TA et al. Mice lacking the metal-loprotease-disintegrin MDC9 (ADAM9) have no evident major abnormalities during development and adult life. Mol Cell Biol 2002; 22: 1537–44.

25 Signaling and transcription factor networks in the human endometrial stroma

Birgit Gellersen and Jan Brosens

Synopsis

Background

- Decidualization is the differentiation of resident endometrial stromal cells into enlarged secretory cells.
- Upon decidualization, endometrial stromal cells acquire new functions that are essential for coordinated trophoblast invasion and placenta formation.

Clinical

- Defective decidualization may predispose to pregnancy complications associated with impaired trophoblast invasion, including miscarriage, preeclampsia, fetal growth restriction, and preterm labor.
- Understanding decidualization will improve the prospects for treatment of dysfunctional uterine bleeding.

Basic Science

- Decidualization in humans (unlike rodent models) is initiated independently of pregnancy.
- Bone marrow-derived cells, especially uterine NK cells and macrophages, are recruited into the uterus during decidualization.
- Differentiation of the resident stromal cells is heterogeneous, so that a population of undifferentiated cells is retained throughout pregnancy.
- The initial decidualizing stimulus is not progesterone, but rather the elevation of intracellular cAMP and sustained activation of the PKA pathway stimulated by ligand binding to G-protein-family receptors and phosphodiesterase inhibition.
- Numerous autocrine and paracrine mediators, including growth factors, cytokines, and protaglandins, modulate the process of decidual differentiation.
- Progestins are essential for enhancing and maintaining the decidual phenotype.
- PR-A is the dominant progesterone receptor isoform.
- Its actions are not predominantly via direct classical transcriptional activation. Rather, it acts as a platform to integrate the activities of numerous other transcription factors by formation of various supramolecular complexes.
- Progestins also act to modulate a variety of cytoplasmic signal transduction pathways.

INTRODUCTION

The success of normal pregnancy depends on the protection, controlled invasion, and growth of the semi-allogenic placenta within the maternal uterine environment. In the endometrium, the maternal response to pregnancy is characterized by influx of specialized uterine natural killer (uNK) cells, remodeling of the spiral arteries, and differentiation of the endometrial stromal cells (ESCs) into decidual cells. In most species, this maternal uterine response, termed decidualization, is triggered by signals derived from the implanting blastocyst. In humans, however, the decidual process occurs independently of pregnancy during the midsecretory phase of each cycle. This apparent switch from embryonic to maternal control of the decidual process has profound consequences for human reproduction. For instance, 'spontaneous' or conceptus-independent decidualization of the endometrium also occurs in the few other species that menstruate, such as Old World monkeys, the elephant shrew (*Elephantus myuras jamesoni*), and certain bats, suggesting that these processes are causally linked.[1] Cyclic decidualization and menstrual shedding occur on average 400 times during the reproductive years of women in developed countries. Consequently, abnormal uterine bleeding is one of the most common disorders in women and a major indication for surgical intervention. Furthermore, emerging evidence suggests that reproductive disorders that affect the preconceptual endometrial milieu predispose to a spectrum of pregnancy complications associated with impaired trophoblast invasion, including miscarriage, preeclampsia, fetal growth restriction, and preterm labor.[2]

A detailed understanding of the decidual process is therefore important from a biological and a clinical perspective. At first glance, decidualization of the endometrial stroma appears to be a straightforward affair, requiring only increased levels of the second messenger cyclic adenosine monophosphate (cAMP) to induce the phenotype and progesterone to maintain the differentiated state.[3] Recent studies have begun to reveal the intriguing complexity of underlying regulatory mechanisms. This chapter summarizes the morphological and biochemical characteristics of decidualizing ESCs and focuses on the signal and transcription factor networks that govern this differentiation process.

DECIDUALIZATION OF THE ENDOMETRIAL STROMAL COMPARTMENT

Morphological differentiation

Endometrial stromal cells are mesenchymal cells that have an elongated spindle-shaped fibroblastic appearance during the proliferative phase of the cycle. The first morphological signs of decidualization become apparent in stromal cells surrounding the terminal spiral arteries of the superficial endometrial layer approximately 10 days after the luteinizing hormone (LH) surge (i.e. LH+10)[4] (Figure 25.1). It is important to note that the onset of the decidual process heralds the end of the limited period of uterine receptivity (LH+6 to LH+10) during which embryo attachment can take place. Ultrastructurally, decidualizing cells are characterized by progressive cell enlargement, rounding of the nucleus with an increase in number and complexity of the nucleoli, expansion of the secretory apparatus with dilatation of the rough endoplasmic reticulum and of the Golgi complex, as well as cytoplasmic accumulation of glycogen and lipid droplets. Multiple club-shaped processes appear on the surface of the predecidual cells, crossing the surrounding basal lamina. These projections

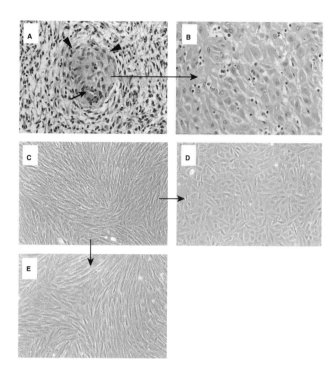

Figure 25.1 Decidual transformation of human endometrial stromal cells (ESCs) in vivo and in vitro. (**A**) Decidualization of the stromal compartment (arrowheads) is initiated in ESCs that surround the terminal portion of the spiral arteries (arrow) of the superficial endometrial layer during the mid secretory phase of the cycle. (**B**) Extensive decidualization of stromal cells during the late luteal phase of the cycle. (**C**) Undifferentiated primary ESCs in culture are characterized by a fibroblastic spindle-shaped appearance. (**D**) Treatment of primary cultures with 8-bromo-cAMP (0.5 mmol/L) for 6 days transforms the spindle-shaped cells into decidual cells, characterized by rounded appearance, abundant cytoplasm, and enlarged nuclei. (**E**) In contrast, treatment of primary cultures with progesterone (250 nmol/L) for 6 days has little effect on cellular morphology.

extend freely into the extracellular matrix (ECM) or indent the cytoplasm of adjacent cells. Between stromal cells, adherens junctions but not true desmosomes are found. In addition, gap junctions may form between processes of the same cell.[5] Interestingly, decidual stromal cells express α-smooth muscle actin, desmin, and vimentin, suggesting they acquire a myofibroblastic phenotype.[6] Extracellular matrix proteins produced by decidualized cells include laminin, type IV collagen, fibronectin, and heparan sulfate proteoglycan.[7]

The decidual reaction continues throughout pregnancy and the extent of this differentiation process often correlates with the degree of trophoblast invasion.[2,8] Wu et al found that morphometric parameters, such as cell size, correlated with the expression of decidual prolactin (PRL), a biochemical hallmark of differentiating ESCs.[9] Not only does the decidual cell size increase throughout pregnancy but also the percentage of stromal cells in the decidua that express PRL mRNA increases from 9.8% in early pregnancy to 57.8% at term. This indicates that a substantial subpopulation of undifferentiated stromal cells persists even in term human decidua. Undifferentiated stromal fibroblasts obtained from term decidua are able to differentiate morphologically and biochemically in vitro.[10]

Biochemical differentiation

The distinct morphological appearance of decidualizing stromal cells is underpinned by biochemical changes. Major secretory products of decidualized stromal cells, such as PRL and insulin-like growth factor binding protein-1 (IGFBP-1), have traditionally been used as markers of the differentiated state.[3] Recently, microarray-based genome-wide expression profiling has identified hundreds of genes that are either up- or down-regulated during the receptive phase of the intact endometrium.[11–17] The same technology has also been applied to interrogate gene expression in purified ESC cultures exposed to a decidualizing stimulus in vitro.[18–21] These studies confirmed that the decidualization process involves sequential reprogramming of functionally related families of genes involved in extracellular organization, cell adhesion, cytoskeletal organization, signal transduction, metabolism, differentiation, and apoptosis. Consequently, upon biochemical reprogramming, decidualizing endometrial stromal cells acquire many new functions that critically govern successful trophoblast invasion and placenta formation. For instance, decidualizing stromal cells surrounding the spiral arteries highly express tissue factor (TF, the initiator of the extrinsic coagulation pathway) and plasminogen activator inhibitor-1 (PAI-1, a fibrinolysis inhibitor), indicating that they play a primary role in maintaining vascular stability prior to menstruation and during endovascular trophoblast invasion.[22] Differentiating ESCs secrete a variety of factors, such as macrophage inflammatory protein-1β, interleukin (IL)-11, IL-15, and PRL, which are thought to provide chemotactic, proliferative, and differentiating signals for uNK cells.[23–25] On the other hand, the decidua also expresses the tryptophan-catabolizing enzyme indoleamine 2,3-dioxygenase (IDO), tumor necrosis factor (TNF)-related apoptosis-inducing ligand (TRAIL), and Fas ligand (FasL), which are implicated in the suppression of T-cell-dependent immune responses to fetal alloantigens.[18,26,27] Remodeling of the extracellular matrix and secretion of growth factors and binding proteins such as IGFBP-1 are thought to critically regulate coordinated trophoblast invasion

and differentiation.[28] Implantation and formation of the placenta are associated with inflammatory processes. Upon differentiation, stromal cells become resistant to inflammatory signals and express enzymes such as manganese superoxide dismutase (MnSOD) that are involved in oxidative stress defenses.[29,30] Decidualized ESCs also show a reduced response to the proinflammatory cytokine IL-1β, a key factor in implantation, signified by a decrease in IL-1β-induced activation of the p38 mitogen-activated protein kinase (MAPK). This is reversed by protein kinase A (PKA) inhibitor and hence is cAMP-dependent.[31]

SIGNALS AND SIGNAL TRANSDUCTION PATHWAYS IN DECIDUALIZATION

The endometrial stroma is exposed to a variety of endocrine, paracrine, and autocrine factors capable of inducing, augmenting, and maintaining the decidual phenotype. Although the postovulatory rise in progesterone levels governs endometrial differentiation, decidual transformation is only first apparent during the mid secretory phase of the cycle, indicating that the expression of decidua-specific genes is unlikely to be under direct transcriptional control of activated progesterone receptor (PR). Overwhelming evidence supports the paradigm that initiation of the decidual process is dependent upon increased cellular cAMP levels and sustained activation of the PKA pathway.[3] Although exposure of primary ESC cultures to progesterone, alone or in combination with estradiol, for 8–10 days will trigger expression of decidual markers, this response is mediated by a gradual increase in intracellular cAMP levels and abrogated in the presence of PKA inhibitor.[32] Induction of the decidual phenotype in cultured ESCs by 6 days of treatment with a cAMP analogue, but not with progesterone, is illustrated in Figure 25.1. With the onset of decidualization, ESCs produce a number of factors capable of propagating this differentiation process in an autocrine or paracrine fashion. Progesterone, on the other hand, plays a pivotal role in modulating and maintaining the decidual response.

cAMP signaling pathway in endometrial stromal cells

Cyclic AMP is a ubiquitous second messenger molecule that is generated from ATP by adenylate cyclase. This enzyme is activated upon binding of ligand to members of the family of G-protein-coupled receptors (GPCRs) which are coupled to a stimulatory heterotrimeric guanine nucleotide-binding protein (G protein).[33] Adenylate cyclase activity in the human endometrium increases during the menstrual cycle and the cAMP content in biopsies obtained from patients during the secretory phase is higher than that in the proliferative phase.[34,35] During the secretory phase of the cycle, local factors are produced capable of increasing cAMP levels in stromal cells, including relaxin, corticotropin-releasing hormone (CRH), and prostaglandin E_2 (PGE$_2$). Expression of these ligands and their respective receptors in the endometrium has been reported.[36-39] Furthermore, the ability of these local endometrial factors to initiate decidualization of ESCs in culture, alone or in combination with progestin, has been demonstrated.[3] There is experimental evidence to suggest that the gonadotropins LH and follicle-stimulating hormone (FSH), as well the β-subunit of human chorionic gonadotropin (hCG), can provide the initial cAMP signal in primary cultures of ESCs, although this remains controversial.[40,41]

The intracellular level of cAMP is determined not only by its production but also by its degradation. Members of the large family of phosphodiesterases (PDEs) convert cAMP to AMP, which no longer stimulates PKA activity.[42] A recent study identified PDE4 and PDE8 as the principal PDE isoforms in ESCs. Interestingly, inhibition of PDE4 was sufficient to induce expression of decidual markers.[43] It has been proposed that the sustained increase in cellular cAMP observed in decidualizing ESC is, at least in part, due to inhibition of PDE activity.

Transcription factors immediately downstream of cAMP signaling

Binding of two cAMP molecules to each of the two regulatory subunits of the cAMP-dependent PKA in its holomeric form leads to release and activation of the two catalytic subunits of the holoenzyme. These catalytic subunits phosphorylate cytoplasmic or nuclear target molecules. Among the major nuclear targets are the cAMP response element binding protein (CREB) and the related cAMP response element modulator (CREM). These transcription factors are activated by PKA phosphorylation, bind to their cognate DNA sequence (cAMP response element, CRE) in cAMP-regulated genes and activate transcription.[44,45] CREB and CREM belong to the family of basic region/leucine zipper (bZIP) transcriptional regulators which dimerize through the leucine zipper and bind to their cognate

DNA sequence through the basic region.[46] Their core region is a bipartite transactivation domain, consisting of one or two glutamine-rich regions, and the central kinase-inducible domain harboring the phosphorylation sites.[45] Due to alternative splicing, alternative translation initiation events, or alternative promoter usage, these transcription factors can be expressed in a multitude of isoforms.[46-48] Depending on the presence or absence of constituents of the transactivation domain, these isoforms are transcriptional activators or repressors.[45] While the expression of CREB is largely constitutive in many systems, its action being tightly regulated by phosphorylation and dephosphorylation events, the CREM gene carries an internal, highly cAMP-inducible promoter P2.[49] Transcripts generated from P2 encode the C-terminal bZIP region but are devoid of the N-terminal transactivation functions. The translation product is known as ICER (inducible cAMP early repressor); through homodimerization or heterodimerization with other CREM/CREB isoforms it functions as a potent repressor and establishes a negative feedback loop to down-regulate transcription of cAMP-induced promoters, including its own. By this mechanism, a cAMP-mediated signal is terminated.[50] However, ESCs represent an exception to this concept. When exposed to long-term treatment with relaxin or cAMP analogue, they do not show the expected transient increase in ICER expression but a persistent up-regulation of ICER, indicating a permissiveness of the cells to the ongoing stimulation of cAMP signaling.[47]

Autocrine/paracrine signals of decidualization

Once the decidual process is initiated, differentiating cells secrete a number of cytokines and growth factors involved in propagating this process (Figure 25.2). In cAMP-treated primary ESC cultures, induction of IL-11 expression parallels that of PRL and IGFBP-1, and inhibition of IL-11 signaling attenuates the expression of these differentiation markers.[51,52] IL-11 and its receptor subunit IL-11Rα are localized in the decidualized stromal cells of the mid–late secretory endometrium.[53] Moreover, female IL-11R-deficient mice are infertile due to a defective post-implantation decidual response.[54,55]

Cyclic AMP signaling also induces expression of heparin-binding epidermal growth factor (HB-EGF), both the soluble form and the transmembrane precursor, as well as its two cognate receptors, EGFR and ErbB4/HER4, in human ESCs. Inhibition of HB-EGF signaling not only attenuates PRL and IGFBP-1 production

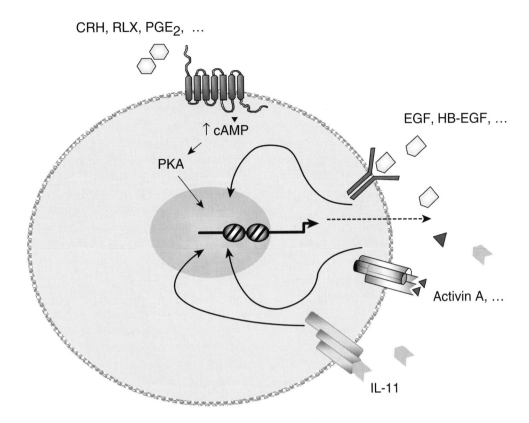

Figure 25.2   Initiation and autocrine control of the decidual process. Activation of various 7-transmembrane G-protein-coupled receptors by local endometrial factors increases intracellular cAMP levels in stromal cells, which in turn leads to the expression and secretion of subsidiary factors, such as HB-EGF, IL-11, and activin-A, that are capable of enhancing the decidual process through binding and activation of their cognate cell surface receptors.

in differentiating ESCs but also sensitizes these cells to apoptosis induced by proinflammatory signals.[56] Notably, HB-EGF induces IL-11 secretion by cultured ESCs.[53]

Members of the transforming growth factor β (TGFβ) superfamily, including inhibins, activins, and follistatin, have also been implicated in the paracrine/ autocrine regulation of the decidual process.[57] Production of activin A, a dimer of βA subunits, is induced in ESCs upon cAMP-induced differentiation. It rises in parallel with PRL secretion between days 2 and 6 of treatment. Conversely, even after 10 days of treatment with estrogen plus progestin, activin A secretion from decidualized cells remains low.[24] It has been shown that activin A itself promotes the expression of decidual markers in vitro, an effect inhibited by co-treatment with the activin-binding protein follistatin.[24] Before the onset of the decidual process in vivo, inhibin and activin dimers are produced by epithelial cells, whereas activin receptors are expressed on stromal cells. As a local stimulus, epithelial activin might initiate the decidual reaction in stromal cells, which is then amplified in a paracrine/autocrine loop as decidual cells themselves assume activin production.[57]

Another TGFβ family member highly expressed upon cAMP stimulation of ESCs is Lefty-A, which was originally identified as an endometrial bleeding-associated factor (EBAF).[20,58] Like other TGFβ members, Lefty-A is expressed as a polypeptide that requires processing for its activity.

Gene profiling of ESCs has revealed that cAMP signaling induces a rapid and marked increase in preprosomatostatin transcripts that encode for the neuropeptide somatostatin.[20] The somatostatin receptor subtype 2 (SSTR2), a GPCR, is also induced by cAMP in ESCs, and SSTR2 has been detected in the endometrium by immunohistochemistry.[20,59]

Subsidiary transcription factors involved in decidualization

Notably, amongst the transcripts that are regulated upon endometrial differentiation, relatively few encode transcription factors. This may reflect the generally low abundance of such mRNAs or the fact that transcription factors are to a large extent regulated at the level of activity, not expression.

Table 25.1 Effect of FOXO1 silencing on the expression of decidual transcripts

Decidual marker	NT siRNA (fold induction by cAMP+MPA)	FOXO1 siRNA (% inhibition)
IGFBP-1	>1000	92.9
PRL	277	84.3
Lefty-A	21	86
SOD-2	7.2	75.2
Bim	2.5	90.9
FOXO1	4.1	83.3

Confluent primary human endometrial stromal cells were transfected with either non-targeting (NT) small interfering RNA (siRNA) or FOXO1 siRNA. Subsequently, the cells remained either untreated or were treated with a decidualizing stimulus, 8-bromo-cAMP (0.5 mmol/L) and medroxyprogesterone acetate (MPA; 1 μmol/L) for 72 hours. Cells were harvested and the expression of specific decidual transcripts determined by real-time quantitative polymerase chain reaction (PCR).

The ability of a transcription factor to modulate gene expression is controlled at multiple levels. First, alternative splicing of the pre-mRNA and utilization of alternative translation initiation codons in the mature mRNA can give rise to a multitude of isoforms with diverse functions. A case in point is the presence of multiple CREM isoforms in decidualizing cells as described above.[47] Secondly, and of eminent importance, are post-translational modifications of transcription factors, such as phosphorylation in response to activation of signal transduction pathways. Phosphorylation occurs by addition of a phosphate group to the hydroxyl group of serine, threonine, or tyrosine residues in an ATP-requiring reaction mediated by two broad families of kinases – serine/threonine protein kinases and tyrosine protein kinases. Like most post-translational modifications, phosphorylation is reversible through the actions of specific phosphatases. Other post-translational modifications include acetylation, glycosylation, sumoylation, and ubiquitinylation, which all can profoundly impact on the stability, degradation, subcellular localization, DNA-binding, and transcriptional activities of nuclear factors. Finally, the ability of a given transcription factor to control expression of a target gene can vary dramatically depending on the presence of interacting proteins, including other transcription factors, co-activators, and co-repressors.

Most of the transcription factors implicated in the regulation of the decidual process have been identified by promoter analyses of decidual marker genes such as PRL, IGFBP-1, and TF. It must be noted that the PRL gene in the decidua is transcribed from an alternative promoter located 6 kilobases upstream of the pituitary PRL promoter and therefore underlies completely different regulatory mechanisms.[60,61] Transcription from the decidual PRL promoter adds a non-coding exon to the PRL mRNA; the resulting protein, however, is identical to that produced in the pituitary.[62]

The forkhead transcription factor FOXO1

The FOXO subfamily of Forkhead transcription factors is a direct downstream target of the phosphatidylinositol 3-kinase (PI3K) signal transduction pathway, which is stimulated by a number of growth factors, including insulin and insulin-like growth factors. PI3K activation results in the phosphorylation of the serine/threonine kinase AKT (also termed PKB), which in turn promotes cellular survival through phosphorylation and inactivation of multiple downstream targets, including FOXO proteins.[63,64]

The three human FOXO proteins, FOXO1, FOXO3a, and FOXO4, are homologues of DAF-16 in *Caenorhabditis elegans*, an important regulator of longevity in this organism.[65] In mammalian cells, FOXO proteins are critical mediators of cell fate decisions, such as cell cycle arrest, senescence, and apoptosis, in response to growth factor, hormonal, and environmental cues.[66] Post-translational modification of FOXO proteins is an important mechanism that regulates the ability of these transcription factors to activate distinct gene sets. Phosphorylation in response to growth factor-mediated activation of the PI3K/AKT signaling pathway results in the cytoplasmic retention of FOXO proteins and, hence, inhibition of forkhead-dependent transcriptional activity. Conversely, targeted phosphorylation of cytoplasmic FOXO factors by Jun N-terminal kinase (JNK) promotes nuclear import.

FOXO proteins are constitutively expressed in many cell types but not in human endometrium. FOXO1 is markedly induced upon decidualization in vivo as well as in vitro and is involved in regulating the expression of endometrial differentiation markers such as PRL and IGFBP-1.[67–69] In addition, as shown in Table 25.1, silencing of FOXO1 in decidualized ESCs profoundly attenuates the expression of a variety of decidual genes, including MnSOD, the proapototic Bcl-2 family member Bim, and Lefty-A. In the presence of the activated cAMP pathway, FOXO1 is predominantly nuclear. However, in the presence of a progestin, FOXO translocates to the cytoplasm, although a fraction remains in the nucleus. Withdrawal of the progestin from differentiated cultures results in rapid nuclear reaccumulation of FOXO1, enhanced expression of Bim, and cell death.[70] Interestingly, silencing of FOXO1 expression in differentiating stromal cells completely abrogates apoptosis induced upon progestin withdrawal, suggesting that decidualizing ESCs become dependent upon progesterone signaling for survival through partial cytoplasmic translocation and inactivation of FOXO1. In contrast to FOXO1, FOXO3a expression is repressed upon endometrial differentiation, whereas FOXO4 appears not to be expressed in this tissue.[70]

Signal transducers and activators of transcription (STATs)

Members of the STAT family of latent transcription factors are implicated in growth and differentiation of many tissues, including adipocytes, hepatocytes, mammary epithelial cells, and endometrium.[71,72] This family comprises seven members, termed STAT1, STAT2, STAT3, STAT4, STAT5a, STAT5b, and STAT6. STATs are activated by numerous cytokines and peptide growth factors. They lack intrinsic kinase activity and, in most cell systems, require targeted phosphorylation by receptor-associated Janus kinases (JAK1, JAK2) for signal transduction. Phosphorylation of a tyrosine residue conserved in all STAT family members induces their dimerization, translocation to the nucleus, and regulation of gene expression. Subsequently, STATs are dephosphorylated and return to their latent site in the cytoplasm.[71]

In humans, two highly related family members, STAT5a and STAT5b, play a critical role in decidualization. STAT5 is selectively expressed in glandular epithelium and a subset of stromal cells during the secretory phase of the cycle.[73] Furthermore, decidualization of stromal cells in culture coincides with the induction, activation and nuclear translocation of STAT5b and, to a lesser extent, STAT5a. Expression of a dominant-negative STAT5b mutant abolishes the activation of the decidual PRL promoter in response to treatment with a cAMP analogue.[72] STAT signal transduction is negatively regulated by a variety of protein tyrosine phosphatases and by suppressor of cytokine signaling (SOCS) family of proteins. Interestingly, SOCS-1, a potent JAK inhibitor, is highly expressed at least in rat decidua.[74]

CCAAT/enhancer-binding protein β (C/EBPβ)

Like CREM and CREB, the C/EBPs are also a subgroup of the class of bZIP transcription factors.[75] Among the six members of the C/EBP family, C/EBPβ has been recognized as an essential factor in female reproductive function. Its expression is required for ovulation and for development and function of the mammary gland.[76–78] During cAMP-induced decidualization of ESCs, C/EBPβ protein is up-regulated and serves as a central mediator of the cAMP stimulus to activate expression of the decidual PRL gene, which carries C/EBP binding sites in its promoter region.[79] Furthermore, there is a striking cycle-dependent increase in C/EBPβ expression in vivo where the protein accumulates in the stromal cell nuclei of the late secretory phase.[67]

There are two isoforms of C/EBPβ: the full-length liver-enriched activating protein (LAP) and the truncated liver-enriched inhibitory protein (LIP). The latter lacks the N-terminal transactivation domains of LAP and acts as a potent repressor of C/EBP-dependent transcription.[80] Western blot analysis studies showed that only LAP is present in normal non-pregnant human endometrium.[67]

Activating protein 1 (AP-1)

The composite transcription factor activating protein 1 (AP-1) integrates various mitogenic signals and is therefore a major regulator of cell proliferation. The AP-1 complex is formed by homo- or heterodimerization of Jun, Fos, and ATF proteins, members of the bZIP family of transcription factors. The Jun family consists of three proteins, c-Jun, JunD, and JunB, while the Fos family contains four proteins, c-Fos, FosB, Fra-1, and Fra-2. In the endometrium, c-Fos and c-Jun expression is estrogen-dependent and confined to proliferative and early- to mid-secretory endometrium.[81] However, JunD and Fra-2 protein expression is markedly increased in secretory phase endometrium and in the decidua of early pregnancy. Furthermore, JunD and Fra-2 have been shown to enhance decidual PRL promoter activity upon binding to AP-1 binding sites in the upstream promoter region.[82]

Ets transcription factors

Ets1 belongs to the ETS (E26) transcription factor superfamily that is defined by a highly conserved 58 amino acid DNA binding motif, called the ETS domain. ETS transcription factors regulate a broad spectrum of cellular processes as they serve as nuclear effectors of multiple signal transduction cascades. Ets1 is highly induced in decidualizing cells in culture and overexpression of Ets has been shown to stimulate decidual PRL gene expression through binding to an ETS motif located in the proximal promoter region.[83]

Homeobox proteins (HOX)

Homeotic genes were first identified as developmental genes in the fruitfly *Drosophila melanogaster*. They are transcription factors characterized by a conserved sequence, the homeobox, and their vertebrate homologues are termed HOX genes. They are divided into four complexes, *HoxA*, *-B*, *-C*, and *-D*, which are clustered in four genomic loci. Genes within a given cluster are expressed sequentially and act on successive segments along the anterior–posterior axis of the developing embryo.[84] Of the 13 paralogues in the *HoxA* cluster, *Hoxa-9*, *-10*, *-11* and *-13* are expressed along the paramesonephric duct in the mouse embryo. After birth, a spatial pattern of *Hox* expression is maintained in the female reproductive tract, with *Hoxa-9* being expressed in the Fallopian tubes, *Hoxa-10* in the uterus, *Hoxa-11* in the uterus and cervix, and *Hoxa-13* in the upper vagina. A corresponding pattern is found in the human.[85] Both *Hoxa-10-* and *Hoxa-11-*deficient mice are sterile.[86,87] The endometrium of mice with a deletion of either gene does not support implantation and shows a defective decidual reaction of the stromal cells.[88,89] These findings have fuelled an interest in the role of these proteins in human uterine function. During the menstrual cycle, highest expression of HOXA-10 and HOXA-11 in the endometrium is seen in the mid-luteal phase, at the time of implantation.[90] In cultured human ESCs, HOXA-10 expression is increased by estrogen or progesterone. The effects of these steroids appear to be additive and are further enhanced by relaxin.[90–92] This observation is contrasted in a different report where combined treatment of ESCs with cAMP plus progestin resulted in a down-regulation of HOXA-10 mRNA and protein.[93]

Sp1

There are four known members of the Sp family of transcription factors, numbered 1–4. Sp1, Sp3, and Sp4 proteins bind with similar affinities to a GC-rich DNA motif that is found in the promoter regions of many genes, including housekeeping genes.[94] Sp1 and Sp3 are ubiquitously expressed and there is evidence that, depending on the promoter context, Sp3 functions as a competitive repressor of Sp1-dependent transcription. In the human endometrium, Sp1 levels have been reported to increase in perivascular stromal cells during the secretory phase when compared with proliferative endometrium. Conversely, Sp3 expression decreases in ESCs upon decidualization.[95] The expression of several decidua-specific genes, such as TF, PAI-1, and IGFBP-1, has been shown to be regulated by the cellular Sp1/Sp3 ratio.[94]

Tumor suppressor p53

The tumor suppressor protein p53 plays a fundamental role in protecting the genome from genotoxic insults. In most normal cells, it is present at very low levels because it is subject to rapid proteasomal degradation under physiological circumstances. In response to stress and DNA damage, the protein is stabilized and rapidly accumulates in the nucleus where it initiates events leading to cell cycle arrest and DNA repair or apoptosis, thus eliminating genotypically aberrant cells from the organism. Structurally, p53 is a transcription factor with an N-terminal transactivation domain, a central DNA binding region, and a C-terminal tetramerization domain. In addition to activating transcription of immediate target genes, p53 exerts its functions also by engaging in protein–protein interactions and suppression of transcription of a different set of target genes.[96,97] In about 50% of all human tumors, p53 is mutated. This results in defective function accompanied by increased protein stability, which makes the mutated p53 immunohistochemically detectable in tumorous cells.[98–100]

Wild-type p53 is massively up-regulated upon cAMP-induced decidualization of ESCs. The kinetics of induction are not those of an acute stress response but parallel the delayed expression of decidual markers after 2–4 days of treatment. Induction of p53 is also observed in vivo in the nuclei of ESCs of the secretory phase. Accumulation of p53 in the nuclei of cultured ESCs is due to protein stabilization as p53 mRNA levels remain unchanged. The presence of p53 is tightly linked to the decidualized status of the cells. Upon withdrawal of the decidualizing stimulus, stromal cells dedifferentiate morphologically and lose expression of decidual PRL and IGFBP-1 along with the disappearance of p53 protein.[101]

GADD45α (growth arrest and DNA-damage-inducible protein 45α), a putative p53 target gene, is also highly expressed in secretory phase endometrium.[12,13] GADD45 proteins are multifaceted factors implicated in the regulation of diverse stress responses, including cell cycle arrest at G_2/M, chromatin remodeling, nucleotide excision repair, and apoptosis. They are presumed to serve as gatekeepers capable of killing cells unable to repair damaged DNA.[102] A potential role of p53 and GADD45α in this system might be to halt proliferation and facilitate differentiation of the stromal compartment. Arguably, p53 and GADD45α could also play a role in safeguarding the genomic stability of endometrial cells during the cyclic process of rapid proliferation, differentiation, menstrual shedding, and regeneration.

Other transcription factors

Recent studies have demonstrated that various members of the TGFβ superfamily, such as activin A and Lefty-A, are likely to be important regulators of the decidual process. While Lefty-A has been shown to signal through the MAPK pathway,[103] members of the TGFβ family generally bind to heteromeric serine/threonine kinase transmembrane receptor complexes which recruit the downstream effectors Smad2 and Smad3. The phosphorylated dimer of the receptor-activated Smads then forms a trimeric complex with Smad4 and translocates to the nucleus where it interacts with Smad-binding elements in target genes and with a large variety of transcription factors, co-activators, or co-repressors to modulate gene expression.[104] In the human endometrial stroma, the expression of Smad3, Smad4, and Smad7, and TGFβ-induced phosphorylation and nuclear translocation of Smad3 have been demonstrated.[105]

Some transcription factors have been implicated in the decidual process on the basis of their expression profiles. One example is the Wilms' tumor suppressor gene (WT1), which encodes a zinc-finger-containing transcription factor that is selectively expressed in the developing urogenital tract and functions as a tissue-specific developmental regulator.[106] In the endometrium, WT is detectable in the nuclei of stromal cells and its expression increases during decidualization both in vivo as well as in vitro.[106] However, the role of WT in regulating stromal cell function is still unknown.

PROGESTERONE SIGNALING IN ENDOMETRIAL STROMAL CELLS

Steroid hormones are small hydrophobic molecules based on a four-membered ring structure.[107] Progesterone, a steroid hormone with 21 carbon atoms, is synthesized by the corpus luteum in the latter half of the menstrual cycle. In the absence of pregnancy, luteolysis and falling circulating progesterone levels during the late secretory phase of the cycle provide the signal for menstrual shedding. In the presence of a conceptus, the corpus luteum will continue to produce progesterone for the first 2–3 months of pregnancy until the placenta takes over steroid biosynthesis.[108] It has long been the paradigm that progesterone exerts its action by passing through the lipophilic plasma membrane and binding to intracellular PRs which function in the nucleus as transcription factors to modulate selectively the expression of target genes. The results of such genomic action, namely modulation of the rate of transcription and ultimately protein synthesis, will only become manifest hours after the initial progesterone signal. However, not all effects of progesterone are genomic and, like other steroid hormones, progesterone has rapid effects on signal transduction pathways independently of transcription.[107] Whether these rapid non-genomic progesterone actions involve the 'classical' PRs or novel unrelated receptor types is a subject of ongoing research.

Genomic progesterone actions

The nuclear PR is a member of the superfamily of ligand-activated transcription factors. Two isoforms exist, PR-A and PR-B, which arise from different promoter usage in a single gene. PR-B differs from PR-A in that it contains an additional 164 amino acids at the N-terminus (B-upstream sequence, BUS).[109] Although the PR isoforms display indistinguishable hormone- and DNA-binding affinities, several studies have shown that, depending on the cell and promoter context, PR-A and PR-B have remarkably different transcriptional activities. In general, the PR-A isoform is transcriptionally much less active and functions as a dominant inhibitor of transcription by PR-B and various other steroid receptors.[110] PR-A shares with PR-B the activation functions AF-1 and AF-2, but lacks AF-3, which is situated in the BUS segment specific to PR-B.[111] AF-1 is a constitutive activation domain N-terminal to the DNA-binding domain while the ligand-dependent activation function AF-2 is located in the ligand-binding domain.[112] The N-terminal segment of PR-A harbors an inhibitory function, termed IF or ID, which represses AF-1 or AF-2, but not AF-3. Removal of IF/ID converts PR-A into a strong transcriptional activator. The BUS domain is thought to repress IF/ID, thereby rendering PR-B a much more potent activator of transcription than PR-A.[113]

Binding of progesterone induces a conformational change in the receptor, resulting in phosphorylation, dissociation from heat shock proteins, dimerization, sumoylation of a subpopulation of receptor molecules, binding and activation of specific response elements in the promoter region of target genes, and recruitment of the basal transcriptional machinery. The latter requires further interaction of the AF-2 region with steroid receptor co-activators (SRCs) resulting in recruitment of other SRC-associated histone acetyltransferases (CREB binding protein and pCAF) and the methyltransferase CARM1 involved in modifying the chromatin template.[114,115] Conversely, silencing of gene expression by steroid hormones or other transcription factors requires binding to co-repressors, such as SMRT and N-CoR, that mediate transcriptional repression.[110] It has been suggested that the lower transactivation potential of PR-A may be a result of its higher affinity for co-repressors and its less efficient recruitment of the co-activator SRC-1.[116] To date, our knowledge on the expression profiles of co-activators and co-repressors, and of their potential hormone dependency, in human endometrium is very limited. However, the endometrium of pseudopregnant mice deficient in SRC-1 fails to decidualize.[117] In humans, SRC-1 is expressed in the various endometrial cellular compartments throughout the menstrual cycle. Furthermore, when overexpressed in differentiating primary ESC cultures, SRC-1 greatly enhances decidual PRL promoter activity.[118]

Non-genomic progesterone actions

The activated PRs can also trigger rapid non-genomic progesterone actions that are independent of transcription. This is mediated, at least in part, by the ability of PR to interact with signaling molecules carrying an Src-homology-3 (SH3) domain, like the Src kinases.[119] In a ligand-dependent fashion, PR can directly associate with Src and convert it to an active state. As a consequence, a rapid and transient activation of the downstream MAP kinases ERK1/2 occurs. Notably, amongst steroid receptors, the ability to interact with SH3 domains of signaling molecules appears to be unique to PR. Progesterone-dependent MAPK activation is effectively inhibited by the PR antagonist RU486. This non-transcriptional activity of PR requires cytoplasmic localization of the receptor and occurs near or at the plasma membrane.[120] How PR, which is predominantly a nuclear protein, interacts with cytoplasmic or cell membrane signaling molecules is not well understood. However, PR, like other steroid receptors, is known to shuttle between the cytoplasmic and nuclear compartments by active import and export mechanisms. This dynamic localization further supports the notion that PRs may have important extranuclear functions.[121]

It is generally believed that not all non-genomic actions of progesterone are mediated by the classical PR but involve progesterone binding to unrelated plasma membrane receptors. In recent years there has been an intense search for such receptors. Hence, the recent cloning of bona fide membrane progestin receptors (mPRs) from fish ovary has been widely considered as a breakthrough in the field.[122,123] Three isoforms – mPRα, mPRβ, and mPRγ – were originally described and found in species ranging from zebrafish to humans. Their amino acid sequence suggested them to be seven transmembrane spanning GPCRs related to the adiponectin receptors. When the mPRα cloned from spotted seatrout was expressed in human breast cancer cells, progestin induced a rapid decrease in cAMP formation, indicating coupling to an inhibitory G protein, and a transient increase in ERK1/2 MAPK activation.[123] The mPRα isoform appeared to be of most relevance to reproductive function, as the mRNA was reported to be predominantly expressed in testis, ovary, and placenta, while mPRβ predominated in the brain and mPRγ in the kidney.[122] The mPRs are also expressed in human endometrium,

albeit at levels much lower than in other tissues such as the placenta.[124] However, evidence that the mammalian homologues of the fish mPR mediate rapid progesterone responses is currently lacking.

Other putative progesterone-binding moieties have been described, including two related proteins (Hpr6.6 and Dg6) which are now named progesterone receptor membrane components 1 and 2 (PGRMC1 and PGRMC2).[125] While little is known about PGRMC2, PGRMC1 is described as a microsomal single transmembrane progesterone-binding protein implicated in progesterone-induced Ca^{2+} influx in sperm.[126] PGRMC1 has recently been shown to interact with PAIRBP1, a protein formerly known as Rda288, which is involved in progesterone-mediated antiapoptotic action in ovarian granulosa cells. Association of PGRMC1 with PAIRBP1 might lead to plasma membrane localization of the complex, with PGRMC1 being the actual progesterone-binding site.[127] Nothing is known as yet regarding protein expression or function of these molecules in the endometrial stroma. It is interesting to note, however, that microarray analyses revealed PGRMC1 mRNA among the most abundant transcripts in the human endometrium although its expression appears to be down-regulated in the mid-secretory phase of the cycle.[12,17]

Progesterone actions in undifferentiated endometrial stromal cells

The endometrial stromal compartment is exposed to progesterone for 9–10 days prior to decidualization. After ovulation, rapid progesterone responses are apparent in the glandular compartment but not in the stroma. In fact, surprisingly few known genes are induced in the endometrial stroma by progesterone with kinetics compatible with direct transcriptional activation by ligand-activated nuclear PR.

One of the early-response genes is that encoding the novel protein Depp (decidual protein induced by progesterone) which was identified in the search for progesterone-responsive genes in ESCs.[128] The mRNA for Depp was up-regulated within 30 minutes of treatment with progesterone and inhibited by RU486. Notably, Depp was also identified as a cAMP-inducible gene in a microarray study.[20] The biological function of Depp has not been elucidated, but it appears to be a nuclear protein, and its overexpression leads to phosphorylation of ERK1/2 and activation of an Elk-1 responsive reporter construct.[128]

Another early-response gene is the promyelocytic leukemia zinc finger protein (PLZF), a member of

Table 25.2   Physical interactions between transcription factors involved in decidual transformation of human endometrial stromal cells

	PR	STAT5	FOXO1	C/EBPβ	Sp1
STAT5	√[153]				
FOXO1	√[68]	?			
C/EBPβ	√[148]	?	√[67]		
Sp1	√[154]	√[155]	?	√[156]	
p53	?	?	?	√[157]	√[158]

the family of Krüppel-like zinc finger proteins, which is a transcriptional repressor involved in cell cycle control.[129] PLZF is induced by progesterone within 2 hours in cultured ESCs. In vivo, there is a marked increase in nuclear PLZF immunoreactivity in the endometrial stromal compartment during the mid to late secretory phase.[130] Interestingly, PLZF was also identified as an androgen-responsive gene in the prostate,[131] and mouse mutants revealed an essential role for this factor in the maintenance of spermatogonial stem cells.[132,133] PLZF confers resistance to apoptosis and does so partly by transcriptional inhibition of the gene encoding the proapoptotic BID protein, a member of the Bcl2 family.[134] The antiproliferative effect of nuclear PLZF is mediated by suppression of cyclin A transcription.[135] This in turn is reversed by HB-EGF-C, the C-terminal soluble fragment resulting from proteolytic cleavage of the membrane-anchored precursor proHB-EGF. While the N-terminal cleavage product HB-EGF is a growth-promoting ligand of the EGF receptor, HB-EGF-C translocates from the membrane to the nucleus, interacts with PLZF, and triggers its nuclear export, leading to reversal of cell cycle inhibition.[136] In the human endometrium, HB-EGF is induced by cAMP, mediates decidualization, and confers resistance to TNFα- and TGFβ-induced apoptosis of ESCs.[56] The role in ESCs of HB-EGF-C, a by-product of HB-EGF formation, has not been assessed but it could conceivably participate in cell fate decision towards the end of the menstrual cycle. Notably, direct transcriptional induction by ligand-activated nuclear PR bound to PREs (progesterone-response elements) in the promoter regions of Depp or PLZF genes has yet to be demonstrated.

Progesterone responses in decidualizing endometrial stromal cells

Although progesterone may not elicit the initial steps of decidual transformation of the stromal compartment,

elevated levels of this hormone are absolutely required to maintain and enhance the differentiated phenotype. Treatment of primary ESC cultures with a cAMP analogue triggers rapid expression of decidual markers but the levels decline upon prolonged exposure. However, addition of progesterone greatly enhances the expression of decidual phenotypic markers such as PRL and supports their maintenance in long-term cultures. Interestingly, this synergy between cAMP and progesterone is apparent only after a lag period of 2–4 days, indicating that paracrine or autocrine signals are involved.[118]

Induction of PR expression or an increase in the PR-B/PR-A ratio would explain how cAMP sensitizes differentiating ESCs to progesterone. However, several studies have shown that in the course of decidualization of the human endometrial stroma, in vivo and in culture, PR-B is down-regulated while PR-A remains expressed and is the dominant isoform.[118,137,138] Consistent with a critical role for PR-A in endometrial stroma, the ablation of this isoform in mice leads to impaired implantation and decidualization, while PR-B-deficient females have no such uterine phenotype.[139]

The classical model of progesterone signaling, which implies that the liganded dimerized PR activates gene expression by binding to specific palindromic DNA-response elements in the promoter region of target genes, is clearly not applicable to decidualizing stromal cells. In recent years an alternative paradigm has emerged which is based on the ability of PR to serve as a platform for interaction with decidua-specific transcription factors[3] (Table 25.2). Within this model, activation of PR is critical for the formation of multiple transcriptional complexes capable of modulating the expression of a large number of gene sets. Furthermore, emerging evidence also suggests an important role for the activated PR in coordinating the activity of various cytoplasmic signal transduction pathways that converge on numerous nuclear proteins.

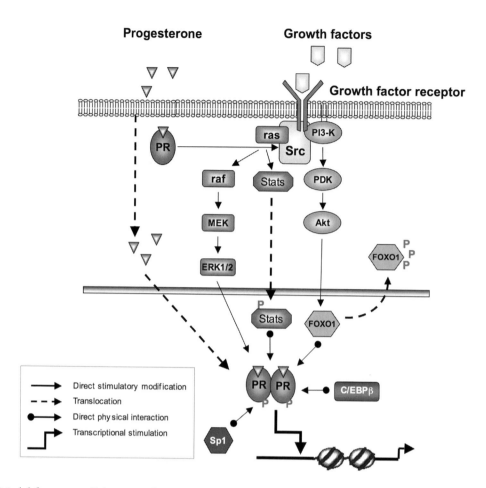

Figure 25.3   Model for cross-talk between the activated PR, cytoplasmic signal cascades, and nuclear transcription factors in decidualizing human ESCs. In the cytoplasm, progesterone-bound PR modulates the activity of MAPK, PI3K, and STAT signaling pathways through interaction with the protein tyrosine kinase c-Src. In the nucleus, the activated PR acquires control of diverse gene sets by recruiting cAMP-induced transcription factors into multimeric transcriptional complexes.[3] For a detailed explanation, see the text.

Cross-talk between progesterone and cytoplasmic signaling cascades

The cross-talk between progesterone and growth factor/cytokine signaling pathways occurs at several levels. For instance, progesterone enhances the expression of various growth factors and their receptors in decidualizing ESCs.[18] On the other hand, progesterone has also been shown to regulate the expression of multiple signal intermediates involved in JAK/STAT and MAPK signaling, at least in breast cancer cells.[140,141] Interestingly, microarray analysis identified JAK1 and JNK1 as two signal molecules down-regulated upon treatment of endometrial explants with the antiprogestin RU486.[142] This suggests that progesterone also sensitizes endometrial cells to the effects of growth factors by modulating the expression of signaling intermediates. Finally, progesterone has rapid effects on cell signaling pathways independently of transcription, as discussed in the 'Nongenomic progesterone actions' section.

The cellular tyrosine kinase c-Src has emerged as a possible focal point for the integration of steroid and growth factor signaling. Decidualization of ESCs in response to estrogen and progesterone is associated with a marked increase in c-Src kinase activity which is reversed upon steroid withdrawal.[143] In vivo, the activated form of c-Src is present predominantly in differentiating stromal cells of the late secretory phase human endometrium and in the decidua of pregnancy.[144] Notably, c-Src null mice have an impaired decidual reaction.[145] c-Src belongs to the Src family of protein tyrosine kinases (SFKs), which are probably best known for their roles downstream of integrin adhesion receptors. SFKs are necessary for the generation of 'outside-in signals' that regulate cytoskeletal organization, cell motility, and gene expression in response to cell adhesion.[146] SFKs play an important role in the activation of several signaling pathways and it is tempting to speculate that in decidualizing cells progesterone regulates the activity of the MAPK, PI3K, and STAT signaling pathways through activation of c-Src (Figure 25.3).

Interestingly, PR itself is one of the downstream targets of those cytoplasmic signaling cascades activated by progesterone. For instance, activation of ERK1/2 results in phosphorylation of the PR at serine 294, which is both a ligand-dependent and a MAPK consensus phosphorylation site. Mutation of this site inhibits the transcriptional activity of PR and blocks cytoplasmic translocation and receptor degradation via the ubiquitin–proteasome pathway.[121,140]

An interesting area is the potential interplay between hormonal and mechanical stimuli. A recent study demonstrated that mechanical stretch markedly enhances IGFBP-1 expression in progesterone-treated ESCs in vitro, suggesting that uterine contraction waves may also play a role in modulating endometrial differentiation in vivo.[147]

Cross-talk between PR and decidua-specific transcription factors

Decidualization of ESCs appears to be dependent upon the induction and activation of diverse and seemingly unrelated transcription factors. However, many of these transcription factors, including STATs, FOXO1, C/EBPβ, and Sp1, have been shown to bind to one another as well as to the activated PR (see Table 25.2). This has led to the suggestion that PR, and in particular the A isoform, has a critical role as a platform for the formation of transcriptional multiprotein complexes.[3] Interaction of two transcription factors has profound and almost always bidirectional consequences for their transcriptional outputs. For instance, PR-A may be a transcriptional inhibitor of PR-B and of other steroid hormone receptors, but, in ESCs, it functions as an enhancer of C/EBPβ-dependent transcription.[148] Consequently, PR-A is more efficient in enhancing PRL or IGFBP-1 promoter activity then PR-B.[149] PR-A also cooperates with AP-1 to enhance progesterone-induced fibronectin promoter activity in cultured ESCs.[150]

Several additional lines of evidence support this model of PR action in decidualizing ESCs. First, few if any decidua-specific genes are regulated through consensus palindromic progesterone-response elements in their promoter regions. In fact, analyses of the decidual PRL, IGFBP-1, and fibronectin promoters identified DNA regions that contain multiple and overlapping response elements which mediate PR actions.[67,68,150] For instance, PR-dependent induction of the fibronectin promoter occurs through a composite CRE/AP1-response element.[150] Recently, Kim and co-workers used the technique of chromatin immunoprecipitation to demonstrate in-vivo interaction between endogenous FOXO1 and PR on the IGFBP-1 promoter as a critical event to regulate IGFBP-1 expression in decidualizing cells.[68] On the other hand, treatment of ESCs with antiprogestins inhibits cAMP-induced PRL expression, indicating that even the unliganded PR may be recruited in a ternary, albeit less-functional, complex.[118] However, in the absence of progesterone, such multimeric transcription complexes or transcriptosomes are likely to be unstable, which can account for the failure of cAMP to maintain the expression of decidua-specific genes in long-term cultures (see Figure 25.3). Finally, transient and stable overexpression of PR-A or PR-B in human ESCs does not enhance but paradoxically inhibits the expression of decidual markers.[118] This suggests that suprastoichiometric PR levels interfere with the assembly of a functional complex through squelching and sequestering of essential transcriptional partners and co-activators. It is indeed striking that upon decidualization in culture, PR as well as HOXA-10 levels gradually decline.[93,118] Similarly, FOXO1 is predominantly nuclear in ESCs treated with a cAMP analogue while addition of progesterone induces a partial translocation of this essential transcription factor to the cytoplasm.[70]

Progesterone has important anti-inflammatory actions in differentiating endometrium. This response is mediated, at least in part, through the ability of the activated PR to interact with and repress transcription factors such as nuclear factor-κB (NFκB) and STAT1 downstream of proinflammatory signaling pathways.[30,151]

CONCLUSIONS AND CLINICAL PERSPECTIVE

Successful implantation of an embryo requires the endometrial stromal compartment to acquire new functions in a matter of days to ensure controlled invasion of the semiallogenic trophoblast. Not surprisingly, decidualization involves extraordinary reprogramming of many cellular functions. In recent years, the number of signals, signal transduction cascades, and transcription factors implicated in this process has grown phenomenally. At first, the complexity of orchestrating the expression of so many diverse gene sets appears startling, if not beyond comprehension. Yet, despite this complexity, a relatively simple and elegant model has emerged. In humans, differentiation of ESCs is initially triggered by local factors capable of elevating cellular cAMP levels and sustained activation of the PKA signaling pathway. This in turn elicits the expression of a number of factors that feedback on the decidualizing cells, thereby activating subsidiary signaling pathways and downstream transcription factors which converge onto the activated PR. By recruiting decidua-specific transcription factors, the activated PR acquires control of the diverse gene sets necessary for cellular differentiation and survival. Consequently, the integrity of the differentiated endometrium, in the presence or absence of pregnancy, becomes entirely dependent upon a single hormone, progesterone.

Defective placenta formation is frequently attributed to intrinsic defects in trophoblast invasiveness. Intuitively, this seems a logical explanation that appears to be supported by experiments in mice demonstrating that ablation of a variety of genes results in impaired trophoblast differentiation along the various cell lineages (for review see Red-Horse et al[152]). However, there is little or no evidence in humans to suggest that primary defects in trophoblast cells are a common cause of defective deep placentation. Instead, increasing evidence indicates that the high incidence of obstetric complications in humans may be a consequence of a hostile endometrial milieu characterized by impaired decidualization.[2] This raises a number of important challenges and opportunities for clinical practice. First, it may be possible to identify women at risk of obstetrical complications on the basis of a biochemical analysis of an endometrial biopsy taken in the mid to late secretory phase of a non-conception cycle. Secondly it emphasizes the importance of periconceptual care for the prevention of not only early pregnancy loss but also late obstetrical complications such as preeclampsia and preterm labor. The corollary implies that medical intervention aimed at preventing late obstetrical complications is likely to be effective only if initiated during the periconceptual period. Finally, by defining the biochemical perturbations in the endometrial milieu prior to pregnancy, it would be possible to target specific underlying defects and tailor treatment to individual patients.

ACKNOWLEDGMENTS

We gratefully acknowledge the work of the members of our groups. We apologize to all those authors whose important work could not be referenced due to space restraints.

REFERENCES

1. Brasted M, White CA, Kennedy TG et al. Mimicking the events of menstruation in the murine uterus. Biol Reprod 2003; 69: 1273–80.

2. Brosens JJ, Pijnenborg R, Brosens IA. The myometrial junctional zone spiral arteries in normal and abnormal pregnancies: a review of the literature. Am J Obstet Gynecol 2002; 187: 1416–23.

3. Gellersen B, Brosens JJ. Cyclic AMP and progesterone receptor cross-talk in human endometrium: a decidualizing affair. J Endocrinol 2003; 178: 357–72.

4. de Ziegler D, Fanchin R, de Moustier B et al. The hormonal control of endometrial receptivity: estrogen (E2) and progesterone. J Reprod Immunol 1998; 39: 149–66.

5. Wynn RM. Ultrastructural development of the human decidua. Am J Obstet Gynecol 1974; 118: 652–70.

6. Oliver C, Montes MJ, Galindo JA et al. Human decidual stromal cells express α-smooth muscle actin and show ultrastructural similarities with myofibroblasts. Hum Reprod 1999; 14: 1599–605.

7. Aplin JD, Charlton AK, Ayad S. An immunohistochemical study of human endometrial extracellular matrix during the menstrual cycle and first trimester of pregnancy. Cell Tissue Res 1988; 253: 231–40.

8. Ramsey EM, Houston ML, Harris JW. Interactions of the trophoblast and maternal tissues in three closely related primate species. Am J Obstet Gynecol 1976; 124: 647–52.

9. Wu W-X, Brooks J, Glasier AF et al. The relationship between decidualization and prolactin mRNA and production at different stages of human pregnancy. J Mol Endocrinol 1995; 14: 255–61.

10. Richards RG, Brar AK, Frank GR et al. Fibroblast cells from term human decidua closely resemble endometrial stromal cells: induction of prolactin and insulin-like growth factor binding protein-1 expression. Biol Reprod 1995; 52: 609–15.

11. Kao LC, Tulac S, Lobo S et al. Global gene profiling in human endometrium during the window of implantation. Endocrinology 2002; 143: 2119–38.

12. Borthwick JM, Charnock-Jones DS, Tom BD et al. Determination of the transcript profile of human endometrium. Mol Hum Reprod 2003; 9: 19–33.

13. Mirkin S, Arslan M, Churikov D et al. In search of candidate genes critically expressed in the human endometrium during the window of implantation. Hum Reprod 2005; 20: 2104–17.

14. Carson DD, Lagow E, Thathiah A et al. Changes in gene expression during the early to mid-luteal (receptive phase) transition in human endometrium detected by high-density microarray screening. Mol Hum Reprod 2002; 8: 871–9.

15. Riesewijk A, Martin J, van Os R et al. Gene expression profiling of human endometrial receptivity on days LH+2 versus LH+7 by microarray technology. Mol Hum Reprod 2003; 9: 253–64.

16. Horcajadas JA, Riesewijk A, Dominguez F et al. Determinants of endometrial receptivity. Ann NY Acad Sci 2004; 1034: 166–75.

17. Talbi S, Hamilton AE, Vo KC et al. Molecular phenotyping of human endometrium distinguishes menstrual cycle phases and underlying biological processes in normo-ovulatory women. Endocrinology 2006; 147: 1097–121.

18. Popovici RN, Kao L-C, Giudice LC. Discovery of new inducible genes in in vitro decidualized human endometrial stromal cells using microarray technology. Endocrinology 2000; 141: 3510–13.

19. Brar A, Handwerger S, Kessler CA et al. Gene induction and categorical reprogramming during in vitro human endometrial fibroblast decidualization. Physiol Genomics 2001; 7: 135–48.

20. Tierney EP, Tulac S, Huang ST et al. Activation of the protein kinase A pathway in human endometrial stromal cells reveals sequential categorical gene regulation. Physiol Genomics 2003; 16: 47–66.

21. Okada H, Nakajima T, Yoshimura T et al. Microarray analysis of gene controlled by progesterone in human endometrial stromal cells in vitro. Gynecol Endocrinol 2003; 17: 271–80.

22. Schatz F, Krikun G, Caze R et al. Progestin-regulated expression of tissue factor in decidual cells: implications in endometrial hemostasis, menstruation and angiogenesis. Steroids 2003; 68: 849–60.

23. Kitaya K, Nakayama T, Okubo T et al. Expression of macrophage inflammatory protein-1β in human endometrium: its role in endometrial recruitment of natural killer cells. J Clin Endocrinol Metab 2003; 88: 1809–14.

24. Dimitriadis E, White CA, Jones RL et al. Cytokines, chemokines and growth factors in endometrium related to implantation. Hum Reprod Update 2005; 11: 613–30.

25. Gubbay O, Critchley HO, Bowen JM et al. Prolactin induces ERK phosphorylation in epithelial and CD56(+) natural killer cells of the human endometrium. J Clin Endocrinol Metab 2002; 87: 2329–35.

26. Kudo Y, Hara T, Katsuki T et al. Mechanisms regulating the expression of indoleamine 2,3-dioxygenase during decidualization of human endometrium. Hum Reprod 2004; 19: 1222–30.

27. Makrigiannakis A, Zoumakis E, Kalantaridou S et al. Endometrial and placental CRH as regulators of human embryo implantation. J Reprod Immunol 2004; 62: 53–9.

28. Giudice LC. Maternal–fetal conflict – lessons from a transgene. J Clin Invest 2002; 110: 307–9.

29. Sugino N, Karube-Harada A, Sakata A et al. Different mechanisms for the induction of copper–zinc superoxide dismutase and manganese superoxide dismutase by progesterone in human endometrial stromal cells. Hum Reprod 2002; 17: 1709–14.

30. Zoumpoulidou G, Jones MC, de Mattos SF et al. Convergence of interferon-γ and progesterone signaling pathways in human endometrium: role of PIASy (protein inhibitor of activated signal transducer and activator of transcription-γ). Mol Endocrinol 2004; 18: 1988–99.

31. Yoshino O, Osuga Y, Hirota Y et al. Endometrial stromal cells undergoing decidualization down-regulate their properties to produce proinflammatory cytokines in response to interleukin-1β via reduced p38 mitogen-activated protein kinase phosphorylation. J Clin Endocrinol Metab 2003; 88: 2236–41.

32. Brar AK, Frank GR, Kessler CA et al. Progesterone-dependent decidualization of the human endometrium is mediated by cAMP. Endocrine 1997; 6: 301–7.

33. Dessauer CW, Posner BA, Gilman AG. Visualizing signal transduction: receptors, G-proteins, and adenylate cyclase. Clin Sci 1996; 91: 527–37.

34. Tanaka N, Miyazaki K, Tashiro H et al. Changes in adenylyl cyclase activity in human endometrium during the menstrual cycle and in human decidua during pregnancy. J Reprod Fertil 1993; 98: 33–9.

35. Bergamini CM, Pansini F, Bettocchi S Jr et al. Hormonal sensitivity of adenylate cyclase from human endometrium: modulation by estradiol. J Steroid Biochem 1985; 22: 299–303.

36. Palejawa S, Tseng L, Wojtczuk A et al. Relaxin gene and protein expression and its regulation of procollagenase and vascular endothelial growth factor in human endometrial cells. Biol Reprod 2002; 66: 1743–8.

37. Ivell R, Balvers M, Pohnke Y et al. Immunoexpression of the relaxin receptor LGR7 in breast and uterine tissues of humans and primates. Reprod Biol Endocrinol 2003; 1: 114.

38. Gravanis A, Stournaras C, Margioris AN. Paracrinology of endometrial neuropeptides: corticotropin-releasing hormone and opioids. Semin Reprod Endocrinol 1999; 17: 29–38.

39. Milne SA, Perchick GB, Boddy SC et al. Expression, localization, and signaling of PGE$_2$ and EP2/EP4 receptors in human nonpregnant endometrium across the menstrual cycle. J Clin Endocrinol Metab 2001; 86: 4453–9.

40. Wolkersdörfer GW, Bornstein SR, Hilbers U et al. The presence of chorionic gonadotrophin β subunit in normal cyclic human endometrium. Mol Hum Reprod 1998; 4: 179–84.

41. Kasahara K, Takakura K, Takebayashi K et al. The role of human chorionic gonadotropin on decidualization of endometrial

42. Mehats C, Andersen CB, Filopanti M et al. Cyclic nucleotide phosphodiesterases and their role in endocrine cell signaling. Trends Endocrinol Metab 2002; 13: 29–35.

43. Bartsch O, Bartlick B, Ivell R. Phosphodiesterase 4 inhibition synergizes with relaxin signaling to promote decidualization of human endometrial stromal cells. J Clin Endocrinol Metab 2004; 89: 324–34.

44. Skålhegg BS, Taskén K. Specificity in the cAMP/PKA signaling pathway, differential expression, regulation, and subcellular localization of subunits of PKA. Front Biosci 2000; 5: d678–93.

45. Mayr B, Montminy M. Transcriptional regulation by the phosphorylation-dependent factor CREB. Nat Rev Mol Cell Biol 2001; 2: 599–609.

46. Walker WH, Habener JF. Role of transcription factors CREB and CREM in cAMP-regulated transcription during spermatogenesis. Trends Endocrinol Metab 1996; 7: 133–8.

47. Gellersen B, Kempf R, Telgmann R. Human endometrial stromal cells express novel isoforms of the transcriptional modulator CREM and up-regulate ICER in the course of decidualization. Mol Endocrinol 1997; 11: 97–113.

48. Gellersen B, Kempf R, Sandhowe R et al. Novel leader exons of the cyclic adenosine 3′,5′-monophosphate response element modulator (CREM) gene, transcribed from promoters P3 and P4, are highly testis-specific in primates. Mol Hum Reprod 2002; 8: 965–76.

49. Molina CA, Foulkes NS, Lalli E et al. Inducibility and negative autoregulation of CREM: an alternative promoter directs the expression of ICER, an early response repressor. Cell 1993; 75: 875–86.

50. Foulkes NS, Borjigin J, Snyder SH et al. Transcriptional control of circadian hormone synthesis via the CREM feedback loop. Proc Natl Acad Sci USA 1996; 93: 14140–5.

51. Dimitriadis E, Stoikos C, Baca M et al. Relaxin and prostaglandin E$_2$ regulate interleukin 11 during human endometrial stromal cell decidualization. J Clin Endocrinol Metab 2005; 90: 3458–65.

52. Karpovich N, Klemmt P, Hwang JH et al. The production of interleukin-11 and decidualization are compromised in endometrial stromal cells derived from patients with infertility. J Clin Endocrinol Metab 2005; 90: 1607–12.

53. Karpovich N, Chobotova K, Carver J et al. Expression and function of interleukin-11 and its receptor α in the human endometrium. Mol Hum Reprod 2003; 9: 75–80.

54. Robb L, Li R, Hartley L et al. Infertility in female mice lacking the receptor for interleukin 11 is due to a defective uterine response to implantation. Nat Med 1998; 4: 303–8.

55. Bilinski P, Roopenian D, Gossler A. Maternal IL-11Rα function is required for normal decidua and fetoplacental development in mice. Genes Dev 1998; 12: 2234–43.

56. Chobotova K, Karpovich N, Carver J et al. Heparin-binding epidermal growth factor and its receptors mediate decidualization and potentiate survival of human endometrial stromal cells. J Clin Endocrinol Metab 2005; 90: 913–19.

57. Jones RL, Salamonsen LA, Findlay JK. Potential roles for endometrial inhibins, activins and follistatin during human embryo implantation and early pregnancy. Trends Endocrinol Metab 2002; 13: 144–50.

58. Kothapalli R, Buyuksal I, Wu SQ et al. Detection of ebaf, a novel human gene of the transforming growth factor β superfamily – association of gene expression with endometrial bleeding. J Clin Invest 1997; 99: 2342–50.

59. Green VL, Richmond I, Maguiness S et al. Somatostatin receptor 2 expression in the human endometrium through the menstrual cycle. Clin Endocrinol (Oxf) 2002; 56: 609–14.

60. Gellersen B, Kempf R, Telgmann R et al. Nonpituitary human prolactin gene transcription is independent of Pit-1 and

stromal cells in vitro. J Clin Endocrinol Metab 2001; 86: 1281–6.

differentially controlled in lymphocytes and in endometrial stroma. Mol Endocrinol 1994; 8: 356–73.

61. Berwaer M, Martial JA, Davis JRE. Characterization of an upstream promoter directing extrapituitary expression of the human prolactin gene. Mol Endocrinol 1994; 8: 635–42.

62. DiMattia GE, Gellersen B, Duckworth ML et al. Human prolactin gene expression. The use of an alternative noncoding exon in decidua and the IM-9-P3 lymphoblast cell line. J Biol Chem 1990; 265: 16412–21.

63. Brunet A, Bonni A, Zigmond MJ et al. Akt promotes cell survival by phosphorylating and inhibiting a Forkhead transcription factor. Cell 1999; 96: 857–68.

64. Kops GJ, de Ruiter ND, De Vries-Smits AM et al. Direct control of the Forkhead transcription factor AFX by protein kinase B. Nature 1999; 398: 630–4.

65. Patterson GI. Aging: new targets, new functions. Curr Biol 2003; 13: R279–81.

66. Accili D, Arden KC. FoxOs at the crossroads of cellular metabolism, differentiation, and transformation. Cell 2004; 117: 421–6.

67. Christian M, Zhang X, Schneider-Merck T et al. Cyclic AMP-induced forkhead transcription factor, FKHR, cooperates with CCAAT/enhancer-binding protein β in differentiating human endometrial stromal cells. J Biol Chem 2002; 277: 20825–32.

68. Kim JJ, Buzzio OL, Li S et al. Role of FOXO1A in the regulation of insulin-like growth factor-binding protein-1 in human endometrial cells: interaction with progesterone receptor. Biol Reprod 2005; 73: 833–9.

69. Kim JJ, Taylor HS, Akbas GE et al. Regulation of insulin-like growth factor binding protein-1 promoter activity by FKHR and HOXA10 in primate endometrial cells. Biol Reprod 2003; 68: 24–30.

70. Labied S, Kajihara T, Madureira PA et al. Progestins regulate the expression and activity of the Forkhead transcription factor FOXO1 in differentiating human endometrium. Mol Endocrinol 2006; 20: 35–44.

71. Darnell JE Jr. STATs and gene regulation. Science 1997; 277: 1630–5.

72. Mak IY, Brosens JJ, Christian M et al. Regulated expression of signal transducer and activator of transcription, Stat5, and its enhancement of PRL expression in human endometrial stromal cells in vitro. J Clin Endocrinol Metab 2002; 87: 2581–8.

73. Jabbour HN, Critchley HOD, Boddy SC. Expression of functional prolactin receptors in nonpregnant human endometrium: Janus kinase-2, signal transducer and activator of transcription-1 (STAT1), and STAT5 proteins are phosphorylated after stimulation with prolactin. J Clin Endocrinol Metab 1998; 83: 2545–53.

74. Barkai U, Prigent-Tessier A, Tessier C et al. Involvement of SOCS-1, the suppressor of cytokine signaling, in the prevention of prolactin-responsive gene expression in decidual cells. Mol Endocrinol 2000; 14: 554–63.

75. Ramji DP, Foka P. CCAAT/enhancer-binding proteins: structure, function and regulation. Biochem J 2002; 365: 561–75.

76. Robinson GW, Johnson PF, Hennighausen L et al. The C/EBPβ transcription factor regulates epithelial cell proliferation and differentiation in the mammary gland. Genes Dev 1998; 12: 1907–16.

77. Seagroves TN, Krnacik S, Raught B, et al. C/EBPβ, but not C/EBPα, is essential for ductal morphogenesis, lobuloalveolar proliferation, and functional differentiation in the mouse mammary gland. Genes Dev 1998; 12: 1917–28.

78. Sterneck E, Tessarollo L, Johnson PF. An essential role for C/EBPβ in female reproduction. Genes Dev 1997; 11: 2153–62.

79. Pohnke Y, Kempf R, Gellersen B. CCAAT/enhancer-binding proteins are mediators in the protein kinase A-dependent activation of the decidual prolactin gene. J Biol Chem 1999; 274: 24808–18.

80. Descombes P, Schibler U. A liver-enriched transcriptional activator protein, LAP, and a transcriptional inhibitory protein, LIP, are translated from the same mRNA. Cell 1991; 67: 569–79.

81. Salmi A, Ammala M, Rutanen EM. Proto-oncogenes c-jun and c-fos are down-regulated in human endometrium during pregnancy: relationship to oestrogen receptor status. Mol Hum Reprod 1996; 2: 979–84.

82. Watanabe K, Kessler CA, Bachurski CJ et al. Identification of a decidua-specific enhancer on the human prolactin gene with two critical activator protein 1 (AP-1) binding sites. Mol Endocrinol 2001; 15: 638–53.

83. Brar AK, Kessler CA, Handwerger S. An Ets motif in the proximal decidual prolactin promoter is essential for basal gene expression. J Mol Endocrinol 2002; 29: 99–112.

84. Favier B, Dollé P. Developmental functions of mammalian Hox genes. Mol Hum Reprod 1997; 3: 115–31.

85. Taylor HS, Vanden Heuvel GB, Igarashi P. A conserved Hox axis in the mouse and human female reproductive system: late establishment and persistent adult expression of the Hoxa cluster genes. Biol Reprod 1997; 57: 1338–45.

86. Satokata I, Benson G, Maas R. Sexually dimorphic sterility phenotypes in Hoxa10-deficient mice. Nature 1995; 374: 460–3.

87. Hsieh-Li HM, Witte DP, Weinstein M et al. Hoxa 11 structure, extensive antisense transcription, and function in male and female fertility. Development 1995; 121: 1373–85.

88. Gendron RL, Paradis H, Hsieh-Li HM et al. Abnormal uterine stromal and glandular function associated with maternal reproductive defects in Hoxa-11 null mice. Biol Reprod 1997; 56: 1097–105.

89. Lim HJ, Ma L, Ma WG et al. Hoxa-10 regulates uterine stromal cell responsiveness to progesterone during implantation and decidualization in the mouse. Mol Endocrinol 1999; 13: 1005–17.

90. Kwon HE, Taylor HS. The role of HOX genes in human implantation. Ann NY Acad Sci 2004; 1034: 1–18.

91. Taylor HS, Arici A, Olive D et al. HOXA10 is expressed in response to sex steroids at the time of implantation in the human endometrium. J Clin Invest 1998; 101: 1379–84.

92. Gui YT, Zhang JN, Yuan LW et al. Regulation of HOXA-10 and its expression in normal and abnormal endometrium. Mol Hum Reprod 1999; 5: 866–73.

93. Qian K, Chen H, Wei Y et al. Differentiation of endometrial stromal cells in vitro: down-regulation of suppression of the cell cycle inhibitor p57 by HOXA10? Mol Hum Reprod 2005; 11: 245–51.

94. Krikun G, Lockwood CJ. Steroid hormones, endometrial gene regulation and the Sp1 family of proteins. J Soc Gynecol Investig 2002; 9: 329–34.

95. Krikun G, Schatz F, Mackman N et al. Regulation of tissue factor gene expression in human endometrium by transcription factors Sp1 and Sp3. Mol Endocrinol 2000; 14: 393–400.

96. Miller LD, Smeds J, George J et al. An expression signature for p53 status in human breast cancer predicts mutation status, transcriptional effects, and patient survival. Proc Natl Acad Sci USA 2005; 102: 13550–5.

97. Mirza A, Wu Q, Wang L et al. Global transcriptional program of p53 target genes during the process of apoptosis and cell cycle progression. Oncogene 2003; 22: 3645–54.

98. Vogelstein B, Lane D, Levine AJ. Surfing the p53 network. Nature 2000; 408: 307–10.

99. Ko LJ, Prives C. p53: puzzle and paradigm. Genes Dev 1996; 10: 1054–72.

100. Ryan KM, Phillips AC, Vousden KH. Regulation and function of the p53 tumor suppressor protein. Curr Opin Cell Biol 2001; 13: 332–7.

101. Pohnke Y, Schneider-Merck T, Fahnenstich J et al. Wild-type p53 protein is up-regulated upon cyclic AMP-induced differentiation of human endometrial stromal cells. J Clin Endocrinol Metab 2004; 89: 5233–44.

102. Zerbini LF, Libermann TA. Life and death in cancer. GADD45α and γ are critical regulators of NF-κB mediated escape from programmed cell death. Cell Cycle 2005; 4: 18–20.

103. Ulloa L, Creemers JW, Roy S et al. Lefty proteins exhibit unique processing and activate the MAPK pathway. J Biol Chem 2001; 276: 21387–96.

104. Feng XH, Derynck R. Specificity and versatility in TGF-signaling through Smads. Annu Rev Cell Dev Biol 2005; 21: 659–93.

105. Luo X, Xu J, Chegini N. The expression of Smads in human endometrium and regulation and induction in endometrial epithelial and stromal cells by transforming growth factor-β. J Clin Endocrinol Metab 2003; 88: 4967–76.

106. Makrigiannakis A, Coukos G, Mantani A et al. Expression of Wilms' tumor suppressor gene (WT1) in human endometrium: regulation through decidual differentiation. J Clin Endocrinol Metab 2001; 86: 5964–72.

107. Norman AW, Mizwicki MT, Norman DPG. Steroid-hormone rapid actions, membrane receptors and a conformational ensemble model. Nat Rev Drug Discov 2004; 3: 27–41.

108. Graham JD, Clarke CL. Physiological action of progesterone in target tissues. Endocr Rev 1997; 18: 502–19.

109. Kastner P, Krust A, Turcotte B et al. Two distinct estrogen-regulated promoters generate transcripts encoding the two functionally different human progesterone receptor forms A and B. EMBO J 1990; 9: 1603–14.

110. Brosens JJ, Tullet J, Varshochi R et al. Steroid receptor action. Best Pract Res Clin Obstet Gynaecol 2004; 18: 265–83.

111. Sartorius CA, Melville MY, Hovland AR et al. A third transactivation function (AF3) of human progesterone receptors located in the unique N-terminal segment of the B-isoform. Mol Endocrinol 1994; 8: 1347–60.

112. Meyer ME, Quirin-Stricker C, Lerouge T et al. A limiting factor mediates the differential activation of promoters by the human progesterone receptor isoforms. J Biol Chem 1992; 267: 10882–7.

113. Hovland AR, Powell RL, Takimoto GS et al. An N-terminal inhibitory function, IF, suppresses transcription by the A-isoform but not the B-isoform of human progesterone receptors. J Biol Chem 1998; 273: 5455–60.

114. Chen H, Lin RJ, Xie W et al. Regulation of hormone-induced histone hyperacetylation and gene activation via acetylation of an acetylase. Cell 1999; 98: 675–86.

115. Wardell SE, Boonyaratanakornkit V, Adelman JS et al. Jun dimerization protein 2 functions as a progesterone receptor N-terminal domain coactivator. Mol Cell Biol 2002; 22: 5451–66.

116. Giangrande PH, Kimbrel EA, Edwards DP et al. The opposing transcriptional activities of the two isoforms of the human progesterone receptor are due to differential cofactor binding. Mol Cell Biol 2000; 20: 3102–15.

117. Xu J, Qiu Y, DeMayo FJ et al. Partial hormone resistance in mice with disruption of the steroid receptor coactivator-1 (SRC-1) gene. Science 1998; 279: 1922–5.

118. Brosens JJ, Hayashi N, White JO. Progesterone receptor regulates decidual prolactin expression in differentiating human endometrial stromal cells. Endocrinology 1999; 140: 4809–20.

119. Boonyaratanakornkit V, Scott MP, Ribon V et al. Progesterone receptor contains a proline-rich motif that directly interacts with SH3 domains and activates c-Src family tyrosine kinases. Mol Cell 2001; 8: 269–80.

120. Leonhardt SA, Boonyaratanakornkit V, Edwards DP. Progesterone receptor transcription and non-transcription signaling mechanisms. Steroids 2003; 68: 761–70.

121. Lange CA. Making sense of cross-talk between steroid hormone receptors and intracellular signaling pathways: Who will have the last word? Mol Endocrinol 2004; 18: 269–78.

122. Zhu Y, Bond J, Thomas P. Identification, classification, and partial characterization of genes in humans and other vertebrates homologous to a fish membrane progestin receptor. Proc Natl Acad Sci USA 2003; 100: 2237–42.

123. Zhu Y, Rice CD, Pang Y et al. Cloning, expression, and characterization of a membrane progestin receptor and evidence it is an intermediary in meiotic maturation of fish oocytes. Proc Natl Acad Sci USA 2003; 100: 2231–6.

124. Fernandes MS, Pierron V, Michalovich D et al. Regulated expression of putative membrane progestin receptor homologues in human endometrium and gestational tissues. J Endocrinol 2005; 187: 89–101.

125. Gerdes D, Wehling M, Leube B et al. Cloning and tissue expression of two putative steroid membrane receptors. Biol Chem 1998; 379: 907–11.

126. Lösel RM, Falkenstein E, Feuring M et al. Nongenomic steroid action: controversies, questions, and answers. Physiol Rev 2003; 83: 965–1016.

127. Peluso J, Pappalardo A, Lösel R et al. Expression and function of PAIRBP1 within gonadotropin-primed immature rat ovaries: PAIRBP1 regulation of granulosa cell and luteal cell viability. Biol Reprod 2005; 73: 261–70.

128. Watanabe H, Nonoguchi K, Sakurai T et al. A novel protein Depp, which is induced by progesterone in human endometrial stromal cells activates Elk-1 transcription factor. Mol Hum Reprod 2005; 11: 471–6.

129. Shaknovich R, Yeyati PL, Ivins S et al. The promyelocytic leukemia zinc finger protein affects myeloid cell growth, differentiation, and apoptosis. Mol Cell Biol 1998; 18: 5533–45.

130. Fahnenstich J, Nandy A, Milde-Langosch K et al. Promyelocytic leukaemia zinc finger protein (PLZF) is a glucocorticoid- and progesterone-induced transcription factor in human endometrial stromal cells and myometrial smooth muscle cells. Mol Hum Reprod 2003; 9: 611–23.

131. Jiang F, Wang Z. Identification and characterization of PLZF as a prostatic androgen-responsive gene. Prostate 2004; 59: 426–35.

132. Buaas FW, Kirsh AL, Sharma M et al. Plzf is required in adult male germ cells for stem cell self-renewal. Nat Genet 2004; 36: 647–52.

133. Costoya JA, Hobbs RN, Barna M et al. Essential role of Plzf in maintenance of spermatogonial stem cells. Nat Genet 2004; 36: 551–3.

134. Parrado A, Robledo M, Moya-Quiles MR et al. The promyelocytic leukemia zinc finger protein down-regulates apoptosis and expression of the proapoptotic BID protein in lymphocytes. Proc Natl Acad Sci USA 2004; 101: 1898–903.

135. Yeyati PL, Shaknovich R, Boterashvili S et al. Leukemia translocation protein PLZF inhibits cell growth and expression of cyclin A. Oncogene 1999; 18: 925–34.

136. Nanba D, Mammoto A, Hashimoto K et al. Proteolytic release of the carboxy-terminal fragment of proHB-EGF causes nuclear export of PLZF. J Cell Biol 2003; 163: 489–502.

137. Wang H, Critchley HOD, Kelly RW et al. Progesterone receptor subtype B is differentially regulated in human endometrial stroma. Mol Hum Reprod 1998; 4: 407–12.

138. Mote PA, Balleine RL, McGowan EM et al. Colocalization of progesterone receptors A and B by dual immunofluorescent histochemistry in human endometrium during the menstrual cycle. J Clin Endocrinol Metab 1999; 84: 2963–71.

139. Mulac-Jericevic B, Conneely OM. Reproductive tissue-selective actions of progesterone receptors. Reproduction 2004; 128: 139–46.

140. Faivre E, Skildum A, Pierson-Mullany L et al. Integration of progesterone receptor mediated rapid signaling and nuclear actions in breast cancer cell models: role of mitogen-activated

protein kinases and cell cycle regulators. Steroids 2005; 70: 418–26.

141. Proietti C, Salatino M, Rosemblit C et al. Progestins induce transcriptional activation of signal transducer and activator of transcription 3 (Stat3) via a Jak- and Src-dependent mechanism in breast cancer cells. Mol Cell Biol 2005; 25: 4826–40.

142. Catalano RD, Yanaihara A, Evans AL et al. The effect of RU486 on the gene expression profile in an endometrial explant model. Mol Hum Reprod 2003; 9: 465–73.

143. Maruyama T, Yoshimura Y, Yodoi J et al. Activation of c-Src kinase is associated with in vitro decidualization of human endometrial stromal cells. Endocrinology 1999; 140: 2632–6.

144. Yamamoto Y, Maruyama T, Sakai N et al. Expression and subcellular distribution of the active form of c-Src tyrosine kinase in differentiating human endometrial stromal cells. Mol Hum Reprod 2002; 8: 1117–24.

145. Shimizu A, Maruyama T, Tamaki K et al. Impairment of decidualization in SRC-deficient mice. Biol Reprod 2005; 73: 1219–27.

146. Shattil SJ. Integrins and Src: dynamic duo of adhesion signaling. Trends Cell Biol 2005; 15: 399–403.

147. Harada M, Osuga Y, Takemura Y et al. Mechanical stretch upregulates IGFBP-1 secretion from decidualized endometrial stromal cells. Am J Physiol Endocrinol Metab 2006; 290: E268–72.

148. Christian M, Pohnke Y, Kempf R et al. Functional association of PR and CCAAT/enhancer-binding protein β isoforms: promoter-dependent cooperation between PR-B and liver-enriched inhibitory protein, or liver-enriched activatory protein and PR-A in human endometrial stromal cells. Mol Endocrinol 2002; 16: 141–54.

149. Gao J, Mazella J, Tang M et al. Ligand-activated progesterone receptor isoform hPR-A is a stronger transactivator than hPR-B for the expression of IGFBP-1 (insulin-like growth factor binding protein-1) in human endometrial stromal cells. Mol Endocrinol 2000; 14: 1954–61.

150. Tseng L, Tang M, Wang Z et al. Progesterone receptor (hPR) upregulates the fibronectin promoter activity in human decidual fibroblasts. DNA Cell Biol 2003; 22: 633–40.

151. Kalkhoven E, Wissink S, van der Saag PT et al. Negative interaction between the RelA(p65) subunit of NF-κB and the progesterone receptor. J Biol Chem 1996; 271: 6217–24.

152. Red-Horse K, Zhou Y, Genbacev O et al. Trophoblast differentiation during embryo implantation and formation of the maternal–fetal interface. J Clin Invest 2004; 114: 744–54.

153. Richer JK, Lange CA, Manning NG et al. Convergence of progesterone with growth factor and cytokine signaling in breast cancer. Progesterone receptors regulate signal transducers and activators of transcription expression and activity. J Biol Chem 1998; 273: 31317–26.

154. Owen GI, Richer JK, Tung L et al. Progesterone regulates transcription of the p21^WAF1 cyclin-dependent kinase inhibitor gene through Sp1 and CBP/p300. J Biol Chem 1998; 273: 10696–701.

155. Too CK. Induction of Sp1 activity by prolactin and interleukin-2 in Nb2 T-cells: differential association of Sp1–DNA complexes with Stats. Mol Cell Endocrinol 1997; 129: 7–16.

156. Lee YH, Yano M, Liu SY et al. A novel cis-acting element controlling the rat CYP2D5 gene and requiring cooperativity between C/EBPβ and an Sp1 factor. Mol Cell Biol 1994; 14: 1383–94.

157. Schneider-Merck T, Pohnke Y, Kempf R et al. Physical interaction and mutual transrepression between CCAAT/enhancer-binding protein β (C/EBPβ) and the p53 tumor suppressor. J Biol Chem 2006; 281: 269–78.

158. Ohlsson C, Kley N, Werner H et al. p53 regulates insulin-like growth factor-I (IGF-I) receptor expression and IGF-I-induced tyrosine phosphorylation in an osteosarcoma cell line: interaction between p53 and Sp1. Endocrinology 1998; 139: 1101–7.

26 Human endometrial hemostasis during the menstrual cycle and gestation

Charles J Lockwood, Graciela Krikun, and Frederick Schatz

REGULATION OF ENDOMETRIAL HEMOSTASIS DURING THE MENSTRUAL CYCLE: THE CRUCIAL ROLE OF DECIDUALIZED STROMAL CELLS

During a woman's reproductive years, the concerted effects of ovarian-derived estradiol (E_2) and progesterone regulate the cyclical changes in the functional endometrial layer that prepare it to receive the implanting blastocyst. In the absence of implantation, the endometrium is sloughed off in the menstrual fluid. Restoration of the endometrium begins in the follicular phase of the next cycle as rising circulating E_2 levels initiate cell proliferation. In the postovulatory period, rising circulating progesterone levels stimulate the E_2-primed endometrial cells together with a second peak of E_2 to stop proliferation and initiate differentiation. Consequently, the glands become tortuous and secrete an array of products that markedly influence the uterine milieu encountered by the implanting blastocyst. The stromal cells undergo decidualization. This process represents the sum total of morphological and biochemical changes that transform precursor stromal cells into decidual cells. The decidualization reaction is initiated around blood vessels and under the glands.[1] Continued stimulation by E_2 and progesterone induces the spread of decidualization throughout the luteal phase and gestational endometrium.[2] An integral component of decidualization is a marked alteration in the expression of proteins that promote hemostasis and enhance vascular stability.

TISSUE FACTOR EXPRESSION BY DECIDUALIZED STROMAL CELLS

TF is the physiological initiator of hemostasis

A member of the class-2 cytokine receptor family, tissue factor (TF) is a cell membrane-bound glycoprotein composed of a hydrophilic extracellular domain, a membrane-spanning hydrophobic domain, and a cytoplasmic tail. Binding of circulating factor VII or its active form VIIa to perivascular cell-bound TF[3] initiates a complex series of proteolytic changes that result in the formation of thrombin from prothrombin and the cleavage of fibrinogen to generate the fibrin clot.[3] The essential role played by TF in preventing bleeding was demonstrated in embryonic lethal TF knockout mice, which develop fragile vessels and die of hemorrhage in utero.[4] Incorporation of the human TF minigene expressed at only 1% of its wild-type level was sufficient to rescue the knockout mice and produce live pups, whereas 40% of pregnancies in which both the mother and the fetus were homozygous low TF expressors experienced intrauterine hemorrhage and intraplacental 'blood pools' in the labyrinth.[5]

Studies of TF expression in human endometrium

Use of in-situ hybridization and immunohistochemistry in human endometrial sections obtained across the menstrual cycle localized elevated levels of TF mRNA and protein to decidualized stromal cells during the mid–late luteal phases.[6–8] The regulation of TF expression was assessed in confluent stromal cell monolayers derived from specimens of predecidualized human endometrium. Figure 26.1 indicates that medroxyprogesterone acetate (MPA) enhanced immunoreactive TF levels in the cell lysates of these cultures. While the stromal cells were unresponsive to E_2 alone, E_2+MPA elicited even greater up-regulation of TF levels.[9] These differential ovarian steroid actions in vitro mimic in-vivo effects in which E_2 primes the endometrium for progesterone-induced decidualization.[10] Figure 26.1 also demonstrates that E_2+MPA, but not MPA alone, significantly elevated TF levels for at least 3 weeks.[9] These observations underscore the relevance of the in-vitro decidualization model for studying TF expression in vivo, since circulating levels of E_2 and progesterone as well as TF expressed by decidualized stromal cells are elevated throughout the luteal phase and gestation. The TF moiety measured by ELISA (enzyme-linked immunosorbent assay) in

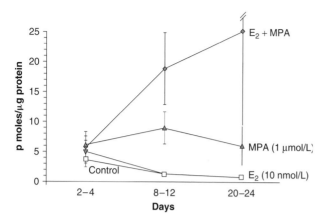

Figure 26.1 Time course of TF induction in human endometrial stromal cells response to estradiol (E₂), medroxyprogesterone acetate (MPA), or E₂ + MPA. Confluent human endometrial stromal cells were incubated in medium containing serum with vehicle control, 10 nmol/L E₂, 1 μmol/L MPA, or E₂+MPA for 2–24 days. Immunoreactive tissue factor content was normalized to the level of culture protein (mean ± SEM for cultures derived from 8 patient specimens; 5 from the proliferative and 3 from the secretory phases). (Reprinted from Lockwood et al,[9] with permission. Copyright 1993, The Endocrine Society.)

the in-vitro decidualized stromal cells proved to be functionally active, as measured by a two-step clotting assay, and to migrate with the mobility of authentic TF, as demonstrated by Western blotting. Additionally, Northern blotting found that changes in steady-state mRNA levels corresponded to those of the TF protein.[6,8]

Prolonged progestin induction of TF mRNA and protein levels in cultured human endometrial stromal cells (HESCs) contrasts with the transient enhancement of TF expression by growth factors, cytokines, and glucocorticoids reported in several cell types in which TF mRNA levels are increased for only a few hours and TF protein levels are generally increased for less than 24 hours.[11] In other cell types, TF is transcriptionally regulated either by activating protein 1 (AP-1), or nuclear factor κB (NF-κB), or early-growth response factor-1 (Egr-1), or the Sp transcription family on the TF gene promoter.[11] However, in HESC monolayers, transient transfections of TF promoter constructs containing overlapping SP and Egr-1 binding sites, or with these sites systematically inactivated by site-directed mutagenesis, or with SP1 overexpressing vectors alone and with a specific blocker of Sp1 binding determined that SP1 mediated basal as well as progestin-enhanced TF transcriptional activity.[12] This conclusion was confirmed by immunostaining of human endometrial sections and cultured stromal cells, which demonstrated that progestin-regulated decidualization in vitro and in vivo involves an increase in the ratio of Sp1 to its Sp3 antagonist.[13]

In monolayers of HESCs, interactions between progestin and epidermal growth factor (EGF) induce proliferation and expression of the decidualization markers prolactin, laminin, and fibronectin,[14] suggesting a role for EGF in progestin-enhanced TF expression in these cells. In confirmation of such an involvement, we observed that immunostaining for the EGF receptor (EGFR) in stromal cells of cycling human endometrium paralleled that previously described for TF.[6–8] Thus, EGFR staining was diffuse in follicular phase HESCs and was more prominent in correspondence with the spread of decidualization in mid–late luteal phase specimens.[15] Levels of EGFR in cultured HESCs changed in accordance with these in-vivo changes. Specifically, Western blotting indicated that EGFR protein levels increased by about three-fold after progestin-induced decidualization of the stromal cells.[16] These in-vitro observations in the stromal cells are consistent with higher EGFR levels reported in endometrial extracts from the progesterone-dominated luteal vs follicular phase.[17] Assessment of EGFR–progestin interactions in regulating TF expression in the stromal cells revealed that augmentation of TF protein and mRNA levels required co-incubation with MPA and an EGFR agonist such as EGF or transforming growth factor α (TGFα).[16]

TISSUE-TYPE PLASMINOGEN ACTIVATOR AND PLASMINOGEN ACTIVATOR INHIBITOR TYPE I EXPRESSION BY DECIDUALIZED STROMAL CELLS

The ratio of tPA to PAI-1 is a crucial determinant of the local hemostatic milieu

While perivascular cell membrane-expressed TF promotes hemostasis via thrombin generation and subsequent fibrin clot formation,[3] this function is kept in check by the activity of tissue-type plasminogen activator (tPA). Specifically, tPA acts as the primary fibrinolytic agent vis-à-vis high-affinity binding of tPA to fibrin where it forms plasmin by cleaving Arg[560]–Val[561] in its preferred substrate, plasminogen. Plasmin is a broad-spectrum serine protease that effectively degrades fibrin.[18] However, the activity of tPA is regulated by its fast inactivator, plasminogen activator inhibitor type 1 (PAI-1).[19]

Studies of tPA and PAI-1 expression in human endometrium

In human endometrial sections across the menstrual cycle, immunoreactive and catalytically active tPA levels

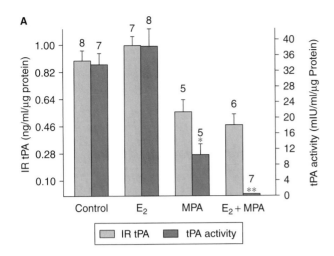

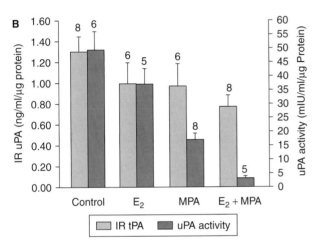

Figure 26.2 Regulation of tissue-type plasminogen activator (tPA) and urokinase-type plasminogen activator (uPA) immunogenic levels vs activity levels in human endometrial stromal cells in response to estradiol (E_2), medroxy progesterone acetate (MPA), or E_2+MPA. Effects of steroids on levels of immunogenic (▨) and catalytic (■) tPA (**A**) and pro-uPA (**B**) in conditioned medium. Individual dishes of confluent cultures were incubated for 3 days in either vehicle control, 10 nmol/L E_2, 100 nmol/L MPA, or E_2+MPA. Specific ELISAs (enzyme-linked immunosorbent assays) were used to measure secreted levels of tPA and uPA antigens; the chromogenic assay was used to measure tPA and uPA activities. Results were normalized to total cell protein. Statistical significance was determined by one-way ANOVA. *, $p < 0.05$; **, $p < 0.005$ (compared to control). (Reprinted from Schatz et al,[21] with permission. Copyright 1995, The Endocrine Society.)

were found to be higher in the late luteal phase compared with either the follicular or early luteal phases. However, we[7] and others[20] also observed elevated PAI-1 levels in endometrial biopsies from the late luteal phase vs biopsies obtained earlier in the menstrual cycle.

Evaluation of the effects of ovarian steroids on tPA and PAI-1 expression in monolayers of HESCs revealed that these proteins are reciprocally regulated in

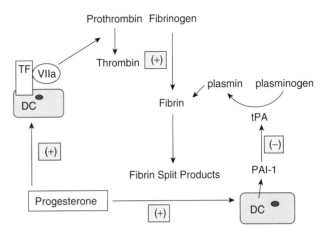

Figure 26.3 Progesterone promotes hemostasis in human endometrium. Following ovulation, progesterone acts on the E_2-primed endometrium to transform stromal cells to decidual cells (DC). Tissue factor (TF) expressed on the DC surface acts as a cofactor for factor VII or its active form VIIa. VIIa promotes cleavage of prothrombin to thrombin. Thrombin cleaves plasma-derived fibrinogen to form the fibrin clot and promote hemostasis. The expression of tissue-type plasminogen activator (tPA), which degrades the fibrin clot via plasmin formation, is inhibited by DC-expressed plasminogen activator inhibitor type 1 (PAI-1).

a decidualization-related manner. Figure 26.2A indicates that MPA lowered HESC-secreted tPA levels as measured by ELISA.[21] Although the cultures were unresponsive to E_2 alone, co-incubation with E_2+MPA greatly augmented this inhibition. Figure 26.2A also demonstrates that MPA preferentially reduced levels of tPA catalytic activity vs immunoreactive (IR) tPA protein levels. This differential inhibition was most pronounced during incubations with E_2+MPA with the conditioned medium containing high IR tPA levels, but barely detectable tPA activity. By contrast, ELISA results indicated that secreted PAI-1 levels were up-regulated by MPA. Incubations with E_2+MPA elicited much greater up-regulation despite an absence of response to E_2 alone.[21] Western blotting confirmed the tPA and PAI-1 ELISA results, and Northern blotting revealed that steady-state PAI-1 mRNA levels were also increased by MPA and further increased by E_2+MPA.[21,22] These changes were specific for PAI-1, since only minute quantities of the potent PA inhibitor PAI-2 were present in the stromal cell conditioned medium under basal conditions or after the addition of steroids.[21] In incubations with E_2+MPA, reciprocal down-regulation of tPA and up-regulation of PAI-1 output produced a marked molar excess of the latter in the conditioned medium.[21] Therefore, preferential inhibition of tPA activity reflects elevated PAI-1 output. Extrapolation of these in-vitro results to the luteal phase endometrium suggests that PAI-1 and TF are key determinants of endometrial hemostasis. The model depicted in Figure 26.3 indicates that progesterone-induced decidualization plays a key role in controlling endometrial hemostasis by modulating TF, tPA, and PAI-1 interactions during the luteal phase of the menstrual cycle.

TURNOVER OF THE EXTRACELLULAR MATRIX REGULATES VASCULAR STABILITY DURING THE MENSTRUAL CYCLE

The role of protease expression by decidualized stromal cells in determining vascular stability

The decidualization reaction is accompanied by a profound and unique change in the composition of the extracellular matrix (ECM). Specifically, the follicular phase endometrial stromal ECM, which is dominated by the presence of fibronectin and collagen types I, III, V, and VI, is converted to a mixture of residual interstitial proteins and new peridecidual basal laminar type components. The latter, which include laminin, heparin sulfate proteoglycan, and collagen type IV, are generally localized to the basement membrane under epithelial cells and are associated with endothelial cells.[23,24] The resulting peridecidual cell ECM modulates trophoblast migration and invasion and mitigates the occurrence of local hemorrhage during endovascular trophoblast invasion by serving as a vascular support and stabilizing scaffolding structure. Transformation of the peridecidual ECM involves the reciprocal synthesis of new proteins and inhibition of proteases that degrade these proteins.

The role of urokinase-type plasminogen activator in regulating turnover of the endometrial extracellular matrix

The urokinase-type plasminogen activator (uPA) is secreted as single-chain pro-uPA. Binding of catalytically inactive pro-uPA to its receptor (uPAR) on the cell surface of cancer cells,[25] trophoblasts,[26] and stromal and decidual cells from cycling and gestational endometrium[27] promotes its conversion to catalytically active double-chain uPA.[19] The latter cleaves plasminogen to plasmin, as described above for tPA. Although plasmin can degrade several ECM proteins directly,[28] it affects ECM degradation primarily by activating the secreted, zymogenic form of matrix metalloproteinases (MMPs), which then degrade the bulk of ECM components.[29]

Studies of uPA and PAI-1 expression in human endometrium

Figure 26.2B illustrates that the pattern of HESC-secreted uPA levels elicited by the addition of steroids was similar to that described for tPA in Figure 26.2A. Specifically, MPA preferentially inhibited secreted levels of catalytically active vs IR uPA with even greater inhibition evident in cultures incubated with $E_2 + MPA$ despite the lack of response to E_2. As is the case for tPA, preferential inhibition of uPA activity is attributable to reciprocal up-regulation of PAI-1, since PAI-1 levels in the culture medium greatly exceeded uPA levels. Previously, progestin was reported to reciprocally up-regulate PAI-1 and down-regulate uPA expression in monolayers of human endometrial stromal cells.[30,31] As is the case with the in-vitro results for tPA shown in Figure 26.2A, the preferential progestin-induced inhibition of uPA activity versus IR uPA levels can be attributed to selective elevation of PAI-1 and is also consistent with the higher IR PAI-1 levels observed in the luteal than in the follicular phase of the menstrual cycle.[7,20]

The role of matrix metalloproteinases in regulating turnover of the endometrial ECM

Despite considerable overlap among the MMPs in their ECM substrate profiles, MMP family members are generally classified on the basis of substrate specificity as collagenases, stromelysins, or gelatinases. Collagenases degrade fibrillar collagens. This class of MMPs is exemplified by interstitial collagenase (MMP-1), which mediates a specific cleavage in the helical structure of fibrillar collagens required for subsequent denaturing to gelatins by other MMPs.[29] Stromelysins degrade the broadest array of ECM components, including proteoglycans, glycoproteins, fibronectin, laminin, type IV and V collagen, both the non-helical amino- and carboxyl-terminal peptides of type II collagen as well as the globular, but not the triple helical regions, of interstitial collagens.[29,32] This class is exemplified by stromelysin 1 (MMP-3), which has the unique capacity of activating the secreted, zymogenic forms of interstitial collagenase (MMP-1), gelatinase B (MMP-9), and collagenase 3 (MMP-13).[32] This versatility places MMP-3 at the focus of an ECM-degrading proteolytic cascade. Gelatinases degrade basement membrane-associated collagens as well as denatured fibrillar collagens (gelatins).[29] Gelatinase A (MMP-2) is unique among the MMPs in that its gene promoter lacks response elements for growth factors, cytokines, reactive oxygen species, and steroids.[33] Instead, the activity of MMP-2 is regulated primarily by activation of pro-MMP-2 via the involvement of membrane type 1 MMP (MT1-MMP),[34,35] and in some cell systems, by transforming growth factor β (TGFβ).[36]

Studies of MMPs in human endometrium

In-situ hybridization measurements in human endometrial sections across the menstrual cycle revealed that mRNA levels of MMP-1 and MMP-3 were markedly lower in the stromal compartment during the progesterone-dominated luteal phase. Both MMP-1 and MMP-3 mRNA levels were increased in correspondence with the steroid withdrawal-initiated menstrual phase. By contrast, MMP-2 mRNA levels, as well as those of the tissue inhibitor of matrix metalloproteinase 1 (TIMP-1), were relatively unchanged.[37] In confluent monolayers of HESCs, addition of E_2, MPA, or E_2+MPA produced a pattern of MMP-1 and MMP-3 mRNA expression that was similar to that shown for tPA and uPA in Figures 26.2A and 26.2B, respectively. Specifically, MPA reduced MMP-1 and MMP-3 mRNA and protein levels, with greater inhibition observed during co-incubations with E_2+MPA despite a lack of response to E_2.[38,39] Moreover, withdrawal of progestin stimulation, as accomplished by switching to a steroid-free medium or by exposure to the antiprogestin mifepristone, reversed the inhibition of MMP-1 and MMP-3 mRNA levels. By contrast, MMP-2 and TIMP-1 mRNA levels were unaffected either by adding progestin or by progestin withdrawal.[38] In cultured HESCs, the absence of a response to progestin exhibited by TIMP-1 was extended to include other TIMP family members.[40]

DYSREGULATION OF ENDOMETRIAL HEMOSTASIS LEADS TO ABNORMAL UTERINE BLEEDING

Abnormal uterine bleeding complicates long-term progestin-only contraception

Because of their safety and prolonged effectiveness, long-term progestin-only contraceptives (LTPOCs) are ideal for use in underdeveloped countries where access to trained medical personnel is limited. Formulations in common use have included Depo-Provera, which involves subdermal injections of MPA; Norplant and Implanon, which consist of subdermally implanted rods that release the active ingredients levonorgestrel (LNG) and etonogestrel, respectively; and Mirena, which releases levonorgestrel from an intrauterine system. The most frequent complication leading to discontinuation of their use is abnormal uterine bleeding (AUB).

Menstrual bleeding and AUB are fundamentally different phenomena. The former represents an organized response to withdrawal of circulating progesterone[41] preceding sloughing into the menstrual fluid of partially degraded endometrial ECM, glands, stroma, and blood vessels.[41] By contrast, during LTPOC-induced AUB, circulating levels of progestin as well as tissue levels of the progesterone receptor isoforms PR-A and PR-B remain elevated, thereby ruling out functional progesterone withdrawal.[42,43] Microscopic examination of endometrial biopsies obtained by camera-directed hysteroscopy obtained 1 year after initiation of Norplant treatment revealed the presence of distinct bleeding and non-bleeding sites. The former contained enlarged, thin-walled vessels that were virtually absent from adjacent non-bleeding sites.[42] This observation is consistent with the hypothesis that AUB associated with LTPOC administration originates from abnormally distended, 'fragile' vessels.[44] That TF is the primary initiator of hemostasis[3] suggested that TF levels would be elevated in decidualized HESCs of non-bleeding sites compared with bleeding sites. Paradoxically, we observed higher IR TF level at the bleeding sites where we estimated that TF levels were comparable to those of normal luteal phase endometrium.[42] Because decidualization-enhanced TF expression involves both the EGFR and PR,[16] we expected differential expression of these receptors at bleeding vs non-bleeding sites. However, no significant differences in EGFR levels or either the PR-A or PR-B isoform were observed at the two sites.[42] Similarly, EGFR and PR-A and PR-B levels were also equivalent at bleeding vs non-bleeding sites of endometrial specimens obtained after Depo-Provera contraception.[45] Equivalent levels of both PR isoforms were also reported after insertion of the Mirena intrauterine system.[46]

Impaired uterine blood flow, dysregulated angiogenesis, and inflammation promote LTPOC-induced AUB

In 2000, Hickey and colleagues observed that Norplant administration to women leads to impaired vasomotion and uterine blood flow.[47] The resulting local hypoxia–reperfusion is the starting point (step 1) for the scheme shown in Figure 26.4 to account for the occurrence of AUB in response to LTPOC treatment.

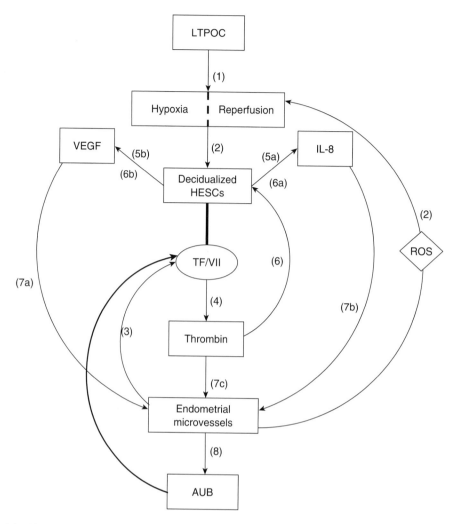

Figure 26.4   Model of long-term progestin-only contraceptive (LTPOC)-induced abnormal uterine bleeding *Step 1*: impaired vasomotion reduces uterine blood flow to induce hyoxia/reperfusion. *Step 2*: hypoxia–reperfusion generates reactive oxygen species (ROS) to directly damage endometrial vessels and increase vascular permeability. *Step 3*: factor VII from the circulation contacts and binds to human endometrial stromal cell (HESC) expressed tissue factor (TF). *Step 4*: thrombin is generated as a result of step 3. *Step 5*: in decidualized HESCs, hypoxia enhances expression of interleukin-8 (IL-8) (5a) and vascular endothelial growth factor (VEGF) (5b). *Step 6*: thrombin acts as an autocrine enhancer on HESCs to further generate IL-8 (6a) and VEGF (6b). *Step 7*: VEGF (7a), IL-8 (7b), and thrombin (7c) induce endothelial cell permeability and angiogenesis via separate endothelial cell-expressed receptors. *Step 8*: Vascular damage arises from the combined effects of ROS and aberrant angiogenesis to promote continued exposure of factor VII to decidual cell-expressed TF to create a feedforward cycle of thrombin, VEGF, and IL-8 generation that results in 'leaky vessels' and AUB.

For clarity, the scheme presents the steps sequentially, although several steps clearly occur concurrently. In step 2, hypoxia–reperfusion generates reactive oxygen species (ROS), which directly damage endometrial microvessels.[48] The resulting increase in vascular permeability increases access of factor VII from the circulation (step 3) to decidual cell-expressed TF to initiate thrombin formation (step 4). Concomitant with step 2, hypoxia enhances expression of interleukin-8 (IL-8)[49] (step 5a) and vascular endothelial growth factor (VEGF)[50,51] (step 5b) in decidualized HESCs. These in-vitro effects are consistent with reports of elevated endometrial levels of IL-8[52] and VEGF[53,54] during LTPOC usage. Our laboratory also found that thrombin, probably acting via the protease-activated membrane receptor 1 (PAR-1) expressed by decidualized HESCs (step 6), augments the expression of IL-8[49] (step 6a) and VEGF[51] (step 6b). Binding of VEGF to endothelial cell-specific surface receptors induces proliferation, migration, protease activity, and vascular permeability,[55] enabling VEGF to act as the primary angiogenic agent. Like VEGF, thrombin promotes angiogenesis and enhances vascular permeability.[56] A member of the CXCL chemokine family and primary neutrophil chemoattractant,[57] IL-8 has also been shown to promote angiogenesis.[58] VEGF (step 7a), IL-8 (step 7b), and thrombin (step 7c) each drive angiogenesis via separate receptors on the endothelial cell surface.[55,56,58] Synergy among these paracrine effectors is expected to elicit abnormal angiogenesis and interfere with vessel maintenance. Interactions of the effects of aberrant angiogenesis with ROS-mediated damage of the microvessels promotes continued exposure of factor VII to decidualized HESC-expressed TF to generate thrombin and create a feedforward cycle that contributes to the onset of AUB (step 8).

Beyond disruption of vascular integrity as a consequence of aberrant angiogenesis, administration of LTPOCs is also likely to destabilize endometrial vessels by inducing expression of proteases in the stroma via the generation of thrombin from decidual cell-expressed TF and by infiltration of leukocytes. Specifically, our laboratory demonstrated that thrombin enhances uPA and MMP expression in decidualized HESCs.[59-61] Since IL-8 is the primary neutrophil chemoattractant and activator, thrombin and hypoxia-enhanced IL-8 production in decidualized HESCs is consistent with the neutrophil infiltration of the endometrium that is reported to complicate Norplant administration.[62] Infiltration of macrophages is also reported to complicate LTPOC treatment.[63] Neutrophils and macrophages express several proteases that degrade ECM components.[64] The concerted effects of decidualized HESC and leukocyte-derived proteases are expected to degrade the basal laminar component-enriched perivascular ECM support scaffolding and help to account for the thin atrophic stroma seen in LTPOC users. The consequent disruption of the integrity of the ECM blood vessel support structure is consistent with exacerbation of AUB.

REGULATION OF ENDOMETRIAL HEMOSTASIS AND VASCULAR STABILITY DURING GESTATION

Human implantation is initiated when the blastocyst adheres to the luminal surface of the endometrial epithelium. Subsequently, blastocyst-derived syncytiotrophoblasts intercalate between adjacent epithelial cells and invade the underlying stroma as cytotrophoblasts, which breach blood vessels enmeshed in a decidualized stromal cell matrix. This process is vital to the development, growth, and survival of the embryo prior to placentation as it provides it with access to oxygen and nutrients and promotes egress of

waste products.[65] That it also risks local hemorrhage is evident from the occurrence of 'chemical pregnancy,' a phenomenon in which trophoblast-derived human chorionic gonadotropin is detected briefly in maternal blood followed by 'spotting' in the decidua.[66,67] The ongoing process of decidualization mitigates the occurrence of this pregnancy-terminating bleeding. Under continued stimulation by progesterone and EGF, decidualization of HESCs promotes hemostasis via enhanced expression of TF[7,9,16] and PAI-1.[7,15,21] Progestin also promotes vascular stabilization via the reciprocal enhanced synthesis and deposition of basal laminar-type proteins in the peridecidual ECM[14,23,24] and inhibited synthesis of the ECM-degrading proteases MMP-1 and MMP-3.[37-40]

Several lines of evidence stress the importance of progesterone-regulated decidualization in determining the depth of cytotrophoblast invasion of the decidua during placentation. Thus, the occurrence of decidualization is limited to species in which the trophoblast invades the stroma. Among species with a hemochorial placenta, the extent of decidualization correlates positively with the degree of trophoblast invasion. Both processes reach their greatest expression in humans, which exhibit the most widespread decidualization reaction and the most invasive trophoblast.[68] The role of decidual cells in restricting this intrinsic invasiveness is clear from the often life-threatening overinvasion that accompanies implantation of the blastocyst at ectopic sites. Sequestration of PAI-1[69] and TGFβ isoforms[70] in the human decidual ECM serve as natural brakes that regulate cytotrophoblast migration and invasion. Expression by cytotrophoblasts of adhesion molecules that recognize basement membrane-type components in the peridecidual ECM determines the depth of invasion.[71] Cytotrophoblasts traverse the decidua, then surround and breach decidual arteries and arterioles to become endovascular trophoblasts that transform the smooth muscle layer and endothelium.[72] This process enhances vascular conductance, increasing blood flow to the intervillous space required for growth and development of the feto–placental unit. However, dysregulation of the normal pattern of adhesion molecule expression impedes cytotrophoblast invasion.[73] Shallow cytotrophoblast invasion results in incomplete uterine vascular conversion and an inadequate fetal blood supply, the primary defect of preeclampsia and intrauterine growth restriction (IUGR).[72,74] Severe thrombophilias,[75] as well as bleeding into the decidua ranging from occult bleeding[76] to frank abruption (decidual hemorrhage),[77] are associated with the occurrence of preeclampsia. Both severe thrombophilias and decidual hemorrhage would generate thrombin from decidual cell-expressed TF. Recently, our laboratory observed that thrombin induced the decidual cells from first trimester, but not term placentas, to synthesize and secrete soluble fms-like tyrosine kinase 1 (sFlt-1).[78] This effect was abrogated by hirudin, a specific thrombin inactivator. Unlike thrombin, neither of the proinflammatory cytokines associated with preeclampsia, tumor necrosis factor-α (TNFα) or interleukin-1β (IL-1β),[79,80] affected s-Flt1 expression in cultured trimester decidual cells. Overexpression of sFlt-1 at the implantation site is postulated to interfere with cytotrophoblast invasion by either impeding this invasion directly and/or indirectly by altering the balance of local angiogenic factors.[81] Extrapolation of our in-vitro results to the events at the human implantation site suggests that thrombin is locally formed in the subset of cases of preeclampsia stemming from underlying decidual hemorrhage or maternal thrombophilias.

ABRUPTIONS OVERCOME PROHEMOSTATIC FACTORS IN THE DECIDUA

Successful human pregnancy requires an increase in hemostatic potential from implantation through delivery.[82] This is accomplished in part by augmented thrombin and fibrin generation across gestation as measured by elevated circulating levels of thrombin–antithrombin (TAT) complexes.[83] The capacity for human decidua to generate thrombin throughout pregnancy is clear from our observations of prominent immunostaining for TF localized to the cell membranes of decidual cells from first trimester as well as term decidua. Moreover, we found that MPA enhanced, and that thrombin further enhanced, TF as well as PAI-1 mRNA and protein expression in cultured decidual cells isolated from term placentas (unpublished results). Abruptions arise when the hemostatic/hemorrhagic equilibrium shifts in favor of the latter. The occurrence of abruptions is a strong predictor of preterm premature rupture of the membranes (PPROM), a leading cause of preterm delivery (PTD). Although PPROM is generally associated with intra-amniotic infections, convincing evidence now links PPROM with placental abruption (i.e. decidual hemorrhage) as manifested by vaginal bleeding.[84] Moreover, occult decidual hemorrhage and retrochorionic hematoma formation as reflected by hemosiderin deposition was reported in nearly 40% of patients with PPROM compared with only about 1% at term ($p < 0.01$), suggesting a much stronger association

between PPROM and abruption than formerly believed.[76] Previously, we showed that thrombin activation, as measured by elevated plasma levels of the TAT complex during the second trimester, predicts the subsequent occurrence of PPROM with high sensitivity and specificity.[85] Moreover, elevated circulating TAT levels during preterm labor were found to predict PTD.[86]

That neutrophil infiltration of the decidua and fetal membranes could play a role in the etiology of prematurity was suggested by a report demonstrating that levels of neutrophil-attracting IL-8 were elevated in the serum, cervicovaginal secretions, and amniotic fluid of women at risk for preterm labor and PPROM.[87] An elevation of IL-8 levels in the amniotic fluid of patients at risk for PTD in the absence of infection[88] suggested that non-infectious mediators may regulate its expression. Although neutrophil infiltration of the cervix and fetal membranes had been associated with PPROM and preterm labor accompanying intra-amniotic infections,[89] our laboratory extended this correlation to include the decidual hemorrhage of abruption. We found that maximum infiltration of neutrophils occurred in the setting of abruption-induced PPROM.[90]

In the fetal membranes, the fibrillar collagen-rich ECM forms a scaffolding that maintains structural integrity and tensile strength.[91] However, it is susceptible to degradation by proteases derived from the decidua or from resident decidual neutrophils. The association between abruption-derived thrombin generation from decidual cell-expressed TF and the onset of PPROM is detailed in the model proposed in Figure 26.5. The capacity of thrombin to act as an autocrine/paracrine inducer of various biological effects via cell surface protease-activated receptors (PARs),[92] taken together with the results of a recent multicenter clinical trial demonstrating that administration of the progestin 17α-hydroxyprogesterone caproate to women conferred protection against PTD,[93] prompted us to evaluate the separate and interactive effects of thrombin and the progestin MPA on MMP and IL-8 expression in cultured term decidual cells. The experimental results demonstrated that thrombin markedly up-regulated mRNA and protein levels of MMP-1, MMP-3, and IL-8. The thrombin inactivator hirudin blocked these effects, indicating the requirement for active thrombin. The addition of MPA to the decidual cell cultures inhibited basal output of MMP-1 and MMP-3 and significantly blunted thrombin-enhanced expression of both MMPs. By contrast, MPA did not significantly affect either basal or thrombin-enhanced expression of IL-8.[90]

Interactions between MMP-1 and MMP-3 play an integral role in degrading fibrillar collagens. A specific

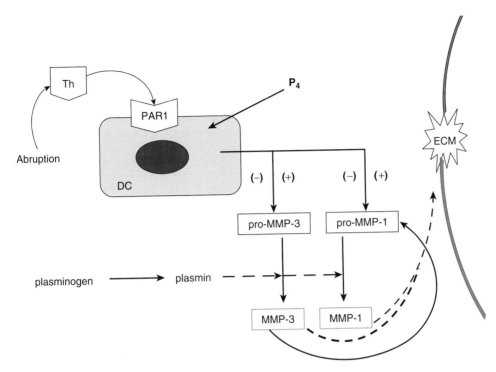

Figure 26.5   Abruption induces preterm premature rupture of membranes (PPROM). During the luteal phase and gestation in human endometrium progesterone (P_4) inhibits (−) the synthesis and secretion of the zymogenic matrix metalloproteinase, (MMP) forms pro-MMP-1 and pro-MMP-3. Abruption-generated thrombin binds to protease-activated receptor 1 (PAR1) on the decidual cell membrane to induce (+) the synthesis and secretion of pro-MMP-1 and pro-MMP-3. Locally generated plasmin activates pro-MMP-1 and pro-MMP-3. Interactions between MMP-1 and MMP-3 degrade extracellular matrix (ECM) of the decidua and the fetal membranes.

cleavage in the helical structure of fibrillar collagens by MMP-1 initiates their denaturation to gelatins, which are then processed further by MMP-3 and MMP-3-activated MMP-9.[29,32] Coordinated changes in the expression of the MMP-1 and MMP-3 genes reflect similarities in their promoters.[32] During normal pregnancies, progesterone inhibits decidual cell-expressed MMP-1 and MMP-3. However, the model depicted in Figure 26.5 indicates that abruption-related thrombin generation overcomes this inhibition to enhance MMP-1 and MMP-3 expression and promote degradation of the decidual ECM as well as that of neighboring fetal membranes. Moreover, the induction by thrombin of IL-8 expression in decidual cells is expected to play a key role in promoting neutrophil infiltration of the decidua during abruptions in the absence of infection. Since neutrophils are also a rich source of ECM-degrading proteases, such as neutrophil elastase, neutrophil MMP-8, and MMP-9,[94,95] these infiltrating decidual neutrophils are expected to augment the effects of thrombin-enhanced MMP-1 and MMP-3 in decidual cells to promote PPROM by contributing to degradation of the ECM of the decidua and fetal membranes.

In summary, extrapolation of the in-vitro results obtained with term decidual cell monolayers to the clinical setting at term indicates that thrombin generated by abruption-induced decidual hemorrhage promotes degradation of the ECM of the decidua and fetal membranes directly by augmenting MMP-1 and MMP-3 expression in decidual cells and indirectly by increasing IL-8 expression in the decidual cells, which then acts as a neutrophil chemoattractant. The concomitant effects of MPA to markedly inhibit both basal and thrombin-induced MMP-1 and MMP-3 expression in cultured term decidual cells[60,61] while augmenting the expression of TF and PAI-1 indicates that in the decidua at term progesterone establishes an antiproteolytic, hemostatic milieu that counteracts the occurrence of decidual thrombin generation that leads to abruption. This mechanism may account for the protection against PTD afforded by administration of 17α-hydroxyprogesterone caproate initiated early in the second trimester.[93] By contrast, MPA did not significantly affect either basal or thrombin-induced IL-8 protein expression in term decidual cells, suggesting a limitation of the clinical efficacy of progesterone therapy in the setting of abruptions.

FUTURE DIRECTIONS

In-vitro studies of human endometrial stromal/decidual cells have generally ignored the presence of immune cells in the cultures. However, immune cells represent a significant portion of the resident endometrial cell population and undergo significant quantitative and qualitative changes during the menstrual cycle and gestation.[96] Moreover, each leukocyte type expresses a specific profile of cytokines and proteases that could exert marked effects on stromal/decidual cell function and phenotype.[40] Specifically, during the first trimester, uterine natural killer (uNK) cells represent an estimated 70–75% of the leukocyte population.[96] Interferon-γ, a major cytokine released by uNK cells,[96] is a potent enhancer of TF expression in cultured HESCs.[97] Recently, we found that TNFα and IL-1β each markedly enhanced IL-8 output in term human decidual cells that were passaged until the cultures were >99% free of the common leukocyte antigen CD 45.[98] By contrast, these proinflammatory cytokines were far less effective in up-regulating IL-8 expression in unpassaged term decidual cells,[99] in which leukocytes constituted about 15% of the cultured cells. These differential responses suggest that the resident immune cells exert inhibitory effects. They emphasize the importance of reevaluating the expression of endpoints regulating hemostasis and vascular stability in leukocyte-free stromal/decidual cell cultures, and then considering carrying out co-culture experiments with the purified stromal/decidual cells and relevant leukocyte subtypes.

ACKNOWLEDGMENTS

This work was supported by the National Institutes of Health grants HL-070004-03 and HD-33937-03. The authors wish to thank all the members of the Lockwood Laboratory, as well as the many researchers in this field, for their contributions to the work reviewed in this chapter. Furthermore, we express our gratitude to all of our colleagues and collaborators for their support.

REFERENCES

1. Bell SC. Decidualization and relevance to menstruation. In: D'Arcangues C, Fraser IS, Newton JR, Odlind V, eds. Contraception and Mechanisms of Endometrial Bleeding. Cambridge: Cambridge University Press, 1990: 188.
2. Tabanelli S, Tang B, Gurpide E. In vitro decidualization of human endometrial stromal cells. J Steroid Biochem Mol Biol 1992; 42(3–4): 337–44.
3. Mackman N. Role of tissue factor in hemostasis, thrombosis, and vascular development. Arterioscler Thomb Vasc Biol 2004; 24: 1015–22.
4. Carmeliet P, Mackman N, Moons L et al. Role of tissue factor in embryonic blood vessel development. Nature 1996; 383: 73–5.
5. Ehrlich JH, Parry GC, Fearns C et al. Tissue factor is required for uterine hemostasis and maintenance of the placental labyrinth during gestation. Proc Natl Acad Sci USA 1999; 96: 8138–43.
6. Lockwood CJ, Nemerson Y, Guller S et al. Progestational regulation of human endometrial stromal cell tissue factor expression during decidualization. J Clin Endocrinol Metab 1993; 76: 231–6.
7. Lockwood CJ, Krikun G, Papp C et al. The role of progestationally regulated stromal cell tissue factor and type-1 plasminogen activator inhibitor (PAI-1) in endometrial hemostasis and menstruation. Ann NY Acad Sci 1994; 734: 57–79.
8. Runic R, Schatz F, Krey L et al. Alterations in endometrial stromal cell tissue factor protein and messenger ribonucleic acid expression in patients experiencing abnormal uterine bleeding while using NORPLANT-2 contraception. J Clin Endocrinol Metab 1997; 82: 1983–8.
9. Lockwood CJ, Nemerson Y, Krikun G et al. Steroid-modulated stromal cell tissue factor expression: a model for the regulation of endometrial hemostasis and menstruation. J Clin Endocrinol Metab 1993; 77(4): 1014–19.
10. Lubbert H, Pollow K, Rommler A et al. Estradiol and progesterone receptor concentrations and 17β-hydroxy-steroid-dehydrogenase activity in estrogen-progestin stimulated endometrium of women with gonadal dysgenesis. J Steroid Biochem 1982; 17: 143–8.
11. Mackman N. Regulation of the tissue factor gene. Thromb Haemost 1997; 78(1): 747–54.
12. Krikun G, Schatz F, Mackman N et al. Transcriptional regulation of the tissue factor gene by progestins in human endometrial stromal cells. J Clin Endocrinol Metab 1998; 83: 926–30.
13. Krikun G, Schatz F, Mackman N et al. Regulation of tissue factor gene expression in human endometrium by transcription factors Sp1 and Sp3. Mol Endocrinol 2000; 14: 393–400.
14. Irwin JC, Utian WH, Eckert RL. Sex steroids and growth factors differentially regulate the growth and differentiation of cultured human endometrial stromal cells. Endocrinology 1991; 129: 2385–92.
15. Lockwood CJ. Progestin–epidermal growth factor interactions regulate plasminogen activator inhibitor-1 expression during decidualization of human endometrial stromal cells. Am J Obstet Gynecol 2001; 184: 798–804.
16. Lockwood CJ, Krikun G, Runic R et al. Progestin–epidermal growth factor regulation of tissue factor expression during decidualization of human endometrial stromal cells. J Clin Endocrinol Metab 2000; 85: 297–301.
17. Imai T, Kurachi H, Adachi K et al. Changes in epidermal growth factor receptor and levels of its ligands during menstrual cycle in human endometrium. Biol Reprod 1995; 52: 928–38.
18. Stassen JM, Arnout J, Deckmyn H. The hemostatic system. Curr Med Chem 2004; 11(17): 2245–60.
19. Mignatti P, Rifkin DB. Biology and biochemistry of proteinases in tumor invasion. Physiol Rev 1993; 73: 161–95.
20. Koh SC, Wong PC, Yuen R et al. Concentration of plasminogen activators and inhibitor in the human endometrium at different phases of the menstrual cycle. J Reprod Fertil 1992; 96(2): 407–13.
21. Schatz F, Aigner S, Papp C et al. Plasminogen activator activity during decidualization of human endometrial stromal cells is regulated by plasminogen activator inhibitor 1. J Clin Endocrinol Metab 1995; 80(8): 2504–10.
22. Schatz F, Lockwood CJ. Progestin regulation of plasminogen activator inhibitor type 1 in cultures of endometrial stromal and decidual cells. J Clin Endocrinol Metab 1993; 77(3): 621–5.
23. Aplin JD. Cellular biology of the endometrium. In: Wynn RM, Jolie WP, eds. Biology of the Uterus, 3rd edn. New York: Plenum Press, 1988: 187–202.

24. Church HJ, Vicovac LM, Williams JDL et al. Laminins 2 and 4 are expressed by human decidual cells. Lab Invest 1996; 74: 21–32.

26. Ossowski L. Invasion of connective tissue by human carcinoma cell lines: requirement for urokinase, urokinase receptor, and interstitial collagenase. Cancer Res 1992; 52(24): 6754–60.

26. Liu J, Chakraborty C, Graham CH et al. Noncatalytic domain of uPA stimulates human extravillous trophoblast migration by using phospholipase C, phosphatidylinositol 3-kinase and mitogen-activated protein kinase. Exp Cell Res 2003; 286: 138–51.

27. Nordengren J, Pilka R, Noskova V et al. Differential localization and expression of urokinase plasminogen activator (uPA), its receptor (uPAR), and its inhibitor (PAI-1) mRNA and protein in endometrial tissue during the menstrual cycle. Mol Hum Reprod 2004; 10(9): 655–63.

28. Bonnefoy A, Legrand C. Proteolysis of subendothelial adhesive glycoproteins (fibronectin, thrombospondin, and von Willebrand factor) by plasmin, leukocyte cathepsin G, and elastase. Thromb Res 2000; 98(4): 323–32.

29. Birkedal-Hansen H, Moore WG, Bodden MK et al. Matrix metalloproteinases: a review. Crit Rev Oral Biol Med 1993; 4(2): 197–250.

30. Casslen B, Urano S, Ny T. Progesterone regulation of plasminogen activator inhibitor 1 (PAI-1) antigen and mRNA levels in human endometrial stromal cells. Thromb Res 1992; 66(1): 75–87.

31. Casslen B, Urano S, Lecander I, Ny T. Plasminogen activators in the human endometrium, cellular origin and hormonal regulation. Blood Coagul Fibrinolysis 1992; 3(2): 133–8.

32. Nagase H. Stromelysins 1 and 2. In: Parks WC, Mecham R, eds. Matrix Metalloproteinases San Diego, CA: Academic Press, 1998: 43–84.

33. Fini ME, Cook JR, Mohan R et al. Regulation of matrix metalloproteinase gene expression. In: Parks WC, Mecham R, eds. Matrix Metalloproteinases San Diego, CA: Academic Press, 1998: 299–356.

34. Zhang J, Hampton AL, Nie G et al. Progesterone inhibits activation of latent matrix metalloproteinase (MMP)-2 by membrane-type 1 MMP: enzymes coordinately expressed in human endometrium. Biol Reprod 2000; 62: 85–94.

35. Suzuki S, Sato M, Senoo H et al. Direct cell–cell interaction enhances pro-MMP-2 production and activation in co-culture of laryngeal cancer cells and fibroblasts: involvement of EMMPRIN and MT1-MMP. Exp Cell Res 2004; 293(2): 259–66.

36. McMahon S, Laprise MH, Dubois CM. Alternative pathway for the role of furin in tumor cell invasion process. Enhanced MMP-2 levels through bioactive TGFbeta. Exp Cell Res 2003; 291(2): 326–39.

37. Rodgers WH, Matrisian LM, Giudice LC et al. Patterns of matrix metalloproteinase expression in cycling endometrium imply differential functions and regulation by steroid hormones. J Clin Invest 1994; 94(3): 946–53.

38. Lockwood CJ, Krikun G, Hausknecht VA et al. Matrix metalloproteinase and matrix metalloproteinase inhibitor expression in endometrial stromal cells during progestin-initiated decidualization and menstruation-related progestin withdrawal. Endocrinology 1998; 139(11): 4607–13.

39. Bruner KL, Eisenberg E, Gorstein F et al. Progesterone and transforming growth factor-beta coordinately regulate suppression of endometrial matrix metalloproteinases in a model of experimental endometriosis. Steroids 1999; 64(9): 648–53.

40. Salamonsen LA, Butt AR, Hammond FR et al. Production of endometrial matrix metalloproteinases, but not their tissue inhibitors, is modulated by progesterone withdrawal in an in vitro model for menstruation. J Clin Endocrinol Metab 1997; 82: 1409–15.

41. Lockwood CJ, Schatz F. A biological model for the regulation of peri-implantational hemostasis and menstruation. Soc Gynecol Investig 1996; 3: 159–65.

42. Runic R, Schatz F, Wan L et al. Effects of norplant on endometrial tissue factor expression and blood vessel structure. J Clin Endocrinol Metab 2000; 85: 3853–9.

43. Critchley HO, Bailey DA, Au CL et al. Immunohistochemical sex steroid receptor distribution in endometrium from long-term subdermal levonorgesterel users and during normal menstrual cycle. Hum Reprod 1993; 8: 1632–9.

44. Rogers PA. Endometrial vasculature in Norplant users. Hum Reprod 1996; 11(2): 45–50.

45. Lockwood CJ, Runic R, Wan L et al. The role of tissue factor in regulating endometrial hemostasis: implications for progestin-only contraception. Hum Reprod 2000; 15: 144–51.

46. Critchley HO, Kelly RW, Wang H et al. Progestin receptor isoforms and prostaglandin dehydrogenase in the endometrium of women using a levonorgesterel-releasing intrauterine system. Hum Reprod 1998; 13(5): 1210–17.

47. Hickey MC, Carati F, Manconi BJ et al. The measurement of endometrial perfusion in Norplant users: a pilot study. Hum Reprod 2000; 15(5): 1086–91.

48. Krikun G, Critchley H, Schatz F et al. Abnormal uterine bleeding during progestin-only contraception may result from free radical-induced alterations in angiopoietin expression. Am J Pathol 2002; 161: 979–86.

49. Lockwood CJ, Kumar P, Krikun G et al. Effects of thrombin, hypoxia, and steroids on interleukin-8 expression in decidualized human endometrial stromal cells: implications for long-term progestin-only contraceptive-induced bleeding. J Clin Endocrinol Metab 2004; 89(3): 1467–75.

50. Sharkey AM, Day K, McPherson A et al. Vascular endothelial growth factor expression in human endometrium is regulated by hypoxia. J Clin Endocrinol Metab 2000; 85: 402–9.

51. Lockwood CJ, Krikun G, Koo AB et al. Differential effects of thrombin and hypoxia on endometrial stromal and glandular epithelial cell vascular endothelial growth factor expression. J Clin Endocrinol Metab 2002; 87(9): 4280–6.

52. Jones RL, Morison NB, Hannan NJ et al. Chemokine expression is dysregulated in the endometrium of women using progestin-only contraceptives and correlates to elevated recruitment of distinct leukocyte populations. Hum Reprod 2005; 20(10): 2724–35.

53. Lau TM, Affandi B, Rogers PA. The effects of levonorgestrel implants on vascular endothelial growth factor expression in the endometrium. Mol Hum Reprod 1999; 5: 57–63.

54. Charnock-Jones DS, Macpherson AM, Archer DF et al. The effects of progestins on vascular endothelial growth factor, oestrogen receptor, and progesterone receptor immunoreactivity and endothelial cell density in human endometrium. Hum Reprod 2000; 15(3): 85–95.

55. Ferrara N. Molecular and biological properties of vascular endothelial growth factor. J Mol Med 1999; 77: 527–43.

56. Tsopanoglou NE, Maragoudakis ME. On the mechanism of thrombin-induced angiogenesis: potentiation of vascular endothelial growth factor activity by up-regulation of its receptors. J Biol Chem 1999; 274: 23969–76.

57. Baggiolini M. Chemokines and leukocyte traffic. Nature 1998; 392: 565–8.

58. Strieter RM, Kunkel SL, Elner VM. Interleukin-8. A corneal factor that induces neovascularization. Am J Pathol 1992; 141: 1279–84.

59. Lockwood CJ, Krikun G, Aigner S et al. Effects of thrombin on steroid-modulated cultured endometrial stromal cell fibrinolytic potential. J Clin Endocrinol Metab 1996; 81: 107–12.

60. Rosen T, Schatz F, Kuczynski E et al. Thrombin-enhanced matrix metalloproteinase-1 expression: a mechanism linking placental abruption with premature rupture of the membranes. J Matern Fetal Neonatal Med 2002; 11(1): 11–17.

61. Mackenzie AP, Schatz F, Krikun G et al. Mechanisms of abruption-induced premature rupture of the fetal membranes: Thrombin enhanced decidual matrix metalloproteinase-3

(stromelysin-1) expression. Am J Obstet Gynecol 2004; 191: 1996–2001.

62. Vincent AJ, Malakooti N, Zhang J et al. Endometrial breakdown in women using Norplant is associated with migratory cells expressing matrix metaloproteinase-9 (gelatinase B). Hum Reprod 1999; 14: 807–15.

63. Hannan NJ, Jones RL, Critchley HO et al. Coexpression of fractalkine and its receptor in normal human endometrium and in endometrium from users of progestin-only contraception supports a role for fractalkine in leukocyte recruitment and endometrial remodeling. J Clin Endocrinol Metab 2004; 89: 6119–29.

64. Vincent AJ, Salamonsen LA. The role of matrix metalloproteinases and leukocytes in abnormal uterine bleeding associated with progestin-only contraceptives. Hum Reprod 2000; 15(3): 135–43.

65. Moore KL. The Developing Human, 4th edn. Philadelphia, PA: WB Saunders, 1988: 40.

66. Levy T, Dicker D, Ashkenazi J, et al. The prognostic value and significance of preclinical abortions in invitro fertilization–embryo transfer programs. Fertil Steril. 1991; 56:71–4.

67. Oka C, Makino T, Itakura I et al. Chemical abortion in patients with recurrent fetal loss. Nippon Sanka Fujinka Gakkai Zasshi 1991; 43: 239–40.

68. Ramsey EM, Houston ML, Harris JW. Interactions of the trophoblast and maternal tissues in three closely related primate species. Am J Obstet Gynecol 1976; 124(6): 647–52.

69. Bauer S, Pollheimer J, Hartmann J et al. Tumor necrosis factor-alpha inhibits trophoblast migration through elevation of plasminogen activator inhibitor-1 in first-trimester villous explant cultures. J Clin Endocrinol Metab 2004; 89: 812–22.

70. Caniggia I, Mostachfi H, Winter J et al. Hypoxia-inducible factor-1 mediates the biological effects of oxygen on human trophoblast differentiation through TGFbeta(3). J Clin Invest 2000; 105: 577–87.

71. Damsky CH, Librach C, Lim KH et al. Integrin switching regulates normal trophoblast invasion. Development 1994; 120(12): 3657–66.

72. Damsky CH, Fisher SJ. Trophoblast pseudo-vasculogenesis: faking it with endothelial adhesion receptors. Curr Opin Cell Biol 1998; 10: 660–6.

73. Zhou Y, Damsky CH, Chiu K et al. Preeclampsia is associated with abnormal expression of adhesion molecules by invasive cytotrophoblasts. J Clin Invest 1993; 91: 950–60.

74. Brosens JJ, Pijnenborg R, Brosens IA. The myometrial junctional zone spiral arteries in normal and abnormal pregnancies: a review of the literature. Am J Obstet Gynecol 2002; 187: 1416–23.

75. Vatten LJ, Skjaerven R. Is pre-eclampsia more than one disease? BJOG 2004; 111: 298–302.

76. Salafia CM, Lopez-Zeno JA, Sherer DM et al. Histologic evidence of old intrauterine bleeding is more frequent in prematurity. Am J Obstet Gynecol 1995; 173: 1065–70.

77. Aoyama K, Suzuki Y, Sato T et al. Cardiac failure caused by severe pre-eclampsia with placental abruption, and its treatment with anti-hypertensive drugs. J Obstet Gynaecol Res 2003; 29: 339–42.

78. Schatz F, Toti P, Arcuri F et al. Thrombin regulates expression of soluble fms-like tyrosine kinase-1 in first trimester decidual cells: implications for preeclampsia. Suppl Soc Gynecol Invest 2006, 53rd Annual Meeting, 13(2): abstract # 674.

79. Rinehart BK, Terrone DA, Lagoo-Deenadayalan S et al. Expression of the placental cytokines tumor necrosis factor alpha, interleukin 1beta, and interleukin 10 is increased in preeclampsia. Am J Obstet Gynecol 1999; 181: 915–20.

80. Hefler LA, Tempfer CB, Gregg AR. Polymorphisms within the interleukin-1 beta gene cluster and preeclampsia. Obstet Gynecol 2001; 97(5): 664–8.

81. Karumanchi SA, Bdolah Y. Hypoxia and sFlt-1 in preeclampsia: the "chicken-and-egg" question. Endocrinology 2004; 145: 4835–7.

82. Clark P. Changes of hemostasis variables during pregnancy. Semin Vasc Med 2003; 3: 13–24.

83. Bremme K, Ostlund E, Almqvist I et al. Enhanced thrombin generation and fibrinolytic activity in normal pregnancy and the puerperium. Obstet Gynecol 1992; 80: 132–7.

84. Harger JH, Hsing AW, Tuomala RE et al. Risk factors for preterm rupture of fetal membranes: a multicenter case-control study. Am J Obstet Gynecol 1990; 163: 130–7.

85. Rosen T, Kuczynski E, O'Neill LM et al. Plasma levels of thrombin–antithrombin complexes predict preterm premature rupture of the fetal membranes. J Matern Fetal Med 2001; 10: 297–300.

86. Elovitz MA, Ascher-Landsberg J, Saunders T et al. The mechanisms underlying the stimulatory effects of thrombin on myometrial smooth muscle. Am J Obstet Gynecol 2000; 183: 674–81.

87. Rizzo G, Capponi A, Vlachopoulou A et al. The diagnostic value of interleukin-8 and fetal fibronectin concentrations in cervical secretions in patients with preterm labor and intact membranes. J Perinat Med 1997; 25: 461–8.

88. Romero R, Ceska M, Avila C et al. Neutrophil attractant/activating peptide-1/interleukin-8 in term and preterm parturition. Am J Obstet Gynecol 1991; 165(4): 813–20.

89. Helmig BR, Romero R, Espinoza J et al. Neutrophil elastase and secretory leukocyte protease inhibitor in prelabor rupture of membranes, parturition and intra-amniotic infection. J Matern Fetal Neonatal Med 2002; 12: 237–46.

90. Lockwood CJ, Toti P, Arcuri F et al. Mechanisms of abruption-induced premature rupture of the fetal membranes: thrombin-enhanced interleukin-8 expression in term decidua. Am J Pathol 2005; 167: 1443–9.

91. Malak TM, Ockleford CD, Bell SC et al. Confocal immunofluorescence localization of collagen types I, III, IV, V and VI and their ultrastructural organization in term human fetal membranes. Placenta 1993; 14: 385–406.

92. Cocks TM, Moffatt JD. Protease-activated receptors: sentries for inflammation? Trends Pharmacol Sci 2000; 21: 103–8.

93. Meis PJ, Klebanoff M, Thom E et al. Prevention of recurrent preterm delivery by 17 alpha-hydroxyprogesterone caproate. N Engl J Med 2003; 348: 2379–85.

94. Maymon E, Romero R, Pacora P et al. Human neutrophil collagenase (matrix metalloproteinase 8) in parturition, premature rupture of the membranes, and intrauterine infection. Am J Obstet Gynecol 2000; 183: 94–9.

95. Vu TH, Web Z. Gelatinase B: structure, regulation, and function. In: Parks WC, Mecham R, eds. Matrix Metalloproteinases. San Diego, CA: Academic Press, 1998: 15–148.

96. Dunn CL, Kelly RW, Critchley HO. Decidualization of the human endometrial stromal cell: an enigmatic transformation. Reprod Biomed Online 2003; 7(2): 151–61.

97. Christian M, Marangos P, Mak I et al. Interferon-gamma modulates prolactin and tissue factor expression in differentiating human endometrial stromal cells. Endocrinology 2001; 142(7): 3142–51.

98. Lockwood CJ, Arcuri F, Toti P et al. Tumor necrosis factor-alpha and interleukin-1 beta regulate interleukin-8 expression in third trimester decidual cells: implications for the genesis of chorioamnionitis. Am J Pathol 2006; 169(4): 1294–302.

99. Dudley DJ, Trautman MS, Mitchell MD. Inflammatory mediators regulate interleukin-8 production by cultured gestational tissues: evidence for a cytokine network at the chorio–decidual interface. J Clin Endocrinol Metab 1993; 76: 404–10.

27 Uterine stromal cell differentiation in non-decidualizing species

Gregory A Johnson

Synopsis

Background

- Embryos of some species, including primates and rodents, are invasive and penetrate the epithelial layer of the endometrium.
- In response, the endometrial stroma undergoes a decidual cell reaction to form the maternal component of the placenta.
- The decidua is a morphologically and functionally distinct tissue that is a source of hormones, promotes embryo nutrition, prevents fetal allograft rejection, and regulates placentation by limiting embryo invasion.
- In other species, including domestic ruminants and pigs, a maternal epithelial barrier is maintained between the fetal placenta and the endometrial microcirculation in what is termed epitheliochorial placentation.
- Because of the lack of stromal invasion, a true decidua does not form, but endometrial stromal changes occur to provide sufficient vascular development to (1) support required nutrient, gas, and metabolic waste exchange; (2) produce hormones and cytokines required to support pregnancy; and (3) limit the movement of inherently invasive embryonic membranes through the uterine wall.

Basic Science

- Features reminiscent of decidualization can be observed in the pregnant endometrial stroma in all implanting species, with most extensive transformation accompanying invasive implantation of rodents and primates, moderate transformation with synepitheliochorial placentation (as in ruminants), and only minor changes occurring in epitheliochorially implanting species such as pigs.
- IFNτ from trophectoderm increases expression of several IFN-stimulated genes (ISGs) in the stroma of the ruminant uterus.
- The best characterized of these, ISG15, is a functional ubiquitin homologue that becomes conjugated to intracellular proteins, either targeting them for degradation in the proteasome, or stabilizing them.
- Altered gene expression in stromal cells during pregnancy correlates with alterations to cytoskeletal composition and cell morphology, and remodeling of extracellular matrix.

Clinical

- Unexplained chronic infertility affects more than six million women in the USA.
- Studies of vascular remodeling and other stromal changes in epitheliochorial species are relevant and helpful both in defining implantation mechanisms in these species and setting hypotheses for why the early events fail so frequently in women.

INTRODUCTION

Implantation of the embryo in the uterus and development of a placental connection to the maternal circulation is a strong evolutionary advantage of eutherian mammals over oviparous animals. The placenta and embryonic/fetal membranes (amnion, chorion, and allantois) form the interface between the microcirculatory systems of the mother and embryo, function for efficient sustained exchange of nutrients, respiratory gases, and metabolic waste, protect the growing embryo/fetus, and are a source of hormones. The membranes are formed by the embryo; however, both the embryo and maternal endometrium begin to form components of the placenta as soon as the embryo implants in the endometrium. Due to its recent appearance in the evolutionary record, a considerable variability exists among species relative to histogenesis and organization of the placenta. Embryos of some species, including primates and rodents, are invasive and penetrate the epithelial layer of the endometrium. In response, the endometrial stroma undergoes a decidual cell reaction to form the maternal component of the placenta. The decidua is a morphologically and functionally distinct tissue that is a source of hormones, promotes embryo nutrition, prevents fetal allograft rejection, and regulates placentation by limiting embryo invasion. Numerous candidate genes have been identified and there has been good progress on identifying gene networks required for development and function of the decidua. In other species, including domestic ruminants and pigs, embryos in the strictest sense do not implant into the uterine wall, but simply attach to the uterus by placental outgrowth. To varying degrees, a maternal epithelial barrier is maintained between the fetal placenta and the endometrial microcirculation in what is termed epitheliochorial placentation. Because of the lack of stromal invasion, a true decidua does not form. As a result, decidualization and the formation of a maternal placenta have not been considered characteristic of epitheliochorial placentation, and endometrial stromal changes in response to placentation have been largely overlooked. However, although classic decidualization is not observed in these species, the endometrium must still provide sufficient vascular development:

* to support required nutrient, gas, and metabolic waste exchange
* to produce hormones and cytokines required to support pregnancy
* to limit the movement of inherently invasive embryonic membranes through the uterine wall.

This chapter highlights some of the new information on uterine stromal cell differentiation in non-decidualizing species, by focusing on observed changes in stromal cells during placentation in domestic ruminants and pigs.

IMPLANTATION AND PLACENTATION

Implantation and placentation are critical events in pregnancy. Implantation failure during the first 3 weeks of gestation is a major cause of infertility in all mammals.[1,2] Some 75% of these pregnancy failures are not clinically recognized as pregnancies because of an inability of the developing conceptus to attach to the uterine endometrial luminal epithelium (LE), implant into the uterine wall, or form a functional placenta.[3–5] Paramount to success of these processes are:

* secretions from the uterine epithelia, i.e. histotroph, to support attachment, development, and growth of the conceptus[6–8]
* remodeling at the uterine mucosal epithelial surface to allow intimate association between conceptus and uterus for implantation[9–11]
* remodeling of the uterine stroma to control movement of the conceptus through the uterine wall during implantation while generating a cytokine-rich environment that directly promotes hematotropic support for the developing conceptus.[12,13]

Dysregulation of these uterine processes is among the primary reasons for infertility.[14]

Implantation is highly synchronized, requiring reciprocal secretory and physical interactions between a developmentally competent conceptus and the uterine endometrium during a restricted period of the uterine cycle termed the 'window of receptivity'.[5,11,15–18] Implantation may be non-invasive (central) or invasive (interstitial or eccentric), depending on whether or not the placental membranes (trophectoderm) invade through uterine LE into the stroma (Figure 27.1). In rodents and man, initial attachment is rapidly followed by invasion of the embryo into the endometrial wall. In contrast, implantation in domestic animals follows a prolonged preattachment period, and does not result in embryo invasion past the basal lamina of the mucosal epithelium. Despite differences in duration of the preimplantation period and degree of conceptus invasiveness, the initial phases of implantation, as defined by Guillomot et al[18] – (1) shedding of the zona pellucida, (2) pre-contact and blastocyst orientation, (3) apposition and (4) adhesion – are common across species (see Figure 27.1). Conceptus attachment first requires loss of antiadhesive molecules in the glycocalyx of LE, comprised largely of mucins that sterically inhibit attachment.[19] This results in 'unmasking' of molecules, including selectins and galectins,[20,21] that contribute to initial attachment of conceptus to uterine LE. These low-affinity contacts are then replaced by a more stable and extensive repertoire of adhesive interactions between integrins and maternal extracellular matrix (ECM), which

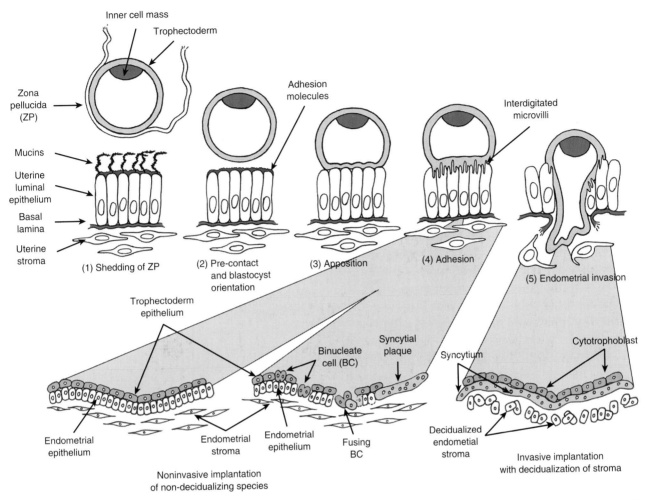

Figure 27.1   Implantation involves five potential phases characterized by increasingly complex interactions between the trophectoderm and the uterine endometrial epithelium or synepitheliochorial type and the stroma. Adhesion is followed by either non-invasive implantation of epitheliochorial or invasive implantation accompanied by endometrial stromal cell decidualization. (Adapted from Guillomot et al.[18])

appear to be the dominant contributors to stable adhesion at implantation.[5,11,16,22] With invasive implanting species, these events are followed by penetration of the endometrial wall by the embryo, necessitating a repertoire of trophectoderm interactions with maternal ECM and stromal cell populations encountered following invasion.[5,20,23] Subsequent cellular interactions involve epithelial–stromal communication that serves to limit invasiveness, establish intimate physical relationships between conceptus and maternal vasculatures, and support numerous additional functions essential to successful development of the conceptus.[12]

Considerable variability exists relative to histogenesis and organization of the placenta; however, trophoblast interaction with maternal tissues remains extensive in all species thus far studied (see Figure 27.1). Pigs demonstrate true epitheliochorial placentation in which there is no displacement or invasion of the maternal

tissues.[24] Ruminants have synepitheliochorial placentas in which binucleate trophectoderm cells migrate, invade, and fuse with uterine LE to form multinucleated syncytia in aglandular areas of the uterus where placentomes form.[25,26] In both epitheliochorial and synepitheliochorial placentation, the conceptus remains within the uterine lumen throughout gestation. The blastocysts of carnivores, rodents, and primates invade and implant deeply into the endometrial stroma and the uterine LE is restored over the site of implantation. The trophoblast layer is highly proliferative and undergoes syncytial formation that establishes extensive contacts with maternal vasculature. Mononuclear cytotrophoblasts underlie syncytiotrophoblasts, and migrate out of the trophoblast layer[27] (see Figure 27.1). Invasive implantation triggers endometrial stromal responses that are collectively known as decidualization.

DECIDUALIZATION

Embryonic membranes are inherently invasive, and can attach to and invade a diverse array of artificial ectopic sites and biological matrices without discrimination or need for hormonal priming.[28,29] Even pig trophectoderm, which does not invade the uterine LE during placentation, will invade and undergo syncytium formation when transplanted to ectopic sites.[30] The endometrial LE is unique in that trophectoderm cannot invade its surface indiscriminantly.[31] The LE remains a barrier to invasion until it is cyclically transformed to a receptive state.[9,10] Invasive implantation is characterized by trophectoderm adhesion to the ECM of LE, local ECM degradation by matrix metalloproteinases (MMPs), trophectoderm migration into endometrial stroma, and eventual inhibition of trophectoderm invasion and migration.[32,33]

Penetration of the LE barrier by invasive trophectoderm triggers a series of stromal responses collectively termed decidualization.[34] During decidualization, hyperplasia and hypertrophy transforms small spindle-like endometrial fibroblast stroma cells into enlarged polygonal epithelial-like cells with extensive cell–cell contacts.[35,36] As they differentiate, these cells express additional or different arrays of cytoskeletal proteins,[37] and exhibit marked accumulation of these proteins, which include microtubules, microfilaments, intermediate filaments, and the microtubular lattice.[38] Two cytoskeletal proteins that have been detected in decidual cells are the intermediate filament desmin,[39,40] and the microfilament α-smooth muscle actin (α-SMA).[41] These cytoskeletal proteins are believed to be physically involved with changes in cell growth, shape, and protein secretion observed during the decidualization process.[42] Functionally, decidualized stroma secretes prolactin[43] and insulin-like growth factor binding protein-1,[44] which probably function in complex gene networks that restrain trophoblast invasion,[45] as well as a rapidly growing list of other endocrine and paracrine factors.[46,47] Decidua also exhibit marked accumulation of ECM proteins, including secreted phosphoprotein-1 (SPP1), laminin, and fibronectin.[34] For SPP1, also known as osteopontin, expression is by decidual natural killer cells in mice,[48] but by stromal cells in humans,[49] and may be involved in angiogenesis within the decidua. The end result is the formation of a morphologically and functionally distinct tissue that is a source of hormones, promotes embryo nutrition, prevents fetal allograft rejection, and regulates placentation by limiting trophoblast invasion through generation of a local cytokine environment which promotes trophoblast attachment over invasion.[50] Decidua constitutes the maternal side of the maternal–fetal interface, and is the site of information exchange between these tissues. As such, it is the tissue in which the intricate balance that ensures successful completion of gestation is most intimately maintained. It is recently becoming apparent that varying degrees of decidualization-like differentiation of endometrial stroma occur in all implanting species, with most extensive transformation accompanying invasive implantation of rodents and primates, moderate transformation with synepitheliochorial placentation, and only minor changes occurring in epitheliochorial implanting pigs.[51]

PREGNANCY-ASSOCIATED ALTERATIONS IN STROMA OF DOMESTIC ANIMALS

Decidualization is characteristic of primates and rodents with invasive implantation, but is not thought to be a property of species with central and non-invasive implantation, including domestic livestock. Because domestic livestock have central non-invasive implantation, few studies have focused on the role of and changes in the uterine stroma that underlie LE. As a result, a considerable gap has developed in knowledge of events in uterine function that may be critical for conceptus survival in these species because, similar to decidua, the endometrial stroma of epitheliochorial and synepitheliochorial placentation serves as the intimate source of hematotropic and hormonal/cytokine support to the LE which directly contacts the fetal placental membranes. Indeed, in the case of the marginally invasive binucleate cells and syncytial formation that occurs in ruminants, stroma potentially regulates placentation by limiting trophoblast invasion through the uterine wall. Certainly, epithelial–stromal interactions have been implicated in development, growth, differentiation, and adult function of the uterus. The stroma is crucial for maintaining hormonal responsiveness, morphogenesis, and secretory function of the uterine epithelium.[52] Uterine epithelial–stromal interactions are also crucial for placental growth and development,[53] and establishment and maintenance of pregnancy in sheep and pigs appears to involve interdependent paracrine conceptus–endometrial and epithelial–stromal interactions.[54–56] Recently, several genes have been shown to be induced in uterine stroma of ruminants in response to conceptus-derived interferon τ (INFτ). The temporal and spatial expression of these genes may be mechanistically involved in a hormonal servomechanism in the sheep uterus, hypothesized to be critical for establishment and maintenance of pregnancy.[56–63] Likewise, changes in ECM and integrin expression within the uterine stroma have been correlated with time of implantation in ruminants, and are believed to be associated with modifications of the composition of the basal lamina that separates LE from underlying stroma.[64–66] Furthermore, observed changes in cell morphology and gene expression indicate that the endometrial stroma of sheep undergoes a program of differentiation that is somewhat similar to decidualization.[51,67]

Cytoskeletal and extracellular matrix molecules

Although decidualization is generally not recognized in domestic livestock, a few early reports suggested that this physiological phenomenon may not be limited to species with invasive implantation. In 1937, Mossman described rounded or polyhedral endometrial connective tissue cells within ovine placentomes.[68] Similar morphological alterations were later reported in 1966 for antelope endometrial stromal fibroblasts.[69] In support of these studies, reported changes in the LE and its supporting basal lamina adjacent to implanting trophectoderm strongly suggest that adhesion to the apical LE causes structural modification of the basal lamina that triggers remodeling of the underlying endometrial stroma of ruminants. In sheep and goats, cytoplasmic processes from the uterine syncytium perforate the basal lamina.[70] Furthermore, in cattle, the basal lamina changes from a strait to a scalloped profile, accompanied by the development of cells within the stratum compactum stroma that stain differently from the other cells of the stroma.[71] It is evident that changes in stromal expression of the ECM molecules type IV collagen and laminin directly result from epithelial modifications; however, reports conflict. In goats, progressive loss of these ECM proteins from the basal lamina and underlying stroma was observed as implantation progressed,[64] and a similar temporal and spatial pattern of expression was reported for cattle.[66] In contrast, MacIntyre et al observed a marked increase in type IV collagen and laminin expression, from a narrow band associated with the basal lamina of the LE to a wide zone of expression extending deep into the stratum compactum stroma of cattle,[65] correlating perfectly with the earlier reports of stromal changes by King et al.[71] Subsequent studies in sheep and goats clearly indicate that endometrial stroma differentiates in response to implantation and placentation.[51,67] A comparison of

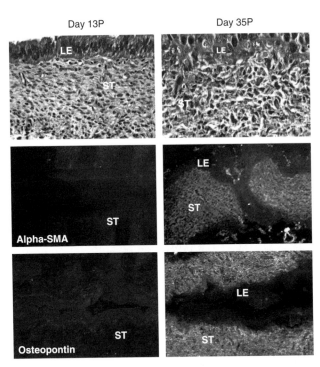

Figure 27.2 Morphological and biochemical differentiation of uterine stroma during the peri-implantation period. Representative photomicrographs of endometrium from day 13 and day 35 pregnant (P) sheep. The top panel shows paraffin-embedded tissues subjected to Masson trichrome stain. This procedure stains nuclei black, cytoplasm and muscle fibers red, and ECM blue. The bottom two panels show OCT-embedded frozen tissues subjected to immunofluorescence staining for α-SMA and SPP1 (osteopontin), respectively. LE, luminal epithelium; ST, stroma.

histoarchitecture between sheep endometrial sections from before implantation (day 13) and after implantation (day 35) showed a decrease in ECM concurrent with the development of fibroblastic cells that exhibited classic morphological characteristics of decidualization, including increased size and rounded or polyhedral shape (Figure 27.2). In addition, the decidualization markers SPP1, desmin, and α-SMA were induced in pregnant uterine stroma of sheep (see Figure 27.2). In goats, increases in stromal expression of both SPP1 and α-SMA were observed during the peri-implantation period.[67]

In contrast to synepitheliochorial sheep, there are no reports of hypertrophy and glycogen accumulation indicative of 'decidualization' within the stratum compactum stroma of true epitheliochorial pigs during pregnancy, and the basal lamina of pigs shows no apparent modification during implantation.[72] It is therefore not surprising that Johnson et al were unable to demonstrate significant morphological or biochemical differentiation in the endometrial stroma of pregnant pigs.[51] This has led to the hypothesis that differential morphology and expression of SPP1, desmin, and α-SMA in the uterine stroma of sheep, goats, and pigs defines a decidualization-like response that correlates with the degree of conceptus invasiveness, and functions to protect and limit trophoblast invasion beyond the compromised LE barrier in ruminants. Transient but direct exposure of stratum compactum stroma to invading embryonic membranes in the form of binucleate cell migration and fusion to form syncytia results in a decidualization-like transformation that restrains further conceptus invasion and maintains superficial implantation in ruminants. There were no obvious morphological changes in porcine uterine stroma through day 40 of pregnancy, because the uterine LE remains intact and placental membranes do not invade the uterine wall. Interestingly, stromal differentiation in goats, as measured by up-regulation of selected genes, was intermediate between sheep and pigs.[67] SPP1 and α-SMA, but not desmin, increased in goat stroma during the latter stages of the peri-implantation period. These results strongly support the hypothesis that endometrial differentiation is common to species with different types of placentation and correlates with the extent of trophoblast interaction with endometrial stroma during implantation. These comparative data are summarized in Table 27.1. Primate and rodent trophectoderm invades the uterine wall to elicit a classical decidualization response.[35] Sheep and goat trophectoderm binucleate cells invade and fuse with LE to form syncytia that terminate at the LE–stromal interface to elicit a decidualization-like differentiation of stromal cells that is slightly less extensive in goats that lack chorionic papilli to anchor conceptus to uterus.[73] And pig trophectoderm simply attaches to the apical surface of LE, eliciting only limited stromal differentiation in response to implantation.

Recently, unilaterally pregnant sheep in which one uterine horn was ligated and the ipsilateral ovary removed to allow comparison between non-gravid and gravid horns have provided strong evidence that stromal differentiation is indeed directly induced by the events of placentation in ruminants (Figure 27.3). When endometrial tissue sections from the gravid and non-gravid horns of the same sheep were subjected to immunofluorescence staining for the cytoskeletal proteins desmin and α-SMA, and the ECM proteins vitronectin and SPP1, each of these markers for decidualization exhibited significantly higher expression in the gravid over the non-gravid horn, with the gravid horn exhibiting extensive expression of SPP1 and vitronectin throughout the stroma, whereas SPP1 protein was detected at lower levels and vitronectin was not detectable in the non-gravid horn (see Figure 27.3).

Table 27.1   Decidualization markers in endometrial stromal fibroblasts

Species	Pre- or post-conceptus attachment	α-SMA	OPN	Desmin
Sheep	Pre	(–)	(–)	(–)
Sheep	Post	(+)	(+)	(+)
Goat	Pre	(–)	(–)	(–)
Goat	Post	(+)	(+)	(–)
Pig	Pre	(–)	(–)	(–)
Pig	Post	(–)	(–)	(–)

α-SMA, α-smooth muscle actin; OPN, osteopontin (SPP1).

Clearly, pregnancy hormones were not sufficient to elicit OPN, vitronectin, and α-SMA in the stroma of non-gravid horns, suggesting that stromal expression of these cytoskeletal and ECM proteins is triggered by the immediate presence of embryonic/placental tissue. The unilaterally pregnant sheep model should provide an excellent opportunity for the assessment of global changes in gene expression of stroma as it undergoes a limited decidual-like transformation. A better understanding of the novel stromal cell differentiation observed in sheep can be exploited to gain insight into the mechanistic nature of the various genes that increase in the decidua of invasive implanting species to coordinate remodeling of the uterine wall for the progressive processes of implantation and placentation.

Interferon-stimulated genes

The peri-implantation period of mammals is complex, involving the overlapping events of pregnancy recognition and remodeling for placentation necessary for conceptus survival during early pregnancy. During early pregnancy in ruminants, the mononuclear cells of the placental trophectoderm synthesize and secrete IFNτ, the signal for maternal recognition of pregnancy.[74] IFNτ acts on the endometrial LE and superficial glandular epithelium to block increases in transcription of estrogen receptor α (ERα) to preclude ERα interactions with (SP1) and/or activating protein 1 (AP-1) that otherwise stimulate oxytocin receptor expression, thereby preventing oxytocin from inducing release of luteolytic pulses of prostaglandin $F_{2\alpha}$.[75] This results in maintenance of the corpus luteum, the source of progesterone required for successful pregnancy.[74] In addition to its antiluteolytic effects, IFNτ also increases expression of several IFN-stimulated genes (ISGs) in the stroma of the ruminant uterus. Over the last 7 years the list of ISGs known to be up-regulated in endometrial

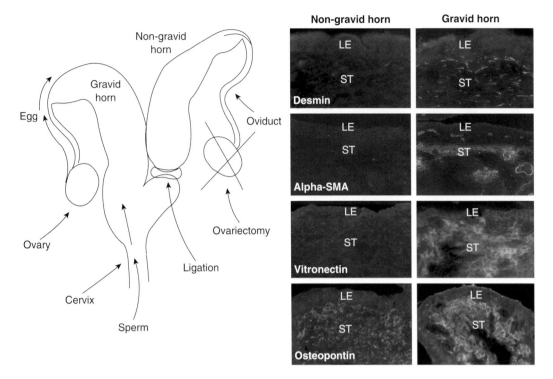

Figure 27.3   Stromal differentiation is directly induced by attachment of the placenta to the uterine LE. (**A**) The ovary ipsilateral to the right uterine horn of a sheep was removed, and a double ligature placed on the base of the right uterine horn at the uterine bifurcation. At the following estrus, the sheep was mated to generate a pregnant gravid and a pregnant non-gravid uterine horn. (**B**) Representative photomicrographs of endometrium from day 145 of gestation. OCT-embedded frozen tissues were subjected to immunofluorescence staining for desmin, α-SMA, vitronectin, and SPP1 (osteopontin), respectively. As expected, increased immunostaining was observed for desmin and α-SMA in the endometrial vasculature of gravid over non-gravid uterine horns, indicating angiogenesis in response to placentation. However, α-SMA also increased in a band of stromal fibroblasts in gravid but not non-gravid horns. Vitronectin expression was induced and SPP1 expression increased in the stroma of gravid horns. LE, luminal epithelium; ST, stroma.

stroma has grown from one (ISG15) to 15. Most of these genes have been characterized in the sheep, and include signal transducer and activator of transcription 1 (STAT1) and STAT2,[60] major histocompatibility complex (MHC) class I and β₂-microglobulin,[76] IFN regulatory factor 1 (IRF1) and IRF9,[60] Mx,[57] 2′,5′-oligoadenylate synthetase (OAS),[77] ubiquitin conjugating enzymes 1-8U and Leu-13,[63,78] cathepsins H and K,[62] ferratin heavy polypeptide 1,[63] prothymosin α,[63] and ISG15.[58,59,61] Although the temporal and spatial expression within the endometrial stroma of pregnant sheep varies slightly between genes, for the most part they follow the expression pattern first described for ISG15 (Figure 27.4). ISG15 mRNA is first detectable in the LE and stratum compactum stroma on day 13 of pregnancy (immediately prior to implantation); then expression extends to the stratum spongiosum stroma by day 15 (time of implantation). Expression is maintained throughout the stroma through day 25, then declines by day 30 of pregnancy, with expression limited to patches of the stratum compactum stroma along the maternal–conceptus interface where it remains throughout pregnancy.[59,61] At present, there

is only speculation on the roles of ISGs within the pregnant endometrium. The best characterized of these genes, ISG15 is a functional ubiquitin homologue that has the C-terminus Leu–Arg–Gly–Gly amino acid sequence common to ubiquitin, allowing conjugation to intracellular proteins.[79] Conjugation of proteins either targets proteins for rapid degradation in the proteasome, or stabilizes proteins for long-term modification.[80] ISG15 does indeed form stable conjugates with endometrial proteins, indicating a biologically active molecule that is responsive to the IFNτ signal from the trophectoderm that can temporally target proteins for pregnancy-associated regulation and/or modification.[61,81] A hallmark of pregnancy in invasive implanting species is the decidualization that uterine stroma undergoes in response to the invading embryo. ISG15 has been shown to be expressed in decidua of mice,[82] baboons,[83] and humans.[84] It is reasonable to project involvement of ISG15 conjugation in decidual roles of hormone secretion, embryo nutrition, fetal allograft protection, uterine remodeling, and limiting of conceptus trophoblast invasion through generation of a local cytokine environment that promotes conceptus attachment over invasion.[34]

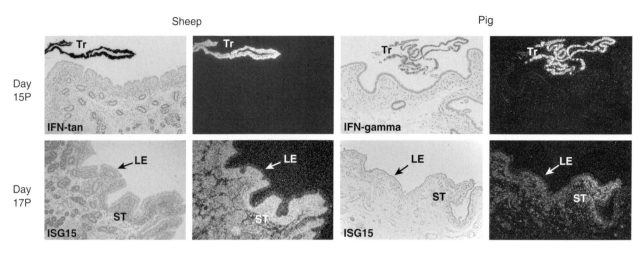

Figure 27.4   Tophoblast interferons increase expression of genes within the endometrial stroma of domestic livestock. In situ hybridization analyses of IFN-τ, IFN-γ, and ISG15 mRNA in cross-sections of sheep and pig uterus and placenta. Corresponding bright- and dark-field images from day 15 and day 17 pregnant (P) sheep and pigs are shown. LE, luminal epithelium; ST, stroma; Tr, trophectoderm.

It may be significant that type I and type II IFNs are produced by the conceptuses of several species, including those that undergo classical stromal decidualization during pregnancy. First-trimester human placental tissues produce the type II IFN γ, with the most intense expression in villous syncytiotrophoblast and extravillous interstitial trophoblast.[85] Stimulation of these tissues with granulocyte–macrophage colony-stimulating factor (GM-CSF), platelet-derived growth factor (PDGF), or Sendai virus results in significant production and secretion of the type I IFNα and IFNβ by invasive extravillous trophoblasts.[86] In mouse placental tissue, antiviral activity consistent with a type I IFN has been detected,[87] but may not be due to a classical IFNα or IFNβ.[88] As stated above, both humans and mice exhibit decidual expression of ISG15, perhaps in response to conceptus IFNs.[82,84] ISGs are also induced in the endometrial stroma of pigs during the peri-implantation period (see Figure 27.4). Similar to in ruminants, these ISGs are expressed by the fibroblasts of the uterine stroma. Because, ISGs do not increase in the endometrium during porcine pseudopregnancy,[89] it is likely that the embryo is involved in the expression of these proteins. Indeed, peri-implantation pig trophectoderm produces type I and type II IFNs, although their physiological role(s) is not clear.[90] The major species is a member of the type II IFN family (IFNγ) and the other is a novel type I IFN (IFNδ).[91] Type I and II IFNs in pigs do not appear to be antiluteolytic during early pregnancy,[92] but paracrine effects for IFNs are suggested by localization of IFN receptors on endometrial epithelial cells.[92] The observation that various species utilizing different factors for maternal recognition of pregnancy express ISGs in endometrial stroma suggests that ISG expression is not merely a consequence of an antiviral state induced by high levels of IFNτ in the lumen of ruminants during pregnancy recognition. Induction of ISGs in stroma may represent one facet of a complex temporal and spatial response of the stroma as its functions change in response to the progressive processes of embryonic development, implantation, and placentation.

Expression of secreted phosphoprotein 1 (osteopontin)

Early reports of SPP1 in the uteri of mice noted high levels in decidua.[93] As such, SPP1 became a marker gene for decidualization.[94] SPP1 mRNA and protein have since been localized in human and baboon decidual cells,[49,95–97] where it is hypothesized that SPP1 may be essential for stromal cell proliferation and differentiation.[95] Global gene profiling using high-density microarray technology has recently identified endometrial genes that either increase or decrease throughout pregnancy in rats.[98] SPP1 gene expression increased 60-fold between day 0 of the estrous cycle and day 20 of pregnancy, the second greatest increase of all genes measured.[98] Due to the prominence of the decidual response in rats, it is likely that much of this increase in SPP1 occurs in the decidua. Indeed, evidence from mice shows significant up-regulation of SPP1 in a population of large granulated uterine natural killer (uNK) cells within the central zone and metrial triangle of decidua, extending to more antimesometrial regions

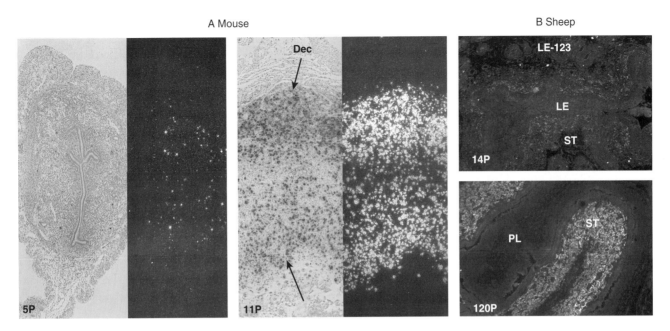

Figure 27.5 SPP1 increases within the stromal compartment adjacent to fetal placenta of mice and sheep. (**A**) In-situ hybridization analysis of SPP1 in cross-sections of mouse uterus. Corresponding bright- and dark-field images from day 5 and 11 pregnant (P) mice are shown. Note APP1 mRNA in uterine NK cells on day 11 of pregnancy. (**B**) Immunofluorescence analysis using anti-SPP1 IgG (LF-123) of OCT-embedded uterine cross-sections from days 14 and 120 of sheep pregnancy. Note SPP1 protein in the stromal fibroblasts on day 120 of pregnancy. Dec, decidua; LE, luminal epithelium; ST, stroma.

adjacent to trophoblast giant cells[48,94] (Figure 27.5). A culmination of studies in mice lacking functional uNK cells indicates that these cells function to support normal development of the decidua and its vasculature.[99,100] Implantation sites from four strains of mice that lack uNK cells (IL null, TG,26, IL-2∃ null × p56[lck], and IL-2R) have anomalies including a lack of lymphocyte aggregation in the mesometrial triangle, hypocellularity and edema of the mesometrial decidua, short decidual spiral arteries with thick walls and reduced luminal diameters, and an overall decrease in size of placenta and fetuses.[100] Significantly, SPP1 null mice exhibit decreases in embryo size on days 10.5, 15.5, and 19.5 of pregnancy similar to those for fetuses of uNK cell-deficient strains of mice,[101] and in mice, uNK cells accumulate and surround the vasculature to supply SPP1 to the decidua in areas correlating spatially and temporally with angiogenic growth of decidual arteries.[100] It is of interest from the comparative physiology perspective that the prominent presence of SPP1 in decidual tissue is conserved despite species differences in localization, i.e. in the decidual stroma of primates, compared to uNK cells of mice[49,94,96,97] (see Figure 27.5). Similar to primates, SPP1 increases in the stratum compactum stroma of pregnant sheep and goats strongly suggests decidual-like transformation of stromal cells in these non-decidualizing species[51,67] (see Figure 27.5).

A comparative examination of SPP1 expression between superficially implanting sheep and pigs may provide valuable insight into the mechanistic nature of the induction of in vivo decidualization. Pig conceptuses undergo true epitheliochorial placentation in which LE remains morphologically intact throughout pregnancy and the conceptus trophectoderm simply attaches to the apical LE surface without contacting the basal lamina or stromal surface.[102] In this species, SPP1 is never expressed in uterine stroma.[51] Synepitheliochorial placentation in sheep involves extensive erosion of the LE due to syncytium formation with trophectoderm binucleate cells. After day 19 of pregnancy, conceptus tissue is apposed to but does not penetrate the uterine stroma.[103] In sheep, expression of SPP1 is low to undetectable in fibroblastic cells of the stratum compactum stroma during the estrous cycle and days 11–20 of pregnancy. However, SPP1 increases in the stratum compactum stroma by day 25, and is detectable in stromal fibroblasts through day 120 of pregnancy.[51] The upregulation of SPP1 within stromal fibroblasts is at least in part the result of placental attachment. When sheep were made unilaterally pregnant to produce pregnant gravid and pregnant non-gravid uterine horns, stromal expression of SPP1 increased significantly in gravid over non-gravid horns (see Figure 27.3). Clearly, pregnancy levels of systemic endocrine factors such as steroid hormones are not sufficient alone to increase SPP1 to maximal level in uterine stroma. However, a role for progesterone, the hormone of pregnancy, to induce SPP1 in stroma cannot be dismissed. The non-gravid horns of unilaterally pregnant sheep have detectable levels of SPP1 above those of uterine tissues from the estrous cycle or early pregnancy (see Figure 27.3). In addition, ovariectomized sheep given daily progesterone injections exhibit low levels of SPP1 that are not observed in the stroma of similar sheep given vehicle in place of progesterone.[104] Collectively, comparative results between sheep and pigs strongly support the hypothesis that stromal differentiation is common to species with different types of placentation and correlates with the extent of trophoblast interaction with endometrial stroma during implantation. Primate and rodent trophectoderm invades the uterine wall to elicit a classical decidualization response. Sheep trophectodermal binucleate cells invade and fuse with LE to form syncytia that terminate at the LE–stromal interface to elicit a decidualization-like stromal differentiation, whereas pig trophectoderm simply attaches to the apical surface of LE, resulting in nominal stromal differentiation in response to implantation.

CONCLUSIONS

Unexplained chronic infertility affects more than six million women in the USA.[105] Although this statistic represents great emotional pain for couples trying to begin families, it is not surprising in light of the fact that, even in fertile women, only 40–50% of babies are estimated to survive beyond the fifth month of pregnancy.[3] Some 75% of these pregnancy failures are not clinically recognized as pregnancies because of an inability of the developing conceptus:

- to attach to the uterine endometrial LE
- to implant into the uterine wall
- to form a functional placenta.

Paramount to success of these processes are

1. Secretions from the uterine epithelia, i.e. histotroph, to support attachment, development, and growth of the conceptus.
2. Remodeling at the uterine mucosal epithelial surface to allow intimate association between conceptus and uterus for implantation.
3. Remodeling of the uterine stroma to control movement of the conceptus through the uterine wall during implantation while generating a cytokine-rich

environment that directly promotes hematotropic support for the developing conceptus.

Essential as this third process is, the physiological, cellular, and molecular interactions between the developing conceptus and the maternal uterine endometrium that result in decidualization remain largely to be defined. During the past decade, knowledge of the mechanisms and factors regulating conceptus implantation in mammals has benefited through insights from domestic animals. However, the focus has been on trophectoderm–epithelial interactions rather than on stromal remodeling for implantation because domestic animals undergo superficial implantation and do not develop a classic decidual response. Recent results highlighted in this chapter strongly suggest that the uterine stroma of many non-decidualizing species undergoes differentiation, but understanding of stromal differentiation in domestic species lags behind what is known about decidualization in mice and humans. The future for advancement of knowledge of this biology is promising. The sequencing of the genomes of domestic animals should generate knowledge and reagents useful for research efforts. Methodologies are now available to mechanistically assess individual stromal factors and their integrative roles by in-vivo, ex-vivo, and in-vitro experiments, global gene array studies, and gain-of-function and loss-of-function studies using promising technologies such as adenoviruses, antisense oligodeoxynucleotides, morpholinos, and small inhibitory RNAs. The limited and graded changes that occur in the stroma of domestic animals offer a unique opportunity to investigate the basic mechanisms underlying conceptus–maternal interactions within the uterine wall. An increased understanding of the mechanisms underlying stromal remodeling for implantation in non-decidualizing species can be used for the rational design of therapies to enhance pregnancy rates in domestic animals and humans.

ACKNOWLEDGMENTS

The author thanks colleagues and the present and past members of the laboratory who contributed much of the research presented in this chapter. In particular, thanks are extended to Dr Robert C Burghardt, Department of Veterinary Integrative Biosciences, Texas A&M University, who has been a daily collaborator in this research. Financial support for these studies was obtained from NIH grants 1-F32-HD08501-0lAl and P30ES0910607.

REFERENCES

1. Flint APF, Saunders PTK, Ziecik AJ. Blastocyst–endometrium interactions and their significance in embryonic mortality. In: Cole DJA Foxcroft GR, eds. Control of Pig Reproduction. London: Butterworth Scientific, 1982: 253–75.

2. Jainudeen MR, Hafez ESE. Reproductive failure in farm animals. In: Hafez ESE, ed. Reproduction in Farm Animals. Philadelphia, PA: Lea and Febiger, 1987: 399–422.

3. Wilcox AJ, Baird DD, Weinberg CR. Time of implantation of the conceptus and loss of pregnancy. N Engl J Med 1999; 340: 1796–9.

4. Norwitz ER, Schust DJ, Fisher SJ. Implantation and the survival of early pregnancy. N Engl J Med 2001; 345: 1400–8.

5. Lessey BA. Adhesion molecules and implantation. J Reprod Immunol 2002; 55: 101–12.

6. Ashworth CJ, Bazer FW. Changes in ovine conceptus and endometrial function following asynchronous embryo transfer or administration of progesterone. Biol Reprod 1989; 40: 425–33.

7. Gray CA, Taylor KM, Ramsey WS et al. Endometrial glands are required for preimplantation conceptus elongation and survival. Biol Reprod 2001; 64: 1608–13.

8. Burton GJ, Watson AL, Hempstock J et al. Uterine glands provide histiotrophic nutrition for the human fetus during the first trimester of pregnancy. J Clin Endocrinol Metab 2002; 87: 2954–9.

9. Glasser SR, Mulholland J. Receptivity is a polarity dependent special function of hormonally regulated uterine epithelial cells. Microsc Res Tech 1993; 25: 106–20.

10. Denker HW. Implantation: a cell biological paradox. J Exp Zool 1993; 266: 541–58.

11. Burghardt RC, Johnson GA, Jaeger LA et al. Integrins and extracellular matrix proteins at the maternal/fetal interface in domestic animals. Cells, Tissues, Organs Special Issue "Molecular Approaches in Cell–Cell Adhesion". Essen Symposium 2002; 172: 202–17.

12. Kliman HJ. Uteroplacental blood flow. The story of decidualization, menstruation, and trophoblast invasion. Am J Pathol 2000; 157: 1759–68.

13. Dosiou C, Giudice LC. Natural killer cells in pregnancy and recurrent pregnancy loss: endocrine and immunologic perspectives. Endocr Rev 2005; 26: 44–62.

14. Cross JC, Werb Z, Fisher SJ. Implantation and the placenta: key pieces of the development puzzle. Science 1994; 266: 1508–18.

15. Carson DD, Bagchi I, Dey SK et al. Embryo implantation. Dev Biol 2000; 223: 217–37.

16. Armant DR. Blastocyts don't go it alone. Extrinsic signals fine-tune the intrinsic developmental program of trophoblast cells. Dev Biol 2005; 280: 260–80.

17. Spencer TE, Johnson GA, Bazer FW et al. Implantation mechanisms: insights from the sheep. Reproduction 2004; 128: 656–68.

18. Guillomot M, Flechon JE, Leroy F. Blastocyst development and implantation. In: Thibault C, Levasseur MC, Hunder RHF, eds. Reproduction in Mammals and Man. Paris: Elipses Press, 1993: 387–411.

19. Aplin JD, Meseguer M, Simon C et al. MUC1, glycans and the cell-surface barrier to embryo implantation. Biochem Soc Trans 2001; 29: 153–6.

20. Kimber SJ, Spanswick C. Blastocyst implantation: the adhesion cascade. Semin Cell Dev Biol 2000; 11: 77–92.

21. Kimber SJ, Illingworth IM, Glasser SR. Expression of carbohydrate antigens in the rat uterus during early pregnancy and after ovariectomy and steroid replacement. J Reprod Fertil 1995; 103: 75–87.

22. Johnson GA, Bazer FW, Jaeger LA et al. Muc-1, integrin, and osteopontin expression during the implantation cascade in sheep. Biol Reprod 2001; 65: 820–8.

23. Salamonsen LA. Role of proteases in implantation. Rev Reprod 1999; 4: 11–22.

24. Burton GJ. Human and animal models: limitations and comparisons. In: Barnea ER, Hustin J, Jainiaux E, eds. The First Twelve Weeks of Gestation. Berlin: Springer Press, 1992: 469–85.

25. Wango EO, Wooding FBP, Heap RB. The role of trophoblast binucleate cells in implantation in the goat; a quantitative study. Placenta 1990; 11: 381–94.

26. Wango EO, Wooding FBP, Heap RB. The role of trophoblastic binucleate cells in implantation in the goat: a morphological study. J Anat 1990; 171: 241–57.

27. van den Brule F, Berndt S, Simon N et al. Trophoblast invasion and placentation: molecular mechanisms and regulation. Chem Immunol Allergy 2005; 88: 163–80.

28. Kirby DR. The development of mouse blastocysts transplanted to the cryptorchid and scrotal testes. J Anat 1963; 97: 119–30.

29. Glasser SR, Mulholland J, Mani SJ et al. Blastocyst–endometrial relationships: reciprocal interactions between uterine epithelial and stromal cells and blastocysts. Trophoblast Res 1991; 5: 229–80.

30. Samuel CA, Perry JS. The ultrastructure of pig trophoblast transplanted to an ectopic site in the uterine wall. J Anat 1972; 113: 139–49.

31. Murphy CR. The cytoskeleton of uterine epithelial cells: a new player in uterine receptivity and the plasma membrane transformation. Hum Reprod Update 1995; 1: 567–80.

32. Damsky CH, Fitzgerald M, Fisher SJ. Distribution patterns of extracellular matrix components and adhesion receptors are intricately modulated during first trimester cytotrophoblast differentiation along the invasive pathway, in vivo. J Clin Invest 1992; 89: 210–22.

33. Bishof P, Campona A. A model for implantation of the human blastocyst and early placentation. Hum Reprod Update 1996; 2: 252–70.

34. Loke YW, King A, Barrows TD. Decidua in human implantation. Hum Reprod 1995; 10: 14–21.

35. Wynn RM. Ultrastructural development of the human decidua. Am J Obstet Gynecol 1974; 118: 652–70.

36. Abrahamsohn PA, Zorn TM. Implantation and decidualization in rodents. J Exp Zool 1993; 266: 603–28.

37. Gard DL, Lazarides E. The synthesis and distribution of desmin and vimentin during myogenesis in vitro. Cell 1980; 19: 263–75.

38. Sananes N, Weiller S, Baulieu E-E et al. In vitro decidualization of rat endometrial cells. Endocrinology 1978; 103: 86–95.

39. Glasser SR, Julian J. Intermediate filament protein as a marker of uterine stromal cell decidualization. Biol Reprod 1986; 35: 463–74.

40. Oliveira SF, Greca CPS, Abrahamsohn PA et al. Organization of desmin-containing intermediate filaments during differentiation of mouse decidual cells. Histochem Cell Biol 2000; 113: 319–27.

41. Christensen S, Verhage HG, Nowak G et al. Smooth muscle myosin II and alpha smooth muscle actin expression in the baboon (Papio anubis) uterus is associated with glandular secretory activity and stromal cell transformation. Biol Reprod 1995; 53: 598–608.

42. Rao KM, Cohen HJ. Actin cytoskeletal network in aging and cancer. Mutant Res 1991; 256: 139–48.

43. Maslar IA, Powers-Craddock P, Ansbacher R. Decidual prolactin production by organ cultures of human endometrium: effects of continuous and intermittent progesterone treatment. Biol Reprod 1986; 34: 741–50.

44. Kim JJ, Jaffe RC, Fazleabas AT. Insulin-like growth factor binding protein-1 expression in baboon endometrial stromal cells: regulation by filamentous actin and requirement for de novo protein synthesis. Endocrinology 1999; 140: 997–1004.

45. Irwin JC, Giudice LC. IGFBP-1 binds to the placental cytotrophoblast $\alpha_5\beta_1$ integrin and inhibits cytotrophoblast invasion into decidualized endometrial stromal cell culture. Growth Horm IGF Res 1998; 8: 21–31.

46. Popovici RM, Kao L-C, Giudice LC. Discovery of new inducible genes in in vitro decidualized human endometrial stromal cells using microarray technology. Endocrinology 2000; 141: 3510–13.

47. Salamonsen LA, Nie G, Findlay JK. Newly identified endometrial genes of importance for implantation. J Reprod Immunol 2002; 53: 215–25.

48. White FJ, Burghardt RC, Croy BA et al. Osteopontin is expressed by endometrial macrophages and decidual natural killer cells during mouse pregnancy. Biol Reprod 2005; 73 (Suppl 1): 155.

49. von Wolff M, Bohlmann MK, Fiedler C, Ursel S, Strowitzki T. Osteopontin is up-regulated in human decidual stromal cells. Fertil Steril 2004; 81(Suppl 1): 741–8.

50. Lee PD, Giudice LC, Conover CA et al. Insulin-like growth factor binding protein-1: recent findings and new directions. Proc Soc Exp Biol Med 1997; 216: 319–57.

51. Johnson GA, Burghardt RC, Joyce MM et al. Osteopontin expression in uterine stroma indicates a decidualization-like differentiation during ovine pregnancy. Biol Reprod 2003; 68: 1951–8.

52. Cunha GR, Bigsby RM, Cooke PS, Sigimura Y. Stromal–epithelial interactions in adult organs. Cell Differ 1985; 17: 137–48.

53. Guillomot M, Flechon J-E, Wintenberger-Torres S. Conceptus attachment in the ewe: an ultrastructural study. Placenta 1981; 2: 169–82.

54. Ka H, Jaeger LA, Johnson GA et al. Keratinocyte growth factor expression is up-regulated by estrogen in porcine uterine endometrium and it functions in trophectodermal cell proliferation and differentiation. Endocrinology 2001; 142: 2303–10.

55. Chen C, Spencer TE, Bazer FW. Fibroblast growth factor-10: a stromal mediator of epithelial function in the ovine uterus. Biol Reprod 2000; 63: 959–66.

56. Spencer TE, Bazer FW. Biology of progesterone action during pregnancy recognition and maintenance of pregnancy. Front Biosci 2002; 7: d1879–98.

57. Ott TL, Spencer TE, Lin JY et al. Effects of the estrous cycle and early pregnancy on uterine expression of Mx protein in sheep (Ovis aries). Biol Reprod 1998; 59: 784–95.

58. Johnson GA, Austin KJ, Collins AM et al. Endometrial ISG17 mRNA and a related mRNA are induced by interferon-tau and localized to glandular epithelial and stromal cells from pregnant cows. Endocrine 1999; 10: 243–52.

59. Johnson GA, Spencer TE, Hansen TR et al. Expression of the interferon-tau inducible ubiquitin cross-reactive protein in the ovine uterus. Biol Reprod 1999; 61: 312–18.

60. Choi YS, Johnson GA, Burghardt RC et al. Interferon regulatory factor two restricts expression of interferon-stimulated genes to the endometrial stroma and glandular epithelium of the ovine uterus. Biol Reprod 2001; 65: 1038–49.

61. Joyce MM, White FJ, Burghardt RC, et al. Interferon stimulated gene 15 (ISG15) conjugates to cytosolic proteins and is expressed at the uterine–placental interface throughout ovine pregnancy. Endocrinology 2005; 146: 675–84.

62. Song G, Spencer TE, Bazer FW. Cathepsins in the ovine uterus: regulation by pregnancy, progesterone, and interferon tau. Endocrinology 2005; 146: 4825–33.

63. Gray CA, Abbey CA, Beremand PD et al. Identification of endometrial genes regulated by early pregnancy, progesterone,

and interferon tau in the ovine uterus. Biol Reprod 2006; 74: 383–94.

64. Guillomot M. Changes in extracellular matrix components and cytokeratins in the endometrium during goat implantation. Placenta 1999; 20: 339–45.

65. MacIntyre DM, Lim HC, Ryan K et al. Implantation-associated changes in bovine uterine expression of integrins and extracellular matrix. Biol Reprod 2002; 66: 1430–6.

66. Yamada O, Todoroki J-I, Takahashi T et al. The dynamic expression of extracellular matrix in the bovine endometrium at implantation. J Vet Med Sci 2002; 64: 207–14.

67. Joyce MM, González JF, Lewis S et al. Caprine uterine and placental osteopontin expression is distinct among epithelio-chorial implanting species. Placenta 2005; 26: 160–70.

68. Mossman HW. Comparative morphogenesis of the fetal membranes and accessory uterine structures. Contrib Embryol 1937; 26: 129–246.

69. Kellas LM. The placenta and foetal membranes of the antelope Ourebia ourebi (Zimmermann). Acta Anat 1966; 64: 390–445.

70. Lawn AM, Chiquoine AD, Amoroso EC. The development of the placenta in the sheep and goat: an electron microscope study. J Anat 1969; 105: 557–78.

71. King GJ, Atkinson BA, Robertson HA. Development of the bovine placentome from days 20 to 29 of gestation. J Reprod Fertil 1980; 59: 95–100.

72. Bowen JA, Bazer FW, Burghardt RC. Spatial and temporal analyses of integrin and Muc-1 expression in porcine uterine epithelium and trophectoderm in vivo. Biol Reprod 1996; 55: 1098–106.

73. Wooding FBP, Staples LD, Peacock MA. Structure of trophoblast papillae on the sheep conceptus at implantation. J Anat 1982; 134: 507–16.

74. Spencer TE, Burghardt RC, Johnson GA et al. Conceptus signals for establishment and maintenance of pregnancy. Anim Reprod Sci 2004; 82–83: 537–50.

75. Fleming JGW, Spencer TE, Safe SH et al. Estrogen regulates transcription of the ovine oxytocin receptor through GC-rich SP1 promoter elements. Endocrinology 2006; 74: 383–94.

76. Choi YS, Johnson GA, Spencer TE et al. Expression of major histocompatibility class I and beta-2-microglobulin genes in the ovine uterus. Biol Reprod 2003; 68: 1703–10.

77. Johnson GA, Stewart MD, Gray CA et al. Effects of the estrous cycle, pregnancy, and interferon tau on 2',5'-oligoadenylate synthetase expression in the ovine uterus. Biol Reprod 2001; 64: 1392–9.

78. Pru JK, Austin KJ, Haas AL et al. Pregnancy and interferon-τ upregulate gene expression of members of the 1–8 family in the bovine uterus. Biol Reprod 2001; 65: 1471–80.

79. Haas AL, Aherns P, Bright PM et al. Interferon induces a 15-kilodalton protein exhibiting marked homology to ubiquitin. J Biol Chem 1987; 262: 11315–23.

80. Wilkinson KD. Ubiquitination and deubiquitination: targeting of proteins for degradation by the proteasome. Cell Develop Biol 2000; 11: 141–8.

81. Johnson GA, Austin KJ, Van Kirk EA et al. Pregnancy and interferon-tau induce conjugation of bovine ubiquitin cross-reactive protein to cytosolic uterine proteins. Biol Reprod 1998; 58: 898–904.

82. Austin KJ, Bany BM, Belden EL et al. Interferon-stimulated gene-15 (Isg15) expression is up-regulated in the mouse uterus in response to the implanting conceptus. Endocrinology 2003; 144: 3107–13.

83. Bebington C, Bell SC, Doherty FJ et al. Localization of ubiquitin and ubiquitin cross-reactive protein in human and baboon endometrium and decidua during the menstrual cycle and early pregnancy. Biol Reprod 1999; 60: 920–8.

84. Bebington C, Doherty FJ, Fleming SD. Ubiquitin cross-reactive protein gene expression is increased in decidualized

endometrial stromal cells at the initiation of pregnancy. Mol Hum Reprod 1999; 5: 966–72.

85. Paulesu L, Romagnoli R, Cintorino M et al. First trimester human trophoblast expresses both interferon-gamma and interferon-gamma-receptor. J Reprod Immunol 1994; 27: 37–48.

86. Aboagye-Mathiesen G, Tóth FD, Zdravkovic M et al. Functional characteristics of human trophoblast interferons. Am J Reprod Immunol 1996; 35: 309–17.

87. Fowler AK, Reed CD, Giron DJ. Identification of an interferon in murine placentas. Nature 1980; 286: 266–7.

88. Cross JC, Farin CE, Sharif SF et al. Characterization of the antiviral activity consitutively produced by murine conceptuses: absence of placental mRNAs for interferon alpha and beta. Mol Reprod Dev 1990; 26: 122–8.

89. Joyce MM, Burghardt RC, Bazer FW et al. Interferon-stimulated genes (ISGs) are induced in the endometrium of pregnant but not pseudopregnant pigs. Biol Reprod 2003; 68(Suppl 1): 230.

90. Bazer FW, Ott TL, Spencer TE. Endocrinology of the transition from recurring estrous cycles to establishment of pregnancy in subprimate mammals. In: Bazer FW, ed. Endocrinology of Pregnancy. New Jersey: Humana Press, 1998: 1–34.

91. Lefevre F, Guillomot M, D'Andrea S et al. Interferon-delta: the first member of a novel type I interferon famile. Biochimie 1998; 80: 779–88.

92. Lefevre F, Martinatbotte F, Locatelli A et al. Intrauterine infusion of high doses of pig trophoblast interferons has no antiluteolytic effect in cyclic gilts. Biol Reprod 1998; 58: 1026–31.

93. Nomura S, Wills AJ, Edwards DR et al. Developmental expression of 2ar (osteopontin) and SPARC (osteonectin) RNA as revealed by in situ hybridization. J Cell Biol 1988; 106: 441–9.

94. Waterhouse P, Parhar RS, Guo X et al. Regulated temporal and spatial expression of the calcium-binding proteins calcyclin and OPN (osteopontin) in mouse tissues during pregnancy. Mol Reprod Devel 1992; 32: 315–23.

95. Fazleabas AT, Bell SC, Fleming S et al. Distribution of integrins and the extracellular matrix proteins in the baboon endometrium during the menstrual cycle and early pregnancy. Biol Reprod 1997; 56: 348–56.

96. Apparao KB, Murray MJ, Fritz MA et al. Osteopontin and its receptor alphavbeta(3) integrin are coexpressed in the human endometrium during the menstrual cycle but regulated differentially. J Clin Endocrinol Metab 2001; 86: 4991–5000.

97. von Wolff M, Bohlmann MK, Fiedler C et al. Osteopontin is up-regulated in human decidual stromal cells. Fertil Steril 2004; 81(Suppl1): 741–8.

98. Girotti M, Zingg HH. Gene expression profiling of rat uterus at different stages of parturition. Endocrinology 2003; 144: 2254–65.

99. Moffett-King A. Natural killer cells and pregnancy. Nat Rev Immunol 2002; 656–63.

100. Croy BA, He H, Esadeg S et al. Uterine natural killer cells: insights into their cellular and molecular biology from mouse modelling. Reproduction 2003; 126: 149–60.

101. Weintraub AS, Lin X, Itskovich VV et al. Prenatal detection of embryo resorption in osteopontin-deficient mice using serial noninvasive magnetic resonance microscopy. Pediatr Res 2004; 55: 419–24.

102. Bjorkman N. Fine structure of the fetal–maternal area of exchange in the epitheliochorial and endotheliochorial types of placentation. Acat Anat 1973; 61(Suppl 1): 1–22.

103. Boshier DP. A histological and histochemical examination of implantation and early placentome formation in sheep. J Reprod Fertil 1969; 19: 51–61.

104. Burghardt RC, White FJ, Greggs SJ et al. The induction of osteopontin in ovine endometrial stroma requires conceptus attachment. Biol Reprod 2005; 73(Suppl1): 586.

105. Smith S, Pfeifer SM Collins JA. Diagnosis and management of female infertility. JAMA 2003; 290: 1767–70.

28a   Implantation of the blastocyst: I. Comparative studies

FB Peter Wooding

Synopsis

Background

- Loss of microvilli from the trophoblast and uterine epithelium and adhesion of the blastocyst are similar in all mammals.
- Four basic patterns of trophoblast/epithelial interactions: simple interdigitation of microvilli, displacement of, fusion with or intrusion through the uterine epithelium.
- The extent of trophoblast invasion and remodeling of the uterine blood vessels and stroma establishes the characteristic placental barrier layers of each species.

Basic Science

- Spacing of blastocysts are possibly regulated by uterine muscular contractions and secretions from the conceptus.
- Fluid intake by the uterine epithelium intiates the intimate contact between the endometrium and blastocyst – adhesion/apposition stage.
- In pigs, camels and whales apposition between the apices of the intact uterine epithelium and trophoblast forms the basis for placental growth.
- In rabbits, ruminants and some marsupials trophoblast cells fuse with maternal endometrial epithelial cells.
- In rats and mice, apposition of trophoblast cells to the uterine epithelium, initiates epithelial cell apoptosis.
- In carnivores, guinea pigs and probably humans trophoblast cells intrude between uterine epithelial cells.

INTRODUCTION

This chapter consists of a brief comparison, with illustrations, of the wide variety of cellular interactions in mammals between maternal uterine epithelium and fetal trophoblast, from the initial contact to the formation of the definitive cellular placental structure between maternal and fetal circulations. This structure differs widely between species but is very constant within a species.

Loss of microvilli from the trophoblast and uterine epithelium and adhesion between them are similar in all mammalian species. Subsequently, there are four basic patterns of trophoblast interaction with the uterine epithelium: simple interdigitation of microvilli, displacement of, fusion with, or intrusion through the uterine epithelium.

Further trophoblast invasion and/or remodeling of the uterine stroma and blood vessels establishes the wide variety of characteristic placental barrier layers between the circulations from the start of placental development. These layers persist, although increasing enormously in area throughout gestation. The second part of this chapter deals in much greater detail with primate implantation.

INITIAL EVENTS: UTERINE ENTRY TO ADHESION

This review considers the structural events occurring in the period from morula or blastocyst entry into the uterus to the formation of an area of the definitive placental membrane layers.

In different species a wide variety of structures are formed: from pigs with simple apposition of uterine epithelium and trophoblast; to deep penetration into, together with loss of, the surface layers and endothelium of the endometrium with syncytial transformation of the trophoblast in guinea pigs and humans. This process is under multifactorial control with growth factors, cytokines, and hormones all directly involved[1–4] (see Chapters in Sections IV and V) This chapter aims to outline the variety of the basic structural changes. The first observation to be explained is that the distribution of blastocyst implantation site(s) in polytocous species is uniform and in monotocous species usually predictable. At this stage the blastocyst is a sphere of cells surrounded by the zona pellucida and usually implants on the antimesometrial side of the uterus. The spacing of the blastocysts is probably achieved roughly by the muscular contractions of the uterus and fine tuned by secretions from the conceptus influencing local contractions and uterine growth.[4] Assuming an initial random mixing stage this would explain how large pig conceptuses randomize colors, evenly spaced, after different colors are introduced into each horn[5] and also the fact that with smaller rat and guinea pig conceptuses, disruption of the myometrial contractions with relaxin alters the normal even distribution.[6] The predominance of the antimesometrial position is said to be due to circular muscle contractions, since the antimesometrial position is more central with respect to the circular muscle in many uteri. Solid pieces of tumor tissue locate antimesometrially in the mouse uterus,[7] whereas deformable oil droplets are randomly positioned.[8] The usefulness of an extracellular membrane during this positioning process is underlined by the production of a second layer to replace the zona after blastocyst swelling in the rabbit and the horse.[9,10]

Generally, the zona pellucida is lost before or just after positioning is established, probably by the action of a combination of enzymes from the uterine glands and conceptus.[11]

At this stage, for example in the pig, conceptus and uterine epithelial surfaces have well-developed microvilli (Figure 28a.1A,B), both with negative charges on their glycocalyces, and there is increasing evidence for changes in the glycocalyx and plasmalemma to facilitate adhesion[4,12] (see Chapters 5 and 22). The uterine lumen is now obliterated at the implantation sites probably as a result of fluid uptake by the uterine epithelium and edematous swelling of the uterine stroma, and at this stage the conceptus may expand considerably. This brings the

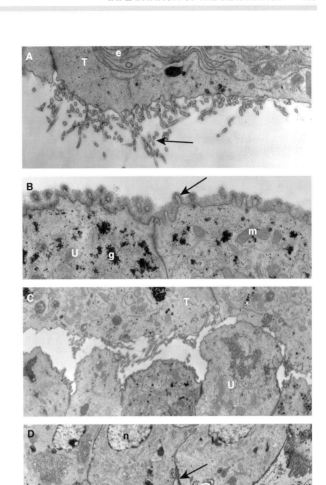

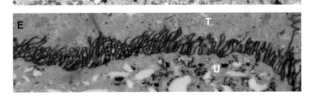

Figure 28a.1 Electron micrographs of early pig implantation. (**A**) 15 days postcoitum (dpc): apex of a trophoblast cell (T) shows elongated microvilli (arrow) characteristic of the free blastocyst, whereas the uterine epithelium (U) at the same stage (**B**) shows blunt microvilli (arrow) with a clear glycocalyx coating all of the plasmalemma surface. (**C**) 16 dpc: the trophoblast (T) is now close to the uterine epithelium (U). The latter has lost its glycocalyx and most of its microvilli and the trophoblast microvilli are considerably reduced. In places (asterisk), the two are in close contact. (**D**) 16 dpc: a different region of the same specimen as in (**C**). Here the trophoblast and the uterine epithelium are in close and flat apposition, with microvillar interdigitation starting in places (arrow). (**E**) 20 dpc to term: the microvillar junction is uniformly developed, maximizing the exchange area between trophoblast (T) and uterine epithelium (U). A,B,×15 000; C,D,E,×8000. Glutaraldehyde/osmium fixation, araldite embedded, uranyl/lead stained (GOAUP); glutaraldehyde fixed, araldite embedded, phosphotungstic acid/uranyl stained (GAPTAU). m, mitochondrion; g, glycogen; e, endoplasmic reticulum; n, nucleus.

conceptus into very close contact with the uterine epithelium and the respective microvilli are modified by apical cytoplasmic changes into a flat apposition between the two apical epithelial plasma membranes (Figure 28a.1C,D).

This is referred to as the adhesion stage since the conceptus(es) cannot be displaced without damage, although there is no definitive freeze fracture evidence for true intercellular junctions (demosomes, tight or spot junctions) between the two membranes. There are definite increases in adhesion between the two surfaces, probably mediated by changes in the molecules of the glycocalyces and the gland secretion of molecules capable of linking the two surfaces[13] (see Chapter 17). This adhesion is also augmented by increased muscle tone in the horse for example.

All species show similar structural changes up to this point, although there are great differences in timing and conceptus size and the adherent trophoblast may be cellular or syncytial.

IMPLANTATION MECHANISMS

Subsequent development can be divided into four categories: interdigitation, fusion, displacement, or intrusion, based on the interaction between trophoblast and uterine epithelial layers (Figure 28a.2)

Interdigitation

The flat apposition develops into mutual interdigitation between trophoblast and uterine epithelial microvilli. These two layers increase in area as pregnancy continues, with considerable thinning but no loss of the epithelia. Examples of this type are from a variety of genera: pig (Figure 28a.1E), camel, lemurs, whales, and dolphins.[4]

Fusion

Maternofetal cellular fusion occurs at some stage in rabbits, ruminants (Figures 28a.2–28a.4), and some marsupials.[4] In the rabbit in a brief initial process, specialized projections or 'knobs' of the syncytial trophoblast fuse with uterine epithelial cells. The rest of the uterine epithelium subsequently turns symplasmic (i.e. not an apoptotic process) and degenerates.[14] The initial maternofetal hybrid tissue is rapidly overgrown by the fetal syncytial trophoblast which is generated

from a cellular cytotrophoblast layer as it penetrates into the stroma to invade the maternal capillaries.

In the ruminants, the first cellular changes are fusions of a population of specialized trophoblast binucleate cells (BNC) with single uterine epithelial cells to form trinucleate cells (see Figures 28a.3 and 28a.4). The cytoplasmic content of the BNC then streams down into the now trinucleate uterine epithelial cell and the numerous granules formed in the BNC are released by exocytosis (see Figure 28a.3B) into the maternal tissue. This is the characteristic feature of ruminant placentation – fetal granules which contain hormones, cytokines, and immunomodulatory molecules are delivered to the maternal circulation from a camouflage of the maternal uterine epithelial plasmalemma.[4] This initiates the maternofetal dialogue essential to a successful pregnancy in this suborder. Continued migration and fusion of BNC into these initially trinucleate cells plus death of adjacent uterine epithelial cells results in maternofetal syncytial plaques replacing the uterine epithelium. In sheep and goats, on the special caruncular areas of the uterus, the cellular trophoblast develops microvillar interdigitations apically with these maternofetal syncytial plaques. These two apposed layers form the definitive placental barrier whose area increases enormously as villi develop to form the characteristic placentomes. The initial uterine epithelial basement membrane persists, although in a much thinner form which is frequently penetrated by processes from the syncytial plaques. The increase in plaque area is fuelled by continuous BNC migration and fusion throughout pregnancy. In cow and deer, the syncytial plaque formation is transient and residual unicellular uterine epithelial cells proliferate to replace it. BNC migration and fusion persists but forming only trinucleate cells in the reformed uterine epithelium. BNC-derived granules are released to the maternal circulation by exocytosis (see Figure 28a.3B) and the trinucleate cells die and are resorbed by the trophoblast and uterine epithelial cells.[4,15]

Some marsupials (Perameles, Isoetes) show fusion of initially separate maternal (uterine epithelium) and fetal (trophoblast) syncytia in the second half of the shortest pregnancy reliably known for any mammal (12.5 days). The definitive placenta thus formed is a thin sheet of maternofetal syncytium deeply indented on both sides by blood vessels;[16] most marsupials have microvillar interdigitation between cellular trophoblast and uterine epithelium throughout pregnancy, although a few show restricted regions where the trophoblast displaces the uterine epithelium.[17]

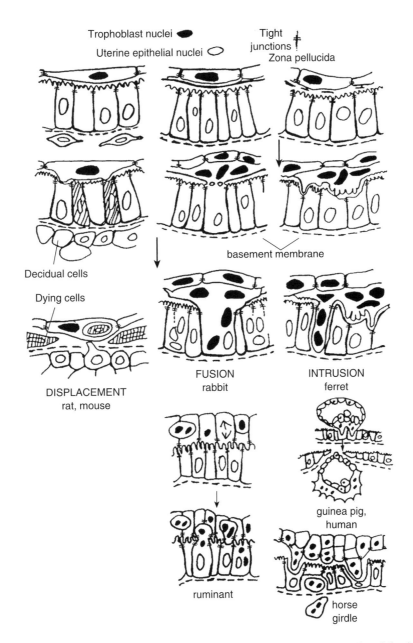

Trophoblast nuclei
Uterine epithelial nuclei
Tight junctions
Zona pellucida
basement membrane
Decidual cells
Dying cells
DISPLACEMENT
rat, mouse
FUSION
rabbit
INTRUSION
ferret
ruminant
guinea pig,
human
horse
girdle

Figure 28a.2   Diagram showing different types of cellular interactions between maternal and fetal tissues at implantation. (Redrawn from Wooding and Flint.[4])

Displacement

In this category, the cellular trophoblast comes into flat apposition with the uterine epithelium, which then dies by apoptosis and is phagocytosed by the cellular trophoblast. This is found in rats and mice.[4] Elimination of the uterine cells requires RNA transcription[18] but is non-specific in that oil droplets can induce the process normally triggered by the trophoblast.[8] Elimination of the uterine epithelium could be one part of the coincident decidualization process whereby uterine stromal changes isolate the

implantation chamber from the maternal vascular system.[12] There is also evidence in the rat that the decidual stromal cells play an important role in disrupting the uterine epithelial basement membrane which has blocked any further trophoblast penetration.[19] Once this basement membrane has been breached, the trophoblast differentiates into primary giant cells, which, by modification of its constituent decidual cells, break through the avascular zone surrounding the conceptus and penetrate the maternal blood sinuses. This allows the maternal blood to irrigate the proliferated surface extensions of these primary giant cells, which

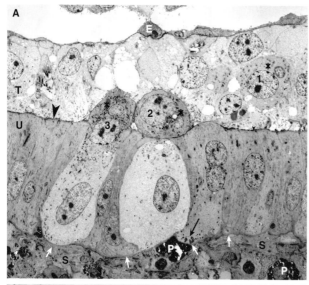

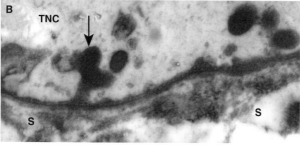

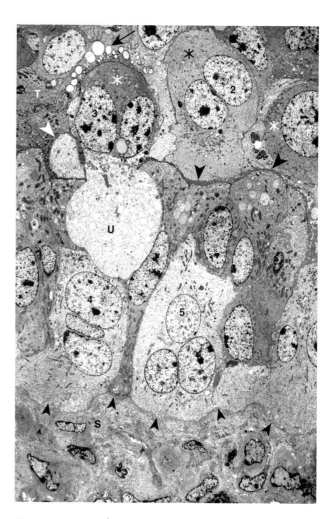

Figures 28a.3 (A,B) Electron micrographs of a 16 dpc ewe implantation site. (**A**) The conceptus (trophoblast [T], endoderm [E]) is closely apposed to the uterine epithelium (U); in places (arrowheads) the microvillar junction is starting to form, and PTA stains this preferentially. Binucleate cells (BNC) develop within the trophoblast epithelium (BNC1), producing their typical complement of PTA staining granules (see white asterisks in BNC1, 2, 3, arrow in 4). They then migrate up to the microvillar junction and fuse apically (BNC2) with a uterine epithelial cell. The content of the BNC is then injected into the uterine epithelial cell (BNC3), the granules streaming down to the base (white arrow) where they exocytose (black arrow in BNC4 and **B**). This forms a trinucleate cell (TNC) such as 4, which has another nucleus out of the plane of this section. P, pigment cell; S, endometrial stroma; white arrows, uterine epithelial cell basement membrane. ×2000, GAPTAU. (**B**) Electron micrograph of the base of a a newly formed TNC showing exocytosis (arrow) of the granules produced in the BNC, releasing their content to the maternal stroma (S). ×24 000, GAPTAU.

form the transient yolk sac placenta.[20] At the same time, the definitive chorioallantoic placenta is forming as a layer of secondary giant cells develop on the surface of the ectoplacental cone, which consists of multilayered unicellular trophoblast cells. There is a considerable loss and remodeling of the mesometrial uterine epithelial cells and stromal decidualized cells immediately above and around the cone in the rat

Figure 28a.4 Electron micrograph of a 20 dpc cow implantation site. The trophoblast (T) forms characteristic granules (asterisks) in the BNC, which are initially (BNC1) within the epithelium. The BNC then migrate up (BNC2) to the microvillar junction (large arrowheads) and eventually fuse (BNC3) with a uterine epithelial cell (U), injecting their cytoplasmic content into the uterine epithelial cell, with the now redundant BNC basolateral plasmalemma blebbing into (arrow), and resorbed by the trophoblast. The TNC so formed (here 4 and 5) have released their granules by exocytosis at the uterine epithelium basement membrane (small arrowheads) to the maternal stroma (S). The BNC granules are less obvious than in Figure 28a.3 with this osmicated preparation. ×2500, GOAUP.

producing finally a large blood sinus into which the cone grows. Once the allantoic sac has reached the base of the ectoplacental cone, considerable growth and differentiation ensue. The secondary giants penetrate the maternal blood sinuses[21] and the cone reorganizes into two closely apposed layers of syncytial trophoblast (Figure 28a.5). This three-layered complex is the basis for the vast increase in area which forms the labyrinthine placenta in the mouse and rat. On the periphery of the cone the trophoblast forms

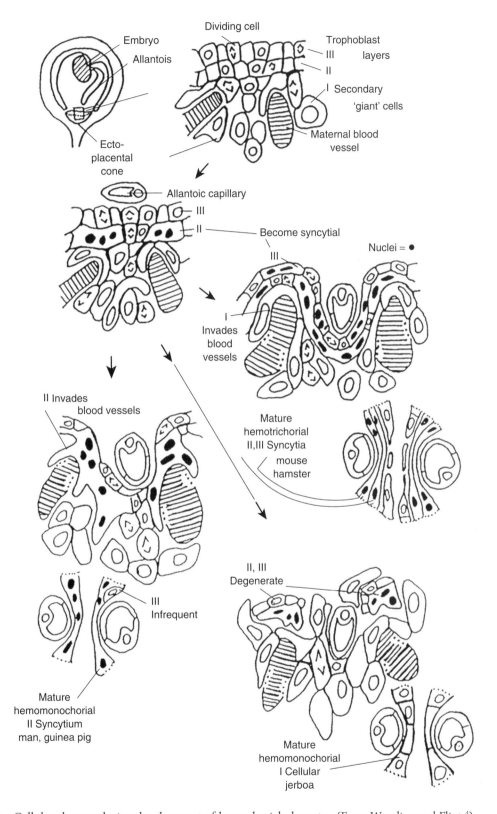

Figure 28a.5   Cellular changes during development of hemochorial placentas. (From Wooding and Flint.[4])

the giants, the cellular spongiotrophoblast layer and cells which migrate into and erode the endothelium of the maternal mesometrial arteries. The allantoic mesoderm vascularizes the proliferating trophoblast layers of the labyrinth whose syncytial components must have considerable unicellular trophoblast interpolations to allow division and growth since nuclei in mammalian syncytia have no capacity for division.[4]

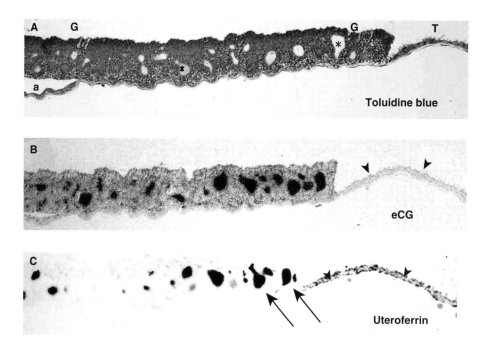

Figure 28a.6 (A–C) Light micrographs of acrylic sections of part of a 37 dpc horse conceptus showing the localized proliferation of the trophoblast (T) cells to form the chorionic girdle (G) around the conceptus. (A) Toluidine blue stained section. The white areas (asterisks) in the girdle are trophoblast cell-lined canaliculi which open at the surface of the girdle. At 'a' notice how easily the girdle BNCs separate from the residual uninucleate trophoblast during processing. (B,C) Adjacent sections processed immunocytochemically to demonstrate equine chorionic gonadotropin (eCG, **B**) and uteroferrin (**C**). (B) Only the girdle cells and canaliculi show localization of eCG immunoreactivity, indicating active synthesis and secretion into the same canaliculi as in **C** (compare at arrows). The non-girdle trophoblast (arrowheads) shows no eCG localization. (C) Uteroferrin (from the maternal uterine glands) is taken up by the non-girdle trophoblast cells (arrowheads) and passively fills the canaliculi, but is not absorbed by the girdle cells. All ×1700.

Not all hemochorial placentas are three layered, but most develop in a similar way, losing one or more layers before forming the definitive structure for that species[4] (see Figure 28a.5).

Intrusion

There are several types of intrusion. In the first, the blastocyst does not expand before apposition but passes through the uterine epithelium, which reforms behind it as found in guinea pigs and humans[22] (see Figure 28a.2). The trophoblast that separates the uterine epithelial cells is syncytial but the detailed ultrastructure of the process of penetration is not yet understood. Once in the stroma, the syncytial trophoblast surrounds the maternal vessels which it eventually disrupts. Other non-human primates implant more superficially after an initial penetration of the uterine epithelium by syncytium (see Chapter 31b for details).

The carnivores show a second type where the enlarged apposed blastocysts extend tongues of syncytial trophoblast between the uterine epithelial cells,

sharing tight and desmosomal junctions with them as the trophoblast pushes down to the uterine epithelial basement membrane[23] (see Figure 28a.2). Trophoblast phagocytoses individual uterine epithelial cells as it spreads, generating syncytium from its backing layer of highly proliferative unicellular cytotrophoblast. These two trophoblast layers surround the maternal blood vessels, which elongate to form the definitive placental membrane structure. This process occurs over the conceptus in the areas that will eventually form the zonary placenta. When the maternal vessels are first surrounded, the trophoblast is backed by the yolk sac, forming a temporary vascular yolk sac placenta. Subsequently, allantoic mesoderm provides the fetal vessels for the equatorial band that constitutes the definitive endotheliochorial allantoic placenta.

In a further intrusive type, seen only in the late implanting equids, a girdle of proliferative trophoblast cells (Figure 28a.6A) forms around the conceptus at about 25 days of pregnancy after loss of both the zona pellucida and the secondary investments or capsule deposited around the subsequently enlarged conceptus.[24,25] At this stage the conceptus is dependent on the uterine secretions for nutrients, as shown by the

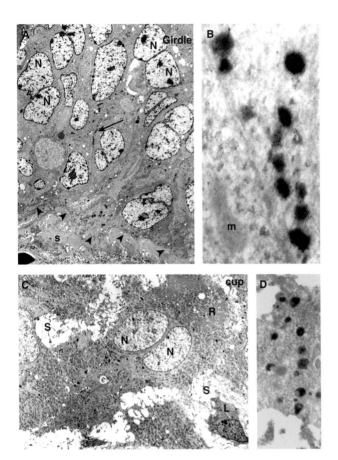

Figure 28a.7 (A–D) Electron micrographs of girdle (**A**) and cup cells (**C**) with immunocytochemical detail (**B,D**). (A) Binucleate (N, N) girdle cells apposed to the original uterine epithelial basement membrane (arrowheads). The small PTA-stained granules (arrow) in the binucleate cells can be shown to contain eCG with immunogold techniques; see the label on the granules in **B**, a higher magnification at the arrow in **A**. (**C**) The girdle cells have now migrated into the endometrial stroma (S) and become cup cells. They have enlarged considerably by proliferation of the rough endoplasmic reticulum (R) and golgi apparatus (G), producing large amounts of eCG in similar size granules (see labeling in **D**) to those in the girdle cells. There is a small maternal lymphocyte (L) between the cup cells in **C**; such cells will eventually accumulate and kill the fetal invaders. **A**, ×22 000; **B**, ×100 000; **D**, ×80 000, GAPTAU; **C** ×35 000, GOAUP. m, mitochondrion; N, nucleus.

uteroferrin uptake by the trophoblast (Figure 28a.6B) The girdle formation is another example of the need for early development of fetomaternal dialogue, since these girdle cells differentiate between 30 and 35 days of pregnancy into binucleate cells capable of equine chorionic gonadotropin (eCG) synthesis (Figure 28a.6C) in flat apposition with uterine epithelial cells.[26] This is an excellent position from which to secrete eCG into the maternal system. Individual girdle cells then protrude pseudopodia into uterine epithelial cell apices (see Figure 28a.2), not into the tight junctions, and

pass through the uterine cells to accumulate on the basement membrane (Figure 28a.7A). As more and more of the BNC migrate, the uterine epithelium is disrupted and replaced by extensive areas of girdle cells with their apices apposed to that basement membrane (see Figure 28a.7A). The trophoblast cells then force their way through the basement membrane into the uterine stroma, forming the endometrial cups. At 50–60 dpc, the cups consist of masses of binucleate trophoblast cells (producing large amounts of eCG; Figure 28a.7B) interspersed with endometrial glands and blood vessels. The lumen of the superficial lymphatic vessels is obliterated by the swelling cup cells, but there are numerous patent deeper lymphatics. The uterine epithelium partially reforms from residual cells and is separated by cup cell secretion from a now uninucleate trophoblast layer on the conceptus – no girdle cells persist in this position. Trophoblast girdle cell differentiation, intrusive migration, cup formation, and hormone secretion are events initiating fetomaternal dialogue in normal equine pregnancy but transient (27–100 dpc, the first third of pregnancy only) and only involve a small area of the conceptus trophoblast surface. Most trophoblast is uninucleate at all times and develops microvillar interdigitation with the uterine epithelium it initially apposes. The definitive placental structure is epitheliochorial as in the pig but with focal membrane proliferation in microcotyledons unlike the diffuse folds seen in the pig.[4]

Implantation in the eventually endotheliochorial elephant placenta shows an interesting variant on the carnivore pattern. The exact method of penetration of the uterine epithelium is as yet unknown, but once a tongue of unicellular trophoblast cells has reached uterine epithelial cell basement membrane, the rest of the epithelium is undermined by spreading trophoblast (Figure 28a.8A) until in what will become the zonary placental region the apex of the trophoblast is apposed to the basement membrane of the uterine epithelium closely adjacent to the maternal endometrial capillaries (Figure 28a.8B). Unlike the carnivore, there is no subsequent syncytium formation and invasion of the endometrium but rather a mutual developmental upgrowth of maternofetal villi of endomonocytochorial structure above the plane of the original endometrium.[27] The fruit bat, Carollia, has also recently been shown to have invasion by cellular trophoblast, initially attaching at the ridges of tight junction on the uterine epithelium and then intruding between the maternal cells while sharing their tight junction.[28] The uterine epithelial cells are removed by phagocytosis by the cellular trophoblast, which only produces a syncytial layer when it reaches the basement membrane of the maternal capillaries. This

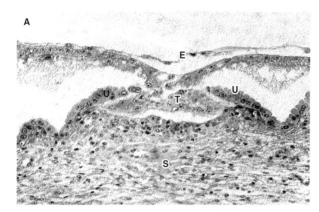

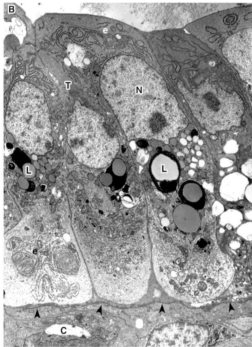

Figure 28a.8 (A) Elephant implantation site, light micrograph. A tongue of trophoblast (T) from the conceptus has penetrated the uterine epithelium and is spreading under (arrowheads) and displacing the intact epithelium (U) at either side. ×250, glutaraldehyde fixation, wax embedding; H & E staining. **(B)** Electron micrograph of a stage subsequent to **A** with the trophoblast (T) now apposed to the original basement membrane of the uterine epithelium (arrowheads), and close to a maternal capillary (C) ×2500, GOAUP. E, fetal endoderm; S, endometrial stroma; c, maternal capillary; N, nucleus; L, lysosome; e, endoplasmic reticulum.

syncytial layer envelopes these capillaries and the mutual growth of these two components then produces the definitive endotheliochorial lamellar placenta characteristic of the carnivores.

The categories interdigitation/fusion/displacement and intrusion are convenient but not exclusive. As more exact observations are made of optimally perfusion-fixed material, recent evidence indicates that maternofetal fusion may be more widespread than initially thought, both in carnivores and rodents. Initial cellular interactions at implantation do not necessarily relate to the definitive placental structure. The horse endometrial cup, maternofetal fusion in carnivores and some ruminants, and plaque formation in primates may be explained more convincingly as transient solutions to the immediate and overriding problem of maternofetal accommodation, the need to minimize immunological intrusion while maximizing nutrient transfer rather than as gradual structural modifications resulting in the definitive placental membrane structures.

REFERENCES

1. Ben Rafael Z, Orvieto R. Cytokines: involvement in reproduction. Fertil Steril 1992; 58: 1093–9.
2. Strickland S, Richards WG. Invasion of the trophoblasts. Cell 1992; 71: 355–7.
3. Wathes DC. Commentary: embryonic mortality and the uterine environment. J Endocrinol 1992; 134: 321–5.
4. Wooding FBP, Flint APF. Placentation. In: Lamming GE, ed. Marshall's Physiology of Reproduction, Vol. III, Part 1, 4th edn. London: Chapman and Hall, 1994: 230–466.
5. Dziuk PJ, Polge C, Rowson LE. Intrauterine migration and mixing of embryos in swine following egg transfer. J Anim Sci 1964; 23: 37–42.
6. Pusey J, Kelly WA, Bradshaw JMC, Porter, DG. Myometrial activity and the distribution of blastocysts in the uterus of the rat: interference by relaxin. Biol Reprod 1980; 23: 394–7.
7. Wilson IB. Tumour tissue analogue of the implanting mouse embryo. Proc Zool Soc Lond 1963; 141: 137–51.
8. Martin L. Early cellular changes and circular muscle contraction associated with the induction of decidualization by intrauterine oil in mice. J Reprod Fertil 1979; 55: 135–9.
9. Betteridge KJ. The structure and function of the equine capsule in relation to embryo manipulation and transfer. Equine Vet J 1989; Suppl 8: 91–100.
10. Oriol JG, Sharom FJ, Betteridge KJ. Developmentally regulated changes in the glycoproteins of the equine trophoblast. J Reprod Fertil 1993; 99: 653–64.
11. Denker HW. Role of trophoblastic factors in implantation. In: Spilman CH, Wilks JW, eds. Novel Aspects of Reproductive Physiology. New York: Spectrum, 1978: 181–2.
12. Parr MB, Parr EL. The implantation reaction. In: Wynn RM, Jollie WP, eds. Biology of Uterus, 2nd edn. New York: Plenum Press, 1989: 233–78.
13. Spencer TE, Johnson GA, Bazer FW, Burghardt RC. Implantation mechanisms: insights from sheep. Reproduction 2005; 128: 657–68.
14. Enders AC, Schlafke S. Implantation in the ferret: epithelial penetration. Am J Anat 1971; 132: 291–316.
15. Wooding FBP. The role of the binucleate cell in ruminant placental structure. J Reprod Fertil 1982; Suppl 31: 31–9.
16. Padykula HA, Taylor JM. Ultrastructural evidence for loss of the trophoblast layer in the chorioallantoic placenta of Australian bandicoots (Marsupialia; Peramelidae). Anat Rec 1976; 186: 357–86.
17. Tyndale-Biscoe H, Renfree M. Reproductive Physiology of Marsupials. Cambridge: Cambridge University Press, 1987.
18. Finn CA, Bredl JCS. Studies on the development of the implantation reaction in the mouse uterus: influence of antinomycin D. J Reprod Fertil 1973; 34: 247–53.

19. Welsh AO, Enders AC. Chorioallantoic placental formation in the rat. I. Luminal epithelial cell death and ECM modifications in the mesometrial region of the implantation chamber. Am J Anat 1991; 192: 215–31.

20. Welsh AO, Enders AC. Chorioallantoic placental formation in the rat. II. Angiogenesis and maternal blood circulation in the mesometrial region of the implantation chamber prior to placental formation. Am J Anat 1991; 192: 346–65.

21. Welsh AO, Enders AC. Trophoblast–decidual cell interactions and establishment of maternal blood circulation in the parietal yolk sac placenta of the rat. Anat Rec 1987; 217: 203–19.

22. Enders AC, Schlafke S. Cytological aspects of trophoblast–uterine interaction in early implantation. Am J Anat 1969; 125: 1–30.

23. Enders AC, Schlafke S. Penetration of the uterine epithelium during implantation in the rabbit. Am J Anat 1971; 132: 219–40.

24. Allen WR, Hamilton DW, Moor RM. Origin of equine endometrial cups. II. Invasion of the endometrium by trophoblast. Anat Rec 1973; 177: 485–502.

25. Enders AC, Liu IKM. Trophoblast–uterine interactions during equine chorionic girdle cell maturation, migration, and transformation. Am J Anat 1991; 192: 366–81.

26. Wooding FBP, Morgan G, Fowden AL, Allen WR. A structural and immunological study of chorionic gonadotropin production by equine trophoblast girdle and cup cells. Placenta 2001; 22: 749–67.

27. Wooding FBP, Stewart F, Mathias S, Allen WR. Placentation in the African elephant, *Loxodonta africanus*: III. Ultrastructural and functional features of the placenta. Placenta 2005; 26: 449–70.

28. Rasweiler JJ 4th, Oliveira SF, Badwaik NK. An ultrastructural study of interstitial implantation in captive-bred, short-tailed fruit bats, *Carollia perspicillata*: trophoblastic adhesion and penetration of the uterine epithelium. Anat Embryol (Berl) 2002; 205: 371–91.

28b   Implantation of the blastocyst: II. Implantation in primates

Allen C Enders

Synopsis

Background

- Anthropoid primates exhibit hemochorial placentation.
- Implantation requires apposition and adhesion of the blastocyst, penetration of uterine epithelium and basal lamina and invasion of the endometrial stroma and maternal vasculature.
- Orientation of the inner cell mass, formation of the trophoplast plate and differentiation of the invasive syncytial trophoblast are common features in these primates.

Basic Science

- The implantation process also differs amongst primates.
- The baboon trophoblast rapidly penetrates the enlarged maternal vessels, the macaque blastocyst establishes a secondary placenta and in the human most of the blastocyst penetrates into the endometrium before establishing continuity with maternal vessels.
- The human endometrium decidualizes more rapidly but unlike the rhesus and baboon, does not initiate a plaque response in the luminal epithelium.
- Endometrial responses to implantation: dilation of superficial capillary plexus, increase in CD56+ large granular lymphocytes, modification of stromal fibroblasts into characteristic decidual cells.

INTRODUCTION

Those primate species in which implantation has been studied extensively share many common features that differ widely from features of implantation in other species. Orientation of the inner cell mass (ICM) towards the uterine epithelium, formation of a trophoblastic plate after epithelial penetration, differentiation of the initial invasive syncytial trophoblast into microvillous absorptive syncytium-lining clefts, and establishment of a lacunar stage followed by formation of primary villi are all common features of implantation in the baboon, macaque, and human. Formation of the amnion by cavitation, formation of a secondary yolk sac, and formation of the exocelom and extraembryonic mesoderm from the primary yolk sac hypoblast are also common features of these species. There are, however, differences among species

involving the amount of the sphere of trophoblast involved in invasion of the endometrium, the rapidity with which superficial vessels are breached, and the distance of invasion into the endometrium before establishing the lacunar stage. In the baboon, trophoblast rapidly establishes communication with enlarged maternal vessels, and consequently forms lacunae by growth above the level of the endometrial surface. The macaque blastocyst, which is the largest of the three, establishes a secondary placenta on the opposite endometrial surface after the initial invasion. In the human, trophoblast appears to invade into the endometrium more deeply before penetrating maternal vessels, all of the sphere of trophoblast is involved in syncytium and cytotrophoblast formation, and individual cytotrophoblast cells invade in great abundance into the endometrial stroma. The human endometrium decidualizes more rapidly than the other species but lacks the plaque response, which is well developed in the macaque and less well developed in the baboon. Understanding both the similarities and dissimilarities is essential in considering whether or not data obtained from one species may be relevant to similar species.

STAGES OF IMPLANTATION IN PRIMATES

In simian primates and the human a hemochorial placenta develops within a uterus simplex. As such, the process of implantation must include apposition and adhesion of the blastocyst to the uterine epithelium, penetration of the uterine epithelium, penetration of the basal lamina of this epithelium, and invasion of the endometrial stroma and maternal vasculature. Although there are differences in some aspects of the way in which implantation is accomplished in these species, the similarities among them are extensive and the differences between this group and other groups are very considerable. Consequently, the general pattern will be considered first, then some of the differences will be highlighted.

Initial association of blastocyst to uterus

In the macaque, baboon, and human, the zona pellucida surrounding the blastocyst is lost prior to implantation. Blastocysts flushed from the uterus of the baboon and rhesus monkey show endoderm formation prior to loss of the zona pellucida. Loss of the zona is sometimes referred to as hatching, which suggests the splitting of an unmodified zona pellucida by expansion of the blastocyst. Although this undoubtedly occurs in vitro, evidence from in-vivo material suggests that the zona pellucida is altered or thins prior to being shed, and that the rupture of an intact zona is probably not a common phenomenon. Therefore loss of the zona pellucida in vivo should be designated shedding rather than hatching.

The blastocyst, when it becomes fixed in position in the uterus, is most commonly situated towards the middle of the slot-like uterine lumen in the upper portion of the body of the uterus where the lumen is widest; i.e. farthest away from the mesometrium. Because this position also places the blastocyst farthest from muscle contractions, it is thought that this location is achieved mechanically. The extent of ciliation of the uterine epithelium appears insufficient to influence blastocyst position, and there is little persuasive evidence that the surface of the endometrium varies by region enough to influence the location of implantation.

Examination of postimplantation blastocysts and of placental attachment shows that in all three species (macaque, baboon, and human) the blastocyst is oriented initially with the ICM towards the uterine luminal epithelium. In the human it also appears that the dorsal surface of the uterus is the preferred attachment site. The orientation of the ICM towards the uterine surface is apparently the result of the formation of patches of syncytial trophoblast in the vicinity of the ICM. Blastocysts flushed from the baboon uterus at about the time of implantation have areas of syncytial trophoblast with blunt projections that could be involved in adhesion in this region.[1] Histological preparations of the earliest implantation site in the rhesus monkey also show syncytium limited to the peri-ICM region.[2] Blastocysts of these three species and the marmoset all have the ability to form syncytial trophoblast in vitro in the absence of uterine influence[3] and to produce chorionic gonadotropins.[4] It has been shown that the amount of chorionic gonadotropin secreted by human blastocysts in vitro increases with attachment of the trophoblast to the substrate;[5,6] this is also the case in the marmoset.[7] Whereas the early differentiation of syncytial trophoblast in the area of the ICM may explain the orientation of the blastocyst, it does not explain the preference for the dorsal endometrial surface seen in human implantations.

Adhesion and epithelial penetration

In none of the higher primates has the stage of blastocyst adhesion prior to epithelial penetration been preserved intact. Some peri-implantation blastocysts have modifications of the surface of syncytial trophoblast of the type that might be expected to participate in adhesion. The study of adhesion molecules on uterine and blastocyst surfaces is currently a topic of considerable interest,[8-11] but is confined to examination of uterine and blastocyst surfaces independently due to the difficulties in obtaining the adhesion stage in primates. Recently Simon and associates[12] have successfully used human blastocysts on uterine tissue in vitro to demonstrate loss of surface mucin glycoprotein 1 (MUC1) from the uterine cells in the region of the blastocyst.

Epithelial penetration by trophoblast has been described by electron microscopy in the macaque[2] and in the marmoset.[13,14] Histological preparations of epithelial penetration in the macaque have appeared previously,[15] but study of the fine structure of this invasion has shown several important features. Initial

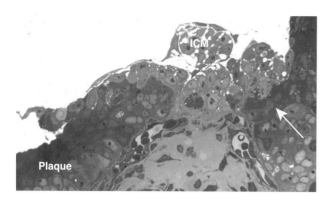

Figure 28b.1 Implantation site of a rhesus monkey 1 day after the onset of implantation (day 10). In this trophoblastic plate stage, trophoblast beneath the inner cell mass (ICM) has invaded into a gland. A cleft (arrow) has developed in the syncytial trophoblast that has invaded the gland on the right. The trophoblast has not penetrated the residual basal lamina of the uterine luminal epithelium or into the underlying capillaries. This is the first stage in which an epithelial plaque reaction is found. ×200. (See also color plate section.)

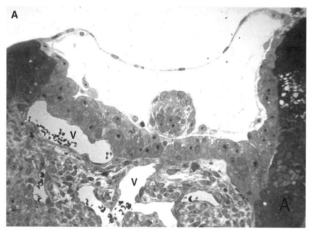

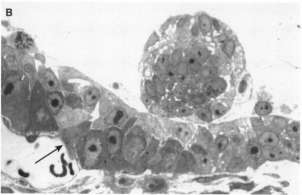

Figure 28b.2 Implantation site of a baboon, trophoblastic plate stage. (A) Note the dilated superficial vessels (v) underlying the trophoblastic plate. (B) Enlargement of an adjacent section, showing where syncytial trophoblast (arrow) has penetrated into the maternal vessel in one area. **A**, ×200; **B**, ×520. (See also color plate section.)

penetration is apparently by intrusion of syncytial trophoblast between uterine luminal epithelial cells. This syncytial trophoblast forms complements of the pre-exisiting apical junctional complex of the epithelial cells, thus both maintaining the permeability barrier of the epithelium and using cell contact as a means of adhesion and orientation. The greater affinity of the syncytial trophoblast for the lateral surfaces of the epithelial cells compared to the apical surfaces has been shown in the secondary implantation site of the macaque.[16] Because of the ability to adhere to lateral surfaces of epithelial cells, the trophoblast tends to dissect the epithelium, flowing around and enveloping individual epithelial cells. It should be noted that this method of penetrating the epithelium is very different from the frequently used term 'erosion' which implies a risk of displacement of the implanting blastocyst during disruption of endometrial epithelial integrity. No human epithelial penetration stage has been described, but the ability of the human blastocyst to form syncytial trophoblast in vitro and the presence of large areas of syncytium in the next stage of implantation suggest that epithelial penetration is similarly accomplished by trophoblast intrusion between uterine epithelial cells in the human as well as in the macaque and marmoset.

Trophoblastic plate stage

Once penetration of the epithelium has been accomplished, trophoblast in the implantation site extends laterally in the plane of the luminal epithelium. In the macaque this expansion takes place entirely within the plane of the epithelium during the day after the onset of implantation (Figure 28b.1), and the basal lamina of the epithelium is not breached until an area several times as large as the initial penetration has been achieved.[17,18] During this time there is proliferation of cytotrophoblast with some fusing to increase the amount of syncytial trophoblast in the initial areas of invasion. This results in a mixed plate of syncytium and cytotrophoblast which has been called the trophoblastic plate stage.[15] In the macaque it is at this stage that a maternal response to implantation can be seen in the epithelial plaque response (hypertrophy of the luminal epithelial cells adjacent to the site of implantation) and also in dilation of the superficial vessels and pronounced edema peripheral to the epithelial plaque.

During the brief trophoblastic plate stage in the baboon, syncytial trophoblast rapidly penetrates through the basal lamina into dilated superficial vessels[19] (Figure 28b.2). In human implantation sites at this

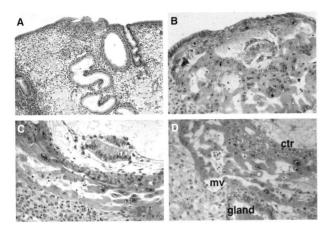

Figure 28b.3 Human implantation sites, photographed from slides in the Carnegie collection. (**A**) In stage 5a, the trophoblast of the trophoblastic plate consists of both cellular and syncytial trophoblast, and is largely above the level of the residual basal lamina of the luminal epithelium. (**B**) Early lacunar stage (stage 5b). At the bottom and right, lacunae with only partially expanded clefts can be seen (*). (**C**) A later lacunar stage (stage 5c). The lacunae are anastomotic, and the beginnings of decidualization can be seen in the underlying endometrial stroma. (**D**) Margin of a late lacunar stage (stage 5c), showing the continuity of the syncytial trophoblast lining the lacunae with the endothelium of a maternal vessel (mv). Note the continuous layer of cytotrophoblast (ctr) adjacent to the forming exocoelom, and the cluster of cytotrophoblast cells (*) initiating a primary villus. **A**, ×80; **B–D**, ×200. (See also color plate section.)

stage, originally described by Hertig and Rock,[20] trophoblast appears not only to have expanded in the plane of the epithelium but also to have penetrated the basal lamina in a few places[17] (Figure 28b.3). However, the human lacks an epithelial plaque reaction, and although there is some uterine edema there appears to be little dilation of the superficial vessels at this early stage.

During the trophoblastic plate stage, syncytial trophoblast contains aggregated nuclei similar to that seen in the syncytium involved in initial epithelial invasion, but in addition a few clefts appear within the syncytium. These clefts are lined by microvilli and have been interpreted as the beginning of differentiation of an absorptive as opposed to an invasive type of syncytial trophoblast.[17,21]

Transition to the lacunar stage

As maternal blood vessels are tapped by trophoblast, maternal blood enters the clefts within trophoblast, expanding them to form lacunae. In the macaque, the lacunar stage is initiated 2–3 days after the onset of implantation. It probably begins a little sooner in the baboon[19] and a little later in the human.[17] A true

lacunar stage does not occur in the marmoset, as trophoblast does not tap maternal vessels until after the fetal circulation is established.[22,23] The syncytial masses that are the first structure to penetrate the maternal vessels adhere to the basolateral aspects of endothelial cells but not to the apical surfaces of these cells. Thus the trophoblast becomes part of the wall of the vessel, and there is a minimum of blood leakage during the process of tapping of maternal vessels. Although this stage has been most intensively studied in the macaque, continuity of the maternal vessels with lacunar spaces can be seen readily in human implantation sites of Carnegie stage 5b[17,24] (see Figure 28b.3B). The earliest known human implantation site to be studied by electron microscopy, a lacunar stage, showed that in this species also syncytial trophoblast shares junctions with endothelial cells in vessels conducting maternal blood to lacunae.[25] It is noteworthy that the tapped vessels are capillaries or venules. No arterioles are invaded at this early stage.

During the lacunar stage there is considerable expansion of the implantation site. In the baboon this expansion results in rapid elevation of the trophoblast above the level of the endometrial surface and protrusion of the margin of the forming placental disk over the surface of the adjacent endometrium.[18,26–28] In the macaque, the extent of elevation is more variable, but rapid expansion of the lacunae elevates most of the trophoblast from the maternal surface. In the human, trophoblast penetrates further into the endometrium before tapping vessels; in addition, all of the trophoblast, including abembryonic trophoblast, forms syncytium and lacunae. This results in an interstitially situated chorionic vesicle. In later lacunar stages, however, there is some elevation from the endometrial surface as the growth of the extraembryonic membranes is greater than their penetration into the endometrium.

In the early lacunar stage the septae between lacunae consist largely of syncytial trophoblast, with cytotrophoblast being located primarily near the cavity of the implanting blastocyst and in occasional patches within the syncytium. As the lacunar stage proceeds, clusters of cytotrophoblast cells accumulate near the base of the interlacunar septae. When such clusters of cytotrophoblast cells are continuous with the layer around the blastocyst cavity they are considered to be primary villi, and the villus stage is initiated (Figure 28b.4). In the human, the lacunar stage lasts from Carnegie stage 5b to 5c (Figure 28b.3B–D), and is probably 3–7 days after the onset of implantation.[24] In the macaque, at the same time that lacunae are forming within the primary placenta, a second implantation

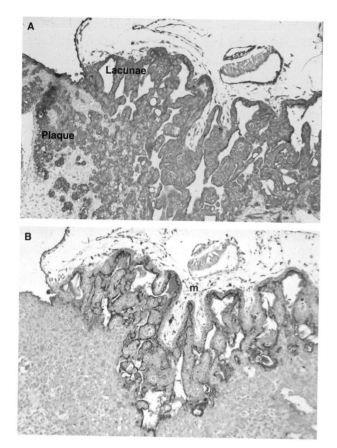

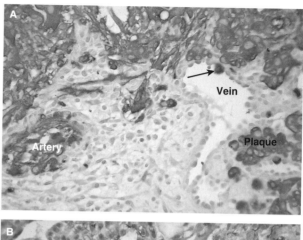

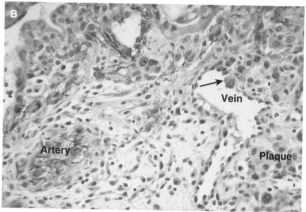

Figure 28b.4 Implantation sites of a cynomolgus macaque at the transition from the lacunar to the villus stage (day 13). (A) This section was immunostained to indicate localization of cytokeratins. Note that the embryo and the trophoblast of the villi stain, and also the uterine epithelium including the epithelial plaque cells. (B) Section adjacent to that in Figure 28b.4A, immunostained for pregnancy-specific β-1 glycoprotein (SP1). This antibody stains syncytial trophoblast but not cellular trophoblast or uterine epithelium. Note the extraembryonic mesenchyme (m) indenting the villi just beneath the embryo. ×80. (See also color plate section.)

Figure 28b.5 Junctional zone of the implantation site shown in Figure 28b.4. (A) This section was immunostained for cytokeratin. Note the multiple cytokeratin-stained cytotrophoblast cells in the artery on the left, and the single cytokeratin-stained cytotrophoblast cell in the vein. (B) Section adjacent to that in Figure 28b.5A, immunostained for NCAM. Note that this cell adhesion molecule marks the surface of migratory cytotrophoblast cells. The lumen of the artery is filled with cytotrophoblast cells, whereas only a single cytotrophoblast cell forms part of the wall of the vein. ×200. (See also color plate section.)

occurs on the opposite wall of the uterus. This usually begins 2–4 days after implantation, although occasionally no secondary implantation occurs.

In the macaque and baboon, soon after lacunae are formed cytotrophoblast cells migrate into the superficial endometrial arterioles.[19] Because of the small size of these arterioles and the large size of cytotrophoblast cells, cytotrophoblast cells appear to block or partially block direct arteriolar blood flow to the lacunae. Such cells have not been found quite this early in the human. On the other hand, interstitial cytotrophoblast cells penetrating into the endometrial stroma around glands and vessels are common in late lacunar stages in the human and are abundant in early villus stages. The situation in the macaque and baboon has not been fully

determined but interstitial cytotrophoblast migration is certainly not as extensive as in the human.[29–31] In the macaque and human, formation of the secondary yolk sac adjacent to the expanding epiblast and conversion of the residual endoderm of the primary yolk sac to mesothelial cells of the exocoelom and extraembryonic mesenchymal cells also occur in the lacunar stage.[32,33]

Villus stage and formation of trophoblastic shell

In the late lacunar stage there is a predominance of syncytial trophoblast not only lining the lacunae but also forming most of the border with the adjacent decidua. After formation of primary villi there is a rapid proliferation of cytotrophoblast within the septae; cytotrophoblast then penetrates through the boundary syncytium into the endometrium. The spread of cytotrophoblast at the junction with the decidua basalis forms the trophoblastic shell (see Figure 28b.4). In the macaque, immunostaining for neural cell adhesion molecule (NCAM) shows strong staining of the margins of these invading cytotrophoblast cells (Figure 28b.5). These migratory cytotrophoblast cells are also platelet–endothelial cell adhesion molecule (PECAM)-positive.[34]

It has been shown that in the macaque there is a brief period of rapid invasion of cytotrophoblast into the endometrium when the trophoblastic shell is being formed. Subsequently, there is differentiation of cytotrophoblast within the shell and the contiguous anchoring villi, and appreciable intercellular matrix material, fibrinoid, appears between cytotrophoblast cells. That the extracellular matrix secreted by cytotrophoblast of the anchoring villi contains components such as laminin, type IV collagen, and fibronectin has been amply documented by immunohistochemistry in the human[35] and macaque,[36] and in vitro in the human.[37,38] As the trophoblastic shell is forming, embryonic mesenchyme invades into the base of the primary villi, converting them to secondary villi. Some of the mesenchymal cells rapidly begin to form blood vessels;[39] however, since no blood circulates in these vessels until the embryonic heart starts pumping about day 21, the villi are not tertiary villi until that time. Generally, the end of the lacunar stage and the beginning of the villus stage is considered the transition from implantation to placentation in primates.

At the time of formation of the trophoblastic shell in the macaque there is a massive invasion of cytotrophoblast into underlying endometrial arteries but not veins.[40–42] The arteries are subsequently modified by formation of pads of cytotrophoblast invading into the arterial wall. As has been shown in the baboon, not all arteries contain intravascular trophoblast.[31] In the human, similar modification of the walls of the spiral arteries is considered to be essential to allow the increase in blood flow necessary in the second half of pregnancy. Without the arterial modification the pregnancy is at risk for high blood pressure (preeclampsia).[30,43] Neither the time sequence of cytotrophoblast migration into the vessels nor the relative participation of intravascular cytotrophoblast as opposed to interstitial cytotrophoblast is as well understood as in the macaque, but a major role for interstitial trophoblast in vessel modification in the human has been suggested.[44] The ways in which cytotrophoblast cells may be modified for participation in this endometrial invasion have been the subject of many studies.[45,46]

ENDOMETRIAL RESPONSES TO IMPLANTATION

In addition to the changes in the endometrium associated with modification of the hormonal milieu, there are local endometrial responses to the presence of an implanting blastocyst. In the macaque, 1 day after the onset of implantation there is a hypertrophy of the luminal epithelial cells and the cells in the necks of glands which is called the epithelial plaque reaction.[47] The cells first hypertrophy, then increase storage of glycogen, then begin to degenerate about 1 week after implantation. Although such cells were not thought to occur in the baboon they are present in this species,[26–28] and it has been shown recently that these cells can be induced in the baboon with chorionic gonadotropin.[48,49] Epithelial plaque cells also form on the opposite side of the macaque uterus prior to formation of the secondary implantation site. They can also be induced by trauma. These features of the cells suggest that they are a normal response of a hormonally receptive uterus to non-specific stimuli. Epithelial plaque cells are not found in the human endometrium.

Another local response of the endometrium to implantation is the dilation of the superficial capillary plexus. This dilation is particularly conspicuous and early in the baboon (see Figure 28b.2). However it is also impressive in the macaque where it results not only in enlargement of vessels immediately underlying the conceptus but also in an edematous ring surrounding the implantation site. The dilation of the superficial vessels converts capillaries to venule-like structures; the endothelial cells of these venules become columnar and react with antibody to transforming growth factor α (TGFα). Such cells can be induced in the properly treated macaque by trauma or by relaxin administration.[50] Dilation of superficial vessels near the implantation site in the human is delayed by several days, and does not reach dramatic proportions until the early villus stage when many venules are extensively dilated and appreciable blood leakage into glands occurs.

The specialized population of T lymphocytes known as large granular lymphocytes (LGLs), which are identified by reaction with antibody to CD56,[51] have been the subject of considerable interest, and are considered elsewhere in this book. They are present in the macaque, baboon, and human, and in all three species they increase during the first trimester of pregnancy. At the time of implantation in the macaque, LGLs in the endometrium are relatively undifferentiated and widely scattered. There is a brief flare of eosinophilic leukocytes near the implantation site, but otherwise the distribution of all classes of leukocytes is similar to the rest of the endometrium. As pregnancy proceeds to the villus stage the LGLs increase in number and cytoplasmic glycogen becomes conspicuous.[47] By the time the trophoblastic shell is formed, three cell types predominate at the interface of the endometrium with trophoblast: decidualizing stromal cells, LGLs, and macrophages.[52]

The distribution of LGLs and macrophages in the macaque endometrium has been reviewed recently[53] and a subset of dendritic cells, the DC-SIGN[+] cells, may be a marker of recognition of pregnancy in this species.[54]

The modification of stromal fibroblasts to form rounded decidual cells occurs after the initiation of implantation in the human, macaque, and baboon. This response occurs most rapidly in the human.[47,55] In all three species, insulin-like growth factor binding protein 1 (IGFBP-1) is an indicator of fibroblast transformation to decidual cells.[56,57] The morphological changes in decidual cells are slower in the macaque and baboon but are essentially similar, including the eventual formation of the peculiar peripheral projections characteristic of mature decidual cells.[28,47]

SUMMARY OF DIFFERENCES AMONG PRIMATES

The general pattern of implantation is quite similar among the higher primates. The variations that occur appear to be the result of differences in timing of differentiation of trophoblast and in the extent of involvement of different areas of the implanting blastocyst. The human blastocyst penetrates further into the endometrium before tapping maternal vessels. During the trophoblastic plate stage, trophoblast spreads not only in the plane of the epithelium but also through the basal lamina and beneath adjacent luminal epithelium. The entire circumference of the trophoblast of the blastocyst forms syncytial trophoblast and lacunae. As such, when maternal blood fills lacunae the expansion is largely within the endometrium, although this may cause the endometrium to bulge into the uterine lumen. In contrast, in the baboon, trophoblast of the implanting blastocyst rapidly invades superficial dilated vessels; lacunae are formed precociously and the conceptus is elevated from the endometrial surface. The macaque

blastocyst is larger than the others at the time of implantation, and the implanting abembryonic trophoblast also forms syncytial trophoblast and clefts. The marmoset, on the other hand, has two or three blastocysts in a simplex uterus. These blastocysts are slow to adhere to and penetrate the luminal epithelium; penetration occurs repeatedly over an extensive area of the uterine lumen[14] extending outward from the area near the ICM of the blastocysts. A peculiarity of marmosets is that trophoblast of adjacent blastocysts eventually fuse.

The epithelial plaque response is highly developed in the macaque, but even in this species it is not as extensive as in New World monkeys.[58] Its role remains poorly understood. The responses by LGLs, macrophages, and decidual cells are more universal features among the primates.

Implantation in prosimians is not considered here, both because this group differs so widely from the simians and anthropoids and because little recent information is available. Luckett[58] and King[59] have reviewed the histology of implantation and epitheliochorial placentation in prosimians.

In addition to the obvious advantage of being able to use non-human primates to model implantation[60] or to compare trauma-induced to blastocyst-induced endometrial changes,[57] the differences in implantation in the different species can be used for analysis of different stages of implantation. The earliest stages, adhesion and infiltration of the uterine epithelium, could be readily studied in the marmoset, where repeated adhesion by trophoblast knobs occurs over several days.[14] Lacuna formation can most readily be studied in the macaque, where the presence of an implantation site can be confirmed by ultrasound as early as day 12 (3 days after initiation of implantation). The invasion of endometrial arterioles can also be studied in this species since invasion starts as early as day 12 and is extensive by day 15, when the implantation site is still small enough to find the invaded vessels readily.[61,62] Consequently, the nature of implantation in non-human primates is interesting not only in showing diversity but also in that it can be used to better understand aspects of human implantation.

ACKNOWLEDGMENTS

Supported by grants HD10342 and HD24491 from the National Institute of Child Health and Human Development (ACE), and NIH RR00169 to the California Regional Primate Research Center.

REFERENCES

1. Enders AC, Lantz KC, Schlafke S. Differentiation of trophoblast of the baboon blastocyst. Anat Rec 1989; 225: 329–40.

2. Enders AC, Hendrickx AG, Schlafke S. Implantation in the rhesus monkey: initial penetration of endometrium. Am J Anat 1983; 167: 275–98.

3. Enders AC, Douglas GC, Meyers S et al. Interactions of macaque blastocysts with epithelial cells in vitro. Hum Reprod 2005; 20: 3026–32.

4. Lopata A, Oliva K, Stanton PG et al. Analysis of chorionic gonadotrophin secreted by cultured human blastocysts. Mol Hum Reprod 1997; 3: 517–21.

5. Dokras A, Sargent L, Ross C et al. The human blastocyst: morphology and human chorionic gonadotropin secretion in vitro. Hum Reprod 1991; 6: 1143–51.

6. Lopata A, Oliva K. Regulation of chorionic gonadotropin secretion by cultured human blastocysts. In: Bavister, ed. Preimplantation Embryo Development. New York: Springer-Verlag, 1993.

7. Hearn JP, Seshagiri PB, Webley GE. Physiology of implantation in primates. In: Wolf DP, Stouffer RL, Brenner RM, eds. In Vitro Fertilization and Embryo Transfer in Primates. New York: Springer-Verlag, 1993: 158–68.

8. Aplin JD. Expression of integrin $\alpha_6\beta_4$ in human trophoblast and its loss from extravillous cells. Placenta 1993; 14: 203–15.

9. Aplin JD. The cell biology of human implantation. Placenta 1996; 17: 269–75.

10. Lopata A. Blastocyst–endometrial interaction: an appraisal of some old and new ideas. Mol Hum Reprod 1996; 2: 519–25.

11. Fazleabas AT, Bell SC, Fleming S et al. Distribution of integrins and the extracellular matrix proteins in the baboon endometrium during the menstrual cycle and early pregnancy. Biol Reprod 1997; 56: 348–56.

12. Meseguer M, Aplin JD, Caballero-Campo P et al. Human endometrial mucin MUC1 is up-regulated by progesterone and down-regulated in vitro by the human blastocyst. Biol Reprod 2001; 64: 590–601.

13. Smith C, Moore HDM, Hearn JP. The ultrastructure of early implantation in the marmoset monkey (Callithrix jacchus). Anat Embryol 1987; 175: 399–410.

14. Enders AC, Lopata A. Implantation in the marmoset monkey: expansion of the early implantation site. Anat Rec 1999; 256: 279–99.

15. Wislocki GB, Streeter GL. On the implantation of the macaque (Macaca mulatta) from the time of implantation until the formation of the definitive placenta. Contrib Embryol, Carnegie Inst 1938; 27: 1–66.

16. Enders AC, Liu IKM, Mead RA et al. Active and passive morphological interactions of trophoblast and endometrum during early implantation. In: Dey SK, ed. Molecular and Cellular Aspects of Periimplantation Processes. New York: Springer-Verlag, 1995: 168–82.

17. Enders AC. Trophoblast differentiation during the transition from trophoblastic plate to lacunar stage of implantation in the rhesus monkey and human. Am J Anat 1989; 186: 85–98.

18. Enders AC. Overview of the morphology of implantation in primates. In: Wolf DP, Stouffer RL, Brenner RM, eds. In Vitro Fertilization and Embryo Transfer in Primates. New York: Springer-Verlag, 1993: 145–57.

19. Enders AC, King BF. Early stages of trophoblastic invasion of the maternal vascular system during implantation in the macaque and baboon. Am J Anat 1991; 192: 329–46.

20. Hertig AT, Rock J. Two human ova of the pre-villous stage, having a developmental age of about seven and nine days respectively. Contrib Embryol Carnegie Inst 1945; 31: 65–84.

21. Enders AC. Transition from lacunar to villous stage of implantation in the macaque, including establishment of the trophoblastic shell. Acta Anat 1995; 152: 151–69.

22. Smith CA, Moore HDM. The morphology of early development and implantation in vivo and in vitro in the marmoset monkey. In: Neubert D, Merker H-J, Hendrickx AG, eds. Nonhuman Primates – Developmental Biology and Toxicology. Berlin: Ueberreuter-Wissenschaft, 1988: 171–87.

23. Merker H-J, Bremer D, Csato W et al. Development of the marmoset placenta. In: Neubert D, Merker H-J, Hendrickx AG, eds. Nonhuman Primates – Developmental Biology and Toxicology. Berlin: Ueberreuter-Wissenschaft, 1988: 245–72.

24. O' Rahilly R, Müller F. Developmental stages in human embryos. Washington, DC: Carnegie Inst, Publ. 1987: 637.

25. Knoth M, Larsen JF. Ultrastructure of a human implantation site. Acta Obstet Gynecol Scand 1972; 51: 385–93.

26. Tarara R, Enders AC, Hendrickx AG et al. Early implantation and embryonic development of the baboon: stages 5, 6 and 7. Anat Embryol 1987; 176: 267–75.

27. Enders AC, Lantz KC, Peterson PE et al. From blastocyst to placenta: the morphology of implantation in the baboon. Hum Reprod Update 1997; 3: 561–73.

28. Jones CJP, Enders AC, Fazleabas AT. Early implantation events in the baboon (Papio anubis) with special reference to the establishment of anchoring villi. Placenta 2001; 22: 440–56.

29. Pijnenborg R. Trophoblast invasion and placentation in the human: morphological aspects. Troph Res 1990; 4: 33–47.

30. Pijnenborg R. Trophoblast invasion. Reprod Med Rev 1994; 3: 53–73.

31. Pijnenborg R, D'Hooghe T, Vercruysse L et al. Evaluation of trophoblast invasion in placental bed biopsies of the baboon, with immunohistochemical localization of cytokeratin, fibronectin, and laminin. J Med Primatol 1996; 25: 272–81.

32. Enders AC, King BF. Formation and differentiation of extraembryonic mesoderm in the rhesus monkey. Am J Anat 1988; 181: 327–40.

33. Bianchi DW, Wilkins-Haug LE, Enders AC et al. The origin of extraembryonic mesoderm in experimental animals: relevance to chorionic mosaicism in humans. Am J Med Genet 1993; 46: 542–50.

34. Blankenship TN, Enders AC. Expression of platelet-endothelial cell adhesion molecule-1 (PECAM) by macaque trophoblast cells during invasion of the spiral arteries. Anat Rec 1997; 247: 413–19.

35. Earl I, Estlin C, Bulmer JN. Fibronectin and laminin in the early human placenta. Placenta 1990; 11: 223–31.

36. Blankenship T, King BF. Developmental changes in the cell columns and trophoblastic shell of the macaque placenta: an immunohistochemical study localizing type IV collagen, laminin, fibronectin and cytokeratins. Cell Tissue Res 1993; 274: 457–66.

37. Aplin JD, Charlton AK. The role of matrix macromolecules in the invasion of decidua by trophoblast: model studies using BeWo cells. Trophoblast Res 1990; 4: 139–58.

38. Vicovac L, Jones CJP, Aplin JD. Trophoblast differentiation during formation of anchoring villi in a model of the early human placenta in vitro. Placenta 1995; 16: 41–56.

39. King BF. Ultrastructural differentiation of stromal and vascular components in early macaque placental villi. Am J Anat 1987; 178: 30–44.

40. Blankenship TN, Enders AC. Modification of uterine vasculature during pregnancy in macaques. Microsc Res Tech 2003; 60: 390–401.

41. Blankenship TN, Enders AC, King BF. Trophoblastic invasion and the development of uteroplacental arteries in the macaque: immunohistochemical localization of cytokeratins, desmin, type IV collagen, laminin, and fibronectin. Cell Tissue Res 1993; 272: 227–36.

42. Enders AC, Lantz KC, Schlafke S. Preference of invasive cytotrophoblast for maternal vessels in early implantation in the macaque. Acta Anat 1996; 155: 145–62.

43. Zhou Y, Damsky CH, Fisher SJ. Preeclampsia is associated with failure of cytotrophoblasts to mimic a vascular adhesion phenotype: one cause of defective endovascular invasion in this syndrome? J Clin Invest 1997; 99: 2152–64.

44. Kaufmann P, Black S, Huppertz B. Endovascular trophoblast invasion: implications for the pathogenesis of intrauterine growth retardation and preeclampsia. Biol Reprod 2003; 69: 1–7.

45. Zhou Y, Fisher SJ, Janatpour M et al. Human cytotrophoblasts adopt a vascular phenotype as they differentiate. A strategy for successful endovascular invasion? J Clin Invest 1997; 99: 2139–46.

46. Genbacev O, Zhou Y, McMaster MT et al. Oxygen regulates human cytotrophoblast proliferation, differentiation, and invasion: implications for endovascular invasion in normal pregnancy and preeclampsia. In: Carson DD, ed. Embryo Implantation: Molecular, Cellular, and Clinical Aspects, New York: Springer-Verlag, 1999: 39–53.

47. Enders A. Structural responses of the primate endometrium to implantation. Placenta 1991; 12: 309–25.

48. Fazleabas AT, Kim JYJ, Donnelly KM et al. Embryo–maternal dialogue in the baboon (*Papio anubis*). In: Carson DD, ed. Embryo Implantation: Molecular, Cellular, and Clinical Aspects, New York: Springer-Verlag, 1999: 202–9.

49. Jones CJ, Fazleabas AT. Ultrastructure of epithelial plaque formation and stromal cell transformation by post-ovulatory chorionic gonadotrophin treatment in the baboon (*Papio anubis*). Hum Reprod 2001; 16: 2680–90.

50. Denker HW, Enders AC, Schlafke S. Bizarre hypertrophy of vascular endothelial cells in rhesus monkey endometrium: experimental induction and electron microscopical characteristics. Verhand Anat Gesell 1985; 79: 545–8.

51. King A, Loke YW. Uterine large granular lymphocytes: a possible role in embryonic implantation? Am J Obstet Gynecol 1990; 162: 308–10.

52. Hunt JS. The role of macrophages in the uterine response to pregnancy. Placenta 1990; 11: 467–75.

53. Slukvin II, Breburda EE, Golos TG. Dynamic changes in primate endometrial leukocyte populations: differential distribution of macrophages and natural killer cells at the rhesus monkey implantation site and in early pregnancy. Placenta 2004; 25: 297–307.

54. Breburda EE, Dambaeva SV, Slukvin II et al. Selective distribution and pregnancy-specific expression of DC-SIGN at the maternal–fetal interface in the rhesus macaque: DC-SIGN is a putative marker of the recognition of pregnancy. Placenta 2006; 27: 11–21.

55. Ramsey EM, Houston ML, Harris JWS. Interactions of the trophoblast and maternal tissues in three closely related primate species. Am J Obstet Gynecol 1976; 124: 647–52.

56. Fazleabas AT, Kim JJ, Srinivasan S et al. Implantation in the baboon: endometrial responses. Semin Reprod Endocrinol 1999; 17: 247–65.

57. Ghosh D, Bell SC, Sengupta J. Immunohistological localization of insulin-like growth factor binding protein-1 in primary implantation sites and trauma-induced deciduomal tissues of the rhesus monkey. Placenta 2004; 25: 197–207.

58. Luckett WP. Comparative development and evolution of the placenta in primates. Contrib Primatol 1974; 3: 142–234.

59. King BF. Development and structure of the placenta and fetal membranes of nonhuman primates. J Exp Zool 1993; 266: 528–40.

60. Fazleabas AT, Kim JJ, Strakova Z. Implantation: embryonic signals and the modulation of the uterine environment – a review. Placenta 2004; 25: S26–31.

61. Enders AC. Trophoblast–uterine interactions in the first days of implantation: models for the study of implantation events in the human. Semin Reprod Med 2000; 18: 255–63.

62. Enders AC. Implantation in the macaque: expansion of the implantation site during the first week of implantation. Placenta 2007; 28: 794–802.

29 Human placental development

John D Aplin and Carolyn JP Jones

Synopsis

Background

- In humans, implantation is interstitial and placentation is hemochorial.
- Trophoblast cells form the outermost layer of the placenta; they originate from the trophectoderm cells of the blastocyst.
- The inner cell mass of the blastocyst gives rise to the embryo as well as non-trophoblast cells of the placenta such as blood vessel and stromal cells.
- By the end of the third week of gestation, the basic cellular organization of the placenta is already in place.
- Initially, placental cell growth is very rapid; development of the placenta is essential for the conceptus to survive.
- The embryonic period ends after 8 weeks.
- From this time the placenta becomes the dominant locus of steroid hormone production.
- At about 4 months' gestation the fetus and placenta are the same size; subsequently, fetal growth exceeds that of the placenta.
- Maternal blood is supplied through spiral arteries to the placenta, while fetal blood circulates in the vessels of the villous placenta which connect via the umbilical cord to the fetus.
- The placenta is an essential immunological barrier; it prevents rejection by maternal immune cells being triggered by paternal antigens on fetal cells.

Basic Science

- The hatched blastocyst first attaches to the uterine luminal epithelium.
- During the first week it penetrates the epithelium and becomes embedded in the underlying stroma.
- Soon after this, the stroma differentiates into decidua.
- Trophoblast develops into villous and extravillous (invasive) lineages.
- Tertiary placental villi form, comprising a surface trophoblast bilayer and inner vascularized stroma.
- Rapid growth and branching lead to elaboration of the villous placenta.
- Embryonic blood circulates in the placenta from about 45 days postconception.
- During the first 10 weeks, maternal blood does not reach the intervillous space; in this period, nutrition is supplied from uterine secretions.
- Thus, the placenta develops at an oxygen tension well below the normal arterial level.
- Syncytiotrophoblast at the villous surface acts to transfer maternal oxygen and nutrients via the placenta to the embryo. Carbon dioxide and waste products are transported in the opposite direction.
- The diffusion distance between maternal and fetal circulations diminishes as pregnancy advances, increasing the efficiency of placental transfer.
- The syncytiotrophoblast is a differentiated, postmitotic compartment that also functions as a barrier to both maternal cells and pathogens, and produces large quantities of steroids, hCG, hCS, hGH, leptin, soluble VEGF receptor (sFlt-1) and many other secretory substances.
- Particulate material is continuously shed from the syncytiotrophoblast into maternal blood.
- Extravillous trophoblast invades the decidual stroma, colonizing and transforming the spiral arteries into expanded non-contractile channels.
- Trophoblast invasion extends as far as the inner third of the myometrium by the 18th week of gestation.

Clinical

- In pathological pregnancies, including miscarriage, preeclampsia, and some types of fetal growth restriction, invasive trophoblast fails to complete the necessary transformation of maternal spiral arteries.
- In miscarriage, there is access of maternal blood to the intervillous space before 10 weeks, when the placenta's resistance to oxidative damage is not yet fully developed.
- In preeclampsia the placenta may sustain damage from chronic ischemia–reperfusion effects.
- Reduced placental vascularization is associated with early pregnancy failure and intrauterine growth restriction.
- Placental amino acid transport efficiency has been shown to be compromised in women carrying a growth-restricted fetus.

INTRODUCTION

The placenta is the first identifiable organ, and its development is a prerequisite for normal development of the embryo into a fetus. It combines in one tissue diverse activities and functions that are separate in the adult, including gas and nutrient transport, waste removal, and hormone biosynthesis. Accounts of early implantation draw on the studies of Hertig and Rock,[1] whose specimens are housed in the Carnegie Collection of the Human Developmental Anatomy Center, Research Collections division of the National Museum of Health & Medicine, in Washington, DC. Human placental development was described in detail by Boyd and Hamilton in their classic book[2] while Fox included information on placental development in a trenchant pathology text.[3] Kaufmann and Benirschke's *Pathology of the Human Placenta*[4] contains much useful information on placental anatomy and development, as well as some molecular aspects. Placentation in diverse species is described elsewhere in Section VI; placental anatomy and transfer are fully discussed in *Knobil and Neill's Physiology of Reproduction*.[5,6] (See also http://medicine.ucsd.edu/cpa/homefs.html.) Studies of the genetic basis of placental development in the mouse are revealing genes that may well be of importance in human placental development[7] (see Chapters 22 and 27). The present account of human placental development is a brief outline and these sources should be consulted for more detailed information.

EARLY STAGES

The apposition and attachment stages of human implantation have not been observed. The earliest described implantation site (Carnegie stage 5a) shows the maternal epithelium to have been penetrated but not yet resealed over the embryo (see Figure 28b.3). A trophoblastic plate comprising a mixed population of syncytio- and cytotrophoblast lies between the inner cell mass (ICM) and the endometrium, which is not yet decidualized. Superficially, a thin monolayer of trophectoderm remains from the blastocyst stage, still in contact with the uterine lumen. At stage 5b, the endometrium has decidualized and the maternal epithelium is spreading over the conceptus. There are now lacunae within the syncytial trophoblast and the amniotic cavity has appeared. By stage 5c, the mixed syncytio- and cytotrophoblast layers have extended around most of the conceptus and the maternal epithelium now forms a complete covering, so that implantation can be said to be complete. Information about these stages in both human and non-human primates can be found in Chapter 31b.

Trophectoderm in the blastocyst gives rise to all trophoblast lineages in the placenta. In contrast, the placental stroma and vasculature arise from extraembryonic mesoderm, which is first apparent at stage 5c, lining the coelomic cavity. This mesoderm appears to originate by delamination from endodermal cells that have spread laterally from the ICM. By Carnegie stage 6 (primitive streak; Figure 29.1), the mesoderm has proliferated to form radially outgrowing tongues of mesenchyme beneath the trophoblast, thus creating secondary villi (Figure 29.1B). A secondary yolk sac is also present. The conceptus, now approximately 7–8 days postattachment, is about 2 mm in diameter. Trophoblast derived human chorionic gonadotropin (hCG) is detectable in maternal blood.

At 20–22 days postconception (pc), the beginnings of vasculogenesis are apparent in the villous mesenchyme, producing the first tertiary villi.[8] These are covered by trophoblast that progressively becomes organized into the bilayer characteristic of the developed placenta, with cytotrophoblast progenitor cells beneath the syncytiotrophoblast, which in turn is covered by a microvillous surface rich in glycoproteins, enzymes, and transporter molecules (Figure 29.2). In the early stages the placenta may have as few as 20 villi, but rapid growth and branching morphogenesis ensue[9,10] to create a villous tree (Figure 29.3).

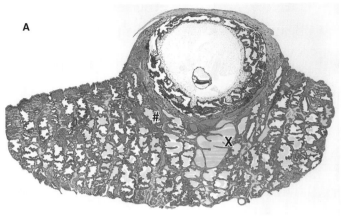

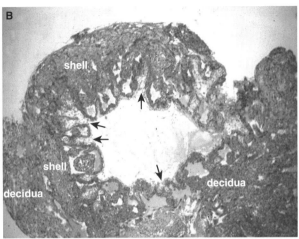

Figure 29.1 (A) Drawing of an early human implantation site (Carnegie stage 6). The superficial uterine epithelium is discontinuous. The conceptus (blue) is about 2 mm in diameter. The embryo is visible and at the bilaminar disc stage and the presumptive intervillous space (*) can be seen within the trophoblast layer. The endometrium comprises a superficial compact layer within which the implantation cavity is located, and a deeper spongiosum. Note the widely dilated secretory uterine glands (e.g. #) which provide histiotrophic nutrition for the growing embryo/placental unit. The stromal cells in this specimen are not markedly decidualized, but endometrial vessels are dilated. On the right of the cavity a large sinus (×) has been invaded by trophoblast. Approximately 7 days after attachment. (Reproduced from Falkiner,[61] with permission.) (B) Placental villi radiate out and begin to invade the decidua. Mesenchymal stroma can be seen in the secondary villi (arrows) and cytotrophoblast cells have grown out from early anchoring villi to form the cytotrophoblast shell from which migratory cytotrophoblast cells originate. The embryo is not in the plane of section. Approximately 8 days after attachment.

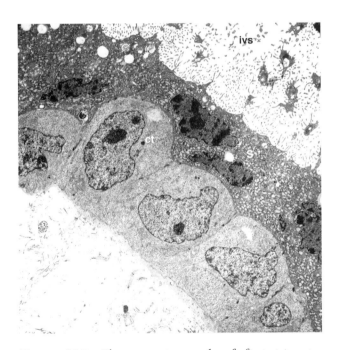

Figure 29.2 Electron micrograph of first trimester trophoblast showing a continuous layer of progenitor cytotrophoblast cells (ct) under the syncytiotrophoblast (s) with its microvillous, scalloped surface and cytoplasm rich in cisternae of endoplasmic reticulum reflecting its intense biosynthetic activity. ivs, intervillous space. (Reproduced from Jones and Fox,[42] with permission.)

Initially, all villi are mesenchymal with a homogeneous, loosely cellular, hyaluronan-rich stroma,[10] but immature intermediate villi soon appear with a swollen

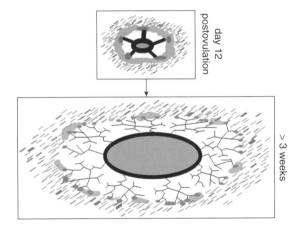

Figure 29.3 The development of anchoring sites connecting the placenta to the uterine wall in the first trimester. Top, 3rd week; bottom, 5th week. The black lines represent chorionic villi which undergo rapid branching morphogenesis. At the periphery of the intervillous space, the tips of villi make contact with the stromal surface of the decidua (red) or the residual cytotrophoblast shell (gray-blue spots); and it is these sites where cytotrophoblast columns (blue spots) form and from where interstitial infiltration of the decidua begins (shown in Figure 29.5). The central area (green) represents the embryo and coelomic cavity. (Reproduced from Aplin et al,[9] with permission.)

stroma that features longitudinally oriented fluid-filled channels lined by sail-shaped mesenchymal cell processes.[11] This transformation appears to be accomplished by the remodeling actions of placental macrophages (Hofbauer cells), which can often be seen

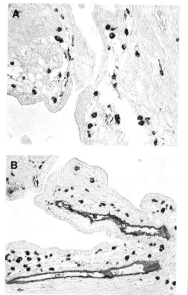

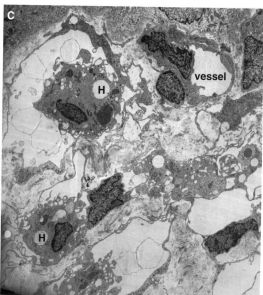

Figure 29.4 Immunocytochemical staining of macrophages with anti-CD68 clearly shows their distribution in a section of first trimester placental villus (A). They are mainly found around the periphery, close to the basal lamina of the trophoblast. (B) Anti-CD34 binding identifies the presence of blood vessels (*); macrophages are stained with anti-CD68. (C) Transmission electron microscopy showing vacuolated macrophages (Hofbauer cells, H) occupying, and spreading their slender processes over the surface of channels in the villous stroma. Hofbauer cells are not seen in blood vessels.

occupying the channels, especially in early pregnancy (Figure 29.4). In turn, immature intermediate villi develop into stem villi with a more fibrous stroma and muscularized arteries.[12] At any later time in first or second trimester, all types of villi are present as the placenta continues to grow, with new peripheral mesenchymal villi developing into intermediate villi, that in turn form new mesenchymal branches. The molecular pathways that control branching are unknown.

Peripheral to the villous placenta is a thick shell largely comprising cytotrophoblast with some syncytial elements. This abuts directly upon the decidual stroma and, from the earliest stages, large numbers of cytotrophoblasts can be seen infiltrating the decidual interstitium and spiral arteries (Figures 29.1 and 29.5). The most superficial portions of endometrial glands and arterial segments become obliterated. Invasive trophoblast is highly phagocytic.

The developing placenta contains many more cells than the embryo (Figure 29.1A), and the early patterns of very rapid trophoblast proliferation, and invasion mediated by syncytium, do not persist as the placenta matures. Embryology texts give useful information for correlating placental and embryonic or fetal stages, but their descriptions of early placental morphology should be viewed with caution, as the trophoblast is often represented inaccurately as a homogeneous syncytium.

MONTHS 2–3

The fetal heart begins to beat at about 22 days pc. However, the connection between developing placental capillaries and the embryonic circulatory system is not established via the connective stalk (forerunner of

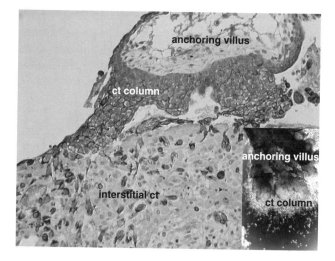

Figure 29.5 Brown-colored cytotrophoblast (ct) cells immunostained to reveal their characteristic cytokeratin filaments can be seen invading the decidua at 12 weeks in vivo. In explant culture (inset), cytotrophoblast cells form a column at the tips of attached villi and migrate into a collagen gel, appearing bright against a dark background.

the umbilical cord) until around day 32, and it is not until 45 days pc that blood circulates in the placenta. By this stage the villous tree is already differentiated, with muscularized vessels appearing in developing stem villi. These more proximal vessels contain nucleated red cells that may have originated from blood islands in the yolk sac, but more peripheral villi (Figure 29.6) contain hemangioblastic cell clusters.[8]

The various pathways of differentiation in the trophoblast lineage have been mapped.[13] The two principal ones are in the villus, from progenitor cytotrophoblast to syncytium, and from villous progenitor cytotrophoblast to migratory extravillous cytotrophoblast (Figure 29.7).

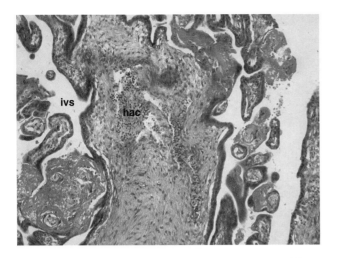

Figure 29.6 This early placental villus contains a central focus of hemangioblastic cells (hac) within the primitive mesenchyme; these will later develop into blood vessels. ivs, intervillous space.

It is still unclear whether all villous cytotrophoblasts retain the potential to differentiate into both lineages. Many of the extravillous cells, which are already postmitotic, and often aneuploid[14] and/or polyploid,[15,16] eventually differentiate further into giant cells of the placental bed (Figure 29.8). These cells develop a microvillous surface and often contain secretory granules, resembling villous syncytium in these respects.[17]

During the first trimester the human placenta is largely deciduochorial (Figure 29.9); i.e. glycogen and other nutrients secreted by decidual glands and stromal cells access the intervillous space (IVS) and are taken up by trophoblast.[18] The mouths of maternal spiral arteries are plugged by aggregates of trophoblast derived from the shell. While some maternal plasma filters into the intervillous space through narrow channels in the plugs, hysteroscopy, Doppler ultrasound, and other methods have demonstrated essentially no maternal blood cells in the IVS before 10 weeks.[19] At this stage the plugs are displaced and maternal arterial blood gains access to the IVS, starting at the periphery where the trophoblastic shell is thinner.[20]

Thus, the placenta develops at an oxygen tension well below the normal arterial level – perhaps 2% or 18 mmHg.[21] This has led to intense interest in the role of the transcriptional regulator hypoxia inducible factor (HIF) in the developing placenta. HIF regulates a large number of genes involved in metabolism, and mice that lack HIF-1β (also known as *arnt*) do not develop a

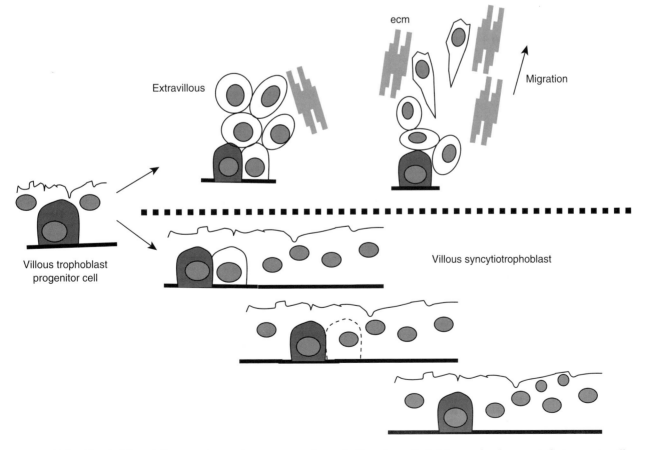

Figure 29.7 Trophoblast differentiation pathways: syncytiotrophoblast by cell division and subsequent fusion; extravillous 'invasive' cytotrophoblast with migrating cells. ecm, extracellular matrix.

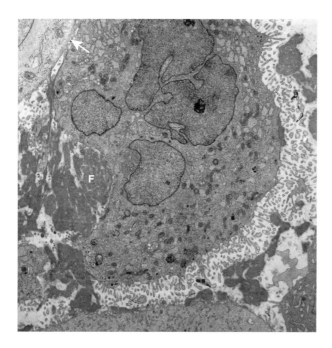

Figure 29.8 Multinucleate placental bed trophoblast giant cell with prominent endoplasmic reticulum and microvillous cell surface. It is attached to another cytotrophoblast in a cell column via desmosomes (arrow) and is surrounded by fibrinoid deposits (F).

normal placenta.[22] However, HIF levels are also strongly influenced by other regulatory factors, including ascorbate and metabolites, and it continues to be expressed in placenta after 12 weeks. Thus, its function at the time of the placental oxygen transition is as yet unclear.

After this time the oxygen level rises progressively, reaching three-fold the earlier value. It has been suggested that in pathological pregnancies, including miscarriage and preeclampsia, insufficient extravillous trophoblast may develop. Ischemia–reperfusion[23] may have a physiological role in triggering the regression of villous tissue in the chorion laeve.[20] If so, velamentous

cord insertion at term is the result of a first trimester developmental malfunction. In miscarriage, there is access of maternal blood to the IVS before 10 weeks, when the placenta's resistance to oxidative damage is not yet fully developed.[20] There is evidence that the preeclamptic placenta may have sustained damage resulting from chronic ischemia–reperfusion effects.[24]

PLACENTAL ANCHORAGE

Anchoring villi are peripheral trophoblastic specializations that attach the placenta to the uterine wall and are fundamental to the establishment of mechanical stability at the feto–maternal junction.[9,17] In addition, they act as feeder sites for migratory cytotrophoblast (see Figures 29.3, 29.5, and 29.7). Anchoring villi are already present as early as 18 days after ovulation, but new villi develop rapidly in the IVS as the placenta grows and ramifies.[10] First trimester mesenchymal floating villi, when confronted with a permissive extracellular matrix (ECM) in explant culture, undergo de-novo development of anchoring sites (see Figure 29.5).[25,26] The cellular and molecular characteristics of these specializations resemble closely those seen in vivo. Thus, it is likely that in the first few weeks of pregnancy, before maternal blood accesses the IVS, a stochastic process occurs in which the tips of mesenchymal villi newly forming at the placental periphery make contact with the decidual surface and develop anchoring columns of cytotrophoblast (see Figures 29.1B, 29.3, and 29.5). In this way the number of attachment sites increases with the surface area of the growing placenta. Development of these multiple sites is important in producing a placental–maternal interface that will be stable to the pulsatile flow of blood in the IVS in the second and third trimesters.[9,25]

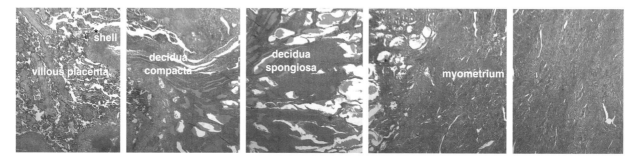

Figure 29.9 Section of the placenta, decidua, and myometrium at about 42 days post-LMP (21 days after implantation). Note the villous placenta (left), superficial decidual glands opening into the intervillous space (*-IVS), and highly expanded vascular spaces in the basal decidua. The distal ends of spiral arteries do not open into the IVS, but are plugged at the level of the cytotrophoblast shell.

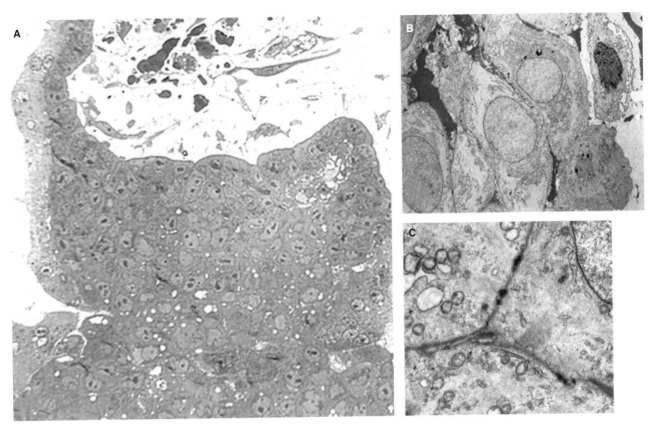

Figure 29.10   (A) Cells at an anchoring villus in a 17-week column. There is a thin layer of syncytiotrophoblast on the left-hand edge and a mesenchymal stroma with sparse cells within the villus core, overlying the mass of cytotrophoblast cells that attach the villus to the decidua; semithin section. (B) Note the differentiated cell with a dark nucleus breaking away from the side of the column (top right). Transmission electron microscopy (TEM) shows dark fibrinoid material between the cells. (C) Desmosomal attachments between cytotrophoblasts, with associated bundles of intermediate filaments in the cytoplasm (TEM).

CYTOTROPHOBLAST INVASION

Hamilton and Boyd[2] had already recognized in 1970 that first trimester cytotrophoblasts break away from anchoring villi (Figure 29.10B) and invade the decidua, and later studies have shown that this is accompanied by dramatic changes in their ultrastructure, including the development of masses of intermediate filaments (Figure 29.10C) and intracellular glycogen deposits.[17,27] The definitive account of invasion, based on serially sectioned pregnancy hysterectomy specimens, was published in 1980[28] and included a description of the physiological transformation of decidual and inner myometrial segments of maternal spiral arteries into flaccid conduits. More recent reviews are available.[29–31]

Cytotrophoblast invasion of the uterine wall begins immediately after implantation (see Figure 29.1) and continues until approximately the 18th week. The early studies lacked the advantage of immunohistochemical markers, making it difficult to recognize the full extent of trophoblastic infiltration (see Figures 29.5 and 29.9). Nonetheless, it was recognized that large numbers of cytotrophoblast infiltrate the decidual stroma and spiral arteries (Figure 29.11). In the second trimester, these cells penetrate as far as the inner one-third of the myometrium and cytokeratin immunohistochemistry with pregnancy hysterectomy specimens show that, in normal pregnancy, cytotrophoblast migrates interstitially about 2 mm into the myometrium (Figure 29.12), and that apoptotic events appear to be frequent, as reported by the presence of activated caspase-3 and cytokeratin-18 cleavage.[32] Cytotrophoblasts in preeclamptic pregnancies migrate only about 0.7 mm into the myometrial interstitium, while in anemia migration is deeper, extending to about 3 mm from the decidual–myometrial interface. These differences appear not to be

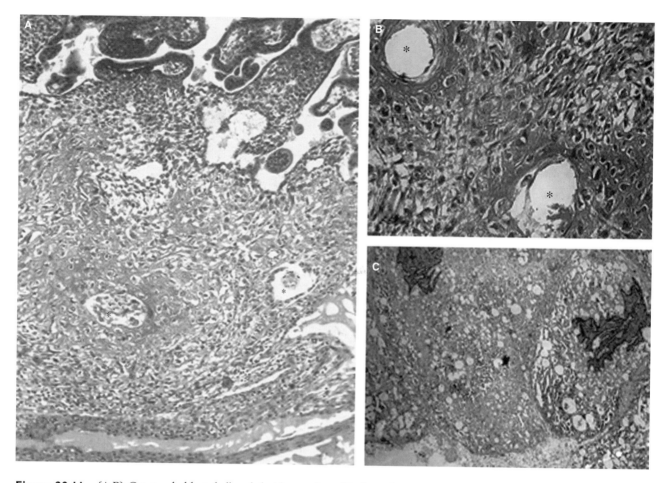

Figure 29.11 (A,B) Cytotrophoblast shell and decidua at about 21 days after implantation, containing the remnants of a spiral artery (*) undergoing transformation by trophoblast with loss of the lining endothelial cells and modification of the intima and smooth muscle cells. (C) Transmission electron microscopy of endovascular trophoblast showing massively developed endoplasmic reticulum and unusually convoluted nuclear profiles.

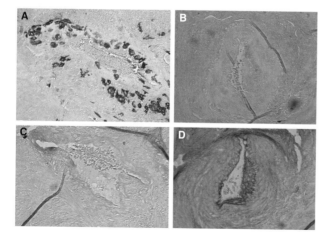

Figure 29.12 Extravillous cytotrophoblast cells immunostained for cytokeratin can be seen in the wall of a transformed artery at term (A), while none are visible in an untransformed artery with narrow lumen (B). Staining for elastin shows its absence in the wall of the transformed artery (C) while it is still present in the untransformed vessel (D).

accounted for by trophoblast apoptosis (e.g. the rate of apoptosis in normal pregnancy is 7% compared to 4% in preeclampsia), although this conclusion must be tempered by the fact that the tissues studied were from near-term. Preeclamptic placentas are characterized by incomplete transformation of the spiral arteries, with muscularized and sometimes atherotic vessels evident, especially in the myometrial segments.

The pathways of cell migration into arterial walls, the factors regulating this phenomenon, the reason why maternal veins are not equally targeted by trophoblast, and the mechanisms that ensure cytotrophoblast migration ceases in the second trimester are all poorly defined; there is evidence that proteases, growth factors, cytokines, components of the ECM, and maternal immune cells are all influential, but detailed discussion lies beyond the scope of this chapter. There is evidence that implantation stimulates the elaboration of local lymphatic drainage in

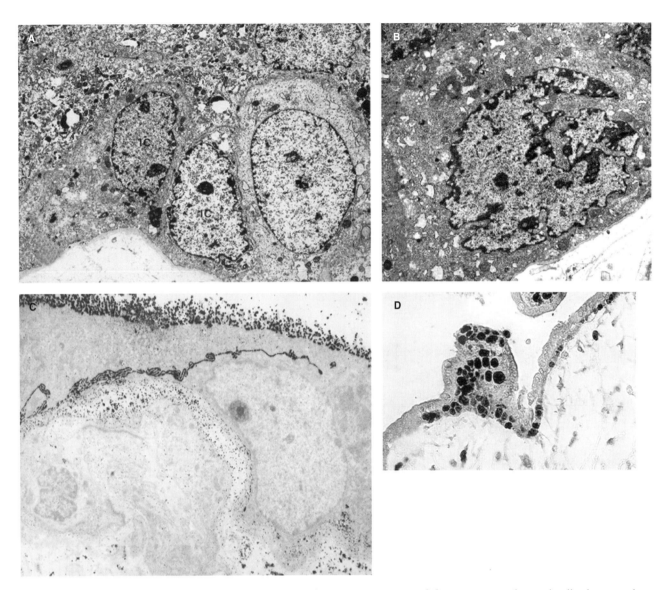

Figure 29.13 Villous trophoblast. (A,B) Transmission electron microscopy of first trimester placental villi showing three intermediate stages of differentiation prior to fusion. (C) A cell labeled for alkaline phosphatase activity showing partial dissolution of the plasma membrane at the cyto–syncytiotrophoblast interface during fusion. (D) Tissue labeled with Ki67 which is expressed in all active phases of the cell cycle, and is found in the cytotrophoblast cell layer. The syncytium is non-proliferative. Note that proliferating cytotrophoblast builds up into a multilayer at sites where sprouting is occurring, and the presence of labeled nuclei in the syncytium reflects locally rapid expansion by incorporation of Ki67-positive cytotrophoblast nuclei. ((B) and (C) reproduced from Jones and Fox;[42] with permission)

decidua.[33] Alterations to endometrial spiral arterial structure (endothelial vacuolation, dilation, disorganized or hypertrophied smooth muscle layers) occur in the late secretory phase of the menstrual cycle as well as in eutopic endometrium during extrauterine implantation, indicating that trophoblast is not required for the initial stages of remodeling.[34] However, the presence of trophoblast in the vessel walls correlates with full transformation, including the loss of vascular smooth muscle and replacement of the normal elastic and collagenous ECM with fibrinoid (see Figure 29.12).[28] This is associated with a trophoblastic phenotype exhibiting large cisternae of rough endoplasmic reticulum (see Figure 29.11C) and expression of matrix metalloproteinases.[35] It has been postulated that factors including insulin-like growth factors (IGFs) produced in the placenta may stimulate migration in a self-limiting fashion such that the signal weakens progressively with distance migrated.[36] There is experimental evidence that

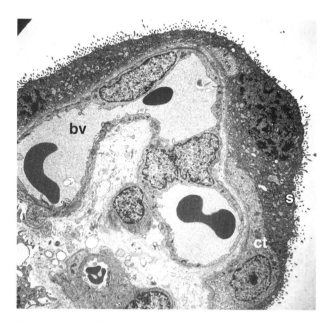

Figure 29.14 A chorionic villus at term. Only occasional cytotrophoblast cells (ct) are present at term, while placental capillaries (bv) dilate to form vasculosyncytial membranes, facilitating diffusion between maternal and fetal blood systems. Note syncytiotrophoblast microvilli which may contribute to microparticle shedding.

arteries in the pregnant uterus are more receptive to trophoblast than in postmenopausal uterus or other vascular beds.[37] The disappearance of vascular smooth muscle is attributed to apoptosis triggered by soluble Fas ligand delivered by trophoblast together with TRAIL (tumor necrosis factor-related apoptosis-inducing ligand) on the trophoblast cell surface and dedifferentiation of smooth muscle cells.[31,33,38–41]

THE DEVELOPING VILLOUS PLACENTA

In first trimester villi, cytotrophoblast forms an essentially continuous layer of cells beneath the syncytium (see Figure 29.2). As pregnancy proceeds, the cytotrophoblast layer becomes discontinuous.[42] Mononucleate cytotrophoblast cells, which continue to show proliferative activity to term, are assumed to undergo an asymmetric cleavage to generate daughter cells, one to maintain the lineage and another that rapidly differentiates to produce an intermediate trophoblast destined to fuse with the overlying syncytium (Figure 29.13). Several molecular participants, including syncytin (HERV-W), an envelope protein derived from an endogenous retrovirus, annexin 5, and externalized phosphatidylserine, play a role in fusion.[43] Before

fusion, the nucleus matures (see Figure 29.13), becoming indistinguishable from syncytially located nuclei.

No DNA synthesis occurs in the syncytium (see Figure 29.13), which functions as a transporting epithelium,[44] a barrier to maternal cells and pathogens, and an endocrine cell, producing large quantities of steroids, hCG, human chorionic somatomammotropin (hCS), human growth hormone (hGH), leptin, soluble vascular endothelial growth factor (VEGF) receptor (sFlt-1), and many other secretory substances.[45]

At the end of the trophoblast life cycle, material is shed from the apical syncytium into maternal blood. Assessed morphologically, the type of material shed differs in first and third trimester. Membrane-bound multinucleate, often multicellular, trophoblast aggregates are seen in maternal uterine venous blood in first trimester, and these appear to have arisen from broken trophoblastic sprouts. Towards term, multinucleate aggregates may shed into maternal circulation from syncytial knots – clusters of nuclei in various stages of degeneration found immediately beneath projections of the syncytial microvillous membrane.[42,46] Other smaller types of shed particle are also found, such as those blebbing off the microvillous surface.[47] In this way a large amount of placental particulate material finds its way into the maternal circulation. Indeed it is estimated that 5% of DNA circulating in maternal blood is of placental origin.[48]

Branching morphogenesis occurs continuously in the placenta throughout pregnancy. It starts with the development of foci of proliferative cytotrophoblasts in mesenchymal or immature intermediate villi that pile up beneath the syncytium and then become invested with stroma. Finally, the stroma is populated by blood vessels.[10]

Mesenchymal villi persist into second trimester as growth and branching continue. From about the 23rd week, mesenchymal villi begin to develop into mature intermediate villi that lack the stromal channels. These in turn give rise not to further mesenchymal villi, but instead to terminal villi. Terminal villi contain the expanded fetal vascular spaces, or sinusoids, and vasculosyncytial membranes where there is found the extreme narrowing of the trophoblast overlying fetal vessels that is characteristic of the term placental exchange surface.[42] This allows a short (approximately 3–5 μm) diffusion distance for gases, nutrients, and waste products to pass between fetal and maternal blood. The maternal–fetal barrier at these vasculosyncytial membranes comprises a thin syncytium, the fused trophoblastic and endothelial basement membranes, and a thin fetal vascular endothelium (Figure 29.14).

VASCULAR DEVELOPMENT

As noted previously, hemangioblastic cords appear from about day 21 pc.[49] These develop a lumen (but no basement membrane – this appears later), giving rise to the first blood vessels, which then move progressively to the villous margins.[50] The hemangioblastic stem cells (see Figure 29.6) appear to arise from pluripotent mesenchymal cells, and are postulated to differentiate into placental macrophages, endothelial cells, and blood cells including erythroblasts.[51,52] Thus, early vasculogenesis does not depend on the angiogenic spread of a network established in the embryo or yolk sac. Similarly, the mouse hemochorial placenta is a major site of hematopoiesis.[53,54]

There follows a phase of uncertain duration when both vasculogenesis and angiogenesis occur, with the latter becoming increasingly dominant, giving rise to a richly branched villous capillary bed with low fetoplacental blood flow impedance. This period is characterized by high placental levels of VEGF but moderate placental growth factor (PlGF) expression. In the second trimester, many larger villi show regression of peripheral capillaries, with the more central capillaries acquiring a tunica media and thus transforming into arteries and veins. Beginning at about week 25 in the newly formed peripheral villi, angiogenesis switches from branching to non-branching and this period is accompanied by a steep drop in VEGF and a slower decline in PlGF expression.[49] As a consequence of this switch, long, poorly branched capillary loops are formed in the periphery of the fetoplacental vascular trees. The capillaries move to the periphery of terminal villi, giving rise to vasculosyncytial membranes (see Figure 29.14). There is increased fetoplacental impedance but blood flow still increases due to rising fetal blood pressure.

Modulation of exchange barrier morphogenesis can occur in response to environmental stimuli; thus, for example, a shorter harmonic mean barrier thickness is observed in placentas developed at high altitude.[55] Reduced vascularization is associated with early pregnancy failure[56] and intrauterine growth restriction.[57] In mouse, imprinted genes, including insulin-like growth factor 2 (*igf2*), can affect fetal growth by modulating the morphogenesis of the placental exchange surface, but also by altering the expression of transporter systems.[58,59] Placental amino acid transport efficiency has been shown to be compromised in women carrying a growth-restricted fetus.[44] Thus, normal vascular morphology, and the efficient transport function required in order for the developing placenta to fulfill the increasing demands of the growing fetus, depend on the precisely coordinated development of the villous tree and its vascular system.[60]

ACKNOWLEDGMENTS

We thank Victoria Cookson for parts of Figures 29.4 and 29.13D and Rebecca Jones and Samantha Smith for part of Figure 29.5.

REFERENCES

1. Adams EC, Hertig AT, Rock J. A description of 34 human ova within the first 17 days of development. Am J Anat 1956; 98: 435–93.
2. Boyd JD, Hamilton WJ. The Human Placenta. Cambridge: Heffer, 1970.
3. Fox H. Pathology of the placenta. 2nd edition, London: WB Saunders; 1997.
4. Benirschke K, Kaufmann P. Pathology of the Human Placenta. New York: Springer, 2000.
5. Burton G, Kaufmann P, Huppertz B. Anatomy and genesis of the placenta. In: Neill JD, ed. Knobil and Neill's Physiology of Reproduction, Vol 1, 3rd edn. Amsterdam: Academic Press, 2006: 189–244.
6. Atkinson DE BR, Sibley CP. Placental transfer. In: Neill JD, ed. Knobil and Neill's Physiology of Reproduction, Vol. 2, 3rd edn. Amsterdam: Academic Press, 2006: 2787–846.
7. Cross JC. How to make a placenta: mechanisms of trophoblast cell differentiation in mice – a review. Placenta 2005; 26(Suppl A): S3–9.
8. Demir R, Kaufmann P, Castellucci M et al. Fetal vasculogenesis and angiogenesis in human placental villi. Acta Anat (Basel) 1989; 136: 190–203.
9. Aplin JD, Haigh T, Vicovac L et al. Anchorage in the developing placenta: an overlooked determinant of pregnancy outcome? Hum Fertil (Camb) 1998; 1: 75–9.
10. Castellucci M, Kosanke G, Verdenelli F et al. Villous sprouting: fundamental mechanisms of human placental development. Hum Reprod Update 2000; 6: 485–94.
11. Martinoli C, Castellucci M, Zaccheo D et al. Scanning electron microscopy of stromal cells of human placental villi throughout pregnancy. Cell Tissue Res 1984; 235: 647–55.
12. Kohnen G, Kertschanska S, Demir R et al. Placental villous stroma as a model system for myofibroblast differentiation. Histochem Cell Biol 1996; 105: 415–29.
13. Aplin JD. Implantation, trophoblast differentiation and haemochorial placentation: mechanistic evidence in vivo and in vitro. J Cell Sci 1991; 99(Pt 4): 681–92.
14. Weier JF, Ferlatte C, Baumgartner A et al. Molecular cytogenetic studies towards the full karyotype analysis of human blastocysts and cytotrophoblasts. Cytogenet Genome Res 2006; 114: 302–11.
15. Zybina TG, Frank HG, Biesterfeld S et al. Genome multiplication of extravillous trophoblast cells in human placenta in the

course of differentiation and invasion into endometrium and myometrium. II. Mechanisms of polyploidization. Tsitologiia 2004; 46: 640–8.

16. Zybina TG, Kaufmann P, Frank HG et al. Genome multiplication of extravillous trophoblast cells in human placenta in the course of differentiation and invasion into endometrium and myometrium. I. Dynamics of polyploidization. Tsitologiia 2002; 44: 1058–67.

17. Enders AC, Blankenship TN, Fazleabas AT et al. Structure of anchoring villi and the trophoblastic shell in the human, baboon and macaque placenta. Placenta 2001; 22: 284–303.

18. Burton GJ, Watson AL, Hempstock J et al. Uterine glands provide histiotrophic nutrition for the human fetus during the first trimester of pregnancy. J Clin Endocrinol Metab 2002; 87: 2954–9.

19. Foidart JM, Hustin J, Dubois M et al. The human placenta becomes haemochorial at the 13th week of pregnancy. Int J Dev Biol 1992; 36: 451–3.

20. Burton GJ, Jauniaux E. Placental oxidative stress: from miscarriage to preeclampsia. J Soc Gynecol Investig 2004; 11: 342–52.

21. Rodesch F, Simon P, Donner C et al. Oxygen measurements in endometrial and trophoblastic tissues during early pregnancy. Obstet Gynecol 1992; 80: 283–5.

22. Kozak KR, Abbott B, Hankinson O. ARNT-deficient mice and placental differentiation. Dev Biol 1997; 191: 297–305.

23. Hung TH, Skepper JN, Charnock-Jones DS et al. Hypoxia-reoxygenation: a potent inducer of apoptotic changes in the human placenta and possible etiological factor in preeclampsia. Circ Res 2002; 90: 1274–81.

24. Jauniaux E, Poston L, Burton GJ. Placental-related diseases of pregnancy: involvement of oxidative stress and implications in human evolution. Hum Reprod Update 2006; 12: 747–55.

25. Aplin JD, Haigh T, Jones CJ et al. Development of cytotrophoblast columns from explanted first-trimester human placental villi: role of fibronectin and integrin alpha5beta1. Biol Reprod 1999; 60: 828–38.

26. Vicovac L, Aplin JD. Epithelial–mesenchymal transition during trophoblast differentiation. Acta Anat (Basel) 1996; 156: 202–16.

27. Enders AC. Fine structure of anchoring villi of the human placenta. Am J Anat 1968; 122: 419–51.

28. Pijnenborg R, Dixon G, Robertson WB et al. Trophoblastic invasion of human decidua from 8 to 18 weeks of pregnancy. Placenta 1980; 1: 3–19.

29. Kaufmann P, Black S, Huppertz B. Endovascular trophoblast invasion: implications for the pathogenesis of intrauterine growth retardation and preeclampsia. Biol Reprod 2003; 69: 1–7.

30. Lyall F. Priming and remodelling of human placental bed spiral arteries during pregnancy – a review. Placenta 2005; 26(Suppl A): S31–6.

31. Pijnenborg R, Vercruysse L, Hanssens M. The uterine spiral arteries in human pregnancy: facts and controversies. Placenta 2006; 27: 939–58.

32. Kadyrov M, Schmitz C, Black S et al. Pre-eclampsia and maternal anaemia display reduced apoptosis and opposite invasive phenotypes of extravillous trophoblast. Placenta 2003; 24: 540–8.

33. Red-Horse K, Rivera J, Schanz A et al. Cytotrophoblast induction of arterial apoptosis and lymphangiogenesis in an in vivo model of human placentation. J Clin Invest 2006; 116: 2643–52.

34. Craven CM, Morgan T, Ward K. Decidual spiral artery remodelling begins before cellular interaction with cytotrophoblasts. Placenta 1998; 19: 241–52.

35. Jones RL, Findlay JK, Farnworth PG et al. Activin A and inhibin A differentially regulate human uterine matrix metalloproteinases: potential interactions during decidualization and trophoblast invasion. Endocrinology 2006; 147: 724–32.

36. Lacey H, Haigh T, Westwood M et al. Mesenchymally-derived insulin-like growth factor 1 provides a paracrine stimulus for trophoblast migration. BMC Dev Biol 2002; 2: 5.

37. Crocker IP, Wareing M, Ferris GR et al. The effect of vascular origin, oxygen, and tumour necrosis factor alpha on trophoblast invasion of maternal arteries in vitro. J Pathol 2005; 206: 476–85.

38. Harris LK, Keogh RJ, Wareing M et al. Invasive trophoblasts stimulate vascular smooth muscle cell apoptosis by a fas ligand-dependent mechanism. Am J Pathol 2006; 169: 1863–74.

39. Keogh RJ HL, Freeman A, Baker PN et al. Fetal-derived trophoblast use the apoptotic cytokine tumor necrosis factor-alpha-related apoptosis-inducing ligand to induce smooth muscle cell death. Circ Res 2007; 100: 834–41.

40. Nanaev AK, Kosanke G, Reister F et al. Pregnancy-induced de-differentiation of media smooth muscle cells in uteroplacental arteries of the guinea pig is reversible after delivery. Placenta 2000; 21: 306–12.

41. Harris LK AJ. Arterial remodelling during pregnancy. Reprod Sci in press, 2007.

42. Jones CJ, Fox H. Ultrastructure of the normal human placenta. Electron Microsc Rev 1991; 4: 129–78.

43. Potgens AJ, Schmitz U, Bose P et al. Mechanisms of syncytial fusion: a review. Placenta 2002; 23(Suppl A): S107–13.

44. Sibley CP, Turner MA, Cetin I et al. Placental phenotypes of intrauterine growth. Pediatr Res 2005; 58: 827–32.

45. Evain-Brion D, Malassine A. Human placenta as an endocrine organ. Growth Horm IGF Res 2003; 13(Suppl A): S34–7.

46. Mayhew TM, Leach L, McGee R et al. Proliferation, differentiation and apoptosis in villous trophoblast at 13–41 weeks of gestation (including observations on annulate lamellae and nuclear pore complexes). Placenta 1999; 20: 407–22.

47. Goswami D, Tannetta DS, Magee LA et al. Excess syncytiotrophoblast microparticle shedding is a feature of early-onset pre-eclampsia, but not normotensive intrauterine growth restriction. Placenta 2006; 27: 56–61.

48. Hahn S, Huppertz B, Holzgreve W. Fetal cells and cell free fetal nucleic acids in maternal blood: new tools to study abnormal placentation? Placenta 2005; 26: 515–26.

49. Kaufmann P, Mayhew TM, Charnock-Jones DS. Aspects of human fetoplacental vasculogenesis and angiogenesis. II. Changes during normal pregnancy. Placenta 2004; 25: 114–26.

50. te Velde EA, Exalto N, Hesseling P et al. First trimester development of human chorionic villous vascularization studied with CD34 immunohistochemistry. Hum Reprod 1997; 12: 1577–81.

51. Demir R, Kayisli UA, Cayli S, Huppertz B. Sequential steps during vasculogenesis and angiogenesis in the very early human placenta. Placenta 2006; 27: 535–9.

52. Challier JC, Galtier M, Cortez A et al. Immunocytological evidence for hematopoiesis in the early human placenta. Placenta 2005; 26: 282–8.

53. Alvarez-Silva M, Belo-Diabangouaya P, Salaun J et al. Mouse placenta is a major hematopoietic organ. Development 2003; 130: 5437–44.

54. Mikkola HK, Gekas C, Orkin SH et al. Placenta as a site for hematopoietic stem cell development. Exp Hematol 2005; 33: 1048–54.

55. Reshetnikova OS, Burton GJ, Milovanov AP. Effects of hypobaric hypoxia on the fetoplacental unit: the morphometric diffusing capacity of the villous membrane at high altitude. Am J Obstet Gynecol 1994; 171: 1560–5.

56. Lisman BA, Boer K, Bleker OP et al. Abnormal development of the vasculosyncytial membrane in early pregnancy failure. Fertil Steril 2004; 82: 654–60.

57. Chen CP, Bajoria R, Aplin JD. Decreased vascularization and cell proliferation in placentas of intrauterine growth-restricted fetuses with abnormal umbilical artery flow velocity waveforms. Am J Obstet Gynecol 2002; 187: 764–9.

58. Sibley CP, Coan PM, Ferguson-Smith AC et al. Placental-specific insulin-like growth factor 2 (Igf2) regulates the diffusional exchange characteristics of the mouse placenta. Proc Natl Acad Sci USA 2004; 101: 8204–8.

59. Constancia M, Angiolini E, Sandovici I et al. Adaptation of nutrient supply to fetal demand in the mouse involves interaction between the Igf2 gene and placental transporter systems. Proc Natl Acad Sci USA 2005; 102: 19219–24.

60. Kingdom JC, Kaufmann P. Oxygen and placental villous development: origins of fetal hypoxia. Placenta 1997; 18: 613–21; discussion 23–6.

61. Falkiner NM. A description of a human ovum 15 days old with special reference to the vascular arrangements and to the morphology of the trophoblast. J Obstet Gynaecol Br Empire 1932; 39: 471–502.

30 Differentiation of the invasive cytotrophoblast lineage in normal pregnancy and in preeclampsia

Virginia D Winn, Kristy Red-Horse, and Susan J Fisher

INTRODUCTION

Following the initial stages of blastocyst implantation and decidualization, formation of the placenta begins in earnest. During this process cells from the trophectoderm, the outer layer of the blastocyst, must proliferate and differentiate into the chorionic villus tree that forms the placenta proper. The human placenta, which is classified as hemochorial, differs from commonly studied animal models such as mice, rats, and rabbits in that it is highly invasive – hemiallogeneic fetal cytotrophoblasts (CTBs) invade uterine tissues, where they reside in an apparently symbiotic fashion for the entirety of gestation. In mammalian species the extent of decidualization correlates with the extent of trophoblast (TB) invasiveness.[1,2] In this regard, the human endometrium, which shows the greatest transformation during pregnancy, plays a critical role by expressing molecules that directly or indirectly govern formation of the placenta. Undoubtedly the converse is true as we also know that invading CTBs induce decidualization and the unique process whereby the maternal vasculature is remodeled into a high-flow system that delivers blood to the placenta. In this chapter, we examine the current state of understanding regarding factors that regulate CTB differentiation and invasion during formation of the human placenta with a particular focus on the maternal–fetal interface (decidua basalis). We also consider aberrations in formation of the placenta and/or the maternal–fetal interface that lead to pregnancy complications of which preeclampsia (PE) is a prime example.

In this context, it is important to understand (at a molecular level) placental development, which in turn, determines the functional capacity of this transient organ. This chapter focuses on one component of this process – differentiation of the subpopulation of CTBs that invade the uterine wall. As discussed below, the trophectoderm layer of the blastocyst is the first embryonic cell type to exhibit highly differentiated functions. At 5–6 days after fertilization,

TBs participate in a complex dialogue with maternal cells that enables implantation, a process that rapidly sequesters the human embryo within the uterine wall. Further embryonic development requires the rapid assembly of the basic building blocks of the placenta–chorionic villi. The unique structure of the human maternal–fetal interface is established when CTBs at the tips of anchoring villi differentiate into invasive cells that anchor the placenta to the uterine wall. The latter process entails many unusual elements. For example, these fetal cells, which are derived from the placenta, form elaborate connections with maternal vessels, thereby diverting uterine blood flow to the placenta. Given the rapid time course during which this organ develops and its many other highly unusual properties, it is not surprising that several pregnancy complications, such as PE, are associated with abnormal placentation.

TROPHOBLAST DIFFERENTIATION AND FORMATION OF THE MATERNAL–FETAL INTERFACE

The placenta is a transient organ with remarkable properties whose progenitors must begin to function within days of fertilization.[3] The mature form arises through the development of specialized subpopulations of chorionic villi, finger-like projections into the intervillous space with blood vessel-containing mesenchymal cores that are surrounded by a TB basement membrane to which a layer of CTBs attaches. In some villi, CTBs fuse to form syncytiotrophoblasts (STBs) that cover the villous surface. These floating villi, so named because they float in maternal blood, are the site of hormone production and the exchange of myriad substances between the mother and the fetus. In the second differentiation pathway (Figure 30.1), CTBs in anchoring chorionic villi, so named because they anchor the fetus to the uterus, form columns of non-polarized single cells that attach to and then

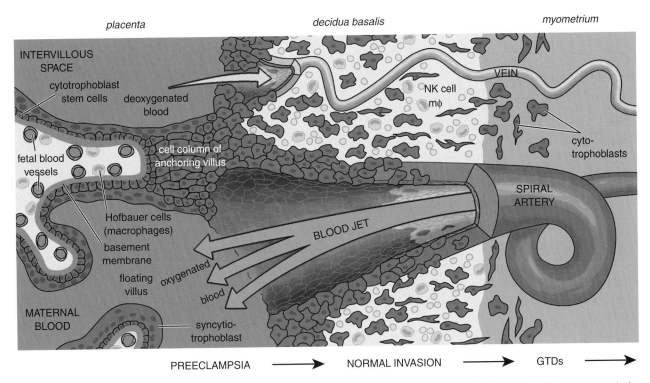

Figure 30.1   The cellular relationships at the human maternal–fetal interface. Floating villi (bottom left) are suspended in maternal blood. Anchoring villi (top left) attach the placenta and embryo/fetus to the uterus. Arrows at the bottom of the diagram indicate the depth of cytotrophoblast invasion in preeclampsia, normal pregnancy, and gestational trophoblast diseases (GTDs).

penetrate the uterine wall, where they give rise to invasive CTBs. During interstitial invasion, a subset of these cells commingles with resident decidual, myometrial, and immune cells. During endovascular invasion, masses of CTBs migrate into the vessels before the lumina eventually recanalize.[4] Together, these two components of CTB invasion anchor the placenta to the uterus and divert uterine blood flow to the intervillous space.

Our focus is on the wide array of molecular processes that regulate CTB invasion, in actuality a complex differentiation program. For example, migration, extracellular matrix dissolution, angiogenesis, adhesion (autocrine and paracrine), and repulsion are involved. Therefore, it is not surprising that CTB invasion involves an equally diverse molecular repertoire: cell cycle regulators, transcription factors, cytoskeleton components, adhesion molecules, degradative enzymes, paracrine hormones, growth and angiogenic factors, chemokines, and small molecules such as oxygen. This chapter highlights a number of the component processes that constitute CTB differentiation and the molecular pathways that are involved.

The generation of mouse TB stem cell lines from early-stage mouse embryos (e.g. prior to day 7.5) has provided important experimental tools for studying

this process, as well as the mechanisms that promote self-renewal of the progenitor stem cell population.[5,6] The actions of fibroblast growth factor (FGF) family members are crucial, as derivations are accomplished by plating disaggregated extraembryonic cells on mouse embryonic fibroblasts in the presence of FGF4, which binds Fgfr2 IIIc, ultimately leading to mitogen-activated protein kinase (MAPK) signaling.[7] It is likely that the yet-to-be-reported derivation of human TB stem cells will also require FGF signals, which may be necessary, but not sufficient. Although bone morphogenetic protein 4 (BMP-4) treatment of human embryonic stem cells results in the expression of TB markers, the cells do not continue to divide.[8] Thus, the majority of what we know about human TB differentiation has come from studies of early-gestation TBs obtained from placentas rather than embryos through the application of in-situ and in-vitro approaches.[9]

CELL CYCLE CONTROL AND CTB DIFFERENTIATION

Early on in pregnancy, CTB progenitors must rapidly expand with proper growth of the placenta requiring the continued proliferation of a subset of the cells.

Therefore, it follows that molecules involved in cell cycle control are highly regulated during placentation. In a comprehensive analysis of CTB expression of 16 cell cycle regulators, dynamic changes in expression patterns were noted both in terms of gestational age and cellular location. In terms of gestation, molecules indicative of proliferation were expressed by more cells in early pregnancy corresponding to the time of most rapid growth. In terms of expression at different stages along the invasive pathway, molecules that regulate every phase of the cell cycle localized to villous CTBs, the progenitor population, and to cells in the proximal column that have begun to differentiate/invade, a finding that is consistent with the fact that these cells are proliferating. In contrast, CTBs in the distal portions of columns expressed cell cycle inhibitors such as p21, p27, and p57, suggesting withdrawal from the mitotic cycle.[10] Given their ability to invade the uterus and numerous ectopic sites, an inability to proliferate is one of the few characteristics that differentiate TBs from tumor cells.

TRANSCRIPTION FACTORS IMPLICATED IN PLACENTATION

As in any differentiation process, transcription factors play a critical role in coordinating alterations in gene expression. Numerous insights into human CTB differentiation have been gained by studying mouse models. Gene deletion studies have either advertently or inadvertently yielded interesting insights into the molecular requirements of normal placentation.[11] Development of the tetraploid rescue technique for giving mutant embryos wild-type placentas has allowed a careful separation of the embryonic and extraembryonic phenotypes.[12,13] As a result, many aspects of murine TB differentiation can now be explained in terms of specific transcriptional regulators.[6,7,14] As to those that control early events, deletion of the T-box gene *Eomesodermin* results in embryonic death soon after implantation due to an arrest in trophectoderm development.[15] Embryos that lack expression of activator protein 2γ (AP-2γ), a member of a family of transcription factors that control cell proliferation, die at embryonic day (E) 7.5 due to malformation of the maternal–fetal interface. The defect is probably attributable to negative effects on the stem cell population, which has reduced expression of *Eomesodermin* and *Cdx2*, two genes that are up-regulated in response to FGF treatment of TB stem cells.[16] Deletion of the orphan receptor, estrogen-receptor-related-receptor

protein β, results in death at day E9.5. Demise is thought to occur secondary to depletion of the TB stem/progenitor population, which is shunted to the giant cell lineage,[17] the murine equivalent of the human CTB population that carries out interstitial and endovascular invasion.[6,18]

Basic helix–loop–helix (bHLH) transcription factors play important roles during the later stages of differentiation. Mash2, a paternally imprinted gene, is required for the production of the precursor population that gives rise to the spongiotrophoblast layer.[19] Interestingly, there is evidence that the polycomb group protein extraembryonic ectoderm development (eed) may be required for lineage-specific Mash2 repression during differentiation.[20] Since bHLH factors function as dimers, their binding partners also need to be expressed at the proper time and location. Finally, their activity can be inhibited by interactions with dominant negative HLH factors that lack DNA-binding sequences: e.g. Id1 and Id2, which are also expressed in the extraembryonic ectoderm.[21]

Many of the same transcription factors demonstrated to be critical for murine placental development are also involved in human CTB differentiation: e.g. human TB progenitors also express Mash2 and Id2, which are down-regulated as the cells differentiate along the invasive pathway.[22] In keeping with the known functions of the latter factors, forced expression of Id2 inhibits CTB differentiation in vitro.[23] This is one example of the many similarities between murine and human placentation at the molecular level. In contrast, another bHLH factor, Hand1, is required for the differentiation of murine primary and secondary giant cells.[24,25] The observation that human TBs beyond the blastocyst stage do not express Hand1 is an example of divergent placental evolution in the two species.[26]

A number of transcription factors also regulate formation of the labyrinth zone, the area of the murine placenta that corresponds to the floating villi of the human placenta (i.e. where the majority of transport activities take place).[6] A screen of human tissues revealed the surprising result that *glial cells missing I* (*Gcm I*), which controls the neuronal to glial transition in *Drosophila*,[27] is solely and constitutively expressed in placental CTBs.[22] Mice that lack expression of this transcription factor die at day E10 due to a block in the branching of the chorioallantoic interface and an absence of the placental labyrinth.[28] Other known regulators of labyrinth development include retinoic acid receptors[29,30] and peroxisome proliferator-activated receptor γ (PPARγ).[31] Wnt2[32] and growth factor (e.g. hepatocyte growth factor[33]) signals are also required.

Aggregation of tetraploid (wild-type) and diploid (mutant) cells is a powerful technique that supplies mutant embryos with normal placentas and, thus, separates a molecule's embryonic and extraembryonic effects.[12,13] The widespread application of this technology has produced many examples of the critical importance of normal placental function to embryonic and fetal development. A startling array of epigenetic effects are propagated downstream from abnormal placentation. For example, targeted mutation of the DNA-binding domain of the Ets2 transcription factor produces numerous defects in the extraembryonic compartment, including a substantial decrease in matrix metalloproteinase-9 production, an attendant failure in extracellular matrix remodeling, and a proliferation defect that involves the ectoplacental cone. The Ets2 null embryos, which are growth-restricted, die before E8.5. Tetraploid rescue resulted in the birth of viable, fertile mice with hair defects – a dramatically different embryonic phenotype than when the entire conceptus lacks Ets2 expression.[34] This general phenomenon has been documented in association with the deletion of many other genes from very diverse molecular families. For example, deletion of JunB, an immediate early gene product and member of the AP-1 transcription factor family, also causes fetal growth restriction, ultimately leading to embryonic death between E8.5 and E10 due to defects in both placental and decidual vessels, the latter receiving improper signals from invading TBs. Again, tetraploid rescue resulted in fetuses that were normally grown.[35]

GROWTH FACTORS INVOLVED IN CTB DIFFERENTIATION

Likewise, fetal growth restriction secondary to defects in the placental labyrinth of the extracellular signal-regulated kinase-2 null mice is rescued by tetraploid aggregation.[36] Similarly, tetraploid rescue results in the birth of mice lacking the hepatocyte growth factor (HGF) receptor c-Met[37] or the suppressor of cytokine signaling 3.[38] In other cases supplying mutant embryos with normal extraembryonic derivatives allows development to progress further than was previously possible. Mice that lack expression of thrombomodulin[39] and desmoplakin[40] fall into this category as do homozygous null mutants that lack expression of Alk2, which encodes a type I transforming growth factor β (TGFβ) family receptor for activins and BMP-7.[41] The latter case provides direct evidence that signals transmitted through this receptor, which is expressed in the extraembryonic region, are required at the time of gastrulation for normal mesoderm formation. Interestingly, deletion of the TGFβ family member Nodal also leads to expansion of the TB giant cell population at the expense of the other subtypes.[42]

CHROMOSOMALLY NORMAL TBS PARTIALLY RESCUE ANEUPLOID EMBRYOS

Interestingly, the impact on embryonic development of aneuploidy involving the fetal membranes can also be alleviated to varying degrees by tetraploid rescue. For example, the development of mice with a t-complex variant of chromosome 17 is sustained for several additional days by wild-type placental cells[43] and tetraploid aggregation allows the birth of mice that carry an additional maternal X chromosome.[44] It is important to note that while in some cases the effects of placental malfunction on the embryo are likely to be directly attributable to defects in the organs' transport functions, in many other instances the connection is likely to involve a higher order of complexity. For example, tetraploid aggregation shows that keratin 8 is a necessary component of the barrier that prevents tumor necrosis factor (TNF)-mediated apoptosis of TB giant cells.[45]

PHYSIOLOGICAL FACTORS INFLUENCE CTB DIFFERENTIATION

Physiological factors also play an important role in formation of the maternal–fetal interface and, consequently, fetal growth. Oxygen tension, a function of uterine blood flow, is a prime example.[46] In recent years a great deal has been learned about the fundamental mechanisms that couple the ability of TBs to sense oxygen levels with their differentiative and metabolic status. Important clues about oxygen effects on the placenta come from several lines of evidence that suggest the early stages of placental (and embryonic) development take place in an environment that is hypoxic relative to the uterus. Specifically, blood flow to the human intervillous space does not begin until 10–12 weeks of pregnancy.[47] Studies in both nonhuman primates[48] and humans[49] suggest that TBs actively limit their access to uterine blood by plugging the lumina of the decidual vessels. Why? Our work shows that CTBs proliferate in vitro under hypoxic conditions that are comparable to those found during early pregnancy in the uterine cavity and the superficial decidua. As TB invasion of the uterus proceeds, the placental cells encounter increasingly higher oxygen levels, which trigger their exit from the cell cycle and subsequent differentiation.[50,51] Hypoxia also regulates cell fate in the murine placenta.[52] We speculate that the paradoxical effects of oxygen in controlling the balance between CTB proliferation and differentiation explain in part why placental mass increases much more rapidly than that of the embryo. Histological sections of early-stage pregnant human uteri show bilaminar embryos surrounded by thousands of TB cells. The fact that hypoxia stimulates CTBs but not most other cells to undergo mitosis[53] could help account for the discrepancy in size between the embryo and the placenta, which continues well into the second trimester of pregnancy.[54] Thus, the structure of the mature placenta is established in advance of the period of rapid fetal growth that occurs during the latter half of pregnancy.

What are the molecular underpinnings of this unusual relationship? Many different lines of evidence suggest that the hypoxia-inducible factor (HIF) system that controls cellular responses to oxygen deprivation is involved (reviewed in Semenza,[55] Safran et al,[56] and Masson and Ratcliffe[57]). HIFs (1–3-α) are bHLH transcription factors that also contain a Per/Arnt/Sim domain that facilitates their dimerization with HIF-1-β (the aryl hydrocarbon receptor nuclear translocator). The heterodimers activate the transcription of numerous downstream targets by binding to a hypoxia responsive promoter element (5′-TACGTG-3′) that is present in a variety of relevant genes, including vascular endothelial growth factor (VEGF), glucose transporter-1, and Stra13, the latter a regulator of murine placental development.[14,58] Because these responses need to be extremely rapid, an important element of control occurs at the protein level. Specifically, enzymatic hydroxylation of certain HIFα proline residues is required for interactions with the von Hippel–Lindau (pVHL) tumor suppressor protein, which under normoxic conditions targets these proteins for polyubiquitination and proteasome degradation. Additionally, hydroxylation of specific HIFα asparagine residues prevents the recruitment of transcriptional co-activators. Interestingly, these enzymatic reactions, which depend on molecular oxygen, do not occur in a low-oxygen environment, providing a direct link between hypoxia, HIF stabilization, and the transcription of downstream target genes. In keeping with the concept that oxygen plays an important role in placental development, deletion of many of the individual components of the cell's machinery for sensing and responding to changes in

oxygen tension leads to prenatal lethality secondary to placental defects. For example, mice that lack expression of either VHL[59] or HIF-1β[60] die in utero as a result of faulty placentation. The lack of heat shock protein 90 (Hsp90), which also controls HIF availability,[61] is associated with placental defects that lead to embryonic death at day 9.0/9.5.[62] Additionally, VHL and HIFs also play important roles in human CTB differentiation/ invasion in vitro.[63] The latter data are in accord with studies of normal and abnormal placentation in vivo. For example, TB remolding of spiral arterioles is restricted at high altitude, suggesting that hypoxia affects placentation in utero.[64] Interestingly, the incidence of PE, which is associated with reduced blood flow to the placenta and deficient arterial invasion,[65,66] increases several-fold at high elevations.[67]

ROLE OF ANGIOGENESIS AND LYMPHANGIOGENESIS FACTORS IN CTB DIFFERENTIATION

Angiogenesis is one well-known consequence of hypoxia.[68] In the special case of placentation, the combined actions of the aforementioned transcriptional and physiological regulators differentiate an unusual subpopulation of CTBs with many vascular-type attributes. The progenitors, which are components of anchoring chorionic villi, leave the placenta proper and attach to the uterine wall, the first step in both the interstitial and endovascular components of uterine invasion (see Figure 30.1). A great deal about these processes has been learned by constructing in-vitro models that allow function perturbation of molecules that are regulated during human uterine invasion. For example, as CTBs transition from the fetal to the maternal compartment they modulate expression of a broad repertoire of adhesion receptors, growth factors and receptors with diverse roles in vasculogenesis, angiogenesis, and lymph angiogenesis.

As CTBs invade the uterine wall they acquire a vascular-like repertoire of adhesion molecules. The onset of CTB differentiation/invasion is characterized by reduced staining for receptors characteristic of polarized CTB epithelial progenitors – integrin $\alpha_6\beta_4$ and E-cadherin – and the onset of expression of adhesion receptors characteristic of endothelium – VE-cadherin, immunoglobulin G (IgG) family members, vascular cell adhesion molecule 1 (VCAM-1) and platelet endothelial cell adhesion molecule 1 (PECAM-1), and integrins $\alpha_V\beta_3$ and $\alpha_1\beta_1$ (reviewed in Damsky and Fisher[69]). Thus, as CTBs from anchoring villi invade and remodel the wall of the uterus, these epithelial cells of ectodermal origin acquire an adhesion receptor repertoire characteristic of endothelial cells. We theorize that this switch permits the heterotypic adhesive interactions that allow fetal and maternal cells to cohabit the uterine vasculature during normal pregnancy.

CTBs also alter their expression of angiogenic factors such as VEGFR1–3 (VEGF receptors 1–3), soluble VEGFR-1 (sFlt1), VEGF-A, VEGF-C, and placental growth factor. Function perturbation experiments show that these ligand–receptor interactions promote CTB differentiation/invasion and survival.[70] We speculate that the expression of regulators of lymphangiogenesis (e.g. VEGFR-3 and VEGF-C[71]) could contribute to the specialized nature of TB-lined uterine vessels, which are able to greatly expand as fetal requirements for maternal blood increase in the latter half of pregnancy. Additionally, the cells express Ang2, a ligand that is also involved in lymphangiogenesis.[72] Since CTBs lack expression of Tie receptors, maternal cells are the likely targets.[73] Recent work using an in-vivo model of human CTB invasion demonstrated that CTBs can remodel arteries and stimulate lymphangiogenesis regardless of the site of ectopic transplantation (e.g. kidney capsule or mammary gland[74]).

PATTERNING CTB INVASION

Interestingly, endovascular invasion and remodeling of uterine vessels observed at the human maternal–fetal interface is skewed toward the arterial side of the circulatory system with minimal modulation of the venous compartment. What molecular signals direct CTBs toward the arteries? Oxygen tension could play a role, with growth factors and chemokines making important contributions.[75,76] Recent work suggests that members of the Eph (receptor) and ephrin (ligand) family of transmembrane signaling molecules may also be involved.[77,78] Specifically, CTB commitment to uterine invasion was accompanied by rapid down-regulation of EphB4 expression, a receptor associated with venous identity, and up-regulation of ephrinB1. Within the uterine wall, the cells also up-regulated expression of ephrinB2, an Eph transmembrane ligand that is associated with arterial identity. In vitro, CTBs avoided EphB4-coated substrates; upon co-culture with 3T3 cells expressing this molecule, their migration was significantly inhibited. As to the mechanisms involved, CTB interactions with EphB4 down-regulated chemokine-induced but not growth factor-stimulated migration. These data suggest that

EphB4/ephrinB1 interactions generate repulsive signals that direct CTB invasion toward the uterus, where chemokines stimulate CTB migration through the decidua. When CTBs encounter EphB4 expressed by venous endothelium, ephrinB-generated repulsive signals and a reduction in chemokine-mediated responses limit their interaction with veins. When they encounter ephrinB2 ligands expressed in uterine arterioles, migration is permitted. The net effect is preferential CTB remodeling of arterioles, a hallmark of human placentation.

CTB INTERACTIONS WITH MATERNAL CELLS

Two recent studies utilized a microarray approach to characterize at a global level interactions between fetal CTBs and maternal decidual cells. The first study utilized an in-vitro model to investigate the influence of CTB-derived secreted factors on decidualized stromal cells.[79] This analysis revealed that paracrine signals from human CTBs dramatically alter decidual expression of immune and angiogenic modulators. The second study characterized the in-situ gene expression profiles at the human maternal–fetal interface as a function of gestational age.[80] Specifically, basal plate biopsy specimens of decidua and invasive CTBs were obtained from 36 placentas (14–40 weeks) at the conclusion of normal pregnancies. RNA was isolated, processed, and hybridized to HG-U133A and HG-U133B Affymetrix GeneChips. Surprisingly, there was little change in gene expression during the 14- to 24-week interval. In contrast, 418 genes were differentially expressed at term (37–40 weeks) as compared to mid gestation (14–24 weeks). Subsequent analyses using quantitative real-time polymerase chain reaction (PCR) and immunolocalization approaches validated a portion of these results. Many of the differentially expressed genes are known in other contexts to be involved in differentiation, motility, transcription, immunity, angiogenesis, extracellular matrix dissolution, or lipid metabolism. At least one-sixth were non-annotated or encoded hypothetical proteins. Modeling based on structural homology revealed potential functions for 31 proteins in this category.

Other important cellular conversations occur in the basal plate region. For example, interactions between decidual natural killer (dNK) cells and invasive CTBs are thought to be critical to pregnancy success.[1] Several studies have provided insights into this unusual dialogue. The unique population of dNK cells, which are CD 56[bright] and CD 16[-], express angiogenic factors and chemokines that directly enhance CTB invasion, as demonstrated by both in-vitro and in-vivo models.[81] The influence of dNK-derived interferon γ (IFN-γ) on CTB invasion was demonstrated in a co-culture system that consisted of concordant villous explants and maternal immune cells.[82] Through the development of these and other model systems that better recapitulate CTB interactions with maternal cells in vivo, we should gain a better understanding of the interplay between these cells that occurs during formation of the maternal–fetal interface.

PREECLAMPSIA AND ABERRANT CTB DIFFERENTIATION AND INVASION

Specific placental defects are associated with PE, especially the most severe cases that occur during the second and early third trimesters of pregnancy. The major alterations affect the anchoring villi that give rise to invasive CTBs. Specifically, the extent of interstitial invasion is variable, but frequently shallow (see Figure 30.2). Endovascular invasion is consistently rudimentary, making it extremely difficult to find any maternal vessels that contain CTBs.[4,83]

Knowledge of the mechanisms that regulate CTB differentiation/invasion in normal pregnancy allows comparative analyses of the analogous processes in pregnancy complications. There is now a great deal of evidence that defects in this pathway are associated with the phenomenon of inadequate endovascular invasion in this syndrome (Figure 30.2). Two basic concepts have emerged. The first is a failure in important aspects of the differentiation process that enables CTB invasion of the uterine wall. Initially, this effect was described in terms of the cells' repertoire of adhesion receptors. Specifically, in pregnancies affected by PE, invasive CTBs, which retain many of their original epithelial characteristics, fail to express a subset of the vascular-type adhesion molecules that we theorize allow them to line uterine arterioles and channel blood to the placenta.[83] In contrast, this switching process is not affected by preterm labor in the absence of infection.[84] Additional proof of this concept is observed at the transcriptional level. For example, in PE, the cells express much higher levels of Id2, a negative regulator of bHLH transcription factors that promote differentiation of the invasive CTB population.[22]

The second concept is that placental production of vasculogenic/angiogenic molecules is abnormal in PE. In this regard, VEGF family members have been a prime area of investigation. In the most severely affected patients, immunolocalization on tissue sections of the placenta showed that CTB VEGF-A and VEGFR-1 staining decreased; however, staining for placental growth factor (PlGF) was unaffected. CTB secretion of soluble Fms-like tyrosine kinase 1 (sFlt-1) in vitro also increased,[70] an observation that gains additional importance in light of the recent discovery that excess sFlt-1 produces a PE-like syndrome in rats.[85] Finally, our group[86] and others have demonstrated the utility of measuring circulating levels of VEGF family members in maternal blood as a potential screening and diagnostic tool for PE (reviewed in Lam et al[87]). Recent work has extended these observations to include other molecules with vasculogenic activities. For example, Karumanchi and co-workers[88] showed that placental production of the soluble form of the TGFβ receptor, endoglin, increases in PE. Interestingly, these investigators also published evidence of the synergistic effects of sFlt and endoglin: in rats, an increase in the circulating levels of both molecules produced a broader spectrum of PE signs that included glomerular endotheliosis. In accord with this finding, there is now evidence that circulating levels of endoglin, PlGF, and sFlt rise before the onset of PE in humans,[89] an observation that could become a clinically useful test. Finally, the work of Caron and co-workers[90] implicates reduced maternal levels of adrenomedullin, another molecule with powerful vasoactive effects, in the pathophysiology of PE.

A very large question that has yet to be answered is exactly how the placenta triggers the maternal signs of PE. In addition to the sFlt-1 mechanism described above, there are several other proposals. For example, in PE, placental debris, including syncytiotrophoblast membrane microparticles that are potentially proinflammatory, is released into the maternal circulation; this could elicit the immunological changes that are observed in these patients.[91] Recently, the same authors reported that this phenomenon is a feature of early-onset PE and not intrauterine growth restriction, an important distinction.[92] Hypoxic stress is also likely to be involved, one factor that could produce CTB apoptosis, which has been observed in PE[93,94] (reviewed in Redman and Sargent[95]). Mechanistic insights are also being described. For example, N-Myc down-regulated gene 1 (Ndrg1) modulates the response of term placental CTBs to hypoxic injury.[96] Very interestingly, a recent report suggests that particular sets of natural killer cell inhibitory receptors and fetal haplotypes are more likely to be associated with the development of PE.[97]

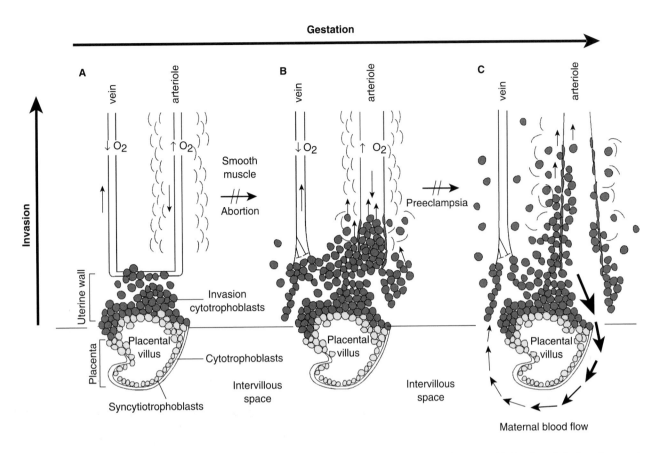

Figure 30.2   Cytotrophoblast invasion and remodeling of the uterine spiral arterioles. It is likely that failed endovascular invasion leads, in some cases, to abortion, whereas an inability to invade to the appropriate depth is associated with preeclampsia and a subset of pregnancies complicated by intrauterine growth restriction.

Finally, genetic studies have also yielded fascinating mechanistic insights. Specifically, in a Dutch family study, a mutated locus associated with PE was identified at 10q22, which encodes *STOX1*, a new member of the winged helix family. Due to imprinting, only the maternal locus is expressed, an explanation for why mutation of one allele leads to development of this pregnancy complication. Although the pathway that links this mutation to the maternal syndrome is not known, interesting speculations are possible; e.g. *STOX1* may play a role in CTB differentiation, possibly through the PI3-K/Akt pathway. The authors note that the one patient who carried the mutation but did not develop PE was treated with heparin therapy in her second pregnancy because she had developed this syndrome in her first. The fact that she had a normal outcome also suggests that coagulation pathways are involved, perhaps triggered by the presence of abnormally differentiated CTBs.[98] At least three other susceptibility loci with significant linkage to PE have been identified – 2p12 (Icelandic[99]); 9p13 (Finnish[100]); and 2p25 (Finnish[101]) – again highlighting the complexity of this syndrome. For this and other reasons, many

investigators have turned to a microarray approach to understand the placental pathophysiology that is associated with PE, work that is discussed in the following section.

The extent to which extraembryonic and embryonic development are linked in humans is an interesting, unresolved question that has gained additional importance due to the realization that the foundation of many aspects of adult health is laid down in utero (i.e. the developmental origins hypothesis[102]). In this context, normal placental function is critical for normal fetal development. At a biochemical level, a great deal of evidence suggests that alterations in placental transport functions are associated with growth restriction.[103,104] However, the actual cause and effect relationship is likely to be much more complicated. For example, uterine blood flow is a critical regulator of placental function and, hence, of fetal growth.[46] Additionally, impaired placental transport is linked to reduced umbilical blood flow and attendant changes in the fetal circulation.[105] Thus, in humans, it is difficult to sort out the primary defect from the ripple effects. This problem is further complicated by the fact that many commonly used drugs (e.g. nicotine) negatively affect TB differentiation and formation of the maternal–fetal interface[106,107] as well as placental transport of amino acids and fetal growth.[108] Additionally, subclinical viral (e.g. cytomegalovirus) and bacterial infections, which are surprisingly common, can inhibit CTB differentiation/invasion.[109,110] Despite the obvious complexity of these interrelationships, it is possible to envision a deterioration in placental function that translates into alterations, at the molecular level, in the fetal circulation that are maintained throughout life, one possible explanation of why a restriction in intrauterine growth is linked to adult cardiovascular disease.

SUMMARY

In recent years a great deal of progress has been made toward identifying the factors that govern TB differentiation and, consequently, implantation and formation of the maternal–fetal interface. One important source of information has been the surprising number of transgenic mice (made for other purposes) that have primary placental defects, a trend that was noted over a decade ago.[11] These analyses have also revealed the critical importance of normal placental function to embryonic development, as there are many examples in which tetraploid aggregation, which supplies a mutant embryo with a normal placenta, either rescues or lessens the severity of the embryonic defects. This principle probably applies to humans, as many aspects of adult health appear to be programmed in utero. Another important source of information has been studies of normal human placental development, which have led, in turn, to a better understanding of the defects that are associated with common pregnancy complications such as PE. In this context, the future challenge is to translate our basic knowledge of factors that govern TB differentiation into clinically useful tests of placental function, a process that will inevitably revolutionize the practice of maternal–fetal medicine. Recently, interesting examples of this type of translational research have been published. For example, as early as the first trimester of pregnancy, increased levels of soluble VEGFR-1 and endoglin and decreased levels of PlGF predict the subsequent development of PE.[76,111] By building on these types of observations, we will greatly increase our understanding of how the placenta impacts maternal physiology in normal and abnormal pregnancies. Along the way, we will also learn a great deal about possible strategies for predicting, preventing, and/or treating pregnancy complications.

ACKNOWLEDGMENTS

The authors thank the past and present members of our laboratory who have made important contributions to this work. Funding sources include: HL64597, The University of California Tobacco-Related Disease Program Grant Number 8DT-0176, The National Institute of General Medical Sciences Minority Biomedical Research Support Research Initiative for Scientific Enhancement (R25 GM59298 and R25 GM56847), U01 HD 42283 (part of the Cooperative Program on Trophoblast–Maternal Tissue Interactions), HD 30367, U54 HD 055764, HD 046744 and the American Association of Obstetricians and Gynecologists Foundation.

REFERENCES

1. Moffett A, Loke C. Immunology of placentation in eutherian mammals. Nat Rev Immunol 2006; 6: 584–94.
2. King A, Loke YW, Chaouat G. NK cells and reproduction. Immunol Today 1997; 18: 64–6.
3. Red-Horse K, Zhou Y, Genbacev O et al. Trophoblast differentiation during embryo implantation and formation of the maternal–fetal interface. J Clin Invest 2004; 114: 744–54.
4. Brosens IA, Robertson WB, Dixon HG. The role of the spiral arteries in the pathogenesis of preeclampsia. Obstet Gynecol Annu 1972; 1: 177–91.
5. Tanaka S, Kunath T, Hadjantonakis AK et al. Promotion of trophoblast stem cell proliferation by FGF4. Science 1998; 282: 2072–5.
6. Rossant J, Cross JC. Placental development: lessons from mouse mutants. Nat Rev Genet 2001; 2: 538–48.
7. Kunath T, Strumpf D, Rossant J. Early trophoblast determination and stem cell maintenance in the mouse – a review. Placenta 2004; 25(Suppl A): S32–8.
8. Xu RH, Chen X, Li DS et al. BMP4 initiates human embryonic stem cell differentiation to trophoblast. Nat Biotechnol 2002; 20: 1261–4.
9. Norwitz ER, Schust DJ, Fisher SJ. Implantation and the survival of early pregnancy. N Engl J Med 2001; 345: 1400–8.
10. Genbacev O, McMaster MT, Fisher SJ. A repertoire of cell cycle regulators whose expression is coordinated with human cytotrophoblast differentiation. Am J Pathol 2000; 157: 1337–51.
11. Cross JC, Werb Z, Fisher SJ. Implantation and the placenta: key pieces of the development puzzle. Science 1994; 266: 1508–18.
12. Nagy A, Gocza E, Diaz EM et al. Embryonic stem cells alone are able to support fetal development in the mouse. Development 1990; 110: 815–21.
13. Nagy A, Rossant J, Nagy R et al. Derivation of completely cell culture-derived mice from early-passage embryonic stem cells. Proc Natl Acad Sci USA 1993; 90: 8424–8.
14. Cross JC, Baczyk D, Dobric N et al. Genes, development and evolution of the placenta. Placenta 2003; 24: 123–30.

15. Russ AP, Wattler S, Colledge WH et al. Eomesodermin is required for mouse trophoblast development and mesoderm formation. Nature 2000; 404: 95–9.

16. Auman HJ, Nottoli T, Lakiza O et al. Transcription factor AP-2gamma is essential in the extra-embryonic lineages for early postimplantation development. Development 2002; 129: 2733–47.

17. Luo J, Sladek R, Bader JA et al. Placental abnormalities in mouse embryos lacking the orphan nuclear receptor ERR-beta. Nature 1997; 388: 778–82.

18. Adamson SL, Lu Y, Whiteley KJ et al. Interactions between trophoblast cells and the maternal and fetal circulation in the mouse placenta. Dev Biol 2002; 250: 358–73.

19. Guillemot F, Nagy A, Auerbach A et al. Essential role of Mash-2 in extraembryonic development. Nature 1994; 371: 333–6.

20. Wang J, Mager J, Schnedier E et al. The mouse PcG gene eed is required for Hox gene repression and extraembryonic development. Mamm Genome 2002; 13: 493–503.

21. Jen Y, Manova K, Benezra R. Each member of the Id gene family exhibits a unique expression pattern in mouse gastrulation and neurogenesis. Dev Dyn 1997; 208: 92–106.

22. Janatpour MJ, Utset MF, Cross JC et al. A repertoire of differentially expressed transcription factors that offers insight into mechanisms of human cytotrophoblast differentiation. Dev Genet 1999; 25: 146–57.

23. Janatpour MJ, McMaster MT, Genbacev O et al. Id-2 regulates critical aspects of human cytotrophoblast differentiation, invasion and migration. Development 2000; 127: 549–58.

24. Riley P, Anson-Cartwright L, Cross JC. The Hand1 bHLH transcription factor is essential for placentation and cardiac morphogenesis. Nat Genet 1998; 18: 271–5.

25. Firulli AB, McFadden DG, Lin Q et al. Heart and extra-embryonic mesodermal defects in mouse embryos lacking the bHLH transcription factor Hand1. Nat Genet 1998; 18: 266–70.

26. Knofler M, Meinhardt G, Vasicek R et al. Molecular cloning of the human Hand1 gene/cDNA and its tissue-restricted expression in cytotrophoblastic cells and heart. Gene 1998; 224: 77–86.

27. Jones BW, Fetter RD, Tear G et al. glial cells missing: a genetic switch that controls glial versus neuronal fate. Cell 1995; 82: 1013–23.

28. Anson-Cartwright L, Dawson K, Holmyard D et al. The glial cells missing-1 protein is essential for branching morphogenesis in the chorioallantoic placenta. Nat Genet 2000; 25: 311–14.

29. Sapin V, Dolle P, Hindelang C et al. Defects of the chorioallantoic placenta in mouse RXRalpha null fetuses. Dev Biol 1997; 191: 29–41.

30. Wendling O, Chambon P, Mark M. Retinoid X receptors are essential for early mouse development and placentogenesis. Proc Natl Acad Sci USA 1999; 96: 547–51.

31. Barak Y, Nelson MC, Ong ES et al. PPAR gamma is required for placental, cardiac, and adipose tissue development. Mol Cell 1999; 4: 585–95.

32. Monkley SJ, Delaney SJ, Pennisi DJ et al. Targeted disruption of the Wnt2 gene results in placentation defects. Development 1996; 122: 3343–53.

33. Schmidt C, Bladt F, Goedecke S et al. Scatter factor/hepatocyte growth factor is essential for liver development. Nature 1995; 373: 699–702.

34. Yamamoto H, Flannery ML, Kupriyanov S et al. Defective trophoblast function in mice with a targeted mutation of Ets2. Genes Dev 1998; 12: 1315–26.

35. Schorpp-Kistner M, Wang ZQ, Angel P et al. JunB is essential for mammalian placentation. EMBO J 1999; 18: 934–48.

36. Hatano N, Mori Y, Oh-hora M et al. Essential role for ERK2 mitogen-activated protein kinase in placental development. Genes Cells 2003; 8: 847–56.

37. Dietrich S, Abou-Rebyeh F, Brohmann H et al. The role of SF/HGF and c-Met in the development of skeletal muscle. Development 1999; 126: 1621–9.

38. Takahashi Y, Carpino N, Cross JC et al. SOCS3: an essential regulator of LIF receptor signaling in trophoblast giant cell differentiation. EMBO J 2003; 22: 372–84.

39. Isermann B, Hendrickson SB, Hutley K et al. Tissue-restricted expression of thrombomodulin in the placenta rescues thrombomodulin-deficient mice from early lethality and reveals a secondary developmental block. Development 2001; 128: 827–38.

40. Gallicano GI, Bauer C, Fuchs E. Rescuing desmoplakin function in extra-embryonic ectoderm reveals the importance of this protein in embryonic heart, neuroepithelium, skin and vasculature. Development 2001; 128: 929–41.

41. Mishina Y, Crombie R, Bradley A et al. Multiple roles for activin-like kinase-2 signaling during mouse embryogenesis. Dev Biol 1999; 213: 314–26.

42. Ma GT, Soloveva V, Tzeng SJ et al. Nodal regulates trophoblast differentiation and placental development. Dev Biol 2001; 236: 124–35.

43. Sugimoto M, Karashima Y, Abe K et al. Tetraploid embryos rescue the early defects of tw5/tw5 mouse embryos. Genesis 2003; 37: 162–71.

44. Goto Y, Takagi N. Tetraploid embryos rescue embryonic lethality caused by an additional maternally inherited X chromosome in the mouse. Development 1998; 125: 3353–63.

45. Jaquemar D, Kupriyanov S, Wankell M et al. Keratin 8 protection of placental barrier function. J Cell Biol 2003; 161: 749–56.

46. Lang U, Baker RS, Braems G et al. Uterine blood flow – a determinant of fetal growth. Eur J Obstet Gynecol Reprod Biol 2003; 110(Suppl 1): S55–61.

47. Jauniaux E, Watson AL, Hempstock J et al. Onset of maternal arterial blood flow and placental oxidative stress. A possible factor in human early pregnancy failure. Am J Pathol 2000; 157: 2111–22.

48. Enders AC, Lantz KC, Schlafke S. Preference of invasive cytotrophoblast for maternal vessels in early implantation in the macaque. Acta Anat (Basel) 1996; 155: 145–62.

49. Jauniaux E, Gulbis B, Burton GJ. The human first trimester gestational sac limits rather than facilitates oxygen transfer to the foetus – a review. Placenta 2003; 24(Suppl A): S86–93.

50. Genbacev O, Joslin R, Damsky CH et al. Hypoxia alters early gestation human cytotrophoblast differentiation/invasion in vitro and models the placental defects that occur in preeclampsia. J Clin Invest 1996; 97: 540–50.

51. Genbacev O, Zhou Y, Ludlow JW et al. Regulation of human placental development by oxygen tension. Science 1997; 277: 1669–72.

52. Adelman DM, Gertsenstein M, Nagy A et al. Placental cell fates are regulated in vivo by HIF-mediated hypoxia responses. Genes Dev 2000; 14: 3191–203.

53. Douglas RM, Haddad GG. Genetic models in applied physiology: invited review: effect of oxygen deprivation on cell cycle activity: a profile of delay and arrest. J Appl Physiol 2003; 94: 2068–83; discussion 84.

54. Boyd JD, Hamilton WJ. Development and structure of the human placenta from the end of the 3rd month of gestation. J Obstet Gynaecol Br Commonw 1967; 74: 161–226.

55. Semenza GL. Targeting HIF-1 for cancer therapy. Nat Rev Cancer 2003; 3: 721–32.

56. Safran M, Kaelin WG Jr. HIF hydroxylation and the mammalian oxygen-sensing pathway. J Clin Invest 2003; 111: 779–83.

57. Masson N, Ratcliffe PJ. HIF prolyl and asparaginyl hydroxylases in the biological response to intracellular O_2 levels. J Cell Sci 2003; 116: 3041–9.

58. Wykoff CC, Pugh CW, Maxwell PH et al. Identification of novel hypoxia dependent and independent target genes of the

von Hippel–Lindau (VHL) tumour suppressor by mRNA differential expression profiling. Oncogene 2000; 19: 6297–305.

59. Gnarra JR, Ward JM, Porter FD et al. Defective placental vasculogenesis causes embryonic lethality in VHL-deficient mice. Proc Natl Acad Sci USA 1997; 94: 9102–7.

60. Kozak KR, Abbott B, Hankinson O. ARNT-deficient mice and placental differentiation. Dev Biol 1997; 191: 297–305.

61. Isaacs JS, Jung YJ, Neckers L. Aryl hydrocarbon nuclear translocator (ARNT) promotes oxygen-independent stabilization of hypoxia-inducible factor-1alpha by modulating an Hsp90-dependent regulatory pathway. J Biol Chem 2004; 279: 16128–35.

62. Voss AK, Thomas T, Gruss P. Mice lacking HSP90beta fail to develop a placental labyrinth. Development 2000; 127: 1–11.

63. Genbacev O, Krtolica A, Kaelin W et al. Human cytotrophoblast expression of the von Hippel–Lindau protein is downregulated during uterine invasion in situ and upregulated by hypoxia in vitro. Dev Biol 2001; 233: 526–36.

64. Tissot van Patot M, Grilli A, Chapman P et al. Remodelling of uteroplacental arteries is decreased in high altitude placentae. Placenta 2003; 24: 326–35.

65. Lunell NO, Nylund LE, Lewander R et al. Uteroplacental blood flow in pre-eclampsia measurements with indium-113m and a computer-linked gamma camera. Clin Exp Hypertens B 1982; 1: 105–17.

66. Naicker T, Khedun SM, Moodley J et al. Quantitative analysis of trophoblast invasion in preeclampsia. Acta Obstet Gynecol Scand 2003; 82: 722–9.

67. Palmer SK, Moore LG, Young D et al. Altered blood pressure course during normal pregnancy and increased preeclampsia at high altitude (3100 meters) in Colorado. Am J Obstet Gynecol 1999; 180: 1161–8.

68. Pugh CW, Ratcliffe PJ. Regulation of angiogenesis by hypoxia: role of the HIF system. Nat Med 2003; 9: 677–84.

69. Damsky CH, Fisher SJ. Trophoblast pseudo-vasculogenesis: faking it with endothelial adhesion receptors. Curr Opin Cell Biol 1998; 10: 660–6.

70. Zhou Y, McMaster M, Woo K et al. Vascular endothelial growth factor ligands and receptors that regulate human cytotrophoblast survival are dysregulated in severe preeclampsia and hemolysis, elevated liver enzymes, and low platelets syndrome. Am J Pathol 2002; 160: 1405–23.

71. Makinen T, Alitalo K. Molecular mechanisms of lymphangiogenesis. Cold Spring Harb Symp Quant Biol 2002; 67: 189–96.

72. Gale NW, Thurston G, Hackett SF et al. Angiopoietin-2 is required for postnatal angiogenesis and lymphatic patterning, and only the latter role is rescued by Angiopoietin-1. Dev Cell 2002; 3: 411–23.

73. Zhou Y, Bellingard V, Feng KT et al. Human cytotrophoblasts promote endothelial survival and vascular remodeling through secretion of Ang2, PlGF, and VEGF-C. Dev Biol 2003; 263: 114–25.

74. Red-Horse K, Rivera J, Schanz A et al. Cytotrophoblast induction of arterial apoptosis and lymphangiogenesis in an in vivo model of human placentation. J Clin Invest 2006; 116: 2643–52.

75. Drake PM, Red-Horse K, Fisher SJ. Reciprocal chemokine receptor and ligand expression in the human placenta: implications for cytotrophoblast differentiation. Dev Dyn 2004; 229: 877–85.

76. Thadhani R, Mutter WP, Wolf M et al. First trimester placental growth factor and soluble fms-like tyrosine kinase 1 and risk for preeclampsia. J Clin Endocrinol Metab 2004; 89: 770–5.

77. Goldman-Wohl D, Greenfield C, Haimov-Kochman R et al. Eph and ephrin expression in normal placental development and preeclampsia. Placenta 2004; 25: 623–30.

78. Red-Horse K, Kapidzic M, Zhou Y et al. EPHB4 regulates chemokine-evoked trophoblast responses: a mechanism for

incorporating the human placenta into the maternal circulation. Development 2005; 132: 4097–106.

79. Hess AP, Hamilton AE, Talbi S et al. Decidual stromal cell response to paracrine signals from the trophoblast: amplification of immune and angiogenic modulators. Biol Reprod 2007; 76: 102–17.

80. Winn V, Haimov-Kochman R, Paquet AC et al. Gene expression profiling of the human maternal–fetal interface reveals dramatic changes between midgestation and term. Endocrinology 2007; 148: 1059–79.

81. Hanna J, Goldman-Wohl D, Hamani Y et al. Decidual NK cells regulate key developmental processes at the human fetal–maternal interface. Nat Med 2006; 12: 1065–74.

82. Hu Y, Dutz JP, MacCalman CD et al. Decidual NK cells alter in vitro first trimester extravillous cytotrophoblast migration: a role for IFN-gamma. J Immunol 2006; 177: 8522–30.

83. Zhou Y, Damsky CH, Fisher SJ. Preeclampsia is associated with failure of human cytotrophoblasts to mimic a vascular adhesion phenotype. One cause of defective endovascular invasion in this syndrome? J Clin Invest 1997; 99: 2152–64.

84. Zhou Y, Bianco K, Huang L et al. Comparative analysis of the maternal–fetal interface in preeclampsia and preterm labor. Cell Tissue Res 2007; 329: 559–69.

85. Maynard SE, Min JY, Merchan J et al. Excess placental soluble fms-like tyrosine kinase 1 (sFlt1) may contribute to endothelial dysfunction, hypertension, and proteinuria in preeclampsia. J Clin Invest 2003; 111: 649–58.

86. Taylor RN, Grimwood J, Taylor RS et al. Longitudinal serum concentrations of placental growth factor: evidence for abnormal placental angiogenesis in pathologic pregnancies. Am J Obstet Gynecol 2003; 188: 177–82.

87. Lam C, Lim KH, Karumanchi SA. Circulating angiogenic factors in the pathogenesis and prediction of preeclampsia. Hypertension 2005; 46: 1077–85.

88. Venkatesha S, Toporsian M, Lam C et al. Soluble endoglin contributes to the pathogenesis of preeclampsia. Nat Med 2006; 12: 642–9.

89. Levine RJ, Lam C, Qian C et al. Soluble endoglin and other circulating antiangiogenic factors in preeclampsia. N Engl J Med 2006; 355: 992–1005.

90. Li M, Yee D, Magnuson TR et al. Reduced maternal expression of adrenomedullin disrupts fertility, placentation, and fetal growth in mice. J Clin Invest 2006; 116: 2653–62.

91. Redman CW, Sargent IL. Pre-eclampsia, the placenta and the maternal systemic inflammatory response – a review. Placenta 2003; 24(Suppl A): S21–7.

92. Goswami D, Tannetta DS, Magee LA et al. Excess syncytiotrophoblast microparticle shedding is a feature of early-onset pre-eclampsia, but not normotensive intrauterine growth restriction. Placenta 2006; 27: 56–61.

93. DiFederico E, Genbacev O, Fisher SJ. Preeclampsia is associated with widespread apoptosis of placental cytotrophoblasts within the uterine wall. Am J Pathol 1999; 155: 293–301.

94. Neale DM, Mor G. The role of Fas mediated apoptosis in preeclampsia. J Perinat Med 2005; 33: 471–7.

95. Redman CW, Sargent IL. Latest advances in understanding preeclampsia. Science 2005; 308: 1592–4.

96. Chen B, Nelson DM, Sadovsky Y. N-myc down-regulated gene 1 modulates the response of term human trophoblasts to hypoxic injury. J Biol Chem 2006; 281: 2764–72.

97. Hiby SE, Walker JJ, O'Shaughnessy KM et al. Combinations of maternal KIR and fetal HLA-C genes influence the risk of preeclampsia and reproductive success. J Exp Med 2004; 200: 957–65.

98. van Dijk M, Mulders J, Poutsma A et al. Maternal segregation of the Dutch preeclampsia locus at 10q22 with a new member of the winged helix gene family. Nat Genet 2005; 37: 514–19.

99. Arngrimsson R, Sigurard ttir S, Frigge ML et al. A genome-wide scan reveals a maternal susceptibility locus for pre-eclampsia on chromosome 2p13. Hum Mol Genet 1999; 8: 1799–805.

100. Lachmeijer AM, Arngrimsson R, Bastiaans EJ et al. A genome-wide scan for preeclampsia in the Netherlands. Eur J Hum Genet 2001; 9: 758–64.

101. Laivuori H, Lahermo P, Ollikainen V et al. Susceptibility loci for preeclampsia on chromosomes 2p25 and 9p13 in Finnish families. Am J Hum Genet 2003; 72: 168–77.

102. Barker DJ. Developmental origins of adult health and disease. J Epidemiol Community Health 2004; 58: 114–15.

103. Bajoria R, Sooranna SR, Ward S et al. Placental transport rather than maternal concentration of amino acids regulates fetal growth in monochorionic twins: implications for fetal origin hypothesis. Am J Obstet Gynecol 2001; 185: 1239–46.

104. Johansson M, Glazier JD, Sibley CP et al. Activity and protein expression of the Na^+/H^+ exchanger is reduced in syncytiotrophoblast microvillous plasma membranes isolated from preterm intrauterine growth restriction pregnancies. J Clin Endocrinol Metab 2002; 87: 5686–94.

105. Battaglia FC. Clinical studies linking fetal velocimetry, blood flow and placental transport in pregnancies complicated by intrauterine growth retardation (IUGR). Trans Am Clin Climatol Assoc 2003; 114: 305–13.

106. Genbacev O, Bass KE, Joslin RJ et al. Maternal smoking inhibits early human cytotrophoblast differentiation. Reprod Toxicol 1995; 9: 245–55.

107. Genbacev O, McMaster MT, Lazic J et al. Concordant in situ and in vitro data show that maternal cigarette smoking negatively regulates placental cytotrophoblast passage through the cell cycle. Reprod Toxicol 2000; 14: 495–506.

108. Pastrakuljic A, Derewlany LO, Koren G. Maternal cocaine use and cigarette smoking in pregnancy in relation to amino acid transport and fetal growth. Placenta 1999; 20: 499–512.

109. Pereira L, Maidji E, McDonagh S et al. Human cytomegalovirus transmission from the uterus to the placenta correlates with the presence of pathogenic bacteria and maternal immunity. J Virol 2003; 77: 13301–14.

110. Yamamoto-Tabata T, McDonagh S, Chang HT et al. Human cytomegalovirus interleukin-10 downregulates metalloproteinase activity and impairs endothelial cell migration and placental cytotrophoblast invasiveness in vitro. J Virol 2004; 78: 2831–40.

111. Levine RJ, Maynard SE, Qian C et al. Circulating angiogenic factors and the risk of preeclampsia. N Engl J Med 2004; 350: 672–83.

31 Mechanisms of trophoblast differentiation and maternal–fetal interactions in the mouse

James C Cross

Synopsis

Background

- Trophoblast–endometrial interactions occur not just at the time of embryo implantation, but throughout pregnancy.
- They influence decidual cell differentiation, vascularization, and immune cell activity.
- Mouse genetics and experimental embryology are powerful tools for dissecting the cellular and molecular pathways involved.
- The trophoblast lineage arises at the blastocyst stage first as a simple epithelium (the trophectoderm) that later goes on to differentiate into a variety of cell subtypes after implantation.
- In rodents, trophoblast giant cells (TGCs) and glycogen trophoblast cells (GlyTCs) are the major cell types mediating postimplantation interactions with the mother.
- The outer layer of the mouse placenta is composed of polyploid TGCs that initially mediate implantation and later invade into the uterus, creating space for the expanding conceptus to grow and also interacting with maternal blood vessels.
- The middle layer of the placenta is called the spongiotrophoblast. In the later stages of gestation, GlyTCs invade diffusely from this layer into the decidua.
- The outer and middle layers together are known as the junctional zone.
- The innermost layer is known as the labyrinth, from where blood vessels feed the umbilical cord.

Basic Science

- Rapid localized trophoblast proliferation in the early postimplantation stage is stimulated by fibroblast growth factor 4 (FGF4) and Nodal from the inner cell mass and embryonic ectoderm.
- Trophoblast stem (TS) cell lines can be derived from blastocysts cultured in the presence of FGF4 and feeder cells that provide Nodal-like growth factors.
- TS cell lines can also be derived from dissected extraembryonic ectoderm up to, but not after, embryonic day (E) 8.5. Later growth of the placenta may be due to more restricted progenitor cells.
- The transcription factor genes *Err2*, *Cdx2*, and *Eomes* are characteristic of TS cells.
- TS cells can contribute to all layers of the placenta.
- There are several subtypes of TGC with distinct patterns of gene expression: parietal TGCs (P-TGCs) at the outer edge of the junctional zone; invasive, smaller, and spindle-like spiral artery-associated TGCs (SA-TGCs); and sinusoidal TGCs (S-TGCs), which are found in the labyrinth.
- TGCs produce a range of hormones, growth factors, matrix-degrading proteinases, angiogenic factors, vasodilators, and anticoagulants.
- P-TGC differentiation depends upon the coordinated activity of several different transcription factors: Mash2, Eed, Hand1, and Stra13.
- P-TGCs induce expression of the interferon (IFN)-inducible gene *Isg15* specifically in the antimesometrial decidua, probably by secreting IFNα.
- Other P-TGC-derived paracrine signals probably induce the genes *Agpt2*, *Dtprp*, and *Prlpa* in decidual cells. These encode secretory polypeptides (angiopoietin 2 and two members of the prolactin family, respectively) that are in turn relayed to maternal endothelial cells, eosinophils, or natural killer (NK) cells.
- GlyTCs invade interstitially into the decidua after E12.5. Their unusually abundant glycogen reserves may indicate a role in the partitioning of glucose between mother, placenta, and fetus.

Clinical

- Several key placental genes initially discovered and characterized in the mouse are also expressed in the human placenta.
- These include *HAND1, MASH2, GCM1*, and several genes encoding cathepsin proteases, providing support for the proposition that mouse studies will reveal pathways that are central to human placental development.
- Discovery of genes whose expression is regulated in the decidua by trophoblast-derived factors may eventually enable identification of a failing conceptus, or an emerging pregnancy pathology, either by measurement of the primary signal or downstream alteration of the maternal response.

INTRODUCTION

Rodents have been used as models for the study of implantation for many years because of the ability to artificially induce and manipulate decidualization. Their use has increased substantially in the last decade, however, because of advances in mouse genetics and experimental embryology. This work has significantly increased our understanding of events after implantation at a molecular level, including the development and functions of the placenta as well as the interactions between trophoblast cells of the placenta and cells within the pregnant uterus. It has become clear that trophoblast–endometrial interactions occur not just at the time of embryo implantation but also after implantation and affect a variety of local changes including decidual cell differentiation, vascularization of the decidua, and immune cell activity. In rodents, specialized subtypes of trophoblast cells, called trophoblast giant cells (TGCs) and glycogen trophoblast cells (GlyTCs), are the major cell types mediating postimplantation interactions with the mother. This chapter reviews current approaches that are used to study trophoblast development and trophoblast–endometrial interactions after implantation and describes molecular pathways that underlie them.

OVERVIEW OF MOUSE PLACENTA STRUCTURE

The mature placenta in mice has three major layers (Figure 31.1) but also a myriad of differentiated cell types within them (for a detailed review, see Simmons and Cross[1]). The outer layer of the placenta is composed of TGCs that initially mediate implantation and later invade into the uterus creating space for the expanding conceptus to grow and also interacting with maternal blood vessels. In the later stages of gestation, GlyTCs also invade diffusely into the decidua. The middle layer of the placenta is called the spongiotrophoblast, the spongy appearance of which is due to the presence of several channels for maternal blood to get into and out of the placenta. This layer is composed exclusively of trophoblast cells, but while they are usually collectively called spongiotrophoblast cells, it is clear that there is some heterogeneity in morphology and gene expression. The outer and middle layers of the placenta are often referred to in the literature as the junctional zone. The inner layer of the placenta is called the labyrinth, which is composed of extensively branched villi that lie in direct contact with small sinusoidal spaces filled with maternal blood. There are several different cell types within the labyrinth layer, including endothelial cells lining the fetal capillaries, two layers of syncytiotrophoblast, and mononuclear cells that are a subtype of TGC. At the fetal surface of the labyrinth where the umbilical cord attaches to the placenta, there is an extensive stroma as well as islands of small, densely packed trophoblast cells that are probably the remnants of the chorionic plate.

TROPHOBLAST STEM CELLS AND ORIGINS OF THE TROPHOBLAST CELL LINEAGE IN MICE

The trophoblast lineage arises at the blastocyst stage first as a simple epithelium (the trophectoderm) that later goes on to differentiate into the variety of cell subtypes after implantation (Figure 31.2).[1] Only ~60 trophectoderm cells are present at the blastocyst stage and, therefore, considerable proliferation occurs after implantation in response to local growth factor cues.[2] The trophectoderm that is not in contact with the inner cell mass of the blastocyst, the mural trophectoderm, stops proliferating and differentiates into 'primary' TGCs. The proliferative trophoblast population is limited to the polar trophectoderm, which represents only ~10 cells lying in immediate contact with the inner cell mass. After implantation and formation of the egg cylinder, the proliferative zone is restricted to those trophoblast cells in immediate contact with the embryonic ectoderm, the so-called extraembryonic ectoderm. The signals from the inner cell mass and embryonic ectoderm that stimulate trophoblast proliferation include fibroblast growth factor 4 (FGF4),[3,4] and Nodal.[5]

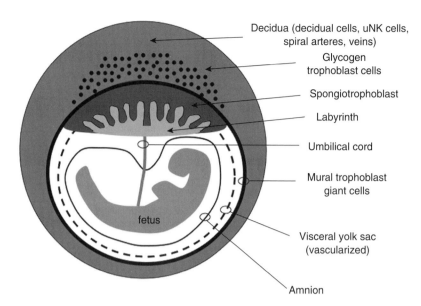

Figure 31.1   Structure of the mature placenta and implantation site in mice at embryonic day 14.5.

Trophoblast stem (TS) cell lines can be derived by culturing blastocysts in the presence of FGF4 and embryonic fibroblasts, or embryonic fibroblast cell conditioned medium, which are a source of Nodal-like growth factors.[4] Nodal is a member of the transforming growth factor β/activin/bone morphogenetic protein (TGFβ/activin/BMP) superfamily of growth factors and, indeed, TS cells can be cultured in the absence of feeder cells using FGF4 and either TGFβ or activin.[6] The transcription factor genes *Err2*, *Cdx2*, and *Eomes*, which are expressed in TS cells in vivo, are responsive to FGF4 in cultured TS cells.[2] Withdrawal of FGF4/Nodal from cultured TS cells results in rapid down-regulation of *Err2*, *Cdx2*, and *Eomes*, and up-regulation of regulatory factors that are specific for specific trophoblast subtypes.[4,5,7]

Because the ~50 mural trophectodermal cells are postmitotic and committed to forming primary TGCs, the polar trophectoderm is thought to give rise to the rest of the trophoblast lineage (see Figure 31.2). However, the next steps in trophoblast lineage development are somewhat more obscure and there are only indirect lineage studies to support the model. Cultured extraembryonic ectoderm[5,8,9] and TS cells[4,6,7] efficiently differentiate into TGCs after withdrawal of growth factors or contact with embryonic ectoderm. During TGC differentiation in vitro, the cells first express genes typical of the ectoplacental cone/spongiotrophoblast layer before expressing TGC-specific genes.[9] The assumption is that during differentiation of TS cells, they first pass through an intermediate stage. Indeed, isolated ectoplacental cone cells rapidly differentiate into TGCs in culture.[9] Moreover, observations from several mouse mutants suggest that spongiotrophoblast cells and TGCs can arise from a common precursor

(for more discussion see Simmons and Cross[1]). By embryonic day (E) 8.5, the implantation site is lined by several hundred TGCs.[10] The substantial increase in TGC number is presumed to be due to differentiation of precursors in the ectoplacental cone, a process called 'secondary' TGC differentiation.

When TS cells are used to make chimeras by injecting them into blastocysts, they can contribute to all layers of the placenta, implying that they are multipotent.[4,6] Similarly, after FGF4 withdrawal, differentiating TS cell cultures begin to express genes characteristic of multiple trophoblast cell subtypes.[7] TS cell lines can be derived from cultured blastocysts and dissected extraembryonic ectoderm tissue up to ~E8.5.[4] Importantly, though, the ability to derive TS cell lines decreases after closure of the ectoplacental cavity during which the extraembryonic ectoderm layer expands and comes into contact with the basal surface of the ectoplacental cone.[11] This suggests that multipotent TS cells may not persist in the developing placenta and implies that later growth of the placenta may be due to more restricted progenitor cells. After closure of the ectoplacental cavity, the extraembryonic ectoderm and the basal layers of the ectoplacental cone come together to form the layers of the chorion. In both the mouse[12] and hamster[13] there appears to be little mingling of these layers and they are thought to persist to become the three different trophoblast cell layers of the labyrinth.

TROPHOBLAST GIANT CELLS

TGCs were first defined as the extremely large cells surrounding the implantation site that are derived

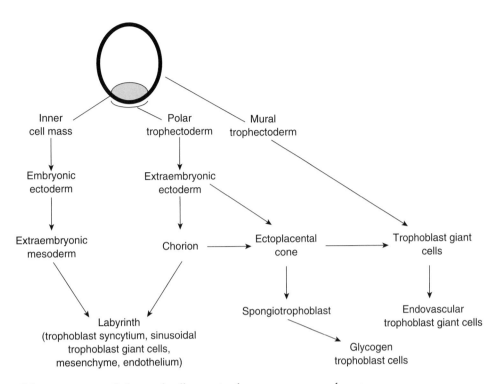

Figure 31.2   Cell lineage origins of placental cell types in the mature mouse placenta.

from the mural trophectoderm. They produce a range of different hormones, growth factors, and angiogenic factors[50,51] They are also inherently invasive in vitro[14] and probably mediate expansion of the implantation site to accommodate growth of the conceptus. The cell adhesion molecules and matrix-degrading proteinases that mediate cytotrophoblast cell invasion in humans are expressed by TGCs in mice.[15] The characteristic feature of rodent TGCs is that they are polyploid,[16] as a result of repeated rounds of DNA replication in the absence of intervening mitoses, an unusual type of cell cycle called endoreduplication.[17] Human extravillous cytotrophoblast[18,19] and bovine binucleate cell nuclei[20] are also polyploid, though ploidy tends to be 4–8C compared with up to 1024C in rodents.[16] This suggests some commonality amongst invasive trophoblast cell subtypes in different species. This may be of evolutionary significance because endoreduplicating cells have lost the ability to undergo mitosis and cell division, a property that would be dangerous for cells that invade into the mother and promote an angiogenic response in the surrounding host. This property makes them different, therefore, from cancer cells.

In the last few years it has become apparent that TGCs are not homogeneous and, moreover, likely that there are multiple subtypes that appear at different times during development and within different parts of the placenta. For example, within the TGC layer lining the implantation site, several genes are not uniformly expressed, including *Mrj*,[21] *thrombomodulin*,[22] and members of the *cathepsin* family.[23] In addition to the TGCs that line the implantation site and form the interface with the maternal decidua, however, there appear to be a variety of other subtypes based on morphological and molecular criteria. For this reason, my laboratory has begun to use terminology that distinguishes them. The TGCs lining the implantation site will be referred to here as parietal TGCs, or P-TGCs. A few years ago we discovered that an endovascular subtype of TGC invades into the maternal spiral arteries to replace endothelial cells.[24] The morphology of the spiral artery associated-TGCs (SA-TGCs) is different to that of P-TGCs as they are smaller and spindle-like, and express different genes.[25] For example, whereas the P-TGCs express *Pl1* and *Plf*, members of the prolactin/placental lactogen gene family (see Chapter 22), the SA-TGCs express *Plf* but not *Pl1*. These cells are also polyploid.[26] A third type of TGC appears in the labyrinth layer. These cells are mononuclear and have historically been referred to as cytotrophoblasts to distinguish them from the multi-nucleated syncytiotrophoblast cells of the labyrinth. However, this name is not appropriate since it implies that they have the same function as cytotrophoblast cells in humans, which are progenitor cells underlying the syncytiotrophoblast. By contrast, the mononuclear trophoblast cells in the rodent labyrinth layer lie outside the syncytiotrophoblast layer and within the maternal blood spaces of the labyrinth called sinusoids. For this reason, we refer to them as sinusoidal TGCs (S-TGCs). They are polyploid[26,27] and appear to be endocrine in function since they express genes of the prolactin/placental lactogen superfamily such as *Pl2/Csh2*.[1] Based on these data, we now assume that there are several subtypes of TGCs.

REGULATION OF TROPHOBLAST GIANT CELL DIFFERENTIATION

TGC differentiation is controlled by a complex interplay of both positive and negative regulators. FGF4 and Nodal, which promote the maintenance of TS cell character, also actively suppress TGC formation and withdrawal of these factors results in rapid TGC differentiation.[4,6,7] Leukemia inhibitory factor (LIF) signaling can also influence TGC differentiation as LIF receptor mutants show diminished TGC-specific gene expression.[28] By contrast, LIF signaling is overactivated by mutation of the *Socs3* gene, which encodes a suppressor of cytokine receptor signaling, and *Socs3* mutant placentas have more TGC cells.[28] Other exogenous factors have been shown to influence TGC differentiation, including parathyroid hormone-related protein (PTHrP),[29,30] the synthetic estrogen diethylstilbestrol (DES) working through the Errβ/Err2 nuclear receptor,[31] and retinoic acid.[32] However, their physiological contexts are not completely clear because their effects have only been shown in vitro and mutant phenotypes have not been described, or because the source of ligand is not clear. Oxygen tension also regulates trophoblast differentiation. Culturing human trophoblast cells in low oxygen alters their proliferation and differentiation potential.[33,34] In mice, mutation of the hypoxia-inducible factor 1β gene (Arnt/HIF1β) results in a lethal placental phenotype in which the labyrinth and spongiotrophoblast layers are diminished and TGC numbers are increased.[35–37] Culturing wild-type TS cells in low oxygen (3%) is sufficient to induce expression of ectoplacental cone/spongiotrophoblast-specific genes but this response is absent in Arnt/HIF1β-deficient cells.[36] These data imply that oxygen tension and HIF regulate alternate trophoblast fate decision-making during normal development.

Within the cell itself, TGC differentiation depends upon the coordinated activity of several different basic helix–loop–helix (bHLH) transcription factors. Mash2 inhibits TGC differentiation[7,10,38,39] and promotes the maintenance of spongiotrophoblast cells.[40–42] Eed, a polycomb group protein, is required for repression of *Mash2* gene expression during TGC differentiation and *Eed* mutants show maintained Mash2 expression and a consequent decrease in secondary TGC differentiation.[43,44] In contrast to Mash2, the Hand[10,38,39] and Stra13[7] bHLH transcription factors can promote differentiation, and deletion of the *Hand1* gene results in a block to TGC formation.[10,45] How the balance between Mash2 vs Hand1 and Stra13 activities is maintained, and whether they act downstream of the cell extrinsic factors described above is still unclear.

It is important to note that essentially everything we know about the regulation of TGC differentiation has come from analysis of what we now call P-TGCs, based on the types of markers that have been used to analyze mutant mouse phenotypes (e.g. *Pl1* is the most commonly used TGC marker gene but its expression in limited to P-TGCs), analysis at early times during development, or from cultures of ectoplacental cones where probably only P-TGCs are formed. Therefore, it remains to be seen whether formation of SA-TGCs and S-TGCs are regulated by similar sorts of molecular pathways as P-TGCs. Clearly, there must be some differences because the different TGC subtypes form at different times, in different locations, and have some differences in gene expression.

ENDOCRINE AND PARACRINE FUNCTIONS OF TROPHOBLAST GIANT CELLS

In addition to mediating invasion of the conceptus into the decidua and interaction with maternal blood vessels, TGCs are also the major endocrine cell type of the rodent placenta and produce a variety of hormones and locally acting growth factors. TGCs produce progesterone,[46] which is thought to help maintain pregnancy, as well as angiogenic factors,[9,47] vasodilators[48,49] and anticoagulants[22] that probably help to promote blood flow to the implantation site. TGCs also express placental lactogens (PL-I and PL-II in mice), which stimulate mammary gland development and luteal production of progesterone by working through the prolactin receptor.[50,51] It has become clear more recently that the luteotropic and mammotropic effects are simply the 'tip of the iceberg'. For example, prolactin/placental lactogen can stimulate hyperplasia of pancreatic islets[52–55] and presumably mediates the increase in islet number and size, as well as the associated metabolic changes during pregnancy.[56–58] Prolactin has also been shown to stimulate neural stem cell proliferation and olfactory neurogenesis during pregnancy in mice.[59]

PL-I and PL-II are encoded by genes that are clustered in the large prolactin/placental lactogen locus on mouse chromosome 13.[60] There are at least 26 genes in the locus, and most appear to be almost exclusively expressed by the placenta and specifically TGCs.[60] The functions of only a few have been described to date. Proliferin (Plf) has been shown to stimulate uterine cell growth[61] and also to regulate angiogenesis.[62] Proliferin-related protein (Prp or Plfr) is a Plf antagonist and Plf and Plfr are expressed in a partially overlapping pattern in the P-TGC and SA-TGC subpopulations of TGCs.[25] Prolactin-like protein E and F (PLP-E/Prlpe and PLP-F/Prlpf) have been shown to stimulate erythropoiesis and thrombopoiesis.[63,64] Prolactin-like protein A (PLP-A or Prlpa) binds to natural killer (NK) cells and suppresses their killing activity.[65] Prlpa-deficient female mice show pregnancy losses, though only when stressed by hypoxia.[66] While the biochemical and knockout mouse data are limited, they imply that the prolactin-related proteins are likely to be involved in a range of biological functions related to maternal adaptations to pregnancy, both local and systemic. More discussion is given in Chapter 22.

GLYCOGEN TROPHOBLAST CELLS

GlyTCs are the second differentiated trophoblast cell type that plays a major role in the dialogue between the mother and fetus during pregnancy. GlyTCs are notable because they accumulate vast amounts of glycogen. Glycogen deposits are a common pathological finding in several different tissues[67] but placental accumulation occurs in all pregnancies in mice. It appears in a subset of cells within the spongiotrophoblast cell layer primarily in the second half of gestation.[24,68] After E12.5, the cells invade interstitially into the decidua.[24] This is a quite different pattern of invasion compared to SA-TGCs whose invasion is restricted to the lumen of spiral arteries. While GlyTCs appear in all pregnancies, the extent of glycogen accumulation can be regulated. For example, it is stimulated by insulin[69] but is increased in diabetic pregnancies,[70,71] arguing that insulin promotes glucose uptake from the maternal circulation and thereby increases glycogen deposition. Glycogen content is reduced in placentas of IGF-II mutant mice.[72] IGF-II is expressed in the placenta and, indeed, knockout of a placental-specific Igf2 gene promoter, called P0,

produces a similar phenotype, suggesting that IGF-II may act in a paracrine manner within the placenta to regulate glucose uptake.[73]

The biggest open question about glycogen trophoblast cells is what is their function? Because the glycogen content of the placenta can be regulated, it is reasonable that the placenta may act as a storage buffer. Some reports have indicated acute glycogenolysis and associated increase in serum glucose following administration of glucagon[69] and catecholamine.[74] However, it is unclear to what extent this contributes to nutrition of the fetus and/or mother. An alternative but not mutually exclusive hypothesis is that since glycogen accumulation increases in diabetic pregnancies, and high glucose levels are toxic to embryos[75] even at the blastocyst stage,[76] it may be that glucose uptake by the placenta from the maternal serum may reduce the amount of glucose transport into the fetal circulation. It would be interesting to explore fetal blood glucose levels and the partitioning of glucose amongst the maternal, fetal, and placental compartments in the $Igf2^{P0}$ mutants as a test of this hypothesis. It is also important to note that in addition to metabolic functions, GlyTCs express several members of the prolactin/placental lactogen gene family (DG Simmons, S Rawn, and JCC, in preparation). Therefore, they may have paracrine and/or endocrine roles as well.

FUNCTIONAL SCREENING FOR TROPHOBLAST–ENDOMETRIAL INTERACTIONS

Exploring the functions of known hormones that are produced by TGCs, and a specific focus on the prolactin/placental lactogen family will continue to be a productive approach to understanding the endocrine and paracrine functions of trophoblast cells. However, there are two inherent limitations. First, there is likely to be considerable redundancy in the prolactin/placental lactogen gene family. For example, aside from the apparent overlapping biological effects of PL-I and PL-II, there are predicted to be three Pl1 genes.[60] Interestingly, the three Pl1 and single Pl2 genes are clustered right next to Prl at one end of the locus, and they are the only prolactin family members that have been shown to function through the prolactin receptor. There are also four predicted Plf genes. Finally, the Prlpe and Prlpf proteins appear to have identical biological effects. One way to investigate function would be to generate mouse mutants in which multiple members of the gene subfamily are deleted.

Secondly, just focusing on known paracrine factors or hormones does not identify new factors. We have tried to address this latter issue by taking a functional approach to identify biological processes that are regulated by trophoblast cells specifically at the implantation site.[77] The initial screen was for differences in gene expression in decidual tissue surrounding a normally implanted conceptus compared to artificially induced deciduoma. As an alternative, we examined gene expression in decidual tissue surrounding a mutant conceptus that had implanted but failed shortly thereafter.

The uterus undergoes dramatic changes in response to an implanting conceptus that, in rodents and primates, includes differentiation of the endometrial stroma into decidual tissue (see Chapter 24). The decidualization process can be induced artificially in rodents by intrauterine injection of oil or lectin-coated beads, indicating that the conceptus is not essential.[78,79] We have conducted gene expression microarray experiments comparing expression of 100 genes that are known to be expressed in the normal decidua compared to an artificially induced 'deciduoma', to determine how the conceptus affects uterine function.[77] We identified several genes that showed lower expression in deciduoma compared to decidua and mapped expression in some cases. The data suggest a complex model for trophoblast–endometrial interactions (Figure 31.3). *Isg15* is an interferon (IFN) inducible gene[80] and *Isg15* mRNA localizes to the antimesometrial decidua, whereas it was undetectable in deciduomas.[81] Conditioned medium from cultured TGCs induced *Isg15* expression in primary endometrial stromal cells showing that TGCs specifically could induce the effect.[77] The response was blocked by depletion with an anti-IFNα antibody, suggesting that TGCs secrete IFNα. *Agpt2*, *Dtprp*, and *Prlpa* mRNA localized to both the antimesometrial and mesometrial decidua, but only mesometrial expression was diminished in deciduomas and IFNα had no effect on their expression, implying that other inducers are involved.

Expression of the conceptus-regulated genes was also examined in decidual tissue surrounding mutant conceptuses that have defects in TGC differentiation or function, including *Ets2*[82] and *Hand1*[10,45] mutants. In *Ets2* mutants, the conceptuses implant but TGCs are unable to penetrate through the basement membrane underlying the uterine epithelium.[82] In *Hand1* mutants, the basement membrane is penetrated but the trophoblast cells fail to undergo normal TGC differentiation. The decidua surrounding both *Ets2* and *Hand1* mutants shows reduced *Prlpa* mRNA whereas

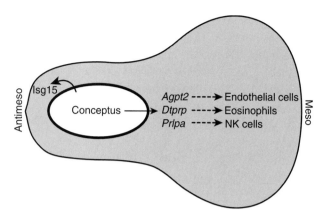

Figure 31.3 Summary of interactions between trophoblast cells and decidual cells after implantation in the mouse as described by Bany and Cross.[77] Within a few days of implantation, the conceptus produces several different types of signal that affect function of the decidua as detected by alterations in gene expression. An interferon-regulated gene, Isg15, is up-regulated within the antimesometrial but not mesometrial decidua. Other genes (*Agpt2*, *Dtprp*, and *Prlpa*) are expressed in both the antimesometrial and mesometrial decidua but the conceptus is only required for up-regulation in the mesometrial domain. *Agpt2*, *Dtprp*, and *Prlpa* have known target cell types as indicated.

expression of *Agpt2*, *Isg15*, *Fgfr1*, *Idb2*, and *Dtprp* is normal.[77]

Thus it is clear that these models can be used to identify biological processes in the endometrium and decidua that are regulated by trophoblast cells. Intriguingly, even though the gene expression microarray studies to date have examined a relatively small subset of genes, they have revealed an unexpected complexity in the signaling that occurs between the placenta and decidua after implantation.[77] First, there is more than one signal and different conceptus-regulated genes may rely on different signals. Secondly, the signals can have very localized effects in the decidua either because the signals are produced asymmetrically or because the decidua is patterned to be differentially responsive. Thirdly, the decidual cells that receive the conceptus-derived signals appear to act as a relay point, translating them into signals for multiple target cell types with the decidua. For example, Agpt2 targets endothelial cells,[83] whereas Dtprp[84] and Prlpa[65] target eosinophils and NK cells, respectively.

CONCLUSIONS AND PERSPECTIVES

At one level the structure and function of the placenta seems simple. No matter the species, placentas are primarily designed to facilitate the exchange of nutrients between the maternal and fetal circulation and as such contain a high surface area to maximize transport with an underlying fetal vasculature. Paracrine and endocrine functions of the placenta help to facilitate uterine blood flow and nutrient delivery to the fetus. However, with increasing study of the placenta at both the morphological and molecular level, it has become apparent that we still have a lot to learn about its structure and functions:

1. The large number of different cell types in the rodent placenta has been apparent for many years based on morphological features. With the discovery and use of molecular markers, these cell types are increasingly being subclassified on the basis of their cell lineage origins and molecular functions.

2. Many of the functions of the known trophoblast cell subtypes are still obscure. For example, as discussed above, there are several different TGC subtypes in the rodent placenta and further subclassification may eventually be required. There can also be circadian differences in function and the placenta itself produces melatonin.[85]

3. The interactions between trophoblast cells in the placenta and endometrium are complex. The identification of genes whose expression is regulated in the decidua by trophoblast cell-derived factors will open the door to new biological processes. Interferon appears to be evolutionarily conserved (see Chapter 17). In addition, the discovery of such genes opens the way to being able to identify a failing conceptus by virtue of alterations in maternal functions. Also, such studies also tell us something about the nature of the paracrine interactions between the placenta and endometrium.

4. Finally, how much of what we have learned in mice can be translated to humans? As described in Chapters 31a and 31b, there are both similarities and differences in the structure of the placenta among diverse mammalian species. At a molecular level, there are several examples of key genes initially discovered and whose function has been described in the mouse that are also expressed in the human placenta. These include *Hand1*,[86] *Mash2*,[87] *Gcm1*,[88] and several genes encoding cathepsin proteases.[89] There are some notable differences, however, reflecting some evolutionary specializations such as the expansion of the prolactin gene locus in rodents but not other species[60] as well as the extra expansion of a placental-specific locus of cathepsin genes in rodents.[90,91]

While there may be species differences in the molecular mechanisms used for placental development or function, it is likely that there are considerable common links in the basic plan. For example, rodents show many of the same maternal physiological adaptations to pregnancy as humans, including increased cardiac output and blood volume but also a mid-gestational decrease in blood pressure due to decreased sensitivity to vasoconstrictors.[92,93] While humans do not have the gene for the placental-specific PLP-E hormone which has erythropoietic activity,[64] the human placenta does express the 'normal' erythropoietic hormone erythropoietin.[94]

ACKNOWLEDGMENTS

Work from my laboratory has been supported by grants from the Canadian Institutes of Health Research, the Alberta Heritage Foundation for Medical Research, and the Stem Cell Network. I would also like to thank the many members of my laboratory who have contributed over the years to the ideas in this chapter and their development.

REFERENCES

1. Simmons DG, Cross JC. Determinants of trophoblast lineage and cell subtype specification in the mouse placenta. Dev Biol 2005; 284: 12–24.

2. Rossant J, Cross JC. Placental development: lessons from mouse mutants. Nat Rev Genet 2001; 2: 538–48.

3. Goldin SN, Papaioannou VE. Paracrine action of FGF4 during periimplantation development maintains trophectoderm and primitive endoderm. Genesis 2003; 36: 40–7.

4. Tanaka S, Kunath T, Hadjantonakis AK et al. Promotion of trophoblast stem cell proliferation by FGF4. Science 1998; 282: 2072–5.

5. Guzman-Ayala M, Ben-Haim N, Beck S et al. Nodal protein processing and fibroblast growth factor 4 synergize to maintain a trophoblast stem cell microenvironment. Proc Natl Acad Sci USA 2004; 101: 15656–60.

6. Erlebacher A, Price KA, Glimcher LH. Maintenance of mouse trophoblast stem cell proliferation by TGF-beta/activin. Dev Biol 2004; 275: 158–69.

7. Hughes M, Dobric N, Scott IC et al. The Hand1, Stra13 and Gcm1 transcription factors override FGF signaling to promote terminal differentiation of trophoblast stem cells. Dev Biol 2004; 271: 26–37.

8. Rossant J, Ofer L. Properties of extra-embryonic ectoderm isolated from postimplantation mouse embryos. J Embryol Exp Morphol 1977; 39: 183–94.

9. Carney EW, Prideaux V, Lye SJ et al. Progressive expression of trophoblast-specific genes during formation of mouse trophoblast giant cells in vitro. Mol Reprod Dev 1993; 34: 357–68.

10. Scott IC, Anson-Cartwright L, Riley P et al. The Hand1 basic helix-loop-helix transcription factor regulates trophoblast giant

cell differentiation via multiple mechanisms. Mol Cell Biol 2000; 20: 530–41.

11. Uy GD, Downs KM, Gardner RL. Inhibition of trophoblast stem cell potential in chorionic ectoderm coincides with occlusion of the ectoplacental cavity in the mouse. Development 2002; 129: 3913–24.

12. Hernandez-Verdun D. Morphogenesis of the syncytium in the mouse placenta. Ultrastructural study. Cell Tissue Res 1974; 148: 381–96.

13. Carpenter SJ. Light and electron microscopic observations on the morphogenesis of the chorioallantoic placenta of the golden hamster (*Cricetus auratus*). Days seven through nine of gestation. Am J Anat 1972; 135: 445–76.

14. Behrendtsen O, Alexander CM, Werb Z. Metalloproteinases mediate extracellular matrix degradation by cells from mouse blastocyst outgrowths. Development 1992; 114: 447–56.

15. Cross JC, Werb Z, Fisher SJ. Implantation and the placenta: key pieces of the development puzzle. Science 1994; 266: 1508–18.

16. Zybina EV, Zybina TG. Polytene chromosomes in mammalian cells. Int Rev Cytol 1996; 165: 53–119.

17. MacAuley A, Cross JC, Werb Z. Reprogramming the cell cycle for endoreduplication in rodent trophoblast cells. Mol Biol Cell 1998; 9: 795–807.

18. Berezowsky J, Zbieranowski I, Demers J et al. DNA ploidy of hydatidiform moles and nonmolar conceptuses: a study using flow and tissue section image cytometry. Mod Pathol 1995; 8: 775–81.

19. Zybina TG, Kaufmann P, Frank HG et al. Genome multiplication of extravillous trophoblast cells in human placenta in the course of differentiation and invasion into endometrium and myometrium. I. Dynamics of polyploidization. Tsitologiia 2002; 44: 1058–67.

20. Klisch K, Hecht W, Pfarrer C et al. DNA content and ploidy level of bovine placentomal trophoblast giant cells. Placenta 1999; 20: 451–8.

21. Hunter PJ, Swanson BJ, Haendel MA et al. Mrj encodes a DnaJ-related co-chaperone that is essential for murine placental development. Development 1999; 126: 1247–58.

22. Weiler-Guettler H, Aird WC, Rayburn H et al. Developmentally regulated gene expression of thrombomodulin in postimplantation mouse embryos. Development 1996; 122: 2271–81.

23. Hemberger M, Himmelbauer H, Ruschmann J et al. cDNA subtraction cloning reveals novel genes whose temporal and spatial expression indicates association with trophoblast invasion. Dev Biol 2000; 222: 158–69.

24. Adamson SL, Lu Y, Whiteley KJ et al. Interactions between trophoblast cells and the maternal and fetal circulation in the mouse placenta. Dev Biol 2002; 250: 358–73.

25. Hemberger M, Nozaki T, Masutani M et al. Differential expression of angiogenic and vasodilatory factors by invasive trophoblast giant cells depending on depth of invasion. Dev Dyn 2003; 227: 185–91.

26. Simmons DG, Fortier AL, Cross JC. Distinct origins and functions of trophoblast giant cells in the mouse placenta. Dev Biol 2007; 304: 567–78.

27. Coan PM, Ferguson-Smith AC, Burton GJ. Ultrastructural changes in the interhaemal membrane and junctional zone of the murine chorioallantoic placenta across gestation. J Anat 2005; 207: 783–96.

28. Takahashi Y, Carpino N, Cross JC et al. SOCS3: an essential regulator of LIF receptor signaling in trophoblast giant cell differentiation. EMBO J 2003; 22: 372–84.

29. El-Hashash AH, Kimber SJ. PTHrP induces changes in cell cytoskeleton and E-cadherin and regulates Eph/Ephrin kinases and RhoGTPases in murine secondary trophoblast cells. Dev Biol 2006; 290: 13–31.

30. El-Hashash AH, Esbrit P, Kimber SJ. PTHrP promotes murine secondary trophoblast giant cell differentiation through induction of endocycle, upregulation of giant-cell-promoting transcription factors and suppression of other trophoblast cell types. Differentiation 2005; 73: 154–74.

31. Tremblay GB, Kunath T, Bergeron D et al. Diethylstilbestrol regulates trophoblast stem cell differentiation as a ligand of orphan nuclear receptor ERR beta. Genes Dev 2001; 15: 833–8.

32. Yan J, Tanaka S, Oda M et al. Retinoic acid promotes differentiation of trophoblast stem cells to a giant cell fate. Dev Biol 2001; 235: 422–32.

33. Genbacev O, Joslin R, Damsky CH et al. Hypoxia alters early gestation human cytotrophoblast differentation/invasion in vitro and models the placental defects that occur in preeclampsia. J Clin Invest 1996; 97: 540–50.

34. Caniggia I, Mostachfi H, Winter J et al. Hypoxia-inducible factor-1 mediates the biological effects of oxygen on human trophoblast differentiation through TGFbeta(3). J Clin Invest 2000; 105: 577–87.

35. Abbott BD, Buckalew AR. Placental defects in ARNT-knockout conceptus correlate with localized decreases in VEGF-R2, Ang-1, and Tie-2. Dev Dyn 2000; 219: 526–38.

36. Adelman DM, Gertsenstein M, Nagy A et al. Placental cell fates are regulated in vivo by HIF-mediated hypoxia responses. Genes Dev 2000; 14: 3191–203.

37. Kozak KR, Abbott B, Hankinson O. ARNT-deficient mice and placental differentiation. Dev Biol 1997; 191: 297–305.

38. Kraut N, Snider L, Chen C et al. Requirement of the mouse I-mfa gene for placental development and skeletal patterning. EMBO J 1998; 17: 6276–88.

39. Cross JC, Flannery ML, Blanar MA et al. Hxt encodes a basic helix-loop-helix transcription factor that regulates trophoblast cell development. Development 1995; 121: 2513–23.

40. Guillemot F, Nagy A, Auerbach A et al. Essential role of Mash-2 in extraembryonic development. Nature 1994; 371: 333–6.

41. Guillemot F, Caspary T, Tilghman SM et al. Genomic imprinting of Mash2, a mouse gene required for trophoblast development. Nat Genet 1995; 9: 235–42.

42. Tanaka M, Gertsenstein M, Rossant J et al. Mash2 acts cell autonomously in mouse spongiotrophoblast development. Dev Biol 1997; 190: 55–65.

43. Wang J, Mager J, Schnedier E et al. The mouse PcG gene seed is required for Hox gene repression and extraembryonic development. Mamm Genome 2002; 13: 493–503.

44. Wang J, Mager J, Chen Y et al. Imprinted X inactivation maintained by a mouse Polycomb group gene. Nat Genet 2001; 28: 371–5.

45. Riley P, Anson-Cartwright L, Cross JC. The Hand1 bHLH transcription factor is essential for placentation and cardiac morphogenesis. Nat Genet 1998; 18: 271–5.

46. Peng L, Arensburg J, Orly J et al. The murine 3beta-hydroxy-steroid dehydrogenase (3beta-HSD) gene family: a postulated role for 3beta-HSD VI during early pregnancy. Mol Cell Endocrinol 2002; 187: 213–21.

47. Voss AK, Thomas T, Gruss P. Mice lacking HSP90beta fail to develop a placental labyrinth. Development 2000; 127: 1–11.

48. Yotsumoto S, Shimada T, Cui CY et al. Expression of adrenomedullin, a hypotensive peptide, in the trophoblast giant cells at the embryo implantation site in mouse. Dev Biol 1998; 203: 264–75.

49 Gagioti S, Scavone C, Bevilacqua E. Participation of the mouse implanting trophoblast in nitric oxide production during pregnancy. Biol Reprod 2000; 62: 260–8.

50. Soares MJ, Muller H, Orwig KE et al. The uteroplacental prolactin family and pregnancy. Biol Reprod 1998; 58: 273–84.

51. Linzer DI, Fisher SJ. The placenta and the prolactin family of hormones: regulation of the physiology of pregnancy. Mol Endocrinol 1999; 13: 837–40.

52. Freemark M, Avril I, Fleenor D et al. Targeted deletion of the PRL receptor: effects on islet development, insulin production, and glucose tolerance. Endocrinology 2002; 143: 1378–85.

53. Fleenor D, Petryk A, Driscoll P et al. Constitutive expression of placental lactogen in pancreatic beta cells: effects on cell morphology, growth, and gene expression. Pediatr Res 2000; 47: 136–42.

54. Vasavada RC, Garcia-Ocana A, Zawalich WS et al. Targeted expression of placental lactogen in the beta cells of transgenic mice results in beta cell proliferation, islet mass augmentation, and hypoglycemia. J Biol Chem 2000; 275: 15399–406.

55. Holstad M, Sandler S. Prolactin protects against diabetes induced by multiple low doses of streptozotocin in mice. J Endocrinol 1999; 163: 229–34.

56. Avril I, Blondeau B, Duchene B et al. Decreased beta-cell proliferation impairs the adaptation to pregnancy in rats malnourished during perinatal life. J Endocrinol 2002; 174: 215–23.

57. Sorenson RL, Brelje TC. Adaptation of islets of Langerhans to pregnancy: beta-cell growth, enhanced insulin secretion and the role of lactogenic hormones. Horm Metab Res 1997; 29: 301–7.

58. Parsons JA, Brelje TC, Sorenson RL. Adaptation of islets of Langerhans to pregnancy: increased islet cell proliferation and insulin secretion correlates with the onset of placental lactogen secretion. Endocrinology 1992; 130: 1459–66.

59. Shingo T, Gregg C, Enwere E et al. Pregnancy-stimulated neurogenesis in the adult female forebrain mediated by prolactin. Science 2003; 299: 117–20.

60. Wiemers DO, Shao LJ, Ain R et al. The mouse prolactin gene family locus. Endocrinology 2003; 144: 313–25.

61. Nelson JT, Rosenzweig N, Nilsen-Hamilton M. Characterization of the mitogen-regulated protein (proliferin) receptor. Endocrinology 1995; 136: 283–8.

62. Jackson D, Volpert OV, Bouck N et al. Stimulation and inhibition of angiogenesis by placental proliferin and proliferin-related protein. Science 1994; 266: 1581–4.

63. Zhou B, Lum HE, Lin J et al. Two placental hormones are agonists in stimulating megakaryocyte growth and differentiation. Endocrinology 2002; 143: 4281–6.

64. Zhou B, Kong X, Linzer DI. Enhanced recovery from thrombocytopenia and neutropenia in mice constitutively expressing a placental hematopoietic cytokine. Endocrinology 2005; 146: 64–70.

65. Muller H, Liu B, Croy BA et al. Uterine natural killer cells are targets for a trophoblast cell-specific cytokine, prolactin-like protein A. Endocrinology 1999; 140: 2711–20.

66. Ain R, Dai G, Dunmore JH et al. A prolactin family paralog regulates reproductive adaptations to a physiological stressor. Proc Natl Acad Sci USA 2004; 101: 16543–8.

67. Cheville NF. Cell Pathology, 2nd edn. Ames, Iowa: The Iowa State University Press, 1983.

68. Bouillot S, Rampon C, Tillet E et al. Tracing the glycogen cells with protocadherin 12 during mouse placenta development. Placenta 2006; 27: 882–8.

69. Goltzsch W, Bittner R, Bohme HJ et al. Effect of prenatal insulin and glucagon injection on the glycogen content of rat placenta and fetal liver. Biomed Biochim Acta 1987; 46: 619–22.

70. Padmanabhan R, Shafiullah M. Intrauterine growth retardation in experimental diabetes: possible role of the placenta. Arch Physiol Biochem 2001; 109: 260–71.

71. Barash V, Gutman A, Shafrir E. Fetal diabetes in rats and its effect on placental glycogen. Diabetologia 1985; 28: 244–9.

72. Lopez MF, Dikkes P, Zurakowski D et al. Insulin-like growth factor II affects the appearance and glycogen content of glycogen cells in the murine placenta. Endocrinology 1996; 137: 2100–8.

73. Constancia M, Hemberger M, Hughes J et al. Placental-specific IGF-II is a major modulator of placental and fetal growth. Nature 2002; 417: 945–8.

74. Barash V, Shafrir E. Mobilization of placental glycogen in diabetic rats. Placenta 1990; 11: 515–21.

75. Chang TI, Loeken MR. Genotoxicity and diabetic embryopathy: impaired expression of developmental control genes as a cause of defective morphogenesis. Semin Reprod Endocrinol 1999; 17: 153–65.

76. Leunda-Casi A, Genicot G, Donnay I et al. Increased cell death in mouse blastocysts exposed to high D-glucose in vitro: implications of an oxidative stress and alterations in glucose metabolism. Diabetologia 2002; 45: 571–9.

77. Bany BM, Cross JC. Post-implantation mouse conceptuses produce paracrine signals that regulate the uterine endometrium undergoing decidualization. Dev Biol 2006; 294: 445–56.

78. Finn CA, Pope MD, Milligan SR. A study of the early morphological changes initiated in the uterine luminal epithelium by substances (oil and carrageenan) which induce the decidual cell reaction in mice. J Reprod Fertil 1989; 86: 619–26.

79. Das RM, Martin L. Uterine DNA synthesis and cell proliferation during early decidualization induced by oil in mice. J Reprod Fertil 1978; 53: 125–8.

80. Ritchie KJ, Zhang DE. ISG15: the immunological kin of ubiquitin. Semin Cell Dev Biol 2004; 15: 237–46.

81. Austin KJ, Bany BM, Belden EL et al. Interferon-stimulated gene-15 (Isg15) expression is up-regulated in the mouse uterus in response to the implanting conceptus. Endocrinology 2003; 144: 3107–13.

82. Yamamoto H, Flannery ML, Kupriyanov S et al. Defective trophoblast function in mice with a targeted mutation of Ets2. Genes Dev 1998; 12: 1315–26.

83. Yancopoulos GD, Davis S, Gale NW et al. Vascular-specific growth factors and blood vessel formation. Nature 2000; 407: 242–8.

84. Wang D, Ishimura R, Walia DS et al. Eosinophils are cellular targets of the novel uteroplacental heparin-binding cytokine decidual/trophoblast prolactin-related protein. J Endocrinol 2000; 167: 15–28.

85. Lee CK, Moon DH, Shin CS et al. Circadian expression of Mel1a and PL-II genes in placenta: effects of melatonin on the PL-II gene expression in the rat placenta. Mol Cell Endocrinol 2003; 200: 57–66.

86. Knofler M, Meinhardt G, Bauer S et al. Human Hand1 basic helix-loop-helix (bHLH) protein: extra-embryonic expression pattern, interaction partners and identification of its transcriptional repressor domains. Biochem J 2002; 361: 641–51.

87. Oudejans C, Alders M, Postmus J et al. Human MASH2 (HASH2) maps to chromosome 11p15 and is expressed in extravillus trophoblast. Placenta 1996; 17: A15.

88. Baczyk D, Satkunaratnam A, Nait-Oumesmar B et al. Complex patterns of GCM1 mRNA and protein in villous and extravillous trophoblast cells of the human placenta. Placenta 2004; 25: 553–9.

89. Varanou A, Withington SL, Lakasing L et al. The importance of cysteine cathepsin proteases for placental development. J Mol Med 2006; 84: 305–17.

90. Deussing J, Kouadio M, Rehman S et al. Identification and characterization of a dense cluster of placenta-specific cysteine peptidase genes and related genes on mouse chromosome 13. Genomics 2002; 79: 225–40.

91. Ishida M, Ono K, Taguchi S et al. Cathepsin gene expression in mouse placenta during the latter half of pregnancy. J Reprod Dev 2004; 50: 515–23.

92. Davisson RL, Hoffmann DS, Butz GM et al. Discovery of a spontaneous genetic mouse model of preeclampsia. Hypertension 2002; 39: 337–42.

93. Wong AY, Kulandavelu S, Whiteley KJ et al. Maternal cardiovascular changes during pregnancy and postpartum in mice. Am J Physiol Heart Circ Physiol 2002; 282: H918–25.

94. Conrad KP, Benyo DF, Westerhausen-Larsen A et al. Expression of erythropoietin by the human placenta. FASEB J 1996; 10: 760–8.

32 Epitheliochorial and endotheliochorial placentas

Vibeke Dantzer, Rudolf Leiser, and Christiane Pfarrer

Synopsis

Background

- Many species, including pigs, horses, ruminants, and some lower primates, develop an epitheliochorial placenta, in which the trophoblast remains in direct contact with maternal uterine epithelium throughout pregnancy.
- Another group of species, including cats, mink, and elephants, undergo endotheliochorial placentation in which the maternal uterine epithelium degenerates upon contact with the outer trophoblast layer, which makes contact with maternal vascular endothelium.
- In both these types of placenta a regulated cellular transfer of nutrients takes place over the maternal epithelium and/or endothelium to be taken up by the trophoblast.
- This emphasizes that different solutions to the problem of maternal–fetal nutrient transfer have been found independently in evolution.

Basic Science

- The endometrium passes through a phase of growth and remodeling in order to achieve an increase in the surface area of well-vascularized tissue.
- A decrease in the physical distance between maternal and fetal blood circulations in the interhemal barrier is also needed in order to obtain the best possible exchange of oxygen and carbon dioxide.
- The subepithelial capillary architecture is altered beneath sites of placental attachment.
- In epithelio- and endotheliochorial species there is close approximation of the capillaries to the overlying epithelium ('intraepithelial capillaries'), well exemplified in the pig and mink. This is regulated by signals from the placenta. Glandar secretions, histotroph, are important in providing special types of nutrients for uptake of the trophoblast.
- Decidual changes of the type and extent seen in human and mouse uterine tissues are not observed in epitheliochorial species. Decidual-like changes are seen in the endotheliochorial species as maternal fibroblasts are transformed into decidual or periendothelial cells.
- There are alterations in maternal immune cell populations in pregnancy in both types of placentation.
- The interaction between the maternal luminal epithelium and allantochorion in epitheliochorial placentas occurs in a highly species-specific manner with variation in the extent and location of the contact and in the degree of folding and branching.
- In cows, sheep, and goats limited invasion takes place when trophoblast and uterine epithelial cells fuse to form various types of multinucleate hybrid cells.
- Despite the above differences in placental anatomy, certain key mediators such as VEGF, MIF, IGFs, HGF, LIF, FGFs, interferons, the renin–angiotensin system, and MMPs seem to be important in the development of the materno–fetal interface in many species.

Clinical

- Where animal models (such as the sheep, which has an epitheliochorial placenta) have been used to model human placental pathology, the different types of placenta and hormonal regulations must be taken into account in extrapolating the findings.

INTRODUCTION

Morphological changes in the endometrium of species with epitheliochorial and endotheliochorial types of placenta are of great interest, as adaptation to an intimate contact between the uterine epithelium and the conceptus has had to evolve in order to meet the needs of the conceptus. The endometrium passes through a phase of growth and remodeling in order to achieve an increase in the surface area of well-vascularized tissue. A decrease in the physical distance between maternal and fetal blood circulations in the interhemal barrier is also needed in order to obtain the best possible exchange of oxygen and carbon dioxide. In these types of placenta a regulated cellular transfer of nutrients takes place over the maternal epithelium and/or endothelium to be taken up by the trophoblast. The genetically foreign conceptus suppresses undesirable maternal immune reactions, whereas the endometrium appears to regulate and control the degree of invasion. The placenta must develop rapidly to achieve the capacity to act as a respiratory, intestinal, and endocrine system. The interplay between regulatory factors that are important for placentation varies among species. Three epitheliochorial systems are considered here:

- the non-invasive diffuse placenta of the pig
- the non-invasive diffuse microcotyledonary placenta of the horse, which exhibits a temporary invasion of the trophoblast into the endometrium for endometrial cup formation
- the cotyledonary synepitheliochorial placenta, where binucleate trophoblast cells invade and fuse with uterine epithelial cells or syncytia, as seen in cow and small ruminants respectively.

The description of the endotheliochorial placenta is mainly confined to that of the mink and the cat, which have an incomplete and complete belt or zonary placenta, respectively.

ENDOMETRIUM OF EPITHELIOCHORIAL AND SYNEPITHELIOCHORIAL PLACENTAS

In epitheliochorial placentation, there is no invasion of the trophoblast of the allantochorion into the maternal endometrium, except for the temporary formation of endometrial cups in horse, and the migration of binucleate trophoblast giant cells which fuse

with uterine epithelial cells in ruminants. The latter placenta is therefore described as synepitheliochorial (see Chapter 31a). These types of allantochorionic placenta maintain all tissue layers – maternal endothelium, connective tissue, uterine epithelium, trophoblast, mesenchyme, and fetal endothelium – and therefore do not develop decidual-like cells. Correspondingly, no maternal tissue layers are released with the afterbirth.

The interaction between the luminal epithelium and allantochorion occurs in a highly species-specific manner with variation in the extent and location of the contact and in the degree of folding and branching.[1] This non-deciduate type of placenta is characteristic for a number of species and can be subdivided into three main categories:

- The mainly diffuse, folded type, found in pig or hog is also present in viviparous squamate reptiles such as the skink *Chalcides chalcides*, lower primates such as the bush babies or Lorisidae, the American mole *Scalopus aquaticus*, and some Artiodactyla such as peccaries and Hippopotamidae.
- The diffuse villous type is seen in Perissodactyla such as horse, donkey, and zebra, and in some cetartiodactyl species such as dolphins (Cetacea), and llamas, camels, and chevrotains (Artiodactyla).
- The multiplex or cotyledonary villous form is found in such animals as cattle, goats and sheep, deer, moose, okapis, giraffes, duikers, gnu, waterbuck, reedbuck, impala, eland, kudu, and bison.[2]

The distinctive events occurring in the endometrium of the most thoroughly investigated species within these three groups (i.e. pig, equine, and ruminants) is described.

Pig

In order to develop the diffuse folded type of placenta, the porcine endometrium undergoes many changes during the establishment of intimate contact with the allantochorion. These adaptations are most likely induced by factors from the blastocyst and estrogens play an especially significant role,[3] as they are first localized at the contact areas, which are close to the embryonic disc.[4,5] The uterine epithelium remains intact and gap junction-mediated intercellular communication seems to be lacking in the uterine epithelium of both pig and equine in contrast to animals exhibiting invasive types of placentation.[6] Endometrial adaptation

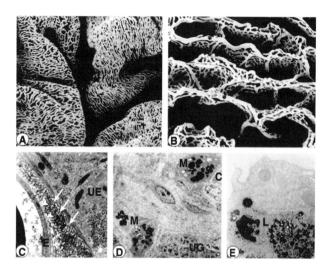

Figure 32.1 Endometrial characteristics of the epitheliochorial pig placenta. (A) Scanning electron micrograph from day 15 postinsemination, showing the subepithelial capillary network, which has now increased in density in some areas. ×77. (B) Scanning electron micrograph of a vascular cast of the subepithelial endometrium from day 99 postinsemination. The vasculature is in an elaborate folded form with wide stem arterioles (*) on the top of the ridges. ×100. (C) Transmission electron micrograph from day 18½ postinsemination, showing the base of a uterine epithelial cell (UE) close to the endothelial (E) wall of a subepithelial capillary. The epithelial basal lamina forms wavy folds into the underlying connective tissue (arrows), whereas the endothelial basal lamina is almost smooth and very narrow (arrowheads). ×15 000. (D) Transmission electron micrograph of iron-loaded macrophages (M) close to uterine gland cells (UG) and a capillary (C) in the porcine endometrium 43 days post-insemination. ×3000. (E) Detail of a macrophage with ferritin particles free in the cytoplasm and in a large lysosome (L). ×50 000.

is reflected by changes in the uterine epithelium (Figure 32.1C) and especially by changes in the architecture of subepithelial capillaries (Figure 32.1A,B),[7] surrounding connective tissue,[8] glycan composition,[9] and the frequency of granulated mast cells and lymphocytes.[10,11]

Vasculature and stroma

During initial placentation, one of the very early processes that gives rise to the typical architecture of the feto–maternal interface is vascular growth, and its displacement and approximation to the overlying uterine epithelium (Figure 32.1A). Folding of the placenta leads to an increase in the surface area of the feto–maternal interface (Figure 32.1B) and a cross- to countercurrent blood flow interrelationship develops

between maternal and embryonic vasculature of the epitheliochorial barrier.[7,12]

Changes in the endometrial stroma are important in the initial development of the interhemal barrier in the pig.[8] The stromal changes comprise a physiological edema, a characteristic increase in vasculature (day 15 pc), and the formation of sling-like extensions of the basal lamina of the uterine epithelium (Figure 32.1C), which develop 1–2 days after the first contact occurs between trophoblast and uterine epithelium (day 13 pc).[8] These extensions appear before the increase in surface area by microscopic folding of the endometrium. At the same time, fine finger-like cellular processes from the endothelial cells of the subepithelial capillaries extend towards the uterine epithelium. These processes appear to penetrate the basal lamina, closely followed by an increase in capillary diameter and approximation to the uterine epithelium.[7,8] In addition, there is an increase in the number of endothelial cell fenestrations,[13,14] especially in the capillary wall facing the uterine epithelium. These rapid changes reflect a well-coordinated epithelial–endothelial interaction with the surrounding connective tissue, including a functional polarization and growth within the capillaries. The endometrial vascular growth seems to be regulated by the conceptus, as straight bred Yorkshire (Y) sows have larger conceptuses than straight bred Meishian (M) sows throughout gestation and at farrowing, but when Y and M conceptuses are together in Y recipient females, the birth weights of M and Y offspring are similar. The placentas of M fetuses, however, remain markedly smaller than those of their Y littermates. This is due to the fetal growth from day 90 to birth in M offspring depending on a progressive increase in the placental blood vessel density, whereas Y conceptuses seems to rely exclusively on placental growth in order to increase the surface area of the feto–maternal interface for nutrient exchange.[15] Keratinocyte growth factor (KGF)/fibroblast growth factor 7 (FGF-7) is an established paracrine mediator of hormone-regulated epithelial growth and differentiation apparently secreted by stromal cells, and in the uterus its up-regulation coincides with a down-regulation in progesterone receptors. KGF is expressed in both luminal and glandular epithelium and shows a great difference between the cycling and pregnant states, being high at days 15 and 12 of gestation, respectively. In glandular epithelium from day 60 to 85 of gestation a high increase in KGF is seen, possibly influencing secretory activity as well as having a role in trophoblast–uterine epithelial interaction.[16]

Carbonic anhydrase may be involved in a variety of functions, such as transport of charged ions (H^+ and HCO_3^-), metabolic CO_2 fixation (for supplying HCO_3^- for pyruvate carboxylation), participation in amino acid synthesis, gluconeogenesis, carbonyl phosphate synthesis, urea cycle generation, acid and base secretion and thus also in intra- and extracellular acid–base balance, as well as in mineralization.[17,18] An additional function for carbonic anhydrase in cell proliferation has been suggested.[19] In the porcine placenta it has been shown by histochemistry that carbonic anhydrase becomes activated in capillaries during the initial stages of placentation and remains up-regulated, although showing a short decline in activity during the period with the most prominent capillary growth and displacement (15–20 days pc) as well as a spatiotemporal variation in its activation in the uterine epithelium.[20] Carbonic anhydrase is most strongly expressed in the pig and although it shows great interspecies variation in its activation at the interhemal barrier the uterine endothelium shows a consistent positive reaction.

Cytoskeleton, integrins, extracellular matrix, and growth factors

The many and complex interactions of the cytoskeleton with the extracellular matrix (ECM) via cell surface receptors and the modulation of these interactions by growth factors are well documented. In the pig endometrium around the time of implantation and early placentation, vimentin is present in cells of mesenchymal origin, and von Willebrand factor has been localized in endothelial cells. Desmin labeling has been seen not only in smooth muscle cells but also in pericytes, pointing to a role of the latter in angiogenesis.[21]

Insulin-like growth factor I (IGF-I) in the porcine uterus is strongest in vascular smooth muscle cells but it is also expressed in the luminal and glandular epithelium.[21] This activity declines markedly after a peak in IGF-I mRNA at days 12–13 with a decrease to a consistently low level after day 14 of gestation. It is remarkable that IGF-I is more abundant during the estrous cycle than during pregnancy. Recent in-vitro studies of porcine uterine glandular epithelium from early pregnancy demonstrated a complex interplay of IGF system components, with IGF-II and IGF binding protein-2 (IGFBP-2) as locally co-expressed uterine epithelial cell mitogens. This suggests a signaling pathway by which IGF-II stimulates epithelial proliferation via the type II receptor.[22] The IGF axis in porcine endometrium and placenta is altered by the exogenous application of recombinant porcine somatotropin in a way that endometrial mRNA levels of IGF-I were low on days 28 and 37, but higher on day 62, while IGF-II was increased in the endometrium. Exposure to somatotropin increased IGFBP-2 mRNA in the endometrium and placenta, while IGFBP-3 mRNA was unchanged.[23] The fact that IGFBP and IGF-II are localized close to each other at the feto–maternal interface suggests an important role for this system in mediating paracrine interactions between fetal and maternal tissues supporting the establishment and maintenance of pregnancy.[24]

Platelet-derived growth factor (PDGF) receptors in the endothelial/perivascular areas of the subepithelial layer from days 24–40 of pregnancy show a stronger expression compared to earlier stages,[21,25] suggesting that PDGF plays a role in the reorganization of the stroma, particularly during maternal placental angiogenesis.

The co-localization of vascular endothelial growth factor (VEGF) and its receptors in endothelial cells and unexpectedly in epithelial and smooth muscle cells during porcine gestation shows spatiotemporal changes in expression during the first half of initial placentation.[26] This suggests that VEGF and both its Flt1 and kinase domain (KDR) receptors have a role in angiogenesis or vascular permeability as well as in cellular differentiation during porcine placentation. However, since radiolabeled VEGF has been detected in porcine placental endothelial cells, but not epithelial cells,[27] additional studies have to confirm the presence of VEGF receptors in the latter.

In addition, selected integrins and ECM components such as laminin, fibronectin, vitronectin, and collagen type IV have been localized by immunohistochemistry from gilts at estrus and at 10–15 days of pregnancy.[28] The authors found no changes in the intensity of staining of any ECM components examined which could be attributed to the day of the cycle or pregnancy status. The stroma, basal lamina of luminal and glandular epithelium, as well as the vasculature all showed intense reactivity for fibronectin, moderate staining for vitronectin and strong staining for laminin and collagen IV. Integrin subunits α_v, α_5, α_4, α_3, β_1, and β_3 were prominent basally in, or adjacent to, the luminal epithelial cells. The use of frozen sections for immunohistochemistry, however, did not permit a more precise localization. Such expression of cytoskeletal filaments and growth factors, integrins, and ECM clearly indicates an area for future research in order to understand the interaction between pregnancy-associated steroids, integrins, cytoskeleton, the activation of enzyme cascades, and participation in various signal transduction processes necessary for the well-organized development of the endometrium.

Cells in the stroma: mast cells

Based on their granular content, mast cells have been reported to decrease in number in the endometrium[11] concomitantly with the establishment of materno–fetal epithelial apposition and the subsequent increase in the subepithelial vascular bed and its approximation to the uterine epithelium. Heparin binding is found to enhance the angiogenic properties of a number of growth factors including the ones mentioned above.[29] Endometrial mast cells may modulate the effects of estrogen on cell growth and proliferation in mice[30] while in humans they stimulate matrix metalloproteinase activity.[31] The role of mast cells in the porcine endometrium during the dramatic morphological changes seen at early placentation is thus of great interest for future research.

Leukocytes

Lymphocyte numbers in the uterine epithelium of the pig are variously reported to remain constant[32] or progressively decrease[33] during the first 3 weeks of gestation. This inconsistency may be due to different tissue sampling: i.e. from the antimesometrial vs the mesometrial side, away from and close to attachment sites, respectively. The conceptus appears to exhibit a local effect on the uterine lymphocyte population, because in cycling animals leukocytes are evenly distributed between epithelium, stroma, and the stromal/epithelial interface, whereas in pregnant animals (days 13–26), leukocytes are abundant in the deep stroma but rare in the epithelium. However, in the pregnant animal a three-fold higher incidence of stromal leukocytes, mainly lymphocytes, is found at attachment sites as compared to the area between them.[10] In vitro, dispersed porcine endometrial cells were lysed by natural killer (NK) cells and this activity is increased at days 10–20 of gestation compared to that found in cycling or pseudopregnant pigs, suggesting stimulation by conceptus-derived factors.[34] Furthermore, this lytic capability is increased by prior incubation of endometrial effectors with interleukin-2 (IL-2). One function of porcine endometrial lymphocytes may be to promote angiogenesis. Recently, it was shown in healthy implantation sites that angiogenic genes were transcribed at a higher rate in endometrial lymphocytes than in trophoblasts. In contrast, uterine lymphocytes in arresting fetal sites had no angiogenic gene transcription and showed rapid elevation in transcription of proinflammatory cytokines Fas and Fas ligand while trophoblasts showed elevated transcription of interferon γ (IFNγ) and Fas.[35] In a more comprehensive study of porcine

endometrial angiogenesis transcripts were compared between endometrial endothelium and lymphocytes from placental of healthy and fetal loss at day 25 and 50. This showed a close interrelation and interplay between VEGF and its two receptors, hypoxia inducible factor-1α (HIF-1α), placental growth factor, IFN-γ and TNF-α, giving further evidence for the importance of lymphocytes in endometrial angiogenesis.[36]

IFN is a major regulator of NK-cell-mediated cytotoxicity. The short porcine type I-IFN, an antiviral conceptus secretion, has been cloned from a day 14–15 embryo.[37] IFN secretion is correlated to endometrial NK-like activity, as it is elevated in the vicinity of the conceptus, suggesting a means by which the porcine trophoblast modulates the maternal immune system and directs its function to the advantage of the offspring (Table 32.1).[10]

Macrophage migratory inhibitory factor (MIF), a proinflammatory cytokine that is suspected to be involved in materno–fetal immunotolerance, has been localized in both trophoblast and uterine epithelium in early gestation as well as in late gestation trophoblast.[38] Two other members of the cytokine family with proposed roles in pregnancy, leukemia inhibitory factor (LIF) and its receptor β-subunit and interleukin-6 (IL-6) mRNA, have been identified in porcine endometrium of early and mid pregnancy, with the greatest steady-state amount at days 36 and 65 of gestation.[39] In contrast, the β_2 microglobulin gene, a potential cytokine responsive target, is present in the endometrium and placenta at the same level during these stages. Further studies throughout gestation are needed to reveal the cell types responsible for the synthesis of, and target for, these interleukins in order to contribute to the understanding of their role in placental growth biology.

Studies of the synthesis of secretory leukocyte proteinase inhibitor (SLPI) have been undertaken in the porcine endometrium from days 16 to 25 of gestation. The results show an up-regulation of SLPI directly beneath the conceptuses, thereby supporting the hypothesis that it may act to prevent trophoblast invasion in species with epitheliochorial placentation.[40,41] Together with other uterine protease inhibitors, SLPI could prevent the enzymatic degradation of the uterine–placental interface taking place in species with invasive placentation. SLPI mRNA is up-regulated by a conceptus-derived low molecular weight protein, possibly transforming growth factor (TGF). SLPI and uterine plasmin/trypsin inhibitor are not only protease inhibitors but also growth factors; their mRNA is present in the endometrium throughout gestation. The

Table 32.1   Uterine lymphocytes proposed to play a role in pregnancy in livestock species

| Species | Morphology | Pregnancy-associated uterine lymphocytes | | | | |
		Phenotype	Proposed lineage	Distribution	Stage of gestation	Proposed role in pregnancy
Sheep	Large, granular	CD8[dim] CD45R+ γδTcR+	γδT	Uterine epithelium at interplacentomal regions	Mid to late	Secretion of cytokines that promote trophoblast development? Defense against infectious pathogens?
Horse	Small	CD4+? CD8+?	T? NK?	Surround fetally derived endometrial cups within uterine stroma	Early	Destruction of endometrial cups
Pig	Large	G7+(NK marker) probably CD2+, CD8+	NK	Uterine stroma	Early	Communication between trophoblast and maternal immune system during early placental development

From Engelhardt and King.[103]

growth-promoting activity of SLPI may additionally be enhanced by heparin, as shown in studies with primary porcine endometrial epithelial cells.[42]

Areolar gland complex

This complex, found in diffuse placentas,[42–44] develops as soon as close contact between the endometrium and the trophoblast is established and can be recognized from day 15 in the pig.[12]

Iron

The secretory activity of the endometrium is of great importance in pig placentation and one of its main functions is to provide iron to the developing embryo/fetus.[46] Iron is secreted as uteroferrin,[47] which constitutes 10–15% of the uterine secretion.[48] Iron bound in ferritin particles accumulates basally in the non-ciliated cells of the uterine glands. The synthesis of uteroferrin follows the common route for glycoprotein secretion, as iron, bound as ferritin, is seen either free in the cytoplasm or accumulated in lysosomes basally in the cells of uterine glands.[49] Uteroferrin has also been identified immunohistochemically in the Golgi complexes and associated secretory granules.[50] The uterine glandular epithelium shows hypertrophy during gestation, reaching its maximum around day 60.[45] The vasculature seems to follow this development, but does not increase around glands to the same extent as seen in the interareolar regions.[12,51] The glandular activity changes from secretion to inhibition, with a subsequent release of the secretory product into the interstitium where

it is taken up by macrophages. It is characteristic that macrophages in the vicinity of the glands are loaded with ferritin and thus contain brownish, highly refractile granules in unstained sections, as in the hemophagous zones of carnivore placentas; at the ultrastructural level, these are seen as electron-dense inclusions (Figure 32.1D). It is thought that their function may be to regulate the iron supply, as the secretion of uteroferrin varies during the cycle and it is sometimes released into the interstitium where it is taken up by macrophages (Figure 32.1D,E), when glandular activity abruptly decreases. Another hypothesis is that macrophages may serve as iron carrier cells between the vasculature and the glandular epithelium,[49] or these two functions may be combined.

Retinol-binding proteins

Recently, it has been found that plasma retinol-binding protein (RBP) immunoreactivity is located in the uterine glands, their secretory products, and in the areolar trophoblast, as well as in the interareolar uterine epithelium, whereas the cellular transport and metabolism of cellular retinol-binding protein-I (CRBP-I) occurs in the interareolar epithelium, and from mid-gestation also in the uterine glandular epithelium and in areolar and interareolar trophoblast. However, cellular retinoic acid binding protein-I (CRABP-I) immunoreactivity, reflecting the metabolically active form supposed to be mainly involved in retinoic acid signaling pathways, is restricted to the interareolar trophoblast. These observations indicate

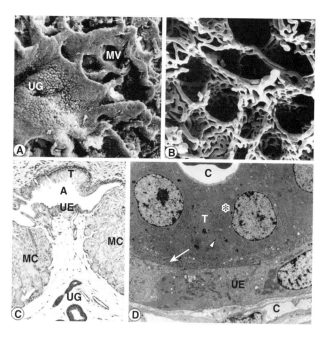

Figure 32.2 Endometrial characteristics of the epithelio-chorial horse placenta. (**A**) Scanning electron micrograph of the endometrial surface showing the opening of a uterine gland (UG) with protruding epithelial cells in close association with crypts normally indented by fetal microvilli (MV). ×500. (**B**) Scanning electron micrograph of the endometrial microvasculature in an area where the villi of fetal microcotyledons are localized ('empty' spots). ×750. (**C**) Histological picture of two microcotyledons (MC) being interrupted by an areola (A). In contrast to the uterine epithelium and microcotyledonary trophoblast, areolar trophoblast (T) is tall and columnar. UG, uterine glands. ×62.5. (**D**) Transmission electron micrograph of the microcotyledonary feto–maternal interface, with darker trophoblast cells (T) and light-colored uterine epithelium (UE) separated from each other by a microvillous interdigitation (arrow). T contains large amounts of rough (*) and smooth (arrowhead) endoplasmic reticulum. C, capillaries. ×8000.

that the transfer of retinoids, necessary for a wide range of processes during embryogenesis, takes place over the areolar gland complex, and that retinoids are important for placental growth and differentiation.[52,53]

Equine

The diffuse, villous, microcotyledonary epitheliochorial placenta of the horse (Figure 32.2A–D) is characterized by late implantation as compared with many other species, namely after day 35 of gestation. The conceptus is kept in a fixed position in utero by myometrial contractions from day 20 pc, shortly before the rupture and loss of the acellular capsule, which has replaced the zona pellucida and thereafter

surrounds the growing spherical blastocyst.[54,55] From days 36 to 44 of gestation there is invasion of the chorionic girdle cells into the uterine endometrium and subsequent formation of endometrial cups,[56] a feature unique to equine placentation. Initial attachment of the non-invasive allantochorion occurs at around day 45,[1,56,57] when developing villi come into close contact with the uterine epithelium and indent the endometrium (Figure 32.2A,B). Decidual or decidual-like cells have not been observed in this species.

Endometrial cup reaction

The formation of endometrial cups by means of trophoblast cell migration and invasion has been described in detail[58] and, in the following, emphasis is placed on the endometrial reaction to the invasion and growth of genetically foreign extraembryonic trophoblast cells, the cup cells, which secrete equine chorionic gonadotrophin (eCG).[56,59,60] These cup cells are able to synthesize metalloproteinase in vitro, probably facilitating their migration in vivo.[61] Following the invasion of cup cells through the epithelial basal lamina, the integrity of the uterine luminal and upper glandular epithelium is rapidly restored,[62] while the superficial blood vessels of the endometrial stroma remain intact. However, at the basal margin of the cups, the migrating trophoblast cup cells intrude through the endothelium of lymphatic vessels.[58] Exocrine secretion by the uterine glands and an endocrine secretion by the fetal trophoblast cup cells take place. Despite these additional functions of the endometrium, there is no evidence of angiogenesis and therefore it is the original endometrial vessels which serve the remaining stroma, the uterine glands, and the high number of clustered endocrine cup cells, which in the light of their endocrine function have a remarkably poor vascularization.[59,63,64] In addition, with age, there seems to be an increasing isolation of the cup vessels, as ECM accumulates in the surrounding stroma.[64]

Uterine glands in endometrial cups

After the invasion of cup cells around day 35, there is enlargement and elongation of the uterine glands as well as hypertrophy of the individual epithelial cells, indicating that the cup cells have a stimulatory effect. This is reflected by differences in glandular secretory activity between non-cup and cup regions, as the neck cells of the glands exhibit specific staining with alcian blue as soon as the cup cells enter the endometrial stroma and remain so when they are in close apposition to cup cells, whereas very little staining is seen in the glands away from the cup.[65] Concomitantly, a change to a heterogeneously viscous secretion that is clearly different in its composition from that of non-cup glands takes place.[65,66] In contrast to alcian blue staining, the reaction of glandular cells with an antibody against TGFα occurred almost entirely in endometrial glands beside the cup region and in glands deep in relation to most of the cup cells. Within the cups, the mid and upper regions of the glands rarely reacted with this antibody, although undilated glands adjacent to cups often stained intensely.[65]

After day 47, the basal regions of the glands deep to the cup cells tend to be highly dilated whereas the gland openings, initially blocked by the girdle cells, and now enclosed by cup cells, remain narrow. It seems to be a consistent feature around day 50, that there is herniation and rupture of the upper portion of the glands so that the glandular secretory product, as visualized by lectin staining, seeps out into the surrounding stroma and may contribute to the nutrition of the cup cells.[66]

The long-lasting regression and eventual sloughing off of the cup cells, which resembles graft rejection,[67] has recently been suggested to be due to impaired vascularization and rupture of glands, thereby inducing necrosis with subsequent leukocyte infiltration, release of foreign antigens to the host mare, and thus eliciting the rejection.[63,64]

Leukocytes

During initial trophoblast invasion there is a burst of small lymphocyte migration into the endometrial stroma which is already rich in lymphocytes, macrophages, and plasma cells, with large granular lymphocytes being numerous in the uterine epithelium (see Table 32.1). However, as soon as the girdle cells enlarge and differentiate into cup cells, the connective tissue components in the stroma decline, leaving only the few blood vessels.[58] At the time of invasion, the endometrial cup cells show a strong expression of major histocompatibility complex (MHC) class I antigen,[56,68] which becomes undetectable by day 60, and by the time the cup cells are hypertrophied, most immune cells have disappeared in the cup area although they remain abundant in the surrounding stroma.[58] A characterization of maternal leukocyte cell types in response to endometrial cups, from their formation to their regression, suggests a complicated cytokine-mediated regulatory network.[69]

The expression of TGFβ$_2$ in maternal leukocytes is undetectable before invasion, but is found in the region of developing cup cells from day 38 to 45 and later from day 78 to 81 in the dense layer of leukocytes at the periphery of cups, where 90% also stained with chromotrope 2e, this being a marker for eosinophils.[70] However, further studies are needed to clarify these findings.

Uterine epithelium and areolar gland complex

Endometrial secretion in the horse is copious in the early stages of gestation, providing histiotroph before intimate feto-maternal contact is established. Thereafter, numerous glands open between the microcotyledons forming the areolar gland subunits (Figure 32.2A,C), which are smaller in size than those of the pig, but occur in high numbers.[71]

The luminal epithelium of the endometrium starts to proliferate after the primary villi of the true epitheliochorial placenta have been formed, and during days 58–70 this effect is only seen in the pregnant horn. During the second half of gestation most of the mitotic activity is confined to the periphery of the microcotyledons.[72]

The glycosylation pattern during gestation shows major variations in the maternal epithelium as well as in the trophoblast only during initial placentation, adhesion, and attachment, up to day 50, whereas the maternal capillaries show very little changes in glycan expression throughout gestation. The maternal epithelium of areolas often shows increased levels of lectin binding at mid gestation, with a gradual decline to low levels at 280 and 300 days.[73] In a comparative study of horse, donkey, and camel glycosylation, it was suggested that glycan diversity between species may be one of the factors preventing implantation and subsequent placental development in interspecies hybrids, as only interbreeding species carry similar glycans in tissues forming the interhemal barrier.[62,74]

The critical enzyme that determines metabolism of primary prostaglandins, 15-hydroxyprostaglandin dehydrogenase, has been localized to the maternal epithelium of microcotyledons and some connective tissue cells but not to the uterine glands at days 150–300 of gestation.[75] Two glucose transport proteins (Glut1 and Glut3) are restricted to the microplacentomes; they are localized differently, as Glut1 is found at the basolateral plasma membrane of both uterine epithelium and trophoblast, whereas Glut3 is restricted to the interdigitating microvilli of the interhemal barrier. This indicates a unique development as a glucose molecule apparently has to use both isoforms to cross from maternal to fetal blood.[76]

The areolar gland complex in the horse transports iron by an iron-binding protein similar to the iron carrier uteroferrin found in the pig.[77] Immunoreactivity to this protein can be seen in Golgi complexes and secretory granules in the uterine glandular epithelium as well as in the luminal content[76] but not in microplacentomes. The binding protein for calcium (calbindin, 9CBP) is confined to the same compartment but uses a different transport mechanism, as the localization differs from that of uteroferrin.[76] This important information sheds new light on the function of the equine areolar gland complex in the transfer of material during gestation, but there are most likely more functions related to this extremely well-developed complex.

Ruminants

The multiplex, villous, synepitheliochorial placenta is a subtype of the epitheliochorial placenta and is characterized by the presence of binucleate trophoblast giant cells (TGCs) (Figure 32.3D–F) which migrate to the uterine epithelium and, in cattle, fuse with single uterine epithelial cells to form a hybrid of the two genetically different cell types. In small ruminants, such as sheep and goats, migration and fusion continue to form multinuclear hybrids in the uterine epithelium, thus contributing to the formation of a uterine or maternal syncytial epithelium.[78] There is no real formation of decidual cells; however, in sheep and goats there are large individual cells, probably residual endometrial fibroblasts or pericytes, located between the maternal epithelial syncytium and the rich maternal vasculature in the crypt walls of the placentomes.[57,79]

Interferons and growth factors

During initial placentation, the conceptus produces interferons τ and α (IFNτ and IFNα). The synthesis of IFNτ is at its maximum between days 15 and 25 in cattle[80] and up to day 18 in goat,[81] and is important in the maintenance of corpus luteum function during early pregnancy by blocking the release of prostaglandin from endometrial epithelial cells;[82,83] this is further discussed in Chapter 17. Experiments during initial placentation indicate that the intercaruncular region seems to be the primary region for oxytocin regulation of prostaglandin $F_{2\alpha}$, whereas the caruncles may be the proliferative site for recognition of the IFNτ signal.[84]

However, in contrast to the inhibitory effect on lymphocytes and oviductal cells,[85,86] neither IFNτ nor IFNα seems to exhibit an antiproliferative effect on endometrial stromal or epithelial cells from days 11–17 after estrus.[87] This indicates that the endometrium is capable of overcoming the antiproliferative effect of IFNτ produced by the conceptus during maternal

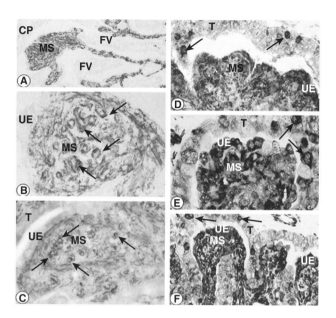

Figure 32.3 Endometrial characteristics of the synepitheliochorial bovine placenta, with special reference to the tips of the maternal septa. (**A–C**) Localization of the cytoskeletal filaments actin and vimentin. (**A**) Overview of the arcade region where the tips of the maternal septa (MS) meet the chorionic plate (CP). Actin immunoreactivity is observed in the MS particularly at the tips, while the trophoblast of fetal villi (FV) and uterine epithelium are both negative. ×31.25. (**B**) Detail of a septal tip (MS) reveals that the microvasculature (arrows) is predominantly positive for actin. UE, uterine epithelium. ×125. (**C**) Septal tips also display immunoreactivity for vimentin in endothelial cells (arrows). ×125. (**D–F**) In-situ hybridization for FGF1 (**D**), FGF2 (**E**), and FGFR (**F**) shows the presence of specific mRNAs in the maternal stroma of septal tips (MS), some caruncular epithelial cells (UE), and single trophoblast giant cells (arrows). **D,F**, ×62.5; **E**, ×125.

recognition of pregnancy. Ovine experiments have shown that the down-regulation of progesterone receptor in uterine glandular epithelium is a prerequisite for progesterone induction of secretory gene expression, and that placental lactogen and growth hormone effects on uterine glands require IFNτ.[87] Furthermore, the deep glandular compartment is the primary target for the action of lactogenic hormones,[88] exhibiting a dramatic increase in prolactin receptor mRNA expression specifically in the ovine glandular compartment, especially in late pregnancy.[89] The interplay of these factors thus participates in the regulation of endometrial gland proliferation and differentiated secretory function.

Furthermore, other results support the hypothesis that progesterone is required for IFNτ induction of type I IFN-responsive genes as, for example, ubiquitin cross-reactive protein in the ovine uterine epithelium.[90] An investigation of the spatiotemporal expression of growth hormone and its receptor in the ovine placenta showed an increase in growth hormone receptor transcripts from days 25 to 43, where the endometrium, placenta, and fetus are all potential targets for placental growth hormone[91] and thus well timed to initiate placentation. It has also been shown that IFNτ stimulates granulocyte–macrophage colony-stimulating factor (GM-CSF) gene expression in bovine uterine stroma as well as in lymphocytes, thus supporting the hypothesis that the conceptus modulates the expression of beneficial cytokines at the feto–maternal interface.[92]

Insulin-like growth factors I and II (IGF-I and IGF-II) are polypeptides with a structural homology with proinsulin. IGF-II plays an especially important role in placental growth and differentiation. The effect of these two IGFs is dependent on their IGF receptors (IGFR1 and IGFR2) and IGF-binding proteins (IGFBP, 1–6), and localization of their respective mRNAs is important to elucidate the regulatory mechanisms for IGF in placentation. Many components of the uterine IGF system, including receptors and binding proteins, are differentially regulated by IGFBP during the estrous cycle and early pregnancy[93–95] and variable IGFBP-5 and -6 gene expression is also found in the ovine uterus of cycling and early pregnant ewes.[96] Hepatocyte growth factor (HGF) and its receptor c-met have also been localized to the ovine uterus[97] and here HGF mRNA is confined to endometrial stroma, whereas the receptor c-met mRNA is exclusively expressed in the luminal and glandular epithelium, giving a strong indication of the participation of HGF in the regulation of epithelial growth.

Integrins and extracellular matrix

Osteopontin (OPN) is an acidic glycoprotein which binds to surface integrins to promote cell–cell attachment and spreading. OPN, being regulated by progesterone, increased between days 11 and 17 during pregnancy in ewes and was localized to luminal and glandular epithelium as well as to trophoblast cells of day 19 blastocysts. Secreted OPN, a ligand for two integrin heterodimers on the trophoblast and uterine epithelium, may induce adhesion at the feto–maternal interface and subsequent placentation.[98] This hypothesis has recently been challenged, since integrin $\alpha_v\beta_3$ did not co-localize with OPN at the feto–maternal interface in the cow and sheep.[99] In bovine placentomes these integrin subunits, together with a variety of other subunits, were found in the caruncular stroma, suggesting that a pool of integrins is present for various signal transduction cascades or functions.[100] During implantation in the goat, a loss of collagen type I and IV and

laminin has been observed in the endometrium adherent to the trophoblast, together with a loss of β_1 integrin and cytokeratins 8, 18, and 19.[101]

During angiogenesis and tissue growth, remodeling is dependent on changes in the ECM, and recently two matrix metalloproteinases (MMPs), type IV collagenases MMP-2 and MMP-9, and tissue inhibitor of metalloproteinase 1 (TIMP-1) have been localized in sheep placenta from the last third of gestation.[102] MMP activity and TIMP were found in uterine intercaruncular epithelium and endothelium, although at lower levels than in the cotyledonary and intercotyledonary trophoblast. Zymography and Western immunoblotting on placental growth-conditioned media, however, gave different results. This inconsistency, which might be due to separation procedures, will require further investigation. It seems likely that trophoblast plays a major role in the maintenance of maternal uterine tissue remodeling during the late stage of ovine gestation. In bovine placentomes in early gestation, MMP-2 occurred abundantly in the maternal septa, whereas in late pregnancy MMP-2 expression was confined to the stromal tissue at the tips of the septa and the trophoblast opposite to these regions.[103] The same authors observed MMP-9 expression in the epithelium and stroma of maternal septa and in mononuclear trophoblast cells, while TIMP-2 was localized in binucleate TGCs, confirming the role of this system in tissue growth, remodeling, and angiogenesis.

Leukocytes

Immediately after the first feto–maternal contact is established, differentiation and migration of binucleate TGCs takes place to form hybrid cells with the uterine epithelium.[78] The complementary surface area is increased by the formation of placentomal villi and crypts.[104] Prior to implantation, intraepithelial lymphocytes are equally distributed, being seen in caruncular as well as intercaruncular epithelium, whereas after implantation intraepithelial lymphocytes are not observed adjacent to hybrid cells or in sheep uterine epithelial syncytium in the placentomes,[105–107] indicating that the binucleate cells suppress lymphocyte migration. In the endometrium between placentomes, numerous leukocytes are found in the stroma and, of these, a band of cells expressing MHC class II is present immediately under the epithelium, whereas in placentomes themselves only a few leukocytes are distributed randomly in the maternal septa and sparse MHC class II+ cells are seen around blood vessels.[105] The distribution of pregnancy-associated lymphocytes in ruminants has been reviewed,[104] and it was stated that the granulated γδ T cells of the pregnant ruminant uterus are morphologically similar to the granulated uterine NK cells found in humans and rodents. However, ruminant γδ T cells are epithelial rather than stromal in location and are absent from the placentomes, the areas most intimately associated with the trophoblast. There is therefore a clear suppression of MHC class IIC and γδ T cells, most likely induced by the trophoblast of the villi of the fetal cotyledons.

In contrast to that of most other mammals, the bovine placenta shows immunoreactivity for MHC I, when investigated at the 4th, 6th, and 8th months of gestation. In the interplacentomal region and at the arcades of the placentomes, MHC I increases towards term both in the trophoblast and in cells of the uterine epithelium, being strongest in the former, whereas no staining for MHC I is observed in the closely related crypt–villus complex seen in placentomes.[108] This may secure the migration of binucleated cells thus being part of a regulatory mechanism to limit trophoblast invasion. MHC I has been detected in the endometrial epithelium of sheep on days 10–12 of early pregnancy, and in the estrous cycle. On days 14–20 of pregnancy, MHC I expression increases only in endometrial stroma and epithelium of the deep glands, but it is absent from the epithelium of the lumen and superficial glands suggesting its involvement in preventing immune rejection of the conceptus allograft.[109]

The renin–angiotensin system and angiogenesis

The presence of the renin–angiotensin system (RAS) in reproductive organs has received increasing attention[110,111] and a great variation in the expression of angiotensin II receptors has been observed. Receptors AT_1 and AT_2 exist across species and thus in different types of placentas.[111] In the bovine placenta, which is rich in the RAS, autoradiographic angiotensin II receptor studies show that there is a high density of receptors throughout gestation.[112] The angiotensin II receptors are mainly of the subtype AT_2 in the fetal and AT_1 in the maternal compartment, being expressed with high intensity in the subepithelial mesenchyme and lamina propria of the fetal and maternal side, respectively, between placentomes. Within the placentomes, the AT_1 receptor is most abundantly localized in the lower-order septa of the maternal crypts but not in the higher-order septa. A similar pattern is seen for AT_2 at the fetal side of the placentomes in the villous tree. Therefore, AT_1 is predominant at the maternal and AT_2 at the fetal side and they are both mainly located around or closely related to the placental stem vessels. Recently, the corresponding enzymes renin (which converts

angiotensinogen to angiotensin I) and angiotensin-converting enzyme (ACE) have also been localized in the bovine uterus and placenta.[113] Renin immunoreactivity was found to occur exclusively in the uterine epithelium and solitary endometrial cells, while ACE was found in fetal and maternal vascular endothelial cells and in the fetal mesenchyme and endometrial stroma. The presence of all system components supports the concept of a local RAS being involved in regulating permeability, angiogenesis, and growth and differentiation processes through angiotensin II and especially the AT_1 receptor.

Vascular development occurs to create a highly efficient cross- to countercurrent interrelationship in the bovine placenta,[114] and VEGF plays an important role in a complex paracrine fashion.[115] In the ovine placenta, VEGF is highly expressed in maternal epithelium and vasculature as well as in trophoblast and amniotic epithelium, even near term.[116] This gives further support to the hypothesis that VEGF has other functions apart from being purely an endothelial mitogen. The potential of VEGF to interact with other factors was recently revealed. The expression of FGF1, FGF2, FGF7, and FGFR, and platelet-activating factor (PAF) receptor and acetylhydrolase was demonstrated in fetal and maternal blood vessels as well as in immature TGCs in bovine placentomes throughout gestation.[117,118] Thus, TGCs may be involved in the paracrine regulation of maternal caruncle functions. Interestingly, after endocrine induction of parturition (resulting from declining progesterone levels), the expression pattern of both growth factor systems changes to the maternal compartment, with high reactivity in the caruncular stroma and epithelium.[117,118] The importance of the expanded, globular tips of the maternal septa as growth zones is highlighted by the fact that cytoskeletal filaments such as actin (Figure 32.3A,B) and vimentin (Figure 32.3C), as well as growth factors and their receptors (Figure 32.3D–F), are associated with the many blood vessels in this area. The accumulation of a pool of stromal integrins[100] and the presence of Ki67 positivity[119] – a marker of proliferative activity – in the septal tips provides further support for this concept.

ENDOTHELIOCHORIAL PLACENTATION

Endotheliochorial placentation is the establishment and development of a placenta in which the chorion, vascularized by the allantois of the conceptus, comes into intimate contact and erodes the maternal or uterine epithelium and associated stroma to the level of the maternal vasculature.[2,56,120,121] The interhemal barrier, comprising three cell layers and two more or less compressed or modified connective tissue layers, consists of, on the fetal side, endothelium, mesenchyme, and trophoblast and, on the maternal side, an interstitial layer and the vascular endothelium. The contact area is increased by the development of villi which may or may not fuse to form folds or lamellae in order to maximize the area available for the exchange of oxygen, carbon dioxide, nutrients, and metabolic products across the interhemal barrier. A labyrinth is formed as the vascularized allantochorionic trophoblast layer envelopes the maternal sinusoids, and this is characterized by hypertrophied maternal endothelial cells (Figure 32.4E) which are most prominent in the mink.[63,122,123] This type of placenta is designated as deciduate.

Endotheliochorial placentation is characteristic of carnivores but is also found among a variety of other species: i.e. Proboscidae (elephant), Phocidae (seal), Tubulidentata (aardvarks), Rodentia (*Dipodomys*, the kangaroo rat), Insectivora (*Talpa*, the European mole), Bradypodidae (the three-toed sloth), and the short-tailed shrew (*Blarina brevicauda*).[2,62] Here, the cat and mink will be taken as examples.

Cat and mink

The allantochorionic placenta develops into a complete (cat) or incomplete (mink) belt or zonary placenta, subdivided into a labyrinth at the fetal side and a transitional or spongy zone towards the endometrial glandular zone.

In the mink, the villous pattern on the fetal side and the complementary maternal vascular crypts derived from the upper part of the uterine glands (Figure 32.4A–C) remain in a complex form throughout gestation. The maternal vessels, stem arteries as well as sinusoids, are enveloped by syncytio- and cytotrophoblast, surrounded and nurtured by a rich fetal capillary network, thus forming the labyrinth,[123] whereas in the cat it develops into the typical lamellar architecture although the initial development is similar to that of the mink.[124] In the mink, placentation is delayed and the termination of embryonic diapause seems to be dependent on LIF, which is expressed in uterine glandular epithelium just prior to implantation and ceases 2 days after implantation.[125]

Decidual-like cells or periendothelial cells

The maternal side of the interhemal barrier is composed of wide capillaries and giant decidual-like cells

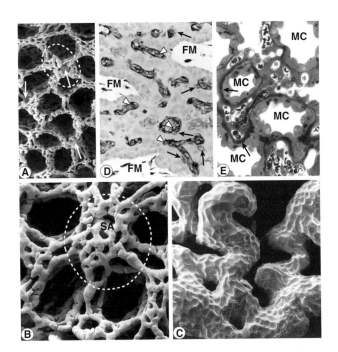

Figure 32.4   Endometrial characteristics of the endotheliochorial mink placenta. (**A,B**) Scanning electron micrographs taken at the same magnification clearly show that even at early stages of placentation the endometrial microvasculature differs between the paraplacental zone (**A**) and the placenta proper (**B**). (**A**) The abundance of endometrial glands leads to a honeycomb-like pattern of vascular supply with lobular complexes (indicated by a dashed line) and stem arteries (arrow). ×1000. (**B**) The same pattern of lobular complexes (dashed line) and stem arteries (SA) is maintained in the placental vascular architecture. However, the diameter of the capillaries and the number of branches has increased. ×1000. (**C**) Detail of the near-term placental labyrinth taken at the same magnification as (**A**) and (**B**) illustrates the extremely wide dimensions of the capillaries with prominent impressions of endothelial cells. ×1000. (**D**) Vimentin immunostaining shows that, apart from endothelial cells (arrowheads), maternal capillaries are surrounded by periendothelial cells (arrows). Capillaries in the fetal mesenchyme (FM) are also positive for vimentin. ×120. (**E**) A semithin section illustrates that maternal capillaries (MC) are delimited by large, protruding endothelial cells. A prominent interstitial layer (arrows) separates the syncytiotrophoblast from maternal endothelial cells. Fetal capillaries (asterisks) deeply indent the syncytiotrophoblast. ×120.

(Figure 32.4d), which are a typical feature in the cat,[126] less frequent in the dog, and smaller in size and only seen in the middle third of pregnancy in the mink.[127,128]

In the mink, these periendothelial cells have been identified by immunohistochemistry and transmission electron microscopy and named according to their location (see Figure 32.4D). They are strongly immunoreactive for α-smooth muscle actin and vimentin (see Figure 32.4D) and a similar reactivity is expressed in the decidual-like cells in cat placenta.[127,128] They are enclosed in the interstitial layer between the maternal endothelium and syncytial trophoblast, often deeply indenting the trophoblast layer. They are mainly present in the middle third of gestation and appear predominantly in the fetal and middle layer of the labyrinth, where they form a cellular ring around the maternal endothelium of the sinusoids. Near term they cannot be recognized. The periendothelial cells but not the endothelial cells of the mink placenta are immunoreactive for retinoid-binding proteins (Johansson, personal communication). The suggested function of the periendothelial cells in mink is therefore to participate in and control maternal placental blood flow and in placental uptake and metabolism of vitamin A.

Uterine vasculature

In the mature placenta, the wide maternal capillaries with prominent endothelial cells, most pronounced in the mink (Figure 32.4C), are delineated by an irregular interstitial layer enclosed by a layer of syncytiotrophoblast, a discontinuous layer of cytotrophoblast, and, at the mesenchymal side, a fine dense fetal capillary network in the placental labyrinth. The interstitial layer (Figure 32.4E), providing a separation between syncytiotrophoblast and maternal endothelium, is bridged in places by extensions from either syncytiotrophoblast or maternal endothelial cells.[127,129] In a review of morphological variations in the interhemal barrier,[63] the interspecies diversity in the thickness of the interstitial layer and bordering trophoblast of the endotheliochorial placenta has been demonstrated. The interstitial layer, typically found in carnivore placentas,[2,43] is presumably the result of a decidual response[130] following an immunological reaction.[130,131] However, decidual or periendothelial cells do not always persist throughout pregnancy, as the cat has giant decidual-like cells throughout gestation, whereas the dog and mink have few decidual-like (dog) or no periendothelial cells (mink) in the last third of gestation when the interstitial layer also increases in thickness. The suggestion that this thickening might be due to an immune response, in which the decidual cells are actively involved, might therefore be relevant to the cat, but not to the dog and mink; alternatively, the immune response may be independent of decidual-like cells in these last two species.

In the mink, the maternal placental stem arteries change abruptly as they pass from the endometrial glandular zone towards the placenta. They lose the smooth muscle cell layer as they grow towards or into

the allantochorion and the endothelial cells enlarge and protrude into the vascular lumen (Figure 32.4E).[122,127] These cells have a well-developed rough endoplasmic reticulum, small to medium-sized Golgi complexes, characteristic lipid droplets, and basally anchored cytoskeletal elements indicative of contractility. The maternal endothelial cells are thus highly differentiated, participating in the interhemal exchange of nutrients, regulation of vascular tone, and possibly protein and hormone synthesis. VEGF and its two receptors, VEGFR-1 (Flt-1) and VEGFR-2 (KDR), are co-localized in the mink placenta in maternal and fetal endothelial cells and uterine glandular epithelium,[133] indicating that VEGF acts on endothelial cells as well as on uterine glandular epithelium. Fibroblast growth factors are localized in endothelial and epithelial cells, while their receptors (FGFR) are detected in endothelial cells of the junctional zone in the placenta of the cat and the dog.[134] Expression of MMP-1, MMP-2, and MMP-13 in the cat placenta[135] indicates that degradation of ECM may allow the release of sequestered growth factors.

Uterine glands

The uterine glands are markedly increased beneath the zonary placenta as compared to when apposed to the smooth part of the allantochorionic sac, which might suggest that factors promoting growth and secretory activity, such as FGFs, are released from the placenta in a paracrine fashion.[134] The mucus produced by the glandular chambers may act as an immunoprotective barrier, since lectin binding demonstrated the presence of sialic acid and a mannose-rich glycoprotein.[136] These authors question the idea that the glandular secretions are a kind of histotroph, because the trophoblast cells neighboring the glandular chambers do not show features of endocytosis.

CONCLUSION

Developmental changes observed during placentation show that there is an interaction between the vasculature and uterine epithelium induced by the conceptus and that this interaction involves adaptations of the basal lamina, stromal cells, extracellular matrix, and immune cells. The regulatory mechanisms that define the distinct extent, shape, interdigitation, and vascular architecture of the materno–fetal interface in different species remain to be clarified. The uterine glands and their secretions seem to play an important role in the transfer of ions and vitamins and deserve special attention in order to understand how placentas with different interhemal barriers solve the transport problems of specific ions and larger molecules.

The role of cell differentiation in protecting the genetically foreign conceptus and providing adequate transfer of nutrients is regulated by a number of growth factors and their receptors. The understanding of how each species selects and utilizes a specific repertoire of factors to secure an efficient, sensitive interplay in the endometrial transformations that occur during placentation might give important information on mechanisms of vascular growth and tissue interaction which may turn out to be essential for research in tumor growth, tissue repair, and acceptance of transplants.

REFERENCES

1. Dantzer V. Epitheliochorial placentation. In: Knobil E, Neill J, eds. Encyclopedia of Reproduction. San Diego: Academic Press, 1999: 18–28.
2. Mossmann HW. Vertebrate Fetal Membranes. Basingstoke, UK: Macmillan, 1987.
3. Bazer FW, Ott TL, Spencer TE. Pregnancy recognition in ruminants, pigs and horses: signals from the trophoblast. Theriogenology 1994; 41: 79–94.
4. Dantzer V. Electron microscopy of the initial stages of placentation in the pig. Anat Embryol (Berl) 1985; 172: 281–93.
5. Stroband HW, Van der Lende T. Embryonic and uterine development during early pregnancy in pigs. J Reprod Fertil Suppl 1990; 40: 261–77.
6. Day WE, Bowen JA, Barhoumi R et al. Endometrial connexin expression in the mare and pig: evidence for the suppression of cell–cell communication in uterine luminal epithelium. Anat Rec 1998; 251: 277–85.
7. Dantzer V, Leiser R. Initial vascularisation in the pig placenta: I. Demonstration of nonglandular areas by histology and corrosion casts. Anat Rec 1994; 238: 177–90.
8. Dantzer V, Svendsen AM, Leiser R. Correlation between morphological events during the initial stages of placentation in the pig. In: Soma H, ed. Placenta: Basic Research for Clinical Application. Basel: Karger, 1991: 188–99.
9. Jones CJ, Dantzer V, Stoddart RW. Changes in glycan distribution within the porcine interhaemal barrier during gestation. Cell Tissue Res 1995; 279: 551–64.
10. Engelhardt H, Croy BA, King GJ. Conceptus influences the distribution of uterine leukocytes during early porcine pregnancy. Biol Reprod 2002; 66: 1875–80.
11. Persson E, Sahlin L, Masironi B et al. Insulin-like growth factor-I in the porcine endometrium and placenta: localization and concentration in relation to steroid influence during early pregnancy. Anim Reprod Sci 1997; 46: 261–81.
12. Leiser R, Dantzer V. Initial vascularisation in the pig placenta: II. Demonstration of gland and areola-gland subunits by histology and corrosion casts. Anat Rec 1994; 238: 326–34.
13. Keys JL, King GJ. Morphological evidence for increased uterine vascular permeability at the time of embryonic attachment in the pig. Biol Reprod 1988; 39: 473–87.
14. Keys JL, King GJ. Morphology of pig uterine subepithelial capillaries after topical and systemic oestrogen treatment. J Reprod Fertil 1995; 105: 287–94.
15. Biensen NJ, Wilson ME, Ford SP. The impact of either a Meishan or Yorkshire uterus on Meishan or Yorkshire fetal and placental development to days 70, 90, and 110 of gestation. J Anim Sci 1998; 76: 2169–76.
16. Ka H, Spencer TE, Johnson GA et al. Keratinocyte growth factor: expression by endometrial epithelia of the porcine uterus. Biol Reprod 2000; 62: 1772–8.
17. Dodgson SJ. Liver mitochondrial carbonic anhydrase, gluconeogenesis, and ureagenesis in the hepatocyte. In: Dodgson SJ, Tashian RE, Carter ND, eds. The Carbonic Anhydrases: Cellular Physiology and Molecular Genetics. New York: Plenum Press, 1991: 297–306.
18. Herbert JD, Coulson RA. A role for carbonic anhydrase in de novo fatty acid synthesis in liver. Ann NY Acad Sci 1984; 429: 525–7.
19. Saarnio J, Parkkila S, Parkkila AK et al. Immunohistochemical study of colorectal tumors for expression of a novel transmembrane carbonic anhydrase, MN/CA IX, with potential value as a marker of cell proliferation. Am J Pathol 1998; 153: 279–85.
20. Ridderstrale Y, Persson E, Dantzer V et al. Carbonic anhydrase activity in different placenta types: a comparative study of pig, horse, cow, mink, rat, and human. Microsc Res Tech 1997; 38: 115–24.
21. Persson E, Rodriguez-Martinez H. Immunocytochemical localization of growth factors and intermediate filaments during the establishment of the porcine placenta. Microsc Res Tech 1997; 38: 165–75.
22. Badinga L, Song S, Simmen RC et al. Complex mediation of uterine endometrial epithelial cell growth by insulin-like growth factor-II (IGF-II) and IGF-binding protein-2. J Mol Endocrinol 1999; 23: 277–85.
23. Freese LG, Rehfeldt C, Fuerbass R et al. Exogenous somatotropin alters IGF axis in porcine endometrium and placenta. Domest Anim Endocrinol 2005; 29: 457–75.
24. Nayak NR, Giudice LC. Comparative biology of the IGF system in endometrium, decidua, and placenta, and clinical implications for foetal growth and implantation disorders. Placenta 2003; 24: 281–96.
25. Rodriguez-Martinez H, Persson E, Hurst M et al. Immunohistochemical localization of platelet-derived growth factor receptors in the porcine uterus during the oestrous cycle and pregnancy. Zentralbl Veterinarmed A 1992; 39: 1–10.
26. Winther H, Ahmed A, Dantzer V. Immunohistochemical localization of vascular endothelial growth factor (VEGF) and its two specific receptors, Flt-1 and KDR, in the porcine placenta and non-pregnant uterus. Placenta 1999; 20: 35–43.
27. Charnock-Jones DS, Clark DE, Licence D et al. Distribution of vascular endothelial growth factor (VEGF) and its binding sites at the maternal–fetal interface during gestation in pigs. Reproduction 2001; 122: 753–60.
28. Bowen JA, Bazer FW, Burghardt RC. Spatial and temporal analyses of integrin and Muc-1 expression in porcine uterine epithelium and trophectoderm in vivo. Biol Reprod 1996; 55: 1098–106.
29. Ahmed A. Heparin-binding angiogenic growth factors in pregnancy: a review. Trophoblast Res 1997; 10: 215–58.
30. Gunin AG, Sharov AA. Role of mast cells in oestradiol effects on the uterus of ovariectomized rats. J Reprod Fertil 1998; 113: 61–8.
31. Zhang J, Nie G, Jian W et al. Mast cell regulation of human endometrial matrix metalloproteinases: a mechanism underlying menstruation. Biol Reprod 1998; 59: 693–703.
32. Bischof RJ, Brandon MR, Lee CS. Cellular immune responses in the pig uterus during pregnancy. J Reprod Immunol 1995; 29: 161–78.
33. King GJ. Reduction in uterine intra-epithelial lymphocytes during early gestation in pigs. J Reprod Immunol 1988; 14: 41–6.
34. Yu Z, Croy BA, King GJ. Lysis of porcine trophoblast cells by endometrial natural killer-like effector cells in vitro does not require interleukin-2. Biol Reprod 1994; 51: 1279–84.

35. Tayade C, Black GP, Fang Y et al. Differential gene expression in endometrium, endometrial lymphocytes, and trophoblasts during successful and abortive embryo implantation. J Immunol 2006; 176: 148–56.

36. Tayade C, Fang Y, Hilchie D et al. Lymphocyte contributions to altered endometrial angiogenesis during early and midgestation fetal loss. J Leukocyte Biol 2007; 82: 877–86. Epub 2007 Jul 18.

37. Lefevre F, Boulay V. A novel and atypical type one interferon gene expressed by trophoblast during early pregnancy. J Biol Chem 1993; 268: 19760–8.

38. Paulesu L, Cateni C, Romagnoli R et al. Variation in macrophage-migration-inhibitory-factor immunoreactivity during porcine gestation. Biol Reprod 2005; 72: 949–53.

39. Modric T, Kowalski AA, Green ML et al. Pregnancy-dependent expression of leukaemia inhibitory factor (LIF), LIF receptor-beta and interleukin-6 (IL-6) messenger ribonucleic acids in the porcine female reproductive tract. Placenta 2000; 21: 345–53.

40. Badinga L, Michel FJ, Fields MJ et al. Pregnancy-associated endometrial expression of antileukoproteinase gene is correlated with epitheliochorial placentation. Mol Reprod Dev 1994; 38: 357–63.

41. Reed KL, Blaeser LL, Dantzer V et al. Control of secretory leukocyte protease inhibitor gene expression in the porcine periimplantation endometrium: a case of maternal–embryo communication. Biol Reprod 1998; 58: 448–57.

42. Badinga L, Michel FJ, Simmen RC. Uterine-associated serine protease inhibitors stimulate deoxyribonucleic acid synthesis in porcine endometrial glandular epithelial cells of pregnancy. Biol Reprod 1999; 61: 380–7.

43. Amoroso EC. Placentation. In: Parkes AS, ed. Marshall´s Physiology of Reproduction. London: Longmans Green, 1952: 127–311.

44. Dantzer V. Scanning electron microscopy of exposed surfaces of the porcine placenta. Acta Anat (Basel) 1984; 118: 96–106.

45. Perry JS, Crombie PR. Ultrastructure of the uterine glands of the pig. J Anat 1982; 134: 339–50.

46. Palludan B, Wegger I, Moustgaard J. Placental transfer of iron. Yearbook, The Royal Veterinary and Agricultural University Copenhagen 1970: 62–91.

47. Buhi WC, Bazer FW, Ducsay CA et al. Iron content, molecular weight and possible function of the progesterone-induced purple glycoprotein of the porcine uterus. Fed Proc 1979; 38: 733.

48. Roberts RM, Bazer FW. The properties, function and hormonal control of synthesis of uteroferrin, the purple protein of the pig uterus. In: Beato M, ed. Steroid Induced Uterine Proteins. Amsterdam: Elsevier North Holland, 1980: 133–49.

49. Dantzer V, Nielsen MH. Intracellular pathways of native iron in the maternal part of the porcine placenta. Eur J Cell Biol 1984; 34: 103–9.

50. Raub TJ, Bazer FW, Roberts RM. Localization of the iron transport glycoprotein, uteroferrin, in the porcine endometrium and placenta by using immunocolloidal gold. Anat Embryol (Berl) 1985; 171: 253–8.

51. Dantzer V, Leiser R. Microvasculature of regular and irregular areolae of the areola-gland subunit of the porcine placenta: structural and functional aspects. Anat Embryol (Berl) 1993; 188: 257–67.

52. Harney JP, Ali M, Vedeckis WV et al. Porcine conceptus and endometrial retinoid-binding proteins. Reprod Fertil Dev 1994; 6: 211–19.

53. Johansson S, Dencker L, Dantzer V. Immunohistochemical localization of retinoid binding proteins at the materno–fetal interface of the porcine epitheliochorial placenta. Biol Reprod 2001; 64: 60–8.

54. Betteridge KJ. The structure and function of the equine capsule in relation to embryo manipulation and transfer. Equine Vet J Suppl 1989; 8: 92–100.

55. Enders AC, Liu IK. Lodgement of the equine blastocyst in the uterus from fixation through endometrial cup formation. J Reprod Fertil Suppl 1991; 44: 427–38.

56. Allen WR. Fetomaternal interactions and influences during equine pregnancy. Reproduction 2001; 121: 513–27.

57. Wooding FB, Flint AP. Placentation. In: Lamming GE, ed. Marshall´s Physiology of Reproduction, 4th edn. London: Chapman and Hall, 1994: 233–460.

58. Enders AC, Liu IK. Trophoblast–uterine interactions during equine chorionic girdle cell maturation, migration, and transformation. Am J Anat 1991; 192: 366–81.

59. Clegg MT, Boda JM, Cole HH. The endometrial cups and allantochorionic pouches in the mare with emphasis on the source of equine gonadotrophin. Endocrinology 1954; 54: 448–63.

60. Wooding FB, Morgan G, Fowden AL et al. A structural and immunological study of chorionic gonadotrophin production by equine trophoblast girdle and cup cells. Placenta 2001; 22: 749–67.

61. Vagnoni KE, Ginther OJ, Lunn DP. Metalloproteinase activity has a role in equine chorionic girdle cell invasion. Biol Reprod 1995; 53: 800–5.

62. Jones CJ, Wooding FB, Abd-Elnaeim MM et al. Glycosylation in the near-term epitheliochorial placenta of the horse, donkey and camel: a comparative study of interbreeding and non-interbreeding species. J Reprod Fertil 2000; 118: 397–405.

63. Enders AC, Blankenship TN, Lantz KC et al. Morphological variation in the interhemal areas of chorioallantoic placentae. A review. Trophoblast Res 1998; 12: 1–19.

64. Enders AC, Lantz KC, Schlafke S et al. New cells and old vessels: the remodeling of the endometrial vasculature during establishment of endometrial cups. Biol Reprod Suppl 1995; 1: 181–90.

65. Enders AC, Lantz KC, Schlafke S et al. Simultaneous exocrine and endocrine secretion: trophoblast and glands of the endometrial cups. J Reprod Fertil Suppl 2000; 56: 615–25.

66. Jones CJ, Enders AC, Wooding FP et al. Equine placental cup cells show glycan expression distinct from that of both chorionic girdle progenitor cells and early allantochorionic trophoblast of the placenta. Placenta 1999; 20: 347–60.

67. Allen WR. Immunological aspects of the endometrial cup reaction and the effect of xenogeneic pregnancy in horses and donkeys. J Reprod Fertil Suppl 1982; 31: 57–94.

68. Donaldson WL, Zhang CH, Oriol JG et al. Invasive equine trophoblast expresses conventional class I major histocompatibility complex antigens. Development 1990; 110: 63–71.

69. Grunig G, Triplett L, Canady LK et al. The maternal leukocyte response to the endometrial cups in horses is correlated with the developmental stages of the invasive trophoblast cells. Placenta 1995; 16: 539–59.

70. Lea RG, Stewart F, Allen WR et al. Accumulation of chromotrope 2R positive cells in equine endometrium during early pregnancy and expression of transforming growth factor-beta 2 (TGF-beta 2). J Reprod Fertil 1995; 103: 339–47.

71. Dantzer V, Leiser R. Areola-gland subunits in the epitheliochorial types of placentae from horse and pig. Micron Microsco Acta 1992; 23: 79–80.

72. Gerstenberg C, Allen WR, Stewart F. Cell proliferation patterns during development of the equine placenta. J Reprod Fertil 1999; 117: 143–52.

73. Jones CJ, Wooding FB, Dantzer V et al. A lectin binding analysis of glycosylation patterns during development of the equine placenta. Placenta 1999; 20: 45–57.

74. Jones CJ, Aplin JD. Glycans as attachment and signalling molecules at the fetomaternal interface. In: Paulesu RL, ed. Signal Molecules in Human and Animal Gestation. Kerala, India: Research Signpost, 2004: 1–21.

75. Han X, Rossdale PD, Ousey J et al. Localisation of 15-hydroxy prostaglandin dehydrogenase (PGDH) and steroidogenic enzymes in the equine placenta. Equine Vet J 1995; 27: 334–9.

76. Wooding FB, Morgan G, Fowden AL et al. Separate sites and mechanisms for placental transport of calcium, iron and glucose in the equine placenta. Placenta 2000; 21: 635–45.

77. Zavy MT, Sharp DC, Bazer FW et al. Identification of stage-specific and hormonally induced polypeptides in the uterine protein secretions of the mare during the oestrous cycle and pregnancy. J Reprod Fertil 1982; 64: 199–207.

78. Wooding FB. Current topic: the synepitheliochorial placenta of ruminants: binucleate cell fusions and hormone production. Placenta 1992; 13: 101–13.

79. Leiser R, Krebs C, Klisch K et al. Fetal villosity and microvasculature of the bovine placentome in the second half of gestation. J Anat 1997; 191: 517–27.

80. Kazemi M, Malathy PV, Keisler DH et al. Ovine trophoblast protein-1 and bovine trophoblast protein-1 are present as specific components of uterine flushings of pregnant ewes and cows. Biol Reprod 1988; 39: 457–63.

81. Guillomot M, Reinaud P, La Bonnardiere C et al. Characterization of conceptus-produced goat interferon tau and analysis of its temporal and cellular distribution during early pregnancy. J Reprod Fertil 1998; 112: 149–56.

82. Bazer FW, Thatcher WW, Hansen PJ et al. Physiological mechanisms of pregnancy recognition in ruminants. J Reprod Fertil Suppl 1991; 43: 39–47.

83. Thatcher WW, Danet-Desnoyers G, Wetzels C. Regulation of bovine endometrial prostaglandin secretion and the role of bovine trophoblast protein-1 complex. Reprod Fertil Dev 1992; 4: 329–34.

84. Asselin E, Drolet P, Fortier MA. In vitro response to oxytocin and interferon-tau in bovine endometrial cells from caruncular and inter-caruncular areas. Biol Reprod 1998; 59: 241–7.

85. Kamwanja LA, Hansen PJ. Regulation of proliferation of bovine oviductal epithelial cells by estradiol. Interactions with progesterone, interferon-tau and interferon-alpha. Horm Metab Res 1993; 25: 500–2.

86. Skopets B, Li J, Thatcher WW et al. Inhibition of lymphocyte proliferation by bovine trophoblast protein-1 (type I trophoblast interferon) and bovine interferon-alpha I1. Vet Immunol Immunopathol 1992; 34: 81–96.

87. Davidson JA, Betts JG, Tiemann U et al. Effects of interferon-tau and interferon-alpha on proliferation of bovine endometrial cells. Biol Reprod 1994; 51: 700–5.

88. Spencer TE, Johnson GA, Burghardt RC et al. Progesterone and placental hormone actions on the uterus: insights from domestic animals. Biol Reprod 2004; 71: 2–10.

89. Cassy S, Charlier M, Guillomot M et al. Cellular localization and evolution of prolactin receptor mRNA in ovine endometrium during pregnancy. FEBS Lett 1999; 445: 207–11.

90. Johnson GA, Spencer TE, Burghardt RC et al. Interferon-tau and progesterone regulate ubiquitin cross-reactive protein expression in the ovine uterus. Biol Reprod 2000; 62: 622–7.

91. Lacroix MC, Devinoy E, Cassy S et al. Expression of growth hormone and its receptor in the placental and feto–maternal environment during early pregnancy in sheep. Endocrinology 1999; 140: 5587–97.

92. Emond V, Asselin E, Fortier MA et al. Interferon-tau stimulates granulocyte–macrophage colony-stimulating factor gene expression in bovine lymphocytes and endometrial stromal cells. Biol Reprod 2000; 62: 1728–37.

93. Han VK, Carter AM. Spatial and temporal patterns of expression of messenger RNA for insulin-like growth factors and their binding proteins in the placenta of man and laboratory animals. Placenta 2000; 21: 289–305.

94. Robinson RS, Mann GE, Gadd TS et al. The expression of the IGF system in the bovine uterus throughout the oestrous cycle and early pregnancy. J Endocrinol 2000; 165: 231–43.

95. Keller ML, Roberts AJ, Seidel GE Jr. Characterization of insulin-like growth factor-binding proteins in the uterus and

96. Gadd TS, Osgerby JC, Wathes DC. Regulation of insulin-like growth factor binding protein-6 expression in the reproductive tract throughout the estrous cycle and during the development of the placenta in the ewe. Biol Reprod 2002; 67: 1756–62.

97. Chen C, Spencer TE, Bazer FW. Expression of hepatocyte growth factor and its receptor c-met in the ovine uterus. Biol Reprod 2000; 62: 1844–50.

98. Johnson GA, Burghardt RC, Bazer FW et al. Osteopontin: roles in implantation and placentation. Biol Reprod 2003; 69: 1458–71.

99. Kimmins S, Lim HC, MacLaren LA. Immunohistochemical localization of integrin $\alpha_V\beta_3$ and osteopontin suggests that they do not interact during embryo implantation in ruminants. Reprod Biol Endocrinol 2004; 2: 19.

100. Pfarrer C, Hirsch P, Guillomot M et al. Interaction of integrin receptors with extracellular matrix is involved in trophoblast giant cell migration in bovine placentomes. Placenta 2003; 24: 588–97.

101. Guillomot M. Changes in extracellular matrix components and cytokeratins in the endometrium during goat implantation. 1999; 20: 339–45.

102. Vagnoni KE, Zheng J, Magness RR. Matrix metalloproteinases-2 and -9, and tissue inhibitor of metalloproteinases-1 of the sheep placenta during the last third of gestation. Placenta 1998; 19: 447–55.

103. Walter I, Boos A. Matrix metalloproteinases (MMP-2 and MMP-9) and tissue inhibitor-2 of matrix metalloproteinases (TIMP-2) in the placenta and interplacental uterine wall in normal cows and in cattle with retention of fetal membranes. Placenta 2001; 22: 473–83.

104. Engelhardt H, King GJ. Uterine natural killer cells in species with epitheliochorial placentation. Nat Immun 1996–97; 15: 53–69.

105. Low BG, Hansen PJ, Drost M et al. Expression of major histocompatibility complex antigens on the bovine placenta. J Reprod Fertil 1990; 90: 235–43.

106. Staples LD, Heap RB, Wooding FB et al. Migration of leucocytes into the uterus after acute removal of ovarian progesterone during early pregnancy in the sheep. Placenta 1983; 4: 339–49.

107. Vander Wielen AL, King GJ. Intraepithelial lymphocytes in the bovine uterus during the oestrous cycle and early gestation. J Reprod Fertil 1984; 70: 457–62.

108. Davies CJ, Hill JR, Edwards JL et al. Major histocompatibility antigen expression on the bovine placenta: its relationship to abnormal pregnancies and retained placenta. Anim Reprod Sci 2004; 82–83: 267–80.

109. Choi Y, Johnson GA, Spencer TE et al. Pregnancy and interferon τ regulate major histocompatibility complex class I and β_2-microglobulin expression in the ovine uterus. Biol Reprod 2003; 68: 1703–10.

110. Kalenga MK, de Gasparo M, Thomas K et al. Angiotensin II and its different receptor subtypes in placenta and fetal membranes. Placenta 1996; 17: 103–10.

111. Nielsen AH, Schauser KH, Poulsen K. Current topic: the uteroplacental renin–angiotensin system. Placenta 2000; 21: 468–77.

112. Schauser KH, Nielsen AH, Winther H et al. Autoradiographic localization and characterization of angiotensin II receptors in the bovine placenta and fetal membranes. Biol Reprod 1998; 59: 684–92.

113. Schauser KH, Nielsen AH, Dantzer V et al. Angiotensin-converting enzyme activity in the bovine uteroplacental unit changes in relation to the cycle and pregnancy. Placenta 2001; 22: 852–62.

114. Pfarrer C, Ebert B, Miglino MA et al. The three-dimensional feto–maternal vascular interrelationship during early bovine

placental development: a scanning electron microscopical study. J Anat 2001; 198: 591–602.

115. Pfarrer C, Ruziwa SD, Winther H et al. Localization of vascular endothelial growth factor (VEGF) and its receptors VEGFR-1 and VEGFR-2 in bovine placentomes from implantation until term. Placenta 2006; 27: 889–98.

116. Bogic LV, Brace RA, Cheung CY. Developmental expression of vascular endothelial growth factor (VEGF) receptors and VEGF binding in ovine placenta and fetal membranes. Placenta 2001; 22: 265–75.

117. Bücher K, Leiser R, Tiemann U et al. Platelet-activating factor receptor (PAF-R) and acetylhydrolase (PAF-AH) are co-expressed in immature bovine trophoblast giant cells throughout gestation, but not at parturition. Prostaglandins Other Lipid Mediat 2006; 79: 74–83.

118. Pfarrer C, Weise S, Berisha B et al. Fibroblast growth factor (FGF)-1, FGF2, FGF7 and FGF receptors are uniformly expressed in trophoblast giant cells during restricted trophoblast invasion in cows. Placenta 2006; 27: 758–70.

119. Schuler G, Wirth C, Klisch K et al. Characterization of proliferative activity in bovine placentomes between day 150 and parturition by quantitative immunohistochemical detection of Ki67-antigen. Reprod Dom Anim 2000; 35: 157–62.

120. Dantzer V. Endotheliochorial placentation. In: Knobil E, Neill J, eds. Encyclodedia of Reproduction. San Diego: Academic Press, 1999: 1078–84.

121. Leiser R, Kaufmann P. Placental structure: in a comparative aspect. Exp Clin Endocrinol 1994; 102: 122–34.

122. Krebs C, Winther H, Dantzer V et al. Vascular interrelationships of near-term mink placenta: light microscopy combined with scanning electron microscopy of corrosion casts. Microsc Res Tech 1997; 38: 125–36.

123. Pfarrer C, Winther H, Leiser R et al. The development of the endotheliochorial mink placenta: light microscopy and scanning electron microscopical morphometry of maternal vascular casts. Anat Embryol (Berl) 1999; 199: 63–74.

124. Leiser R, Kohler T. The blood vessels of the cat girdle placenta. Observations on corrosion casts, scanning electron microscopical and histological studies. I. Maternal vasculature. Anat Embryol (Berl) 1983; 167: 85–93.

125. Song JH, Houde A, Murphy BD. Cloning of leukemia inhibitory factor (LIF) and its expression in the uterus during embryonic diapause and implantation in the mink (*Mustela vison*). Mol Reprod Dev 1998; 51: 13–21.

126. Leiser R, Koob B. Development and characteristics of placentation in a carnivore, the domestic cat. J Exp Zool 1993; 266: 642–56.

127. Winther H, Leiser R, Pfarrer C et al. Localization of micro- and intermediate filaments in non-pregnant uterus and placenta of the mink suggests involvement of maternal endothelial cells and periendothelial cells in blood flow regulation. Anat Embryol (Berl) 1999; 200: 253–63.

128. Winther H, Pfarrer C, Leiser R et al. Variation in expression of cytoskeleton filaments of the interhemal barrier in epithelio- and endotheliochorial placenta types. Placenta 1998; 19: A38.

129. Bäcklin BM, Persson E, Jones CJ et al. Polychlorinated biphenyl (PCB) exposure produces placental vascular and trophoblastic lesions in the mink (*Mustela vison*): a light and electron microscopic study. APMIS: Acta Pathol Microbiol Immunol Scand 1998; 106: 785–99.

130. Enders RK. Reproduction in the mink (*Mustela vison*). Proc Am Philos Soc 1952; 96: 696–741.

131. Malassine A. Evolution ultrastructurale du labyrinthe de placenta de chatte. Anat Embryol (Berl) 1974; 146: 1–20.

132. Wynn RM. Noncellular components of the placenta. Am J Obstet Gynecol 1969; 103: 723–39.

133. Winther H, Dantzer V. Co-localization of vascular endothelial growth factor and its two receptors flt-1 and kdr in the mink placenta. Placenta 2001; 22: 457–65.

134. Pfarrer C, Schuler G, Allen WR et al. Localisation of fibroblast growth factors (FGF) in placentae with differing degrees of trophoblast invasiveness. In: Sibbons PD, Wade JF, ed. Comparative Placentology. Victoria, Canada: R & W Communications, 2005: 8–11.

135. Walter I, Schonkypl S. Extracellular matrix components and matrix degrading enzymes in the feline placenta during gestation. Placenta 2006; 27: 291–306.

136. Grether BM, Friess AE, Stoffel MH. The glandular chambers of the placenta of the bitch in the second third of pregnancy (day 30–44): an ultrastructural, ultrahistochemical and lectinhistochemical investigation. Anat Histol Embryol 1998; 27: 95–103.

33 Innate and adaptive immunity in the human female reproductive tract: influence of the menstrual cycle and menopause on the mucosal immune system in the uterus

Charles R Wira, John V Fahey, Todd M Schaefer, Patricia A Pioli,
Charles L Sentman, and Li Shen

Synopsis

Background

- The mucosal surfaces of the female reproductive tract (FRT) defend it against pathogenic organisms.
- The reproductive tract is an inductive as well as a reactive site for immune responses.
- Immune protection must deal with sexually transmitted or opportunistic bacterial, fungal, and viral pathogens, while responding differently to allogeneic spermatozoa, and the immunologically distinct fetus.
- The mucosal defense function combines innate (antigen non-specific) and adaptive (antigen-specific) characteristics.
- The uterus contains immune cell types, including T and B cells, neutrophils, macrophages, dendritic cells, and natural killer (uNK) cells. Endometrial glandular and luminal epithelial cells also play an important role in immune defense.
- Cells of the innate immune system such as macrophages, dendritic cells, and uNK cells regulate the local adaptive immune system by presenting antigen and producing chemokines and cytokines. Epithelial cells can play similar roles.
- Neutrophils are also present (even in the absence of inflammatory change) and produce cytokines and remodeling enzymes. There is a large influx of neutrophils immediately prior to menstruation.

Basic Science

- Oval lymphoid aggregates, comprising B cells, T cells, and macrophages, are present in endometrial stroma. They arise by cell trafficking and are at their largest (3000–4000 cells) in the secretory phase, and absent after the menopause.
- Mature lymphoid aggregates contain a core of CD19+ B cells, surrounded by CD3+/CD4–/CD8+ – T cells and an outer mantle of CD14+ macrophages.
- The antigen-independent cytolytic activity of these T cells decreases in the secretory phase, suggesting hormonal or microenvironmental regulation.
- Secretory IgA traffics across the endometrial epithelium into the lumen where it increases in secretory phase and contributes to antimicrobial protection.
- IgG is also present: for example, instillation of attenuated polio vaccine into the uterus and vagina leads to the appearance of specific IgG in uterine secretions.
- Other epithelial apical secretions with known bactericidal effects are defensins, secretory leukocyte protease inhibitor (SLPI), the enzymes lysozyme and lactoferrin, and tracheal antimicrobial peptide.
- Production of these factors by epithelial cells can be stimulated by LPS-activated macrophages.
- Epithelial cells express toll-like receptors (TLR) that detect microbial pathogens, leading to the production of cytokine and chemokine secretions to attract inflammatory cells.
- Uterine epithelial cells recognize an analogue of viral dsRNA, probably through TLR3, and respond by both secreting and expressing intracellularly antiviral factors expected to inhibit HIV infection.

- Thus, for example, epithelial IL-8 and GM-CSF act synergistically to attract neutrophils.
- Macrophages and dendritic cells sample the lumen for microbes, thus contributing to immune surveillance.
- These factors contribute to making the normal uterine cavity a predominantly sterile environment.
- uNK cells seem to play multiple roles, contributing to tissue remodeling during pregnancy, interacting with migratory trophoblast, and producing cytokines to stimulate cell-mediated immunity.

Clinical

- The FRT is the target of more than 20 pathogens that are transmissible through sexual intercourse. Each year there are an estimated 340 million new cases of sexually transmitted infections (STIs).
- STIs include bacteria (group B streptococcus, *Neisseria gonorrhoeae*, *Chlamydia trachomatis*, *Treponema pallidum*), parasites (*Trichomonas vaginalis*), and viruses (herpes simplex virus, human papilloma virus, human immunodeficiency virus).
- With the recognition that the endometrium is an inductive site, the potential now exists to immunize the reproductive tract, as well as other mucosal sites, to obtain optimal T and B immune protection against STIs.
- A significant but as yet poorly defined proportion of infertility cases is likely to have an underlying immunological causation.

INTRODUCTION: INNATE AND ADAPTIVE IMMUNITY

The mucosal immune system in the female reproductive tract (FRT) and at other mucosal surfaces is the first line of defense against pathogenic organisms.[1–4] Of all the mucosal surfaces in the body, the FRT has unique requirements for regulation of immune protection since it must deal with sexually transmitted bacterial and viral pathogens, allogeneic spermatozoa, and the immunologically distinct fetus.[5–7] To accomplish this, the FRT has evolved immune mechanisms to protect against potential pathogens without compromising fetal survival. Failure of the immune system either to rid the reproductive tract of pathogens or to resist attacking allogeneic sperm and fetus significantly compromises procreation, as well as the health of the mother.

The immune system in mammals consists of innate and adaptive components that work cooperatively to protect the host from microbial (viral, bacterial, and fungal) infections. Innate immunity comprises antigen non-specific mechanisms that are inherent or act within the first few hours of encountering antigen. Examples include the physical barriers of the skin and mucous membranes that line the inner surfaces of the body (i.e. lungs, intestine, reproductive tract), the chemical barrier of pH, the proteins and lipids elaborated upon initial infection by infected or injured cells, and the leukocytes other than T and B cells that ingest and/or destroy pathogens. As seen in Figure 33.1, the innate immune system differs from the adaptive immune system in the cells involved (macrophages, dendritic cells [DCs], neutrophils, natural killer [NK] cells and epithelial cells), the type and specificity of receptors for antigen, the immediacy of response, and the nature of the response to antigenic challenge. This system is now recognized as the first line of defense, through which the body attempts to prevent and control the invasion of pathogens. Beyond immediate protection, cells of the innate immune system regulate the adaptive immune function through the production of chemokines and cytokines, as well as Class I, II, and co-stimulatory molecules for antigen presentation.

The innate immune system has evolved to recognize foreign structures that are not normally found in the host. It relies on conserved germ-line-encoded receptors that recognize conserved pathogen-associated microbial patterns (PAMPs) found in groups of microorganisms.[8,9] The pattern recognition receptors (PRRs) of the host that recognize PAMPs are expressed on cells of the innate immune system. Toll-like receptors (TLRs) are one group of PRRs that are essential mediators expressed on macrophages, DCs, and, as more recently shown, neutrophils, NK cells, and epithelial cells. Signaling through TLRs in response to PAMPs involves a number of adaptors and other molecules that lead to immune responses.[10] Members of the TLR family, of which at least 11 have been identified, recognize distinct PAMPs produced by various bacterial, fungal, and viral pathogens.[11–19]

Adaptive immunity encompasses pathogen (bacterial, viral, fungal)-specific defense mechanisms. An effective immune response to pathogens requires that antigen presenting cells (APCs) process antigen from the pathogen and present it to T cells, thereby inducing T-cell activation. Following antigen presentation,

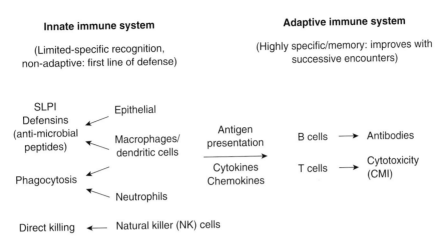

Figure 33.1   Elements of the mucosal immune system: innate and adaptive immunity.

lymphocyte effector functions, including cytokine production, cytotoxicity, and antibody synthesis, are activated. Protection is mediated, either through specific antibodies produced by B cells (humoral immunity) or the destruction of specific pathogens directly or indirectly by T cells (cell-mediated immunity). Cell surface proteins have been identified on T cells and are used routinely to identify all T cells (CD3) or T-cell subgroups that either help in the production of antibodies (CD4) or in the killing of infected cells (CD8). Re-exposure to a specific antigen results in a quicker response due to memory cells created during the clonal expansion.

Innate and adaptive immunity rarely operate singularly, but have evolved a variety of interactive mechanisms to protect the host from pathogens. For example, leukocytes (neutrophils, monocytes, macrophages, DCs) ingest, process, and present antigen to the T cells. In addition, lymphocytes and leukocytes have developed extensive lines of communication by the elaboration of soluble factors called chemokines (that attract immune cells to the site of infection) and cytokines (that stimulate and regulate the immune response) by which they help one another respond to viral and bacterial pathogens. The coordinated and complementary interplay between the cells of the immune system often determines the potential for and the extent of disease.

Although these cells are found in blood and in most tissues throughout the body, their presence has more recently been demonstrated in the human reproductive tract. While the emphasis on mucosal immunity has concentrated on the immune responses in the intestinal tract, recent studies have shown unequivocally that the FRT is an inductive site for specific and non-specific immune responses. Understanding the innate and adaptive immune systems in the reproductive tract[20] is essential because sexually transmitted infections (STIs) are a major worldwide health problem.[21,22] Despite

extensive efforts at control, only limited success has been achieved in dealing with a growing list of STIs, including herpes simplex virus type 2 (HSV-2), *Chlamydia trachomatis*, group B streptococcus, and acquired immunodeficiency syndrome (AIDS),[23] which devastate both adult and newborn. Recent studies indicate that heterosexual transmission of human immunodeficiency virus (HIV) is the major route of infection on a worldwide basis with documentation of male to female and female to male spread.[24,25] With the identification of HIV in semen and cervical secretions,[26–29] AIDS is recognized as a life-threatening STI.[30,31] By defining the mucosal immune system in the FRT and how the endocrine system controls mucosal immunity, a means may be devised to more effectively treat STIs.

Understanding the immune system in the FRT has particular importance in human infertility. Within the population of couples unable to have children, approximately 10% have underlying immunological problems.[32] A clear understanding of the regulation of the immune system in the FRT should provide a background against which immune problems can be resolved by endocrine therapy to permit a return to fertility. Alternatively, the immune system has potential for preventing fertilization. Of particular interest is the report of decreased fertility in female rats following oral feeding of sperm.[33,34] By choosing appropriate antigens and immunization protocols, the potential exists for using the immune system of the FRT to interfere with any number of stages throughout the reproductive process (gametogenesis to fertilization).

The following sections describe the mucosal immune system in the human FRT and its regulation by sex hormones and cytokines. Our focus will be to identify what is known about innate immunity in the uterus and to define the regulatory influences

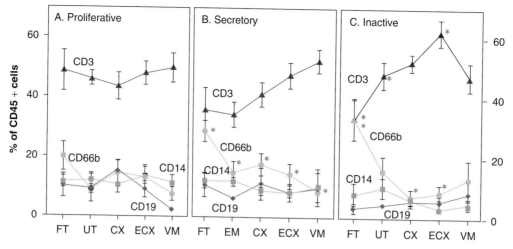

Figure 33.2   T cells (CD3), neutrophils (CD66b), monocytes (CD14), and B cells (CD19) at different stages of the cycle.[46] FT, Fallopian tube; UT, uterine endometrium; CX, endocervix; ECX, ectocervix; VM, vaginal mucosa.

that occur during the menstrual cycle and following menopause that contribute to protection from and susceptibility to potential pathogens. Each section is self-contained to include background information, significant new findings, and conclusions that can be drawn. We review the adaptive immune system (humoral and cellular responses) and then focus on the innate immune system to define the role of epithelial cells, macrophages, DCs, neutrophils, and NK cells, their functions and regulation during the menstrual cycle, and means of communication with the adaptive immune system. Lastly, emphasis will be placed on innate immunity as it relates to STIs, including HIV-1, the causative agent of AIDS.

OVERVIEW OF ADAPTIVE IMMUNITY IN THE UTERUS

Immune cells in the uterus

Leukocytes in the FRT play a central role in providing cellular, humoral, and innate immune protection against bacterial and viral invasion. Histological sections reveal immune cells that are sparsely and non-uniformly distributed in both the stromal layer and the epithelium.[35–38] Tissues can be dispersed by enzymatic or mechanical means for more quantitative flow cytometric or functional analyses. Past studies on dispersed cells from the FRT have emphasized the uterine endometrium.[39–41] Lymphocytes are a large proportion of the uterine endometrial leukocyte population.[36,39,40,42–45] In particular, NK cells and CD3+ T lymphocytes, including the CD4+ T helper cells and CD8+ T cytotoxic/suppressor cells, are the two major

leukocyte subsets, present at approximately 25% and 35–50%, respectively. Givan et al[46] extended the studies of others[36,39,40,42,45] to show that CD3+ T lymphocytes were present in substantial numbers, not only in the uterine endometrium but also throughout the FRT, including the ovary, Fallopian tube, uterine endometrium, endocervix, ectocervix, and vagina. Three-color FACS (fluorescence-activated cell sorter) analysis permitted the identification of the CD3+ T-cell subset as a percentage of leukocytes. Leukocytes were found to be 6–20% of the total number of cells within the FRT, where the uterine endometrium and Fallopian tube contained a higher proportion of leukocytes (mean of 14±2% in the uterine endometrium) relative to other sites within the FRT. As seen in Figure 33.2, T lymphocytes were a major constituent of reproductive tract leukocytes from all tissues. The Fallopian tube contained granulocytes as a second major constituent. Granulocytes were significantly less numerous in the other tissues. All tissues contained B lymphocytes and monocytes as clearly detectable but minor components. The proportions of leukocyte subsets in tissues from premenopausal women show only small differences related to stage of the menstrual cycle. Numbers of leukocytes were decreased in inactive endometrial samples relative to premenopausal samples, when analyzed on a percentage of total cells or per gram basis, possibly reflecting, in part, a decreased cellularity in postmenopausal endometrium.

Organization of immune cells in the uterus

Discrete lymphoid aggregates (follicles) in the uterine endometrium have been recognized by

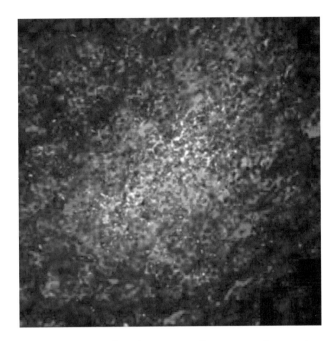

Figure 33.3 Triple-color immunofluorescent phenotyping of the cells in a uterine lymphoid aggregate. This photoplate consists of a single optical section through the center of a lymphoid aggregate in the uterine endometrium at the proliferative stage of the menstrual cycle. The three fluorochromes are T cells (Cy3-anti CD3, red), B cells (FITC anti CD19, green) and macrophages (Cy5-anti CD14, blue). (Adapted from Yeaman et al[48].) (see also Color Plate Section.)

histopathologists over many years (reviewed in Dahlenbach-Hellwig[35]) and were thought to occur in response to infection. Only recently[47,48] have these structures been shown to develop during the menstrual cycle independent of infection or malignancy. They are composed of predominantly B cells, T cells, and macrophages. Confocal scanning laser microscopy of vibratome-prepared endometrial tissue sections revealed aggregates of T cells. These aggregates were oval in shape and located between glands in the functionalis region. Lymphoid aggregates were composed of a B-cell core surrounded by T cells and an outer halo of macrophages. The B-cell core (CD19+) was most often seen in large aggregates present in the late proliferative and secretory stages of the cycle. Phenotypic analysis indicated that T cells are almost exclusively CD3+, CD8+, and CD4−. Cells of the CD3+CD4+ phenotype were also present but were usually located outside the aggregates in the stroma. Monocytes/macrophages (CD14+ cells) were found as a mantle around the T cells. The size of lymphoid aggregates was found to vary with the stage of the menstrual cycle.[48] As shown in Figure 33.3, aggregates were significantly larger during the secretory

(3000–4000 cells) than the proliferative stage (300–400 cells). The absence of aggregates in uteri from postmenopausal women provided further evidence that these aggregates are under hormonal control. The distribution and frequency of CD8+ T cells in aggregates using expression of Vβ2 or Vβ8 as markers of clonality and Ki-67 as marker of dividing cells was investigated,[49] leading to the conclusion that lymphoid aggregates form largely by the trafficking of cells to nucleation sites within the endometrium, rather than by division of precursor cells.

Humoral immunity

The humoral immune system in the FRT has evolved to protect against potential pathogens without compromising fetal survival. Immunoglobulins (Igs) and plasma cells are present in the female reproductive tract of various species.[6,50] In the human, lymphocytes and/or plasma cells are distributed throughout the reproductive tract with low numbers present in the uterus and vagina.[51–53] Depending on the tissue analyzed and the species involved, IgA and IgG may be either synthesized locally and/or of serum origin.[52,54] Levels of IgA and IgG in the rat uterus and vagina are regulated by female sex hormones.[55–58] These effects are tissue specific in that levels of IgA and IgG were elevated in the uterus and lowered in cervical–vaginal secretions in response to estradiol.[58–61] In humans, the amount of IgA and IgG in the uterus varies with the stage of the menstrual cycle, as well as with anatomical location.[62] IgG levels in secretions from the uterine mucosa were highest during the periovulatory phase, whereas levels in the Fallopian tube were lowest at that time. IgA and IgG levels in cervical secretions also vary with the stage of the menstrual cycle, with lowest levels measured at mid cycle.[63] Suppression of IgA and IgG throughout the menstrual cycle was observed when women were treated with oral contraceptives.

Polarized epithelial cells synthesize the polymeric immunoglobulin receptor (pIgR) which traffics to the basolateral surface where it binds polymeric IgA and IgM. Following endocytosis, the pIgR–Ig complex translocates to the apical surface and undergoes proteolytic cleavage. Polymeric Ig bound with secretory component (SC), the external domain of pIgR, is released into secretions.[64] In the uterus, endometrial gland cells stain strongly for IgA and SC.[54,65] SC action at mucosal surfaces results in immunological protection in the FRT because secretory IgA (IgA bound to SC) prevents microbial invasion.[66] It has been suggested that SC may also be capable of immunological suppression by inhibiting both lymphocyte proliferation[67] and immunoglobulin production.[68] The female sex hormones estradiol and progesterone have profound effects on the local immunoglobulin production and transport in the rodent[69,70] and human reproductive tracts.[71,72] When cultured human endometrial cells are incubated with interleukin-4 (IL-4) and interferon γ (IFNγ), the presence of estrogen increases the expression of pIgR, thereby increasing the transport of IgA into the lumen.[57,73] Normal epithelial cells produce SC, which accumulates preferentially in the apical compartment and correlates with increased transepithelial resistance.[61,74,75] Epithelial cells from endocervix and ectocervix, but not the vagina, also showed preferential production and release of SC into the apical chamber. These results suggest that uterine and cervical epithelial cells play a key regulatory role in the control of IgA transcytosis from tissue into secretions.

In concert with these SC variations, uterine intraepithelial content of IgA is also known to rise during the secretory phase of the menstrual cycle.[52–54,76] This IgA accumulation is most likely regulated by SC, which binds specifically to polymeric IgA.[64] However, uterine secretion of IgA appears to peak at around the time of ovulation,[63] whereas we have demonstrated that luminal SC levels remain relatively elevated throughout the secretory phase. Since SC controls IgA movement into external secretions, one might expect enhanced IgA secretion throughout the latter half of the menstrual cycle. One possible reason for this apparent discrepancy involves the availability of uterine IgA for transfer. In normal endometria, the numbers of IgA-containing plasma cells are low.[52–54,76] During the time of ovulation, though, levels of stromal IgA increase.[53] This process appears to be due to the estrogen-induced transudation of serum IgA into the uterus.[77,78] Thus, with increased levels of both IgA and SC at ovulation, IgA secretion would be expected to ensue. Our data from a rat uterine model support this hypothesis.[57,79]

Cell-mediated immune responses

Antiviral cytotoxic T-lymphocyte (CTL) responses in the lower female genital tract were first reported using the rhesus macaque model.[80] In humans, Musey et al[81] used cervical cytobrush specimens from HIV-1 infected women to develop T-cell lines. These studies demonstrated that cervical class I major histocompatibility complex (MHC)-restricted CD8+ and class II MHC-restricted CD4+ CTL could lyse autologous targets made to express HIV-1 proteins. This study demonstrated antigen-specific CTL responses within the human endometrium.

White et al[82] used hysterectomy specimens that contained CD3+CD8+ T lymphocytes to demonstrate cytolytic function in the Fallopian tube, uterine endometrium, endocervix, ectocervix, and vagina. Cytolytic function was demonstrable when freshly isolated unfractionated cell populations from the reproductive tract were cultured overnight in medium containing low concentrations of IL-2 prior to use in an antigen-independent anti-CD3 mAb-mediated lysis assay system to measure cytolytic potential. Cytolytic activity was specific for CD3+ T cells and was distinct from NK cell or FcγRIII+ cell-mediated cytolytic activity.[82,83] Selective antibody-mediated lysis of lymphocyte populations indicated that CTL activity is mediated by CD8+ T cells. To determine the potential for hormonal control, CTL activity was analyzed in tissues from patients at various stages of the menstrual cycle and following menopause. Women at the proliferative stage (low–increasing levels of estradiol, low levels of progesterone) of the menstrual cycle at the time of hysterectomy displayed uterine CTL activity that was low but significantly higher than the barely detectable activity found in uterine samples during the secretory phase (high levels of estradiol and progesterone) of the cycle.[82] In contrast, CTL activity in uteri from postmenopausal women was significantly greater than that seen in premenopausal tissues irrespective of stage of the menstrual cycle. These studies led to the conclusion that CTL activity in the uterus is under hormonal control since CTL activity was highest when levels of hormones were low; conversely, CTL activity was either low or not detectable during the secretory stage of the cycle when estradiol and progesterone are elevated in blood. The absence of CD8+ T-cell lytic activity in the uterus occurred at a time when fertilization and implantation would take place and thus may be a mechanism by which allogeneic fetal cells at the maternal–fetal interface avoid recognition and rejection by maternal uterine CD8+ T cells. The presence of CD3+CD8+ T cells in the uterus throughout the menstrual cycle suggested that estradiol and/or progesterone down-regulate CTL activity by means other than cell trafficking. The finding that down-regulation of CTL activity occurred at a time when uterine lymphoid aggregates were largest suggested that localized suppression of CTL function is a consequence of lymphoid aggregate formation; this, however, remains to be established. In contrast to the uterine endometrium, CTL activity remained high in the cervix and vagina regardless of endocrine state.[82,83] This discrete compartmentalization of CTL activity led to the hypothesis that the continued presence of high lytic potential serves as a protective immunological barrier.[82,83]

INDUCTION OF IMMUNE RESPONSES IN THE UTERUS

Background

The maintenance of health is dependent on local immune responses at mucosal surfaces to potentially infectious and toxic agents. Innate mucosal immune responses can lead to antigen processing and presentation of potential pathogens in the local environment to confer adaptive immune protection. Ogra and Ogra made the seminal observation that instillation of attenuated polio vaccine into the uterus and vagina leads to specific IgG antibody in uterine and cervical secretions.[84]

Initial steps in the development of an adaptive immune response are the uptake, processing, and presentation of antigenic fragments by antigen-presenting cells (APCs) to T cells (see Trombetta and Mellman[85] for review). At mucosal surfaces, APCs such as DCs can contact antigen by extending podia between epithelial cells to sample the luminal contents for potential pathogens.[86] Antigen can also be taken up by epithelial cells and, with or without processing to antigenic fragments, extruded to APCs below the epithelial barrier. Once inside an APC, antigen is 'processed' by enzymes to produce fragments that are transported to the cell surface where they are presented to T cells in association with MHC class I, class II, or CD1 molecules to T lymphocytes.[87–89] Activated T cells regulate the humoral immune response to antigen, often by stimulating, directly and indirectly, B cells to produce antigen-specific immunoglobulins. Interactions among APCs, T cells, and B cells are enhanced by accessory molecules as well as cytokines. In addition to DCs, APCs in the endometrium include macrophages, B cells, and epithelial cells.[46]

The innate and adaptive immune systems are linked by several mechanisms, particularly via TLRs. For example, innate immune cells, including epithelial cells, have TLRs that bind to potential pathogens and stimulate the synthesis and secretion of chemokines and cytokines that attract and activate APCs, T cells, and B cells. In the absence of TLR-induced inflammatory cytokines, T-cell activation does not occur.[90] TLRs are also responsible for the induction of DC maturation,[91] which is required for processing and presentation of antigen. Another mechanism of TLR-mediated activation of T-cell responses is the blocking of suppression by regulatory T cells.[90] Pesare and Medzhitov recently showed that T-dependent antigen-specific antibody responses require activation of TLRs in B cells.[92] Thus, TLR involvement in adaptive immunity is mediated through several mechanisms and involves several cells. For this reason, inclusion of TLR ligands in vaccines has been invaluable.[93]

Among mucosal tissues, the uterus is unique in that sex steroid hormones modulate both efferent and afferent immune responses. Therefore, immune responses such as those engendered by APCs and other various immune reactions dependent upon cell interaction are modulated by stage of the reproductive cycle and pregnancy. In the rat, antigen presentation is under endocrine control and varies with the stage of the reproductive cycle. When given to ovariectomized rats, estradiol enhanced antigen presentation in the uterus[94,95] and inhibited antigen presentation in the vagina.[96] Estradiol inhibited antigen presentation in the vagina without affecting the number of class II positive cells and at a time when macrophages/DCs/granulocytes increase in response to estradiol treatment.[97] In response to estradiol, isolated uterine and vaginal epithelial cells inhibit stromal antigen presentation by secreting transforming growth factor β (TGFβ).[98,99] More recently, we extended these studies by using T cells from transgenic mice specific for the class II MHC-restricted OVA[323–339] peptide and found that freshly isolated uterine epithelial, uterine stromal, and vaginal APCs present ovalbumin to naïve and memory T cells.[100] Estradiol given to ovariectomized rats and mice inhibits antigen presentation by stromal APCs from the uterus and vagina. In contrast, whereas mouse uterine epithelial cell antigen presentation is inhibited, rat epithelial cell antigen presentation is stimulated by estradiol.[101] Several studies have shown that human and murine uterine epithelial and stromal cells express class II molecules, which are essential for class II-mediated presentation of antigen, and that class II expression is modulated by sex hormones.[95,102–104] In other studies, we found that IL-6 enhances antigen presentation by epithelial and mixed stromal cells when placed in the lumen of ovariectomized rats[94] and that hepatocyte growth factor or stromal conditioned media increases antigen presentation by polarized mouse epithelial cells in culture. These results demonstrate that antigen presentation in the female reproductive tract is regulated by sex hormones and soluble factors of stromal origin.

In previous studies, we examined mixed cell suspensions from throughout the human female reproductive tract and found that they contained cells capable of presenting antigen to autologous T cells.[105] Uterine cells isolated from several patients at different stages of the menstrual cycle and at menopause demonstrated significant antigen presentation. In contrast to the uterus, mixed cell populations isolated from Fallopian tube, cervix, and ectocervix were less likely to present antigen. One explanation for why antigen presentation occurs in some tissues and not in others may be that APCs migrate in and out of the FRT in a pattern that is hormonally dependent. To more fully characterize the immune system in the human FRT, uterine epithelial and stromal cells from a hysterectomy patient were purified to assess the capacity of these cells to present antigen. Irradiated epithelial cells or stromal cells co-cultured with T cells and tetanus toxoid induced autologous T-cell proliferation in comparison to cultures without tetanus toxoid.[104] Proliferation was significant, suggesting that both purified epithelial cells and stromal cells were capable of antigen presentation to autologous T cells.

New findings

Antigen presentation by human uterine epithelial cells

Endometrial epithelial cells were purified after hysterectomy, irradiated, and co-cultured with autologous T cells isolated from peripheral blood and with or without tetanus toxoid (TT), a common immunization protein, for 4 days. The uptake of a 1-day pulse of ^{3}H-thymidine into activated T cells was measured as an indication of antigen presentation. The epithelial cells presented TT to T cells as shown by an increase in radiolabeled thymidine in co-cultures incubated with tetanus compared to those cultured without the toxoid. In the absence of antigen, T-cell proliferation was present but well below the level seen with TT. The antigen-presenting ability of myeloid cells was compared with that of the endometrial epithelial cells. Peripheral blood mononuclear cells (PBMCs) were irradiated and incubated with the autologous purified T cells and TT and incorporation of radiolabeled thymidine was assessed. Antigen presentation was typically 10-fold greater for myeloid APCs compared to that of the epithelial cells. Results shown in Figure 33.4 are representative of the patients in this study.[106]

Expression of CD40 and CD1d on human uterine epithelial cells

MHC class II is up-regulated by IFNγ in human uterine epithelial cells,[104] in addition to which there

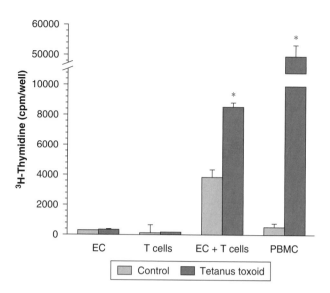

Figure 33.4 Antigen presentation by human uterine epithelial cells. Uterine epithelial cells (EC) were isolated and purified from the proliferative phase endometrium of a hysterectomy patient and irradiated. T cells were isolated from the blood of the same patient and purified over a T-cell column. EC and/or T cells were incubated with or without 10 μg/ml tetanus toxoid for 4 days; ^{3}H-thymidine was added to the wells for the last 24 hours of each incubation. The increase in radiolabeled thymidine uptake in the co-incubation with toxoid compared to without the antigen represents antigen presentation by the EC to autologous T cells. Antigen presentation by peripheral blood mononuclear cells (PBMC) is included as a relative comparison to the EC antigen presentation. Values shown represent the mean and SEM of quadruplicate cultures. *, Significantly ($p < 0.01$) different from EC + T cells without tetanus toxoid. (Adapted from Fahey et al[106].)

is expression of other molecules needed for antigen presentation. CD40–CD40 ligand interactions function in the adaptive immune response to enhance inflammatory response markers, including cell adhesion molecules, cytokines, matrix-degrading enzymes, and apoptotic mediators.[107] In addition, CD40 on DCs can bind to CD154 on T cells and induce increased expression of MHC on the DC surface. Using confocal microscopy, we have found expression of CD40 on human uterine epithelial cells, which suggests that the epithelial cells can activate T cells for antigen presentation. Epithelial CD40 has been shown to be up-regulated in certain cancers and with IFNγ treatment.[108] Interestingly, innate immune activation induced by CD40 ligation has been implicated in early pregnancy loss, and was related to endocrine dysfunction.[109] CD1 proteins are another family of antigen-presenting molecules that bind bacterial and lipid antigens for presentation to T cells.[89] The CD1 gene family encodes non-polymorphic MHC class I molecules that present primarily non-peptide antigens to T cells. One member of the CD1 family, CD1d, interacts with an effector T-cell subset that may promote the development of Th2-mediated responses associated with pregnancy.[110] CD1d has been shown to be expressed on dendritic cells, B cells, hepatocytes, intestinal epithelial cells,[111] trophoblast cell lines,[110] and mouse endometrial epithelial cells.[112] Cultured human uterine epithelial cells also express CD1d, suggesting they have the potential to present lipid antigens and interact with CD8 + or double-negative T cells.

Conclusions

The endometrium is an inductive site for mucosal immune responses. The antigen presentation results may have particular importance from the standpoint of inducing protection against STIs, including HIV. With the growing interest in vaccines to enhance mucosal immune responses, our findings suggest that potential pathogens or vaccines in the reproductive tract may be important determinants in eliciting immune protection. With the recognition that the endometrium is an inductive site, the potential now exists to immunize the reproductive tract, as well as other mucosal sites, to obtain optimal T and B immune protection. The diversity of APCs, antigen-presentation molecules, and T cells in the endometrium enables a variety of immune responses to protect the host against the plethora of antigens and antigen types. The ability of uterine epithelial cells to present antigen to T cells further demonstrates that these multitasking cells are vital for health and reproduction.

ROLE OF UTERINE EPITHELIAL CELLS IN IMMUNE PROTECTION

Background

Mucosal epithelial cells contribute in many ways to immune protection in the endometrium (see Wira et al[101] and Wira and Fahey[113] for review). Uterine epithelial cells form an uninterrupted mucosal barrier between the lumen and underlying cells and prevent pathogenic microbes from infiltrating the body. Disruption of the tight junctions or damage to the epithelial layer can lead to infection. With an apical surface to the lumen and a basolateral surface to the basement membrane and underlying cells, epithelial cells have a structurally and functionally polarized

orientation. The tight junction prevents the mixing of apical and basolateral contents, and permits the epithelial cells to respond to different stimuli and serve as a directional conduit. For example, SC and pIgR traverse the epithelium from the basolateral to the apical side to release IgA into the lumen.[20] In addition, uterine epithelial cells reportedly secrete cytokines such as TGFβ preferentially at the basolateral surface and tumor necrosis factor α (TNFα) at the apical surface.[114]

Since the adaptive immune system at mucosal surfaces may take days to be activated and effective against pathogens, initial innate protective mechanisms are available and essential for health.[101] One such mechanism is the production of soluble factors by FRT epithelial cells that inhibit the growth of microorganisms. Among the epithelial cell secretions with known bactericidal effects are defensins, secretory leukocyte protease inhibitor (SLPI), the enzymes lysozyme and lactoferrin, tracheal antimicrobial peptide, and numerous other small peptides (for review, see Ganz and Lehrer[115]). Human α-defensin-5 was shown with an apical orientation on uterine epithelial cells, suggesting secretion mode.[116] Human β-defensin 1 (HBD1) expression has also been shown in situ[117] and in cultured epithelial cells.[118] HBD3 mRNA is highest during the secretory phase of the menstrual cycle, while HBD4 mRNA levels peak in the proliferative phase.[119] Other studies showed that SLPI varies in cervical mucus during the menstrual cycle, increases in amniotic fluid during gestation and labor,[120] and is secreted by cervical tissue in response to progesterone.[121] The primary site of SLPI synthesis in the endometrium and decidua was the glandular epithelium, and tissues derived from women in late secretory phase produced higher SLPI levels than tissues obtained from women in the proliferative phase.[122,123] The expression of endometrial SLPI has been shown to be up-regulated by estrogen in the rat,[124] and by progesterone in the Rhesus monkey[125] and human.[121] Perhaps one reason that the endometrium maintains a predominantly sterile environment is due to the production of antimicrobial factors such as defensins and SLPI.[101,126]

The endometrium is characterized by progressive tissue growth and remodeling which occurs during each menstrual cycle, and cell proliferation, apoptosis, and cell migration are essential for reproductive tract renewal to occur. Growth in preparation for fertilization, implantation, and successful pregnancy is mediated by a changing pattern of chemokine, cytokine, and adhesion molecule expression that is regulated by the sex steroid hormones.[127–129] Kaysili and associates reported on the importance of IL-8 and monocyte chemotactic protein 1 (MCP-1) in normal uterine physiology, particularly in proliferation, angiogenesis, menstruation, implantation, cervical ripening, and parturition.[130] The chemokines and cytokines regulate production of themselves and other chemokines/cytokines by autocrine and paracrine mechanisms. Also, sex hormones exert control over many chemokines/cytokines in the FRT. For example, progesterone withdrawal results in up-regulation of MCP-1 and IL-8, leading to chemotaxis and activation of monocytes and neutrophils, which results in release and activation of matrix metalloproteinases (MMPs) for initiation of menstruation.[131] Thus, concentrations of chemokines and cytokines will vary in the endometrium during normal physiological processes, as well as pathological conditions such as infection. Excessive production of chemokines and cytokines by uterine epithelial cells may contribute to pathological conditions during pregnancy. A correlation between elevated concentrations of IL-6, IL-8, and MCP-1 and amniotic microbial infection has been found in cervicovaginal fluid and amniotic fluids from patients in preterm labor and premature rupture of membranes.[132–134] Romero and colleagues reported on the association between bacterial vaginosis and preterm birth and demonstrated compelling evidence for TNFα in preterm parturition associated with infection.[135] Simhan and colleagues found that low cervical fluid concentrations of IL-1β, IL-8, and IL-6 correlated with clinical chorioamnionitis in early pregnancy.[136] They concluded that low concentrations of multiple cytokines indicated a broad immune hyporesponsiveness that could create a permissive environment for ascending infection. Indeed, they further suggested that concentration ranges of some immune factors in female reproductive tract fluids are necessary for a healthy pregnancy; too low indicates susceptibility to infection and too high suggests that there is a dangerous infection.

New findings

We have explored the potential for primary human uterine epithelial cells to produce endogenous microbicides. TLR stimulation of uterine epithelial cells induces the mRNA expression of the antimicrobial peptides HBD1 and HBD2[137] and IL-1β stimulates HBD2.[138] In addition, the inhibition by estradiol of the IL-1β-induced HBD2 increase was due to the down-regulation of IL-receptor type 1. Estradiol reduction

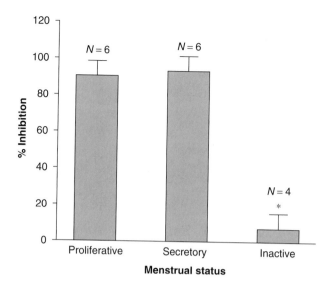

Figure 33.5 Effect of menstrual status on the antibacterial activity of human uterine epithelial cells derived from 16 women. Epithelial cells were grown to confluence and high transepithelial resistance in cell inserts and then cultured for 24 hours without medium in the apical chamber. Rinses of the apical chamber were then incubated for 1 hour with *Staphylococcus aureus* before plating to count bacterial colonies. The mean colony-forming units from 4 cell inserts from each patient were compared with controls to determine percent inhibition for that patient. The mean inhibition ±SD of each menstrual group is shown. *, Significantly ($p < 0.001$) lower than antibacterial activity of proliferative and secretory groups.[139]

of IL-1β responses may be important for dampening proinflammatory responses during ovulation or pregnancy. In other studies, as shown in Figure 33.5, apical secretions from polarized epithelial cells recovered from women at the proliferative and secretory stages of the menstrual cycle, but not from postmenopausal women, were equally effective in killing *Staphylococcus aureus*; similar results were obtained when *Escherichia coli* was used.[139] Further, SLPI production correlated with bactericidal activity with respect to menstrual status and time in culture, and anti-SLPI antibody significantly decreased bactericidal activity from premenopausal epithelial cells.

Human uterine epithelial cell lines express TLR capable of recognizing specific structural components of bacterial, fungal, and viral pathogens.[137,140–142] Addition of the TLR2 and TLR5 agonists zymogen and flagellin to ECC-1 endometrial epithelial cells stimulated the production of the chemokines IL-8 and MCP-1, respectively, as well as the cytokine IL-6.[140] Cultured primary human uterine epithelial cells express TLR 1 through 9, indicating the potential to respond to a wide range of potential pathogens.[137] The TLR3 agonist poly (I:C) and/or LPS stimulated the uterine epithelial cells to secrete several proinflammatory cytokines and chemokines. In addition to cytokines and chemokines, the TLR3-mediated stimulation with poly (I:C) of uterine epithelial cells induced the mRNA expression of IFNβ and the IFNβ-stimulated antiviral genes myxovirus resistance gene 1 and 2′,5′-oligoadenylate synthetase.[137] The chemokine/cytokine response to double-stranded RNA viruses, which can be nuclear factor κB (NF-κB)-independent, suggests that uterine epithelial cells possess the inherent capability to respond to RNA viruses.

We have demonstrated the secretion of the chemokines IL-8, MCP-1, macrophage inflammatory protein 1β (MIP-1β), and the cytokines IL-6, TNFα, granulocyte colony-stimulating factor (G-CSF), granulocyte–macrophage colony-stimulating factor (GM-CSF), and macrophage migration inhibitory factor (MIF) by uterine epithelial cell lines and primary cells.[137,140,143,144] Figure 33.6 shows the constitutive secretion of seven chemokines and cytokines by human uterine female reproductive tract epithelial cells.[143] Unsolicited chemokines and cytokines in secretions of the female reproductive tract tissues would allow, for immediate responsiveness to pathogenic microbes, both as microbicides and activators of immune cells, should a breech of the epithelial barrier occur. In addition, several chemokines and cytokines have effects on proliferation and apoptosis that may contribute to maintenance of normal FRT architecture and environments. Also, the epithelial factors may contribute to the quantity and type of immune cells trafficking in FRT tissues,[46] the formation of uterine lymphoid aggregates,[48] and the sampling of luminal fluids for pathogenic microbials by leukocytes.[86]

Several epithelial cell secreted factors are predominantly known for their chemotactic effect on leukocytes. For example, IL-8 and MCP-1 are potent chemokines for neutrophils[145] and monocytes,[146] respectively. Most pertinent is that we have demonstrated that the secretions from the cultured uterine epithelial cells characterized in this study have been shown to attract neutrophils[147] and monocytes.[148] The concentrations of IL-8 and MCP-1 in the FRT epithelial cell secretions were sufficient to achieve maximum effects in standard chemotaxis assays compared to recombinant chemokine. In addition, the chemotactic activity for neutrophils or monocytes was effectively removed by preincubation of the epithelial secretions with specific neutralizing antibodies to either IL-8 or MCP-1, respectively.

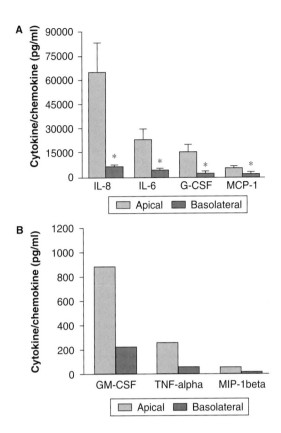

Figure 33.6 The 48 hour accumulation of chemokines and cytokines secreted by polarized human uterine epithelial cells grown to confluence and high transepithelial resistance in cell inserts from six patients. The apical and basolateral conditioned media from a minimum of 4 inserts derived from each patient were collected separately and analyzed by Luminex technology. The mean values for (A) IL-8, IL-6, G-CSF, and MCP-1 and (B) GM-CSF, TNFα, and MIP-1β from each patient's cells were then used to determine the mean concentrations ±SEM. *, Significantly ($p < 0.05$) different from apical values.[143]

Conclusions

Uterine epithelial cells produce a variety of microbicidal substances (β-defensins, MIP-3α, SLPI, etc.) that serve links between the adaptive and innate immune systems.[143] Furthermore, epithelial cells express TLRs that detect microbial pathogens.[137,140–142] Finally, uterine epithelial cells are involved, through their cytokine and chemokine secretions, in normal physiological processes such as menstruation and receptivity. Therefore, these cells act as sentinels against pathogenic assault, promote normal reproductive tract physiology, and play an essential role in regulating immunity to provide for a healthy mother and allogeneic conceptus/fetus.

Uterine epithelial cells show a preferential secretion of most proinflammatory chemokines and cytokines to the apical compartment of cell inserts. There are several potential benefits. Luminal secretions of natural microbicides in the upper FRT tissues can wash down to protect the cervix and vagina. These epithelial factors, which are modulated by sex hormones, undoubtedly contribute to the resident and temporary populations of immune cells in the subepithelial layers of the endometrium. For example, the chemokines produced by the epithelial cells could account for the influx of leukocytes and lymphocytes that form lymphoid aggregates observed during the secretory phase of normal endometrium.[48] The immune cells, also under hormonal control, participate in histological changes that occur during the menstrual cycle, as well as interacting with trophoblast in the presence of a conceptus. Also, should a breech in the epithelial lining occur, chemokines and cytokines will fill the injured area and have immediate effects on immune cell trafficking and activation. Finally, chemokines and cytokines attract macrophages and DCs to the epithelial lining to sample the lumen for microbes, thus contributing to immune surveillance.

NEUTROPHILS AT MUCOSAL SURFACES

Background

Neutrophils are prototypical innate immune leukocytes that provide a first line of defense against infection. When tissue cells are damaged by injury and infection, adjacent endothelial cells up-regulate expression of adhesion molecules, initiating neutrophil transmigration between endothelial cells and into the subcellular space. As they cross the endothelial barrier, neutrophils begin to exocytose granules, releasing collagen-degrading enzymes that ease the cells' passage through the basement membrane.[149] Neutrophil migration through tissues is orchestrated by chemokines, small chemoattractant peptides that are produced by many types of tissue cells.[150] At sites of infection, neutrophils eliminate bacteria by phagocytosis,[151] production of toxic oxidative compounds by the cytoplasmic and membrane-bound NADPH oxidase system,[152] and release of potent microbicides such as defensins and serine proteases from intracellular granules.[153,154]

During most of the menstrual cycle, neutrophils are present in endometrium in low numbers.[155] That they are present at all is somewhat surprising since it is generally maintained that neutrophils enter tissues in response to infections or tissue damage.[156] It is likely that the constitutive production by endometrium of

IL-8, a major neutrophil chemoattractant, is responsible for the presence of neutrophils at this site.[150,157] While these tissue neutrophils do not produce an inflammatory condition, they may be poised to intercept any incoming microorganisms that show invasive tendencies.[158] Indeed, it is possible though not proven that the high secretion of IL-8 at the apical surface of uterine epithelial cells may serve to attract neutrophils into the uterine lumen, which is connected to the nonsterile, external environment.[147]

The phenotype and function of neutrophils in normal, non-infected, non-inflamed human endometrium have not been extensively studied, although a majority produce IFNγ.[159] The presence of IFNγ-positive neutrophils did not appear to differ with stage of cycle or menopause. Binding of IFNγ to endometrial extracellular matrix was noted. These cells may therefore contribute to an endometrial environment favorable to Th-1 responses.

Immediately prior to menses, the number of neutrophils in endometrium rises dramatically.[160] Production of the chemoattractant IL-8 by endometrial epithelium increases throughout the menstrual cycle and is highest at late secretory phase.[161] This production appears to be hormonally controlled, as evidenced by a study of women receiving progesterone therapy. Endometrial IL-8 increased significantly after progesterone was withheld.[162] Hormones, in particular progesterone, orchestrate the rise in MMPs in stromal and epithelial cells that culminates in menses.[155,163] These connective tissue-degrading enzymes are produced as inactive precursors and are converted to their active form by other MMPs and by elastase from neutrophil intracellular granules.[164–166] Neutrophils also contain latent MMPs[167] and when endometrial stromal cells and blood neutrophils were co-cultured, the MMPs released by the mixed cells became activated.[168] At menses, endometrial neutrophils localize to regions of tissue breakdown;[42] thus it is likely that neutrophils contribute to the shedding of the functionalis at foci of tissue degradation. Since the integrity of the protective epithelial layer is destroyed during menses, the presence of high numbers of neutrophils would also serve to defend the endometrium against pathogens during this vulnerable phase.

Interestingly, endometrial repair commences while tissue breakdown is still in progress.[168] At this time high numbers of neutrophils still persist in the endometrium. Although short-lived in the circulation, neutrophil longevity is prolonged by cytokines in the tissue environment.[169] Neutrophils that have migrated into tissue down-regulate receptors mediating chemotaxis

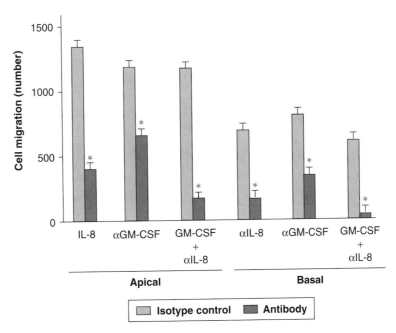

Figure 33.7   Apical or basolateral (Basal) supernatants from primary cultures of endometrial epithelial cells were treated for 1 hour with non-specific isotype control immunoglobulin or neutralizing antibodies to IL-8 or GM-CSF, singly or mixed. Chemotaxis to the treated CM were then measured in the under-agarose chemotaxis assay.[308] While both anti-IL-8 and anti-GM-CSF reduced migration, neutralization of both chemokines together resulted in greater reduction. *, Significantly ($p < 0.01$) different from isotype control.

and microbicidal activity and up-regulate genes encoding products that induce fibroblast migration and promote angiogenesis.[170] Indeed, intense intravascular foci of VEGF (vascular endothelial growth factor) in microvessels of proliferative phase endometrium were found to be contained within neutrophils that were adherent to the endothelia.[171] Additionally, this study demonstrated a positive correlation between vessels containing VEGF-positive foci and vessel proliferation in the subepithelial endometrial layer. Further evidence that neutrophils may contribute to endometrial regeneration came from observations on estrogen-stimulated endometrial angiogenesis in mice, in which depletion of neutrophils in vivo reduced endothelial proliferation.[172] Together, these studies suggest that endometrial neutrophils are not only a first line of innate immune defense but also are important contributors to normal endometrial physiology.

New findings

To obtain more insight into factors that promote neutrophil chemotaxis into endometrial tissue we conducted chemotaxis studies comparing conditioned media (CM) from endometrial epithelial cells in a system where secretions may be harvested from both apical and basal sides of the monolayer. The monolayers displayed high electrical resistance characteristic of healthy confluent epithelia, and were unstimulated. We found that apical CM was a more potent inducer of chemotaxis than basal CM. We also compared the IL-8 content of CM with their ability to induce chemotaxis and found that IL-8 did not account for all of the activity (Figure 33.7). Studies using specific neutralizing antibodies showed that the high chemoattractant activity of epithelial CM resulted from synergistic action between IL-8 and GM-CSF secreted by epithelial cells.[147] These results indicate that relatively low concentrations of GM-CSF can potentiate the activity of CXC chemokines in induction of neutrophil chemotaxis in endometrium, and suggest that future studies of chemokine production in FRT tissue should also consider the secretion of GM-CSF.

It is known that neutrophils preferentially cross monolayers of cultured epithelial cells from the basal to apical side[173] and that very few neutrophils cross unless IL-8 is applied to produce a basal to apical gradient.[174] Our studies suggest that unstimulated epithelial cells in the FRT secrete chemokines basally to attract neutrophils to the epithelium. In addition, they produce a higher amount of chemoattractant on the luminal side that might induce neutrophils to cross the epithelium and enter the lumen, where they would proactively remove microorganisms at the epithelial surface. Indeed,

Mikamo and coworkers showed a positive correlation between IL-8 concentration in the uterine lumen of women and the number of luminal neutrophils.[175]

GM-CSF produced in endometrium augments many neutrophil functions and may thus be important in boosting innate immune protection.[176] We therefore examined the chemotactic function of neutrophils after exposure to GM-CSF at a concentration typical of that found in CM of non-activated epithelial cells.[147] Although the number of IL-8 receptors was unchanged by GM-CSF treatment, neutrophils lost much of their chemotactic responsiveness to IL-8 while retaining chemotaxis to fMLP (N-formylmethionyl-leucyl-phenylalanine), a bacterial chemoattractant[177] (Figure 33.8). Additionally, we found that GM-CSF-treated neutrophils demonstrated a significant diminution of IL-8-mediated signaling and a slight increase in fMLP-mediated signaling. This suggests that functionally different neutrophil populations may arise as a result of exposure to cytokines. It is noteworthy that in the endometrium most GM-CSF protein is made by epithelial cells.[178] It is possible that one of the many actions of GM-CSF on neutrophils could be to down-regulate responses when they are no longer necessary to the role of the cell. In crossing the epithelium, the neutrophil would encounter high levels of GM-CSF, and then enter the lumen of the FRT. In this locale the only purpose of the neutrophil would be to destroy microorganisms and responsiveness to IL-8 could be counterproductive.

While neutrophils in endometrium and in other female reproductive tissues are thought to contribute significantly to normal physiology, these neutrophils have yet to be characterized in any detail. One of the reasons is that neutrophils in endometrium are very difficult to obtain in sufficient numbers. However, a much richer source of FRT neutrophils is found in Fallopian tube (FT) tissue. We have begun to explore the biology of FRT neutrophils by characterizing the surface receptors, cytoplasmic granules,[153] and intracellular cytokines[179] of neutrophils in single cell suspensions of dispersed FT tissue. Relative to neutrophils from peripheral blood (PB), FT neutrophils express higher levels of the CD15 adhesion determinant, also known as Lewis X.[180] FT neutrophils appear to have undergone some degranulation as a lower percent were positive for MMP-9 (a tertiary granule marker), lactoferrin (a secondary granule marker), and myeloperoxidase (a primary granule marker) vs PB cells. However, FT neutrophils that retained secondary and primary granules had significantly higher intracellular levels of lactoferrin and myeloperoxidase than did

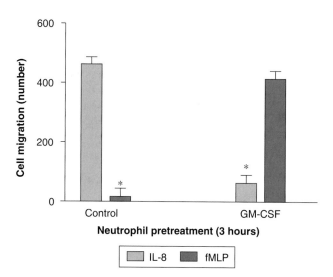

Figure 33.8 Chemotaxis of neutrophils after 3 hour culture in medium or GM-CSF. While freshly isolated neutrophils migrated to both stimuli, neutrophils cultured with medium lost ability to migrate to fMLP but retained chemotaxis to IL-8. However, when cells were cultured with GM-CSF, chemotaxis to IL-8 was lost while migration to fMLP was retained. *, Significantly ($p < 0.01$) different from control value.

PB neutrophils. This is surprising since it is widely believed that granule proteins are produced only in immature cells during granulopoiesis and not in circulating neutrophils, which are considered terminally differentiated.[153] This observation suggests that factors in the environment of FRT tissue are able to stimulate microbicide synthesis in mature neutrophils.

Another striking finding was that FT neutrophils express human leukocyte anitgen (HLA)-DR, unlike their PB counterparts. HLA-DR may be induced on blood neutrophils in culture by the cytokines GM-CSF, IFNγ, and IL-3.[181] Neutrophils expressing HLA-DR and the appropriate co-stimulatory molecules are reported to induce T cell proliferation in response to superantigen as well as in a class II restricted manner. This suggests that neutrophils within the FRT have potential to regulate local adaptive immunity.

Intracellular levels of inflammatory cytokines IL-12, IFNγ, and TNFα, and of the vascular growth factor VEGF were also significantly higher in FT than blood neutrophils. The cytokines may augment immune defense by activating or priming other innate cell types. Neutrophil-derived VEGF may influence endothelial cell proliferation and other VEGF-modulated functions such as microvascular permeability.[182] These data indicate that neutrophils from the FT exhibit a phenotype, distinct from their PB precursors, that indicates both physiological and innate immune roles within FRT tissue.

Conclusions

Neutrophils contain an array of prepackaged enzymes and microbicides that enable them to penetrate tissues in order to mediate innate immunity. In the absence of infection or inflammation these cells infiltrate tissues of the endometrium in low numbers during most of the menstrual cycle. However, neutrophil numbers increase dramatically prior to and during menses. The influx of neutrophils at this time correlates with production of higher levels of IL-8 in endometrial tissue. An interaction between neutrophils, stromal, and epithelial cells appears to help in converting latent MMPs into active tissue-degrading enzymes at menses. Cytokines made by endometrial cells, in particular GM-CSF, serve to prolong the neutrophil life span in endometrial tissue. Neutrophils are also reported to congregate at sites of tissue repair and vascular growth during endometrial regeneration. This appears related to high levels of VEGF in neutrophils at these sites. Our results indicate significant differences between neutrophils in reproductive tract tissue and PB that suggest they contribute both to tissue physiology and innate defense.

Cytokines within endometrial tissue may enhance the innate immune potential of neutrophils by altering receptor expression and cell function. GM-CSF, for instance, strongly up-regulates many neutrophil functions in addition to delaying neutrophil apoptosis. Our studies suggest that GM-CSF produced at the endometrial epithelial surface acts synergistically with the potent chemoattractant IL-8 to bring neutrophils towards the epithelium, or even to induce them to cross into the lumen. Moreover, GM-CSF may skew the chemotactic responses of neutrophils towards bacterial chemotactic factors. The hormonal effects on chemokine production by endometrial tissues regulate the influx of neutrophils into the endometrium in the process of menstruation. It is likely that hormonally regulated cytokines and growth factors also modulate the innate immune functions of neutrophils within this tissue and in the uterine lumen.

ROLE OF NK CELLS AT MUCOSAL SURFACES

Background

NK cells are a major population of leukocytes within the human endometrium. These uterine NK (uNK) cells have a unique phenotype compared to blood NK cells, and their presence in the endometrium may be regulated by sex hormones during the menstrual cycle. NK cells are particularly prominent in the first trimester decidua and much of the research on uNK cells has focused on their function during pregnancy. For many years it has been theorized that uNK cell interactions with fetal trophoblasts result in the inactivation of NK cells via recognition of HLA-G, and this was one reason for the subsequent down-regulation of maternal immunity against paternal antigens. However, data have been reported that HLA-G recognition may induce NK cell cytokine production.[183,184] Elegant studies in murine models have produced evidence that NK cell IFNγ is important for proper restructuring of maternal spiral arteries in the decidua.[185] Thus, a more nuanced view of NK cell function in the endometrium is required, and these new data support a complex regulation of NK cell recruitment and activation within the endometrium. The interplay of NK cells with maternal cells and trophoblasts is probably a well-orchestrated interaction involving activation and regulation of all cells. One must not forget that NK cells are innate immune cells that have a role in activation of adaptive immunity and cell-mediated immunity. The role of uNK cells in local mucosal immunity is beginning to be explored.

New findings

NK cells are innate immune cells that express a variety of receptors that recognize self- and non-self proteins.[186,187] Data have demonstrated roles for NK cells in immune defense against a variety of pathogens.[188–190] NK cells have been shown to produce many different cytokines that have the ability to activate immune responses and promote destruction of pathogens. More in-depth molecular analysis of NK cell subpopulations has revealed differences between blood NK cells and NK cells within the uterus.[191–193] Human blood NK cells can be broadly defined into two major subsets. One subset is CD56^{dim}, CD16+, CD57+, and express many killer immunoglobulin-like receptors (KIRs), while the other NK cell subset is CD56^{bright}, CD16^{low}, CD57−, and express CD94 and few KIRs. CD56^{dim} NK cells have high lytic activity, and the CD56^{bright} NK cell subset produces more cytokines upon monokine stimulation.[194] Uterine NK cells have been described as a unique NK cell subset that express a different set of markers than those on NK cells in the blood. NK cells in the endometrium are CD56^{bright}, CD16$^{low/−}$, CD57−, CD94+, and KIRs. These uNK cells also express CD9 and CD69.[192] Decidual NK cells expressed 278 genes that were unique compared to blood NK cells.[191] These data suggest that as NK cells enter the endometrium, specific genes are up-regulated, and the process of decidualization and trophoblast invasion probably induces new gene expression.

In human endometrium, NK cell numbers increase as the menstrual cycle progresses.[46,195,196] These findings suggest that sex hormones may regulate NK cell migration into the endometrium, and recent reports support this idea.[197–201] Chemokines found in human endometrium have been shown to induce NK cell migration in vitro. CXCR3 ligands, CXCL9, CXCL10, and CXCL11, are implicated in the recruitment of NK cells into non-pregnant endometrium, and CXCL10 and CXCL11 are induced by estrogen and progesterone in human endometrium.[198] The induction of CXCL10 and CXCL11 was observed using fresh tissue pieces and could be blocked by a specific estrogen receptor antagonist. CXCL12 is produced by human trophoblasts, and there is preferential expression of its receptor, CXCR4, on blood CD56[bright] NK cells, supporting a role for CXCL12 in recruitment of NK cells to the decidua.[202,203] Data from studies with mice that lack specific chemokine receptors demonstrate that CCR2 and CCR5 are not required for recruitment of NK cells to implantation sites.[204] CXCR3-deficient mice appear to have near normal numbers of uNK cells during pregnancy, but they do have a reduced recruitment of cells to the decidua.[205] CXCR3 mice also have a defective recruitment of NK cells into lung, liver, and blood.[206] Caution must be taken when using murine data to extrapolate to humans because of the many differences in NK cell localization and numbers in humans compared to mice.[193] The chemokines involved in the recruitment of NK cells near trophoblasts may also be different to those involved in recruitment of NK cells to non-pregnant endometrium.

Blood NK cells have been shown to express several TLRs at the mRNA level and respond to TLR agonists.[207–209] There is controversy about whether blood NK cells respond directly via TLRs or whether resting NK cells require contact with other cells (e.g. DCs) in order to respond to TLR agonists. uNK cells express a number of TLRs (Table 33.1). Initial studies support the idea that resting uNK cells do not respond directly to TLR agonists, but they require signals from other cells, such as APCs (Eriksson and Sentman, unpublished data). Activated uNK cell clones can respond directly to TLR agonists, although responses are weaker than when uNK cells are in the presence of other endometrial cells. These data support the idea

Table 33.1   Uterine NK cells expression of Toll-like receptors

TLR	uNK	Blood NK
1	+	+
2	+++	−
3	+/−	+
4	++	+
5	−	−
6	+	+
7	+	+/−
8	−	−
9	−	−
10	++	+

Toll-like receptors (TLRs) expression on uterine NK (uNK) cell clones and blood NK cell clones. Data were analyzed by quantitative real-time PCR (polymerase chain reaction). Relative amounts of mRNA expression are indicated as high expression (+++), moderate expression (++), low expression (+), only in some samples (+/−), or no expression (−).

that cell surface molecules or cytokines induced by TLR triggering on various stromal cells in the endometrium help to stimulate uNK cell activity. This need for stimulation from other cells may help regulate uNK cells to avoid unwanted activation unless a sufficiently large infection is present.

Endometrium has other ways of regulating uNK cell function. TGFβ is a powerful anti-inflammatory cytokine that has been shown to down-regulate many immune functions.[210,211] The uNK cells produce a variety of cytokines upon stimulation (Figure 33.9), including IFNγ, IL-8, and GM-CSF.[211a] Many of these cytokines activate macrophages and induce cellular immunity. Blockade of endogenous TGFβ is sufficient to enhance uNK cell responses to cytokines.[192] In a similar manner, blood NK cell IFNγ responses are also increased upon blockade of endogenous TGFβ or the TGFβ type 1 receptor kinase, ALK5.[212] The increased cytokine production was due to both an increase in the number of NK cells producing IFNγ and in the amount of IFNγ produced per cell. This increase was observed for both monokine and TLR agonist stimulation of blood NK cells. These data, along with data from a murine genetic model,[213] suggest that blockade of TGFβ by pharmacological means may be one way to increase NK cell activity and promote cell-mediated immunity.

Conclusions

NK cells can be found throughout the FRT. Endometrial NK cells may account for up to 70% of all leukocytes at late stages in the menstrual cycle. During

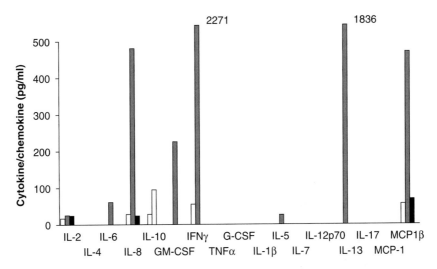

Figure 33.9 Cytokine production by uNK cells is inhibited by TGFβ. A uNK cell clone was stimulated by IL-12/IL-15, and cytokine production was determined after 3 days. NK cells were stimulated by IL-12/IL-15 (gray bars), IL-12/IL-15/TGFβ (black bars), or medium only (white bars). Adapted from Sentman et al.[211a]

pregnancy, NK cell–trophoblast interactions may be important for reorganization of spiral arteries. Combinations of NK cell KIRs and their HLA-C ligands have been associated with increases in preeclampsia in humans.[214] Collectively, these data support a role for NK cells in the remodeling of the vasculature during placental development.

In addition to their role during pregnancy, uNK cells probably play a role in immune defenses within the endometrium. NK cells isolated from the endometrium have the capacity to make a variety of potent cytokines and stimulate cell-mediated immunity. They may be triggered via cytokine signals, cell–cell interactions, or perhaps directly via TLRs. These uNK cell responses are tightly regulated by TGFβ so that a sufficiently large stimulus must be provided to activate uNK cell cytokine release. As uNK cell interactions with other endometrial cells are explored and the nature of NK cell-activating ligands determined within the human endometrium, it should be possible to understand how these innate lymphocytes influence both mucosal immune defense and fetal implantation.

REGULATION OF MACROPHAGES AND DENDRITIC CELLS AT MUCOSAL SURFACES

Background

Monocytes and macrophages

Monocytes circulate throughout the periphery, mediating recognition and clearance of pathogens and cellular debris and extravasate into tissues, where they differentiate into macrophages. Macrophages function as key effectors of both innate and humoral immunity, as they actively phagocytose foreign molecules and display antigens on their surface to T lymphocytes.[215] These processes are regulated through the expression of surface receptors for complement components, carbohydrates, Fc receptors for immunoglobulins, and importantly, through the expression of MHC class I and II.[216] The phenotype of tissue macrophages is affected by and uniquely dependent on the cellular milieu to which it is exposed, including local cytokines, chemokines, and other biological effector molecules, as well as extracellular matrix and cellular components.

Regulation of uterine macrophage localization

Macrophages constitute approximately 10% of the total leukocyte population in tissues of the human FRT, and are most highly represented in the endometrial stroma and myometrial connective tissue of the cycling uterus.[38,46] Steroid hormones modulate the recruitment of uterine macrophages, as migration of macrophages to the endometrium is affected by cyclic variations in estrogen and progesterone levels.[217,218] Macrophages are most numerous in the endometrial stroma just prior to menstruation, concurrent with depressed expression of estrogen and progesterone as the result of luteolysis.[42] These fluctuations in macrophage localization are probably attributable to hormonal regulation of cytokine and chemokine expression. In support of this, treatment of endometrial stromal cells with estradiol has been reported to inhibit expression of MCP-1, which correlates with decreased macrophage chemotaxis.[219] Furthermore, gene array analysis of RNA extracted from human endometrial tissue cells indicates that expression of the macrophage chemoattractants MDC, MCP-3, FKN, and MIP-1β is up-regulated perimenstrually.[220]

Influence of hormonal regulation on macrophage immune function

Sexual dimorphism in immune function suggests that steroid hormones are involved in modulating immune responses in vivo. Estrogen has been reported to have pleiotropic effects on cytokine and chemokine production by human macrophages. The ability of estrogen to induce either pro- or anti-inflammatory mediator production is largely concentration- and context-dependent. For example, while treatment of PMA (phorbal myristate acetate)-differentiated U937 cells with estradiol elicits production of the proinflammatory cytokine TNFα,[221] incubation of microglia with estradiol inhibits proinflammatory cytokine synthesis.[222] While it is clear that estrogen exerts complex heterogeneous effects on macrophage function, recent data attribute a predominantly immunosuppressive role to estrogen in the modulation of innate immune responses. This response, mediated by estrogen receptor α (ERα), was demonstrated by studies in which peritoneal macrophages from ERα-deficient mice were challenged with two TLR agonists: lipopolysaccharide (LPS) and *Mycobacterium avium*.[223] Treatment of these macrophages with both bacterial stimuli resulted in increased secretion of TNFα and decreased bacterial load when compared with responses elicited from peritoneal macrophages derived from wild-type mice.[223]

Dendritic cells

As professional APCs, dendritic cells bridge the gap between innate and adaptive immunity through stimulation of naive T cells. Immature dendritic cells (iDCs) reside in the periphery, acquire antigen, and mature in response to inflammatory and/or pathogenic stimulation.[224] This process leads to the up-regulation of MHC II and the co-stimulatory molecules CD80 and CD86.[224] DCs migrate into T-cell areas of secondary lymphoid tissues, and undergo terminal maturation via ligation of CD40 with CD154 (CD40L) on antigen-specific T lymphocytes.[225]

Hormonal regulation of dendritic cell function

Dendritic cell function is subject to hormonal regulation, as estradiol treatment of iDCs increases secretion of IL-6 and the inflammatory chemokines IL-8 and MCP-1.[226] Moreover, estrogen modulates mature dendritic cell effector functions, as mature DCs pretreated with estradiol (E$_2$) demonstrate an enhanced ability to stimulate naive CD4+ T cells when compared with untreated controls.[226] In addition, estradiol mediates migration of mature dendritic cells toward the chemokine CCL-19, most likely through activation of the cyclic AMP/protein kinase A (cAMP/PKA) signal transduction pathway.[226,227] Collectively, these data implicate a role for estradiol in the regulation of DC effector function and, consequently, in the induction and resolution of the inflammatory response.

Localization of dendritic cells in reproductive tract tissues and influence on uterine homeostasis

The identification of DCs within tissues of the human FRT has significant implications for the progression of disease and inflammation, as well as for the maintenance of successful pregnancy. In this regard, DCs are resident in early human pregnancy decidua, where they have been proposed to mediate tolerance to the human conceptus, and assist in the development of the maternal immune response to pathogenic challenge.[228]

In the context of infection, DCs have been demonstrated to transmit HIV from mucosal sites to secondary lymphoid organs via expression of the type II integral membrane protein DC-SIGN, which binds the envelope of HIV-1.[229,230] DC-SIGN+ dendritic cells have been identified in the human uterus, cervix, and vagina.[231,232] In the vaginal mucosa, DC-SIGN+ dendritic cells are localized to the subepithelial lamina propria, and are thus protected from infectivity in most instances due to the physical barrier provided by the epithelium.[232] However, hormonal changes (such as altered progesterone levels) or exposure to microbes may result in thinning of the vaginal epithelium, and thus potentially increase the incidence of vaginal HIV transmission.[232]

New findings

Recent studies have focused on determining the influence of hormonal regulation on macrophage innate immune function.

Uterine macrophages and epithelial cells modulate innate defense cooperatively

Previous studies have demonstrated that although human uterine epithelial cells express the endotoxin receptor TLR4, treatment of these cells with LPS fails

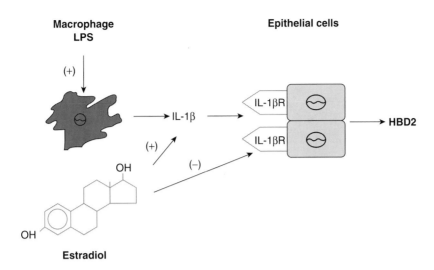

Figure 33.10   Model of the dynamic interaction of uterine macrophages and epithelial cells. Estrogen enhances the LPS-induced secretion of IL-1β by macrophages. IL-1β then binds to receptors on the surface of uterine epithelial cells and induces the secretion of HBD2.

to induce secretion of soluble factors involved in mediating innate responses.[137] In contrast, stimulation of macrophages with LPS results in copious production of proinflammatory cytokines, including IL-1β.[233] As recent work has shown that stimulation of uterine epithelial cells with IL-1β induces secretion of the antimicrobial peptide human β-defensin 2 (HBD2),[138] we postulated that the response to bacterial stimulation in the human endometrium is mediated cooperatively through the dynamic interaction of macrophages and epithelial cells. To test this hypothesis, human peripheral blood monocytes and primary uterine macrophages were stimulated with LPS, and supernatants derived from these cells were co-cultured with uterine epithelial cells. Real-time PCR (polymerase chain reaction) and ELISA (enzyme-linked immunosorbant assay) data demonstrated that both monocytes and uterine macrophages up-regulate mRNA and protein expression of biologically active IL-1β upon activation with LPS. Pretreatment of blood-derived monocytes with high doses of estradiol augments expression of IL-1β in an ER-dependent manner. Moreover, LPS-stimulated monocyte and uterine macrophage-derived IL-1β induces secretion of HBD2 by human uterine epithelial cells. These data indicate dynamic immunological interaction between uterine macrophages and epithelial cells (Figure 33.10) and implicate a role for estradiol in the regulation of the immune response.

Estradiol attenuates LPS-induced IL-8 expression by primary human monocytes

Given the exquisite sensitivity of human peripheral blood monocytes to microbial stimulation[234] and the

determination that these cells express both ER message and protein,[235,236] the effect of estradiol on production of IL-8 was investigated. IL-8 is acutely up-regulated by exposure to LPS and mediates the recruitment of leukocytes to sites of inflammation.[234,237] Pretreatment of primary human monocytes with estradiol attenuates LPS-induced IL-8 production. This inhibition is both time- and dose-dependent, as reflected by reduced levels of IL-8 message and protein (Figure 33.11). Moreover, the effect is mediated through the ER, as incubation with the ER antagonist ICI 182,780 abrogates it. Notably, expression of the LPS-inducible antimicrobial molecule SLPI is unaffected by estradiol pretreatment of these cells, indicating the attenuation of IL-8 expression is specific.

Conclusions

In accordance with previously published work, our data demonstrate that estradiol exerts pleiotropic effects on monocyte and macrophage effector function, and thus have broad implications when considered in the context of human uterine homeostasis. Significantly, we have shown that treatment of uterine macrophages with LPS, the major surface component of Gram-negative bacteria, increases expression of proinflammatory IL-1β, which subsequently induces uterine epithelial cell production of HBD2. These data suggest a mechanism whereby uterine epithelial cells may combat pathogenic challenge through cooperative interaction with monocytes and uterine macrophages. Thus, although uterine epithelial cells do not produce HBD2 directly when stimulated with

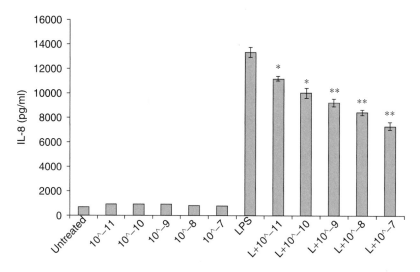

Figure 33.11   Estradiol attenuation of LPS-induced IL-8 production by human peripheral blood monocytes. Monocytes were incubated with indicated concentrations of 17β-estradiol for 24 hours, and then stimulated with 10 ng/ml LPS for an additional 12 hours, after which supernatants were collected and analyzed for IL-8. *, Significantly ($p < 0.05$) different from LPS alone; **, significantly ($p < 0.01$) different from LPS alone.[309]

LPS, production of uterine epithelial HBD2 is invoked by macrophage-derived IL-1β, thereby conferring protection to the human FRT against Gram-negative bacterial invasion.

Moreover, it is noteworthy that LPS-induced IL-1β expression is augmented only in the context of high concentrations of estradiol. Intriguingly, the dose of estradiol that mediated this effect (100 nmol/L) has physiological relevance during pregnancy.[238,239] These data suggest that during periods of regular menstrual cycling, estradiol has little influence on the ability of macrophages to mediate proinflammatory cytokine production. However, during pregnancy, when estradiol levels are elevated and fetal protection is paramount, myeloid effector function is heightened, and consequently microbicide release by epithelial cells is increased.

In addition, the ability of estradiol to attenuate LPS-induced IL-8 production in primary human monocytes may provide an important means of modulating the inflammatory response. Given its role in promoting inflammation, tight regulation of this chemokine is essential to the maintenance of a controlled immune reaction. In this regard, it is notable that premenopausal women have a selective survival advantage over men and postmenopausal women when challenged with endotoxic shock.[240] Thus, attenuation of inflammation by estrogen may present a mechanism for combating pathogenic challenge while ensuring protection from septic shock.

Collectively, these data implicate a role for estrogen in the modulation of macrophage effector function and may lead to an enhanced understanding of inflammatory control mechanisms within the human FRT.

INFECTION OF UTERINE EPITHELIAL CELLS BY HIV-1

Background

The FRT is the target of more than 20 pathogens that are transmissible through sexual intercourse. Each year throughout the world there are an estimated 340 million new cases of STI, including those of bacterial (*Neisseria gonorrhoeae*, *Chlamydia trachomatis*, *Treponema pallidum*), parasitic (*Trichomonas vaginalis*), and viral origin (herpes simplex virus [HSV], human papillomavirus [HPV], human immunodeficiency virus [HIV]) (Table 33.2).[241] STI of females is one of the leading causes of morbidity worldwide. It is associated with bacterial vaginosis, pelvic inflammatory disease, decreased fertility, preterm birth, and increased perinatal morbidity and mortality.[242] While numerous pathogenic organisms have a major impact on women's health and fertility, there is little argument that HIV/AIDS is currently the world's most devastating public health concern, particularly with regard to women's health. This section will focus on the mechanisms by which HIV-1 is transmitted through sexual contact and the relevant host defenses.

HIV/AIDS is unique in human history in its rapid spread, its extent, and the depth of its impact. Since the first AIDS case was diagnosed in 1981, the world has struggled to come to grips with its extraordinary dimensions. Having eclipsed the 20 million deaths caused by the 1918–1919 influenza pandemic and the 25 million deaths incurred by the 1346–1352 bubonic plague, HIV/AIDS is one of the world's worst pandemics.[243–245] The total number of people living with HIV worldwide has risen to an estimated 40.3 million people, with more than 1 million in the United States.[243] With every passing year the HIV/AIDS pandemic is becoming more a female disease. Women are approximately twice as likely as men to contract HIV infection during vaginal intercourse.[246,247] Each year brings an increase in the number of women infected with HIV. In particular, women and girls make up nearly 57% of those newly infected with HIV in Sub-Saharan Africa, where a striking 76% of young people (aged 15–24 years) living with HIV are female.[248] In the United States, the proportion of AIDS cases reported among women increased from 7% in 1985 to nearly 28% in 2003. In fact, from 1999 through 2003, the annual number of estimated AIDS diagnoses increased 15% among women and increased 1% among men.[247]

HIV-1 infection of the female reproductive tract

Heterosexual transmission is now the source of 80% of new HIV-1 infections. Transmission of HIV-1 to a female host occurs when the FRT mucosal epithelial surface is exposed to cell-free or cell-associated HIV-1 present in genital secretions (e.g. semen). Transmission of HIV-1 is directly related to the viral load in peripheral blood of the infected host[249] and preexistence of other STI increases the likelihood of transmitting and acquiring HIV-1.[250] HIV-1 crosses epithelial cells by transcytosis with or without infection, then is released as infectious virus from the basolateral surface, spreading to the susceptible cells (T lymphocytes, macrophages, and DCs) of the submucosa.[251,252] In ex-vivo FRT organ cultures, the first cells targeted by HIV-1 were intraepithelial memory CD4 + T cells.[253,254] HIV-1-infected cells form a virally mediated synapse with mucosal FRT epithelial cells, resulting in efficient transcytosis of HIV through the epithelial barrier and gaining access to the submucosa.[255] On the contrary, cell-free transcytosis of HIV-1 probably occurs non-selectively by fluid phase transcytosis.[256]

Whereas HIV-1 recovered from individuals undergoing primary infection is largely R5/M-tropic and of the non-syncytium-inducing (NSI) phenotype,[257,258] both X4/T-tropic syncytium-inducing (SI) variants and R5/M-tropic NSI variants are found in blood and genital secretions of HIV-1-seropositive individuals at

Table 33.2 Incidence of sexually transmitted pathogens worldwide per year.

Pathogen	New infections worldwide per year
Bacterial	
Neisseria gemorrhoeae	62 million
Chlamydia trachomatis	92 million
Treponema pallidum	12 million
Parasite	
Trichomonas vaginalis	174 million
Viral	
HSV	21 million: prevalence rate: USA (20%), Sub-Saharan Africa (50%)
HPV	660 million: most common STP
HIV	5 million: total number of people living with HIV is 40.3 miilion

STP, sexually transmitted pathogen; HSV, herpes simplex virus; HPV, human papillomavirus; HIV, human immunodeficiency virus.

a later stage of disease.[259,260] Thus, a selection process favoring R5/M-tropic NSI phenotypes occurs during or soon after transmucosal penetration of the virus. This phenomenon may partly be explained by the observation that X4/T-tropic HIV-1 readily infects uterine epithelial cells, while R5/M-tropic HIV-1 is sequestered by the epithelial cell and transmitted to underlying T cells, macrophages, or DCs.[261,262]

While the site in the FRT where HIV-1 penetrates the mucosal epithelium and thereby infects the host is not known, both the upper and lower FRT (vagina and cervix) have been implicated. In the vagina and ecto-cervix, thinning and breaks in the mucosa caused by STI and bacterial vaginosis have been associated with enhanced HIV-1 transmission.[250,263–265] In the upper FRT, it has been proposed that the single layer of epithelium of the upper FRT, as opposed to the multilayer stratified squamous epithelium of the vagina and ectocervix, may be more easily traversed by HIV-1.[266] This is in part supported by the finding that a higher concentration of simian immunodeficiency virus (SIV)-infected cells is found in the endocervical mucosa after intravaginal inoculation.[267]

Other recent observations have suggested that the uterus and Fallopian tube might be a portal of entry for HIV-1 following sexual intercourse. Labeled-albumin macrospheres and dyes enter the uterus and Fallopian tubes within 2 minutes of placement in the vagina.[268–271] Within minutes after insemination, spermatozoa can be found in the uterus and Fallopian tubes.[268,272] Because spermatozoa bind HIV-1 gp120,[273] it is likely that virus could be transported to the upper FRT by piggybacking on sperm. In other studies, both bacterial and viral pathogens, including HIV-1,[274] have been found to travel freely in FRT secretions. This suggests that HIV-1 may reach the upper FRT within minutes of deposition in the vagina. Epithelial cells of the FRT have been shown to be susceptible to HIV-1 infection.[275–277] This includes uterine epithelial cells, which are susceptible to HIV-1 infection, integration, and propagation of infectious virions.[261,262,276] Co-receptors used by HIV-1, including CD4, CXCR4, CCR5, and galactosylceramide (GalC), are expressed on uterine and cervical epithelial cells and expression varies with the menstrual cycle.[278,279] Epithelial cell expression of CD4, CCR5, and CXCR4 was highest during the proliferative phase of the cycle when estradiol is present. In contrast, expression of GalC (an alternative HIV infectivity receptor) on endometrial glands was higher during the secretory than the proliferative phase. Variation in expression of these receptors may indicate regulation by estradiol and progesterone.

Innate immunity in the human FRT and the role of mucosal epithelium

The estimated rate of HIV-1 transmission per sexual encounter is 1:122 to 1:1000, indicating that the probability of becoming infected with HIV is quite low.[280,281] This suggests that there exists within the FRT effective immunity that protects from HIV and probably other STIs. In the following section, we review our current knowledge of the innate immune factors expressed by the FRT mucosal epithelium that are known to inhibit HIV-1, as well as present several new findings detailing the innate immune responses generated by epithelial cells that may inhibit infection of the FRT by HIV-1.

The FRT is immunologically unique in that the endometrium must protect itself from STIs, while allowing for the presence of allogeneic sperm and the immunologically distinct fetus. Epithelial cells throughout the FRT play a pivotal role in the innate response to pathogen challenge and probably represent the first line of defense against viruses such as HIV-1.[101] That being said, little is known about the innate immune defense that epithelial cells exert when faced with a viral pathogen. Understanding what role FRT epithelial cells play in immune surveillance and host defense is crucial for the development of effective mucosal vaccines as well as therapies for ongoing infections.

The main attribute by which epithelial cells protect the FRT from STIs is generally thought to be their barrier function. However, other mechanisms exist by which epithelial cells defend the FRT from HIV-1 and thereby contribute to the low rate of HIV-1 transmission. Secreted antimicrobial factors including α-defensin-5 (HD5), β-defensins 1–4 (HBD1–4), and SLPI exhibit potent anti-HIV-1 activity[116,139,282] as well as being active against Neisseria gonorrhoeae, Chlamydia trachomatis, Candida albicans, and herpes simplex virus-2.[139,241,283–295] Other factors found within epithelial cell secretions exhibiting anti-HIV-1 activity are the chemokines CCL3/MIP-1α, CCL4/MIP-1β, CCL5/RANTES, and CXCL12/SDF-1α.[296,297] These inhibit HIV-1 infection of target host cells by interfering with the ability of HIV-1 to bind co-receptors CCR5 and CXCR4 found on host cells. It is important to note that while these antimicrobials exhibit antiviral activity toward HIV-1, the tropism of HIV-1 influences its susceptibility. For example, while HBD2 and HBD3 are potent inhibitors of CXCR4/T-Tropic HIV-1 isolates, their antiviral effects on the CCR5/M-Tropic HIV-1 isolates are greatly reduced.[290] Likewise, the CCR5 agonists CCL3, CCL4, and CCL5 are inhibitors of CCR5/M-Tropic HIV-1, not CXCR4/T-Tropic HIV-1, whereas CXCL12 inhibits CXCR4/T-Tropic HIV-1 but has no effect on CCR5/M-Tropic HIV-1. It is important to note that the expression of many of these innate immune factors appear to be regulated by sex hormones. Levels of HBD1, HBD2, and HD5 peak during the secretory phase, HBD4 during the proliferative phase, HBD2 during menstruation, and SLPI during the mid–late secretory phase of the menstrual cycle.[116,119,122,123] Moreover, the secretion of SLPI by polarized uterine epithelial cells in culture from premenopausal women is significantly higher than seen with cells from postmenopausal women.[139] The mechanisms driving hormonal regulation of antimicrobial expression and secretion have yet to be elucidated.

A second level of innate immune defense against HIV-1 is mediated by the expression of intracellular viricidal factors. These factors are often the by-product of type I IFN production by infected epithelial cells, which, in turn, is crucial for limiting early replication and viral spread.[298] Type I IFNs, known also as viral IFNs, exert their activity through the IFNα/β receptor and include IFNα and β. Type I IFNs induce the expression of intracellular viricidal factors, such as 2′,5′-oligoadenlyate synthetase (2′,5′-OAS) and RNA-dependent protein kinase (PKR), both of which inhibit HIV-1 replication[299–302] by shutting down protein synthesis.[303,304]

New findings

While the constitutive expression of secreted and intracellular antiviral factors provides a foundation for protecting the FRT from invading viral pathogens, their augmented expression may be essential for preventing HIV-1 infection. Indeed, expression of antiviral factors could be induced following exposure to conserved pathogen-associated molecular patterns (PAMPs) synthesized by microorganisms,[137,140,141,305] and recognized by TLRs. Primary uterine epithelial cells grown on cell inserts were treated both apically and basolaterally with agonists to TLR2, TLR3, TLR4, TLR5, and TLR9, after which conditioned apical and basolateral media were collected and examined for the secretion of CCL4/MIP-1β and the mRNA expression of HBD1 and HBD2. Only treatment with the TLR3 agonist poly (I:C) induced an innate immune response. TLR3 recognizes double-stranded RNA, which is synthesized by most viruses during their replication cycle.[306] As shown in Figure 33.12, poly (I:C) significantly induced the apical and basolateral secretion of CCL4/MIP-1β and mRNA encoding HBD1 and HBD2. It also induced mRNAs endoding IFNβ and the antiviral gene 2′,5′-OAS 70-fold and 96-fold, respectively (Figure 33.13). PKR mRNA expression was also significantly induced (4.4-fold). Thus, uterine epithelial cells are poised to respond to viral infection. Enhanced production of CCL4/MIP-1β and HBD1 and HBD2 would have inhibitory effects on viral entry into susceptible cells and therefore help protect against HIV-1 infection. Production of IFNβ by uterine epithelial cells may induce the expression of intracellular antiviral factors that would inhibit HIV-1 replication in infected epithelial cells. Furthermore, the secretion of CCL4/MIP-1β, β-defensins, and IFNβ may help protect the mucosal surfaces of the lower FRT, since it is known that epithelial cell secretions of the upper FRT continuously bathe the lower tract.[307]

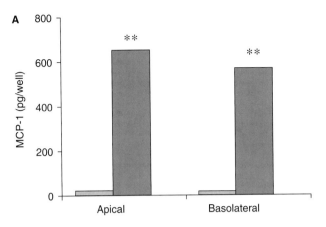

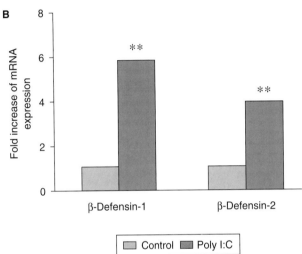

Figure 33.12 Secretion of CCL4/MIP-1β and mRNA expression of β-defensins by poly (I:C)-treated uterine epithelial cells. (**A**) Cultured medium was collected following 24-hour poly (I:C) stimulation and analyzed for the presence of CCL4/MIP-1β protein expression by ELISA. (**B**) Real-time RT-PCR was used to determine the relative levels of expression of HBD1 and HBD2 mRNA, normalized against an endogenous control, CD71. The data were normalized by using values from the control for calibration. *, Significantly different ($p<0.05$). **, Significantly different ($p<0.01$) from control. (Adapted from Schaefer et al[137].)

Conclusions

Uterine epithelial cells are capable of recognizing an analogue of viral dsRNA, probably through TLR3, and respond by secreting enhanced levels of antiviral factors and inducing the expression of intracellular antiviral factors that probably inhibit or slow HIV-1 infection at the FRT mucosa. Heterosexual contact is now the predominant source of new HIV-1 infections and women have become the main targets of HIV/AIDS. Understanding how the mucosal immune system in the female reproductive tract can innately inhibit the transmission of HIV as well as how it recognizes and responds to this virus are essential to the development of efficacious vaccines and therapeutics. This basis of knowledge will be essential for not only protecting the host from HIV-1 infection but also from bacterial, fungal, and other viral pathogens which compromise reproductive health and threaten the lives of women worldwide.

ACKNOWLEDGMENT

This work was supported by a National Institutes of Health grant AI51877 (CRW), AI13541 (CRW).

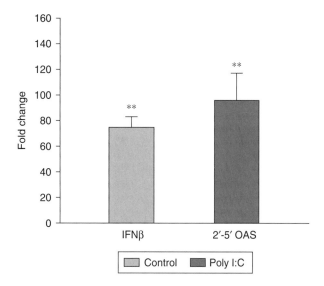

Figure 33.13 Expression of antiviral genes by uterine epithelial cells treated with the TLR3 agonist poly (I:C). Real-time RT-PCR was used to determine the relative levels of expression of IFNβ and 2′,5′-OAS, normalized against CD71. The data were normalized by using values from the control for calibration. **, Significantly different ($p < 0.01$) from control. (Adapted from Schaefer et al.[137])

REFERENCES

1. Ogra P, Yamanaka T, Losonsky GA. Local immunologic defenses in the genital tract. In: Fleicher N, ed. Reprod Immunol. New York: Alan R Liss, 1981: 381–94.
2. Underdown BJ, Schiff JM. Immunoglobulin A: strategic defense initiative at the mucosal surface. Annu Rev Immunol 1986; 4: 389–417.
3. Mestecky J, McGhee JR. Immunoglobulin A (IgA): molecular and cellular interactions involved in IgA biosynthesis and immune response. Adv Immunol 1987; 40: 153–245.
4. Wira CR, Fahey JV, White HD et al. The mucosal immune system in the human female reproductive tract: influence of stage of the menstrual cycle and menopause on mucosal immunity in the uterus. In: Glasser S, Aplin J, Guidice L, Tabibzadeh S, eds. The Endometrium. New York: Taylor and Francis, 2002: 371–404.
5. Grossman CJ. Interactions between the gonadal steroids and the immune system. Science 1985; 227: 257–61.
6. Wira CR, Richardson J, Prabhala R. Endocrine regulation of mucosal immunity: effect of sex hormones and cytokines on the afferent and efferent arms of the immune system in the female reproductive tract. In: Ogra PL, Mestecky J, Lamm ME et al, eds. Handbook of Mucosal Immunology. New York: Academic Press, 1994: 705–18.
7. Kutteh WH, Mestecky J, Wira CR. Mucosal immunity in the human female reproductive tract. In: Mestecky J, Bienenstock J, Lamm ME eds. Mucosal Immunology. New York: Academic Press, 2005: 1631–47.
8. Medzhitov RM, Janeway CJ. Innate immunity. N Engl J Med 2000; 343: 338–44.
9. Janeway CAJ, Medzhitov R. Innate immune recognition. Annu Rev Immunol 2002; 20: 197–216.
10. Akira S, Takeda K. Toll-like receptor signaling. Nat Rev Immunol 2004; 4: 499–511.
11. Lien E, Sellati TJ, Yoshimura A et al. Toll-like receptor 2 functions as a pattern recognition receptor for diverse bacterial products. J Biol Chem 1999; 247: 33419–25.
12. da Silva Correia J, Soldau K, Christen U et al. Lipopolysaccharide is in close proximity to each of the proteins in its membrane receptor complex. Transfer from CD14 to TLR4 and MD-2. J Biol Chem 2001; 267: 21129–2135.
13. Hayashi F, Smith KD, Ozinsky A et al. The innate immune response to bacterial flagellin is mediated by Toll-like receptor 5. Nature 2001; 410: 1099–103.
14. Muroi M, Ohnishi T, Azumi-Mayuzumi S et al. Lipopolysaccharide-mimetic activities of a Toll-like receptor 2-stimulatory substance(s) in enterobacterial lipopolysaccharide preparations. Infect Immun 2003; 71: 3221–6.
15. Takeuchi O, Hoshino K, Kawai T et al. Differential roles of TLR2 and TLR4 in recognition of gram-negative and gram-positive bacterial cell wall components. Immunity 1999; 11: 443–51.
16. Alexopoulou L, Holt AC, Medzhitov R et al. Recognition of double-stranded RNA and activation of NF-kappaB by Toll-like receptor 3. Nature 2001; 413: 732–8.
17. Hemmi H, Kaisho T, Takeuchi O et al. Small anti-viral compounds activate immune cells via the TLR7 MyD88-dependent signaling pathway. Nat Immunol 2002; 3: 196–200.
18. Jurk M, Heil F, Vollmer J et al. Human TLR7 or TLR8 independently confer responsiveness to the antiviral compound R-848. Nat Immunol 2002; 3: 499.
19. Hemmi H, Takeuchi O, Kawai T et al. A Toll-like receptor recognizes bacterial DNA. Nature 2002; 408: 740–5.
20. Wira CR, Stern J. Endocrine regulation of the mucosal immune system in the female reproductive tract: control of IgA, IgG, and secretory component during the reproductive cycle, at implantation and throughout pregnancy. In: Pasqualini JR, Scholler R, eds. Hormones and Fetal Pathophysiology. New York: Marcel Dekker, 1992: 343–68.
21. Cates W. Priorities for sexually transmitted diseases in the late 1980s and beyond. Sex Trans Dis 1986; 13: 114–17.
22. Piot P, Plummer FA, Mhalu FS et al. AIDS: an international perspective. Science 1988; 239: 573–9.
23. Peterman TA, Curran JW. Sexual transmission of human immunodeficiency virus. JAMA 1986; 256: 2222–6.
24. Harris C, Small CB, Klein RS et al. Immunodeficiency in female sexual partners of men with the acquired immunodeficiency syndrome. N Engl J Med 1983; 308: 1181–4.
25. Calabrese LH, Gopalakrishna KV. Transmission of HTLV-III infection from man to woman to man. N Engl J Med 1986; 314: 987.
26. Ho DD, Schooley RT, Rota TR et al. HTLV-III in the semen and blood of a healthy homosexual man. Science 1984; 226: 451–3.
27. Vogt MW, Witt DJ, Craven DE et al. Isolation of HTLV-III/LAV from cervical secretions of women at risk for AIDS. Lancet 1986; 1: 525–7.
28. Vogt MW, Witt DJ, Craven DE et al. Isolation patterns of the human immunodeficiency virus from cervical secretions during the menstrual cycle of women at risk for AIDS. Ann Intern Med 1987; 106: 380–2.
29. Wofsy CB, Cohen JB, Hauer LB et al. Isolation of AIDS-associated retrovirus from genital secretions of women with antibodies to the virus. Lancet 1986; 1: 527–9.
30. McDonough PG. Comment. Fertil Steril 1987; 48: 704.
31. Alexander NJ, Anderson DJ. Immunology of semen. Fertil Steril 1987; 47: 192–205.
32. Bronson RA. Immunology. In: Seibel MM, ed. Infertility: A Comprehensive Text. Norwalk, CT: Appleton and Lange, 1990: 217–34.
33. Allardyce RA. Effect of ingested sperm on fecundity in the rat. J Exp Med 1984; 159: 1548–53.

34. Allardyce R, Rademaker M. Female genital tract immunity and infertility after oral vaccination with sperm antigens in mice. Adv Exp Med Biol 1987; 216B: 1807–13.

35. Dahlenbach-Hellweg G. Histopathology of the Endometrium. New York: Springer-Verlag, 1975.

36. Morris H, Edwards J, Tiltman A et al. Endometrial lymphoid tissue: an immunohistological study. J Clin Pathol 1985; 38: 644–52.

37. Bulmer JN, Earl U. The expression of class II MHC gene products by fallopian tube epithelium in pregnancy and throughout the menstrual cycle. Immunology 1987; 61: 207–13.

38. Hunt JS. Immunologically relevant cells in the uterus. Biol Reprod 1994; 50: 461–6.

39. Chen CK, Huang SC, Chen CL et al. Increased expressions of CD69 and HLA-DR but not of CD25 or CD71 on endometrial T lymphocytes of nonpregnant women. Human Immunol 1995; 42: 227–32.

40. Lachapelle MH, Miron P, Hemmings R et al. Flow-cytometric characterization of hematopoietic cells in non-pregnant human endometrium. Am J Reprod Immunol 1996; 35: 5–13.

41. Lachapelle MH, Miron P, Hemmings R et al. Endometrial T, B, and NK cells in patients with recurrent spontaneous abortion. Altered profile and pregnancy outcome. J Immunol 1996; 156: 4027–34.

42. Kamat BR, Isaacson PG. The immunocytochemical distribution of leukocytic subpopulations in human endometrium. Am J Pathol 1987; 127: 66–73.

43. Hameed A, Fox WM, Kurman RJ et al. Perforin expression in endometrium during the menstrual cycle. Int J Gynecol Pathol 1995; 14: 143–50.

44. Loke YW, King A. Human Implantation: Cell Biology and Immunology. Cambridge: Cambridge University Press, 1995.

45. Bulmer JN. Cellular constituents of human endometrium in the menstrual cycle and early pregnancy. In: Bronson RA, Alexander NJ, Anderson D, Branch DW, Kutteh WH, eds. Reprod Immunol. Cambridge, MA: Blackwell Science, 1996: 212–39.

46. Givan AL, White HD, Stern JE et al. Flow cytometric analysis of leukocytes in the human female reproductive tract: comparison of Fallopian tube, uterus, cervix, and vagina. Am J Reprod Immunol 1997; 38: 350–9.

47. Tabibzadeh S. Proliferative activity of lymphoid cells in the human endometrium throughout the menstrual cycle. J Clin Endocrinol Metab 1990; 70: 437–43.

48. Yeaman GR, Guyre PM, Fanger MW et al. Unique CD8 + T cell-rich lymphoid aggregates in human uterine endometrium. J Leuk Biol 1997; 61: 427–35.

49. Yeaman GR, Collins JE, Fanger MW et al. CD8 + T cells in human uterine endometrial lymphoid aggregates shows no clonal restriction: evidence that uterine lymphoid aggregates arise by cell trafficking. Immunology 2001; 102: 434–40.

50. Parr MB, Parr EL. Mucosal immunity in the female and male reproductive tracts. In: Ogra PL, Mestecky J, Lamm ME et al, eds. Handbook of Mucosal Immunology. New York: Academic Press, 1994: 677–89.

51. Lippes J, Ogra S, Tomasi TBJ et al. Immunohistochemical localization of γG, γA, γM, secretory piece and lactoferrin in the human female genital tract. Contraception 1970; 1: 163.

52. Rebello R, Green F, Fox H. A study of the secretory immune system of the female genital tract. J Obstet Gynecol 1975; 82: 812–16.

53. Kelly JK, Fox H. The local immunological defense system of the human endometrium. J Reprod Immunol 1979; 1: 39–45.

54. Tourville DR, Ogra SS, Lippes J, Tomasi TB. The human female reproductive tract: immunohistological localization of γA, γG, γM, secretory 'piece' and lactoferrin. Am J Obstet Gynecol 1970; 108: 1102–8.

55. Wira CR, Sandoe CP. Sex steroid hormone regulation of IgA and IgG in rat uterine secretions. Nature 1977; 268: 534–6.

56. Wira CR, Hyde E, Sandoe CP et al. Cellular aspects of the rat uterine IgA response to estradiol and progesterone. J Steroid Biochem 1980; 12: 451–9.

57. Sullivan DA, Underdown BJ, Wira CR. Steroid hormone regulation of free secretory component in the rat uterus. Immunology 1983; 49: 379–86.

58. Wira CR, Sullivan DA. Estradiol and progesterone regulation of IgA, IgG and secretory component in cervico-vaginal secretions of the rat. Biol Reprod 1985; 32: 90–5.

59. Wira CR, Sandoe CP. Hormone regulation of immunoglobulins: influence of estradiol on IgA and IgG in the rat uterus. Endocrinology 1980; 106: 1020–6.

60. Kaushic C, Richardson JM, Wira CR. Regulation of polymeric immunoglobulin. A receptor messenger ribonucleic acid expression in rodent uteri: effect of sex hormones. Endocrinology 1995; 136: 2836–44.

61. Kaushic C, Frauendorf E, Wira CR. Polymeric immunoglobulin. A receptor in the rodent female reproductive tract: expression in vagina and tissue specific mRNA regulation by sex hormones. Biol Reprod 1997; 57: 958–66.

62. Tauber PF, Wettich W, Nohlen M et al. Diffusible proteins of the mucosa of the human cervix, uterus, and fallopian tubes: distribution and variations during the menstrual cycle. Am J Obstet Gynecol 1985; 15: 1115–25.

63. Schumacher GFB. Humoral immune factors in the female reproductive tract and their changes during the cycle. In: Dinsda D, Schumacher G, eds. Immunological Aspects of Infertility and Fertility Control. North Holland: Elsevier, 1980: 93–141.

64. Brandtzaeg P. Transport models for secretory IgA and IgM. Clin Exp Immunol 1981; 44: 221–32.

65. Vaerman J-P, Férin J. Local immunological response in the vagina, cervix and endometrium. Acta Endocrinol 1974; 194: 281–305.

66. Ganguly RCD, Waldman RH. Local immunity and local immune responses. Prog Allergy 1980; 27: 1–68.

67. South MS. In: Ogra PL, Dayton DH, eds. Immunology of Breast Milk. New York: Raven Press, 1979: 193.

68. Crago SS, Kulhavy R, Prince SJ et al. Inhibition of the pokeweed mitogen-induced response of normal peripheral blood lymphocytes by humoral components of colostrum. Clin Exp Immunol 1981; 45: 386–92.

69. Wira CR, Sandoe CP. Origin of IgA and IgG antibodies in the female reproductive tract: regulation of the genital response by estradiol. Adv Exp Med Biol 1987; 216A: 403–12.

70. Richardson J, Kaushic C, Wira CR. Estradiol regulation of secretory component: expression by rat uterine epithelial cells. J Steroid Biochem 1993; 47: 143–9.

71. Menge AC, Mestecky J. Surface expression of secretory component and HLA class II DR antigen on glandular epithelial cells from human endometrium and two endometrial adenocarcinoma cell lines. J Clin Immunol 1993; 13: 259–64.

72. Menge AC, Naz RK. Immunoglobulin (Ig) G, IgA, and IgA subclass antibodies against fertilization antigen-1 in cervical secretions and sera of women of infertile couples. Fertil Steril 1993; 60: 658–63.

73. Wira CR, Stern JE, Colby E. Estradiol regulation of secretory component in the uterus of the rat: evidence for involvement of RNA synthesis. J Immunol 1984; 133: 2624–8.

74. Richardson JM, Kaushic C, Wira CR. Polymeric immunoglobulin (Ig) receptor production and IgA transcytosis in polarized primary cultures of mature rat uterine epithelial cells. Biol Reprod 1995; 53: 488–98.

75. Fahey JV, Humphrey SL, Stern JE et al. Secretory component production by polarized epithelial cells from the human female reproductive tract. Immunol Invest 1998; 27: 167–80.

76. Hurlimann J, Dayal R, Gloor E. Immunoglobulins and secretory component in endometrium and cervix: influence of inflammation and carcinoma. Virch Arch Path Anat Histol 1978; 377: 211–23.

77. Sullivan DA, Wira CR. Hormonal regulation of immunoglobulins in the rat uterus: uterine response to a single estradiol treatment. Endocrinology 1983; 112: 260–8.

78. Sullivan DA, Wira CR. Hormonal regulation of immunoglobulins in the rat uterus: Uterine response to multiple estradiol treatments. Endocrinology 1984; 114: 650–8.

79. Sullivan DA, Wira CR. Variations in free secretory component levels in mucosal secretions of the rat. J Immunol 1983; 130: 1330–5.

80. Lohman BL, Miller CJ, McChesney MB. Antiviral cytotoxic T lymphocytes in vaginal mucosa of simian immunodeficiency virus-infected rhesus macaques. J Immunol 1995; 155: 5855–60.

81. Musey L, Hu Y, Eckert L et al. HIV-1 induces cytotoxic T lymphocytes in the cervix of infected women. J Exp Med 1997; 185: 293–303.

82. White HD, Crassi KM, Givan AL et al. CD3 + CD8 + CTL activity within the human female reproductive tract: influence of stage of the menstrual cycle and menopause. J Immunol 1997; 158: 3017–27.

83. White HD, Crassi K, Wira CR. Cytolytic functional activities of NK cells and cytotoxic T lymphocytes (CTL) are coordinately regulated in the human female reproductive tract. In: Husband AJ, Beagley KW, Clancey RL et al, eds. Mucosal Solutions: Advances in Mucosal Immunology. Sydney, Australia: The University of Sydney, 1997; 1: 385–91.

84. Ogra PL, Ogra SS. Local antibody response to poliovaccine in the human female genital tract. J Immunol 1973; 110: 1307–11.

85. Trombetta ES, Mellman I. Cell biology of antigen processing in vitro and in vivo. Annu Rev Immunol 2005; 23: 975–1028.

86. Rescigno M, Urbano M, Valzasina B et al. Dendritic cells express tight junction proteins and penetrate gut epithelial monolayers to sample bacteria. Nat Immunol 2001; 2: 361–7.

87. Lechler R, Aichinger G, Lightstone L. The endogenous pathway of MHC class II antigen presentation. Immunol Rev 1996; 151: 51–79.

88. Reyes VE, Ye G, Ogra PL et al. Antigen presentation of mucosal pathogens: the players and the rules. Int Arch Allergy Immunol 1997; 112: 103–14.

89. Lawton AP, Kronenberg M. The third way: progress on pathways of antigen processing and presentation by CD1. Immunol Cell Biol 2004; 82: 295–306.

90. Pasare C, Medzhitov R. Toll-dependent control mechanisms of CD4 T cell activation. Immunity 2004; 21: 733–41.

91. Pasare C, Medzhitov R. Toll-like receptors: linking innate and adaptive immunity. Adv Exp Med Biol 2005; 560: 11–18.

92. Pasare C, Medzhitov R. Control of B-cell responses by Toll-like receptors. Nature 2005; 438: 364–8.

93. van Duin D, Medzitov R, Shaw AC. Triggering TLR signaling in vaccination. Trends Immunol 2006; 27: 49–55.

94. Prabhala RH, Wira CR. Sex hormone and IL-6 regulation of antigen presentation in the female reproductive tract mucosal tissues. J Immunol 1995; 155: 5566–73.

95. Wira CR, Rossoll RM. Antigen presenting cells in the female reproductive tract: influence of the estrous cycle on antigen presentation by uterine epithelial and stromal cells. Endocrinology 1995; 136: 4526–34.

96. Wira CR, Rossoll RM. Antigen presenting cells in the female reproductive tract: influence of sex hormones on antigen presentation in the vagina. Immunology 1995; 84: 505–8.

97. Wira CR, Rossoll RM, Kaushic C. Antigen-presenting cells in the female reproductive tract: influence of estradiol on antigen presentation by vaginal cells. Endocrinology 2000; 141: 2877–85.

98. Wira CR, Roche MA, Rossoll RM. Antigen presentation by vaginal cells: role of TGFbeta as a mediator of estradiol inhibition of antigen presentation. Endocrinology 2002; 143: 2872–9.

99. Wira CR, Rossoll RM. Oestradiol regulation of antigen presentation by uterine stromal cells: role of transforming growth factor-beta production by epithelial cells in mediating antigen-presenting cell function. Immunology 2003; 109: 398–406.

100. Wira C, Rossoll R, Young R. Polarized uterine epithelial cells preferentially present antigen at the basolateral surface: role of stromal cells in regulating class II-mediated epithelial cell antigen presentation. J Immunol 2005; 175: 1795–804.

101. Wira CR, Grant-Tschudy KS, Crane-Godreau M. Epithelial cells in the female reproductive tract: a central role as sentinels of immune protection. Am J Reprod Immunol 2005; 53: 1–12.

102. Head JR, Gaede SD. Ia antigen expression in the rat uterus. J Reprod Immunol 1986; 9: 137–53.

103. Bjercke S, Brandtzaeg P. Glandular distribution of immunoglobins, J chain, secretory component, and HLA-DR in the human endometrium throughout the menstrual cycle. Hum Reprod 1993; 8: 1420–5.

104. Wallace PK, Yeaman GR, Johnson K et al. MHC class II expression and antigen presentation by human endometrial cells. J Steroid Biochem Mol Biol 2001; 76: 203–11.

105. Fahey JV, Prabhala RH, Guyre PM et al. Antigen-presenting cells in the human female reproductive tract: analysis of antigen presentation in pre- and post-menopausal women. Am J Reprod Immunol 1999; 42: 49–57.

106. Fahey JV, Wallace PK, Johnson K et al. Antigen presentation by human uterine epithelial cells to autologous T cells. Am J Reprod Immunol 2006; 55: 1–11.

107. Biancone L, Cantaluppi V, Camussi G. CD40–CD154 interaction in experimental and human disease (review). Int J Mol Med 1999; 3: 343–53.

108. Young LS, Eliopoulos AG, Gallagher NG et al. CD40 and epithelial cells: across the great divide. Immunol Today 1998; 19: 502–6.

109. Erlebacher A, Zhang D, Parlow AF et al. Ovarian insufficiency and early pregnancy loss induced by activation of the innate immune system. J Clin Invest 2004; 114: 39–48.

110. Jenkinson HJ, Wainwright SD, Simpson KL et al. Expression of CD1D mRNA transcripts in human choriocarcinoma cell lines and placentally derived trophoblast cells. Immunology 1999; 96: 649–55.

111. Mayer LF, Blumberg RS. Role of epithelial cells in mucosal antigen presentation. In: Mestecky J, Lamm ME, Strober W et al, eds. Mucosal Immunology. Boston, MA: Elsevier Academic Press, 2005; 1: 435–50.

112. Sallinen K, Verajankorva E, Pollanen P. Expression of antigens involved in the presentation of lipid antigens and induction of clonal anergy in the female reproductive tract. J Reprod Immunol 2000; 46: 91–101.

113. Wira CR, Fahey JV. The innate immune system: gatekeeper to the female reproductive tract. Immunology 2004; 111: 13–15.

114. Grant KS, Wira CR. Effect of mouse uterine stromal cells on epithelial cell transepithelial resistance (TER) and TNFalpha and TGFbeta release in culture. Biol Reprod 2003; 69: 1091–8.

115. Ganz T, Lehrer RI. Defensins. Pharmacol Ther 1995; 66: 191–205.

116. Quayle AJ, Porter EM, Nussbaum AA et al. Gene expression, immunolocalization, and secretion of human defensin-5 in human female reproductive tract. Am J Pathol 1998; 152: 1247–58.

117. Valore EV, Park CH, Quayle AJ et al. Human β-defensin-1, an antimicrobial peptide of urogenital tissues. J Clin Invest 1998; 101: 1633–42.

118. King AE, Fleming DC, Critchley HO et al. Regulation of natural antibiotic expression by inflammatory mediators and mimics of infection in human endometrial epithelial cells. Mol Hum Reprod 2002; 8: 341–9.

119. King AE, Fleming DC, Critchley HO et al. Differential expression of the natural antimicrobials, beta-defensins 3 and 4, in human endometrium. J Reprod Immunol 2003; 59: 1–16.

120. Denison FC, Kelly RW, Calder AA et al. Secretory leukocyte protease inhibitor concentration increases in amniotic fluid with the onset of labour in women: characterization of sites of release within the uterus. J Endocrinol 1999; 161: 299–306.

121. King AE, Morgan K, Sallenave JM et al. Differential regulation of secretory leukocyte protease inhibitor and elafin by progesterone. Biochem Biophys Res Commun 2003; 310: 594–9.

122. King AE, Critchley HO, Kelly RW. Presence of secretory leukocyte protease inhibitor in human endometrium and first trimester decidua suggests an antibacterial protective role. Mol Hum Reprod 2000; 6: 191–6.

123. Fleming DC, King AE, Williams AR et al. Hormonal contraception can suppress natural antimicrobial gene transcription in human endometrium. Fertil Steril 2003; 79: 856–63.

124. Chen D, Xu X, Cheon YP et al. Estrogen induces expression of secretory leukocyte protease inhibitor in rat uterus. Biol Reprod 2004; 71: 508–14.

125. Ace CI, Okulicz WC. Microarray profiling of progesterone-regulated endometrial genes during the rhesus monkey secretory phase. Reprod Biol Endocrinol 2004; 2: 54–60.

126. Quayle AJ. The innate and early immune response to pathogen challenge in the female genital tract and the pivotal role of epithelial cells. J Reprod Immunol 2002; 57: 61–79.

127. Tabibzadeh S. Evidence of T-cell activation and potential cytokine action in human endometrium. J Clin Endocrinol Metab 1990; 71: 645–9.

128. Tabibzadeh S. The signals and molecular pathways involved in human menstruation, a unique process of tissue destruction and remodelling. Mol Hum Reprod 1996; 2: 77–92.

129. Dominguez F, Pellicer A, Simon C. Paracrine dialogue in implantation. Mol Cell Endocrinol 2002; 186: 175–81.

130. Kayisli UA, Mahutte NG, Arici A. Uterine chemokines in reproductive physiology and pathology. Am J Reprod Immunol 2002; 47: 213–21.

131. Critchley HO, Kelly RW, Brenner RM et al. The endocrinology of menstruation – a role for the immune system. Clin Endocrinol (Oxf) 2001; 55: 701–10.

132. Jacobsson B, Holst RM, Wennerholm UB et al. Monocyte chemotactic protein-1 in cervical and amniotic fluid: relationship to microbial invasion of the amniotic cavity, intra-amniotic inflammation, and preterm delivery. Am J Obstet Gynecol 2003; 189: 1161–7.

133. Matsuda Y, Kouno S, Nakano H. Effects of antibiotic treatment on the concentrations of interleukin-6 and interleukin-8 in cervicovaginal fluid. Fetal Diagn Ther 2002; 17: 228–32.

134. Goepfert AR, Goldenberg RL, Andrews WW et al. The Preterm Prediction Study: association between cervical interleukin 6 concentration and spontaneous preterm birth. Am J Obstet Gynecol 2001; 184: 483–8.

135. Romero R, Chaiworapongsa T, Kuivaniemi H et al. Bacterial vaginosis, the inflammatory response and the risk of preterm birth: a role for genetic epidemiology in the prevention of preterm birth. Am J Obstet Gynecol 2004; 190: 1509–19.

136. Simhan HN, Caritis SN, Krohn MA et al. Decreased cervical proinflammatory cytokines permit subsequent upper genital tract infection during pregnancy. Am J Obstet Gynecol 2003; 189: 560–7.

137. Schaefer TM, Fahey JV, Wright JA et al. Innate immunity in the human female reproductive tract: antiviral response of uterine epithelial cells to the TLR3 agonist poly(I:C). J Immunol 2005; 174: 992–1002.

138. Schaefer TM, Wright JA, Pioli PA et al. IL-1beta-mediated proinflammatory responses are inhibited by estradiol via down-regulation of IL-1 receptor type 1 in uterine epithelial cells. J Immunol 2005; 175: 6509–16.

139. Fahey JV, Wira CR. Effect of menstrual status on antibacterial activity and secretory leukocyte protease inhibitor production by human uterine epithelial cells in culture. J Infect Dis 2002; 185: 1606–13.

140. Schaefer TM, Desouza K, Fahey JV et al. Toll-like receptor (TLR) expression and TLR-mediated cytokine/chemokine production by human uterine epithelial cells. Immunology 2004; 112: 428–36.

141. Young SL, Lyddon TD, Jorgenson RL et al. Expression of Toll-like receptors in human endometrial epithelial cells and cell lines. Am J Reprod Immunol 2004; 52: 67–73.

142. Hirata T, Osuga Y, Hirota Y et al. Evidence for the presence of toll-like receptor 4 system in the human endometrium. J Clin Endocrinol Metab 2005; 90: 548–56.

143. Fahey JV, Schaefer TM, Channon JY et al. Secretion of cytokines and chemokines by polarized human epithelial cells from the female reproductive tract. Hum Reprod 2005; 20: 1439–46.

144. Schaefer TM, Fahey JV, Wright JA et al. Migration inhibitory factor secretion by polarized uterine epithelial cells is enhanced in response to the TLR3 agonist poly (I:C). Am J Reprod Immunol 2005; 54: 193–202.

145. Baggiolini M. Activation and recruitment of neutrophil leukocytes. Clin Exp Immunol 1995; 101(Suppl 1): 5–6.

146. Yoshimura T, Leonard EJ. Human monocyte chemoattractant protein-1: structure and function. Cytokines 1992; 4: 131–52.

147. Shen L, Fahey JV, Hussey SB et al. Synergy between IL-8 and GM-CSF in reproductive tract epithelial cell secretions promotes enhanced neutrophil chemotaxis. Cell Immunol 2004; 230: 23–32.

148. Meter RA, Fahey JV, Wira CW. Secretion of monocyte chemotactic protein (MCP)-1 by polarized human uterine epithelium directs monocyte migration in culture. Fertil Steril 2005; 84: 191–201.

149. Lomas DA, Stone SR, Llewellyn-Jones C et al. The control of neutrophil chemotaxis by inhibitors of cathepsin G and chymotrypsin. J Biol Chem 1995; 270: 23437–43.

150. Gale LM, McColl SR. Chemokines: extracellular messengers for all occasions? Bioessays 1999; 21: 17–28.

151. Brown EJ. The role of extracellular matrix proteins in the control of phagocytosis. J Leukoc Biol 1986; 39: 579–91.

152. Nathan CF. Neutrophil activation on biological surfaces. Massive secretion of hydrogen peroxide in response to products of macrophages and lymphocytes. J Clin Invest 1987; 80: 1550–60.

153. Faurschou M, Borregaard N. Neutrophil granules and secretory vesicles in inflammation. Microbes Infect 2003; 5: 1317–27.

154. Faurschou M, Sorensen OE, Johnsen AH et al. Defensin-rich granules of human neutrophils: characterization of secretory properties. Biochim Biophys Acta 2002; 1591: 29–35.

155. Salamonsen LA, Woolley DE. Menstruation: induction by matrix metalloproteinases and inflammatory cells. J Reprod Immunol 1999; 44: 1–27.

156. Nathan C. Points of control in inflammation. Nature 2002; 420: 846–52.

157. Kelly RW, Illingworth P, Baldie G et al. Progesterone control of interleukin-8 production in endometrium and chorio-decidual cells underlines the role of the neutrophil in menstruation and parturition. Hum Reprod 1994; 9: 253–8.

158. Godaly G, Bergsten G, Hang L et al. Neutrophil recruitment, chemokine receptors, and resistance to mucosal infection. J Leukoc Biol 2001; 69: 899–906.

159. Yeaman GR, Collins JE, Currie JK et al. IFN-gamma is produced by polymorphonuclear neutrophils in human uterine

endometrium and by cultured peripheral blood polymorphonuclear neutrophils. J Immunol 1998; 160: 5145–53.

160. Poropatich C, Rojas M, Silverberg SG. Polymorphonuclear leukocytes in the endometrium during the normal menstrual cycle. Int J Gynecol Pathol 1987; 6: 230–4.

161. Arici A, Seli E, Senturk LM et al. Interleukin-8 in the human endometrium. J Clin Endocrinol Metab 1998; 83: 1783–7.

162. Critchley HO, Jones RL, Lea RG et al. Role of inflammatory mediators in human endometrium during progesterone withdrawal and early pregnancy. J Clin Endocrinol Metab 1999; 84: 240–8.

163. Salamonsen LA, Lathbury LJ. Endometrial leukocytes and menstruation. Hum Reprod Update 2000; 6: 16–27.

164. Okada Y, Nakanishi I. Activation of matrix metalloproteinase 3 (stromelysin) and matrix metalloproteinase 2 ('gelatinase') by human neutrophil elastase and cathepsin G. FEBS Lett 1989; 249: 353–6.

165. Salamonsen LA, Zhang J, Hampton A et al. Regulation of matrix metalloproteinases in human endometrium. Hum Reprod 2000; 15(Suppl 3): 112–19.

166. Owen CA, Campbell EJ. Neutrophil proteinases and matrix degradation. The cell biology of pericellular proteolysis. Semin Cell Biol 1995; 6: 367–76.

167. Daimon E, Wada Y. Role of neutrophils in matrix metalloproteinase activity in the preimplantation mouse uterus. Biol Reprod 2005; 73: 163–71.

168. Lathbury LJ, Salamonsen LA. In-vitro studies of the potential role of neutrophils in the process of menstruation. Mol Hum Reprod 2000; 6: 899–906.

169. Klein JB, Rane MJ, Scherzer JA et al. Granulocyte-macrophage colony-stimulating factor delays neutrophil constitutive apoptosis through phosphoinositide 3-kinase and extracellular signal-regulated kinase pathways. J Immunol 2000; 164: 4286–91.

170. Theilgaard-Monch K, Knudsen S, Follin P et al. The transcriptional activation program of human neutrophils in skin lesions supports their important role in wound healing. J Immunol 2004; 172: 7684–93.

171. Gargett CE, Lederman F, Heryanto B et al. Focal vascular endothelial growth factor correlates with angiogenesis in human endometrium. Role of intravascular neutrophils. Hum Reprod 2001; 16: 1065–75.

172. Heryanto B, Girling JE, Rogers PA. Intravascular neutrophils partially mediate the endometrial endothelial cell proliferative response to oestrogen in ovariectomized mice. Reproduction 2004; 127: 613–20.

173. Liu L, Mul FP, Lutter R et al. Transmigration of human neutrophils across airway epithelial cell monolayers is preferentially in the physiologic basolateral-to-apical direction. Am J Respir Cell Mol Biol 1996; 15: 771–80.

174. Kidney JC, Proud D. Neutrophil transmigration across human airway epithelial monolayers: mechanisms and dependence on electrical resistance. Am J Respir Cell Mol Biol 2000; 23: 389–95.

175. Mikamo H, Kawazoe K, Izumi K et al. Effects of long-term administration of roxithromycin on neutrophil count and interleukin-8 level in endometrial cavity subjected to pyometra. Chemotherapy 1997; 43: 148–52.

176. Kumaratilake LM, Ferrante A, Jaeger T et al. GM-CSF-induced priming of human neutrophils for enhanced phagocytosis and killing of asexual blood stages of *Plasmodium falciparum*: synergistic effects of GM-CSF and TNF. Parasite Immunol 1996; 18: 115–23.

177. Shen L, Smith JM, Shen Z et al. Differential regulation of neutrophil chemotaxis to IL-8 and fMLP by GM-CSF: lack of direct effect of oestradiol. Immunology 2006; 117: 205–12.

178. Giacomini G, Tabibzadeh SS, Satyaswaroop PG et al. Epithelial cells are the major source of biologically active granulocyte macrophage colony-stimulating factor in human endometrium. Hum Reprod 1995; 10: 3259–63.

179. Cassatella MA, Gasperini S, Russo MP. Cytokine expression and release by neutrophils. Ann NY Acad Sci 1997; 832: 233–42.

180. Kerr MA, Stocks SC. The role of CD15-(Le(X))-related carbohydrates in neutrophil adhesion. Histochem J 1992; 24: 811–26.

181. Gosselin EJ, Wardwell K, Rigby WF et al. Induction of MHC class II on human polymorphonuclear neutrophils by granulocyte/macrophage colony-stimulating factor, IFN-gamma, and IL-3. J Immunol 1993; 151: 1482–90.

182. Roberts WG, Palade GE. Increased microvascular permeability and endothelial fenestration induced by vascular endothelial growth factor. J Cell Sci 1995; 108 (Pt 6): 2369–79.

183. van der Meer A, Lukassen HG, van Lierop MJ et al. Membrane-bound HLA-G activates proliferation and interferon-gamma production by uterine natural killer cells. Mol Hum Reprod 2004; 10: 189–95.

184. Rajagopalan S, Fu J, Long EO. Cutting edge: induction of IFN-gamma production but not cytotoxicity by the killer cell Ig-like receptor KIR2DL4 (CD158d) in resting NK cells. J Immunol 2001; 167: 1877–81.

185. Ashkar AA, Black GP, Wei Q et al. Assessment of requirements for IL-15 and IFN regulatory factors in uterine NK cell differentiation and function during pregnancy. J Immunol 2003; 171: 2937–44.

186. Lanier LL. NK cell recognition. Annu Rev Immunol 2005; 23: 225–74.

187. Kumar V, McNerney ME. A new self: MHC-class-I-independent natural-killer-cell self-tolerance. Nat Rev Immunol 2005; 5: 363–74.

188. Biron CA, Nguyen KB, Pien GC et al. Natural killer cells in antiviral defense: function and regulation by innate cytokines. Annu Rev Immunol 1999; 17: 189–220.

189. Ferlazzo G, Morandi B, D'Agostino A et al. The interaction between NK cells and dendritic cells in bacterial infections results in rapid induction of NK cell activation and in the lysis of uninfected dendritic cells. Eur J Immunol 2003; 33: 306–13.

190. Scott MJ, Hoth JJ, Gardner SA et al. Natural killer cell activation primes macrophages to clear bacterial infection. Am Surg 2003; 69: 679–86; discussion 686–7.

191. Koopman LA, Kopcow HD, Rybalov B et al. Human decidual natural killer cells are a unique NK cell subset with immunomodulatory potential. J Exp Med 2003; 198: 1201–12.

192. Eriksson M, Meadows SK, Wira CR et al. Unique phenotype of human uterine NK cells and their regulation by endogenous TGF-beta. J Leukoc Biol 2004; 76: 667–75.

193. Moffett-King A. Natural killer cells and pregnancy. Nat Rev Immunol 2002; 2: 656–63.

194. Cooper MA, Fehniger TA, Caligiuri MA. The biology of human natural killer-cell subsets. Trends Immunol 2001; 22: 633–40.

195. King A, Wellings V, Gardner L et al. Immunocytochemical characterization of the unusual large granular lymphocytes in human endometrium throughout the menstrual cycle. Hum Immunol 1989; 24: 195–205.

196. Bulmer JN, Lash GE. Human uterine natural killer cells: a reappraisal. Mol Immunol 2005; 42: 511–21.

197. Kitaya K, Nakayama T, Okubo T et al. Expression of macrophage inflammatory protein-1beta in human endometrium: its role in endometrial recruitment of natural killer cells. J Clin Endocrinol Metab 2003; 88: 1809–14.

198. Sentman CL, Meadows SK, Wira CR et al. Recruitment of uterine NK cells: induction of CXC chemokine ligands 10 and 11 in human endometrium by estradiol and progesterone. J Immunol 2004; 173: 6760–6.

199. Kitaya K, Nakayama T, Daikoku N et al. Spatial and temporal expression of ligands for CXCR3 and CXCR4 in human endometrium. J Clin Endocrinol Metab 2004; 89: 2470–6.

200. Daikoku N, Kitaya K, Nakayama T et al. Expression of macrophage inflammatory protein-3beta in human endometrium throughout the menstrual cycle. Fertil Steril 2004; 81(Suppl 1): 876–81.

201. Chantakru S, Miller C, Roach LE et al. Contributions from self-renewal and trafficking to the uterine NK cell population of early pregnancy. J Immunol 2002; 168: 22–8.

202. Hanna J, Wald O, Goldman-Wohl D et al. CXCL12 expression by invasive trophoblasts induces the specific migration of CD16- human natural killer cells. Blood 2003; 102: 1569–77.

203. Wu X, Jin LP, Yuan MM et al. Human first-trimester trophoblast cells recruit CD56bright CD16- NK cells into decidua by way of expressing and secreting of CXCL12/stromal cell-derived factor 1. J Immunol 2005; 175: 61–8.

204. Chantakru S, Kuziel WA, Maeda N et al. A study on the density and distribution of uterine natural killer cells at mid pregnancy in mice genetically-ablated for CCR2, CCR 5 and the CCR5 receptor ligand, MIP-1 alpha. J Reprod Immunol 2001; 49: 33–47.

205. Xie X, Kang Z, Anderson LN et al. Analysis of the contributions of L-selectin and CXCR3 in mediating leukocyte homing to pregnant mouse uterus. Am J Reprod Immunol 2005; 53: 1–12.

206. Jiang D, Liang J, Hodge J et al. Regulation of pulmonary fibrosis by chemokine receptor CXCR3. J Clin Invest 2004; 114: 291–9.

207. Chalifour A, Jeannin P, Gauchat JF et al. Direct bacterial protein PAMP recognition by human NK cells involves TLRs and triggers alpha-defensin production. Blood 2004; 104: 1778–83.

208. Sivori S, Falco M, Della Chiesa M et al. CpG and double-stranded RNA trigger human NK cells by Toll-like receptors: induction of cytokine release and cytotoxicity against tumors and dendritic cells. Proc Natl Acad Sci USA 2004; 101: 10116–21.

209. Hart OM, Athie-Morales V, O'Connor GM et al. TLR7/8-mediated activation of human NK cells results in accessory cell-dependent IFN-γ production. J Immunol 2005; 175: 1636–42.

210. Schmidt-Weber CB, Blaser K. Regulation and role of transforming growth factor-beta in immune tolerance induction and inflammation. Curr Opin Immunol 2004; 16: 709–16.

211. Chen W, Wahl SM. Manipulation of TGF-beta to control autoimmune and chronic inflammatory diseases. Microbes Infect 1999; 1: 1367–80.

211a. Sentman CL, Wira CR, Ericksson M. NK cell function in the human female reproductive tract. Am J Reprod Immunol 2007; 57: 108–15.

212. Meadows SK, Eriksson M, Barber A et al. Human NK cell IFN-gamma production is regulated by endogenous TGF-beta. Int Immunopharmacol 2006; 6: 1020–8.

213. Laouar Y, Sutterwala FS, Gorelik L et al. Transforming growth factor-beta controls T helper type 1 cell development through regulation of natural killer cell interferon-gamma. Nat Immunol 2005; 6: 600–7.

214. Hiby SE, Walker JJ, O'Shaughnessy KM et al. Combinations of maternal KIR and fetal HLA-C genes influence the risk of preeclampsia and reproductive success. J Exp Med 2004; 200: 957–65.

215. Stein-Streilein J, Sonoda KH, Faunce D et al. Regulation of adaptive immune responses by innate cells expressing NK markers and antigen-transporting macrophages. J Leukoc Biol 2000; 67: 488–94.

216. Adams DO, Hamilton TA. The cell biology of macrophage activation. Annu Rev Immunol 1984; 2: 283–318.

217. DeLoia JA, Stewart-Akers AM, Brekosky J et al. Effects of exogenous estrogen on uterine leukocyte recruitment. Fertil Steril 2002; 77: 548–54.

218. Jones RL, Kelly RW, Critchley HO. Chemokine and cyclooxygenase-2 expression in human endometrium coincides with leukocyte accumulation. Hum Reprod 1997; 12: 1300–6.

219. Arici A, Senturk LM, Seli E et al. Regulation of monocyte chemotactic protein-1 expression in human endometrial stromal cells by estrogen and progesterone. Biol Reprod 1999; 61: 85–90.

220. Jones RL, Hannan NJ, Kaitu'u TJ et al. Identification of chemokines important for leukocyte recruitment to the human endometrium at the times of embryo implantation and menstruation. J Clin Endocrinol Metab 2004; 89: 6155–67.

221. Carruba G, D'Agostino P, Miele M et al. Estrogen regulates cytokine production and apoptosis in PMA-differentiated, macrophage-like U937 cells. J Cell Biochem 2003; 90: 187–96.

222. Vegeto E, Bonincontro C, Pollio G et al. Estrogen prevents the lipopolysaccharide-induced inflammatory response in microglia. J Neurosci 2001; 21: 1809–18.

223. Lambert KC, Curran EM, Judy BM et al. Estrogen receptor-alpha deficiency promotes increased TNF-alpha secretion and bacterial killing by murine macrophages in response to microbial stimuli in vitro. J Leukoc Biol 2004; 75: 1166–72.

224. Banchereau J, Steinman RM. Dendritic cells and the control of immunity. Nature 1998; 392: 245–52.

225. Cella M, Scheidegger D, Palmer-Lehmann K et al. Ligation of CD40 on dendritic cells triggers production of high levels of interleukin-12 and enhances T cell stimulatory capacity: T-T help via APC activation. J Exp Med 1996; 184: 747–52.

226. Bengtsson AK, Ryan EJ, Giordano D et al. 17beta-estradiol (E2) modulates cytokine and chemokine expression in human monocyte-derived dendritic cells. Blood 2004; 104: 1404–10.

227. Driggers PH, Segars JH. Estrogen action and cytoplasmic signaling pathways. Part II: the role of growth factors and phosphorylation in estrogen signaling. Trends Endocrinol Metab 2002; 13: 422–7.

228. Kammerer U, Schoppet M, McLellan AD et al. Human decidua contains potent immunostimulatory CD83(+) dendritic cells. Am J Pathol 2000; 157: 159–69.

229. Cameron P, Pope M, Granelli-Piperno A et al. Dendritic cells and the replication of HIV-1. J Leukoc Biol 1996; 59: 158–71.

230. Grouard G, Clark EA. Role of dendritic and follicular dendritic cells in HIV infection and pathogenesis. Curr Opin Immunol 1997; 9: 563–7.

231. Geijtenbeek TB, Kwon DS, Torensma R et al. DC-SIGN, a dendritic cell-specific HIV-1-binding protein that enhances trans-infection of T cells. Cell 2000; 100: 587–97.

232. Jameson B, Baribaud F, Pohlmann S et al. Expression of DC-SIGN by dendritic cells of intestinal and genital mucosae in humans and rhesus macaques. J Virol 2002; 76: 1866–75.

233. Dinarello CA. Interleukin-1 and interleukin-1 antagonism. Blood 1991; 77: 1627–52.

234. Dentener MA, Bazil V, Von Asmuth EJ et al. Involvement of CD14 in lipopolysaccharide-induced tumor necrosis factor-alpha, IL-6 and IL-8 release by human monocytes and alveolar macrophages. J Immunol 1993; 150: 2885–91.

235. Phiel KL, Henderson RA, Adelman SJ et al. Differential estrogen receptor gene expression in human peripheral blood mononuclear cell populations. Immunol Lett 2005; 97: 107–13.

236. Ashcroft GS, Mills SJ, Lei K et al. Estrogen modulates cutaneous wound healing by downregulating macrophage migration inhibitory factor. J Clin Invest 2003; 111: 1309–18.

237. Liebler JM, Kunkel SL, Burdick MD et al. Production of IL-8 and monocyte chemotactic peptide-1 by peripheral blood monocytes. Disparate responses to phytohemagglutinin and lipopolysaccharide. J Immunol 1994; 152: 241–9.

238. Adeyemo O, Jeyakumar H. Plasma progesterone, estradiol-17 beta and testosterone in maternal and cord blood, and maternal human chorionic gonadotropin at parturition. Afr J Med Med Sci 1993; 22: 55–60.

239. Sarda IR, Gorwill RH. Hormonal studies in pregnancy. I. Total unconjugated estrogens in maternal peripheral vein, cord vein, and cord artery serum at delivery. Am J Obstet Gynecol 1976; 124: 234–8.

240. Merkel SM, Alexander S, Zufall E et al. Essential role for estrogen in protection against *Vibrio vulnificus*-induced endotoxic shock. Infect Immun 2001; 69: 6119–22.

241. WHO. Global Prevalance and Incidence of Selected Curable Sexually Transmitted Infections. Overview and Estimates. Geneva: WHO, 2001.

242. Moodley P, Sturm AW. Sexually transmitted infections, adverse pregnancy outcome and neonatal infection. Semin Neonatol 2000; 5: 255–69.

243. UNAIDS/WHO 2005. AIDS Epidemic Update: Special Report on HIV Prevention. Geneva: WHO, 2005.

244. McEvedy C. The bubonic plague. Sci Am 1988; 258: 118–23.

245. Webster RG. The importance of animal influenza for human disease. Vaccine 2002; 20(Suppl 2): S16–20.

246. Comparison of female to male and male to female transmission of HIV in 563 stable couples. European Study Group on Heterosexual Transmission of HIV. BMJ 1992; 304: 809–13.

247. CDC. HIV/AIDS Surveillance Report 2003. Atlanta: US Department of Health and Human Services, CDC; 2003.

248. UNAIDS 2004. AIDS epidemic update. Geneva: UN, 2004.

249. Quinn TC, Wawer MJ, Sewankambo N et al. Viral load and heterosexual transmission of human immunodeficiency virus type 1. Rakai Project Study Group. N Engl J Med 2000; 342: 921–9.

250. Fleming DT, Wasserheit JN. From epidemiological synergy to public health policy and practice: the contribution of other sexually transmitted diseases to sexual transmission of HIV infection. Sex Transm Infect 1999; 75: 3–17.

251. Hu J, Gardner MB, Miller CJ. Simian immunodeficiency virus rapidly penetrates the cervicovaginal mucosa after intravaginal inoculation and infects intraepithelial dendritic cells. J Virol 2000; 74: 6087–95.

252. Spira AI, Marx PA, Patterson BK et al. Cellular targets of infection and route of viral dissemination after an intravaginal inoculation of simian immunodeficiency virus into rhesus macaques. J Exp Med 1996; 183: 215–25.

253. Collins KB, Patterson BK, Naus GJ et al. Development of an in vitro organ culture model to study transmission of HIV-1 in the female genital tract. Nat Med 2000; 6: 475–9.

254. Gupta P, Collins KB, Ratner D et al. Memory CD4(+) T cells are the earliest detectable human immunodeficiency virus type 1 (HIV-1)-infected cells in the female genital mucosal tissue during HIV-1 transmission in an organ culture system. J Virol 2002; 76: 9868–76.

255. Alfsen A, Yu H, Magerus-Chatinet A et al. HIV-1-infected blood mononuclear cells form an integrin- and agrin-dependent viral synapse to induce efficient HIV-1 transcytosis across epithelial cell monolayer. Mol Biol Cell 2005; 16: 4267–79.

256. Bomsel M, Prydz K, Parton RG et al. Endocytosis in filter-grown Madin-Darby canine kidney cells. J Cell Biol 1989; 109: 3243–58.

257. van't Wout AB, Kootstra NA, Mulder-Kampinga GA et al. Macrophage-tropic variants initiate human immunodeficiency virus type 1 infection after sexual, parenteral, and vertical transmission. J Clin Invest 1994; 94: 2060–7.

258. Zhu T, Mo H, Wang N et al. Genotypic and phenotypic characterization of HIV-1 patients with primary infection. Science 1993; 261: 1179–81.

259. Delwart EL, Mullins JI, Gupta P et al. Human immunodeficiency virus type 1 populations in blood and semen. J Virol 1998; 72: 617–23.

260. Zhu T, Wang N, Carr A et al. Genetic characterization of human immunodeficiency virus type 1 in blood and genital secretions: evidence for viral compartmentalization and selection during sexual transmission. J Virol 1996; 70: 3098–107.

261. Asin SN, Fanger MW, Wildt-Perinic D et al. Transmission of HIV-1 by primary human uterine epithelial cells and stromal fibroblasts. J Infect Dis 2004; 190: 236–45.

262. Asin SN, Wildt-Perinic D, Mason SI et al. Human immunodeficiency virus type 1 infection of human uterine epithelial cells: viral shedding and cell contact-mediated infectivity. 2003; 187: 1522–33.

263. Cohn MA, Frankel SS, Rugpao S et al. Chronic inflammation with increased human immunodeficiency virus (HIV) RNA expression in the vaginal epithelium of HIV-infected Thai women. J Infect Dis 2001; 184: 410–17.

264. Martin HL, Richardson BA, Nyange PM et al. Vaginal lactobacilli, microbial flora, and risk of human immunodeficiency virus type 1 and sexually transmitted disease acquisition. J Infect Dis 1999; 180: 1863–8.

265. Sewankambo N, Gray RH, Wawer MJ et al. HIV-1 infection associated with abnormal vaginal flora morphology and bacterial vaginosis. Lancet 1997; 350: 546–50.

266. Pope M, Haase AT. Transmission, acute HIV-1 infection and the quest for strategies to prevent infection. Nat Med 2003; 9: 847–52.

267. Zhang Z, Schuler T, Zupancic M et al. Sexual transmission and propagation of SIV and HIV in resting and activated CD4+ T cells. Science 1999; 286: 1353–7.

268. Kunz G, Beil D, Deiniger H et al. The uterine peristaltic pump. Normal and impeded sperm transport within the female genital tract. Adv Exp Med Biol 1997; 424: 267–77.

269. Kunz G, Beil D, Deininger H et al. The dynamics of rapid sperm transport through the female genital tract: evidence from vaginal sonography of uterine peristalsis and hysterosalpingoscintigraphy. Hum Reprod 1996; 11: 627–32.

270. Kunz G, Noe M, Herbertz M et al. Uterine peristalsis during the follicular phase of the menstrual cycle: effects of oestrogen, antioestrogen and oxytocin. Hum Reprod Update 1998; 4: 647–54.

271. Parsons AK, Cone RA, Moench TR. Uterine uptake of vaginal fluids: implications for microbicides. Presented at Microbicides 2002, Antwerp, Belgium, 2002. Abstract B-175: 36.

272. Settlage DS, Motoshima M, Tredway DR. Sperm transport from the external cervical os to the fallopian tubes in women: a time and quantitation study. Fertil Steril 1973; 24: 655–61.

273. Bagasra O, Freund M, Weidmann J et al. Interaction of human immunodeficiency virus with human sperm in vitro. J Acquir Immune Defic Syndr 1988; 1: 431–5.

274. Brogi A, Presentini R, Solazzo D et al. Interaction of human immunodeficiency virus type 1 envelope glycoprotein gp120 with a galactoglycerolipid associated with human sperm. AIDS Res Hum Retroviruses 1996; 12: 483–9.

275. Gosselin EJ, Howell AL, Schwarz L et al. Infectivity by HIV-1 of human uterine endometrial carcinoma cells. Adv Exp Med Biol 1995; 371B: 1003–6.

276. Howell AL, Edkins RD, Rier SE et al. Human immunodeficiency virus type 1 infection of cells and tissues from the upper and lower human female reproductive tract. J Virol 1997; 71: 3498–506.

277. Tan X, Phillips DM. Cell-mediated infection of cervix derived epithelial cells with primary isolates of human immunodeficiency virus. Arch Virol 1996; 141: 1177–89.

278. Yeaman GR, Asin S, Weldon S et al. Chemokine receptor expression in the human ectocervix: implications for infection by the human immunodeficiency virus-type I. Immunology 2004; 113: 524–33.

279. Yeaman GR, Howell AL, Weldon S et al. Human immunodeficiency virus receptor and coreceptor expression on human uterine epithelial cells: regulation of expression during the menstrual cycle and implications for human immunodeficiency virus infection. Immunology 2003; 109: 137–46.

280. Mastro TD, de Vincenzi I. Probabilities of sexual HIV-1 transmission. AIDS 1996; 10(Suppl A): S75–82.

281. Wawer MJ, Gray RH, Sewankambo NK et al. Rates of HIV-1 transmission per coital act, by stage of HIV-1 infection, in Rakai, Uganda. J Infect Dis 2005; 191: 1403–9.

282. Ganz T. Defensins: antimicrobial peptides of innate immunity. Nat Rev Immunol 2003; 3: 710–20.

283. Duits LA, Nibbering PH, van Strijen E et al. Rhinovirus increases human beta-defensin-2 and -3 mRNA expression in cultured bronchial epithelial cells. FEMS Immunol Med Microbiol 2003; 38: 59–64.

284. Ganz T. Defensins and host defense. Science 1999; 286: 420–1.

285. Lehrer RI, Ganz T. Defensins of vertebrate animals. Curr Opin Immunol 2002; 14: 96–102.

286. Porter E, Yang H, Yavagal S et al. Distinct defensin profiles in *Neisseria gonorrhoeae* and *Chlamydia trachomatis* urethritis reveal novel epithelial cell–neutrophil interactions. Infect Immun 2005; 73: 4823–33.

287. Beppu Y, Imamura Y, Tashiro M et al. Human mucus protease inhibitor in airway fluids is a potential defensive compound against infection with influenza A and Sendai viruses. J Biochem (Tokyo) 1997; 121: 309–16.

288. Gropp R, Frye M, Wagner TO et al. Epithelial defensins impair adenoviral infection: implication for adenovirus-mediated gene therapy. Hum Gene Ther 1999; 10: 957–64.

289. Hiemstra PS, Maassen RJ, Stolk J et al. Antibacterial activity of antileukoprotease. Infect Immun 1996; 64: 4520–4.

290. Quinones-Mateu ME, Lederman MM, Feng Z et al. Human epithelial beta-defensins 2 and 3 inhibit HIV-1 replication. AIDS 2003; 17: F39–48.

291. Tomee JF, Hiemstra PS, Heinzel-Wieland R et al. Antileukoprotease: an endogenous protein in the innate mucosal defense against fungi. J Infect Dis 1997; 176: 740–7.

292. Virella-Lowell I, Poirier A, Chesnut KA et al. Inhibition of recombinant adeno-associated virus (rAAV) transduction by bronchial secretions from cystic fibrosis patients. Gene Ther 2000; 7: 1783–9.

293. Hocini H, Becquart P, Bouhlal H et al. Secretory leukocyte protease inhibitor inhibits infection of monocytes and lymphocytes with human immunodeficiency virus type 1 but does not interfere with transcytosis of cell-associated virus across tight epithelial barriers. Clin Diagn Lab Immunol 2000; 7: 515–18.

294. McNeely TB, Dealy M, Dripps DJ et al. Secretory leukocyte protease inhibitor: a human saliva protein exhibiting anti-human immunodeficiency virus 1 activity in vitro. J Clin Invest 1995; 96: 456–64.

295. Shugars DC, Sauls DL, Weinberg JB. Secretory leukocyte protease inhibitor blocks infectivity of primary monocytes and mononuclear cells with both monocytotropic and

lymphocytotropic strains of human immunodeficiency virus type I. Oral Dis 1997; 3(Suppl 1): S70–2.

296. Bleul CC, Farzan M, Choe H et al. The lymphocyte chemoattractant SDF-1 is a ligand for LESTR/fusin and blocks HIV-1 entry. Nature 1996; 382: 829–33.

297. Cocchi F, DeVico AL, Garzino-Demo A et al. Identification of RANTES, MIP-1 alpha, and MIP-1 beta as the major HIV-suppressive factors produced by CD8+ T cells. Science 1995; 270: 1811–15.

298. Le Bon A, Tough DF. Links between innate and adaptive immunity via type I interferon. Curr Opin Immunol 2002; 14: 432–6.

299. Player MR, Maitra RK, Silverman RH et al. Targeting RNase L to human immunodeficiency virus RNA with 2-5A-antisense. Antivir Chem Chemother 1998; 9: 225–31.

300. Roy S, Katze MG, Parkin NT et al. Control of the interferon-induced 68-kilodalton protein kinase by the HIV-1 tat gene product. Science 1990; 247: 1216–19.

301. Schroder HC, Kelve M, Muller WE. The 2-5A system and HIV infection. Prog Mol Subcell Biol 1994; 14: 176–97.

302. Sobol RW, Fisher WL, Reichenbach NL et al. HIV-1 reverse transcriptase: inhibition by 2',5'-oligoadenylates. Biochemistry 1993; 32: 12112–18.

303. Clemens MJ, Williams BR. Inhibition of cell-free protein synthesis by pppA2'p5'A2'p5'A: a novel oligonucleotide synthesized by interferon-treated L cell extracts. Cell 1978; 13: 565–72.

304. Farrell PJ, Balkow K, Hunt T et al. Phosphorylation of initiation factor eIF-2 and the control of reticulocyte protein synthesis. Cell 1977; 11: 187–200.

305. Jorgenson RL, Young SL, Lesmeister MJ et al. Human endometrial epithelial cells cyclically express Toll-like receptor 3 (TLR3) and exhibit TLR3-dependent responses to dsRNA. Hum Immunol 2005; 66: 469–82.

306. Jacobs BL, Langland JO. When two strands are better than one: the mediators and modulators of the cellular responses to double-stranded RNA. Virology 1996; 219: 339–49.

307. Koch JU. Sperm migration in the human female genital tract with and without intrauterine devices. Acta Eur Fertil 1980; 11: 33–60.

308. Nelson RD, Quie PG, Simmons RL. Chemotaxis under agarose: a new and simple method for measuring chemotaxis and spontaneous migration of human polymorphonuclear leukocytes and monocytes. J Immunol 1975; 115: 1650–6.

309. Pioli PA, Weaver LK, Schaefer TM et al. Lipopolysaccharide-induced IL-1β production by human uterine macrophages upregulates uterine epithelial cell expression of human β-defensin 2. J Immunol 2006; 176: 6647–55.

34 Molecular immunology of the maternal–fetal interface

Joan S Hunt and Margaret G Petroff

Synopsis

Background

- The components of the maternal–fetal interface include, from the fetus, the placenta, fetal blood, and extraplacental membranes and, from the mother, the decidualized endometrium and circulating maternal blood.
- During pregnancy the local immune environment of the uterus must be modified so as to prevent maternal rejection of the semiallogeneic fetus(es) while concurrently permitting immune system components to provide host defense and participate in the reproductive process.
- During gestation, cells constituting the adaptive immune system that normally inhabit the uterine mucosa are replaced by cells of the innate immune system that confer less-effective protection against disease, incurring a certain vulnerability to infection.

Basic Science

- During pregnancy, the placenta and extraplacental membranes interface directly with maternal blood and tissue.
- The placenta, a tissue of fetal origin, is adapted for multiple functions, one of which is avoidance of immune rejection of paternally inherited antigens.
- Molecular adaptations identified in placentas that contribute to immune privilege include replacement of the highly polymorphic major histocompatibility complex (MHC) antigens that stimulate graft rejection with MHC antigens, including HLA-G, that have little variation on fetal cells interfacing directly with maternal blood and tissues.
- The placenta also preferentially expresses immunoinhibitory co-stimulatory molecules such as B7-H1 rather than immunostimulatory members of this family and produces an abundance of soluble molecules such as interleukin-10 (IL-10) that facilitate tolerance and immune privilege in pregnancy.
- The results of expression analysis in the human placenta together with functional studies in the mouse strongly suggest that B7-H1 serves as a molecular shield against lymphocytes, and that human pregnancy is dependent upon B7-H1 expression in trophoblast.
- Because of the abundance of complement components in serum and the potential for both auto- or alloantibody-mediated and spontaneous activation of this potent pathway, the trophoblast must employ universally effective mechanisms to counter its activation.
- Leukocyte subpopulations in maternal blood are changed in pregnancy, with a rise in the number of circulating, activated mononuclear phagocytes.
- The most prominent leukocyte subpopulations that remain in the postimplantation uterus are NK cells, antigen-presenting cells including dendritic cells and macrophages, and a few T lymphocytes (regulatory or cytotoxic). This restructuring permits introduction and safe harbor for new, non-self elements, i.e. fetally derived cells and their products.
- An emerging concept is that the altered local environment, where acquired immunity is dampened and the innate immune system prevails, is programmed mainly by the placenta and its products, thus introducing the required feature of pregnancy specificity.

Clinical

- Many normal pregnancies are characterized by formation of antipaternal antibodies, with no apparent consequence.
- Antiphospholipid autoantibodies often preexist in maternal serum, particularly in women with lupus; these antibodies are strongly associated with thrombosis and increased incidence of miscarriage.
- Antibodies from aPL-positive, but not aPL-negative patients, induce fetal loss and growth retardation after passive transfer to mouse in a complement-dependent manner.
- Heparin is clinically important in the treatment of women experiencing antibody-associated recurrent miscarriage, and may mediate its antiabortive effect in mice through inhibition of complement rather than solely by its antithrombotic effects.
- Uterine NK cells bearing KIR receptors may receive activatory signals from HLA-C on invasive trophoblast to assist in spiral artery modification. Recent data suggest that preeclampsia may be associated with specific combinations of alleles of KIR and HLA-C (on invading trophoblast), resulting in failure of this NK cell function.
- Better knowledge of placental function will eventually allow earlier diagnosis of pregnancy problems and new approaches for treating subfertile women.

ABSTRACT

Successful mammalian pregnancy is characterized by the introduction of new patterns of gene expression in the female reproductive organs. In the case of pregnancy in outbred species where the fetus is internalized and maternal and fetal tissues are in direct contact, one major change is in the local immune environment, which must be modified so as to prevent maternal rejection of the semiallogeneic fetus(es) while concurrently permitting immune system components to provide host defense and participate in the reproductive process. Decades of experimentation have shown that pregnancy is well protected by overlapping and redundant protective mechanisms supplied by both the mother and the fetus. An emerging concept is that the altered local environment, where adaptive immunity is dampened and the innate immune system prevails, is programmed mainly by the placenta and its products. A second major emerging concept is that placental products have dual or multiple roles, participating in placental organogenesis and function as well as providing immune privilege. These and other recent insights on placental functions may lead to earlier diagnosis of pregnancy problems and to new approaches for treating women with less than optimal fertility.

INTRODUCTION

As with essentially all tissue remodeling and associated biological processes, successful pregnancy requires orchestration of multiple, interconnected networks and is achieved by modulation of gene expression that changes patterns of synthesis of messenger RNAs and proteins. In the case of pregnancy in outbred mammalian species where the fetus is internalized and maternal and fetal tissues are in direct contact, the local immune environment must be modified so as to prevent maternal immune rejection of the semiallogeneic fetus(es) while concurrently supporting its growth and development. Decades of experimentation have shown that in humans and other species, pregnancy is well protected by overlapping and redundant mechanisms supplied by both the mother and the fetus.[1–3]

The fetal components of the maternal–fetal interface include the extraplacental membranes and the placenta, whereas maternal components include the decidualized endometrium and circulating blood. The placenta, an organ that only temporarily inhabits the uterus, is uniquely designed for multiple functions, one of which is avoidance of immune rejection. Molecular adaptations identified in placentas that contribute to immune privilege include replacement of the highly polymorphic major histocompatibility complex (MHC) antigens that stimulate graft rejection with MHC antigens that have little variation on fetal cells interfacing directly with maternal blood and tissues. The placenta also preferentially expresses immunoinhibitory co-stimulatory molecules such as B7H1 rather than immunostimulatory members of this family and produces an abundance of soluble molecules such as interleukin-10 (IL-10) that facilitate tolerance and immune privilege in pregnancy. These and other rejection-avoiding features of the placenta and extraplacental fetal membranes markedly resemble those of tumor cells that successfully evade the host immune system.[4]

The maternal components, the endometrium and maternal blood, are altered with the onset of pregnancy. In decidualized endometrium, adaptive immunity is dampened and the innate immune system prevails. Because cells constituting the adaptive immune system that normally inhabit this mucosal site are dispersed and are replaced by cells of the innate immune system that confer less effective protection against disease, a certain vulnerability to infection is incurred during gestation. In the maternal blood circulation, proportions of leukocyte subpopulations are changed, with a rise in the number of circulating, activated mononuclear phagocytes being the most notable.

The events taking place in the endometrium during preparation for pregnancy and maintenance of the fetus rely, for the most part, on signals from fetal tissues. The altered local immune environment is programmed mainly by the placenta and its products, thus permitting alterations to the uterine immunological environment only during pregnancy. Also, newly recognized is that the placental products programming maternal immune cells have dual or multiple roles, thus improving the efficiency of resource utilization. For example, tumor necrosis factor (TNF) gene family proteins contributing to immune privilege and deviation of the maternal immune response into beneficial channels appear also to participate in placental organogenesis. This chapter explores these new concepts, focusing on human pregnancy but highlighting insights developed in experimental animal models.

ANATOMICAL FEATURES OF THE HUMAN PLACENTA

The fetal portion of the maternal–fetal interface is composed of the placenta and extraplacental membranes. Figure 34.1 illustrates the critical point that, in normal pregnancies, the placenta and extraplacental membranes interface directly with maternal blood and tissue and therefore carry the major responsibility for preventing the mother from summarily rejecting the 'foreign object', the fetus. Special mechanisms allow placental cells, which may express 'foreign' paternal antigens, to survive and enjoy nourishment from the mother. The fetal placenta and its continuing membranes contain two major types of cells, trophoblast cells and stromal cells. These differ embryologically and functionally.

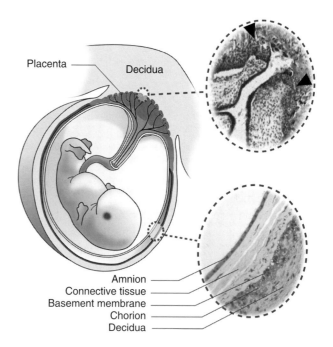

Figure 34.1 The maternal–fetal interface. The fetus is entirely surrounded and encased by trophoblast cells in the placenta and chorion membrane. The mother's cells and fetal cells are intermixed at the border between the placenta and decidua basalis (top inset) and between the chorion membrane and decidua parietalis (bottom inset). In the upper inset, arrowheads point to invading extravillous cytotrophoblast cell and the white spaces represent maternal blood lacunae. Original magnifications: upper, ×200; lower, ×200. (Modified from Figure 1, reference 1)

Placental trophoblast cells

The human placenta contains many types of cells and exerts multiple functions throughout its short-lived residency in the uterus. Of these cells, reproductive immunologists focus primarily on trophoblast cells because they are the major fetal cell type interfacing with maternal blood and decidua and are an entirely unique lineage not found in men or in women other than during pregnancy. Trophoblast cells arise from the trophectoderm, which is the outermost layer of the blastocyst. After implantation, the giant trophoblasts derived from this layer differentiate into structurally and functionally distinct subpopulations of trophoblast cells.[5] The mouse is an excellent model for studying these events, as the sequences of changes are demonstrable hourly and are readily evaluated in histological tissue sections by using light microscopy. A strong case for parallels between differentiation of trophoblast cells in the placentas of mice and women that justifies use of the mouse for many if not all types of functional studies has been made by Rossant and Cross.[6]

Trophoblast precursor cells in human placentas, which are the villous cytotrophoblast (CTB) cells, choose one of two pathways of differentiation. Throughout gestation, these cells merge with the syncytium that forms the outermost later of the floating villi to increase the size of the placenta as the fetus grows. In early to middle stages of gestation, the villous CTB cells may proliferate, emerge from the villi and form columns that contact the maternal decidua (see Figure 34.1, top inset). A recent study from James et al[7] suggests that the tips of the floating villi may contain a special population designed for proliferation and invasion. The general subpopulations in early to middle gestation are (1) villous CTB cells, (2) syncytium, and (3) migrating CTB cells. The migrating extravillous CTB cells have additional special designations. Those in the distal column are termed the trophoblastic shell, those located in the decidual stroma are termed interstitial CTB cells, those lining the maternal spiral arteries are termed the endovascular CTB cells.

By the third trimester, CTB cells in floating villi have been heavily depleted and the syncytiotrophoblast layer predominates. Regression of the extravillous CTB cells has taken place and this subpopulation is now located exclusively in the basal plate, a collagenous layer between the villous placenta and the decidua, and in the chorion membrane.

Subpopulation status dictates specific functions. For example, only villous CTB cells are capable of merging with the syncytiotrophoblast cell layer as it expands to accommodate the needs of the growing fetus. Syncytiotrophoblast is responsible for providing defense against immune cells and their potentially destructive products in maternal blood, facilitating bidirectional transport of nutrients and wastes between the mother and the embryo/fetus, producing pregnancy-specific hormones, serving as a structural barrier to maternal–fetal cell traffic, and protecting against environmental toxicants.[1,2,8] By contrast, the extravillous CTB cells exhibit migratory properties as they drive into the decidua to anchor the placenta to the mother and replace the endothelial cells of the spiral arteries. Endothelial cell replacement is critical to expanding the maternal vasculature so that maternal blood can flow over the floating villi, an event that takes place in human placentas around the 10th–12th week of gestation.[9] The migrating CTB cells have special immune protective devices, many of which are regulated by O_2 levels in the decidua. Oxygen levels are low in the early placenta and higher during the middle to late stages of gestation. The regulated CTB cell molecules include certain members of the B7 family of co-stimulatory molecules and human leukocyte antigen (HLA)-G proteins, both of which have immunotolerizing properties.[1-3,10]

Placental stromal cells

The placental stroma is derived from the extraembryonic mesoderm of the inner cell mass and is contiguous with the umbilical cord. It contains endothelial cells, smooth muscle cells, fibroblasts and macrophages. The endothelial cells and smooth muscle cells generate the placental vasculature, with activity highest in the tips of the villi. The fibroblasts may include not only classic cells with high production of growth factors but also undifferentiated fibroblastic-like cells with the ability to transform into these or other cell types. In early-gestation placentas, the resident macrophages are termed Hofbauer cells. These cells are highly phagocytic. Their cell surface molecules, including HLA class II molecules and macrophage markers, as well as their patterns of cytokine production, increase in diversity and develop sophistication during the course of gestation.[11,12] The placental macrophages become involved in defense of the semiallogeneic embryo when the trophoblast cell layer is breached. This condition, called villitis, is a common occurrence. The denuded villi contain not only fetal macrophages but also maternal macrophages and lymphocytes.[13]

Extraplacental membranes

Following implantation and throughout gestation, the developing fetus resides in a fluid-filled amniotic sac, where it is entirely sequestered from maternal cells (see Figure 34.1). In mammals, the amniotic fluid contains many cells, among which are macrophages. The macrophages reportedly migrate into the myometrium and influence pregnancy termination in mice.[14] The amniotic sac or membrane is formed of a single epithelial cell layer joined by tight junctions. As is the case with other cells derived from the inner cell mass, amnion epithelial cells in the amnion membrane display a normal spectrum of HLA class Ia antigens that can be enhanced by interferon γ (IFNγ).[15]

Underlying the amnion membrane is an area of connective tissue that contains no vasculature but is sparsely populated with fetal fibroblasts and macrophages that are interconnected to form a three-dimensional network.[16] These cells may communicate through the collagenous zone, an idea as yet unexplored experimentally. The next cell layer is the chorion laeve, which is composed of the remaining extravillous CTB cells that were derived from the trophectoderm (see Figure 34.1, bottom inset). Atrophic villi containing connective tissue and macrophages are readily identified throughout this four- to six-cell-deep membrane. Although the chorionic CTB cells retain many characteristics of extravillous CTB cells, the cells have limited ability to migrate near the conclusion of pregnancy.

Immunological interactions between maternal decidual leukocytes and the chorion membrane CTB cells are essentially the same as between maternal and fetal cells in the decidua during early to middle stages of pregnancy. Chorion membrane CTB cells exhibit the same immunologically critical cell surface and soluble antigen profiles as do their extravillous CTB cell counterparts in early pregnancy. Expression of HLA-G illustrates this point as chorion membrane CTB cells directly adjacent to the decidua express HLA-G5, and a few of these cells express HLA-G1 and HLA-G2/G6. This is also the case with their counterparts in the distal trophoblast column during early pregnancy.[1–3,17]

ENDOMETRIAL LEUKOCYTES

Both cycling and pregnant uteri contain cells derived from the bone marrow that provide immune protection. At the site of implantation, the uterus is temporarily flooded with neutrophils and other inflammatory cells, a process best documented in the mouse.[18] This is believed to be mainly the consequence of destruction of the uterine lining and release of debris to which neutrophils are attracted. Thereafter, the uterine cells promoting adaptive immunity are removed to the outer reaches of the uterus, i.e. into the myometrium, whereas populations of cells constituting the innate immune system are retained and even more are attracted into the decidual environment. This switch from the adaptive to the innate immune system, which is likely to be critical to the maintenance of semiallogeneic pregnancy, seems to be programmed first by ovarian estrogens and then by hormones and chemokines produced in the placenta. The chemokines include monocyte inflammatory protein-1β (MIP-1β), RANTES, monocyte chemotactic protein-1 (MCP-1), HCC-1 and SLC, which bind to CCR receptors, and interleukin-8 (IL-8), GCP-2, CXCL1, ITAC (CXCL11) IP-10 (CXCL10), SDF-1, CXCL16, and fractalkine, which bind to CXCR receptors.[1–3]

Cycling uterus

T and B lymphocytes form functional aggregates in the cycling uterine endometrium just as they do at other mucosal surfaces. Antigen-presenting cells (APCs), which include macrophages and their close relatives, dendritic cells, are distributed through the endometrial stroma and are threaded through the connective tissue in the myometrium. Natural killer (NK) cells are also inhabitants of the cycling uterus, and mast cells are prominent near the end of the cycle. Although the macrophages, dendritic cells, and NK cells provide host defense against pathogens, the mast cells have been implicated in driving menstruation.[19,20]

Many uterine leukocytes respond to and depend on ovarian hormones. For example, macrophages are attracted into the cycling uterus when levels of estrogens are high and human NK cell populations have prolactin receptors and also depend on progesterone for maintenance and proliferation.[11,12,21,22] These effects may be either direct or indirect as hormones influence both cell behavior and cellular production of a broad spectrum of cytokines. For example, estrogens up-regulate production of IFNγ, a proinflammatory cytokine that is critical to activation of macrophages. Oppositely, progesterone has a calming effect on immune cells similar to that of corticosteroids. At high levels progesterone may act through the glucocorticoid receptor to down-regulate production of inflammatory cytokines.[23]

Uterine leukocytes also respond to chemoattractants, production of which may be dependent upon female steroid hormones. An example is progesterone enhancement of the chemoattractants IL-8 and MCP-1, during the window of implantation.[24] At least two chemokines, IP-10 and ITAC, have been reported to respond to steroid hormones. At times of embryo implantation and menstruation, chemokine patterns are highly predictable.[1,2]

Pregnant uterus

B and T lymphocytes generate antigen-specific, adaptive immunity. If these cells were present in the pregnant uterus, they might recognize paternally derived fetal MHC or other antigens expressed in the placenta as foreign and mount an attack. In this case, if activated, maternal immune cells could be a significant danger to the semiallogeneic fetus. It is therefore not surprising that, concurrently with implantation, dramatic changes take place in the uterus, including restructuring into a site of innate immunity. B cells and most T cells almost entirely disappear from the decidualizing endometrium.[25–27] The most prominent leukocyte subpopulations that remain in the postimplantation uterus are NK cells, APCs, and a few T lymphocytes. This restructuring permits introduction and safe harbor for new, non-self elements, i.e. fetally derived cells and their products.[27]

Although not all of the factors leading to these environmental alterations have been uncovered, products of trophoblast cells forming the leading edge of the invasive implant are important. Chemokines and their receptors found in gestational tissues that interact in complex pathways to alter leukocyte subpopulations include MIP-1β, which attracts monocytes and NK cells into the human uterus, and IL-8, which may influence neutrophil and other leukocyte populations.[1-3] Reprogramming of resident and incoming leukocytes for immune suppression is essential; with implantation, genetically dissimilar, highly specialized CTB cells from the implanted blastocyst drive directly toward these leukocytes and must be protected. Importantly, the maternal leukocytes may not be simply anergic (unresponsive) but may have positive functions that benefit pregnancy.[28]

Natural killer cells

The imagination of many investigators has been captured by decidual NK cells because of their unusual structural and functional characteristics and their high densities in the early human decidua.[21,22] These cells have a defined chronological profile where the cells are extremely numerous during the first two trimesters of human pregnancy, constituting 20–40% of the decidual stromal cells. Levels decline dramatically as termination of pregnancy approaches. NK cells in human uteri (uNK cells) are small cells of the lymphoid lineage. They contain distinct granules and express a defined pattern of cell surface markers, CD56[bright]CD16[-]. These markers distinguish them from NK cells in the blood, most of which are CD56[dim]CD16[+]. Mouse and rat uNK cells are readily identified throughout pregnancy by their exceptionally large size relative to human uNK cells, and their prominent granules. The life cycle of the mouse uNK cell has been extensively documented, and includes degranulation in the last trimester and replenishment from the spleen.[28]

NK cells serve an immune surveillance function at most mucosal surfaces, killing infected and abnormal cells they encounter. However, uNK cells are not cytotoxic, despite having readily detectable reservoirs of killer molecules such as granzymes and TNFα in their granules, a surprising condition identified in the mouse by Parr et al.[29] The cytokine profiles of the uNK cells are generally but not invariably consistent with their functional anomalies; they produce both T helper cell type 1 (Th1-type) cytokines such as IFNγ that are associated with inflammation and cell activation, and T helper cell type 2 (Th2-type) cytokines such as interleukin-10 (IL-10) that drive the immune system into anti-inflammatory pathways.[30]

Immune surveillance is a major function of NK cells; these cells recognize and destroy aberrant host cells which fail to exhibit normally expressed HLA. One major reason why CTB cells migrating into the uNK-filled decidua choose to exhibit cell surface HLA class I antigens may be to avoid this danger. The HLA molecules expressed by these cells, which are the HLA class I molecules HLA-G, -E, and C,[1-3,31] are likely to program the uNK cells away from the killing mode and into a protective role. King and colleagues have offered evidence in support of the idea that binding of trophoblast cell HLA-E to uNK CD94/NKG2 inhibitory receptors effects loss of killer function in human uNK cells[32] although HLA-G has not been eliminated as a modulator of uNK activity.

The role(s) that uNK cells play in pregnancy remain unclear despite considerable experimentation.[33] Yet the general principle that in normal pregnancies uNK cells may function as pregnancy promoters rather than as cytotoxic killer cells that comprise a danger is developing support. Two popular ideas for which experimental support has been developed in the mouse are that the uNK cells participate in modification of maternal vasculature via production of IFNγ and promote placental growth and development.[34] Because of the major ways in which uNK cells differ from both blood NK cells and NK cells in other mucosa, diagnostic tests for their functions must be assessed by testing those that are resident in the uterus rather than those that circulate in maternal blood. Testing of blood NK cells to predict events in gestation in patients with suboptimal reproductive capacity is insupportable.

Macrophages

Macrophages and dendritic cells, which are two of the cell types capable of presenting antigen to lymphocytes, are normal inhabitants of the pregnant uterus. Macrophages are extremely numerous, whereas the dendritic cells are few in number. The two types of cells are closely related but differ morphologically and have different pathways of development and differentiation from precursor cells in the bone marrow.

Uterine macrophages, unlike uNK cells, are a constant feature of the decidua throughout the course of pregnancy, averaging 15–20% of the decidual stromal cells.[25,27] Macrophages in human decidua are frequently located close to invading CTB cells, adjacent to the uterine glandular epithelium and proximal to uterine blood vessels. Uterine macrophages resemble their counterparts in other organs in that they are highly versatile and multifunctional. These cells are proposed to be critical to host defense, uterine homeostasis, and local immune modulation.[11,12,35,36]

Environmental programming, which was first proposed for macrophages in the uterus by Hunt and Robertson,[12] shifts the functional phenotype of resident and incoming hematopoietic cells into immune inhibitory profiles consistent with their roles as mediators of the tolerogenic environment required to sustain semiallogeneic pregnancy. Human decidual macrophages are in a state of activation, as evidenced by their expression of HLA class II, CD11c, and CD86 antigens[1-3] and would therefore be expected to present microbial or other exogenous antigens to antigen-specific T lymphocytes. However, the immune inhibition exerted by these cells suggests a different state.

Gordon[37] has defined five categories of macrophage activation/deactivation: innate, humoral, classical, alternative, and innate/adaptive deactivation. These states are stimulated by signaling through, respectively, Toll-like receptors (TLRs), Fc and complement receptors, IFNγ receptors, IL-4/IL-13 receptors, and IL-10, transforming growth factor β (TGFβ)/IFNα/β or macrophage colony-stimulatinig factor (M-CSF) receptors. In normal pregnancies, decidual macrophages would fall into the category of 'alternative activation' with production of potent immunoinhibitory cytokines such as IL-10 and TGFβ$_1$[38,39] but the decidual macrophages also display features of innate/adaptive deactivation, including high expression of HLA class II antigens. Evidence exists for reversibility of these states depending upon cytokine signals.

Soluble HLA-G produced in placentas programs macrophages into the states that are consistent with tolerance in pregnancy.[39] Thus, levels of HLA-G may dictate whether or not the fetus resides in an immune privileged environment. Other markers associated with immune evasion and activation for suppression are expressed by human decidual macrophages. These may include B7-H1,[40] an inhibitory member of the B7 family of co-stimulatory molecules, as well as ILT3, DC-SIGN, MS-1, and factor 13.[1-3]

Dendritic cells

Dendritic cells, small numbers of which are found in the human decidua are powerful APC.[41] Dendritic cells fall into two categories: mature cells that are CD83$^+$ and represent approximately 1% of decidual stromal cells,[41] and CD83$^-$ cells, which are an immature population. Mature CD83$^+$ decidual dendritic cells display an immunosuppressive phenotype;[42] they secrete less IL-12, a promoter of T-cell activation,

than monocyte-derived dendritic cells, and induce Th2-producing T cells when co-cultured with naive CD4$^+$ T cells. Immature (CD83$^-$) dendritic cells appear to induce T-cell anergy. This category is composed of an assortment of related cells, some of which display classical dendritic cell markers (DC-SIGN$^+$CD14$^+$) and others of which are DC-SIGN$^-$CD14$^-$DEC-205$^+$. DC-SIGN$^+$ cells may be a precursor population that differentiates into either macrophages or dendritic cells when programmed by certain cytokines. The cell surface marker DC-SIGN is utilized for immune evasion by several viral and bacterial pathogens, and binding alters both cytokine production and antigen presentation in ways that benefit the pathogen.[43] If this is also a feature of pregnancy, endometrial DC-SIGN$^+$ cells targeted by immunosuppressive molecules from the placenta could be central players in the development of the pregnant uterus as an immune privileged site benefiting the fetus.

Regulatory T cells (T$_{reg}$)

T lymphocytes comprise only about 10% of the decidual leukocytes.[44] Of the CD3$^+$ subpopulation, most are CD8$^+$, i.e. belong to the cytotoxic T-cell group. However, some are mucosal T cells bearing TcRγ/δ and others are CD4$^+$ helper T lymphocytes. Within the CD3$^+$CD4$^+$ subpopulation are regulatory T cells (T$_{reg}$), which are characterized by display of CD4$^+$CD25$^+$ and Foxp3. Proliferation of these cells is stimulated by estrogen.[45] The T$_{reg}$ cells constitute approximately 14% of CD4$^+$ cells in early decidua,[44] so altogether represent only a small fraction of decidual leukocytes.

Decidual T$_{reg}$ cells appear to be very similar to T$_{reg}$ cells in other locations. The decidual T$_{reg}$ cells express intracellular cytotoxic T lymphocyte antigen-4 (CTLA-4), GITR, and OX40, all of which are markers for this subset.[44] Percentages of CD4$^+$CD25$^+$ cells in the peripheral blood increase during early pregnancy,[46] suggesting that cells circulating in blood may migrate into the uterus to increase their numbers in the decidualized endometrium. TGFβ, a cytokine that is ubiquitous in the pregnant uterus and placenta, induces the CD4$^+$CD25$^+$ regulatory phenotype from normally CD4$^+$CD25$^-$ mouse T lymphocytes.[47] Induction is via enhancement of the winged helix/forkhead transcription factor, Foxp3, and down-regulation of Smad 7. T$_{reg}$ cells are highly influential negative regulators of immunity. They maintain peripheral tolerance when autoreactive T-cell clones have arisen or have escaped from thymic selection.[48,49] Their major products are IL-10 and TGFβ, which are important immunosuppressive cytokines at the maternal–fetal interface, as discussed below. It would

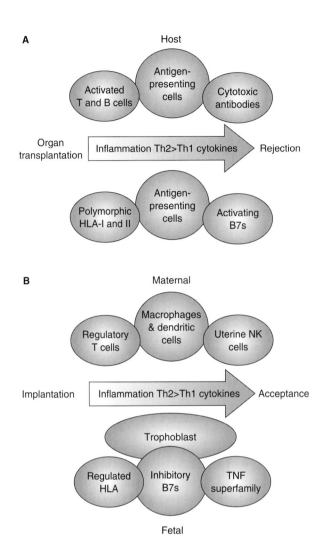

Figure 34.2 Features of transplantation and implantation. Although both processes are characterized by inflammation, transplantation (**A**) involves more extensive tissue damage and a predominance of inflammation-associated (Type 1) cytokines. Immune cells involved in recognition and rejection of grafted organs and tissues that are genetically different from the host include activated lymphocytes and APC interaction, which can lead to production of cytotoxic antibodies and T-cell-mediated cytolysis. Polymorphic HLA, and co-stimulatory molecules can exacerbate this process and lead to graft rejection. (**B**) Implantation results in limited tissue damage, mainly of the uterine epithilium and adjacent stroma. Pregnancy is characterized by a predominance of anti-flammatory (type 2) cytokines, although pro-inflammatory cytokines are present at comparatively low levels. Maternal APC are present, but are programmed into an immunosuppressive mode; similarly, T cells appear to be of a regulatory phenotype. Trophoblast cells contribute greatly to ensuring inhibition of maternal lymphocytes through expression of inhibitory cell surface molecules and production of soluble immunosuppressive molecules.

not be surprising to learn that, as in the mouse,[50] CD4+CD25+ T lymphocytes constitute a critical subpopulation of suppressor cells in the human decidua.[50]

MECHANISMS OF GRAFT REJECTION

Because the paradox of the fetal allograft was originally recognized in the context of rejection of transplanted tissue, it is appropriate to keep in mind the parallels and differences between these phenomena as we learn more about the mechanisms of each. Figure 34.2 illustrates these points; many of the details with regard to pregnancy are discussed in the following paragraphs.

Ischemia is a major barrier to successful transplantation because it precipitates a vigorous feedback loop leading to rejection. Cellular damage resulting from lack of oxygenation induces injury, leading to inflammation characterized by production of cytokines and chemokines. This effectively attracts cells of both the innate and adaptive immune systems to the site of transplantation. Likewise, implantation is an event characterized by inflammatory mediators; however, it is also highly controlled such that inflammation is held in check by negative regulatory molecules.[51] In addition to the anti-inflammatory cytokines produced at the site of implantation, the blastocyst may produce soluble factors that actively control potentially harmful leukocytes.

Antibodies can play a major role in graft rejection, although B cells do not necessarily act in isolation to effect rejection, since, regardless of the timing of antibody production, T-cell help is usually required. However, recognition of alloantigens by host T cells themselves is not necessarily required, since preexisting antibodies can be devastating to transplant survival. These antibodies arise as a result of previous transplantation, blood transfusion, or pregnancy and most often are directed against donor HLA and ABO blood group antigens.[52] The antibodies target donor endothelium and cause destruction within minutes as a consequence of activation of the complement cascade. Ultimately, the result is rampant inflammation as well as insertion of pore-forming proteins into the membranes of target cells. Complement-independent death of cells can also occur, resulting from antibody-mediated activation of endothelial cells and ensuing inflammation.[53]

Complement also probably plays a major role in fetal loss that is associated with the presence of certain antibodies in maternal serum. As discussed below, preexisting antibodies that could target trophoblast cells are thought to be a significant cause of miscarriage. In contrast, de-novo generation of antipaternal HLA antibodies is a frequent occurrence that is not thought to be problematic to fetal survival.[54] Complement regulatory proteins, which include decay accelerating factor (DAF, or CD55), membrane cofactor protein

(MCP or CD46), and CD59, play a role in acceptance or 'accommodation' of grafts.[53] As it turns out, these proteins probably also play a critical role in protection of the fetal allograft from spontaneous and/or antibody-mediated activation of complement.

In the clinic, steps are rigorously followed to assure avoidance of hyperacute transplant rejection mediated by preexisting antibodies. Unfortunately, T-cell-mediated events that occur later are equally menacing. These events critically involve both CD4+ and CD8+ T cells. Early inflammatory events activate cellular and molecular processes, leading to recognition of donor antigen by host T cells. This can occur via direct antigen presentation, indirect antigen presentation, or both.[52] In direct antigen presentation, donor-derived APCs (i.e. endothelial cells) are recognized by recipient T cells. The antigen is thought to be the donor's MHC molecule itself. Recognition of donor antigen can also occur indirectly following phagocytosis and presentation of donor antigen (again, probably MHC). These are the grounds for extensive 'tissue typing' between donor and recipient in the clinic. In either scenario, the result is initial activation of CD4+ T cells, followed by activation of B cells (which may subsequently produce harmful antibody), CD8+ T cells, or both. When activated CD8+ T cells recognize their cognate antigen on cells, those cells become targets of granzyme- or perforin-mediated 'kiss of death'.

In the pregnant mother, T lymphocytes are tolerized to fetal major and minor histocompatibility antigens.[55] Antigen presentation is a critical event in T-cell activation, as discussed above, but is also a central event in tolerance.[56] However, the molecular and cellular interactions involved in generation of fetal tolerance remain unknown. One possibility is that tolerance is induced via the unique HLA molecules that are expressed by trophoblast cells; another is the phagocytosis of dying tolerogenic fetal trophoblast or parenchymal cells by maternal tolerogenic APCs to lymphocytes. What is clear, however, is that should maternal T-cell tolerization fail due to lack of specific immunosuppressive elements, the fetus cannot survive.[57]

MOLECULAR DEFENSE SYSTEMS IN THE PLACENTA PREVENTING REJECTION

The cells of the placenta that are directly exposed to maternal blood and tissues require protection against maternal adaptive and innate immune systems. In human pregnancies, highly sophisticated evasive strategies provide this protection. These invariably rely on unique expression patterns for genes encoding immunologically important ligands and receptors by fetal cells interfacing directly with maternal tissues, i.e. migrating extravillous CTB cells and maternal decidua, and fetal cells interfacing directly with maternal blood, i.e. syncytiotrophoblast. These patterns may be the same or different for trophoblast cells in these two different situations.

Figure 34.2 compares the immune pathway that takes place during pregnancy which leads to uneventful gestation and the pathway that takes place in transplanted organs resulting in graft rejection. The pathway toward rejection might also be followed in pregnancy if protective mechanisms were overcome, which is the case in infections during pregnancy. Although it is possible that the rejection pathway might be taken in pregnancy as a consequence of maternal immune recognition of paternally derived fetal 'transplantation antigens', this remains undocumented.

Protection against antigen-specific immunity

Multiple mechanisms protect fetal cells from attack by the antigen-specific components of the maternal immune system. These include exclusion of potentially attacking T and B lymphocytes from the decidua, as described above, and special molecular adaptations taken by the placenta. Unique strategies in the placenta include down-regulation of the transplantation antigens that are primarily responsible for graft rejection, secreting immunosuppressive co-stimulatory molecules, and displaying molecules that interfere with complement activation.

Regulation of major histocompatibility complex antigens

Of the defense mechanisms identified in placentas, regulated display of the MHC antigens may be among the most important. There are no reports of viable human fetuses whose placentas have failed entirely to follow the predicted patterns of antigen display. The MHC antigens (first known as 'transplantation antigens' because of their central roles in graft rejection) are termed, in humans, the human leukocyte antigens (HLAs). Human chromosome 6p21 (mouse chromosome 17) contains a cluster of these genes (Figure 34.3).[1–3] The class I genes that are expressed by cells are subdivided into the highly polymorphic class Ia, which include HLA-A, -B, and -C genes, and the poorly polymorphic class Ib genes, which include HLA-E, -F, and -G genes. HLA class II (HLA-D) genes are also highly polymorphic. Expression of the antigens encoded by

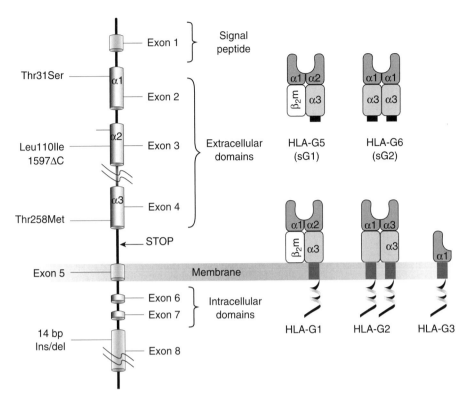

Figure 34.3   The HLA-G gene and 5 of its 7 protein isoforms. The various protein isoforms are derived by alternative splicing of a single message. HLA-G1, -G2 and -G3 (all shown) and -G4 (not shown) molecules are bound to the cell membrane and have short cytoplasmic tails. Two of the soluble isoforms have two sets of identifiers. In this chapter, we use the HLA-G5, (soluble HLA-G1), -G6 (soluble HLA-G2) (both shown), and -G7 (not shown) designations. These molecules circulate as soluble isoforms because they lack the transmembrane and cytoplasmic domains present in HLA-G1, -G2, and -G3. Portions of intron 4 are found tailing the HLA-G5 and -G6 molecules and a portion of intron 2 tails the HLA-G7 molecule. Bolded nucleotides identify HLA-G alleles. β_2m, β_2-microglobulin light chain.

these three groups differs greatly, being highly cell- and tissue-specific as well as related to cell differentiation and activation. The antigens are functionally versatile, driving either immunostimulatory or immunoinhibitory pathways.

Class I HLA antigens and expression patterns in trophoblast cells.   Individual cells express many HLA class I antigens on their surfaces since maternal and paternal MHC genes are co-dominant. Although these antigens may be cleaved from the cell surface as cells die and disintegrate, the usual circumstance is that they exist primarily as membrane-bound molecules. Their expression is not cell type-restricted; to a greater or lesser degree, the HLA class Ia antigens, HLA-A, -B, and -C are expressed by all somatic cells. These antigens are unique markers of individual identity because each gene is highly polymorphic. For example, nearly 350 alleles are known for *HLA-B*.[1]

Protein products of the class Ib genes differ markedly from those derived from the class Ia genes. The numbers of alleles are low for *HLA-E* and *HLA-F*, and of these only two alleles of each gene encode proteins with differing amino acids. *HLA-G* has only five alleles. The class Ib proteins have restricted distribution, with expression being cell type-, tissue-, or organ-specific and/or related to stage of cell differentiation and activation. The glycoproteins associated with class Ia and class Ib antigens are also significantly different.

Trophoblast cells in human placentas either fail entirely to express HLA antigens or select specific genes with special non-immunogenic properties for expression.[1,58,59] Unexpressed antigens include HLA-A and -B, which, in other contexts, are highly effective stimulators of graft rejection, and HLA class II antigens,[60] which are used for stimulation of the T helper cell subset. Trophoblast cells in explants of term placental villi cannot be induced to express either set of antigens,[61] yet when released from their normal environment, some of the antigens are inducible.[62] Thus, intrinsic elements of the placental stroma influence expression of HLA in trophoblast cells.

Certain subpopulations of human trophoblast, specifically the extravillous CTB cells, express one of the class Ia antigens, HLA-C, and all three class Ib molecules, HLA-E, -F, and -G. *HLA-C* is moderately polymorphic, and could stimulate maternal antifetal adaptive immunity if paternal alleles differed from maternal. Although allelic disparity at the *HLA-C* locus has not been identified as a causal factor in infertility or termination of pregnancy, Hiby and coworkers have reported that special genetic combinations of maternal HLA-C killer inhibitory receptors (KIRs) and fetal *HLA-C* genes somehow influence the risk of preeclampsia.[63] Thus, the products of this gene have potential importance to pregnancy.

HLA-E, -F, and -G are the other HLA class I antigens expressed by trophoblast cells. The relevance of HLA-E is discussed above in the uNK section. Although there was some early confusion, it now seems clear that HLA-E, which binds to the CD94/NKG2 receptor, is of prime importance in preventing uNK cells from killing their normal targets. Yet HLA-G might have a role; the uNK cells express immunoglobulin-like transcript-2 (ILT2, LILRB1) receptors and KIR2/DL4, which signal inhibition but via different pathways. HLA-F is present on invading CTB cells[64] but its activities remain unknown.

HLA-G was the first HLA class Ib molecule identified in placentas.[58] Its major receptors are LILRB1 (leukocyte immunoglobulin-like receptor B1; also known as ILT2) and LILRB2 (ILT4).[65] Leukocytes in human decidua and placentas express these receptors in vitro[1] and in situ (RM McIntire and JS Hunt, unreported data).

The structure of HLA-G and expression in trophoblast cells.
HLA-G has unique physical properties that profoundly influence its regulation and functions. First, the promoter region of the gene has a large deletion that precludes enhancement of expression by the usual modulators, i.e. interferons and TNFα. Further, the single HLA-G transcript is alternatively spliced to yield seven different messages, of which four encode membrane-bound proteins and three encode soluble proteins (see Figure 34.3).[1–3]

HLA-G was the first of the class Ib antigens to be identified in/on trophoblast cells and remains an antigen of great interest and focus of experimental evaluation. Expression patterns for HLA-G have been the subject of numerous reviews.[1–3,58,59] Briefly, HLA-G was first identified on the remnants of extravillous CTB cells that populate the chorion membrane in late gestation. Subsequently, HLA-G was demonstrated on the extravillous CTB cells forming CTB cell columns, islands, interstitial CTB, and endovascular CTB in early to middle stages of pregnancy. More recent

experiments suggest that the isoforms derived from the *HLA-G* gene by alternative splicing may have specific expression patterns. The distal column CTB forming the trophoblastic shell as well as other invasive subpopulations of CTB cells express HLA-G1 and probably also HLA-G2 and -G6.[17] HLA-G5, a soluble isoform, is ubiquitous in placentas and membranes taken from all three trimesters of pregnancy.[17]

HLA-G1 and HLA-G5. The functions of the HLA-G1 membrane-bound isoform have not been thoroughly elucidated but its target could be uNK cells through LILRB1 (ILT2) or KIR2/DL4 receptors. However, this isoform might also interact with LILRB1 or LILRB2 receptors on normal macrophages and/or T$_{reg}$ cells. Studies on mononuclear phagocytes would be difficult because this lineage is also believed to synthesize HLA-G under certain conditions of activation.[66] In vitro, monocyte HLA-G inhibits autologous CD4 T-cell activation and production of both Th1-type (IFNγ, IL-2) and Th2-type (IL-10) cytokines. Furthermore, HLA-G1-transfected APC lines have been shown to display enhanced levels of receptors such as KIR2DL4, LILRB1, ILT3, and LILRB2, which could comprise a feedforward pathway for secretion of cytokines or alteration of other APC activities.

HLA-G5 might function similarly to HLA-G1, as their structures are identical except that HLA-G5 is missing the transmembrane and cytoplasmic domains and is therefore a soluble protein. This molecule has clearly documented immunosuppressive properties. HLA-G5 influences on leukocytes include but are not limited to (1) stimulation of death of phytohemagglutinin (PHA)-treated lymphocytes through the Fas/FasL cell death pathway, (2) reduction of expression of lymphocyte CD8α, a co-receptor involved in linking CTL with APC, and (3) driving mononuclear phagocytes into an immunosuppressive profile where the cells produce high levels of TGFβ.[1–3] Soluble HLA-G appears to be selective in its enhancement of suppressive cytokines; there is no relation, for example, between levels of HLA-G and IL-10 in serum.[67] The major receptor for HLA-G5 on mononuclear phagocytes may be LILRB2, but studies in U937 cells, a histiocytic cell line, indicate that both the LILRB1 and LILRB2 receptors on these phagocytes bind HLA-G5.[39]

Isoform-specific functions. HLA-G isoforms may have similar or distinctly different functions. Regarding redundancy in function, studies have shown that in the absence of HLA-G1 and -G5 due to a deletion in the *HLA-G* gene, women have demonstrable HLA-G proteins in their placentas and produce viable offspring.[68,69] In this condition, other isoforms probably provide functional compensation. An early report suggested that the smaller isoforms such as HLA-G6 and -G7 were not synthesized in or released by trophoblast cells[70] but more recent studies show that these molecules are not only present but also are functional in placentas.[17,71–73] The idea that isoforms have specific functions is supported by the finding of differential distribution in trophoblast subpopulations. For example, both HLA-G1 and -G2/G6 are expressed exclusively in the extravillous CTB cells, whereas HLA-G5 is readily detected in multiple trophoblast subpopulations and in maternal blood.[74,75] The functions of HLA-G2, -G3, and -G4 remain poorly explored with the exception of a report from Riteau and coworkers showing that, as with HLA-G1, all of these isoforms protect transfected cells from effector cell lysis.[73] HLA-G7 activities are unknown.

Immunogenicity of HLA-G. Because alleles that differ structurally from one another have been identified, the question arises as to whether or not HLA-G produced in placentas might be immunogenic to the mother. Anti-HLA-G is produced in approximately 9% of women but the antibodies are not allele-specific and do not harm the fetus or placenta; mothers who produce anti-HLA-G have multiple successful pregnancies.[76] Thus, antibodies may be produced but do no damage, as is normally the case with antibodies generated to paternal HLA class I and class II.

HLA-G and reproductive performance in women. Attempts to establish relationships between HLA-G and common problems of pregnancy have had mixed results, possibly as a consequence of different diagnostic criteria and/or laboratory techniques. Unexplained recurrent miscarriage has been tested,[77–79] with recent data emerging that relate miscarriage rates with variation in the HLA-G promoter region.[79] However, Patel and coworkers report that HLA-G on cell membranes is not associated with idiopathic recurrent pregnancy loss.[80] Preeclampsia is marked by abnormal invasion of CTB cells into the decidua,[81] suggesting a role for HLA-G, which is prominent in invasive CTB cells. Reports have emerged indicating that the cells in the decidua of preeclampic women have reduced levels of HLA-G.[82,83]

Recent studies focusing on associations between HLA-G alleles and isoforms or combinations thereof and preeclampsia are now appearing in the scientific literature.[84–87] Le Bouteiller et al have reviewed some of the recent observations on HLA-G and preeclampsia.[88]

Although less attention has been paid to intrauterine growth retardation, it has been definitively shown that this condition is not associated with loss of the ability of a mother to synthesize HLA-G1 and -G5.[68] The major point in these experiments is that specific *HLA-G* DNA sequences, whether in the promoter or coding region, appear to control the amounts of HLA-G protein that are produced.[89] Reduced levels may be associated with disease. Yet when the changes result mainly in reduction of specific isoforms, other isoforms may substitute and compensate, permitting pregnancy to proceed.[68]

Finally, the scientific literature now holds many reports of successful pregnancies following transfer of embryos fertilized in vitro that secrete high levels of soluble HLA-G,[90–95] indicating a role for this protein in implantation.

Selective expression of B7 family members

Following the identification of the hallmark members of the B7 family, B7-1 (CD80) and B7-2 (CD86), and their shared receptors, CD28 and CTLA-4, it became apparent that these proteins serve as central regulators of the adaptive immune response. Naive T cells do not respond to antigen effectively in the absence of engagement of the CD28 receptor by B7-1 or B7-2. Conversely, the loss of functional CTLA-4 signaling, which is mediated by the same ligands, results in fatal lymphoproliferative disease early in life.[96,97] It is now well-accepted that B7-1 and/or B7-2 on APCs deliver the requisite 'second signal' to T cells through CD28, along with the MHC/antigen 'first signal' to effect T-cell activation. In fact, the absence of the second signal leads to the opposite effect: rather than being activated, lymphocytes may become tolerant. The restriction of B7-1 and B7-2 expression to professional APCs ensures that only these cells can initiate an adaptive immune response.

The dynamic nature of tissues and organs as they undergo development, restructuring, and aging necessitates mechanisms to thwart potentially self-reactive lymphocytes from attacking self-tissue. While the limited expression of the aforementioned B7s is probably critical in passive avoidance of unwanted lymphocyte activation, mechanisms to actively induce lymphocyte tolerance must also be in place. Through inspection of nucleotide sequence homology to B7-1 and B7-2, seven additional members of the B7 family, and four CD28 family members, have recently been discovered.[98] Functional studies of these new molecular pathways have afforded us a much better appreciation of the pivotal importance of B7 proteins in positive

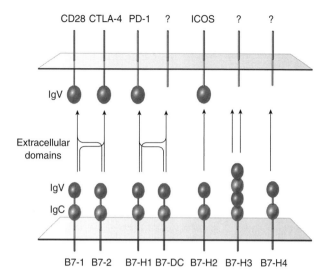

Figure 34.4 The B7 family of co-stimulatory and co-inhibitory molecules. B7 family proteins serve as ligands for respective CD28 family members. The latter are expressed by lymphocytes and intracellular domains mediate downstream signal transduction leading to the appropriate cellular response. Several B7 proteins share one or two CD28 receptors, which may mediate differential responses. Red arrows denote stimulatory responses, while black arrows denote inhibitory responses.

and negative regulation of the immune response, particularly in peripheral tissues, including the placenta.

Both B7 proteins and their CD28 family receptors are type I transmembrane proteins belonging to the immunoglobulin (Ig) superfamily (Figure 34.4). Like B7-1 and B7-2, the new members of the B7 family are not constitutively expressed on most cells. However, they can be induced on APCs, endothelial cells, lymphocytes, and parenchymal cells. In contrast, CD28 family receptors are expressed almost exclusively on lymphocytes and myeloid cells. The functional consequences of receptor ligation are determined by both the ligand–receptor specificity and the nature of their intracellular signaling domains, which dictate the subsequent downstream signaling pathways (see Figure 34.4).

The human placenta is unique among other tissue systems in that B7-H1, -DC, -H2, and -H3 are constitutively expressed by trophoblast cells.[99,100] This finding alone implies that trophoblast cells uniquely regulate their expression in vivo, through as-yet unknown mechanisms. B7-H1 and -DC share the inhibitory receptor, PD-1, and possibly a second as-yet unidentified activating receptor. B7-H1 is expressed on all populations of trophoblast cells throughout pregnancy, and is especially high from the second trimester onwards. This may be due to elevated oxygen in the latter two trimesters.[101] B7-DC, interestingly, is expressed only by syncytiotro-

phoblast of the early placenta, but its expression is shifted to the fetal endothelium by term. B7-H2 and B7-H3, on the other hand, are expressed mainly by extravillous trophoblast cells, although some degree of villous trophoblast expression is evident. Although the function(s) of most of the B7s in the placenta is unknown, compelling evidence points to a crucial role for B7-H1.

Genetic mutation of the genes for B7-H1 and PD-1 in mice unequivocally reveals that the major in-vivo function of these proteins is to maintain immunological self-tolerance. Mutation of *PD-1* results in fatal autoimmune disease.[102,103] These murine models have been authenticated by the finding in humans that polymorphisms in the *PD-1* gene are associated with autoimmune diseases, including lupus, rheumatoid arthritis, and type I diabetes.[104–107]

Mutation of *B7-H1* in mice also results in immune dysregulation, although the phenotypes are less severe than the PD-1 knockouts.[108,109] Specifically, whereas the PD-1 knockout mice develop spontaneous autoimmune disease, B7-H1 null mice exhibit increased susceptibility to autoimmunity when presented with a specific challenge, such as autoimmune hepatitis or experimental autoimmune encephalomyelitis (EAE). One study suggests that allogenic pregnancy may represent such a challenge, as fetuses were lost when dams were treated with B7-H1 antibody.[110]

Indoleamine-2-3-dioxygenase (IDO)

The idea that indoleamine-2,3-dioxygenase (IDO), a tryptophan catabolic enzyme, might play an important immunological role is not new, but much enthusiasm was generated upon the finding that a competitive inhibitor of this enzyme induces T-cell-mediated rejection of allogeneic, but not syngeneic fetuses in pregnant mice.[111] Since this landmark report, a rush of reports has followed in which this enzyme has been implicated as a central player in tolerance not only to the fetus but also to self and tumor antigens.[112–114]

IDO is expressed by many cell types at the maternal–fetal interface, including trophoblast cells, glandular epithelial cells, and macrophages.[115–118] Although expression of the enzyme can occur constitutively, its activity is induced by IFNγ; this has been confirmed in placental explants.[118] The molecular mechanisms by which IDO mediates suppression of T cells are not completely clear, but are thought to occur by depletion of tryptophan and/or accumulation of toxic metabolites, or alternatively, through alteration of antigen presentation and T$_{reg}$ cells.[114] Deposition of complement factors, which in independent studies has also been shown to be highly embryotoxic (see discussion below), is thought to be the ultimate effector of embryonic death in the murine IDO model of fetal rejection, although the molecular pathway leading to this result has not been completely elucidated.[119]

Chemical inhibition of IDO clearly has catastrophic effects on fetal viability in mice but genetic deletion of IDO has no effect.[116] The reasons for the discrepancy in the two models are unclear, but could be due to differential molecular compensation in an acutely vs a chronically inhibited model. Alternatively, others have suggested cytotoxic effects of the inhibitor used in the studies, and still others have found it to have non-specific (IDO-independent) effects on stimulation of T-cell proliferation.[120,121] Clearly, the role of IDO at the maternal–fetal interface is controversial; further studies will likely tease out the conflicting nature of the data thus far.

Complement regulatory proteins and antigen–antibody-activated complement

As noted above, complement is a set of humoral components that straddle adaptive and innate immunity insofar as the cascade leading to cell death can be activated by either branch of the immune system. Complement factors circulate in plasma, serving to protect against invading pathogens via the promotion of phagocytosis, the generation of inflammation, and the formation of lytic complexes that can be deposited on the surface of target cells. Activation of this pathway occurs through at least three mechanisms:

- the classical pathway, which involves deposition of complement-fixing antibodies onto antigen
- the alternative pathway, in which a low level of spontaneous activation occurs continuously in plasma
- the lectin pathway, in which carbohydrate moieties associated with antigens are bound by a lectin, which are in turn bound by complement.

Because of the abundance of complement components in plasma and the potential for both auto- or alloantibody-mediated and spontaneous activation of this potent pathway, the trophoblast must employ universally effective mechanisms to counter activation of this cascade.

The continual washing of placental villi in maternal blood renders them, like endothelial cells, erythrocytes, and leukocytes, particularly vulnerable to plasma complement factors. That the fetus is allogeneic in relation to the mother only increases the potential for complement-fixing alloantibody that might be generated during pregnancy. Indeed, many normal pregnancies are

characterized by formation of antipaternal antibodies, fortunately, with no apparent consequence.[54] However, antiphospholipid autoantibodies often preexist in maternal plasma, particularly in women with lupus; these antibodies are strongly associated with thrombosis and increased incidence of miscarriage.[122]

As with the adaptive immune system where self-reactive lymphocytes are deleted, the innate immune system has developed clever strategies to protect cells from damage by immune mechanisms such as the complement system. Indeed, all cells utilize complement regulatory proteins to avoid susceptibility to spontaneously activated complement as well as susceptibility to bystander damage in the event of an infection. In this context, human trophoblast cells strongly express several complement inhibitory proteins.[123–125] These include DAF (also called CD55; a competitive inhibitor of C3 convertase), MCP (also called CD46; a cofactor in cleavage/activation of a complement protein), and CD59 (inhibits formation of the porous membrane attack complex). In-vitro studies show that antibody-mediated inhibition of complement regulatory proteins increases susceptibility to killing of trophoblast cells by complement, illustrating the functional significance of these proteins.[126]

The importance of protection of the fetus from complement-mediated damage is underscored by elegant studies showing that murine embryos lacking the complement regulatory protein Crry, a rodent-specific protein with functional properties paralleling human MCP and DAF, universally succumb to maternal complement-mediated damage by mid gestation.[127] Protection was only afforded when Crry–/– embryos were implanted in C3–/– mothers, thus providing proof that fetal complement inhibitors must inhibit maternally derived complement if lethal consequences are to be avoided.

The role of maternal antibodies and complement in human disease is coming to light thanks to an interesting model in which normal pregnant mice are treated with IgG from either antiphospholipid antibody (aPL)-positive or -negative human patients. Antibodies from aPL-positive, but not aPL-negative patients, induce fetal loss and growth retardation in this model in a complement-dependent manner. These results suggest that these antibodies may play a similarly harmful role in aPL-positive women experiencing recurrent pregnancy loss. Indeed, aPL antibodies in general, and antibody against β_2-glycoprotein I (GPI) in particular, can bind to and inhibit functions of trophoblast cells in vitro.[128] Other studies suggest the involvement of complement activation, thrombosis, and functional blocking of placental GPI in antibody-mediated fetal loss.[129–131] Interestingly, a recent report suggested that heparin, which is clinically important treatment for women experiencing antibody-associated recurrent miscarriage, mediates its antiabortive effect in mice through inhibition of complement rather than solely by its antithrombotic effects.[132] Thus, intersection of the basic and clinical sciences has shown promise of aiding our ability to document and improve the prognosis of recurrent miscarriage that is associated with the presence of potentially harmful autoantibodies.

Protection against the innate immune system

Protection against adaptive immunity is clearly critical to the initiation and maintenance of semiallogeneic pregnancy. The failure of experimentalists to identify women entirely lacking in the ability to synthesize HLA-G proteins or all of the complement regulatory proteins points to the essential nature of the expression of these proteins in human placentas.

However, the maternal leukocytes in the most intimate and long-term relationship with extraembryonic fetal cells are those of the innate immune system. These are the uNK cells and macrophages that populate the decidua. Both cell types contain toxic molecules and are fully capable of destruction. As described above, it is likely that HLA-E and perhaps also HLA-G bind to uNK inhibitory receptors, LILRB1 and LILRB2, to block activating signals. In macrophages, placental HLA-G appears to bind both receptors but to have a preference for LILRB2.[1,39]

Hormones produced in placentas are also critical to down-regulation of uterine immune cell cytotoxicity. These include progesterone, which interferes with activation via nuclear factor-κB (NF-κB)[23] and chorionic gonadotropin, although the latter remains a subject of debate. Prostaglandins from decidual cells or macrophages themselves are also capable of diminishing toxicity, and other autocrine pathways that include IL-10 and TGF-β_1 operate in decidua and placentas.

It is clear that these pathways are effective; uNK cells cannot kill,[22] and uterine macrophages are in an immunotolerant state.[1–3]

MULTIPLE TASKS FOR IMMUNE SYSTEM-RELATED MOLECULES IN PLACENTAS: THE TNF SUPERFAMILY

Because of its limited natural life span, the placenta serves as a model for studying the varied and diverse processes of organogenesis, programmed cellular function, and, finally, pathways for cell death and discard of unwanted tissue. Surprisingly, life span influences on the birth, maturation/differentiation, and demise of placental cells include novel use of molecules first identified in the immune system. One of the first of these to be discovered was macrophage colony stimulating factor (M-CSF also known as colony stimulating factor-1, CSF-1), a hematopoietic system growth and differentiation factor that is abundant in the pregnant uterus and may program both trophoblast cell and decidual macrophage functions.[12,133] Others soon followed.

In the paragraphs below the TNF family of ligands is used to illustrate the point that, although first identified in inflammation and tissue destruction, TNF ligands are not universally toxic and may even benefit pregnancy. The *TNF* gene family contains at least 17 functionally distinct ligands. Of these, nine interact with receptors containing death domains; eight interact with receptors that do not include death domains in their signaling apparatus but may mediate apoptosis through other pathways. The 17 ligands interact with at least 24 receptors. A notable feature of ligand:receptor interactions in the TNF family is that many ligands recognize more than one receptor. TRAIL and LIGHT top the list with four and three receptors respectively.

TNF ligands fall into two general categories: i.e. those that are capable of signaling apoptosis and those that are not. Within the apoptosis category, whether or not a cell dies may be determined by which receptor and/ or what type of cell binds the ligand. The ability to induce apoptosis may be a critical developmental function of TNFα, which, together with essentially all of the apoptosis-inducing TNF ligands, is found in the placenta.[134,135] Yui and colleagues have posited that TNFα assists in facilitating maternal–fetal transport across the syncytiotrophoblast layer by killing villous CTB cells in order to allow the syncytium to come into closer proximity to fetal vessels.[136] Interestingly, TNFα induces apoptosis in normal villous CTB cells[136] but is used as a growth factor by tumorigenic trophoblast cells.[137] This dichotomy clearly illustrates how normal growth and differentiation molecules are subverted in cancer.

TRAIL (CD253) is a second TNF ligand capable of inducing apoptosis via death domain-containing receptors (DR4, DR5). However, CTB cells use multiple inhibitors of apoptosis to resist killing by this molecule.[138] LIGHT is a third ligand of interest. This molecule does not signal CTB cell death.[139,140] Instead, it appears to play a role in placental cell differentiation (RM Gill and JS Hunt, unreported data). In adult lymphoid tissues, lymphotoxins (LT), LIGHT, and TNFα

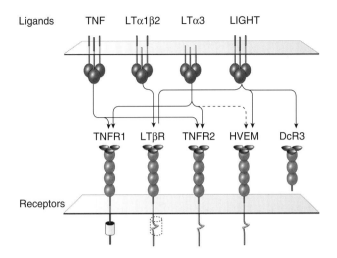

Ligands   TNF   LTα1β2   LTα3   LIGHT

TNFR1   LTβR   TNFR2   HVEM   DcR3

Receptors

Figure 34.5 Apoptosis-inducing members of the TNF families of ligands and receptors present in human placentas that may be involved in immune regulatory networks. TNF, tumor necrosis factor; LT, lymphotoxin in two different configurations ($\alpha_1\beta_2$, α_3); LIGHT, homologous to *l*ymphotoxins, exhibits *i*nducible expression, competes with herpes simplex virus *g*lycoprotein D for *H*VEM, a receptor expressed by *T* lymphocytes; DcR3, decoy receptor-3. Note that intracellular sequences of the receptors may include a classical death domain (solid cylinder) or alternate pathways to cell death.

(Figure 34.5) constitute an integrated signaling network necessary for innate and adaptive immune responses.[141] Its disruption alleviates autoimmune inflammation and decreases resistance to pathogens. It is, therefore, of great interest to learn about potential networks in placentas, where all three genes and their proteins as well as their receptors are expressed.

The presence of these cytokines raises the question of how normal bystander cells are protected against killing. Soluble TNFα receptors,[142] decoy TRAIL receptors,[138] and lack of functional Fas receptors on placental cells[143] may be important, but placentas also contain many apoptosis-inhibiting proteins.[144,145]

Even though mRNAs and proteins of the non-apoptosis-inducing TNF ligands are readily identified in human placentas, specific messages encoding their receptors are absent.[146] Thus, these molecules may participate in paracrine pathways, stimulating maternal rather than fetal cells. Phillips et al[146] have postulated that BAFF and APRIL, both important to antibody production, may assist mothers in generating the large volumes of Ig required for transport into the fetus, but this remains to be determined experimentally. At present, little or nothing is known of the reproductive functions of the T-cell co-stimulatory molecules 4-1BBL (TNFSF9), CD30L (TNFSF8), CD40L, CD27L (TNFSF7, CD70), OX40L (TNFSF4), or GITRL

(TNFSF18, AITRL). The potential power of these molecules to influence both placental growth and development and fetal interactions with the mother indicates that more experimentation should be done in this area.

DISEASES OF PREGNANCY

Common complications of pregnancy that may cause premature labor and/or delivery include infections that may be ascending or hematogenous, preeclampsia, and intrauterine growth restriction (IUGR). The paragraphs below discuss potential mechanisms underlying the first two. IUGR is frequently associated with preeclampsia or may be due to multiple other causes.

Infections and uterine leukocytes

In the pregnant uterus, support of embryonic development is preferred to maintenance of host defense. This is undoubtedly a consequence of the cellular changes and programming for anti-inflammatory rather than pro-inflammatory responses required for avoiding rejection of the antigenically 'foreign' fetus. In the cycling uterus, defensins and other antimicrobials are abundant but this is not the case in the pregnant uterus.[147] Infection-associated preterm labor is an unfortunate consequence, as discussed by Caucheteux and colleagues.[148]

Microenvironmental factors that normally drive decidual macrophages into an immune suppressive mode during pregnancy may be overcome or bypassed in certain conditions such as Gram-negative infections. In these conditions, the cells assume a proinflammatory profile, as first proposed in 1989 by Hunt[149] and modified more recently,[150] with activation signals arising through toll-like receptors (TLR) (innate activation) and/or IFNγ receptors (classical activation). When confronted with Gram-negative organisms, decidual macrophages produce high levels of TNFα, other inflammatory cytokines, and prostaglandin E_2 (PGE_2), which may ultimately induce labor.[151–153]

NK cells may be similarly prone to reprogramming when facing an inflammatory insult at the maternal–fetal interface. While most evidence highlights the beneficial role of NK cells on uterine decidualization and vascular remodeling (see discussions above), recent data suggest that the hierarchical Th2 cytokine IL-10 keeps these cells at bay during an inflammatory response.[154] When IL-10 was absent, fetal demise occurred in association with abnormally high invasion and acquisition of cytolytic ability by uNK cells. Interestingly, fetal viability was restored upon functional inhibition of TNFα, but not IFNγ, the latter being a well-known product of uNK cells. These are the first data to suggest that uNK cells might indeed be harmful to pregnancy if not controlled by the appropriate cytokine milieu.

Preeclampsia

Preeclampsia, a disease of pregnant women characterized by vascular dysfunction and systemic inflammation, places the lives of both mother and baby in jeopardy. The disease is caused by poor cytotrophoblast invasion. Failure of fetal cells to properly colonize the decidua ultimately leads to inadequate transformation of uterine spiral arteries from the narrow vasoactive vessels of the first trimester to flaccid conduits of the second trimester onwards. Through poorly understood sequelae, the disease culminates in systemic vasoconstriction, inflammation, endothelial dysfunction, and thrombosis.[155] Unfortunately, maternal and/or fetal mortality, could result should the preeclamptic mother not receive treatment; the only cure for preeclampsia is delivery.

The cause of defective trophoblast invasion is not known, but is probably influenced by both maternal and fetal factors.[156] Genetic contribution by both may be a major determinant; as mentioned above, certain allelic combinations of fetal HLA-C and maternal KIRs are risk factors in preeclampsia.[63] In this newly proposed model, uterine NK cells receiving activating signals from trophoblast HLA-C respond by assisting in spiral artery modification. When inappropriate alleles of KIR and HLA-C alleles are combined, however, the result can be excessive inhibition of uNK cells and thus their inability to perform their requisite functions properly.

The decidual macrophage may also be of consequence in limiting trophoblast invasion. This hypothesis is supported by the observation that excessively activated macrophages in the decidua of preeclamptic patients gather around spiral arteries, possibly inducing trophoblast apoptosis via TNFα, before they reach their intended destination.[157,158] The underlying mechanisms of inappropriate macrophage activation remain unknown.

The events linking improper trophoblast invasion and maternal preeclampsia are not understood, but are assumed to arise from lowered placental perfusion.[155,159] Fluctuating oxygen tension can lead to high oxidative stress, a well-known cause of apoptosis. Higher than normal shedding of syncytial microfragments into the maternal circulation may result, in turn leading to endothelial damage, leukocyte activation, and inflammation in the preeclamptic mother.[156,160]

Although spontaneously occurring preeclampsia is a human-specific disease, animal models have proven to be useful in determining the causes of preeclampsia. Administration of the soluble form of the vascular endothelial growth factor receptor 1 (VEGFR-1 or soluble Fms-like tyrasine kinase 1 [sFlt-1]) causes preeclampsia-like symptoms in pregnant rats, and elevated concentrations of this molecule circulate in pregnant women destined to develop preeclampsia.[161,162] Affected women also have reduced concentrations of bioactive VEGF and a second sFlt-1 ligand, placental growth factor (PlGF).[163] Flt-1 is sensitive to regulation by oxygen, and trophoblast cells enhance its production when exposed to hypoxic conditions.[164] This observation may translate into the in-vivo situation; should there be a failure of spiral artery transformation, abnormally low oxygen concentration may cause enhanced secretion of sFlt-1 by trophoblast cells. The mechanisms by which these high concentrations cause the maternal symptoms in the animal model is unknown, but may relate to their inhibition of VEGF and/or PlGF action.[164,165]

These promising areas of research have provided some of the much needed insights as to the causes and consequences of preeclampsia. However, the ways by which the genetic, cellular, and molecular events that have been discovered to date are tied together to lead to preeclampsia syndrome is an area that will require further investigation.

SUMMARY AND SPECULATION

The maternal–fetal interface is a highly complex environment where networks designed to protect the fetal 'foreigner' develop and function efficiently on a routine basis. So effective are these networks that rejection of the fetus as a consequence of maternal immune cell recognition of paternal HLA is undocumented. At the same time, implantation is risky, and it is estimated that nearly 50% of human pregnancies fail at this stage. Whether defective immunological mechanisms account for any of this loss in women remains unknown.

Protective strategies are by far the most numerous and sophisticated in humans. For example, even the closely related primates, monkeys, and baboons do not demonstrate all of the isoforms of the HLA-G-like proteins they produce in their placentas. Humans have three different genes encoding the complement regulatory proteins; mice have one. Thus, evolution has made special accommodation for successful pregnancy in women, which could positively impact the success of the species. Transgenic and knockout mouse models where factors believed to have critical roles in both human and mouse pregnancy were studied have provided much intriguing information on the potential of many of these factors to contribute to human losses or reduced fertility. These include investigations of the complement regulatory proteins, Fas, IL-11, B7H1, and T_{reg} cells. Other studies in rodents have investigated families of genes, prolactin being an example, which are very different in humans and may therefore be of lesser value. Translation into human models is the final difficult step. Yet a full understanding of the immunological aspects of pregnancy and identification of therapeutic measures requires imaginative pursuit of this aim.

ACKNOWLEDGMENTS

These studies are supported in part by grants from the National Institutes of Health to JSH (HD24212; PO1 HD39878, Project III; HD33994, Project IV) and MGP (HD045611). The authors appreciate the assistance and contributions of their many students, fellows, and colleagues, the U54 Reproductive Sciences Image Analysis core laboratory (PF Terranova, P.I., U54 HD33994) and the Kansas INBRE (P20 RR16475, JS Hunt, P.I.).

REFERENCES

1. Hunt JS, Petroff MG, McIntire RH et al. HLA-G and immune tolerance in pregnancy. FASEB J 2005; 19: 681–93.
2. Hunt JS, McIntire RH, Petroff MG. Immunobiology of human pregnancy. In: Neill JD, ed. Knobil and Neill's Physiology of Reproduction, 3rd edn. St Louis, MO: Elsevier/Academic Press, 2006; 2: 2759–85.
3. Hunt JS, Langat D, McIntire RH et al. The immunology of human pregnancy: an overview. Reprod Biol Endocrinol 2006.
4. Rouas-Freiss N, Moreau P, Ferrone S et al. HLA-G proteins in cancer: do they provide tumor cells with an escape mechanism? Cancer Res 2005; 65: 10239–44.
5. Burton GJ, Kaufmann P, Huppertz B. Anatomy and genesis of the placenta. In: Wassarmen PM, ed. Knobil and Neill's Physiology of Reproduction, 3rd edn. Amsterdam: Elsevier/Academic Press, 2006; 1: 189–244.
6. Rossant J, Cross JC. Placental development: lessons from mouse mutants. Nat Rev Genet Rev 2001; 2: 538–48.
7. James JL, Stone PE, Chamley LW. Cytotrophoblast differentiation in the first trimester of pregnancy: evidence for separate progenitors of extravillous trophoblasts and syncytiotrophoblast. Reproduction 2005; 130: 95–103.
8. Audus KL, Soares MJ, Hunt JS. Characteristics of the fetal/maternal interface with potential usefulness in the development of future immunological and pharmacological strategies. J Pharmacol Exp Ther 2002; 301: 402–9.
9. Burton GJ, Hempstock J, Jauniaux E. Oxygen, early embryonic metabolism and free radical-mediated embryopathies. Reprod BioMed Online 2002; 6: 84–96.
10. Holets ML, Hunt JS, Petroff MG. Trophoblast CD274 (B7-H1) is differentially expressed across gestation: influence of oxygen concentration. Biol Reprod 2006; 74: 352–8.
11. Hunt JS. Current topic: the role of macrophages in the uterine response to pregnancy. Placenta 1990; 11: 467–75.
12. Hunt JS, Robertson SA. Uterine macrophages and environmental programming for pregnancy success. J Reprod Immunol 1996; 32: 1–25.
13. Boyd TK, Redline RW. Chronic histiocytic intervillositis: a placental lesion associated with recurrent reproductive loss. Hum Pathol 2000; 32: 1022–3.
14. Condon JC, Jeyasuria P, Faust JM, Mendelson CR. Surfactant protein secreted by the maturing mouse fetal lung acts as a hormone that signals the initiation of parturition. Proc Natl Acad Sci USA 2004; 101: 4978–83.
15. Hunt JS, Wood GW. Gamma interferon induces class I HLA and beta-2-microglobulin expression by human amnion cells. J Immunol 1986; 136: 364–7.
16. Ockleford C, Malak T, Hubbard A et al. Confocal and conventional immunofluorescence and ultrastructural localization of intracellular strength-giving components of human amniochorion. J Anat 1993; 183: 483–505.
17. Morales PJ, Pace JL, Platt JS et al. Placental cell expression of HLA-G2 isoforms is limited to the invasive trophoblast phenotype. J Immunol 2003; 171: 6215–24.
18. Wang H, Dey SK. Roadmap to embryo implantation: clues from mouse models. Nat Rev Genet 2006; 7: 185–99.
19. Salamonsen LA, Lathbury LJ. Endometrial leukocytes and menstruation. Hum Reprod Update 2000; 6: 16–27.
20. Salamonsen LA, Zhang J, Brasted M. Leukocyte networks and human endometrial remodeling. J Reprod Immunol 2002; 57: 95–108.
21. Moffett-King A. Natural killer cells and pregnancy. Nat Rev Immunol 2002; 2: 656–63.
22. Trundley A, Moffett A. Human uterine leukocytes and pregnancy. Tissue Antigens 2004; 63: 1–12.
23. Miller L, Hunt JS. Sex steroid hormones and macrophage function. Life Sci 1996; 59: 1–14.
24. Caballero-Campo P, Dominguez F, Coloma J et al. Hormonal and embryonic regulation of chemokines IL-8, MCP-1 and RANTES in the human endometrium during the window of implantation. Mol Hum Reprod 2002; 8: 375–84.
25. Bulmer JN, Pace D, Ritson A. Immunoregulatory cells in human decidua: morphology, immunohistochemistry and function. Reprod Nutr Dev 1988; 28: 1599–613.
26. Vassiliadou N, Bulmer JN. Quantitative analysis of T lymphocyte subsets in pregnant and nonpregnant human endometrium. Biol Reprod 1996; 55: 1017–22.
27. Hunt JS, Petroff MG, Burnett TG. Uterine leukocytes: key players in pregnancy. Semin Cell Dev Biol 2000; 11: 127–37.
28. Croy BA, He H, Esadeg S et al. Uterine natural killer cells: insights into their cellular and molecular biology from mouse modeling. Reproduction 2003; 126: 149–60.
29. Parr EL, Chen HL, Parr MB et al. Synthesis and granular localization of tumor necrosis factor-alpha in activated NK cells in the pregnant mouse uterus. J Reprod Immunol 1995; 28: 31–40.
30. Eriksson M, Meadows SK, Wira CR et al. Unique phenotype of human uterine NK cells and their regulation by TGF-β. J Leukoc Biol 2004; 76: 667–75.
31. Le Bouteiller P, Mallet V. HLA-G and pregnancy. Rev Reprod 1997; 2: 7–13.
32. King A, Allan DS, Bowen M et al. HLA-E is expressed on trophoblast and interacts with CD94/NKG2 receptors on decidual NK cells. Eur J Immunol 2000; 30: 1623–31.
33. Bulmer JN, Lash GE. Human uterine natural killer cells: a reappraisal. Mol Immunol 2005; 42: 511–21.

34. Ashkar AA, Di Santo JP, Croy BA. Interferon γ contributes to initiation of uterine vascular modification, decidual integrity, and uterine natural killer cell maturation during normal murine pregnancy. J Exp Med 2000; 192: 259–70.

35. Vince GS, Starkey PM, Jackson MC et al. Flow cytometric characterisation of cell populations in human pregnancy decidua and isolation of decidual macrophages. J Immunol Methods 1990; 132: 181–9.

36. Hunt JS. Immunologically relevant cells in the uterus. Biol Reprod 1994; 50: 461–6.

37. Gordon S. Alternative activation of macrophages. Nat Rev Immunol 2003; 3: 23–35.

38. Heikkinen J, Mottonen M, Komi J et al. Phenotypic characterization of human decidual macrophages. Clin Exp Immunol 2003; 131: 498–505.

39. McIntire RH, Morales PJ, Petroff MG et al. Recombinant HLA-G5 and -G6 drive U937 myelomonocytic cell production of TGF-β₁. J Leukocyte Biol 2005; 76: 1220–8.

40. Petroff MG, Chen L, Phillips TA et al. B7 family molecules are favorably positioned at the human maternal–fetal interface. Biol Reprod 2003; 68: 1496–504.

41. Gardner L, Moffett A. Dendritic cells in the human decidua. Biol Reprod 2003; 69: 1438–46.

42. Miyazaki S, Tsuda H, Sakai M et al. Predominance of Th2-promoting dendritic cells in early human pregnancy decidua. J Leukoc Biol 2003; 74: 514–22.

43. van Kooyk Y, Geijtenbeek TB. Dendritic cell-SIGN: escape mechanism for pathogens. Nat Rev Immunol 2003; 3: 697–709.

44. Heikkinen J, Mottonen M, Alanen A et al. Phenotypic characterization of regulatory T cells in the human decidua. Clin Exp Immun 2004; 136: 373–8.

45. Polanczyk MJ, Carson BD, Subramanian S et al. Cutting edge: estrogen drives expansion of the CD4+CD25+ regulatory T cell compartment. J Immunol 2004; 173: 2227–30.

46. Somerset DA, Zheng Y, Kilby MD et al. Normal human pregnancy is associated with an elevation in the immune suppressive CD25+CD4+ regulatory T-cell subset. Immunology 2004; 112: 38–43.

47. Fantini MC, Becker C, Monteleone G et al. TGF-β induces a regulatory phenotype in CD4+CD25− T cells through Foxp3 induction and down-regulation of Smad7. J Immunol 2004; 172: 5149–53.

48. Sakaguchi S. Regulatory T cells: key controllers of immunologic self-tolerance. Cell 2000; 101: 455–8.

49. Read S, Powrie F. CD4 (+) regulatory T cells. Curr Opin Immunol 2001; 13: 644–9.

50. Aluvihare VR, Kallikourdis M, Betz AG. Regulatory T cells mediate maternal tolerance to the fetus. Nature Immunol 2004; 5: 266–71.

51. Pijneneborg R. Implantation and immunology: maternal inflammatory and immune cellular responses to implantation and trophoblast invasion. Reprod Biomed Online 2002; 4(Suppl 3): 14–17.

52. Lu C, Jaramillo A. Tissue and solid organ allograft rejection. In: Austen F, Frank MM, Atkinson JP, Cantor H, eds. Samter's Immunologic Diseases, 6th edn. Philadelphia, PA: Lippincott, Williams and Wilkins, 2001.

53. Colvin RB, Smith RN. Antibody-mediated organ-allograft rejection. Nature Rev Immunol 2005; 5: 807–17.

54. Choudhury SR, Knapp LA. Human reproductive failure I: immunological factors. Hum Reprod Update 2001; 7: 113–34.

55. Vacchio MS, Jiang SP. The fetus and the maternal immune system: pregnancy as a model to study peripheral T-cell tolerance. Crit Rev Immunol 1999; 19: 461–80.

56. Redmond WL, Sherman LA. Peripheral tolerance of CD8 T lymphocytes. Immunity 2005; 22: 275–84.

57. Petroff MG. Immune interactions at the maternal–fetal interface. J Reprod Immunol 2005; 68: 1–13.

58. Hunt JS, Orr HT. HLA and maternal–fetal recognition. FASEB J 1992; 6: 2344–8.

59. Le Bouteiller P. HLA class I chromosomal region, genes, and products: facts and questions. Crit Rev Immunol 1994; 14: 89–129.

60. Murphy SP, Choi JC, Holtz R. Regulation of major histocompatibility complex class II gene expression in trophoblast cells. Reprod Biol Endocrinol 2004; 2: 52.

61. Hunt JS, Andrews GK, Wood GW. Normal trophoblasts resist induction of class I HLA. J Immunol 1987; 138: 2481–7.

62. Lenfant F, Fort M, Rodriguez AM et al. Absence of imprinting of HLA class Ia genes leads to coexpression of biparental alleles on term human trophoblast cells upon IFN-γ induction. Immunogenetics 1998; 47: 297–304.

63. Hiby SE, Walker JJ, O'Shaughnessy KM et al. Combinations of maternal KIR and fetal HLA-C genes influence the risk of preeclampsia and reproductive success. J Exp Med 2004; 200: 957–65.

64. Ishitani A, Sageshima N, Lee N et al. Protein expression and peptide binding suggest unique and interacting functional roles for HLA-E, F, and G in maternal–placental immune recognition. J Immunol 2003; 171: 1376–84.

65. Brown D, Trowsdale J, Allen R. The LILR family: moderators of innate and adaptive immune pathways in health and disease. Tissue Antigens 2004; 64: 215–25.

66. Yang Y, Chu W, Geraghty DE et al. Expression of HLA-G in human mononuclear phagocytes and selective induction by interferon-γ. J Immunol 1996; 156: 4224–31.

67. Hviid TV, Rizzo R, Christiansen OB et al. HLA-G and IL-10 in serum in relation to HLA-G genotype and polymorphisms. Immunogenetics 2004; 56: 135–41.

68. Ober C, Aldrich C, Rosinsky R et al. HLA-G1 protein expression is not essential for fetal survival. Placenta 1998; 19: 127–32.

69. Castro MJ, Morales P, Rojo-Amigo R et al. Homozygous HLA-G*0105N healthy individuals indicate that membrane-anchored HLA-G1 molecule is not necessary for survival. Tissue Antigens 2000; 56: 232–329.

70. Bainbridge DR, Ellis SA, Sargent I. The short forms of HLA-G are unlikely to play a role in pregnancy because they are not expressed at the cell surface. J Reprod Immunol 2000; 47: 1–16.

71. Menier C, Riteau B, Dausset J et al. HLA-G truncated isoforms can substitute for HLA-G1 in fetal survival. Hum Immunol 2000; 61: 1118–25.

72. Riteau B, Rouas-Freiss N, Menier C et al. HLA-G2, -G3, and -G4 isoforms expressed as nonmature cell surface glycoproteins inhibit NK and antigen-specific CTL cytolysis. J Immunol 2001; 166: 5018–26.

73. Moreau P, Dausset J, Carosella ED et al. Viewpoint on the functionality of the human leukocyte antigen-G null allele at the maternal–fetal interface. Biol Reprod 2002; 67: 1375–8.

74. Hunt JS, Jedhav L, Chu W, Geraghty DE, Ober C. Soluble HLA-G circulates in mothers during pregnancy. Am J Obstet Gynecol 2000; 183: 682–8.

75. Solier C, Aquerre-Girr M, Lenfant F et al. Secretion of pro-apoptotic intron 4-retaining soluble HLA-G1 by human villous trophoblast. Eur J Immunol 2002; 32: 3576–86.

76. Hunt JS, Pace JL, Morales P et al. Immunogenicity of the soluble isoforms of HLA-G. Mol Hum Reprod 2003; 9: 729–35.

77. Aldrich CL, Stephenson MD, Karrison T et al. HLA-G genotypes and pregnancy outcome in couples with unexplained recurrent miscarriage. Mol Hum Reprod 2001; 7: 1162–72.

78. Pfeiffer KA, Fimmers R, Engels G et al. The HLA-G genotype is potentially associated with idiopathic recurrent spontaneous abortion. Mol Hum Reprod 2001; 7: 373–8.

79. Ober C, Aldrich CL, Chervoneva I et al. Variation in the HLA-G promoter region influences miscarriage rates. Am J Hum Genet 2003; 72: 1425–35.

80. Patel RN, Quack KC, Hill JA et al. Expression of membrane-bound HLA-G at the maternal–fetal interface is not associated with pregnancy maintenance among patients with idiopathic recurrent pregnancy loss. Mol Hum Reprod 2003; 9: 551–7.

81. Lim KH, Zhou Y, Janatpour M et al. Human cytotrophoblast differentiation/invasion is abnormal in pre-eclampsia. Am J Pathol 1997; 151: 1809–18.

82. Colbern GT, Chiang MH, Main EK. Expression of the non-classic histocompatibility antigen HLA-G by preeclamptic placenta. Am J Obstet Gynecol 1994; 170: 1244–50.

83. Goldman-Wohl DS, Ariel I, Greenfield C et al. Lack of human leukocyte antigen-G expression in extravillous trophoblasts is associated with pre-eclampsia. Mol Hum Reprod 2000; 6: 88–95.

84. Rebmann V, van der Ven K, Passler M et al. Association of soluble HLA-G plasma levels with HLA-G alleles. Tissue Antigens 2001; 57: 15–21.

85. Aldrich C, Verp MS, Walker MA et al. A null mutation in HLA-G is not associated with preeclampsia or intrauterine growth retardation. J Reprod Immunol 2000; 47: 41–8.

86. Hviid TV, Hylenius S, Rorbye C et al. HLA-G allelic variants are associated with differences in the HLA-G mRNA isoform profile and HLA-G mRNA levels. Immunogenetics 2003; 55: 63–79.

87. Emmer PM, Joosten I, Schut MH et al. Shift in expression of HLA-G mRNA splice forms in pregnancies complicated by preeclampsia. J Soc Gynecol Investig 2004; 11: 220–6.

88. Le Bouteiller P, Pizzato N, Barakonyi A et al. HLA-G, pre-eclampsia, immunity and vascular events. J Reprod Immunol 2003; 59: 219–34.

89. Ober C, Billstrand C, Kuldanek S et al. The miscarriage-associated HLA-G-725 allele influences transcription rates in JEG-3 cells. Hum Reprod 2006; 21: 1743–8.

90. Menicucci A, Noci I, Fuzzi B et al. Non-classic sHLA class I in human oocyte culture medium. Hum Immunol 1999; 60: 1054–7.

91. Pfeiffer KA, Rebmann V, Passler M et al. Soluble HLA levels in early pregnancy after in vitro fertilization. Hum Immunol 2000; 61: 559–64.

92. Sher G, Keskintepe L, Nouriana M et al. Expression of sHLA-G in supernatants of individually cultured 46-h embryos: a potentially valuable indicator of 'embryo competency' and IVF outcome. Reprod Biomed Online 2004; 9: 74–8.

93. Noci I, Fuzzi B, Rizzo R et al. Embryonic soluble HLA-G as a marker of developmental potential in embryos. Hum Reprod 2005; 20: 138–46.

94. Yie S, Balakier H, Motamedi BRT et al. Secretion of human leukocyte antigen-G by human embryos is associated with a higher in vitro fertilization pregnancy rate. Fertil Steril 2005; 83: 30–6.

95. Hviid TVF, Hylenius S, Lindhard A et al. Association between human leukocyte antigen-G genotype and success of in vitro fertilization and pregnancy outcome. Tissue Antigens 2004; 64: 66–9.

96. Waterhouse P, Penninger JM, Timms E et al. Lympho-proliferative disorders with early lethality in mice deficient in CTLA-4. Science 1995; 270: 985–8.

97. Tivol EA, Borriello F, Schweitzer AN et al. Loss of CTLA-4 leads to massive lymphoproliferation and fatal multiorgan tissue destruction, revealing a critical negative role of CTLA-4. Immunity 1995; 3: 541–7.

98. Greenwald RJ, Freeman GJ, Sharpe AH. The B7 family revisited. Annu Rev Immunol 2005; 23: 515–48.

99. Petroff MG, Chen L, Phillips TA et al. B7 family molecules are favorably positioned at the human maternal–fetal interface. Biol Reprod 2003; 68: 1496–504.

100. Petroff MG, Kharatyan E, Torry DS et al. The immunomodulatory proteins B7-DC, B7-H2, and B7-H3 are differentially expressed across gestation in the human placenta. Am J Pathol 2005; 167: 465–73.

101. Holets LM, Hunt JS, Petroff MG. Trophoblast CD274 (B7-H1) is differentially expressed across gestation: influence of oxygen concentration. Biol Reprod 2006; 74: 352–8.

102. Nishimura H, Nose M, Hiai H et al. Development of lupus-like autoimmune diseases by disruption of the PD-1 gene encoding an ITIM motif-carrying immunoreceptor. Immunity 1999; 11: 141–51.

103. Nishimura H, Okazaki T, Tanaka Y et al. Autoimmune dilated cardiomyopathy in PD-1 receptor-deficient mice. Science 2001; 291: 319–22.

104. Nishimura H, Honjo T. PD-1: an inhibitory immunoreceptor involved in peripheral tolerance. Trends Immunol 2001; 22: 265–8.

105. Prokunina L, Castillejo-López C, Oberg F et al. A regulatory polymorphism in PDCD1 is associated with susceptibility to systemic lupus erythematosus in humans. Nat Genet 2002; 32: 666–9.

106. Nielsen C, Hansen D, Husby S et al. Association of a putative regulatory polymorphism in the PD-1 gene with susceptibility to type 1 diabetes. Tissue Antigens 2003; 62: 492–7.

107. Kong EK, Prokunina-Olsson L, Wong WH et al. A new haplotype of PDCD1 is associated with rheumatoid arthritis in Hong Kong Chinese. Arthritis Rheum 2005; 52: 1058–62.

108. Dong H, Zhu G, Tamada K et al. B7-H1 determines accumulation and deletion of intrahepatic CD8+ T lymphocytes. Immunity 2004; 20: 327–36.

109. Latchman YE, Liang SC, Wu Y et al. PD-L1-deficient mice show that PD-L1 on T cells, antigen-presenting cells, and host tissues negatively regulates T cells. Proc Natl Acad Sci USA 2004; 101: 10691–6.

110. Guleria I, Khosroshahi A, Ansari MJ et al. A critical role for the programmed death ligand 1 in fetomaternal tolerance. J Exp Med 2005; 202: 231–7.

111. Munn DH, Zhou M, Attwood JT et al. Prevention of allogeneic fetal rejection by tryptophan catabolism. Science 1998; 281: 1191–3.

112. Friberg M, Jennings R, Alsarraj M et al. Indoleamine-2,3-dioxygenase contributes to tumor cell evasion of T cell-mediated rejection. Int J Cancer 2002; 101: 151–5.

113. Sakurai K, Zou JP, Tschetter JR et al. Effect of indoleamine 2,3-dioxygenase on induction of experimental autoimmune encephalomyelitis. J Neuroimmunol 2002; 129: 186–96.

114. Mellor AL, Munn DH. IDO expression by dendritic cells: tolerance and tryptophan catabolism. Nat Rev Immunol 2004; 4: 762–74.

115. Sedlmayr P, Blaschitz A, Wintersteiger R et al. Localization of indoleamine 2,3-dioxygenase in human female reproductive organs and the placenta. Mol Hum Reprod 2002; 8: 385–91.

116. Baban B, Chandler P, McCool D et al. Indoleamine 2,3-dioxygenase expression is restricted to fetal trophoblast giant cells during murine gestation and is maternal genome specific. J Reprod Immunol 2004; 61: 67–77.

117. Honig A, Rieger L, Kapp M et al. Indoleamine 2,3-dioxygenase (IDO) expression in invasive extravillous trophoblast supports role of the enzyme for materno–fetal tolerance. J Reprod Immunol 2004; 61: 79–86.

118. Kudo Y, Boyd CAR, Spyropoulou I et al. Indoleamine 2,3-dioxygenase: distribution and function in the developing human placenta. J Reprod Immunol 2004; 61: 87–98.

119. Mellor AL, Jayabalan S, Chandler P et al. Prevention of T cell-driven complement activation and inflammation by tryptophan catabolism during pregnancy. Nat Immunol 2001; 2: 64–8.

120. Bonney EA, Matzinger P. Much IDO about pregnancy. Nat Med 1998; 4: 1128–9.

121. Terness P, Chuang JJ, Opelz G. The immunoregulatory role of IDO-producing human dendritic cells revisited. Trends Immunol 2006; 27: 68–73.

122. Tincani A, Balestrieri G, Danieli E et al. Pregnancy complications of the antiphospholipid syndrome. Autoimmunity 2003; 36: 27–32.

123. Holmes CH, Simpson KL, Okada H et al. Complement regulatory proteins at the feto–maternal interface during human placental development: distribution of CD59 by comparison with membrane cofactor protein (CD46) and decay accelerating factor (CD55). Eur J Immunol 1992; 22: 1579–85.

124. Hsi BL, Hunt JS, Atkinson JP. Differential expression of complement regulatory proteins on subpopulations of human trophoblast cells. J Reprod Immunol 1991; 19: 209–23.

125. Holmes CH, Simpson KL, Wainwright SD et al. Preferential expression of the complement regulatory protein decay accelerating factor at the fetomaternal interface during human pregnancy. J Immunol 1990; 144: 3099–105.

126. Tedesco F, Narchi G, Radillo O et al. Susceptibility of human trophoblast to killing by human complement and the role of the complement regulatory proteins. J Immunol 1993; 151: 1562–70.

127. Xu C, Mao D, Holers VM et al. A critical role for murine complement regulatory crry in fetomaternal tolerance. Science 2000; 287: 498–501.

128. Di Simone N, Raschi E, Testoni C et al. Pathogenic role of anti-beta 2-glycoprotein I antibodies in antiphospholipid associated fetal loss: characterization of beta 2-glycoprotein I binding to trophoblast cells and functional effects of anti-beta 2-glycoprotein I antibodies in vitro. Ann Rheum Dis 2005; 64: 462–7.

129. Girardi G, Bulla R, Salmon JE et al. The complement system in the pathophysiology of pregnancy. Mol Immunol 2006; 43: 68–77.

130. Bose P, Black S, Kadyrov M et al. Adverse effects of lupus anticoagulant positive blood sera on placental viability can be prevented by heparin in vitro. Am J Obstet Gynecol 2004; 191: 2125–31.

131. Robertson SA, Roberts CT, van Beijering E et al. Effect of β2-glycoprotein I null mutation on reproductive outcome and antiphospholipid antibody-mediated pregnancy pathology in mice. Mol Hum Reprod 2004; 10: 409–16.

132. Girardi G, Redecha P, Salmon JE. Heparin prevents antiphospholipid antibody-induced fetal loss by inhibiting complement activation. Nat Med 2004; 10: 1222–6.

133. Guleria I, Pollard JW. The trophoblast is a component of the innate immune system during pregnancy. Nat Med 2000; 6: 589–93.

134. Hunt JS, Phillips TA, Rasmussen CA et al. Apoptosis-inducing members of the tumor necrosis factor supergene family: potential functions in placentas. Trophoblast Res 1999; 13: 243–57.

135. Phillips TA, Ni J, Hunt JS. Death-inducing tumor necrosis factor (TNF) superfamily ligands and receptors are transcribed in human placentas, cytotrophoblasts, placental macrophages and placental cell lines. Placenta 2001; 22: 663–72.

136. Yui J, Garcia-Lloret M, Wegmann TG et al. Cytotoxicity of tumour necrosis factor-alpha and gamma-interferon against primary human placental trophoblasts. Placenta 1994; 5: 819–35.

137. Yang Y, Yelavarthi KK, Chen H-L et al. Molecular, biochemical and functional characteristics of tumor necrosis factor-α produced by human placental cytotrophoblastic cells. J Immunol 1993; 150: 5614–24.

138. Phillips TA, Ni J, Pan G et al. TRAIL (Apo-2L) and TRAIL receptors in human placentas: implications for tumor protection and immune privilege. J Immunol 1999; 162: 6053–9.

139. Gill RM, Ni J, Hunt JS. Differential expression of LIGHT and its receptors in human placentas and amniochorion membranes. Am J Pathol 2002; 161: 2011–17.

140. Gill RM, Ka H, Hunt JS. TRAIL, LIGHT and the expanding tumor necrosis factor superfamily in human placentas. Proc Indian Nat Acad Sci 2003; B69(4): 469–84.

141. Ware C. Network communications: lymphotoxins, LIGHT, and TNF. Ann Rev Immunol 2005; 23: 787–819.

142. Arntzen KJ, Liabakk NB, Jacobsen G et al. Soluble tumor necrosis factor receptor in serum and urine throughout normal pregnancy and at delivery. Am J Reprod Immunol 1995; 34: 163–9.

143. Payne SG, Smith SC, Davidge ST et al. Death receptor Fas/Apo-1/CD95 expressed by human placental cytotrophoblasts does not mediate apoptosis. Biol Reprod 1999; 60: 1144–50.

144. Ka H, Hunt JS. Temporal and spatial patterns of expression of inhibitors of apoptosis (IAP) in human placentas. Am J Pathol 2003; 63: 413–22.

145. Ka H, Hunt JS. FLICE-inhibitory protein: expression and in early and late gestation human placentas. Placenta 2006; 27: 626–34.

146. Phillips TA, Ni J, Hunt JS. Cell-specific expression of B lymphocyte- (APRIL, BLyS) and Th2- (CD30L/CD153) promoting tumor necrosis factor superfamily ligands in human placentas. J Leukocyte Biol 2003; 74: 81–7.

147. King AE, Critchley HO, Kelly RW. Innate immune defences in the human endometrium. Reprod Biol Endocrinol 2003; 1: 116.

148. Caucheteux SM, Kanellopoiulos-Langevin C, Ojcius DM. At the innate frontiers between mother and fetus: linking abortion with complement activation. Immunity 2003; 18: 169–72.

149. Hunt JS. Cytokine networks in the uteroplacental unit: macrophages as pivotal regulatory cells. J Reprod Immunol 1989; 16: 1–17.

150. Hunt JS, McIntire RH. Inflammatory cells and cytokine production. In: Peebles DM, Myatt L, eds. Inflammation and Pregnancy. London: Informa Healthcare, 2006: 1.

151. Gomez R, Ghezzi F, Romero R et al. Premature labor and intra-amniotic infection. Clinical aspects and role of cytokines in diagnosis and pathophysiology. Clin Perinatol 1995; 22: 281–342.

152. Gomez R, Romero R, Edwin SS et al. Pathogenesis of preterm labor and preterm premature rupture of membranes associated with intraamniotic infection. Infect Dis Clin North Am 1997; 11: 135–76.

153. Ruiz RJ, Fullerton J, Dudley DJ. The interrelationship of maternal stress, endocrine factors and inflammation on gestational length. Obstet Gynecol Surv 2003; 58: 415–28.

154. Murphy SP, Fast LD, Hanna NN et al. Uterine NK cells mediate inflammation-induced fetal demise in IL-10-null mice. J Immunol 2005; 175: 4084–90.

155. Roberts JM, Gammill HS. Preeclampsia: recent insights. Hypertension 2005; 46: 1243–9.

156. Redman CW, Sargent IL. Placental debris, oxidative stress and preeclampsia. Placenta 2000; 21: 597–602.

157. Reister F, Frank HG, Heyl W et al. The distribution of macrophages in spiral arteries of the placental bed in preeclampsia differs from that in healthy patients. Placenta 1999; 20: 229–33.

158. Reister F, Frank HG, Kingdom JC et al. Macrophage-induced apoptosis limits endovascular trophoblast invasion in the uterine wall of preeclamptic women. Lab Invest 2001; 81: 1143–52.

159. Redman CW, Sargent IL. Latest advances in understanding preeclampsia. Science 2005; 308: 1592–4.

160. Hung TH, Skepper JN, Charnock-Jones DS et al. Hypoxia-reoxygenation: a potent inducer of apoptotic changes in the human placenta and possible etiological factor in preeclampsia. Circ Res 2002; 90: 1274–81.

161. Maynard SE, Min JY, Merchan J et al. Excess placental soluble fms-like tyrosine kinase 1 (sFlt1) may contribute to endothelial dysfunction, hypertension, and proteinuria in preeclampsia. J Clin Invest 2003; 111: 649–58.

162. Koga K, Osuga Y, Yoshino O et al. Elevated serum soluble vascular endothelial growth factor receptor 1 (sVEGFR-1) levels in women with preeclampsia. J Clin Endocrinol Metab 2004; 88: 2348–51.

163. Levine RJ, Maynard SE, Qian C et al. Circulating angiogenic factors and the risk of preeclampsia. N Engl J Med 2004; 350: 672–83.

164. Nagamatsu T, Fujii T, Kusumi M et al. Cytotrophoblasts up-regulate soluble fms-like tyrosine kinase-1 expression under reduced oxygen: an implication for the placental vascular development and the pathophysiology of preeclampsia. Endocrinology 2004; 145: 4838–45.

165. Ahmad S, Ahmed A. Elevated placental soluble vascular endothelial growth factor receptor-1 inhibits angiogenesis in preeclampsia. Circ Res 2004; 95: 884–91.

35 Cytokine and chemokine regulation of endometrial immunobiology

Sarah A Robertson

Synopsis

Background

- Cytokines are a family of several hundred small diffusible glycoproteins that act as soluble intercellular signaling agents.
- Chemokines are a subset of the cytokine family distinguished by their chemotactic properties towards leukocytes.
- Cytokine binding to high-affinity receptors on target cells activates tyrosine kinases of the JAK–STAT family.
- Soluble receptor isoforms act as extracellular antagonists. Intracellular SOCS proteins act to damp down cytokine-activated signaling pathways.
- A cytokine can elicit widely diverse responses in target cells, depending on the combined effect of intrinsic and extrinsic environmental cues.
- There is overlap of function between different cytokines.
- Cytokines are not expressed constitutively, being produced in response to specific stimuli such as other cytokines, bacterial or viral products, immunoglobulin, hormones, or neurotransmitters.

Basic Science

- Cytokines and their receptors are expressed in all uterine and placental cell populations.
- Cytokines in the endometrium act to support a cellular environment that discriminates between the conceptus and infectious pathogens, and initiates immune responses of a character and extent appropriate to these discrete antigenic stimuli.
- Cytokine expression is regulated primarily by ovarian steroid hormones, but also by local factors secreted by adjacent endometrial cells or emanating from microorganisms, semen, the conceptus, or the placenta.
- Further influences on endometrial cytokine expression occur in the form of stress and neuroendocrine signals, nutritional status, and polymorphisms in cytokine and cytokine receptor genes.
- Chemokines play an integral role in regulating leukocyte recruitment by promoting extravasation of specific populations of leukocytes from peripheral blood. The cervical and uterine inflammatory response to seminal fluid is an important example of this phenomenon.
- Pathogens in the upper reproductive tract bind to toll-like receptors on epithelial cells, leading to the production of cytokines that in turn attract immune cells to the site. In this way, immune–epithelial cell communication is established.
- Epithelial and trophectodermal cytokines are responsible for the preimplantation maternal–embryonic dialogue, and this in turn influences profoundly the eventual outcome of the pregnancy.
- Stromal cytokines, especially IL-11, are required for decidual differentiation and placental development.
- Cytokine secretion is important in the capacity of macrophages and dendritic cells to engage in immunoregulatory and tissue remodeling processes including vascular development in the cycling and pregnant uterus.
- In pregnancy, decidual macrophages produce anti-inflammatory and tolerance-inducing cytokines, but this phenotype (associated with *immune deviation*) may alter to a more conventional activated state if infection sets in.
- Antigen-specific T cells, despite being sparse in the uterus, are a potentially important source of cytokines, because their products, particularly IFNγ, are extremely potent. T_{reg} cells have an important immunosuppressive function in pregnancy, linked to their synthesis of copious TGFβ and IL-10.

- Uterine NK cells become common in decidua. They require IL-15 for survival. IL-12 and IL-18 regulate their production of IFNγ, which in mice is important in modifying spiral arteries that supply the placenta. They produce many other cytokines.

Clinical

- Cytokine networks operating in the uterus before and after insemination, and before and after implantation, are crucial for optimal pregnancy outcome.
- Disturbances of immune function and cytokine balance are evident in endometriosis, infertility, and disorders of pregnancy.
- Inflammatory changes appear to play an important role in the persistence and expansion of endometriotic implants and the resulting morbidity. Cytokine antagonists and other anti-inflammatory strategies may be useful treatment options.
- An imbalance in cytokine networks may affect uterine receptivity, leading to failed implantation.
- Dysregulated cytokine networks may provoke a hostile decidual environment in recurrent miscarriage.
- It remains unclear whether such alterations cause these pathologies, or arise as the consequence of other lesions.

INTRODUCTION

The endometrium is remarkable in two respects – first, in its capacity to undergo regular and extensive tissue growth, breakdown, and repair; and, secondly, as a mucosal tissue able to discriminate between and respond appropriately to foreign agents as disparate as semen, the conceptus, and sexually transmitted pathogens. Cytokines and chemokines have central roles in these immune and tissue remodeling processes that are essential for normal endometrial function. They provide the intercellular communication signals that govern leukocyte recruitment and regulate induction of immune responses. Through targeting cell lineages other than leukocytes, including cells in the preimplantation embryo and placenta, cytokines are also key mediators of the tissue restructuring that accompanies the menstrual cycle and pregnancy (Figure 35.1). Disruption or imbalance in the endometrial cytokine–leukocyte axis is a principal factor in the etiology of infertility, endometriosis, and uterine bleeding disorders, and in diseases of pregnancy related to 'shallow' placentation.[1–4]

This chapter reviews the synthesis of endometrial cytokines and chemokines and their roles in the immunobiology of this tissue, focusing on data from the interstitial implanting species, particularly the mouse and human. Two principal communication pathways are highlighted – regulation of endometrial leukocyte populations by cytokines derived from other uterine cell lineages and the conceptus; and conversely, regulation of uterine epithelial and stromal cells, and cells of the pre- and postimplantation embryo, by cytokines of leukocyte origin. Preceding this is a brief description of the cytokine family of molecules, with emphasis on those characteristics that are of special relevance to the physiology of the endometrium.

CYTOKINES, CHEMOKINES, AND CELL COMMUNICATION

Cytokines were originally described on the basis of their actions in the lymphohematopoietic system, but have since been shown to have a wide range of activities with many different cell types producing and responding to these molecules. Thus, cytokines are a somewhat arbitrary subdivision of the large growth factor family, which together with neurotransmitters and hormones constitute the body's armory of soluble intercellular signaling agents. Chemokines are a subset of the cytokine family distinguished by their chemotactic properties. They act to regulate the recruitment of leukocytes from the blood, as well as their directional movement within tissues and their exodus via the lymphatic system. Cytokines, chemokines, and related molecules such as cytokine inhibitors, are typically low in molecular weight (<80 kDa) but otherwise are made up of a heterogeneous array of glycoproteins, now numbering several hundred in total, that are highly diverse in structure and amino acid sequence.

Cytokines are usually named after the biological function for which they were first discovered, and so their nomenclature can be misleading and even anomalous. On the basis of structural similarities, gene organization, chromosomal location, and receptor usage

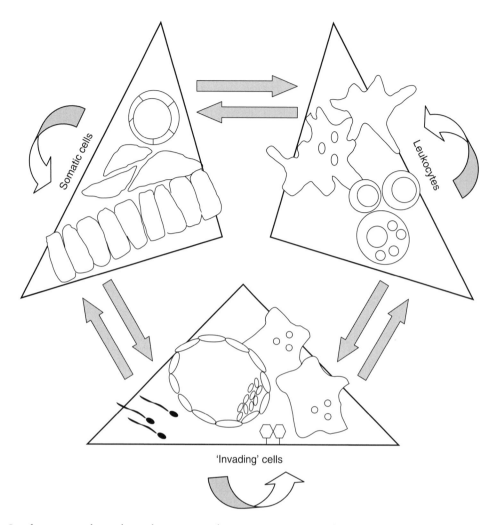

Figure 35.1   Cytokine networks in the endometrium. The unique properties of cytokines facilitate their roles as mediators of cell communication within and between non-hematopoietic cells (epithelial cells, stromal fibroblasts, and endothelial cells), infiltrating leukocyte populations (macrophages and dendritic cells, granulocytes, and lymphocytes) and 'invading' cells associated with semen, the conceptus and placenta, or microorganisms. The cellular sources and functions in the endometrium of many individual cytokines and chemokines are given in Tables 35.4 and Table 35.5, respectively.

Table 35.1   Structural families of cytokines and receptors expressed in the endometrium

Family	Members	Receptor type
Hematopoietins	IL-2, IL-3, IL-4, IL-5, IL-6, IL-11	
	IL-15, GM-CSF, LIF, G-CSF	hematopoietin receptor type I
	IL-10, IFNα, IFNβ, IFNγ, IFNτ	hematopoietin receptor type II
	CSF-1, SCF	tyrosine kinase
β-trefoil	IL-1α, IL-1β, IL-1Rα, IL-18	IL-1 receptor
β-jelly roll	TNFα, TNFβ, fas ligand	TNF receptor
Cysteine knot	TGFβ1, TGFβ2, TGFβ3	serine/threonine kinase
	PDGF	tyrosine kinase
Chemokines	IL-8, eotaxin, MCP-1, MIP-1α, etc.	G-protein-coupled superfamily

they can be classified into six families: the hematopoietins (including the colony-stimulating factors [CSFs], interferons [IFNs], and most of the interleukins), epidermal growth factors, β-trefoils (fibroblast growth factors and interleukin [IL]-1), the tumor necrosis factors (TNFs), the cysteine knot cytokines (including the transforming growth factor [TGF]-β family) and the chemokines (Table 35.1).[5]

Despite their structural diversity, this family of molecules share a number of common properties

Table 35.2 Comparison of the properties and functions of cytokines and ovarian steroid hormones

Cytokine	Ovarian steroid hormones	Cytokines
Cellular origins	few	many
Biological redundancy	low	high
Biological pleiotrophy	low	high
Presence in the circulation	yes	rarely
Sphere of influence	endocrine (distant)	autocrine, paracrine, juxtacrine (local)
Inducers	gonadotropins, cytokines	sex steroid hormones, cytokines, prostaglandins
Influence of microenvironment on biological effect	low	high
Effector action in target cells	often indirect	usually direct
Receptor location	nuclear	cell surface
Naturally occurring antagonists	no	yes

that contrast with those of the endocrine hormones (Table 35.2). Generally, cytokines are produced in relatively small quantities and exert their actions at nanomolar or picomolar concentrations. Most cytokines are secreted into the extracellular fluid, but some can be sequestered into the extracellular matrix through binding with glycosaminoglycans, or produced in alternative isoforms which may be anchored to the cell membrane. Together with the transient existence conferred by their short half-life, this usually restricts their sphere of influence to autocrine, paracrine, or juxtacrine actions within the immediate neighborhood of production. These properties can complicate the detection and quantification of cytokine proteins and messenger RNA (mRNA) sequences in tissues, so that extremely sensitive and precise techniques are required to investigate their synthesis and function.

Cytokines do not act as effector molecules directly, but rather bind to specific, high-affinity receptors on the surface of the target cell. Binding triggers a cascade of intracellular events that ultimately cause changes in the pattern of gene expression and protein synthesis. In this way, cytokines provide the signals that promote or inhibit multiple aspects of cell behavior, including survival, proliferation, and reversible and irreversible transitions in phenotype, secretory profile, and motility. Many cytokines bind to a single cognate receptor, while others share receptor components or whole receptors. Amongst chemokines, an individual receptor may bind one or more ligands, and each chemokine can bind several alternative receptors with different affinities.[6]

Activation of cytokine-responsive gene expression in target cells occurs as the end result of complex cascades of intracellular signal transduction pathways involving protein tyrosine kinases of the Janus family (JAK1, JAK2, JAK3, and Tyk2) and signal transducer and activation of transcription (STAT) molecules.[7–9] Initially, ligand binding catalyses receptor subunit oligomerization in the cell membrane, causing

transphosphorylation and activation of JAKs. This in turn leads to phosphorylation of receptors to allow docking of STAT molecules, which dimerize and translocate into the nucleus to initiate transcription of cytokine responsive genes. Different combinations of JAKs and STATs are utilized by different cytokine receptors to generate cytokine-specific responses.

Key concepts: context, pleiotrophy, and redundancy

The response of a cell to a given cytokine is dependent not only on its lineage and differentiation state but also on the local microenvironment, particularly the concentration of other cytokines and growth factors, and the extracellular matrix.[10] Thus, cytokines do not work in isolation, but rather interact within a network to amplify, modulate, or antagonize each other's activities. Appreciation of the importance of context in cytokine signaling led to the view that cytokines are best regarded as individual elements of a code or alphabet,[11] with the ultimate reaction of a cell depending on the sum total of signals converging at the cell surface. Cytokines are remarkably promiscuous and pleiotropic in their actions. A single factor can elicit extraordinarily diverse and sometimes apparently opposite responses in a range of different target cells, exerting key functions in tissues as disparate as the bone marrow, the brain, and the reproductive tract.

Cytokines are also notable for the considerable degree of overlap in activity between family members. The capacity for duplication of function between individual cytokines is clearly borne out by the surprising lack of severe phenotypic consequences of null mutation of many cytokine genes in mice. An individual cytokine is usually found to be absolutely essential in only a small proportion of the repertoire of cellular events in which it participates, presumably because most biological

Table 35.3   The reproductive phenotypes of mice genetically deficient in endometrial cytokines (see text for details)

Cytokine	Ligand/receptor	Phenotype of null mutation	Reference
CSF-1	ligand	severely reduced fertility, macrophage deficiency, gametogenesis dysregulated	Pollard et al[91]
GM-CSF	ligand	increased fetal resorption, fetal growth impairment, placental abnormality	Robertson et al[168]
IFNγ	ligand	uNK cells dysregulated, decidual necrosis, increased fetal resorption	Ashkar and Croy[144]
IL-1Rt1	receptor	implantation normal, slightly reduced litter size	Abbondanzo et al[135]
IL-2Rγc	receptor[a]	uNK deficiency, irregular estrous cycles, normal fertility	Miyazaki et al[189]
IL-4	ligand	normal fertility	Svensson et al[190]
IL-5	ligand	normal fertility, eosinophil deficiency	Robertson et al[113]
IL-6	ligand	increased fetal resorption	
IL-10	ligand	normal fertility; altered placental structure	White et al[192]
IL-11Rα	receptor	infertile; implantation failure	Robb et al[55] and Bilinski et al[192]
IL-12	ligand	implantation normal, increased fetal resorption	Zhang et al[118]
IL-15	ligand	uNK deficiency, implantation normal, slight fetal growth impairment	Barber et al[119]
LIF	ligand	infertile; implantation failure	Stewart et al[129]
LIFR	receptor	infertile; placental abnormality	Ware et al[163]
TGFβ₁	ligand	severely reduced fertility, impaired oocyte and embryo development	Ingman et al[167]

[a]IL-2Rγc is the common γ chain shared by receptors for IL-2, IL-4, IL-7, IL-8, and IL-15.

responses can be achieved by more than one cytokine. Rather than suggesting that many cytokines are therefore essentially dispensable, cytokine 'knockout' experiments indicate that critical cellular functions are usually backed up by 'fail-safe' mechanisms where the loss of one cytokine can be compensated by another factor with similar activities. This principle is particularly evident in the reproductive system, where null mutations in only a few cytokines lead to complete infertility (Table 35.3). However, it is important to interpret data from cytokine-deficient mice with caution, since mutations showing negligible effects in the rarefied environment of an animal research facility can prove to have more profound effects in outbred populations or when mice are challenged by infection, nutritional deprivation, or other environmental stressors. Furthermore, while deletion of individual cytokines may be consistent with viable pregnancy, the resulting perturbation in maternal tract cytokine balance can compromise the quality of placental and fetal development, leading to fetal growth retardation and reduced health of offspring in neonatal and adult life (see Table 35.3).

Regulation of cytokine synthesis and activity

Cytokines are not expressed constitutively and are produced only in response to specific excitants such as other cytokines, bacterial or viral products (via ligation of Toll-like receptors, TLRs), immunoglobulin,

hormones, or neurotransmitters. Different cell lineages can produce different combinations of cytokines in response to a given stimulus, and within an individual cell, distinct patterns of cytokine expression result when different intracellular pathways are triggered. Induction of cytokine release in most instances is achieved by increased de-novo synthesis of cytokine mRNA, accompanied in some cases by an increase in mRNA stability. Less commonly, cytokine secretion may result from up-regulated translation of existing mRNA, or from release of protein stored within cytoplasmic granules.

A variety of elaborate extracellular and intracellular control mechanisms exist to limit the duration and spread of a cytokine response.[12] These ensure that the potent effects of cytokines are confined to the immediate vicinity of the producing cell, and limit the life span of the response in the target cell. When stimulation for cytokine expression abates, a reduction in transcription rate and rapid degradation of mature transcripts rapidly follows. Down-regulation of cytokine receptors on responding cells is achieved through a reduction in the rate of synthesis, or by internalization and subsequent degradation of receptor–ligand complexes. Targeted secretion of cytokine towards the direction of the eliciting stimulus occurs in leukocytes and in polarized epithelial and endothelial cells, and acts to further limit the inadvertent activation of bystander cells.

Cytokine activities are further counterbalanced and modulated by other cytokines that oppose their effects, as well as by naturally occurring cytokine antagonists. These factors act to restore homeostasis and to prevent the exponential proliferation of consequences that would ensue if a response were left unchecked. Cytokine inhibitors arise from alternatively spliced mRNA transcripts and act by interfering with binding of a cytokine to its cell surface receptor.[13] They may take the form either of soluble receptors that compete with surface receptors by binding cytokine, for example gp130 or TNFα soluble receptors, or may be non-signal transducing isoforms of the cytokine, such as IL-1 receptor antagonist.

Suppressors of cytokine signaling (SOCS) are another family of molecules that terminate excessive cytokine receptor signaling.[14,15] This family of small intracellular proteins act as feedback inhibitors by interfering with the JAK–STAT signal transduction pathways. Their effects are elicited by direct binding to components of the cytokine signaling cascade, or by preventing access of JAKs or STATS to the signaling complex. Transgenic mice in which SOCS proteins are overexpressed or deleted show that members of the SOCS family have essential roles in regulating cytokine responses in leukocytes and other tissues.[14]

CYTOKINE AND CHEMOKINE SYNTHESIS IN THE ENDOMETRIUM

Interest in the origins and roles of cytokines in the endometrium began when uterine and placental tissues were discovered as potent sources of lymphohematopoietic cytokine activity.[16] The first significant advance in the field occurred in the late 1980s when it was shown that colony-stimulating factor 1 (CSF-1) in the uterus is synthesized by uterine epithelial cells, as opposed to resident leukocyte populations.[17] Subsequently, endometrial tissues, in particular the uterine epithelium, were identified as the source of an array of cytokines.[18,19] Several hundred studies are now published detailing the expression patterns of a wide range of cytokines and their receptors in the endometrium of women and animal species.[20–25] Cytokines and their receptors are expressed in distinct spatial and temporal patterns during the estrous cycle and pregnancy, regulated primarily by ovarian steroid hormones, but also by local factors secreted by adjacent endometrial cells or emanating from semen, the conceptus, or microorganisms. Further influences on endometrial cytokine expression occur in the form of stress and neuroendocrine signals, nutritional status, and polymorphisms in cytokine and cytokine receptor genes (Figure 35.2). The best-characterized endometrial cytokines, their cellular origins, regulators of synthesis, and target cells are listed in Table 35.4, while the most important chemokines and their regulators are shown in Table 35.5.

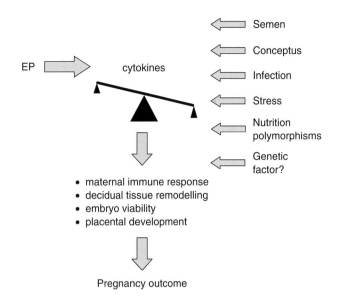

Figure 35.2 Normal endometrial function, and in particular a decidual environment conducive to optimal growth and development of the conceptus, is dependent on finely balanced cytokine equilibria, orchestrated primarily by ovarian steroid hormones, but also influenced by factors derived from semen, the preimplantation embryo and placental cells, and infectious microorganisms. Less well understood are the effects on endometrial cytokine expression of stress, nutritional status, and genetic factors such as cytokine gene polymorphisms.

The intention of this chapter is not to provide a comprehensive review of every endometrial cytokine but rather to highlight central and emerging concepts, using selected studies to illustrate common themes. The discussion will focus on studies in women, together with information from animal models. Experiments in rodents and other animals generally precede and inform human research, and studies in mice with null mutations in cytokine genes provide particularly useful insight. In the human, the physiological roles of cytokines in the endometrium are more difficult to define and often must be inferred from descriptive studies or in-vitro experiments with cells harvested from placentas and uterine tissues.

Cytokine production by endometrial epithelial and mesenchymal cells

Lymphocytes and macrophages are often assumed to be the principal source of tissue cytokines. However, in the endometrium, the range and output of cytokines synthesized by uterine epithelial and stromal cells often exceeds that of the leukocyte compartment. In-situ hybridization and immunohistochemical studies demonstrate that uterine epithelial cells lining the luminal cavity and constituting the endometrial glands

Table 35.4 The cellular origins, regulators, and potential target cells of key cytokines synthesized in the murine and human endometrium

Cytokine	Cellular source (species)	Regulators	Target cells	Key references
CSF-1	epithelial cells (m,h) uNK, lymphocytes (m,h) fibroblasts (h)	↑E, ↑P, ↑decidual factors	Mac pre-embryo trophoblast cells	Arceci et al[17] Pollard et al[91] Daiter and Pollard[26]
GM-CSF	epithelial cells (m,h) uNK, lymphocytes (m,h) mast cells (m)	↑E, ↓P ↓IFNγ ↑LPS ↑TGFβ ↑Seminal plasma ↑IgE ± substance P	Mac DC, Ne, Eo pre-embryo trophoblast cells endothelial cells	Robertson et al[122] Robertson et al[168] Giacomini et al[42] Sjoblom et al[151]
G-CSF	mac (h) decidual cells uNK, lymphocytes (m,h)		Ne endothelial cells trophoblast cells	Shorter et al[193] McCracken et al[194]
IFNγ	uNK, lymphocytes, Mac, neutrophils (m,h)	↑IL-12, IL-2, LPS ↑TNFα	Mac epithelial cells uNK cells pre-embryo trophoblast cells	Bulmer et al[195] Tabibzadeh et al[127] Chen et al[144] Ashkar and Croy[144] Yeaman et al[87]
IL-1	Mac (m, h) endothelial cells (m, h)	↑E, ↑P ↑LPS ↑GM-CSF	Mac, Ne, Eo lymphocytes endothelial cells epithelial cells	McMaster et al[70] Tabibzadeh and Sun[19] Simon et al[196]
IL-4	lymphocytes (h)	↑P	Mac, DC	Saito et al[77] Piccinni and Romagnani[81]
IL-6	epithelial cells (m,h) fibroblast cells (m,h) Mac (m) endothelial cells (m)	↑E ↑Seminal plasma ↑IL-1 ↑LPS ↑CD40 ligand	Mac lymphocytes NK cells endothelial cells pre-embryo	Robertson et al[122] Tabibzadeh and Sun[19] Koumas et al[57]
IL-10	epithelial cells (m,h) decidual cells (h) uNK cells (m,h) T lymphocytes (h)	↑LPS ↑IL-1	Mac trophoblast cells smooth muscle cells	Lin et al[197] Kimatrai et al[198] Trautman et al[199]
IL-11	epithelial cells (h) fibroblast cells (m,h)	↑IL-1 ↑TNFα ↑TGFβ	decidual cells	Robb et al[55] Dimitriadis et al[29] Cork et al[30]
IL-15	Mac (m,h) epithelial cells (h) perivascular stromal cells (h)	↑P, ↑PGE$_2$, ↑IFNγ ↓IL-1	uNK cells	Ye et al[116] Kitaya et al[32] Verma et al[65] Dunn et al[201]
IL-18	epithelial cells (m,h) uNK cells (m,h)		uNK cells T cells	Yoshino et al[33] Zhang et al[118] Ostojic et al[202]
LIF	epithelial cells (m, h) uNK, lymphocytes (m,h) fibroblasts (h)	↑E, ↑P ↑IL-1 ↑TNFα ↑TGFβ ↓IFNγ	epithelial cells Mac pre-embryo trophoblast cells	Bhatt et al[40] Stewart et al[129] Charnock-Jones et al[41] Cullinan et al[131] Arici et al[202]
TGFβ	epithelial cells (m) uNK, lymphocytes (m,h)	↑E,↑P	epithelial cells Mac, DC pre-embryo trophoblast cells	Shull and Doetschman[203]
TNFα	epithelial cells (m,h) Mac (m,h) uNK, lymphocytes (m,h) Mast cells (m)	↑E, ↑P ↑LPS ↑GM-CSF ↑IgE ± substance P	Mac, DC, Ne endothelial cells epithelial cells pre-embryo trophoblast cells	Hunt[27] McMaster et al[70] Pampfer et al[153]

The cellular source and regulators (↑ increase/up-regulation; ↓ decrease/down-regulation) of the best-studied cytokines known to be produced in the murine (m) or human (h) endometrium are shown, together with the likely cellular targets of those cytokines in the uterus and conceptus. uNK, uterine natural killer cells; Mac, macrophages, Ne, neutrophils; Eo, eosinophils; DC, dendritic cells. Key references are given, but for additional detail see reviews and references cited in the text.

Table 35.5 The cellular origins, regulators, and potential target cells of central chemokines synthesized in the murine and human endometrium

Cytokine	Cellular source (species)	Regulators	Target cells	Key references
6Ckine	epithelial cells (h) decidual cells (h) Mac, uNK (h)		T and B cells NK cells, DC	Nakayama et al[204] Jones et al[49]
eotaxin	epithelial cells (h) decidual cells (h)	↑E, ↓P	Eo, Ba T cells	Zhang et al[48] Robertson et al[95] Jones et al[49]
fractalkine	epithelial cells (h) decidual cells (h)		Mo, DC NK cells Ne, T cells	Jones et al[49]
IL-8	fibroblast cells (h) epithelial cells (h)	↓P ↑IL-1 ↑CD40 ligand	Ne, T cells, Ba endothelial cells stromal cells	Jones et al[97] Arici et al[136] Koumas et al[57]
MCP-1	perivascular stroma (h) epithelium (h)		Mo, T cells, Ba NK cells	Jones et al[97] Hampton et al[205]
MCP-3	epithelium (h) epithelial cells (h)		Mo, T cells Eo, Ba NK cells, DC	Jones et al[49]
MIP-1α	epithelial cells (h) decidual cells (h)	↑IL-1 ↑TNFα ↑IL-4	Mo, T cells Eo, Ba NK cells, DC	Dudley et al[206] Akiyama et al[207]
MIP-1β	epithelial cells (h) decidual cells (h)		Mo, T cells NK cells, DC	Kitaya et al[208] Jones et al[49]
RANTES	stromal cells (h)	↑IL-1 ↑TNFα ↑LPS ↓IL-4	T cells, Eo, Ba NK cells, DC	Hornung et al[209] Arima et al[210]

The cellular source and regulators (↑ increase/up-regulation; ↓ decrease/down-regulation) of the best-studied chemokines known to be produced in the murine (m) or human (h) endometrium are shown, together with the likely cellular targets of those cytokines in the uterus and conceptus. uNK, uterine natural killer cells; Mo, monocytes; Mac, macrophages, Ne, neutrophils; Eo, eosinophils; Ba, basophils; DC, dendritic cells. Key references are given, but for additional detail see reviews and references cited in the text.

secrete an extensive repertoire of cytokines. The first factors identified include CSF-1, granulocyte–macrophage colony-stimulating factor (GM-CSF), leukemia inhibitory factor (LIF), TNFα, IL-6, and TGFβ.[18,20,22–24,26–28] The known epithelial cell cytokine repertoire is now expanded to include IL-11,[29,30] IL-13,[31] 1L-15,[32,33] and IL-18.[33] Tissue localization studies also identify epithelial cells as the predominant uterine source of an array of chemokines that include IL-8, monocyte chemotactic protein (MCP)-1, MCP-3, macrophage inflammatory protein (MIP)-1α, MIP-1β, regulated on activation, normal T cell expressed and secreted (RANTES), eotaxin, fractalkine, hemofiltrate CC chemokine (HCC)-1, HCC-4, 6Ckine, and macrophage-derived chemokine (MDC).[23,24,34,35]

Epithelial cytokine synthesis is regulated over the course of the reproductive cycle by ovarian sex steroids acting at the transcriptional level. Individual cytokine genes show different temporal patterns, suggesting their independent regulation or sequential activation, by mechanisms that are not fully defined but likely to involve cross-talk between cytokine-activated transcription factors and steroid hormone receptors.[36,37]

Local regulatory factors other than steroid hormones – such as cytokines, growth factors, prostaglandins, and other agents – can further modulate epithelial cell cytokine expression (see Table 35.4). In this way diverse and dynamic cytokine microenvironments are generated at different locations within the endometrium during the estrous cycle and pregnancy. In mice, a surge in expression of proinflammatory cytokines, including GM-CSF, IL-6, and an array of chemokines, is induced in estrogen-primed uterine epithelial cells after the introduction of specific seminal factors at mating, particularly TGFβ derived from the seminal vesicle gland.[38] The secretion pattern alters again prior to implantation, when increasing concentrations of circulating progesterone inhibit GM-CSF and chemokine synthesis,[39] and drive a switch to epithelial cell CSF-1 and LIF expression.[17,40]

There appear to be similarities between steroid-hormone regulated cytokine secretion patterns in the rodent and human uterine epithelium. Estrogen-regulated cytokines including CSF-1, GM-CSF, and TNFα increase in abundance over the course of the proliferative phase in women. A secretory phase decline in GM-CSF, and further increase in CSF-1, TNFα, and LIF, match patterns occurring early in murine pregnancy.[26,27,41,42] Seminal factors including TGFβ and prostaglandin E$_2$ (PGE$_2$) are capable of inducing expression of IL-8, GM-CSF, IL-6, and other cytokines and chemokines in human cervical epithelial cells[43,44] which drive the leukocytosis that accompanies insemination in women.[45] Whether cytokine changes in the endometrium can also occur as a consequence of interaction between endometrial cells and the smaller quantity of seminal material that accesses the human uterus remains to be evaluated, but seems likely based on in-vitro studies.[46] In the event of implantation of an embryo, CSF-1, LIF, and other progesterone-induced epithelial cytokines are up-regulated and then predominate for the duration of the pregnancy for as long as circulating progesterone remains high.[47] In the absence of pregnancy, a switch back to expression of proinflammatory cytokines, including several chemokines, is afforded by premenstrual progesterone withdrawal.[48,49]

Factors associated with microorganisms can induce proinflammatory cytokine expression in uterine and endocervical epithelial cells. Cervical epithelial cells respond to *Chlamydia* infection with increased mRNA expression and secretion of IL-1, IL-8, growth-related oncogene (GRO)α, GM-CSF, and IL-6,[50] and lipo-oligosaccharides from *Escherichia coli* or *Neisseria gonorrhoeae* similarly induce inflammatory cytokine expression.[51] It is likely that cytokine networks induced after infection act in an amplifying cascade, with factors such as IFNγ and TNFα elicited in endometrial leukocytes implicated as potent stimulators of cytokine and chemokine expression in cervical epithelial cells.[52] Members of the TLR family of pattern recognition receptors are expressed by epithelial cells in the cervix[51] and uterus[53,54] and play central roles in recognizing the presence of infection and eliciting the cytokines necessary to activate a protective immune response.

Stromal fibroblasts and endothelial cells constituting the mesenchymal compartment also secrete a range of cytokines and chemokines, including GM-CSF, TNFα, IL-6, TGFβ (reviewed in Robertson et al[20] and Tabibzadeh[21]), IL-11,[30,55] and IL-8,[56] and IL-15.[32] Distinct spatial patterns in cytokine secretion are evident: for example IL-8 and IL-15 are preferentially expressed in stromal cells adjacent to spiral arteries.[32] Heterogeneity in the functional phenotypes of uterine fibroblasts appears to account for this, with perivascular cells distinguished by their expression of Thy1 and responsiveness to activation via CD40 ligation to induce IL-6 and IL-8 synthesis.[57] Stromal fibroblast cytokine expression is differentially regulated depending on the stage of the cycle or pregnancy. Increased expression of IL-11 and IL-15 accompanies the differentiation of stromal fibroblasts into rounded decidual cells in the secretory phase of the human cycle or at implantation in rodents.[30,32,58]

Cytokine production by endometrial leukocytes

The endometrium is richly populated with morphologically and phenotypically heterogeneous leukocyte populations, particularly macrophages, dendritic cells, granulocytes, lymphocytes, and mast cells, all of which are important sources of a variety of cytokines. The secretory profile of leukocytes is highly variable depending on their activation state.

Macrophages are exceptionally versatile in this regard.[59–61] Like macrophages in other mucosal tissues, endometrial macrophages can secrete an array of cytokines in patterns that are flexible and responsive to external environmental cues.[62] Cytokine secretion is a key property in the capacity of endometrial macrophages to engage in immunoregulatory and tissue remodeling processes in the cycling and pregnant uterus. There is evidence of a close lineage relationship between endometrial macrophages and dendritic cells,[63,64] raising the possibility of trans-differentiation between the two lineages and collaboration in antigen processing for the activation of immune responses.

Uterine and decidual macrophages can secrete cytokines with immune-activating or immune suppressive properties. In the proliferative phase of the cycle, macrophages are the predominant uterine source of IL-15.[65] In healthy pregnancies decidual macrophages synthesize anti-inflammatory and tolerance-inducing cytokines TGFβ and IL-10[66,67] and IL-1 receptor antagonist.[19] Exposure to human leukocyte antigen (HLA)-G expressed by fetal trophoblast cells may provide environmental 'programming' signals to decidual macrophages, resulting in increased TGFβ synthesis.[68,69] Conventional activation phenotypes, characterized by expression of IL-1 (α and β) and TNFα mRNAs, are evident in uterine macrophages during the inflammatory response to insemination[70] and during the process of fetal resorption in mice.[71] Bacterial lipopolysaccharide (LPS) also profoundly alters the secretory profile of decidual macrophages in mice, activating expression of IFNγ and IL-12.[72]

A high proportion of the lymphocytes found in the uterus and decidua are uterine natural killer (uNK) cells. Following implantation, they differentiate into large cells with a characteristic granulated appearance and accumulate in the metrial gland and decidua basalis where they associate closely with placental tissue.[73] Human uNK cells also express NK cell markers and are distributed throughout the decidua in pregnancy.[74] Messenger RNA transcripts and/or bioactivity for several factors are present in murine uNK cells (CSF-1, IL-1, LIF, TNFα, TGFβ, IFNγ, and IL-18)[75,76] and human uNK cells (IL-4, IL-5, IL-10, IL-13, GM-CSF, granulocyte-CSF [G-CSF], CSF-1, TNFα, IFNγ, and LIF).[77] Heterogeneity in the patterns of expression of these cytokines indicates that a variety of subsets of uNK cells exist in the decidua and that uNK cells expressing immunosuppressive cytokines predominate.[78]

Antigen-specific T lymphocytes are potentially very important sources of cytokines, because their cytokine products, particularly IFNγ, are extremely potent. Conventional α/β T lymphocytes are sparsely distributed in endometrial tissues, but cells expressing γ/δ T-cell receptors are more plentiful. Secretion patterns characteristic of type 1 and type 2 polarization are evident in both α/β and γ/δ T cells, with distinct populations of TGFβ/IL-10 secreting cells and TNFα/IFNγ secreting cells appearing to have opposing functional activity.[79] Helper (CD4+) and suppressor/cytotoxic (CD8+) T lymphocytes aggregating in the human endometrium and decidua[74,80] can secrete an array of cytokines, including all of those listed for uNK cells, plus IL-4 and IL-2.[81,82] A key T-lymphocyte population in conferring maternal immune tolerance in pregnancy is CD4+CD25+ T-regulatory (T$_{reg}$) cells.[83] The suppressive function of this population is linked to their synthesis of copious TGFβ and IL-10.[84,85]

Eosinophils, neutrophils, and mast cells exist in varying abundance in the cycling and pregnant endometrium. In the rodent uterus, their numbers peak at estrus and during the inflammatory response of early pregnancy, but despite increasing evidence from other tissues that they can synthesize a variety of different cytokines and chemokines in a regulated manner, their secretory activity in the endometrium has not been described. Recent studies in the human endometrium have begun to address this; mast cells and eosinophils found to be especially prominent immediately prior to and during menstruation are implicated in the synthesis of matrix metalloproteinases (MMPs) and other tissue degrading and remodeling enzymes.[86] Somewhat surprisingly, neutrophils have been identified as a potent source of IFNγ in the human endometrium, with expression regulated by LPS, IL-12, and TNFα.[87] In the mouse, recent studies suggest that uterine mast cells may contribute significantly to local GM-CSF and TNFα content, with release during early pregnancy being induced by the neuropeptide substance P and unidentified embryo-derived factors.[88]

CYTOKINE AND CHEMOKINE REGULATION OF ENDOMETRIAL LEUKOCYTES

Leukocyte trafficking

In many respects, the abundant leukocyte populations in the endometrium are comparable in composition and function to their counterparts in other mucosal epithelia. However, the endometrial leukocyte populations are distinguished by their responsiveness to the ovarian steroid hormones estrogen and progesterone. Fluctuations in the number and distribution of macrophages and granulocytes accompany the demise and regeneration of endometrial tissue across the menstrual cycle and the decidual differentiation required for early pregnancy, and are likely effector cells in these processes.[62,74,89] The kinetics of T- and B-lymphocyte and uNK cell recruitment also fluctuate in a cyclic manner,[74,90] in tandem with the immunological demands of accommodating insemination and possible pregnancy, and maintaining defense against infection. At times of maximal tissue remodeling, during embryo implantation, and immediately prior to menstrual shedding, leukocytes constitute approximately 40% of the total endometrial stromal cells.

Cytokines, in particular the chemokine subfamily, play an integral role in regulating leukocyte recruitment, through orchestrating the molecular events that promote extravasation of specific populations of leukocytes from the peripheral blood into the tissue. Attachment and transmigration of leukocytes across the endothelial cell barrier, and their subsequent movement through the tissue, occurs in response to chemokine gradients. In the endometrium, these movements are driven by changing patterns of cytokines and chemokines emanating from uterine epithelial and stromal cells. Complex amplification networks may evolve after the further release of cytokines and chemokines from recruited leukocytes. For some lymphocyte lineages, proliferation in situ may further boost the number of cells in endometrial tissue.

Studies in mice have been particularly illuminating in identifying the active factors in recruiting and regulating the position and behavior of endometrial macrophages. A key role for CSF-1 in maintaining endometrial macrophages during the estrous cycle was shown using genetically CSF-1-deficient *csfm^{op}/csfm^{op}* mice.[91] However, other factors compensate for the absence of this cytokine at estrus and during early pregnancy.[92] These observations led to detection of several chemokines expressed during the estrous cycle in steroid hormone-regulated patterns that parallel macrophage recruitment.[92-95] Chemokines identified in the mouse uterus include RANTES, MIP-1α, MIP-1β, MCP-1, and C10. Each of these fluctuates in abundance across the cycle and all are maximally induced during early pregnancy, resulting in the further infiltration and activation of inflammatory cells that precedes embryo implantation. Transcripts encoding granulocyte chemokines MIP-2 and KC are also expressed in the mouse uterus, initially at ovulation and increasing substantially after insemination.[94,95] Inhibition by progesterone causes their expression to drop and a parallel reduction in inflammatory leukocyte invasion occurs as embryo implantation is initiated.[95]

Chemokines clearly mediate regulation of leukocyte recruitment in the human endometrium. The first described were IL-8 and MCP-1, both of which localize to perivascular cells of blood vessels, consistent with a role in eliciting extravasation of blood-borne neutrophils and monocytes, respectively, into endometrial tissue[56,96,97] during the proliferative and particularly the premenstrual phase of the cycle.[97] Decidual IL-8 and MCP-1 expression is negatively regulated by progesterone, since mifepristone administration in early pregnancy causes leukocyte influx in association with elevated chemokine synthesis.[96] Eosinophil accumulation in the endometrium is also a feature of the late secretory phase of the menstrual cycle, and expression patterns of both eotaxin and its receptor CCR3 are consistent with eosinophil regulation by this chemokine.[48]

The range of chemokines identified in human endometrium now includes IL-8, MCP-1, MCP-3, MIP-1α, MIP-1β, RANTES, eotaxin, fractalkine, HCC-1, HCC-4, 6Ckine, and MDC[23,24,34,35] (see Table 35.5).

Several of these were identified in an elegant gene-array study, which, by providing quantitative comparison of expression levels of 21 chemokines across the menstrual cycle, revealed a clear hierarchy in their relative abundance in endometrial tissue.[49] Tightly regulated synthesis of a group of nine prominent chemokines is implicated in precisely regulating the spatial and temporal fluctuations in each endometrial leukocyte lineage, with combinations of chemokines at different cycle stages targeting different cell lineages. In this manner, distinct chemokine expression profiles during early pregnancy compared with the premenstrual period can account for the uNK cell recruitment required for pregnancy as opposed to the macrophage, eosinophil, and neutrophil recruitment implicated in tissue breakdown and menstrual shedding.[49] The study pinpoints three decidual factors – 6Ckine, MIP-1β, and MCP-3 – as principal agents for directing migration of precursor uNK cells into the implantation site. While the precise nature of the factors driving the homing and/or infiltration of other lymphocytes remains to be defined, many of the identified endometrial chemokines have T-lymphocyte as well as NK-cell chemotactic activity.

Leukocyte activation and function

Maturation into the correct functional state is essential for the appropriate behavior of leukocytes in mediating their indispensable functions in the endometrium. Like recruitment patterns, the differentiation and activation phenotypes of endometrial macrophages, dendritic cells, granulocytes, and lymphocytes are governed by local environmental signals. Most important in this regard is the cytokine milieu prevailing in the tissue once chemokine-mediated recruitment is accomplished.

Heterogeneity is most evident in tissue macrophages, which, depending on the environmental signals they encounter in the tissue after recruitment, can give rise to a variety of specialized phenotypes.[59-61] Macrophages are pivotal regulators of local immunological events, and through their ability to transdifferentiate into dendritic cells, are important accessory cells in the activation and suppression of lymphocyte activity. These cells also actively participate in tissue remodeling processes, a role for which they are well equipped by their armory of secreted cytokines, prostaglandins, vasoactive amines, and matrix remodeling enzymes. The local concentration of regulatory cytokines, including TNFα and IFNγ, IL-4 and IL-13, CSF-1, and GM-CSF, is the principal determinant of which of three known phenotypes tissue macrophages assume; IFNγ and TNFα give rise to 'classically activated' macrophages, IL-4 and IL-13 generate 'alternatively activated' macrophages, and 'type 2-activated' macrophages occur after ligation of the immunoglobulin receptor FcγR.[59–61] These cells have differing predispositions to tissue remodeling and repair, contribution to host defense, differentiation into dendritic cells, and cytokine secretion, with the alternative and type 2 macrophages having anti-inflammatory properties through their secretion of IL-10. The balance between GM-CSF and CSF-1 also influences the immunoaccessory properties of macrophages[98,99] while all macrophage phenotypes are susceptible to the classical 'deactivating' signals of IL-10 and TGFβ.[59,60]

In view of the cycle and pregnancy-related fluctuations in macrophage-regulating cytokines in the uterus, it is unsurprising that evidence is emerging for heterogeneity in resident uterine macrophage phenotypes. In mice, variation occurs in their expression of activation markers, including F4/80, MHC class II, macrosialin, scavenger receptor A, and sialoadhesin, plus a range of dendritic cell markers, consistent with both mature macrophages and dendritic cells differentiating from recruited immature undifferentiated macrophage precursors.[63] During the inflammatory response to mating, uterine macrophages are exposed to high levels of GM-CSF, TNFα, and IL-1 and appear to participate in the removal of debris and induction of immune responses to seminal antigens[62] (SA Robertson, unpublished data). In contrast, macrophages recovered from the pregnant uterus are highly immunosuppressive and implicated in maintaining tolerance of the conceptus.[100–102] This is consistent with their exposure to cytokines CSF-1, IL-4, and IL-13, which are up-regulated in the progesterone-dominated pregnant uterus, or might be due to direct effects of progesterone on macrophage gene expression.[103] Macrophages in the pregnant uterus may be poised to assume a fully activated, 'defensive' phenotype in the event of infection, since IFNγ receptor mRNA is up-regulated in uterine macrophages at the onset of pregnancy and remains high until term.[104] Importantly, LIF has also been identified as a key regulator and possibly chemokine for uterine macrophage populations, with disturbances in their abundance and tissue distribution in LIF null mutant mice.[105]

In women, decidual macrophages recovered in early pregnancy produce high levels of IL-10[106] and express mRNAs encoding stabilin-1 and coagulation factor XIIIa,[107] which together are markers consistent with an alternative activation phenotype. However, like mouse decidual macrophages, they remain responsive to signaling through TLRs[108] and this indicates a capacity to switch to a conventionally activated phenotype in the

event of infection. Dendritic cells in the non-pregnant endometrium and in decidual tissue in pregnancy display heterogeneic marker expression patterns consistent with a monocyte-derived, immature phenotype.[63,109–111] Once implantation is established, differential expression of IFNγ, IL-4, and other macrophage-regulating cytokines in different compartments of the decidual and placental tissues at the fetal–maternal interface would be expected to induce further heterogeneity in local macrophage and dendritic cell populations.

The functions of granulocytes and their regulating cytokines in the endometrium are less clear than those of macrophages. In women, menstruation is preceded by an accumulation of eosinophils, neutrophils, and mast cells in the superficial layers and their expression of enzymes which activate MMPs implicates these cells in tissue degradation at menstruation.[112] It might be speculated that these cells also have a protective role in defending the tract from opportunistic invaders while the integrity of the endometrial barrier is compromised. In mice, eosinophils and neutrophils are most prominent at ovulation and after insemination, when participation in immune responses to semen-associated antigens occurs. Cytokines identified as regulating uterine eosinophils include IL-5[113,114] and GM-CSF,[115] and IL-8, TNFα, and IL-1 are additional likely candidates for granulocyte regulation.

Local cytokines also orchestrate the activation phenotype and secretory behavior of uNK cells and the populations of T lymphocytes found in the decidualized endometrium. IL-15 is an essential survival factor for uNK cells.[116,117] IL-12 and IL-18, derived from decidual cells, macrophages, and via autocrine production in uNK cells, act in concert to regulate normal uNK production of IFNγ and other cytokines.[118] Genetic deletion of these cytokines impairs the spiral artery modifications normally mediated by uNK-cell-derived IFNγ.[117–119] Macrophages and uNK cells appear to interact in a reciprocal regulation network, since the macrophage cytokines IL-12 and TNFα stimulate uNK activation, and macrophages respond to the ensuing increase in uNK-cell-derived IFNγ.[120]

Immune deviation and tolerance

The primary function of the endometrium is to nurture the growth and development of the semiallogeneic conceptus, but at the same time there is a need to maintain vigilant protection from viral and bacterial infections of the reproductive tract. Thus, the immune system servicing the endometrium must discriminate between the conceptus and infectious pathogens, and be able to initiate immune responses of a character and extent appropriate to each antigenic stimulus. An important role for the rich complexity of cytokines found in the endometrium is to support this special immunological attribute, since the prevailing cytokine environment at the time and location where antigen is first perceived is the paramount determinant of the subsequent immune outcome.

This influence of cytokines in the selective induction of permissive or antagonistic immune responses is effected principally through professional antigen-presenting cells: i.e. dendritic cells and activated (major histocompatibility complex) MHC class II+ macrophages. These cells have the discretionary capacity to take up and process antigen, migrate to draining lymph nodes, and express surface molecules involved in the differential activation of various regulatory T-lymphocyte populations.[121] Like all other mucosal tissues, the endometrium is richly endowed with dendritic cells as well as macrophages. In cycling human and mouse endometrium these cells form a dense network in the endometrial stroma subjacent to the luminal epithelial surface.[63,110] In pregnancy, large populations of dendritic cells persist in the decidua and in the non-decidualized endometrial tissues.[109–111]

Dendritic cells purified from decidual tissue exhibit an immature phenotype, maintained in in-vitro experiments by GM-CSF and IL-4.[110] These cells show the capacity to be efficiently matured by exposure to inflammatory cytokines IL-1, IL-6, TNFα, and prostaglandin E (PGE). This phenotypic change is characterized by increased expression of MHC class II and co-stimulatory molecules and efficient capacity to stimulate allogenic T cells.[110] Dendritic cell-activating cytokines are expressed in the endometrium in temporally variable patterns during the estrous cycle and pregnancy, and fluctuations in their expression are likely to contribute to the cycle stage-specific capacity of the uterus to act as an inductive site for immune responses.[90] In rodents, the mating-induced surge in GM-CSF expression in epithelial cells,[122] reinforced by TNFα and IL-1 secretion from recruited macrophages,[70] triggers enhanced MHC class II and CD86 expression and increased dendritic cell emigration to lymph nodes.[95] This environment is likely to be more conducive to antigen uptake and processing than the relatively immunosuppressive environment afforded by the progesterone-induced CSF-1 and IL-10-dominated cytokine milieu of implantation and placental development.

Activation of T-lymphocyte populations in the uterus is directly dependent on the phenotype of dendritic cells,

which, together with the cytokine milieu at the site of antigen uptake, is the major determinant of whether immune activation, as opposed to tolerance, is induced. Thus TGFβ, IL-10, IL-6, and IL-4 facilitate the induction of 'type 2' (humoral) immunity and/or tolerance, and IFNγ and IL-12 are associated with induction of 'type 1' (cell-mediated) immunity.[121,123] Human decidual dendritic cells express less IL-12 than peripheral blood dendritic cells and activate type 2 biased T-cell responses.[124] A similar situation is evident in the mouse, where decidual dendritic cells are predominantly CD8– and biased towards IL-10 and against IL-12 expression, consistent with a predisposition to activate type 2 immune responses.[109] Furthermore, the copious amounts of TGFβ and IL-6 present during exposure to male antigens at insemination, and TGFβ, IL-4, and IL-10 in the developing placenta, would be further likely to bias against type 1 immunity to the conceptus, which is likely to be important for mediating immune tolerance to paternal antigens present in semen and shared by the conceptus.[125] However, to protect against reproductive tract or placental infection, mechanisms must exist to override this bias and ensure that effective cellular immunity can be induced. The detrimental consequences of this for the viability of the pregnancy are commonly seen in women infected with cytomegalovirus or *Listeria monocytogenes*, and in mouse models of *Leishmania major* infection.[126] Inhibition of type 1 immunity appears to be essential for maintaining maternal immune tolerance in pregnancy, and the immunosuppressive properties of T_{reg} cells are now known to be pivotal cells in achieving this.[83] The uterine cytokine environment is likely to be of central importance in driving the activation and expansion of these cells, with TGFβ a major candidate cytokine in this role.[85]

CYTOKINE REGULATION OF ENDOMETRIAL EPITHELIAL CELLS

While leukocytes are generally viewed as the main target for endometrial cytokines, non-hematopoietic cells also respond to their autocrine and paracrine effects, in a manner that can lead to modulation of growth factor responses. For example, IFNγ and TGFβ antagonize the proliferative effects of epidermal growth factor and insulin-like growth factor (IGF)-1 and are implicated in the postovulatory switch to secretory epithelium.[127] Both of these cytokines are induced by progesterone and exert their antiproliferative effects through binding to specific receptors on epithelial cells. Cytokines targeting the epithelium probably originate in infiltrating leukocytes which accumulate immediately beneath the glandular and luminal epithelium to varying extents over the course of the estrous cycle, such that spatial and temporal regulation of epithelial function could be mediated by the proximity and abundance of infiltrating cells. For example in the human endometrium, IFNγ produced by scattered lymphoid aggregates acts together with IL-6 to induce MHC class II expression in adjacent glandular epithelial cells.[90] Cytokines synthesized by stromal cells are also implicated in regulating production of secretory component and polymeric immunoglobulin (Ig) receptor,[128] required for epithelial cell translocation of IgA into the luminal compartment. Together with the aforementioned leukocyte changes, these fluctuations in the immunological function of epithelial cells at least partially explain why ovarian steroid hormones influence the capacity of the endometrium to both induce and exert immune responses to local antigens.[90]

An essential role for LIF in implantation, indicated by the complete infertility of genetically LIF-deficient mice, is likely to be mediated through an autocrine or paracrine effect in endometrial epithelial cells.[129] A peak in glandular epithelial LIF expression at implantation is accompanied by expression of the LIF receptor and its co-receptor gp130 in the luminal epithelium, in mice and in women.[40,41,130,131] This conservation in pattern of expression across species, together with the finding that implantation failure is independent of the genotype of the embryo, suggests that LIF may exert a transforming influence in luminal epithelial cells, perhaps resulting in their capacity to transduce a decidualization-inducing signal.

Macrophages are particularly abundant during the pre- and peri-implantation period when these cells interdigitate between luminal epithelial cells. This spatial association raises the question of whether macrophage-derived cytokines might have a role in influencing epithelial cell phenotype, particularly adhesion molecule expression, in readiness for embryo implantation. Leukocyte regulation of epithelial adhesive properties has been shown in human uterine epithelial cells in vitro.[132] The ability of macrophages to alter transport properties and affect epithelial barrier integrity[133] might assist at implantation by facilitating trophoblast breaching of the epithelial surface, and potentially contributes to the epithelial apoptosis which subsequently occurs. Whether cytokines mediate these effects and the identity of the signaling agents remains to be determined.

Epithelial cells may also respond to cytokines released by the pre-implantation embryo. For example, human blastocysts can induce expression of the putative embryo attachment factor $\alpha_v\beta_3$ integrin in human endometrial epithelial cells in vitro through the release of IL-1.[134] This function may be physiologically relevant since IL-1R antagonist can block the implantation of blastocysts in mice,[134a] although the findings that normal implantation rates and pregnancies occur in mice genetically deficient in IL-1R type 1[135] suggests that any role for IL-1 is not essential.

CYTOKINE REGULATION OF ENDOMETRIAL FIBROBLAST/DECIDUAL CELLS

Stromal fibroblasts provide an additional target for cytokine action throughout the estrous cycle and especially during the process of decidualization. Macrophage-derived cytokines including IL-1, TNFα, and TGFβ can influence stromal fibroblast cell proliferation and/or secretion of prostaglandins and cytokines, such as IL-8, heparin-binding epidermal growth factor (HB-EGF), hepatocyte growth factor (HGF), and RANTES.[136–139] The same regulatory factors are postulated to participate in differentiation of stromal fibroblasts into decidual cells. However, none of these factors is indispensable since endometrial structure is normal and decidualization proceeds unimpaired in mice deficient in each of these cytokines. In contrast, mice deficient in the receptor for IL-11 exhibit implantation failure due to disrupted decidual cell transformation and consequent dysregulated proliferation and invasion of trophoblast tissue.[55] IL-11 is also a key cytokine during decidualization in humans, with ligand and receptor expression mapping studies, together with culture experiments, suggesting that IL-11 of epithelial or endothelial origin initiates decidual transformation, prior to decidual cells activating autocrine IL-11 release to amplify the process.[58] Activin A, a member of the TGFβ family of cytokines, may be another essential factor in the decidualization process, potentially acting via induction of factors including PGE$_2$, MMP-2, and fibronectin.[58]

At menstruation, cytokines are implicated as the communication molecules linking leukocytes with resident cells in the processes of extracellular matrix degradation and stromal cell apoptosis. TNFα and IL-1 secreted by the leukocytes that accumulate in the endometrium late in the secretory phase act in an autocrine and paracrine manner to stimulate the release of macrophage and stromal cell MMPs that catalyze matrix breakdown.[112] Members of the TGFβ family of cytokines are particularly well represented in decidual tissue and may play important roles in decidual regression at menstruation or after implantation failure.[140]

CYTOKINE REGULATION OF ENDOTHELIAL CELLS

The cyclical changes in endometrial structure are matched by profound changes in the local vascular architecture. Angiogenesis is an obligatory aspect of endometrial growth after menstruation, in preparation for and in response to implantation, and during development of the placenta. Tissue macrophages are thought to be key cells in influencing each phase of the angiogenic process, including alterations of the local extracellular matrix, induction of endothelial cells to migrate and proliferate, and formation of capillaries.[141] Macrophages and other cells in the local environment can modulate endothelial cell function through cytokines, including TNFα, TGFβ, IL-6, GM-CSF, and G-CSF,[142,143] as well as the vascular endothelial growth factor (VEGF) family. Each of these cytokines is expressed at appropriate times and locations in endometrial and decidual tissue to exert positive and negative influences on developing vascular networks. Cytokines secreted by uNK cells, particularly IFNγ, play a major role in regulating the dilation of uterine spiral arteries required for normal placental development during early pregnancy.[117,144] Similar pathways may contribute to the increased vascular permeability leading to endometrial edema at estrus and prior to embryo implantation.[145] Furthermore, leukocyte recruitment into the endometrium is regulated by distinct patterns of expression of vascular adhesion molecules,[146] and several of these adhesion molecules are regulated in endothelial cells by the local cytokine environment.

CYTOKINE REGULATION OF THE CONCEPTUS

The cytokine/preimplantation embryo axis

Cytokines originating from the oviductal and endometrial epithelium target the developing embryo as it traverses the reproductive tract prior to implantation. Through both positive and negative effects on the timing and extent of blastomere survival, proliferation, and differentiation, these factors have important roles in synchronizing embryo growth with the maternal changes that lead to uterine receptivity. This concept

has emerged from studies in several species, including humans, showing that the preimplantation embryo produces and responds to a range of cytokines[147,148] produced by the uterine and oviduct epithelium during early pregnancy. LIF, CSF-1, GM-CSF, and TGFβ have each been shown to improve secretory activity, the rate of proliferation and viability of blastomeres, and/or the proportion of embryos that develop to the blastocyst stage and beyond, in rodents and more recently in humans.[147,149–151] In each case cognate receptors are synthesized by the embryo. The actions of cytokines are dependent on the developmental stage of the embryo, and can vary slightly between species and even among strains of mice. Attainment of an 'adhesive' phenotype in trophectoderm cells at implantation is a further differentiation event likely to be influenced by cytokines, perhaps including GM-CSF and CSF-1, which, in other cell lineages can both induce expression of integrins implicated in blastocyst attachment.

Effects of epithelial cytokines on blastocyst development may be revealed by detailed examination of cytokine-deficient mice. In GM-CSF null mutant mice, blastocyst development is retarded due to diminished viability of inner cell mass (ICM) cells.[152] Some cytokines have detrimental effects on blastocyst development – TNFα can reduce the viability of cells in the ICM of murine embryos[153] while IFNγ also has embryotoxic effects, limiting trophectoderm proliferation.[154] These interactions are of considerable physiological significance, since even small perturbations in blastomere number and ICM/trophectoderm allocation in the blastocyst are associated with metabolic disturbances influencing growth trajectory and viability later in gestation and after birth.[155] This is well illustrated in embryos cultured in the presence or absence of GM-CSF, where addition of cytokine alleviates the adverse consequences of culture on fetal and placental development, and influences the postnatal growth trajectory and metabolic status of offspring in adult life.[156] Overabundance of detrimental cytokines in the tract prior to implantation can have similar consequences to lack of embryotrophic factors, with TNFα exposure during preimplantation development implicated in the fetal growth retardation seen in diabetic rats.[157] These studies suggest that the pre- and peri-implantation cytokine environment experienced by the embryo has profound consequences for fetal and postnatal development, perhaps through influencing genomic imprinting or otherwise activating gene expression pathways in the embryo which later impact placental development.

The embryo itself has been found to synthesize cytokines, including IL-1, LIF, TGFβ, and IL-6, which potentially have autocrine roles or provide signals to maternal tissues. Embryo-derived IL-1 may function in signaling events preceding implantation (discussed previously). Another example is IFNτ, produced by the preimplantation embryo in sheep and cattle, which acts to mediate maternal recognition of pregnancy through preventing regression of the corpus luteum.[158] Each of these cytokines is active in the immune compartment and it is conceivable that their release from the embryo may attenuate the maternal immune axis to promote maternal tolerance at implantation.[159]

The cytokine/placental trophoblast axis

As pregnancy proceeds, the potential roles for decidual cytokines expand in parallel with the increasing structural complexity of the interacting uterine and placental tissues. Abundant evidence indicates that placental trophoblast cells actively participate in local cytokine networks, by secreting copious quantities of several cytokines, and responding to many others that are released by decidual cells and particularly leukocytes in maternal tissues.

Tissues at the placental/decidual interface synthesize a plethora of cytokines, of which the most functionally important in trophoblast differentiation and invasion are likely to be CSF-1, TGFβ, TNFα, GM-CSF, LIF, IFNγ, IL-6, and IL-10 (reviewed by Robertson et al,[20] Pollard,[22] Daiter and Pollard,[26] and Hunt[27]). As previously described, the development and function of the placenta is also integrally dependent on cytokines involved in decidual transformation, uNK recruitment and function, and regulation of maternal immune tolerance. The interactions and balance between these factors act in concert with other growth factors to both promote and constrain invasion of maternal tissues by placental trophoblast cells.[160,161] Further complexity is afforded by attenuating molecules, including soluble receptors for TNFα, GM-CSF, and unusual isoforms of cytokines such as CSF-1 and IL-2.

Leukocytes are a major source of trophoblast-regulating cytokines once the implantation site is established, although for many factors secretion is also seen in decidual mesenchymal cells and placental cells. Thus, the various leukocyte lineages present in the implantation site, and their secretory phenotypes, can modulate placental development and function. Uterine NK cells are particularly important in this regard, as the most abundant leukocyte lineage within close proximity to the invading trophoblast cells. Their

essential role in normal placental development is demonstrated by the finding of small, poorly developed placentas in uNK-cell-deficient mice.[117] Cytokine secretion by other leukocyte subpopulations impacts placental development indirectly: e.g. macrophages and dendritic cells secrete cytokines implicated in uNK cell support,[110,118] and T$_{reg}$ cells inhibit maternal immune rejection through their secretion of immunosuppressive TGFβ.[83,85]

Patterns of receptor expression in specific trophoblast cell layers together with data from in-vitro models suggest that individual cytokines have specific roles in driving sequential waves of trophoblast proliferation and differentiation, and in regulating functional parameters corresponding to the invasive, adhesive, secretory, and antigenic properties of different trophoblast lineages. For example, cytokines are clearly implicated in controlling the highly invasive properties of undifferentiated cytotrophoblast cells early in placental development, through regulating their expression of the MMP family of enzymes. Certain cytokines, including IL-1, IL-6, IL-15, and TNFα, act to promote MMP activity, while others such as IL-10, LIF, and TGFβ inhibit MMP secretion and/or stimulate expression of tissue inhibitors of matrix metalloproteinases (TIMPs).[162] The relative proportions of these factors in the implantation site is thus of crucial importance in determining the structure and hence the eventual functional capacity of the growing placenta. Hormones secreted by placental trophoblast cells, including human chorionic gonadotropin (hCG), placental lactogen, and aromatase, are also cytokine responsive.[22,161]

Studies in mice genetically deficient in individual cytokines or their receptors or regulators identify the IL-6 family of cytokines as particularly important in placental development. Most notably, LIF has an essential role in regulating differentiation of cytotrophoblasts into extravillous anchoring cells. This was first suggested by studies in mice with a null mutation in the LIF receptor (LIFR) gene, which produce grossly abnormal placentas with a greatly diminished capacity to support embryonic development to term.[163] Null mutation in SOCS3, a negative regulator of signaling through the gp130 receptor subunit shared by IL-6 family cytokines, results in disordered placental development, with reduced spongiotrophoblasts and increased trophoblast giant cells.[164] Uncontrolled LIF signaling appears to be the mechanism underpinning the placental lesion in SOCS3 null mutant mice, since genetic deletion of this cytokine or its receptor largely reverses the SOCS3 placental phenotype.[164,165]

The TGFβ family is strongly implicated in trophoblast regulation, as an inhibitor of differentiation, proliferation, and invasion of human cytotrophoblast cells.[165a] The difficulty in maintaining TGFβ null mutants to reproductive age has hampered investigation of the importance of TGFβ in placental development. Fetuses homozygous for TGFβ$_2$ and TGFβ$_3$ null mutations die in utero of fetal abnormalities,[166] but TGFβ$_1$ null mutant mice can survive to adulthood if bred on an immunodeficient background to prevent systemic inflammatory demise. Recently, it has been shown that female mice deficient in TGFβ$_1$ can carry fetuses to term.[167] These experiments show that neither fetal nor maternal TGFβ$_1$ is essential for development of a functional placenta, but the outcome of deficiency in both compartments has not been reported.

Several other cytokines have less crucial roles in placental morphogenesis, with cytokine null mutants showing their deletion attenuates, but does not completely prevent, development of a functional placenta. The pattern of CSF-1 and CSF-1R expression at the placental–decidual interface in humans and mice is well-documented,[26] and is consistent with CSF-1 having a significant role in the regulation of early placental development, particularly in promoting differentiation and invasion of the anchoring trophoblast lineages. However, any role of CSF-1 in placental development is largely redundant since only a small amount of fetal wastage is evident in CSF-1-deficient mice,[91] and whether this is associated with any placental malformation is not clear. Decidual cells also secrete GM-CSF throughout gestation and proliferating cytotrophoblast cells express receptors for this cytokine. Physiological roles for GM-CSF and IL-10 in placental development are confirmed by the alterations in placental architecture seen in mice with null mutations. Enlargement of the spongiotrophoblast region at the expense of the labyrinth is seen in GM-CSF null mutants[168] and the reverse effect, with an expanded structure, occurs in mice deficient in IL-10.[169] Decidual cytokines can traverse the placental membranes and enter the fetal circulation where they may influence development of the fetus directly, particularly in the lymphohematopoietic compartment. This is clearly borne out by the finding that maternal G-CSF influences fetal granulopoiesis in rats.[170]

Cytokine-mediated cell communication at the placental–decidual interface is a two-way interaction, with placental trophoblast cells secreting a plethora of cytokines that influence the composition and function of cell populations in the maternal compartment. Cytokines synthesized in greatest abundance by the placenta and placental membranes are the type 2 cytokines TGFβ, IL-4, and IL-10.[159,171] These cytokines are notable for their immunoregulatory properties and

have been proposed to contribute to an immune environment favoring tolerance of the conceptus. Their actions would be fortified by secretion of the same factors from decidual leukocytes, particularly uNK cells and 'suppressor' lymphocyte populations, including T cells. One beneficial effect of this type 2 cytokine bias at the fetal–maternal interface is likely to be inhibition of the induction and expansion of cytotoxic leukocytes reactive with trophoblast antigens. These effects are exerted locally, through maintaining type 2 phenotypes in antigen-presenting cells patrolling the uterine environment,[124] and distally in lymph nodes draining the uterus to regulate the phenotypes of any expanding lymphocyte populations. In addition, placental cytokines suppress inappropriate activation of macrophages and uNK cells in the decidua, which when exposed to TNFα or IFNγ, respectively, can cause placental failure through induction of thrombosis and interruption of the maternal uteroplacental blood supply.[172] Further reinforcement of this immune deviation is mediated through a direct effect of progesterone in lymphocytes, acting to induce the release of an immunomodulatory protein (pregnancy-induced blocking factor, PIBF) that influences the cytokine output of any regulatory T lymphocytes activated during pregnancy.[173]

The sensitivity to perturbation of this cytokine–leukocyte equilibrium is demonstrated by a series of studies in mice. Administration of exogenous type 1 cytokines (IL-2, IFNγ, TNFα, and TNFβ), which antagonize the influence of placental type 2 cytokines, is detrimental to pregnancy outcome.[174] Incomplete immune deviation appears to be the cause of pregnancy loss in the abortion-prone, CBA × DBA/2 mating combination in mice,[175] since fetal loss can be averted by prior immunization with paternal antigen or use of immune adjuvants,[176] or provision of exogenous T$_{reg}$ cells.[177] Abortion is also precipitated by stress and abundance of infectious microorganisms in the environment, situations which lead to elevated type 1 cytokine expression through the effects of the neurotransmitter substance P and endotoxin, respectively.[178,179] Importantly, each of these detrimental influences can be reversed by the administration of type 2 cytokines, a treatment which down-regulates deleterious type 1 cytokine expression in the decidua.[174,179]

DYSREGULATION OF CYTOKINE NETWORKS IN REPRODUCTIVE PATHOLOGIES

The widespread and integral roles of cytokines in regulating endometrial homeostasis and accommodation of pregnancy raise the question of their contribution to the pathophysiology of endometriosis, infertility, and disorders of pregnancy. Disturbances of immune function and cytokine balance have been implicated in each of these conditions, but their precise roles in etiologies of disease are difficult to define. This is largely because in the absence of appropriate animal models, it is extremely difficult to establish the causal sequence of events and determine whether immune and cytokine disturbances are the cause of the pathology or arise as the consequence of another underpinning lesion.

In endometriosis, cycles of tissue breakdown and repair are regulated by inflammatory leukocytes, and their cytokine products occur in ectopic endometrium in a manner comparable to those in eutopic tissue.[4] Abnormal synthesis of proinflammatory cytokines and chemokines occurs in endometriotic tissue, together with activated macrophages and elevated angiogenesis. The extent to which these changes are a cause or response to the disease is now being addressed in model systems whereby human endometrial tissue is transplanted into immunocompromised mice. Either way, the inflammatory changes appear to play an important role in the persistence and expansion of endometriosis implants and the morbidity of the disease.[180] Using the explant approach it has been possible to demonstrate the efficacy of chemokine antagonists in limiting progression of endometriotic tissue outgrowth,[181] raising the future prospect of using cytokine antagonists and other anti-inflammatory strategies to treat this disease.

Endometrial cytokine disturbances are implicated in forms of unexplained infertility where implantation fails, or where implantation is successful but miscarriage occurs in a recurrent manner in the first trimester despite chromosomal normality in the conceptus. Several studies have examined potential differences in endometrial cytokine synthesis between normal fertile women and women experiencing infertility or recurrent miscarriage.[182] The usefulness of some studies is confounded by the necessity for investigating rigorously defined patient populations and examining only tissue collected at precisely timed, mid-secretory stage of the cycle. However, there are several studies linking compromised fertility with altered endometrial expression of cytokines from the IL-6 family. Reduced LIF,[183,184] reduced IL-11,[185] and, paradoxically, reduced expression of the IL-6 and LIF antagonist soluble gp130[186] are evident in unexplained infertility. In recurrent miscarriage, endometrial tissues show diminished expression of IL-6[187] and decreased IL-11 protein,[188] implying that dysregulated decidual transformation may be at fault.

SUMMARY

There is compelling evidence for the existence in the endometrium of a complex cytokine network with the principal role of mediating communication between leukocytes, non-hematopoietic cells, and the conceptus. Cytokines are therefore pivotal in orchestrating appropriate immune responses to the various challenges posed by reproductive events and in regulating the structural remodeling to epithelial cells, stromal cells, and endothelial cells required for embryo implantation and placental development. A vast amount of information is accumulating on the cellular origin, spatial location, and regulation of a large repertoire of cytokines and their receptor subunits in the endometrium. In many instances descriptive studies are corroborated by functional experiments indicating essential or supporting roles for several cytokines in mediating pivotal endometrial processes. However, attempts to construct models for causal sequences in cytokine signaling in vivo are still constrained by incomplete knowledge of functional overlap and the significance of soluble receptors, specific antagonists, and other factors that attenuate cytokine signaling. Importantly, the notion of 'context' in cytokine function limits confident extrapolation from in-vitro experiments or with cells from other tissues or from other species, since it is virtually impossible to replicate the full range of environmental influences to which cells are exposed in vivo.

Genetic models will continue to provide the most valuable experimental tools in this endeavor. Studies in mice with cytokine gene disruptions have proven very informative in defining specific functions in vivo, and will be of even greater benefit as tissue-specific promoters and RNA inhibitor technology, permitting precise control of the location and timing of factor depletion, becomes more widespread. Transgenic strategies using reporter genes to inform on cytokine-specific signaling cascades also offer promise in reproductive tissues. Null mutant experiments would be greatly facilitated by discovery of uterus-specific promoters to allow distinction between local effects of cytokines in the uterus and indirect effects mediated through other tissues. In the meantime, there is useful information to be gained by investigating reproductive tract immune parameters in existing cytokine-deficient mice in the face of 'real-world' challenges such as allogeneic pregnancy, infection, and nutritional or environmental stress. Mice with null mutations in two or more cytokine genes will assist in identifying functional overlap between cytokines and unraveling compensatory mechanisms.

The lessons learnt from animal models are beginning to find application in human and veterinary medicine. Increasingly, clinical studies implicate aberrant cytokine patterns with endometriosis, implantation failure, miscarriage, and impaired fetal development resulting from 'shallow' placentation. As our understanding of the local regulation of endometrial function advances, so do the prospects for novel therapeutic interventions, based on using cytokine agonists or antagonists, to treat these disorders.

REFERENCES

1. Bulmer JN. Immune aspects of pathology of the placental bed contributing to pregnancy pathology. Baillieres Clin Obstet Gynaecol 1992; 6: 461–88.
2. Raghupathy R. Th1-type immunity is incompatible with successful pregnancy. Immunol Today 1997; 18: 478–82.
3. Conrad KP, Benyo DF. Placental cytokines and the pathogenesis of preeclampsia. Am J Reprod Immunol 1997; 37: 240–9.
4. Rier SE, Yeaman GR. Immune aspects of endometriosis: relevance of the uterine mucosal immune system. Semin Reprod Endocrinol 1997; 15: 209–20.
5. Callard RE, Gearing AJH. The Cytokine Facts Book. London: Academic Press, 1994.
6. Vaddi K, Keller M, Newton RC. The Chemokine Factsbook: Ligands and Receptors. London: Academic Press, 1997.
7. Ihle JN. Cytokine receptor signalling. Nature 1995; 377: 591–4.
8. Gadina M, Hilton D, Johnston JA et al. Signaling by type I and II cytokine receptors: ten years after. Curr Opin Immunol 2001; 13: 363–73.
9. Ihle JN. The Stat family in cytokine signaling. Curr Opin Cell Biol 2001; 13: 211–17.
10. Nathan C, Sporn M. Cytokines in context. J Cell Biol 1991; 113: 981–6.
11. Sporn MB, Roberts AB. Peptide growth factors are multifunctional. Nature 1988; 332: 217–19.
12. Yasukawa H, Sasaki A, Yoshimura A. Negative regulation of cytokine signalling pathways. Annu Rev Immunol 2000; 18: 143–64.
13. Burger D, Dayer JM. Inhibitory cytokines and cytokine inhibitors. Neurology 1995; 45: S39–43.
14. Alexander WS, Hilton DJ. The role of suppressors of cytokine signaling (SOCS) proteins in regulation of the immune response. Annu Rev Immunol 2004; 22: 503–29.
15. Ilangumaran S, Ramanathan S, Rottapel R. Regulation of the immune system by SOCS family adaptor proteins. Semin Immunol 2004; 16: 351–65.
16. Burgess AW, Wilson EMA, Metcalf D. Stimulation by human placental conditioned medium of hemopoietic colony formation by human marrow cells. Blood 1977; 49: 573–83.
17. Arceci RJ, Shanahan F, Stanley ER et al. Temporal expression and location of colony-stimulating factor 1 (CSF-1) and its receptor in the female reproductive tract are consistent with CSF-1 regulated placental development. Proc Natl Acad Sci USA 1989; 86: 8818–22.
18. Robertson SA, Seamark RF. Granulocyte–macrophage colony stimulating factor (GM-CSF): one of a family of epithelial cell-derived cytokines in the preimplantation uterus. Reprod Fertil Dev 1992; 4: 435–48.
19. Tabibzadeh S, Sun XZ. Cytokine expression in human endometrium throughout the menstrual cycle. Hum Reprod 1992; 7: 1214–21.
20. Robertson SA, Seamark RF, Guilbert LJ et al. The role of cytokines in gestation. Crit Rev Immunol 1994; 14: 239–92.
21. Tabibzadeh S. Role of cytokines in endometrium and at the fetomaternal interface. Reprod Med Rev 1994; 3: 11–28.
22. Pollard JW. Role of cytokines in the pregnant uterus of interstitial implanting species. In: Bazer FW, ed. The Endocrinology of Pregnancy. Totowa, NJ: Humana Press, 1998: 59–82.
23. Salamonsen LA, Dimitriadis E, Robb L. Cytokines in implantation. Semin Reprod Med 2000; 18: 299–310.
24. Dimitriadis E, White CA, Jones RL et al. Cytokines, chemokines and growth factors in endometrium related to implantation. Hum Reprod Update 2005; 11: 613–30.
25. Kelly RW, King AE, Critchley HO. Cytokine control in human endometrium. Reproduction 2001; 121: 3–19.
26. Daiter E, Pollard JW. Colony stimulating factor-1 (CSF-1) in pregnancy. Reprod Med Rev 1992; 1: 83–97.
27. Hunt JS. Expression and regulation of the tumour necrosis factor-alpha gene in the female reproductive tract. Reprod Fertil Dev 1993; 5: 141–53.
28. Kimber SJ. Leukaemia inhibitory factor in implantation and uterine biology. Reproduction 2005; 130: 131–45.
29. Dimitriadis E, Salamonsen LA, Robb L. Expression of interleukin-11 during the human menstrual cycle: coincidence with stromal cell decidualization and relationship to leukaemia inhibitory factor and prolactin. Mol Hum Reprod 2000; 6: 907–14.
30. Cork BA, Li TC, Warren MA et al. Interleukin-11 (IL-11) in human endometrium: expression throughout the menstrual cycle and the effects of cytokines on endometrial IL-11 production in vitro. J Reprod Immunol 2001; 50: 3–17.
31. Chegini N, Ma C, Roberts M et al. Differential expression of interleukins (IL) IL-13 and IL-15 throughout the menstrual cycle in endometrium of normal fertile women and women with recurrent spontaneous abortion. J Reprod Immunol 2002; 56: 93–110.
32. Kitaya K, Yasuda J, Yagi I et al. IL-15 expression at human endometrium and decidua. Biol Reprod 2000; 63: 683–7.
33. Yoshino O, Osuga Y, Koga K et al. Evidence for the expression of interleukin (IL)-18, IL-18 receptor and IL-18 binding protein in the human endometrium. Mol Hum Reprod 2001; 7: 649–54.
34. Garcia-Velasco JA, Arici A. Chemokines and human reproduction. Fertil Steril 1999; 71: 983–93.
35. Kayisli UA, Mahutte NG, Arici A. Uterine chemokines in reproductive physiology and pathology. Am J Reprod Immunol 2002; 47: 213–21.
36. van der Burg B, van der Saag PT. Nuclear factor-kappa-B/steroid hormone receptor interactions as a functional basis of anti-inflammatory action of steroids in reproductive organs. Mol Hum Reprod 1996; 2: 433–8.
37. Kawana K, Kawana Y, Schust DJ. Female steroid hormones use signal transducers and activators of transcription protein-mediated pathways to modulate the expression of T-bet in epithelial cells: a mechanism for local immune regulation in the human reproductive tract. Mol Endocrinol 2005; 19: 2047–59.
38. Tremellen KP, Seamark RF, Robertson SA. Seminal transforming growth factor beta1 stimulates granulocyte–macrophage colony-stimulating factor production and inflammatory cell recruitment in the murine uterus. Biol Reprod 1998; 58: 1217–25.
39. Robertson SA, Mayrhofer G, Seamark RF. Ovarian steroid hormones regulate granulocyte–macrophage colony-stimulating factor synthesis by uterine epithelial cells in the mouse. Biol Reprod 1996; 54: 183–96.
40. Bhatt H, Brunet LJ, Stewart CL. Uterine expression of leukemia inhibitory factor coincides with the onset of blastocyst implantation. Proc Natl Acad Sci USA 1991; 88: 11408–12.
41. Charnock-Jones DS, Sharkey AM, Fenwick P et al. Leukaemia inhibitory factor mRNA concentration peaks in human endometrium at the time of implantation and the

blastocyst contains mRNA for the receptor at this time. J Reprod Fertil 1994; 101: 421–6.

42. Giacomini G, Tabibzadeh SS, Satyaswaroop PG et al. Epithelial cells are the major source of biologically active granulocyte macrophage colony-stimulating factor in human endometrium. Hum Reprod 1995; 10: 3259–63.

43. Denison FC, Grant VE, Calder AA et al. Seminal plasma components stimulate interleukin-8 and interleukin-10 release. Mol Hum Reprod 1999; 5: 220–6.

44. Sharkey DJ, Jasper MJ, Tremellen KP et al. Pro-inflammatory cytokine mRNA expression is induced within the human cervix following insemination. Biol Reprod 2004; 37th Annual Meeting of the Society for the Study of Reproduction: 221.

45. Thompson LA, Barratt CL, Bolton AE et al. The leukocytic reaction of the human uterine cervix. Am J Reprod Immunol 1992; 28: 85–9.

46. Gutsche S, von Wolff M, Strowitzki T et al. Seminal plasma induces mRNA expression of IL-1beta, IL-6 and LIF in endometrial epithelial cells in vitro. Mol Hum Reprod 2003; 9: 785–91.

47. Kelly RW. Inflammatory mediators and parturition. Rev Reprod 1996; 1: 89–96.

48. Zhang J, Lathbury LJ, Salamonsen LA. Expression of the chemokine eotaxin and its receptor, CCR3, in human endometrium. Biol Reprod 2000; 62: 404–11.

49. Jones RL, Hannan NJ, Kaitu'u TJ et al. Identification of chemokines important for leukocyte recruitment to the human endometrium at the times of embryo implantation and menstruation. J Clin Endocrinol Metab 2004; 89: 6155–67.

50. Rasmussen SJ, Eckmann L, Quayle AJ et al. Secretion of proinflammatory cytokines by epithelial cells in response to Chlamydia infection suggests a central role for epithelial cells in chlamydial pathogenesis. J Clin Invest 1997; 99: 77–87.

51. Fichorova RN, Cronin AO, Lien E et al. Response to Neisseria gonorrhoeae by cervicovaginal epithelial cells occurs in the absence of toll-like receptor 4-mediated signaling. J Immunol 2002; 168: 2424–32.

52. Fichorova RN, Anderson DJ. Differential expression of immunobiological mediators by immortalized human cervical and vaginal epithelial cells. Biol Reprod 1999; 60: 508–14.

53. Young SL, Lyddon TD, Jorgenson RL et al. Expression of Toll-like receptors in human endometrial epithelial cells and cell lines. Am J Reprod Immunol 2004; 52: 67–73.

54. Schaefer TM, Desouza K, Fahey JV et al. Toll-like receptor (TLR) expression and TLR-mediated cytokine/chemokine production by human uterine epithelial cells. Immunology 2004; 112: 428–36.

55. Robb L, Li R, Hartley L et al. Infertility in female mice lacking the receptor for interleukin 11 is due to a defective uterine response to implantation. Nat Med 1998; 4: 303–8.

56. Critchley HO, Kelly RW, Kooy J. Perivascular location of a chemokine interleukin-8 in human endometrium: a preliminary report. Hum Reprod 1994; 9: 1406–9.

57. Koumas L, King AE, Critchley HO et al. Fibroblast heterogeneity: existence of functionally distinct Thy 1(+) and Thy 1(−) human female reproductive tract fibroblasts. Am J Pathol 2001; 159: 925–35.

58. Salamonsen LA, Dimitriadis E, Jones RL et al. Complex regulation of decidualization: a role for cytokines and proteases – a review. Placenta 2003; 24 (Suppl A): S76–85.

59. Gordon S. Alternative activation of macrophages. Nat Rev Immunol 2003; 3: 23–35.

60. Gordon S, Taylor PR. Monocyte and macrophage heterogeneity. Nat Rev Immunol 2005; 5: 953–64.

61. Mosser DM. The many faces of macrophage activation. J Leukoc Biol 2003; 73: 209–12.

62. Hunt JS, Robertson SA. Uterine macrophages and environmental programming for pregnancy success. J Reprod Immunol 1996; 32: 1–25.

63. Hudson-Keenihan SN, Robertson SA. Diversity in phenotype and steroid hormone dependence in dendritic cells and macrophages in the mouse uterus. Biol Reprod 2004; 70: 1562–72.

64. McIntire RH, Hunt JS. Antigen presenting cells and HLA-G – a review. Placenta 2005; 26 (Suppl A): S104–9.

65. Verma S, Hiby SE, Loke YW et al. Human decidual natural killer cells express the receptor for and respond to the cytokine interleukin 15. Biol Reprod 2000; 62: 959–68.

66. Chen HL, Yelavarthi KK, Hunt JS. Identification of transforming growth factor-beta 1 mRNA in virgin and pregnant rat uteri by in situ hybridization. .J Reprod Immunol 1993; 25: 221–33.

67. Heikkinen J, Mottonen M, Komi J et al. Phenotypic characterization of human decidual macrophages. Clin Exp Immunol 2003; 131: 498–505.

68. Petroff MG, Sedlmayr P, Azzola D et al. Decidual macrophages are potentially susceptible to inhibition by class Ia and class Ib HLA molecules. J Reprod Immunol 2002; 56: 3–17.

69. McIntire RH, Morales PJ, Petroff MG et al. Recombinant HLA-G5 and -G6 drive U937 myelomonocytic cell production of TGF-beta1. J Leukoc Biol 2004; 76: 1220–8.

70. McMaster MT, Newton RC, Dey SK et al. Activation and distribution of inflammatory cells in the mouse uterus during the preimplantation period. J Immunol 1992; 148: 1699–705.

71. Baines MG, Duclos AJ, Antecka E et al. Decidual infiltration and activation of macrophages leads to early embryo loss. Am J Reprod Immunol 1997; 37: 471–7.

72. Haddad EK, Duclos AJ, Antecka E et al. Role of interferon-gamma in the priming of decidual macrophages for nitric oxide production and early pregnancy loss. Cell Immunol 1997; 181: 68–75.

73. Croy BA, Kiso Y. Granulated metrial gland cells: a natural killer cell subset of the pregnant murine uterus. Microsc Res Tech 1993; 25: 189–200.

74. Bulmer JN, Morrison L, Longfellow M et al. Granulated lymphocytes in human endometrium: histochemical and immunohistochemical studies. Hum Reprod 1991; 6: 791–8.

75. Croy BA, Guilbert LJ, Browne MA, et al. Characterization of cytokine production by the metrial gland and granulated metrial gland cells. J Reprod Immunol 1991; 19: 149–66.

76. Xie X, He H, Colonna M et al. Pathways participating in activation of mouse uterine natural killer cells during pregnancy. Biol Reprod 2005; 73: 510–18.

77. Saito S, Nishikawa K, Morii T et al. Cytokine production by CD16-CD56 bright natural killer cells in the human early pregnancy decidua. Int Immunol 1993; 5: 559–63.

78. Higuma-Myojo S, Sasaki Y, Miyazaki S et al. Cytokine profile of natural killer cells in early human pregnancy. Am J Reprod Immunol 2005; 54: 21–9.

79. Arck P, Dietl J, Clark D. From the decidual cell internet: trophoblast-recognizing T cells. Biol Reprod 1999; 60: 227–33.

80. Yeaman GR, Guyre PM, Fanger MW et al. Unique CD8 + T cell-rich lymphoid aggregates in human uterine endometrium. J Leukoc Biol 1997; 61: 427–35.

81. Piccinni MP, Romagnani S. Regulation of fetal allograft survival by a hormone-controlled Th1- and Th2-type cytokines. Immunol Res 1996; 15: 141–50.

82. Jokhi PP, King A, Sharkey AM et al. Screening for cytokine messenger ribonucleic acids in purified human decidual lymphocyte populations by the reverse-transcriptase polymerase chain reaction. J Immunol 1994; 153: 4427–35.

83. Aluvihare VR, Kallikourdis M, Betz AG. Regulatory T cells mediate maternal tolerance to the fetus. Nat Immunol 2004; 5: 266–71.

84. Sakaguchi S, Sakaguchi N, Shimizu J et al. Immunologic tolerance maintained by CD25 + CD4 + regulatory T cells: their

common role in controlling autoimmunity, tumor immunity, and transplantation tolerance. Immunol Rev 2001; 182: 18–32.

85. von Boehmer H. Mechanisms of suppression by suppressor T cells. Nat Immunol 2005; 6: 338–44.

86. Jeziorska M, Salamonsen LA, Woolley DE. Mast cell and eosinophil distribution and activation in human endometrium throughout the menstrual cycle. Biol Reprod 1995; 53: 312–20.

87. Yeaman GR, Collins JE, Currie JK et al. IFN-gamma is produced by polymorphonuclear neutrophils in human uterine endometrium and by cultured peripheral blood polymorphonuclear neutrophils. J Immunol 1998; 160: 5145–53.

88. Cocchiara R, Albeggiani G, Azzolina A et al. Effect of substance P on uterine mast cell cytokine release during the reproductive cycle. J Neuroimmunol 1995; 60: 107–15.

89. Salamonsen LA, Woolley DE. Menstruation: induction by matrix metalloproteinases and inflammatory cells. J Reprod Immunol 1999; 44: 1–27.

90. Wira CR, Kaushic C, Richardson J. Role of sex hormones and cytokines in regulating the mucosal immune system in the female reproductive tract. In: Ogra PL, Mestecky J, Lammet ME et al. Handbook of Mucosal Diseases. New York: Academic Press, 1998.

91. Pollard JW, Hunt JS, Wiktor-Jedrzejczak W et al. A pregnancy defect in the osteopetrotic (op/op) mouse demonstrates the requirement for CSF-1 in female fertility. Dev Biol 1991; 148: 273–83.

92. Pollard JW, Lin EY, Zhu L. Complexity in uterine macrophage responses to cytokines in mice. Biol Reprod 1998; 58: 1469–75.

93. Baggiolini M, Dewald B, Moser B. Human chemokines: an update. Annu Rev Immunol 1997; 15: 675–705.

94. Wood GW, Hausmann E, Choudhuri R. Relative role of CSF-1, MCP-1/JE, and RANTES in macrophage recruitment during successful pregnancy. Mol Reprod Dev 1997; 46: 62–9.

95. Robertson SA, Allanson M, Mau VJ. Molecular regulation of uterine leukocyte recruitment during early pregnancy in the mouse. Trophoblast Res 1998; 11: 101–20.

96. Critchley HO, Kelly RW, Lea RG et al. Sex steroid regulation of leukocyte traffic in human decidua. Hum Reprod 1996; 11: 2257–62.

97. Jones RL, Kelly RW, Critchley HO. Chemokine and cyclooxygenase-2 expression in human endometrium coincides with leukocyte accumulation. Hum Reprod 1997; 12: 1300–6.

98. Willman CL, Stewart CC, Miller V et al. Regulation of MHC class II gene expression in macrophages by hematopoietic colony-stimulating factors (CSF). Induction by granulocyte/macrophage CSF and inhibition by CSF-1. J Exp Med 1989; 170: 1559–67.

99. Bilyk N, Holt PG. Cytokine modulation of the immunosuppressive phenotype of pulmonary alveolar macrophage populations. Immunology 1995; 86: 231–7.

100. Hunt JS, Manning LS, Wood GW. Macrophages in murine uterus are immunosuppressive. Cell Immunol 1984; 85: 499–510.

101. Chang MD, Pollard JW, Khalili H et al. Mouse placental macrophages have a decreased ability to present antigen. Proc Natl Acad Sci USA 1993; 90: 462–6.

102. Munn DH, Zhou M, Attwood JT et al. Prevention of allogeneic fetal rejection by tryptophan catabolism. Science 1998; 281: 1191–3.

103. Hunt JS, Miller L, Roby KF et al. Female steroid hormones regulate production of pro-inflammatory molecules in uterine leukocytes. J Reprod Immunol 1997; 35: 87–99.

104. Chen H-L, Kamath R, Pace JL et al. Gestation-related expression of the interferon-gamma receptor gene in mouse uterine and embryonic hemopoietic cells. Placenta 1994; 15: 109–21.

105. Schofield G, Kimber SJ. Leukocyte subpopulations in the uteri of leukemia inhibitory factor knockout mice during early pregnancy. Biol Reprod 2005; 72: 872–8.

106. Lidstrom C, Matthiesen L, Berg G et al. Cytokine secretion patterns of NK cells and macrophages in early human pregnancy decidua and blood: implications for suppressor macrophages in decidua. Am J Reprod Immunol 2003; 50: 444–52.

107. Cupurdija K, Azzola D, Hainz U et al. Macrophages of human first trimester decidua express markers associated to alternative activation. Am J Reprod Immunol 2004; 51: 117–22.

108. Singh U, Nicholson G, Urban BC et al. Immunological properties of human decidual macrophages – a possible role in intrauterine immunity. Reproduction 2005; 129: 631–7.

109. Blois SM, Alba Soto CD, Tometten M et al. Lineage, maturity, and phenotype of uterine murine dendritic cells throughout gestation indicate a protective role in maintaining pregnancy. Biol Reprod 2004; 70: 1018–23.

110. Kammerer U, Eggert AO, Kapp M et al. Unique appearance of proliferating antigen-presenting cells expressing DC-SIGN (CD209) in the decidua of early human pregnancy. Am J Pathol 2003; 162: 887–96.

111. Gardner L, Moffett A. Dendritic cells in the human decidua. Biol Reprod 2003; 69: 1438–46.

112. Salamonsen LA, Zhang J, Brasted M. Leukocyte networks and human endometrial remodelling. J Reprod Immunol 2002; 57: 95–108.

113. Robertson SA, Mau VJ, Young IG et al. Uterine eosinophils and reproductive performance in interleukin 5-deficient mice. J Reprod Fertil 2000; 120: 423–32.

114. Sferruzzi-Perri AN, Robertson SA, Dent LA. Interleukin-5 transgene expression and eosinophilia are associated with retarded mammary gland development in mice. Biol Reprod 2003; 69: 224–33.

115. Robertson SA, O'Connell AC, Hudson SN et al. Granulocyte–macrophage colony-stimulating factor (GM-CSF) targets myeloid leukocytes in the uterus during the post-mating inflammatory response in mice. J Reprod Immunol 2000; 46: 131–54.

116. Ye W, Zheng LM, Young JD et al. The involvement of interleukin (IL)-15 in regulating the differentiation of granulated metrial gland cells in mouse pregnant uterus. J Exp Med 1996; 184: 2405–10.

117. Guimond MJ, Luross JA, Wang B et al. Absence of natural killer cells during murine pregnancy is associated with reproductive compromise in TgE26 mice. Biol Reprod 1997; 56: 169–79.

118. Zhang JH, He H, Borzychowski AM et al. Analysis of cytokine regulators inducing interferon production by mouse uterine natural killer cells. Biol Reprod 2003; 69: 404–11.

119. Barber EM, Pollard JW. The uterine NK cell population requires IL-15 but these cells are not required for pregnancy nor the resolution of a *Listeria monocytogenes* infection. J Immunol 2003; 171: 37–46.

120. Marzusch K, Buchholz F, Ruck P et al. Interleukin-12- and interleukin-2-stimulated release of interferon-gamma by uterine CD56++ large granular lymphocytes is amplified by decidual macrophages. Hum Reprod 1997; 12: 921–4.

121. Moser M, Murphy KM. Dendritic cell regulation of TH1-TH2 development. Nat Immunol 2000; 1: 199–205.

122. Robertson SA, Mayrhofer G, Seamark RF. Uterine epithelial cells synthesize granulocyte–macrophage colony-stimulating factor and interleukin-6 in pregnant and nonpregnant mice. Biol Reprod 1992; 46: 1069–79.

123. Coffman RL, von der Weid T. Multiple pathways for the initiation of T helper 2 (Th2) responses. J Exp Med 1997; 185: 373–5.

124. Miyazaki S, Tsuda H, Sakai M et al. Predominance of Th2-promoting dendritic cells in early human pregnancy decidua. J Leukoc Biol 2003; 74: 514–22.

125. Robertson SA, Mau VJ, Hudson SA, Tremellen KP. Cytokine–leukocyte networks and the establishment of pregnancy. Am J Reprod Immunol 1997; 37: 438–42.

126. Krishnan L, Guilbert LJ, Russell AS et al. Pregnancy impairs resistance of C57BL/6 mice to Leishmania major infection and causes decreased antigen-specific IFN-gamma response and increased production of T helper 2 cytokines. J Immunol 1996; 156: 644–52.

127. Tabibzadeh SS, Satyaswaroop PG, Rao PN. Antiproliferative effect of interferon-gamma in human endometrial epithelial cells in vitro: potential local growth modulatory role in endometrium. J Clin Endocrinol Metab 1988; 67: 131–8.

128. Richardson JM, Wira CR. Uterine stromal cell suppression of pIgR production by uterine epithelial cells in vitro: a mechanism for regulation of pIgR production. J Reprod Immunol 1997; 33: 95–112.

129. Stewart CL, Kaspar P, Brunet LJ et al. Blastocyst implantation depends on maternal expression of leukaemia inhibitory factor. Nature 1992; 359: 76–9.

130. Yang ZM, Le SP, Chen DB et al. Leukemia inhibitory factor, LIF receptor, and gp130 in the mouse uterus during early pregnancy. Mol Reprod Dev 1995; 42: 407–14.

131. Cullinan EB, Abbondanzo SJ, Anderson PS et al. Leukemia inhibitory factor (LIF) and LIF receptor expression in human endometrium suggests a potential autocrine/paracrine function in regulating embryo implantation. Proc Natl Acad Sci USA 1996; 93: 3115–20.

132. Kosaka K, Fujiwara H, Tatsumi K et al. Human peripheral blood mononuclear cells enhance cell–cell interaction between human endometrial epithelial cells and BeWo-cell spheroids. Hum Reprod 2003; 18: 19–25.

133. Zareie M, McKay DM, Kovarik GG et al. Monocyte/macrophages evoke epithelial dysfunction: indirect role of tumor necrosis factor-alpha. Am J Physiol 1998; 275: C932–9.

134. Simon C, Gimeno MJ, Mercader A et al. Embryonic regulation of integrins beta 3, alpha 4, and alpha 1 in human endometrial epithelial cells in vitro. J Clin Endocrinol Metab 1997; 82: 2607–16.

134a. Simon C, Frances A, Piquette GN et al. Embryonic implantation in mice is blocked by interleukin-1 receptor antagonist. Endocrinology 1994; 134: 521–8.

135. Abbondanzo SJ, Cullinan EB, McIntyre K et al. Reproduction in mice lacking a functional type 1 IL-1 receptor. Endocrinology 1996; 137: 3598–601.

136. Arici A, Seli E, Senturk LM et al. Interleukin-8 in the human endometrium. J Clin Endocrinol Metab 1998; 83: 1783–7.

137. Lebovic DI, Chao VA, Taylor RN. Peritoneal macrophages induce RANTES (regulated on activation, normal T cell expressed and secreted) chemokine gene transcription in endometrial stromal cells. J Clin Endocrinol Metab 2004; 89: 1397–401.

138. Chobotova K, Karpovich N, Carver J et al. Heparin-binding epidermal growth factor and its receptors mediate decidualization and potentiate survival of human endometrial stromal cells. J Clin Endocrinol Metab 2005; 90: 913–19.

139. Khan KN, Masuzaki H, Fujishita A et al. Interleukin-6- and tumour necrosis factor alpha-mediated expression of hepatocyte growth factor by stromal cells and its involvement in the growth of endometriosis. Hum Reprod 2005; 20: 2715–23.

140. Moulton BC. Transforming growth factor-beta stimulates endometrial stromal apoptosis in vitro. Endocrinology 1994; 134: 1055–60.

141. Sunderkotter C, Steinbrink K, Goebeler M et al. Macrophages and angiogenesis. J Leukoc Biol 1994; 55: 410–22.

142. Mantovani A, Bussolino F, Dejana E. Cytokine regulation of endothelial cell function. FASEB J 1992; 6: 2591–9.

143. Naldini A, Carraro F. Role of inflammatory mediators in angiogenesis. Curr Drug Targets Inflamm Allergy 2005; 4: 3–8.

144. Ashkar AA, Croy BA. Interferon-gamma contributes to the normalcy of murine pregnancy. Biol Reprod 1999; 61: 493–502.

145. Rockwell LC, Pillai S, Olson CE et al. Inhibition of vascular endothelial growth factor/vascular permeability factor action blocks estrogen-induced uterine edema and implantation in rodents. Biol Reprod 2002; 67: 1804–10.

146. Kruse A, Martens N, Fernekorn U et al. Alterations in the expression of homing-associated molecules at the maternal/fetal interface during the course of pregnancy. Biol Reprod 2002; 66: 333–45.

147. Pampfer S, Arceci RJ, Pollard JW. Role of colony stimulating factor-1 (CSF-1) and other lympho-hematopoietic growth factors in mouse pre-implantation development. Bioessays 1991; 13: 535–40.

148. Stewart CL, Cullinan EB. Preimplantation development of the mammalian embryo and its regulation by growth factors. Dev Genet 1997; 21: 91–101.

149. Sharkey AM, Dellow K, Blayney M et al. Stage-specific expression of cytokine and receptor messenger ribonucleic acids in human preimplantation embryos. Biol Reprod 1995; 53: 974–81.

150. Dunglison GF, Barlow DH, Sargent IL. Leukaemia inhibitory factor significantly enhances the blastocyst formation rates of human embryos cultured in serum-free medium. Hum Reprod 1996; 11: 191–6.

151. Sjoblom C, Wikland M, Robertson SA. Granulocyte–macrophage colony-stimulating factor promotes human blastocyst development in vitro. Hum Reprod 1999; 14: 3069–76.

152. Robertson SA, Sjoblom C, Jasper MJ et al. Granulocyte–macrophage colony-stimulating factor promotes glucose transport and blastomere viability in murine preimplantation embryos. Biol Reprod 2001; 64: 1206–15.

153. Pampfer S, Moulaert B, Vanderheyden I et al. Effect of tumour necrosis factor alpha on rat blastocyst growth and glucose metabolism. J Reprod Fertil 1994; 101: 199–206.

154. Cameo M, Fontana V, Cameo P et al. Similar embryotoxic effects of sera from infertile patients and exogenous interferon-gamma on long-term in-vitro development of mouse embryos. Hum Reprod 1999; 14: 959–63.

155. Thompson JG, Kind KL, Roberts CT et al. Epigenetic risks related to assisted reproductive technologies: short- and long-term consequences for the health of children conceived through assisted reproduction technology: more reason for caution? Hum Reprod 2002; 17: 2783–6.

156. Sjöblom C, Roberts CT, Wikland M, Robertson SA. GM-CSF alleviates adverse consequences of embryo culture on fetal growth trajectory and placental morphogenesis. Endocrinology 2005; 146: 2142–53.

157. Wuu YD, Pampfer S, Becquet P et al. Tumor necrosis factor alpha decreases the viability of mouse blastocysts in vitro and in vivo. Biol Reprod 1999; 60: 479–83.

158. Bazer FW, Spencer TE, Ott TL. Interferon tau: a novel pregnancy recognition signal. Am J Reprod Immunol 1997; 37: 412–20.

159. Chaouat G, Assal Meliani A, Martal J et al. IL-10 prevents naturally occurring fetal loss in the CBA × DBA/2 mating combination, and local defect in IL-10 production in this abortion-prone combination is corrected by in vivo injection of IFN-tau. J Immunol 1995; 154: 4261–8.

160. Saito S. Cytokine cross-talk between mother and the embryo/placenta. J Reprod Immunol 2001; 52: 15–33.

161. Bowen JM, Chamley L, Keelan JA et al. Cytokines of the placenta and extra-placental membranes: roles and regulation during human pregnancy and parturition. Placenta 2002; 23: 257–73.

162. Bischof P, Meisser A, Campana A. Control of MMP-9 expression at the maternal–fetal interface. J Reprod Immunol 2002; 55: 3–10.

163. Ware CB, Horowitz MC, Renshaw BR et al. Targeted disruption of the low-affinity leukemia inhibitory factor receptor gene causes placental, skeletal, neural and metabolic defects and results in perinatal death. Development 1995; 121: 1283–99.

164. Takahashi Y, Carpino N, Cross JC et al. SOCS3: an essential regulator of LIF receptor signaling in trophoblast giant cell differentiation. EMBO J 2003; 22: 372–84.

165. Robb L, Boyle K, Rakar S et al. Genetic reduction of embryonic leukemia-inhibitory factor production rescues placentation in SOCS3-null embryos but does not prevent inflammatory disease. Proc Natl Acad Sci USA 2005; 102: 16333–8.

165a. Lala PK, Graham GH, Lysiak JJ, Khso NK, Hamilton GS. TGFβ regulation of trophoblast function. Trophoblast Res 1998; 11: 149–57.

166. Ingman WV, Robertson SA. Defining the actions of transforming growth factor beta in reproduction. Bioessays 2002; 24: 904–14.

167. Ingman WV, Robker RL, Woittiez K et al. Null mutation in transforming growth factor β_1 disrupts ovarian function and causes oocyte incompetence and early embryo arrest. Endocrinology 2006; 147: 835–45.

168. Robertson SA, Roberts CT, Farr KL et al. Fertility impairment in granulocyte–macrophage colony-stimulating factor-deficient mice. Biol Reprod 1999; 60: 251–61.

169. Roberts CT, White CA, Wiemer NG et al. Altered placental development in interleukin-10 null mutant mice. Placenta 2003; 24 (Suppl A): S94–9.

170. Novales JS, Salva AM, Modanlou HD et al. Maternal administration of granulocyte colony-stimulating factor improves neonatal rat survival after a lethal group B streptococcal infection. Blood 1993; 81: 923–7.

171. Wegmann TG, Lin H, Guilbert L et al. Bidirectional cytokine interactions in the maternal–fetal relationship: is successful pregnancy a TH2 phenomenon? Immunol Today 1993; 14: 353–6.

172. Clark DA, Chaouat G, Arck PC et al. Cytokine-dependent abortion in CBA × DBA/2 mice is mediated by the procoagulant fgl2 prothrombinase. J Immunol 1998; 160: 545–9.

173. Szekeres Bartho J and Wegmann TG. A progesterone-dependent immunomodulatory protein alters the Th1/Th2 balance. J Reprod Immunol 1996; 31: 81–95.

174. Chaouat G, Menu E, Clark DA et al. Control of fetal survival in CBA × DBA/2 mice by lymphokine therapy. J Reprod Fertil 1990; 89: 447–58.

175. Tangri S, Wegmann TG, Lin H et al. Maternal anti-placental reactivity in natural, immunologically-mediated fetal resorptions. J Immunol 1994; 152: 4903–11.

176. Baines MG, Duclos AJ, de Fougerolles AR et al. Immunological prevention of spontaneous early embryo resorption is mediated by non-specific immunosimulation. Am J Reprod Immunol 1996; 35: 34–42.

177. Zenclussen AC, Gerlof K, Zenclussen ML et al. Abnormal T-cell reactivity against paternal antigens in spontaneous abortion: adoptive transfer of pregnancy-induced CD4 + CD25 + T regulatory cells prevents fetal rejection in a murine abortion model. Am J Pathol 2005; 166: 811–22.

178. Arck PC, Merali FS, Stanisz AM et al. Stress-induced murine abortion associated with substance P-dependent alteration in cytokines in maternal uterine decidua. Biol Reprod 1995; 53: 814–19.

179. Krishnan L, Guilbert LJ, Wegmann TG et al. T helper 1 response against Leishmania major in pregnant C57BL/6 mice increases implantation failure and fetal resorptions. Correlation with increased IFN-gamma and TNF and reduced IL-10 production by placental cells. J Immunol 1996; 156: 653–62.

180. Berkkanoglu M, Arici A. Immunology and endometriosis. Am J Reprod Immunol 2003; 50: 48–59.

181. Berkkanoglu M, Zhang L, Ulukus M et al. Inhibition of chemokines prevents intraperitoneal adhesions in mice. Hum Reprod 2005; 20: 3047–52.

182. Laird SM, Tuckerman EM, Cork BA et al. A review of immune cells and molecules in women with recurrent miscarriage. Hum Reprod Update 2003; 9: 163–74.

183. Delage G, Moreau JF, Taupin JL et al. In-vitro endometrial secretion of human interleukin for DA cells/leukaemia inhibitory factor by explant cultures from fertile and infertile women. Hum Reprod 1995; 10: 2483–8.

184. Laird SM, Tuckerman EM, Dalton CF et al. The production of leukaemia inhibitory factor by human endometrium: presence in uterine flushings and production by cells in culture. Hum Reprod 1997; 12: 569–74.

185. Karpovich N, Klemmt P, Hwang JH et al. The production of interleukin-11 and decidualization are compromised in endometrial stromal cells derived from patients with infertility. J Clin Endocrinol Metab 2005; 90: 1607–12.

186. Sherwin JR, Smith SK, Wilson A et al. Soluble gp130 is up-regulated in the implantation window and shows altered secretion in patients with primary unexplained infertility. J Clin Endocrinol Metab 2002; 87: 3953–60.

187. Lim KJ, Odukoya OA, Ajjan RA et al. Profile of cytokine mRNA expression in peri-implantation human endometrium. Mol Hum Reprod 1998; 4: 77–81.

188. Linjawi S, Li TC, Tuckerman EM et al. Expression of interleukin-11 receptor alpha and interleukin-11 protein in the endometrium of normal fertile women and women with recurrent miscarriage. J Reprod Immunol 2004; 64: 145–55.

189. Miyazaki S, Tanebe K, Sakai M et al. Interleukin 2 receptor gamma chain (gamma(c)) knockout mice show less regularity in estrous cycle but achieve normal pregnancy without fetal compromise. Am J Reprod Immunol 2002; 47: 222–30.

190. Svensson L, Arvola M, Sallstrom MA et al. The Th2 cytokines IL-4 and IL-10 are not crucial for the completion of allogeneic pregnancy in mice. J Reprod Immunol 2001; 51: 3–7.

191. White CA, Johansson M, Roberts CT et al. Effect of interleukin-10 null mutation on maternal immune response and reproductive outcome in mice. Biol Reprod 2004; 70: 123–31.

192. Bilinski P, Roopenian D, Gossler A. Maternal IL-11Ralpha function is required for normal decidua and fetoplacental development in mice. Genes Dev 1998; 12: 2234–43.

193. Shorter SC, Vince GS, Starkey PM. Production of granulocyte colony-stimulating factor at the materno–foetal interface in human pregnancy. Immunology 1992; 75: 468–74.

194. McCracken S, Layton JE, Shorter SC et al. Expression of granulocyte-colony stimulating factor and its receptor is regulated during the development of the human placenta. J Endocrinol 1996; 149: 249–58.

195. Bulmer JN, Morrison L, Johnson PM, Meager A. Immunohistochemical localization of interferons in human placental tissues in normal, ectopic, and molar pregnancy. Am J Reprod Immunol 1990; 22: 109–16.

196. Simon C, Frances A, Piquette GN et al. Embryonic implantation in mice is blocked by interleukin-1 receptor antagonist. Endocrinology 1994; 134: 521–8.

197. Lin H, Mosmann TR, Guilbert L et al. Synthesis of T helper 2-type cytokines at the maternal–fetal interface. J Immunol 1993; 151: 4562–73.

198. Kimatrai M, Blanco O, Munoz-Fernandez R et al. Contractile activity of human decidual stromal cells. II. Effect of interleukin-10. J Clin Endocrinol Metab 2005; 90: 6126–30.

199. Trautman MS, Collmer D, Edwin SS et al. Expression of interleukin-10 in human gestational tissues. J Soc Gynecol Investig 1997; 4: 247–53.

200. Dunn CL, Critchley HO, Kelly RW. IL-15 regulation in human endometrial stromal cells. J Clin Endocrinol Metab 2002; 87: 1898–901.

201. Ostojic S, Dubanchet S, Chaouat G et al. Demonstration of the presence of IL-16, IL-17 and IL-18 at the murine feto–maternal interface during murine pregnancy. Am J Reprod Immunol 2003; 49: 101–12.

202. Arici A, Engin O, Attar E et al. Modulation of leukemia inhibitory factor gene expression and protein biosynthesis in human endometrium. J Clin Endocrinol Metab 1995; 80: 1908–15.

203. Shull MM, Doetschman T. Transforming growth factor-beta 1 in reproduction and development. Mol Reprod Dev 1994; 39: 239–46.

204. Nakayama T, Kitaya K, Okubo T et al. Fluctuation of 6Ckine expression in human endometrium during the menstrual cycle. Fertil Steril 2003; 80: 1461–5.

205. Hampton AL, Rogers PA, Affandi B, Selamonsen LA. Expression of the chemokines, monocyte chemotactic protein (MCP)-1 and MCP-2 in endometrium of normal women and Norplant users, does not support a central role in macrophage infiltration into endometrium. J Reprod Immunol 2001; 49: 115–32.

206. Dudley DJ, Spencer S, Edwin S et al. Regulation of human decidual cell macrophage inflammatory protein-1 alpha (MIP-1 alpha) production by inflammatory cytokines. Am J Reprod Immunol 1995; 34: 231–5.

207. Akiyama M, Okabe H, Takakura K et al. Expression of macrophage inflammatory protein-1alpha (MIP-1alpha) in human endometrium throughout the menstrual cycle. Br J Obstet Gynaecol 1999; 106: 725–30.

208. Kitaya K, Nakayama T, Okubo T et al. Expression of macrophage inflammatory protein-1beta in human endometrium: its role in endometrial recruitment of natural killer cells. J Clin Endocrinol Metab 2003; 88: 1809–14.

209. Hornung D, Ryan IP, Chao VA et al. Immunolocalization and regulation of the chemokine RANTES in human endometrial and endometriosis tissues and cells. J Clin Endocrinol Metab 1997; 82: 1621–8.

210. Arima K, Nasu K, Narahara H et al. Effects of lipopolysaccharide and cytokines on production of RANTES by cultured human endometrial stromal cells. Mol Hum Reprod 2000; 6: 246–51.

36 Endometrial complement: physiology and pathophysiology

Steven L Young

Synopsis

Background

- Complement was amongst the first immune system components described by immunologists.
- The complement system participates in both humoral and cellular components of the innate and adaptive immune responses.
- Complement components are expressed in the endometrium of rodents and humans in a cycle dependent manner.

Basic Science

- Many complement components are endoproteinases which are activated by proteolytic cleavage to activate a cascade reaction.
- Complement has three main functions: recognition and lyses of pathogens; opsonization and stimulation of pathogen phagocytoses; promotion of inflammation.
- Complement components C3, factor B and DAF are maximally expressed during the mid to late secretory phases of the menstrual cycle.
- Possibly functions as host defense mechanisms within the endometrium.

Clinical

- Paroxysmal noctural hemoglobinuria caused by a deficiency in glycophosphatidylinositol (GPI) which regulates the function of DAF and CD59, is associated with poor fertility.
- Ablation of Crry, a specific component regulator in a mouse models results in embryonic lethality.
- Limited clinical evidence provides correlative data to support a role for complement in human pregnancy loss.
- Limited evidence for a potential role in endometrial cancer and endometriosis.

INTRODUCTION AND HISTORICAL PERSPECTIVE

The complement system is an evolutionarily ancient facet of the human immune system that plays a profound and pleiotropic role in the immune response. Complement was among the first immune system components described by the first experimental immunologists, working in the late 19th century. The most important contributor to complement's discovery and characterization was Jules Bordet, whose work on the two major components of humoral immunity led to the Nobel Prize in 1919.[1] Bordet described two distinct components of animal serum responsible for bacterial cell wall rupture.[2,3] The two serum components differed as to whether they maintained function after heating and whether prior antigen exposure was necessary. The first component, later termed antibodies, was heat resistant and was found only in animals with previous exposure to the same pathogen. A second component, originally termed 'alexin' was shown to be distinct from antibodies since it was heat-labile and was found in all animals, regardless of prior pathogen exposure. Alexin was later renamed 'complement' by Paul Ehrlich, because it 'complemented' the action of antibodies. It would be decades later before a primary action of complement directly on cell membranes would be experimentally described, although Baumgartner proposed direct membrane action, without evidence, as early as 1919.[2,3]

Experimental observations during the last 50 years have revealed a multitude of functions for the complement components in both humoral and cellular components of both innate and adaptive immune responses. It is now understood that complement factors play key roles in direct and antibody-mediated killing of pathogens and abnormal host cells, promotion of phagocytosis, mediation of inflammation, enhancement of humoral immunity, modulation of T-cell immunity, alteration of cytokine production, stimulation of specific immune cell proliferation, and regulation of immune tolerance.[4] The complement system is also involved in the pathogenesis of ischemic, inflammatory, and autoimmune diseases.[5,6] If uncontrolled, complement can lead to systemic inflammation, tissue destruction, and shock.[7] Because the complement system is involved in so many processes and because unregulated complement activation can be lethal, a complex network of regulatory mechanisms exist that limit activation of complement proteins.

Expression of complement by endometrial tissues was first noted by Weed and Arquembourg in endometriosis lesions.[8] Production of complement components by eutopic human endometrium was first described in 1987, suggesting a local function.[9] Later findings that complement proteins were not only synthesized but also secreted by endometrial stroma and epithelium further supported a physiological role.[10,11] More recently, experiments in mice and humans have suggested that endometrial complement expression is cycle-regulated and that activation of endometrial complement at the maternal–fetal interface can cause reproductive failure. Further evidence suggests additional roles for the complement system in other aspects of endometrial physiology and pathophysiology. This chapter provides an overview of the basic biochemistry and immunology of the complement system as well as a review of the literature regarding the endometrial expression, regulation, and function of complement components.

COMPLEMENT NOMENCLATURE

In order to understand the effects of complement in the endometrium, it is necessary to first understand the nomenclature, function, and interactions of components that constitute the complement system.

Complement components are designated with the letter 'C' followed by a number specifying the order in which they were discovered (e.g. C3). Many complement components are endoproteases, which are themselves activated by proteolytic cleavage. Thus, these components form a cascade of proteases, each activating the next. As each complement component is cleaved, two fragments are formed. The smaller fragment is named by appending an 'a' (e.g. C3a), while the larger fragment is indicated by appending a 'b' (e.g. C3b). Each of the primary fragments can be further cleaved and are given later letters of the alphabet (e.g. C3c, C3d). Some activating components unique to the alternative pathway are named after other letters of the alphabet (e.g. factor B). These non-'C' factors utilize the same additional naming conventions as the factors whose names begin with 'C' (e.g. factor B is cleaved to form factor Ba and Bb). Complement regulatory proteins, which prevent excessive or inappropriate actions of complement, are named either as another letter (e.g. factor I) or as another name entirely (e.g. decay accelerating factor or DAF). Membrane-bound, cell-surface proteins in the complement system also have a 'cluster of differentiation' (CD) designation used to describe all lymphocyte surface proteins (e.g. DAF is CD55). The complement components which have been described in the human endometrium are listed in Table 36.1.

COMPLEMENT COMPONENTS, ACTIVATION, AND REGULATION

The functional organization of the human complement system can be described as three separate activation pathways leading to a final common endpoint, the generation of a C3 convertase (Figure 36.1). A C3 convertase is an enzyme complex which can cleave C3 into C3a and C3b. C3b binds to an antigenic surface, resulting in tagging the cell for phagocytosis (opsonization) and/or direct killing by formation of a membrane attack complex (MAC). In order to form an MAC, a C3b-containing C5 convertase cleaves inactive C5 to C5b, which combines with C6–9. The resulting MAC lyses cells by forming membrane pores. C3b, C3a, and C5a also induce specific immune responses (see below). Regulatory proteins prevent MAC assembly on the body's own cells. CD59 (protectin) binds C8 and C9 and prevents MAC formation. Vitronectin (S-protein) and clusterin (apolipoprotein J or sulfated glycoprotein 2) can also prevent MAC

Table 36.1 Complement components described in the endometrium

Component	Cyclic endometrial expression?	Relevant cleavage products	Primary function(s)
Part A. Complement activation pathway and effectors			
C1q	Yes	None	Recognizes antibody–antigen complexes, component of C1
C1r	Yes	None	Component of C1, classical pathway initiation
C1s	Yes	None	Component of C1, classical pathway initiation
C2	Yes	C2b	Component of classical C3 convertase
		C2a	Component of classical C3 convertase
		C3a	Anaphylatoxin
C3	Yes	C3b	Opsonin and a component of both classical and alternative C3 convertases
C4	Yes	C4b	Opsonin, component of classical C3 convertase
		C4a	Anaphylatoxin
C5	No	C5b	Initiates formation of membrane attack complex (MAC)
		C5a	Anaphylatoxin
C6	Yes	None	Component of MAC, cell lysis
C7	Yes	None	Component of MAC, cell lysis
C8	Yes	None	Component of MAC, cell lysis
C9	Yes	None	Component of MAC, cell lysis
Factor B	Yes	C3b	Alternative pathway initiation
		C3a	Can inhibit proliferation of pre-B lymphocytes
Factor D	Yes	None	Alternative pathway initiation, cleaves factor B
Part B. Complement regulatory proteins			
Decay accelerating factor (DAF, CD55)	Yes	None	Accelerates breakdown of C2 and factor B and disassociation of C2a and Bb from cell surface, prevents complement attack
Membrane cofactor protein (MCP, CD46)	No	None	Cleaves C3b and C4b, prevents complement attack
Protectin (CD59)	No	None	Binds C8 and/or C9, inhibiting MAC assembly, prevents complement attack
C4 binding protein (C4BP)	Yes	None	Cofactor in factor I-mediated cleavage of C4b to C4d (inactive) accelerates breakdown of C2 and disassociation of C2a from cell surface, protects gonococci from complement-mediated killing
Part C. Complement receptors			
Complement receptor 1 (CR1, CD35)	No	None	Receptor for C3b and C4b, triggers phagocytosis
C5a receptor (C5aR, CD88)	No	None	Receptor for C5a, stimulates chemotaxis and release of inflammatory mediators

activity, although the physiological relevance is poorly characterized.

The three complement pathways – classical, lectin, and alternative – are classified according to the mechanism of activation (Figure 36.1). Activation of either the classical or lectin pathway results in formation of an identical C3 convertase, termed the classical C3 convertase (see Figure 36.1). The classical pathway takes its name from the fact that it was the first discovered, although it may be the most recently evolved.[12] The classical pathway is initiated by C1q binding to clustered Fc portions of immunoglobulin M (IgM) or complement-fixing IgG antibodies, as found in antigen–antibody complexes. The order of potency of antibody types in activating the classical pathway is IgM > IgG3 > IgG1 > IgG2 >> IgG4, with IgM being about 1000 times more potent than IgG3.[4] Other proteins can also activate C1q independently of antibody, including serum amyloid protein, an HIV (human immunodeficiency virus) coat protein, and C-reactive protein.

The lectin pathway can be triggered by complex carbohydrate moieties characteristic of many pathogens, including bacteria, fungi, and viruses.[4] Activation is initiated by either mannose-binding lectin (MBL or collectin) or ficolin, either of which, after binding to specific carbohydrate moieties, bind and activate two specific proteases, MASP1 and MASP2. The MBL–MASP

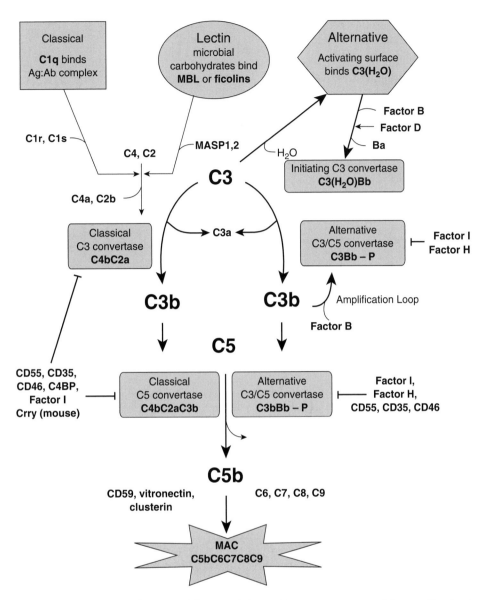

Figure 36.1 Complement activation pathways and their modulators. Factors in gray are inhibitors of activation at the pathway level indicated.

complex is structurally and functionally analogous to the C1q-C1r-C1s of the classical pathway.[12]

Inappropriate or excessive activation of the lectin and classical pathways is prevented by the action of complement regulatory proteins, including the membrane-bound proteins, CD55 (DAF), CD35 (complement receptor 1 or CR1), CD46 (membrane cofactor protein or MCP), as well as soluble proteins, including C4b-binding protein (C4BP), and factor I. DAF acts primarily by inhibiting the association (and promoting the disassociation) of C2 and C4b, while MCP acts primarily as a cofactor in the factor I-mediated proteolytic breakdown of C3b. CR1 can act in a fashion analogous to that of both DAF and MCP. The mouse has an additional regulatory molecule not found in humans,

complement receptor related protein (Crry) that can function in a similar fashion to DAF, CR1, and MCP.

The alternative pathway is initiated directly by an activating surface of a cell. Direct activation can occur because C3 continually undergoes a limited amount of spontaneous hydrolysis, a process known as tickover, to form $C3(H_2O)$, also known as C3i (C3i should not be confused with iC3b, an intermediate product of C3b breakdown). $C3(H_2O)$ can bind to an activating surface and to factor B. The binding of $C3(H_2O)$ to factor B results in a conformational change in factor B, which allows proteolytic cleavage of factor B by the constitutively active factor D, resulting in factor Ba and Bb. The $C3(H_2O)Bb$ complex can then cleave C3 to C3a and C3b, generating C3bBb, itself a potent C3 and C5 convertase. Another alternative pathway factor, properdin, can stabilize the interaction between factor B and C3 forms, thus increasing the efficiency of C3b and C5b formation. Interestingly, the alternative pathway can serve as an amplification loop of the classical and lectin pathways, since fixed C3b produced by those pathways can bind factor B, making it accessible to factor D and thus activating the alternative pathway. In either method of activation, a positive feedback amplification loop is generated because C3 breakdown to C3b leads to more C3Bb, which can generate more C3b. Clearly, this pathway must be under tight regulation to avoid spontaneous or excessive complement activation. Additional factors can also activate the alternative pathway, including zymosan, a yeast cell-wall component, C3 nephritic factor, an autoantibody, and cobra venom factor.

The ability to bind and activate factor H is one of the major determinants of whether a cell surface is an 'activating' surface. Factor H acts as a cofactor in the factor I-mediated proteolytic breakdown of C3b in the alternative pathway C3/C5 convertase. Thus, a surface binding to factor H is generally not a target of alternative pathway attack. Additionally, evidence suggests that CD55, CD46, and CD35 may inhibit alternative pathway activation in a fashion analogous to that of the classical and lectin pathways. Of course any factor that inhibits alternative pathway activation can dampen the classical and lectin pathways by preventing alternative pathway amplification of the other pathways.

Although not commonly recognized as a complement-activation pathway, proteases released by activated leukocytes can also cleave C5, resulting in anaphylatoxin C5a and as well as C5b production. The neutrophil enzyme responsible for C5 cleavage is elastase, but the identity of the macrophage enzyme remains unclear. Interestingly, complement can also be activated by ischemia. Each of the three pathways (classical, lectin, and alternative) has also been shown to be a key component of ischemia–reperfusion damage in one or more of the following organs: heart, skeletal muscle, liver, and kidneys.[7]

IMMUNOLOGICAL EFFECTS OF COMPLEMENT COMPONENTS

The traditional view of complement function included three functions: (1) recognition and direct lysis of pathogens, (2) opsonization and stimulation of pathogen phagocytosis, and (3) promotion of inflammation. Opsonization is the process of coating a target cell

with complement fragments (primarily C3b and iC3b, although C1q can also serve the purpose) that serve to identify the cell as a target for phagocytosis. Phagocytes, including monocytes, macrophage, and neutrophils, recognize the complement fragments using complement receptors, CR1 (CD35), CR3 (CD18/11b), and possibly CR4 (CD18/11c). Upon binding of a complement fragment to a complement receptor, the phagocyte is activated to ingest the target cell.

Activation of the complement cascade is a potent inflammatory stimulus and the complement cascade plays an important role in abnormal inflammatory states, including septic shock. The inflammatory actions of complement are due primarily to C5a and C3a, the so-called anaphylatoxins. C5a is generally the most potent of these, followed by C3a. C3a and C5a can cause mast cell and eosinophil chemotaxis and degranulation, resulting in histamine release, edema, and smooth muscle constriction. C5a is also an important stimulator of neutrophil and macrophage chemotaxis.

Direct killing of pathogens is accomplished by assembling an MAC on the surface of a target cell. The part of the complex made by polymers of up to 14 C9 monomers forms a pore, which allows free ion flux, resulting in cell killing. The MAC complex can also act to stimulate cytokine and chemokine production, further promoting inflammation.

Interestingly, complement factors are also involved in regulating immunological tolerance by the adaptive branch of the immune system. One example of this is a result of complement opsonization of apoptotic cells, which modulates phagocytosis by dendritic cells and macrophages. The phagocytes are responsible for directing T-cell reactivity. Thus, complement components are important in promoting autoantigen tolerance.[6,13] The ability of complement components to play multiple roles in pathogen elimination as well as alter adaptive immune reactivity and tolerance has obvious theoretical implications for a role in immune function. In the next section, the data supporting a role for complement in endometrial functions such as host defense and embryonic and fetal tolerance are reviewed.

EXPRESSION AND REGULATION OF ENDOMETRIAL COMPLEMENT COMPONENTS

Complement components known to be produced by the endometrium (see Table 36.1) include C3, C4, and factor B as well as CD55 (DAF), CD46 (MCP), CD35

(CR1), and CD59 (protectin). The components of the MAC (C5–C9) have also been found on the uterine epithelium using immunohistochemistry. Clear evidence has been presented that C3, factor B, and DAF are highly cycle-regulated, with maximal expression in the mid to late secretory phase in humans. The mechanisms by which cyclic regulation is achieved are unclear, but in-vitro experiments suggest the possibility that progesterone-induced heparin-binding epidermal growth factor (HB-EGF) could be a factor in stimulation of DAF expression in the mid secretory phase. It should also be noted that at least one complement component, C3, is highly up-regulated by estradiol in mice. Furthermore, expression of complement components C2, C3, C4, and C6, as well as uterine complement activity against bacteria, is induced by estradiol and inhibited by dexamethasone.[14] The mouse C3 promoter contains a classical estrogen response DNA element, which the human promoter lacks (unpublished observation) and C3 protein is maximally expressed during the secretory phase, not the proliferative.[15] Thus, significant up-regulation of the human C3 gene by estradiol is not likely.

Recent microarray experiments suggest a similar up-regulation in the mid to late secretory phase for C1r, C1s, C2, factor D, CR1, C5a receptor (CD88), C4BP, and C4.[16] The same microarray experiments suggest an interesting divergence of regulation between components in the late as compared to mid secretory phases. C1q CR1, C5a receptor, and CD59 are all increased from mid to late secretory, while factor D, DAF, C1r, C1s, and C4BP are all decreased in the late secretory vs mid secretory phases. These differences could have many causes, as they are based only on microarray analysis of mRNA. For example, DAF protein levels, as assessed by immunohistochemistry, do not fall from mid to late secretory phases, but do increase from early to mid secretory.[17] Expression of C3 and factor B proteins is also cycle-dependent, with maximal expression in the secretory phase.[11,15,18] Thus, complement components are cycle-regulated in normal human endometrium, suggesting a possible cycle-dependent function.

PHYSIOLOGICAL FUNCTION OF ENDOMETRIAL COMPLEMENT

The role of complement proteins in the endometrium remains unclear. Clues to potential functions of endometrial complement come from demonstrated functions in other systems as well as the nature of cyclic regulation in endometrium. It is highly likely that endometrial complement can function in host defense against pathogens, as complement does in other systems. However, demonstration of a protective role for complement against ascending genital pathogens has not been experimentally confirmed. Despite some uncertainty in detail, complement component expression in the endometrium is markedly cyclic (see above and Table 36.1). Complement component expression in other tissues is not generally described as regulated by hormonal stimulus or any other non-infectious or non-inflammatory stimuli. Thus, it is valid to ask what changing role endometrial complement components may play in cycling endometrium.

If the primary purpose of complement is host defense, one must speculate that the needs for host defense fluctuate with the menstrual cycle. One could postulate an increased demand for uterine-based host defense at the late proliferative and at menstruation based on the following arguments. Cervical defenses may be reduced in the late proliferative phase, when cervical mucus becomes watery and allows easier entry of foreign cells, including sperm and sperm-bound microbes. Also, at menstruation, the cervix becomes more dilated, and defensive functions of mucus may be overcome by blood, a potential nutrient medium. If these physical alterations in host defense were the reason for cyclic expression, then maximal expression of complement factors would be predicted to be in late proliferative and menstrual phase, not in the mid and late secretory phases. Thus, complement may play additional roles in endometrial function.

Complement components may be involved in early events of embryo implantation. Mid secretory increases in expression of a number of complement components parallel the acquisition of endometrial receptivity. Complement activation produces C5a, which can induce adhesion molecule expression, including β_1 integrin subunit (CD29), β_2 integrin subunit (CD18), E-selectin, intracellular adhesion molecule 1 (ICAM-1), and vascular cell adhesion molecule 1 (VCAM-1) in neutrophils and endothelial cells.[5,19] Furthermore, C5a can signal via the EGF receptor by stimulating the expression of HB-EGF, a component thought to be involved in regulating endometrial receptivity.[20] Further data suggest that HB-EGF can, in turn, stimulate expression of a complement protective factor in endometrial cells.[17]

The endometrial cavity has very low oxygen tension, and menstruation is thought to involve a series of ischemia–reperfusion events due to spasm of spiral arteries. Hypoxia and reperfusion are well-described triggers for complement activation.[7] Thus, it is attractive to speculate that complement mediated lysis is one of the mechanisms involved in lysis of endometrial cells at the time of menstruation, but, as with implantation, there are no experimental data to support this conjecture.

Anaphylatoxins C5a and C3a act via specific receptors to stimulate or inhibit expression and release of cytokines by neutrophils and macrophages.[5,7,21] Since the receptor for C5a is expressed and cycle-regulated in human endometrium (see above), C5a may also regulate endometrial cytokine expression. Since cytokines act as paracrine regulators of multiple endometrial functions (e.g. chemotaxis of cyclically regulated immune cell populations and possibly chemotaxis of trophoblasts at implantation), activation of endometrial complement could regulate endometrial functions via its effects on cytokine expression.

One could also speculate that cyclic regulation of complement results from unique immunological demands of embryo implantation and/or menstruation. Perhaps the relative suppression of adaptive immunity thought to occur in the endometrium in the mid secretory phase[22] could lead to an increased need for innate defense, one component of which is the alternative pathway. This hypothesis is consistent with the findings that the alternative-pathway specific factors, factors B and D, as well as some other necessary factors (C3 and C4) are cyclically expressed. The maximal phase of protein expression of these factors is not well established, but evidence supports major increases in RNA for all of these factors in the mid secretory phase, the time of receptivity to embryo implantation. Interestingly, along with up-regulation of components of the complement cascade, there is up-regulation of the complement regulatory proteins DAF and CD59, suggesting the need for protection of endometrial cells against complement attack. DAF has been shown to specifically protect trophoblast from complement-mediated lysis.[23] Further data in other systems demonstrate the ability of complement components to regulate T-cell and B-cell function as well as mediate rejection of an allograft.[24–26] The ability to regulate adaptive immunity and allograft rejection has obvious importance in the regulation of a systemic and local immune response to the semiallogeneic fetal trophoblast.

Thus, complement components might play a role in regulation of implantation, clearance of cells during menstruation, regulation of endometrial cytokines, regulation of immune cell and/or trophoblast chemotaxis, or alterations in innate vs adaptive immune balance.

Additional functions and potential roles in pathogenesis may be revealed by studies of complement component deficiency states as described below.

PATHOLOGICAL EFFECTS OF ENDOMETRIAL COMPLEMENT ON PREGNANCY

If complement components have important roles in endometrial physiology, it seems likely that qualitative and quantitative deficiencies in complement components would result in significant pathology. Although deficiencies and polymorphisms of many complement components have been described in humans, only one association has been reported between a uterine function and a complement system deficiency. Paroxysmal nocturnal hemoglobinuria (PNH), caused by a deficiency in glycophosphatidylinositol (GPI), is associated with poor fertility and reproductive outcomes.[27,28] GPI is used to anchor both DAF (CD55) and CD59 to cell membranes and the absence of GPI leads to lack of function for DAF and CD59.[29] The lack of DAF, and especially CD59, leads to complement-mediated lysis of red blood cells, resulting in paroxysmal hematuria.

It is unclear if reproductive problems in women with PNH can be attributed to abnormalities in implantation, as many pregnancy complications, including maternal morbidity and mortality as well as fetal wastage, have been described.[27,28] Maternal morbidity with PNH derives primarily from anemia, infections, thrombocytopenia, and venous thrombosis. Although some women with PNH can become pregnant, pregnancy seems uncommon as less than 100 cases of pregnancy in PNH patients are described in the literature. Given the built-in redundancy of the complement system, it is possible that loss or dysfunction of one factor may not be enough to cause clear pathology. Thus, it is interesting that loss of two complement regulatory proteins (DAF and CD59) is the only abnormality to demonstrate an obvious reproductive phenotype. Further complicating interpretation is the fact that GPI deficiency in many cases of PNH is partial and that there are at least 28 GPI-linked proteins beside DAF and CD59 that are deficient.[28] Furthermore, the mutation responsible for PNH is somatic and variably present in each cell lineage. Thus, each PNH is unique in the degree of GPI defect and the set of cells with the GPI defect.

While data from human complement deficiencies and pregnancy complications remain unclear, compelling evidence that the complement system plays an important role in pregnancy physiology is found in four distinct mouse models of pregnancy loss (summarized in Table 36.2).

The first clear indication that complement activation may be critical for pregnancy loss was genetic ablation of a mouse-specific complement regulator, Crry, which resulted in 100% wastage of Crry[-/-] embryos.[30] Complement deposition and activation are seen at the placenta of Crry[-/-] embryos and no embryonic losses occur if C3 is also knocked out. Interestingly, neither classical components (C1, C4, and C2), antibodies, nor the MAC components (C5b-9) appear necessary for fetal loss.[31] Thus, loss appears to be mediated via alternative pathway activation and probably via the actions of C3 fragments, possibly via binding to receptors such as CR3, CR4, or C3a receptor.[32] The relevance of this to humans remains theoretical. The Crry gene does not have an exact human homologue, but Crry is similar in both structure and function to DAF (CD55) and MCP (CD46). In mouse embryos, the only complement regulator expressed on the early trophoblast cells is Crry, but in humans at least three complement regulators (DAF, MCP, and CD59), are expressed by first trimester trophoblasts.[33] Thus, deficiency of a single regulatory factor is unlikely to be critical in human placental cells.

Interestingly, complement activation also appears to underlie antiphospholipid antibody (APA)-dependent fetal loss in murine model systems.[34] In this model system, C4, C5, C5a receptor, and factor B were all critical for fetal loss, but neither C6 (critical for MAC assembly) nor Fc receptor deficiency could rescue the fetal loss.[35] Thus, as in the Crry[-/-] mice, fetal loss due to APA syndrome depends upon an alternative pathway member as well as C3, but not on MAC formation. The mechanism of APA-dependent loss differs from that of Crry[-/-] mice in that it requires both a classical pathway factor (C4) and C5.

Another mouse model of fetal loss also appears to depend on complement activation, although it has been less well characterized. In this model of immunological fetal loss, allogeneic embryos are rejected by mothers treated with an inhibitor of indoleamine 2,3-dioxygenase (IDO), a substance which inhibits T-cell activation.[36] The mechanism appears to be antibody independent and T-cell dependent, involving both inflammation and complement activation.[37] Interestingly, syngeneic mating does not result in fetal loss, suggesting that loss depends on T-cell recognition of alloantigens.

More recently, a long-studied model of immune-mediated fetal loss was also shown to require complement components.[38] It has long been established that matings between two inbred mouse strains CBA/J and DBA/2 result in an increased frequency of fetal loss as well as fetal growth restriction.[39] In the recent study, the fetal growth restriction and fetal loss were shown to depend on C3 convertase, C5, and C5aR. Interestingly, the paper also provided evidence suggesting that the placentas of affected pregnancies were deficient in free vascular endothelial growth factor (VEGF) levels and that complement activation was the cause via C5 stimulation of soluble VEGF receptor 1 production.[38]

Thus, four different mouse models appear to depend on complement activation as a mediator of fetal loss, but the models require distinct subsets of complement components for pregnancy loss to occur. It is possible, then, that complement is an important mediator of fetal loss in humans, which would suggest a potential for pharmacological inhibitors of complement production, activation, or function in the prevention of miscarriage.

Investigators have already begun to study the role of complement inhibition in mouse models. In the APA-treated mouse, heparin prevents fetal loss.[40] Furthermore, the ability for other anticoagulants to prevent fetal loss in the mouse model depends entirely on their ability to inhibit complement activation and not on their anticoagulant activity.[40] Thus, heparin, a mainstay of treatment in women with APA syndrome because of its anticoagulant effect, may have a more important effect as a complement inhibitor in the prevention of pregnancy loss.

Taken together, evidence for complement as an important cause of fetal loss in mouse model systems provides an attractive hypothesis that complement is a factor in human fetal loss. Only three papers in the currently available literature have provided data relevant to this question in humans. Tichenor et al reported that among women who later had a spontaneous loss, 20% of primiparas and 30% of recurrent aborters demonstrated complement prior to signs and symptoms of fetal loss.[41] Depletion of circulating C3 and factor B in these women suggests the involvement of the alternative pathway. Another study demonstrated low C4 levels in recurrent spontaneous aborters who were positive for anticardiolipin antibody.[42] Finally, some women with pregnancy loss have been shown to have complement-fixing antibodies that are cytotoxic to syncytiotrophoblasts.[43] Thus, limited correlational data exist to support the role of complement activation in human pregnancy loss.

Other evidence suggests a potential role for complement in endometrial cancer and endometriosis. Although there is no clear relationship between endometrial cancer pathogenesis or progression and the

Table 36.2 Complement components in mouse and human reproductive disorders

Disease	Species	Molecular lesion	Immune factors required for disease expression	Immune factors not required for disease expression	Comments
Recurrent pregnancy loss	Mouse	Crry gene knockout	C3, factor B	Ag:Ab complex, C4, C5, neutrophils, B lymphocytes, T lymphocytes	1. Crry is not expressed in humans, but is similar to both CD55 and CD46, which are expressed at the human maternal–fetal interface 2. 100% fetal loss 3. Placental C3 deposition
	Mouse	Antiphospholipid antibodies	C3, factor B, C4, C5, neutrophils (some effect of C5 and TNFα)		1. Placental C3 deposition 2. Decreased VEGF production 3. Rescued by anticoagulants only if they also act as complement inhibitors
	Mouse	CBA/J × DBA/2	C3, C5, C5aR		1. C3 deposition on placenta 2. Decreased free VEGF
	Mouse	IDO inhibitor	T lymphocytes	Antibody	C3 deposition on placenta
	Human	Antiphospholipid antibodies	?	?	Prevented by heparin, which acts as a complement inhibitor
	Human	?	?	?	In some cases preceded by systemic complement activation
Endometriosis	Human	?	?	?	Increased synthesis of C3, C7, and C4BP in endometriotic lesions and eutopic endometrium of women with endometriosis
Paroxysmal nocturnal hemoglobinuria	Human	GPI deficiency, leading to lack CD55 and CD46 of cell-surface	?	?	Multiple reproductive abnormalities, unclear if due to systemic illness

complement system, a few pertinent observations are worthy of reflection. The rationale of an association between complement system activity and endometrial cancer pathogenesis comes from observations suggesting that overexpression of complement regulatory proteins might protect cancer cells from immune attack.[44,45] Malignant endometrium was shown to overexpress CD35, CD46, CD55, and CD59 relative to benign endometrium.[46] Furthermore, CD55 was overexpressed in cells derived from a cell line derived from a metastatic endometrial adenocarcinoma vs one derived from a well-differentiated primary tumor.[47] Thus, complement protective proteins appear to be overexpressed in endometrial cancer, providing a potential mechanism to escape immune surveillance and a potential barrier to immunotherapy.

The association between complement expression patterns and endometriosis is also modest. Endometriosis lesions overproduce complement component C3[11,48] and peritoneal fluid from women with endometriosis demonstrates much higher levels of C3 than peritoneal fluid of women without endometriosis.[49] Microarray analysis has also suggested that implants overexpress C1 (s subcomponent).[50] Complement is also overexpressed in human endometrial explants cultured in SCID mice, which is used as an endometriosis model.[51] Since endometriosis lesions also express high levels of complement protective proteins (DAF and MCP), the lack of complement deposition is explained.[52] Interestingly, complement components are involved in tolerance vs sensitization to autoantigens of apoptotic cells.[6] Since endometriosis is correlated with autoimmunity, it is possible that complement dysregulation is either cause or effect.

CONCLUSIONS

The complement system is an important aspect of host defense and probably plays that role in the endometrial cavity. Compelling evidence suggests that endometrial complement plays a role in fetal loss from APA syndrome and possibly other causes. Circumstantial evidence suggests a possible role for endometrial complement in embryo implantation, menstruation, and/or immunological adaptations to each. Further research in this field has the promise of application to a number of diseases in the endometrial cavity.

REFERENCES

1. Petterson A. The Nobel Prize in Physiology or Medicine 1919: presentation speech by Professor A Petterson. 1920, Nobelprize.org.
2. Chaplin H Jr. Review: the burgeoning history of the complement system 1888–2005. Immunohematol 2005; 21: 85–93.
3. Volanakis J, Frank M, eds. The Human Complement System in Health and Disease. New York: Marcel Dekker, 1998: 672.
4. Walport M, Complement. In Roitt I, Brostoff J, Male D, eds. Immunology. Mosby: London, 1998.
5. Guo RF, Ward PA. Role of C5a in inflammatory responses. Annu Rev Immunol 2005; 23: 821–52.
6. Roos A, Xu W, Castellano G et al. Mini-review: a pivotal role for innate immunity in the clearance of apoptotic cells. Eur J Immunol 2004; 34: 921–9.
7. Arumugam TV, Shiels JA, Woodruff TM et al. The role of the complement system in ischemia–reperfusion injury. Shock 2004; 21: 401–9.
8. Weed JC, Arquembourg PC. Endometriosis: can it produce an autoimmune response resulting in infertility? Clin Obstet Gynecol 1980; 23: 885–93.
9. Bartosik D, Damjanov I, Vicarello RR, Riley JA. Immunoproteins in the endometrium: clinical correlates of the presence of complement fractions C3 and C4. Am J Obstet Gynecol 1987; 156: 11–15.
10. Bischof P, Planas-Basset D, Meisser A, Campana A. Investigations on the cell type responsible for the endometrial secretion of complement component 3 (C3). Hum Reprod 1994; 9: 1652–9.
11. Isaacson KB, Galman M, Coutifaris C, Lyttle R. Endometrial synthesis and secretion of complement component-3 by patients with and without endometriosis. Fertil Steril 1990; 53: 836–41.
12. Matsushita M, Matsushita A, Endo Y et al. Origin of the classical complement pathway: Lamprey orthologue of mammalian C1q acts as a lectin. Proc Natl Acad Sci USA 2004; 101: 10127–31.
13. Nauta AJ, Roos A, Daha MR. A regulatory role for complement in innate immunity and autoimmunity. Int Arch Allergy Immunol 2004; 134: 310–23.
14. Rhen T, Cidlowski JA. Estrogens and glucocorticoids have opposing effects on the amount and latent activity of complement proteins in the rat uterus. Biol Reprod 2006; 74: 265–74.
15. Hasty LA, Lambris JD, Lessey BA et al. Hormonal regulation of complement components and receptors throughout the menstrual cycle. Am J Obstet Gynecol 1994; 170(1 Pt 1): 168–75.
16. Talbi S, Hamilton AE, Vo KC et al. Molecular phenotyping of human endometrium distinguishes menstrual cycle phases and underlying biological processes in normo-ovulatory women. Endocrinology 2006; 147: 1097–121.
17. Young SL, Lessey BA, Fritz MA et al. In vivo and in vitro evidence suggest that HB-EGF regulates endometrial expression of human decay-accelerating factor. J Clin Endocrinol Metab 2002; 87: 1368–75.
18. Hasty LA, Brockman WW, Lambris JD, Lyttle CR. Hormonal regulation of complement factor B in human endometrium. Am J Reprod Immunol 1993; 30: 63–7.
19. Albrecht EA, Chinnaiyan AM, Varambally S et al. C5a-induced gene expression in human umbilical vein endothelial cells. Am J Pathol 2004; 164: 849–59.
20. Schraufstatter IU, Trieu K, Sihora L et al. Complement c3a and c5a induce different signal transduction cascades in endothelial cells. J Immunol 2002; 169: 2102–10.
21. Hawlisch H, Belkaid Y, Boelder R et al. C5a negatively regulates toll-like receptor 4-induced immune responses. Immunity 2005; 22: 415–26.
22. Sacks G, Sargent I, Redman C. An innate view of human pregnancy. Immunol Today 1999; 20: 114–18.
23. Cunningham DS, Tichenor JR Jr. Decay-accelerating factor protects human trophoblast from complement-mediated attack. Clin Immunol Immunopathol 1995; 74: 156–61.
24. Cai J, Terasaki PI. Humoral theory of transplantation: mechanism, prevention, and treatment. Hum Immunol 2005; 66: 334–42.

25. Carroll MC. The complement system in regulation of adaptive immunity. Nat Immunol 2004; 5: 981–6.

26. Carroll MC. The complement system in B cell regulation. Mol Immunol 2004; 41: 141–6.

27. Bjorge L, Ernst P, Haram KO. Paroxysmal nocturnal hemoglobinuria in pregnancy. Acta Obstet Gynecol Scand 2003; 82: 1067–71.

28. Parker C, Omine M, Richards S et al. Diagnosis and management of paroxysmal nocturnal hemoglobinuria. Blood 2005; 106: 3699–709.

29. Inoue N, Murakami Y, Kinoshita T. Molecular genetics of paroxysmal nocturnal hemoglobinuria. Int J Hematol 2003; 77: 107–12.

30. Xu C, Mao D, Helers VM et al. A critical role for murine complement regulator crry in fetomaternal tolerance. Science 2000; 287: 498–501.

31. Mao D, Wu X, Deppong C et al. Negligible role of antibodies and C5 in pregnancy loss associated exclusively with C3-dependent mechanisms through complement alternative pathway. Immunity 2003; 19: 813–22.

32. Molina H. Complement regulation during pregnancy. Immunol Res 2005; 32: 187–92.

33. Girardi G, Bulla R, Salmon JE, Tedesco F. The complement system in the pathophysiology of pregnancy. Mol Immunol 2006; 43: 68–77.

34. Holers VM, Girardi G, Mo L et al. Complement C3 activation is required for antiphospholipid antibody-induced fetal loss. J Exp Med 2002; 195: 211–20.

35. Girardi G, Berman J, Redecha P et al. Complement C5a receptors and neutrophils mediate fetal injury in the antiphospholipid syndrome. J Clin Invest 2003; 112: 1644–54.

36. Munn DH, Zhou M, Attwood JT et al. Prevention of allogeneic fetal rejection by tryptophan catabolism. Science 1998; 281: 1191–3.

37. Mellor AL, Sivakumar J, Chandler P et al. Prevention of T cell-driven complement activation and inflammation by tryptophan catabolism during pregnancy. Nat Immunol 2001; 2: 64–8.

38. Girardi G, Yarilin D, Thurman JM et al. Complement activation induces dysregulation of angiogenic factors and causes fetal rejection and growth restriction. J Exp Med 2006; 203: 2165–75.

39. Clark DA, Chaouat G, Arck PC et al. Cytokine-dependent abortion in CBA x DBA/2 mice is mediated by the procoagulant fgl2 prothrombinase. J Immunol 1998; 160: 545–9.

40. Girardi G, Redecha P, Salmon JE. Heparin prevents antiphospholipid antibody-induced fetal loss by inhibiting complement activation. Nat Med 2004; 10: 1222–6.

41. Tichenor JR, Bledsoe LB, Opsahl MS, Cunningham DS. Activation of complement in humans with a first-trimester pregnancy loss. Gynecol Obstet Invest 1995; 39: 79–82.

42. Unander AM, Norbery R, Hahn L, Arfors L. Anticardiolipin antibodies and complement in ninety-nine women with habitual abortion. Am J Obstet Gynecol 1987; 156: 114–19.

43. Tedesco F, Pausa M, Nardon E et al. Prevalence and biological effects of anti-trophoblast and anti-endothelial cell antibodies in patients with recurrent spontaneous abortions. Am J Reprod Immunol 1997; 38: 205–11.

44. Loberg RD, Day LL, Dunn R et al. Inhibition of decay-accelerating factor (CD55) attenuates prostate cancer growth and survival in vivo. Neoplasia 2006; 8: 69–78.

45. Spendlove I, Ramage JM, Bradley R et al. Complement decay accelerating factor (DAF)/CD55 in cancer. Cancer Immunol Immunother 2006; 55: 987–95.

46. Murray KP, Mathure S, Kaul R et al. Expression of complement regulatory proteins – CD 35, CD 46, CD 55, and CD 59 – in benign and malignant endometrial tissue. Gynecol Oncol 2000; 76: 176–82.

47. Nowicki S, Nowicki B, Pham T et al. Expression of decay accelerating factor in endometrial adenocarcinoma is inversely related to the stage of tumor. Am J Reprod Immunol 2001; 46: 144–8.

48. Isaacson KB, Coutifaris C, Garcia CR, Lyttle CR. Production and secretion of complement component 3 by endometriotic tissue. J Clin Endocrinol Metab 1989; 69: 1003–9.

49. Tao XJ, Sayegh RA, Isaacson KB. Increased expression of complement component 3 in human ectopic endometrium compared with the matched eutopic endometrium. Fertil Steril 1997; 68: 460–7.

50. Eyster KM, Boles AL, Brannian JD, Hansen KA. DNA microarray analysis of gene expression markers of endometriosis. Fertil Steril 2002; 77: 38–42.

51. Awwad JT, Seyegh RA, Tao XJ et al. The SCID mouse: an experimental model for endometriosis. Hum Reprod 1999; 14: 3107–11.

52. D'Cruz OJ, Wild RA. Evaluation of endometrial tissue specific complement activation in women with endometriosis. Fertil Steril 1992; 57: 787–95.

37 Endometrial paradigms

Kathy L Sharpe-Timms, Breton F Barrier, and Susan C Nagel

Synopsis

Background

- Controlled in-vivo investigations of endometrial function in women are restricted by ethical considerations and limited accessibility of human endometrial tissue.
- In-vivo paradigms include direct observation or imaging of human endometrium, and primate and rodent models that provide the opportunity to study and modulate gene expression.
- In-vitro paradigms include human and animal whole tissue perfusion, tissue fragment explant culture, isolated cell cultures, and 3D cell culture models.
- Mathematical models, stereology, and image reconstruction have also been developed to predict correlations between clinical observations and laboratory analyses.

Clinical

- MRI and TV-US may be effective in evaluating treatment strategies for endometriosis and anatomical or physiological anomalies such as placentation defects associated with recurrent pregnancy loss or uterine fibroids.
- The baboon develops spontaneous endometriosis in captivity, with associated infertility, and has been used for the development of novel therapies for endometriosis.
- Surgically transplanted uterine tissue in rodents grows and behaves similarly to human endometriotic lesions. It elicits infertility and pain and responds to a variety of chemical and herbal therapeutic approaches and is useful for examining molecular profiles of lesions and identifying therapeutic targets.
- The rhesus monkey has been useful in the preclinical stages of testing of reproductive pharmaceutical agents: treatment and prevention of *Chlamydia* and especially the development of contraceptive agents.
- The patas monkey is the only monkey known to develop preeclampsia, in which pregnant dams develop new-onset proteinuria (although no hyperuricemia) and hypertension with perineal edema that spontaneously resolves after delivery.
- Transgenic reporter mice have proved very useful in revealing effects on steroid-activated pathways of environmental contaminants such as bisphenol A or drugs such as tamoxifen.
- In-vivo gene transfer technologies are showing promise in animal models of uterine function.

ABSTRACT

Despite the pivotal role of the endometrium in the establishment of pregnancy and the significant human health problems associated with endometrial disease, the mechanisms controlling these processes are poorly understood and confounded by in-vivo complexity. In general, controlled investigations of endometrial function in women are restricted by ethical considerations and limited accessibility of human endometrial tissue. Hence, various paradigms to study endometrial function and disease have been developed. In-vivo paradigms include direct visualization and imaging of the endometrium in women and in-vivo primate and rodent animal models to study and modulate endometrial function. In-vitro paradigms include human and animal whole tissue perfusion, tissue fragment explant culture, isolated cell culture, and three-dimensional (3D) cell culture models. Mathematical models have also been developed to study various facets of endometrial function and disease. These various paradigms may enhance our understanding of endometrial function and disease and translate into therapeutic use in humans. This chapter was designed to provide an appreciation of endometrial paradigms, along with their assets and putative deficits, for investigations in normal and pathological endometrial function and disease.

INTRODUCTION

The endometrium is primarily composed of luminal and glandular epithelium, stroma, resident immune cells, and endothelial cells. Endometrial function is modulated by sex steroid hormones, cytokines, chemokines, and growth factors, as well as paracrine interactions.[1-4] Remarkably, the endometrium undergoes dramatic cyclic remodeling each month during the non-pregnant reproductive cycle and functional remodeling to assure uterine receptivity and successful placentation at the time of embryo implantation.[5-12]

Endometrial research has been designed to evaluate clinically significant, often paradoxical topics including reproductive cyclicity and menopause, fertility and infertility, implantation and spontaneous abortion, and assisted reproductive technologies and contraception. Endometrial research has also addressed various other pathologies such as abnormal uterine bleeding, endometriosis, inadequate placental growth and function, preterm labor, and endometrial cancer as well as the effects of environmental exposures, such as xenobiotics, on reproduction.

Most controlled in-vivo investigations of endometrial function in women are restricted by ethical considerations and limited accessibility of human endometrial tissue. Therefore, endometrial paradigms have been developed to study the endometrium. In-vivo paradigms include direct observation or imaging of human endometrium and primate and rodent models which provide the opportunity to study and modulate gene expression. In-vitro paradigms include human and animal whole tissue perfusion, tissue fragment explant culture, isolated cell cultures, and 3D cell culture models. Mathematical models have also been developed to predict correlations between clinical observations and laboratory analyses.

These various paradigms may provide insight and enhance our understanding of endometrial cell biology, including various aspects of cell proliferation and differentiation, steroid hormone, growth factor, and cytokine responsiveness and action, autocrine and paracrine communication within and between endometrial cells and the embryo, interactions between endometrial cells and extracellular matrix (ECM), tumorigenesis including attachment, migration, and invasion, and various pharmacological, immunomodulatory, xenobiotic, and gene therapy effects on endometrial function at the molecular, cellular, and proteomic levels, most with a similar translational goal for therapeutic use.

This chapter was designed to provide an appreciation of endometrial paradigms, along with their assets and putative deficits, for investigations in normal and pathological endometrial function. Specific examples have been provided for each paradigm.

IN-VIVO HUMAN PARADIGMS

Direct observation or imaging of human endometrium

In humans, experimental results can be generated by direct observation of endometrial tissue in vivo, utilizing hysteroscopy and hysterography or by imaging technologies such as magnetic resonance imaging (MRI) or transvaginal ultrasonography (TV-US). MRI and TV-US have become cost-effective tools in the evaluation of endometrial anomalies in women.[13-15] They are non-invasive and reliably differentiate uterine anatomy. Although the potential is great for imaging technologies in the preoperative evaluation of women, imaging has yielded varying results between studies.

For example, TV-US has shown that in women with endometriosis, the halo surrounding the uterine endometrium and representing the subendometrial myometrium is significantly enlarged compared with disease-free women.[16] The expansion is more pronounced in older women, yet, it is not correlated with the severity of the endometriotic disease. In these women, MRI furnished similar data in that the endometrial junctional zone was expanded compared to controls.[16] While the sensitivity (83%) and specificity (98%) of MRI for detection of ovarian endometriosis are good, the sensitivity and specificity of MRI for the more common focal peritoneal endometriotic lesions are generally low.[16,17] Thus, imaging of the eutopic endometrium may be a more valuable tool in women who suffer from peritoneal endometriosis. MRI and TV-US may be more effective in evaluating treatment strategies where anatomical or physiological anomalies such as placentation defects associated with recurrent pregnancy loss or uterine fibroids exist.

Studies of human endometrium collected by biopsy

Another approach to studying the human endometrium includes analyses of human endometrial tissues collected by biopsy at various points of the menstrual cycle or before and after therapeutic intervention. Molecular, cellular, and proteomic studies may be performed with the endometrial tissues as they are collected or studied after in-vitro manipulation of tissues and/or isolated cells.

IN-VIVO ANIMAL PARADIGMS

Primate models of endometrial physiology and disease

Primates provide an excellent model of human endometrial physiology. Apes have a reproductive physiology quite similar to the human, but are not generally available for reproductive research. Monkeys are commonly used in reproductive research. Some monkeys have monthly menses, spontaneous ovulation, hemochorial discoid placentation, and singleton gestations remarkably similar to the human. Thus, the primate model is an important asset useful for testing the efficacy and safety of beneficial medications and devices prior to the initiation of human trials.

The primary disadvantage of working with primates is cost, both absolute animal cost and especially the cost of maintaining them in captivity for use in research. Other costs are intangible. Certain monkeys, such as the rhesus, are capable of transmitting lethal infections to humans. The cost can also be high for the animal, and ethics dictates that primates, by virtue of their similarity to man, be used for research only when the information to be gained is very important and not attainable through the use of other animal models or requiring them to suffer unnecessarily in the process.

Primates used for reproductive research include both Old and New World monkeys. The Old World monkeys are more commonly used and include the macaques (*Macaca mulatta*, a.k.a. rhesus monkey; *Macaca nemestrina*, a.k.a. pigtail macaque; and *Macaca fascicularis*, a.k.a. cynomolgus monkey), baboons (*Papio anubis*, a.k.a. olive baboon; *Papio hamadryas*, a.k.a. Egyptian baboon; and *Papio cynocephalus*, a.k.a. yellow baboon), African green monkey (*Chlorocebus aethiops* or vervet money), and African red monkey (*Erythrocebus patas* or patas monkey) amongst others. The macaques and baboons are used for the bulk of endometrial research, while the African green monkey and especially the patas monkey are rarely employed. The even less commonly used marmoset (*Callithrix jacchus*) is a New World monkey, originating in South America. Each primate species boasts benefits and disadvantages, and has developed its own respective niche in reproductive research.

Rhesus monkeys and baboons are closely related, each animal containing a complement of 42 chromosomes per somatic cell and each demonstrating a reproductive physiology similar to that of the human. These monkeys have been experimentally interbred in the past to producing a viable sterile hybrid offspring dubbed a 'rheboon' with a normal life span.[18] Many reagents (i.e. antibodies, primers, probes, etc.) have been developed for one or the other species, and may be useful in both types of monkeys. Although the homology of various cytokines, growth factors, and other proteins in the endometrium is similar between rhesus and baboon, they can occasionally be significantly dissimilar from the human.

The rhesus monkey (*Macaca mulatta*) is the most popular primate model for endometrial and early pregnancy research. The rhesus reaches sexual maturity at age 3 and is capable of breeding until its late teens. The rhesus menstrual cycle typically lasts 26–28 days with visible menses, and ovulation is spontaneous. Although they are seasonal breeders in the wild, in captivity rhesus breed year-round. The rhesus monkey does not display the marked anogenital sex skin swelling as do other Old World primates, although their perineum does redden as ovulation approaches. By comparison, the pigtail macaque (*Macaca nemestrina*) is a year-round breeder and spontaneously ovulates and experiences marked sex skin changes.

The rhesus monkey has been used successfully in vast numbers of reproductive investigations, the scope of which precludes comprehensive review in this chapter. Ovulation induction and in-vitro fertilization is well described in this primate.[19-21] Endometrial physiology has been extensively explored, including the role in endometrial function of matrix metalloproteinases (MMPs),[22] integrins,[23] growth factors,[24] prostaglandins[25] and steroid hormones,[10,26-28] and relaxin.[29] The groundwork is also being laid for evaluation of the immunology of the maternal–fetal interface in the rhesus monkey.[30]

The rhesus monkey has been useful in the preclinical stages of testing of reproductive pharmaceutical agents. Treatment and prevention of *Chlamydia*[31-33] and especially in the development of contraceptive agents[34-39] using this primate have yielded fruitful data.

A significant disadvantage in working with monkeys of the genus *Macaca* is that many are chronic carriers of the herpes B virus. Susceptibility of man to clinical herpes B infection is low, but contact with monkey saliva, tissues, or tissue fluids may lead to transmission of the virus. If the herpes encephalitis occurs in the human, the mortality rate is high, and the few survivors almost universally suffer profound and permanent neurological injury.[40]

The baboon is a substantially larger (and more expensive) relative of the macaque and therefore amenable to serial procedures such as laparoscopy or blood sampling. It is also a comparably docile primate, and unable to contract the herpes B infection. The baboon reaches sexual maturity at age 4, and is able to breed until approximately age 20, carrying a singleton pregnancy to term in 164–186 days. In captivity, baboons are year-round spontaneous ovulators. Their menstrual cycle has a mean duration of 36 days, with 1–3 days of visible menses. Ovulation occurs similarly to the human, and endometrial receptivity to implantation occurs between postovulatory days 6–10. The menstrual cycle stage is discernible by a dramatic change in the anogenital sex skin as it responds to ovarian steroids. At ovulation, the sex skin reaches maximum turgescence, a bright red and bulbous display for the male, and then it deturgesces under the influence of luteal progesterone. The swelling correlates well with sex steroid concentrations and can be used as a surrogate for them for many experiments.

At laparoscopy the baboon uterus is shaped similar to that of the human, although the lower uterine segment is less well developed. The uterosacral ligaments and pubocervical fascial support is all but absent, and the uterus falls flat into the posterior cul-de-sac during laparoscopy, causing difficulty in elevation of the fundus unless an intrauterine manipulator is used.

Baboon endometrium has been obtained through transcervical aspiration biopsy. This process is effective in multiparous dams and allows retrieval of tissue for intraperitoneal inoculation for induction of endometriosis.[41,42] Transcervical endometrial biopsy is difficult in the nulliparous female baboon because the vagina is long and tortuous and the cervix is small and fleshy. Because of the smaller size and lack of central stability, the baboon uterus is perhaps more prone to lateral perforation during transcervical sampling than is the human uterus.

Another technique for obtaining a large amount of endometrial tissue from both baboon and rhesus is through laparotomy with fundal hysterotomy and endometrectomy using a small sterile reagent spatula.[43] In order to prevent significant blood loss, a tourniquet consisting of an elastic band is placed around the lower uterine segment and held around the uterine vasculature with a small hemostat. The cervix is clamped via the vagina. After the procedure, the uterus is closed with a running locking absorbable suture. The endometrial basalis is not removed in this procedure, and the endometrium regenerates without harm. Uterine cavity flushing for fluid analysis can be accomplished prior to endometrectomy using hollow-bore phlebotomy needles for flushing with a sterile isotonic solution.[44]

Molecular mechanisms controlling endometrial decidualization have been well described in the baboon,[45–47] as has elucidation of precise events surrounding implantation.[48–50] The effect of estrogen on vascular endothelial growth/permeability factor expression by glandular epithelial and stromal cells in the baboon endometrium has been described.[51]

The baboon has been well developed as a model for the study of the pathophysiology of both spontaneous[52,53] and induced[54,55] endometriosis, and for the development of novel therapies for endometriosis.[41,56,57] The baboon develops spontaneous endometriosis in captivity, with associated infertility. In a large breeding colony of baboons, endometriosis is found at the time of laparoscopy in 60% of reproductive-aged females with primary infertility.[56] By comparison, it has been previously reported that endometriosis occurs in 25% of all otherwise normal captive reproductive-aged females.[58]

Endometriosis may be induced in the baboon by placing biopsied endometrium directly into the peritoneal cavity under direct visualization at the time of laparoscopy. Results are most consistent during the menstrual phase.[42,52] Endometriosis can also be induced by occlusion of the cervix.[57]

The baboon can be housed in individual cages or groups of four for a short period of time in order to obtain non-anesthetized real-time samples of blood or other body fluids, vital signs including blood pressure, and to administer medications.[59] The tether is harnessed to the animal's back and secured in place out of the animal's reach. A reinforced cable containing lines connects the backpack to the cage roof.

The green monkey (vervet; *Chlorocebus aethiops*) is a seasonal breeder in the wild but may breed year-round in captivity. The vervet endometrium has been studied little compared with the rhesus and baboon. A recent study reported the expression of β_3 integrin and insulin-like growth factor binding protein 1 (IGFBP-1) in the endometrium at different phases of the menstrual cycle and also provided a limited description of endometrial architecture which was found to be similar to that of the human.[60] Light and electron microscopy of placentation and placental bed have been described in this primate.[61] The presence of estrogen receptors (ERs) and progesterone receptors (PRs) has also been described at different stages of the menstrual cycle and in abnormal cycles.[62] The advantage of the vervet may be its small size and inability to develop herpes B infection, but, comparably, the rhesus monkey has been much better studied and remains the model of choice.

The patas monkey (*Erythrocebus patas*) deserves mention due to its potential as a model for abnormal placentation as a cause of preeclampsia. The patas monkey is the only monkey known to develop human identical preeclampsia, in which pregnant dams develop new-onset proteinuria and hypertension with perineal edema that spontaneously resolves after delivery.[63] Placental changes from a stillbirth delivered by an affected dam included atherosis of decidual vessels.[64] One difference between patas and human preeclampsia is the lack of hyperuricemia in the former. Unfortunately, the availability of patas monkeys for research in the United States has consistently declined over the last decade.

Finally, the marmoset (*Callithrix jacchus*) has been the subject of extensive research regarding hypothalamic–pituitary–ovarian endocrinology yet boasts only a small number of investigations of endometrial function. The emphasis on ovarian research is due to this primate's pattern, unique among primates, of routine multiple (up to four) ovulation events per cycle. Marmosets do not have visible menses but have a 28-day ovarian cycle that consists of an 8- to 10-day follicular phase and an 18- to 20-day luteal phase.[65] The follicular phase is characterized by low levels of circulating progesterone, a day 2 follicle-stimulating hormone (FSH) peak similar to humans and Old World primates, and a prominent preovulatory LH surge.[66,67] In contrast with other primates, the marmoset experiences a mid-phase FSH peak, multiple dominant follicles, and an abundance of non-ovulatory antral follicles.

Endometrial investigations in the marmoset have included an anatomical survey of the structural differentiation of endometrial zones in response to ovarian steroids[68] and immunohistochemical studies exploring endometrial staining patterns of leukemia inhibitory factor (LIF),[69] the prolactin receptor,[70] relaxin,[71] and ERs and PRs.[72] Microvascular development of the marmoset endometrium during early pregnancy has recently been described.[73]

In summary, primate models offer an important experimental tool to obtain a greater understanding of human endometrial function. The advantages of physiological similarity are somewhat offset by cost, and therefore these models are only available for use in studies in which similarity to the human is essential for satisfactory answers to important experimental questions. Further, ethics dictates that these animals, by virtue of their similarity to man, be used for research only when the information to be gained is very important, not attainable through the use of other animal models, and not requiring the monkey to suffer unnecessarily in the process. Also as mentioned, a significant disadvantage in working with monkeys of the genus *Macaca*, including the rhesus monkey, is that many are chronic carriers of the herpes B virus.[40] And while quite similar, the non-human primate endometrium and human endometrium are not identical. For example, differences have been noted in cyclically regulated endometrial epithelial glycan expression, with abundant expression in the baboon in proliferative and early secretory phases, but expression is delayed in the human until the mid to late secretory phases.[74]

Rodent models of endometrial physiology and disease

Other types of in-vivo animal endometrial paradigms are abundant in the literature. Beyond primate studies, these animal paradigms for human disease are primarily conducted with mice and rats. They have provided important insights into normal and pathological endometrial function. Due to the impracticalities of studying implantation in humans, these animal models are essential to our understanding of the molecular and mechanical events of this process. In addition, these models have successfully been used in pharmacological, toxicological, and gene therapy studies.

Although rodent models have provided valuable information about endometrial biology and pathophysiology on a per-species basis, the data are difficult to extrapolate across species. A major hurdle in cross-species comparisons of endometrial biology is that humans and some non-human primates menstruate, whereas other species exhibit an estrous cycle, which is fundamentally different from a menstrual cycle.

The decidual transformation of the endometrial stroma is critical to implantation. In rodents, decidualization can be induced artificially, indicating that the conceptus may not be essential for a proper maternal response in early pregnancy. Using a murine model, Bany and Cross[75] tested the hypothesis that presence of the conceptus differentially affects uterine gene expression as compared to artificially induced decidualization. They found five genes (*Angpt1*, *Angpt2*, *Dtprp*, *G1p2*, and *Prlpa*) whose steady-state expression in the decidualizing uterus depended on the presence of a conceptus. Decidual Prlpa expression was reduced in the uterus adjacent to Hand1- and Ets2-deficient embryos, providing evidence that normal trophoblast giant cells in the placenta are required for the conceptus-dependent effects on Prlpa expression in the mesometrial decidua.

Lee and DeMayo[76] have published an excellent review comparing differences in implantation between animal models and describe how these differences might be utilized to investigate discrete implantation stages. They also reviewed factors that have been shown to be involved in implantation in the human and animal models, including growth factors, cytokines, cell adhesion, and developmental factors.

Tranguch et al[77] have published an excellent review of mouse models for studying the molecular complexity in establishing uterine receptivity and implantation. They focused on defined signaling cascades involved in this dialogue, specifically on cyclooxygenase 2 (COX-2)-derived prostaglandins, endocannabinoids, Wnt proteins, homeotic transcription factors, and immunophilins.

Describing all studies performed with rodent models for endometrial function and diseases would probably result in an entire book itself. Thus, we have focused on three examples: mouse models of sex steroid function; rodent models for endometriosis; and gene-targeting paradigms in rodents.

Mouse endometrial models of sex steroid function

Knockout mice

Targeted disruption of specific genes (knockout, KO) in mice has aided in defining the function of many genes and gene pathways in the uterus. For example, during development, estrogen receptor α or β (ERα or ERβ) is required for normal development of the uterus. In adulthood, ERα is required for the normal maturation and complete functioning of the uterus, whereas ERβ is required for neither.[78,79] However, mice lacking both ERα and β (double KO) have two-fold narrower uteri (with equal reductions in cell size and number distributed between cell types) than ERαKO mice, demonstrating a physiological role of ERβ in the uterus.[80] Elegant tissue recombination studies have been performed between uterine stromal and epithelial cells from wild-type and ERKO tissue. These studies have definitively shown that it is ERα expression in the stroma that drives proliferation in uterine epithelial cells.[81]

Mice with targeted disruption of the cyp19 gene, which codes for the principal estrogen synthesizing enzyme, aromatase, are viable and grow to adulthood but exhibit hypoplastic uteri.[82,83]

Female aromatase knockout (ArKO) mice are infertile due to disrupted folliculogenesis and an inability to ovulate.[83] Importantly, serum estradiol levels are reduced in ArKO mice, but still circulate low levels of estrogens.

Progesterone receptor knockout (PRKO) mice have yielded important advances in our understanding of PR action in the uterus. PR null mice (lacking both isoforms, which share the same gene) are viable, but exhibit many defects in reproductive tissues. Females are unable to ovulate and exhibit uterine hyperplasia.[84] In isoform-specific KO mice, PR-A and PR-B function as independent transcription factors.[84,85] In PR-A knockout (PRAKO) mice, progesterone induced uterine epithelial proliferation via PR-B. Importantly, these studies have also shown that tissue specificity is largely conferred by the target gene promoter as opposed to differences in tissue-specific expression of PR isoform.

Nuclear hormone receptors require co-activators for full transcriptional activation. It has been suggested that tissue specificity in steroid hormone action may be due in part to the tissue-specific expression of nuclear receptor co-modulatory proteins. Steroid receptor co-activator 1 (SRC-1) is a co-activator for members of the nuclear receptor superfamily.[86] SRC-1 null mice appear phenotypically normal; however, they exhibit mild steroid hormone resistance. For example, estrogen-stimulated uterine weight gain is reduced 35% in SRC-1 knockout mice.[87] Interestingly, steroid receptor co-activator-3 (SRC-3) is not expressed in the endometrium; however, SRC-3 knockout mice have 40% lower circulating estradiol levels.[88]

Transgenic reporter mice

Several investigators have exploited the use of steroid receptor response elements to generate hormone responsive transgenic reporter mice to monitor genomic signaling through these receptors. Several ER reporter mice have been developed by linking two or more estrogen response elements (EREs) to a reporter gene, such as β-galactosidase (estrogen receptor action indicator (ERIN) mouse)[89] or luciferase.[90,91]

Estrogen-induced reporter gene activity was measured in a variety of classical and non-classical estrogen target tissues, including the uterus, pituitary, brain, liver, kidney, thyroid, adipose tissue, and adrenal glands in ERIN mice.[89] Ciana et al[90] found estrogen-induced expression by a total of 15 different tissues in ERE-luciferase mice.

An important use of reporter mice is the ability to examine the effect of cell context on estrogen action, as the specific promoter is unchanged. For example, in ovariectomized ERIN mice the pituitary was 25-fold more sensitive to the synthetic estrogen diethylstilbestrol than the uterus in the same mouse at the identical time. These studies affirm that cell context is a major determinant of endpoint responsiveness to estrogens.[89]

Another example of the use of reporter mice to uncover new aspects of estrogen actions is the analysis of xenobiotic estrogens like bisphenol A (BPA). BPA has been examined in both the ERIN mouse and the ERE-luciferase mouse and these studies have led to increased understanding not only of the mechanism of action of this endocrine disrupting chemical but also to the basic estrogen biology. BPA is a monomer that is polymerized to make polycarbonate plastic. After repeated use or exposure to heat or extremes in pH, bisphenol A leaches into food and beverages from polycarbonate containers.

Bisphenol A is also a xenobiotic estrogen that can bind to and activate ER. Relative to its affinity for ER, BPA has a limited ability to stimulate uterine wet weight gain. Whereas BPA is a poor stimulator of uterine weight gain, it is a much more potent stimulator of ERIN activity. Conversely, tamoxifen showed considerable stimulation of uterine weight gain, but it showed no stimulation of ERIN activity.[89] Tamoxifen is a selective estrogen receptor modulator and functions as a full antagonist in the breast; however, it functions as a partial agonist in the uterus. The agonist activity in the uterus results primarily from stimulation of non-ERE-dependent genes: e.g. signaling through ER bound to activating protein 1 (AP-1) via the AP-1 response element.[92,93] These data indicate that:

- non-ERE-dependent pathways, at least in part, mediate estrogen-stimulated uterine weight gain
- BPA may only be active in classical ERE-mediated signaling.

In-vivo imaging of estrogen-stimulated ERE-luciferase activity allows for analysis of ER activity in real time. Lemmen et al[94] showed that when BPA was administered to pregnant dams estrogenic activity could be detected in the fetuses. In utero stimulated ERE-luciferase activity was visualized in living fetuses where BPA was more active (its potency was 1% of diethylstilbestrol) than would have been predicted from in-vitro assays of its estrogenic activity.[94] Taken together, the above studies predicted that BPA would be more active in the animal than originally reported and this prediction has been confirmed in over 100 studies of the low-dose activity of BPA.[95]

Recently, Harris et al[96] showed that the ERβ selective agonist ERB-041 induced the complete regression of all intraperitoneal endometriotic lesions in nude mice. This effect appeared to be systemic, probably on the immune system, as the lesions did not express ERβ.

Rodent models of endometriosis

Vernon and Wilson[97] first described induction of endometriosis by autotransplantation of uterine squares into the peritoneal cavity in rats and this method was modified by Cummings et al in mice.[97,98] This model consists of obtaining several equal-size pieces of uterine tissue from ablation of one of the two uterine horns. Mice have a bicornuate uterus, consisting of two equal parts; thus, endometriotic implants can be compared to the remaining intact uterine tissue (eutopic endometrium). The uterine squares, called implants, are autotransplanted to the arterial cascade of the intestinal mesentery, where all implants develop into endometriotic lesions. Surgically transplanted uterine tissue in rodents grows and behaves similarly to human endometriotic lesions. It elicits infertility[99] and pain,[100,101] and responds to a variety of chemical and herbal therapeutic approaches.[102–108]

Our laboratory has identified several genes and protein products that are differentially expressed by eutopic and ectopic endometrium in humans and in a rodent model of endometriosis.[109–114] Intriguingly, established rodent and human endometriotic lesions (and eutopic endometrium in women with endometriosis) express haptoglobin mRNA and protein in vivo, whereas eutopic endometrium from rats and women without endometriosis does not.[109,114] Endometriotic haptoglobin has immunomodulatory properties that favor the development of endometriosis.[116,117]

Many studies have implicated MMPs and their tissue inhibitors of metalloproteinases (TIMPs) are reported to play a significant role in the pathogenesis of endometriosis.[118–123] MMPs and TIMPs regulate normal and pathological remodeling of the ECM. Using the rat model for endometriosis, we have shown that MMP-3, MMP-7, and TIMP-1, which are temporally and spatially regulated in eutopic endometrium, are anomalously expressed in endometriosis.[109,115]

Using the athymic immunodeficient or nude mouse model for endometriosis,[124,125] Bruner-TranL and colleagues[126] reported the down-regulation of endometrial MMP-3 and MMP-7 expression in vitro. Furthermore, therapeutic regression of experimental endometriosis in vivo was elicited by a novel non-steroidal progesterone receptor agonist, tanaproget. Osteen and colleagues[123] have further hypothesized that a defect in PR signaling may, in part, mediate the misexpression of MMPs and TIMPs in women with endometriosis.

Recently, Somigliana et al[127,128] reported successful implantation of injected endometrial tissue in immunocompetent mice. Endometriosis was induced by injection of donor endometrial scrapings into syngenic recipient mice. Furthermore, this study demonstrated that intraperitoneal administration of interleukin 12 (IL-12) significantly prevented ectopic endometrial implantation. Subsequently, this method has been modified using transgenic C57BL6 mice that constitutively express green fluorescent protein (GFP) for donor endometrium.[129,130] These modifications greatly improved the ease and reliability of identifying ectopic fluorescent lesions. Endometrial scrapings were retrieved from one donor mouse (GFP+/−) and injected into two recipient (GFP−/−) ovariectomized mice. In this study, ovariectomized recipient mice received either vehicle control or estrogen supplementation. Subsequently, control-treated mice developed an average of two lesions per mouse, whereas estrogenized mice developed five lesions per mouse, replicating prior studies of the estrogen-stimulated growth of endometriotic lesions.[129]

This approach was also undertaken by injection of human endometrium transduced in vitro by adenoviral infection with the GFP cDNA into nude mice.[131] Fluorescent endometrial fragments implanted in the nude mice formed endometriotic-like lesions and could be directly visualized through the skin of live mice with a simple imaging device. This model provides the opportunity for non-invasive and dynamic studies of lesion implantation and development. In addition to providing insights into the pathophysiology of the disease, this model represents a potential preclinical tool for testing the efficacy of new drugs targeting endometriosis.

Defrere et al[132] have recently developed a method of fluorimetric evaluation combined with morphometric analysis of endometriosis-like lesions in a nude mouse model. This method permits objective and reliable recording of endometriosis development. This type of quantification could therefore be useful for future pharmacological and toxicological studies.

The nude mouse model has been used to demonstrate the effects of the antiangiogenic agent nimesulide, a COX-2 inhibitor; it was not capable of reducing the size and number of ectopic human endometrial lesions as predicted.[133] However, in a subsequent study, they found that the soluble truncated receptor (flt-1) and an affinity-purified antibody to human vascular endothelial growth factor (VEGF) significantly inhibited the growth of nude mouse explants.[134] Nap et al[135] found that the effect of the angiostatic compounds antihuman VEGF, TNP-470, endostatin, and anginex, effectively interfered with the maintenance and growth of endometriosis in this model.

To assess the timing of endometrial lesion revascularization, Eggermont et al[136] performed a time course of pelvic endometriotic lesion revascularization in the nude mouse model. They found that platelet endothelial cell adhesion molecule 1 (PECAM-1) is a reliable endothelial cell marker to evaluate the role of angiogenesis in the nude mouse model. They reported that revascularization of human endometrial implants in the nude mouse occurred between 5 and 8 days after implantation and involved the disappearance of native graft vessels, coinciding with the invasion of the interface and then the stroma by murine vessels.

The nude mouse model has further been used to evaluate the histological response of normal human endometrium to steroid hormones.[137] As there was a gap in our knowledge of the histological and biological effects of individual sex steroids on human endometrium, combined with the widespread use of hormonal therapy for menopausal symptoms, oral contraception, and treatment of metastatic breast carcinoma, the ovariectomized athymic mouse was investigated as a host for human endometrium in which the hormonal was manipulated and the histological response determined. Proliferation of endometrial gland cells occurred in the transplanted endometrium of estradiol-treated mice and the complete sequence of secretory phase events, including subnuclear vacuolization, luminal secretion, and decidualization of stroma, were observed during a 14-day period of treatment with estradiol and progestin (medroxyprogesterone acetate). Progestin treatment alone also caused lesser secretory phase changes. The endometrium transplanted into nude mice that did not receive steroid hormones appeared to be inactive.

Bruner-Tran et al[138] have reviewed the potential role of environmental toxins in the pathophysiology of endometriosis. They have shown that 2,3,7,8-tetrachlorodibenzo-p-dioxin (TCDD or dioxin) can disrupt steroid regulation of endometrial MMPs, which are necessary for formation of endometriosis lesions in the nude mouse. TCDD exposure promoted establishment of endometriosis by interfering with the ability of progesterone to suppress endometrial MMP expression.

Numerous investigators have used the nude mouse model to study development, progression, and effects of therapies for various types of cancer. For example, Satyaswaroop et al[139] studied human endometrial carcinomas of different histological grade and steroid receptor characteristics in the nude mouse system.

Biologically and clinically important information on the role of steroid receptors in eliciting hormonal responses in these tumors was obtained. Furthermore, the model was also used to study hormonal therapy and chemotherapeutic compounds for human endometrial adenocarcinoma.[140,141] These studies form the basis for designing and testing various treatment strategies for endometrial carcinomas of different histological grade and receptor content. The potential use of the nude mouse for development of a preclinical model for hormonal therapy of human endometrial carcinomas was reviewed by Satyaswaroop.[142]

Gene-targeting paradigms in rodents

The use of animal models has provided access to evaluation of gene-targeting approaches, the introduction of an exogenous DNA (or RNA) into cells, that would not be immediately feasible in humans. Gene targeting may be developed in vivo by several methods. Daftary and Taylor[143] have reviewed and performed studies of endometrial gene transfer in the in-vivo rat uterus, ex-vivo human uterus, and human endometrial cancer cell lines. In general, they reported that the primary hurdle in in-vivo gene transfer is achieving reliable levels of transgene expression in target tissues. Compared to viral vectors or liposome-mediated gene transfer, lipofection was reportedly more efficient, rapid, and reproducible with fewer complications. Kimura et al[144] have recently provided an excellent review regarding in-vivo gene-targeting strategies to elucidate the function of specific genes in the endometrium in several animal models.

Complete gene knockout studies in mice often result in a normal reproductive phenotype or embryonic lethality, making them inadequate models for investigating endometrial physiology.[145] Transfer of macromolecules, including glycoproteins and recombinant peptides, into the uterine cavity is very expensive, and the rate of metabolism of these exogenously introduced proteins is generally high. On the contrary, gene transfer has been more efficient and provided interesting strategies for modulating normal endometrial cell function in a sequence-specific manner. These methods hold significant promise for development of novel therapeutics for human endometrial dysfunction.[144]

In-vivo gene transfer (or transfection) may introduce specific exogenous cDNA sequences, decoy antisense oligodeoxynucleotides (ODNs), and interfering RNA sequences (RNAi) for modulating endometrial function and dysfunction at the molecular level in a gene-specific manner. Vectors are required to facilitate transfer of the gene DNA (or RNA) through the cell membrane. Vectors are classified as viral and non-viral.

The viral vectors include retrovirus, adenovirus, adeno-associated virus (AAV), and lentivirus-derived vectors. Retroviral vectors impart long-term expression of exogenous genes as they are transfected into actively dividing cells and the gene is incorporated into the host chromosome. It is, however, possible that insertion of the exogenous gene may disturb the normal physiology of the host cells. Adenoviral transfections are transient in nature as the vector does not integrate into the host genome, but rather the vector expresses the transgene from a non-chromosomal location. Beyond the transient nature, use of the adenovirus has potentially problematic immunogenicity to the host. The AAV is a non-pathogenic modified parvovirus in which the viral genome integrates into host chromosome and allows long-term expression of the transgene. Recombinant lentiviruses are derived from human, feline, and simian immunodeficiency viruses. These viruses are more successful in a wider range of tissues and cells than conventional retroviruses.[143]

Although numerous protocols have been developed for gene therapy or in-vivo gene transfer experiments with these viral vectors, successful examples of gene transfer into the uterus with these viruses has not been reported.[144] However, gene transfer into reproductive tissues has been successful with non-viral vectors.[143,144]

Non-viral vectors are generally based on lipid particle–DNA complexes. In-vivo gene transfer of β-galactosidase into mouse endometrium using cationic liposomes showed clear β-galactosidase staining in endometrial epithelial cells.[145,146] Cationic liposomes have also been used for transfection of ODNs into rat endometrium; some successful results causing alterations in implantation physiology are as follows.

The first successful modulation of implantation physiology by in-vivo gene transfer has been reported by using antisense ODNs. Calcitonin, a 32 amino acid peptide hormone primarily synthesized and secreted by the thyroid gland which regulates calcium metabolism, is dramatically up-regulated in the pregnant rat uterus just prior to implantation.[147] Zhu et al[148] designed antisense ODNs, containing phosphorothioate linkages and C5-propynyl modifications at the uridine and cytidine residues for calcitonin. The antisense ODNs were transferred into rat pregnant uterus at day 2 of gestation (postcoitum) with cationic liposomes. The calcitonin ODNs were distributed in the glandular endometrial cells and calcitonin mRNA and protein were suppressed in the day 4 of gestation uterus. Furthermore, implantation sites were less than half the size as compared with those in control rats.[148]

Mice with a targeted mutation of the Hoxa10 gene demonstrate uterine factor infertility.[147] HOXA10 is a member of a family of genes that serve as transcription factors during development and have been shown to be important for uterine function.[149] Hoxa10 gene expression has critical functions for murine implantation.[143,150,151] HOXA 10 is also expressed in human endometrium at the time of implantation in response to sex steroid hormone.[152] The importance of maternal Hoxa10 expression was assessed by injecting the uteri of day 2 pregnant mice with a DNA–liposome complex containing constructs designed to alter maternal Hoxa10 expression before implantation. Transfection with a Hoxa10 antisense ODN significantly decreased the number of implantation sites. Conversely, transfection with a plasmid which constitutively expresses Hoxa10 optimized survival of implanted embryos and resulted in an increased litter size. These results demonstrate that maternal Hoxa10 expression is essential for implantation. Alteration of human endometrial HOXA10 via liposome-mediated gene transfection is a potential contraceptive agent or fertility treatment.[147]

Hoxa11 is also an essential regulator of the cyclic development of endometrium and is required for female fertility, as evidenced by targeted mutation. Chau et al.[153] identified a naturally occurring Hoxa11 (mouse)/HOXA11 (human) antisense transcript present in the adult mouse and human endometrium which varied during the menstrual cycle. Transfection of the murine uterus with Hoxa11 antisense ODNs did not, however, block Hoxa11 function, suggesting that Hoxa11 antisense does not regulate Hoxa11 mRNA by formulation of sense/antisense duplexes. The authors concluded that HOXA11 antisense functions by transcriptional interference, repressing HOXA11 expression by competing for transcription of the common gene, rather than by sense/antisense interaction.[153]

Nuclear factor κB (NFκB) is a transcription factor that is involved in many types of inflammatory and immune responses. Some genes whose expression is closely related to implantation in the mouse and human, such as COX-2, LIF, and colony-stimulating factor (CSF)-1, are under the transcriptional control, at least in part, of the NFκB system.[154,155] Kimura et al[144] introduced a mutant form of inhibitor IκBαM (IκBαM; a nuclear factor κB (NFκB) super-repressor) cDNA into the mouse uterus on day 1.5 post coitus (pc). This mutant IκBαM is resistant to phosphorylation and degradation and thereby hence blocks NFκB activity. NFκB activities, as measured by electrophoretic mobility shift assay (EMSA) at 3.5 and 4.5 days post coitus were suppressed as compared to controls.[156] IκBαM cDNA transfection

was associated with fewer implantation sites and also significantly altered fetal weight gain and development and delayed the date of parturition. The expression level of LIF in the whole uterus was also suppressed by IκBαM cDNA transfection and the number of implantation sites was significantly rescued after co-transfection with IκBαM and LIF cDNA.[156] These observations provide evidence that activation of NFκB in the uterine endometrium determined the timing of implantation, partly via activation of LIF expression.

Reportedly, the use of cationic lipids instead of anionic lipids as a liposome component dramatically reduces the in-vivo transfection efficiency,[157] despite the fact that cationic liposomes show excellent entrapment of negatively charged macromolecules such as DNA and highly efficient transfection of in-vitro cultured cells, whose plasma membranes are negatively charged. To circumvent the reduced in-vivo transfection efficiency, fusigenic non-viral particles were constructed by incorporating fusion proteins of HVJ (hemaglutinating virus of Japan; Sendai virus) into cDNA-loaded liposomes. These HVJ-liposomes showed higher efficiency of exogenous gene transfection in vivo.[157] More recently, macromolecules have been directly incorporated into inactivated HVJ particles without the use of mediating liposomes.[158]

GenomONE-NEO™ is a commercially available, inactivated HVJ-E vector purified by ion-exchange column chromatography supplied from Ishihara Sangyo Co. Ltd. (Osaka, Japan). This vector system has successfully been used to transfect exogenous genes such as luciferase cDNA into various organs in vivo with excellent transfection efficiency.[144,159]

Nakamura et al[160] introduced the HVJ-E vector into the murine uterine cavity on day 1.5 pc. Very strong luciferase activity was noted 24 hours after luciferase cDNA transfection, reportedly 120 times higher than the luciferase activity obtained by lipofectamineTM transfection. The luciferase activity continued for 3 days, suggesting exogenous cDNA may be expressed by this method at the opening of the implantation window of the mouse endometrium. Furthermore, after HVJ-E vector transfer, no difference in pregnancy rate, duration of pregnancy, litter size, birth weight, or crown–rump length of pups was noted and immunoreactivity of HVJ F-protein disappeared after 72 hours of transfection. Transfected DNA could not be detected in the fetus by polymerase chain reaction (PCR).

Collectively, these studies suggest that methods used for in-vivo gene transfer into the endometrium to study implantation physiology should have high efficiency of gene transfer into the endometrium, not interfere with the physiology of pregnancy, and the exogenous gene should not be transferred to the fetus. In-vivo gene transfer into mouse pregnant endometrium with HVJ-E vector satisfied these conditions.[157,159,160]

Other clinicians have designed promoter-specific, expression plasmid ligated cDNA when introducing exogenous cDNA with a non-viral vector system. Charnock-Jones et al,[145] Bagot et al,[145] and Hsieh et al[161] used plasmids driven by a cytomegalovirus (CMV) promoter. Yet other researchers have tested the Epstein–Barr (EB) virus replicon-based plasmid,[162] a plasmid containing the chicken β-actin promoter and enhancer called pAct-NII,[157] pEBAct (a fusion plasmid of the above two), and the CMV promoter-driven plasmid pcDNA3 (Invitrogen) with luciferase cDNA, and found that pcDNA3 showed the highest luciferase activity in the uterus within 24 hours of the transfection.

GenePORTER® (Gene Therapy Systems, Inc., San Diego, CA) is an example of a commercially available system that has also been used successfully in many tissues and cells. For example, in the mouse uterus, luciferase activity was identified after transfection of a CMV-driven luciferase cDNA.[161]

In the future, administration of such therapy in humans may be intrauterine via the cervix, thereby avoiding potential problems associated with systemic administration and the need for specific endometrial targeting. Gene transfer therapies hold significant promise for future medical applications.

IN-VITRO ANIMAL PARADIGMS

Extracorporeal paradigms

Extracorporeal perfusion of whole uteri through catheterization of the arterial vessels with hysterectomy specimens has been performed to evaluate actions of test agents added to the perfusion medium, to monitor endometrial synthetic and metabolic activities, and to study interactions with trophoblast cells.[163,164] Perfusions have been prolonged for 48–72 hours with retention of endometrial viability, as determined by evaluation of morphological and biochemical parameters. A potential limitation of this technique may be the availability of non-pathological uteri collected at hysterectomy.

Richter et al[165] performed extracorporeal perfusion of the human uterus collected after standard hysterectomy. The uteri were subjected to an isovolumetric exchange of perfusion medium at different intervals from 1 to 6 hours and examined for pH, pO_2, pCO_2, lactate, lactate dehydrogenase, and creatine kinase by taking arterial and venous samples every hour for 24 hours, while maintaining flow rates at 15–35 ml/min and at pressures ranging from 70 to 130 mmHg. Isovolumetric exchange of the perfusate every 3–4 hours was the maximum interval to keep pH, the arteriovenous gradients of pO_2 and pCO_2, and the other biochemical parameters in physiological ranges. Examination by light and electron microscopy showed well-preserved features of myometrial and endometrial tissue. However, a 6-hour exchanging interval led to increasing hypoxic and cytolytic parameters during the whole perfusion period. X-ray studies using digital subtraction angiography and perfusion studies with methylene blue demonstrated the homogeneous distribution of the perfusion fluid throughout the entire organ.

Analyses made from whole tissue have the advantage of maintaining their in-vivo spatial relationships; however, deciphering information about specific interactions of the various cell populations of the endometrium is challenging. It is well known that paracrine interactions between endometrial epithelial and stromal cells affect endometrial function, blastocyst implantation, and trophoblast invasion.

Endometrial tissue explant/organ culture paradigms

In-vitro tissue explant/organ culture has been used to study endometrial and placental function since as early as the 1920s. A historic review of studies utilizing intact endometrial tissue explants, maintained in vitro for several months, has been reviewed elsewhere.[166] Human endometrial tissues have been shown to remain viable and responsive to steroid, growth factor, and cytokine treatment for 1–2 weeks.[167–171]

A wide variety of experiments have been performed with endometrial tissue explants to study both normal and pathogenic events in the endometrium.[172,173]

Like extracorporeal perfusion of whole uteri, an advantage of tissue explant culture is that cellular elements are maintained in their in-situ organization, which facilitates paracrine interaction. Explant culture systems provide the opportunity to study mRNA extracted from the tissue explants and can be studied by Northern blot analysis, real-time quantitative PCR, or microarray analysis. The origin of these genes and the localization of their protein products can be determined by in-situ hybridization and immunohistochemistry, respectively. De-novo synthesis and secretion of endometrial products in the culture medium may also be identified by MALDI-TOF (matrix assisted laser desorption/ionization-time of flight) approaches. Tissue explant cultures may also be used to study several aspects of chemical carcinogenesis that cannot be contemplated in vivo.

The disadvantages of tissue explant culture include limited and variable viability during prolonged culture as a result of restricted nutrient flow and gas exchange. Furthermore, cellular heterogeneity of the explants confounds assignment of function to specific cell types. Choice of culture media and gas phase may also alter hormone synthesis and secretion by tissue explants and confound results. Damaged tissues release hydrolytic enzymes, which may lead to spurious results.

Tan et al[177] developed a model to study embryo implantation by co-culturing blastocysts with intact uterine endometrium from mice. In previous studies, embryos were cultured on a monolayer of either uterine epithelial cells or ECM substratum on which embryos could adhere and outgrow. These models failed to demonstrate embryonic invasion, probably due to the absence of critical structural and molecular supports that are available in vivo. Tan et al[174] demonstrated day 4 murine embryos co-cultured on intact mouse uterine endometrium collected on day 4 of pregnancy attached to the uterine endometrium and displayed partial invasion into the endometrial stroma. Interestingly, no outgrowth of trophoblasts on the surface of uterine endometrium was seen, while embryos exhibited a pole-specific attachment. As opposed to prior cell monolayer studies, this model demonstrated a true invasion of the blastocyst within the endometrial stroma and may be useful for studies of early embryo implantation.[174]

Endometrial cell culture paradigms

Endometrial cell culture models have provided a reasonable alternative to circumvent the challenges of whole tissue analyses. Endometrial cell culture models first appeared in the scientific literature around the 1970s, with dramatic advances in the culture paradigms occurring in the 1980s and 1990s. Using in-vitro models, regulators of endometrial function may be independently defined, free from confounding in-vivo interferences, and may be used to develop novel diagnostic and therapeutic treatment regimens for gynecological problems such as recurrent bleeding, spontaneous abortion, or inadequate placental growth and function.

Well-designed laboratory models that focus on molecular, cellular, and proteomic processes may be used to probe cause and effect relationships not otherwise accessible. In-vitro culture models also allow integration of molecular, cellular, and proteomic techniques to identify cell-specific, stage-specific markers that may focus on the mechanism of these disorders. In addition, more recent demands from animal protectionists may be satisfied by cell cultures and tissue models in biological, pharmacological, and toxicological assays.[171]

Endometrial epithelial cells grown on ECM, which start as monolayers of tadpole-shaped cells with prominent off-centered nuclei and whirling cell–cell processes that wrap around adjacent cells in vitro, form 3D mounds of epithelial cells that appear connected by tubular processes resembling glandular-like structures.[174–179]

Endometrial stromal cells display a homologous, cobblestone mosaic-like, single-cell monolayer pattern with centrally located nuclei, distinct cytoplasmic borders which do not overlap or demonstrate cell–cell processes. Endometrial stromal can be treated with physiological doses of ovarian hormones to induce characteristics of decidualization in vitro.[181] In general, the ultrastructural, proliferative, and biochemical changes induced by such treatment are characteristic of decidualization in vivo, providing an in-vitro model for human decidualization.

The literature now contains numerous publications reporting development of 3D cell culture models. Typical 3D models utilize human endometrial epithelial and stromal cells from hysterectomy specimens. Three-dimensional paradigms are established by overlaying a bottom collagen gel containing an endometrial stromal cell layer with an upper layer of Matrigel (BD BioSciences, San Jose, CA) containing endometrial epithelial cells.

While designing 3D models, it is also important to consider appropriate nutritive and adhesive factors, to allow access to components of optimal matrix, and to enable cell contacts in 3D. An interesting example of the importance for optimal cell contact is the finding that the ectopic implantation of embryonic cells transforms them into malignant tissue while the same cells located in the uterus undergo normal embryogenesis.[171]

In comparison with conventional cultures, structural and molecular analyses clearly showed that spatial cultures resemble the in-vivo situation with regard to cell shape and biological behavior, tissue differentiation, and paracrine interactions between the epithelial and stromal cell types, which are of paramount importance in vivo. Interactions of mesenchymal and epithelial cells have previously been shown to alter both morphological and functional characteristics of these cell types.[182,183] Critical endometrial stromal–epithelial cell interactions mediate steroid and growth factor-regulated expression of endometrial tissue factor as well as members of the plasminogen activator/inhibitor family, various members of the MMP/TIMP family, expression of integrins, and cyclooxygenases;[184–188] as such, these interactions mediate peri-implantation homeostasis and menstruation. Interactions between cultures of human endometrial cells and trophoblast cells have also provided insights into differential gene expression when the trophoblast cells are present.[189]

Yang et al[188] performed an ultrastructural examination of such cultures at 48 hours and found monolayered columnar epithelial cells with microvilli on the stromal cell collagen layer. The epithelial cells had tight junctions and desmosomes between the cells, a cell layer closely resembling the native endometrium. The endometrial epithelial cells showed a strong immunoreactivity for cytokeratin, integrin α_1, α_4, and β_3 subunits, COX-1 and -2, MMPs-1, -2, -3, and -9, and TIMPs-1 and -2 comparable to the native endometrial epithelium. The endometrial stromal cells showed stronger immunoreactivity for cyclooxygenases, integrins, and MMPs, but less for cytokeratin. Zymographic analyses of the media from the reconstructed endometrium model showed gelatinase activity bands at 57, 60, 72, 92, and 97 kDa molecular weight, respectively. Typically, when endometrial epithelial or stromal cells are cultured directly on plastic-ware, such responses are not found or diminished in nature.

In defining an in-vitro cell paradigm for embryo implantation, Negami[190] studied the importance of choosing the correct ECM. Type IV collagen and other ECM components were necessary mainly below the epithelial layer, whereas the stromal layer was diffusely located in type I and III collagens. A lower stromal layer and superficial myometrial layer consisting of, primarily, type V collagen was present. With this paradigm, human and rabbit endometrial epithelial cells underwent re-epithelialization following glandular formation. Estrogen added to the culture media stimulated the glandular formation. Progesterone administration after estrogen priming did not affect the glandular formation; however, the proliferation of the superficial epithelium and the re-epithelialized area were increased.

Rabbit blastocysts successfully attached and implanted into the reconstructed endometrium and development of the implanted embryos was morphologically normal. Human cultured trophoblast cells attached, invaded, and penetrated into the ECM components. Using type V collagen-coated dishes, trophoblast cells could invade the stromal layer; however, the type V collagen layer did not permit the trophoblast cells to invade into the

collagen layer. In vivo, type V collagen, expressed in the lower stromal layer and the surface of the myometrium, may play a role to limit early embryo invasion to the decidual compartment.[190]

Other clinicians have used 3D models to study the disease of endometriosis. Proliferative and morphogenic changes were identified when uterine epithelial and stromal cells and peritoneal mesothelial and subserosal cells were co-cultured with homologous cell types, heterologous cell types, or as isolated populations using a bicameral chamber design.[191] It was found that peritoneal mesothelial cells augmented proliferation and induced cellular aggregation of uterine stromal cell monolayers while peritoneal subserosal cells amplified proliferation and induced an irregular, compacted morphology in uterine epithelial cells. The proliferation and morphology of the two peritoneal cell types was not altered by uterine cell co-culture.

Fasciani et al[192] used endometrial samples in a 3D fibrin matrix culture system to study the degree of proliferation of stromal cells and invasion of the fibrin matrix, gland, and stroma formation, vessel sprouting, and immunohistochemical characterization of various cellular components. They observed that endometrial cells proliferated and invaded the fibrin matrix in vitro, and that new glands, stroma, and vessels were generated as consistent with endometriosis.

Immortalized cells

Collection of endometrial cells for culture from hysterectomy specimens limits control of the type and normalcy of specimen arriving in the laboratory. Furthermore, primary cells often dedifferentiate in culture within 1–2 weeks. Therefore, immortalized endometrial cells have been developed and validated as more controlled experimental paradigms.

Brosens et al[193] immortalized human endometrial fibroblasts by infection with simian virus 40 large T antigen and established as a permanent cell line, St-2. Differentiation of this cell line was maintained as demonstrated and thoroughly validated by the ability of a decidualizing stimulus, 8-bromo-cAMP + medroxyprogesterone acetate, to induce prolactin secretion and increase the enzymatic activity of estrone sulfatase.

Kyo et al[194] established immortalized human endometrial glandular cells that retain normal functions and characteristics of primary cells. Because the Rb/p16 and p53 pathways are known to be critical elements of epithelial senescence in early passages, human papillomavirus E6/E7 was used to assess these pathways. The combination of human papillomavirus-16 E6/E7 expression and telomerase activation by the introduction of human telomerase reverse transcriptase (hTERT) led to successful immortalization of the endometrial glandular cells. E6/E7 expression alone was sufficient to extend their life span more than 20 population doublings, but the telomerase activation was further required to enable the cells to pass through the subsequent replicative senescence at 40 population doublings. No chromosomal abnormalities or only non-clonal aberrations were noted, responsiveness to sex steroid hormones was retained, the cells exhibited glandular structure on 3D culture, and lacked transformed phenotypes on soft agar or in nude mice. Endometrial stromal cells have also been immortalized by transfection of cells with vectors expressing the catalytic subunit of hTERT.[195]

MATHEMATICAL MODELS

Computer-generated mathematical models have been used to generate 3D reconstruction of histological parallel serial sections displaying microvascular and glandular structures in human endometrium.[196] High-resolution 3D images of microvasculature structures in curettage, hysterectomy, or endometrial resection biopsies using parallel histological serial sections were assessed. Tissues were stained with mouse anti-human QBEnd-10, using a streptavidin–biotin–alkaline phosphatase method and visualized by using diaminobenzidine. The images were directly digitized from a light microscope into the KS400 Universal Image Processing and Analysis software via a CCD color camera; binary images of the structures were created and the binary images were exported into VoxBlast 3D rendering software to view still and rotating 3D images on a computer monitor. This in turn enabled hard copies of the full sequence to be printed.

Blumenson and Bross[198] described a mathematical model to bridge the relationship between the observations in the clinic and underlying movements of the individual tumor cells. The model was used to assess the efficacy of preoperative radiation treatment in reducing the visible size of endometrial tumors, thereby providing a quantitative estimate of the radiation effect. The model was also used to estimate the motility of tumor cells in vivo and this was compared with measurements obtained in the laboratory. Other clinicians have also applied mathematical models to a clinical study of the local spread of endometrial cancer and to bridge the clinic–laboratory gap[197,198] and for light dosimetry in photodynamic destruction of human endometrium.[199]

SUMMARY

In summary, as controlled investigations of endometrial biology in women are restricted due to ethical considerations and limited accessibility of human endometrial tissue, a variety of paradigms have been developed to study endometrial function and pathology. Non-human primates are the most closely related animal model for studying events related to the human endometrium. Unfortunately, studies involving primates are limited by cost, by the number of animals available for such procedures, and the same ethical problems of performing repetitive surgical procedures as in humans.

Beyond the primate, the majority of in-vivo endometrial paradigms have been developed in rodents. Knockout mice, transgenic reporter mice, and surgical models have provided important insights into normal and pathological endometrial function. Due to the limits imposed on in-vivo endometrial studies in women, these animal models are essential to our understanding of the molecular and mechanical events of normal endometrial function, embryo implantation, and endometrial disease including endometriosis. In addition, these animal models have successfully been used in pharmacological, toxicology and gene therapy studies.

In-vitro model systems have also been developed including whole tissue perfusion, tissue fragment explant culture, isolated cell and 3D cell models. In addition to clinically relevant information, these models have provided insight and enhanced our understanding of endometrial cell biology, physiology, biochemistry, and pathophysiology.

While extracorporeal perfusion and tissue explant culture paradigms provide a more in situ relationship of endometrial components, they provide little information regarding the interactions of the various cell populations of the endometrium. In-vitro 3D endometrial cell culture models resemble the in-vivo situation with regard to cell shape and biological behavior, tissue differentiation and paracrine interactions between the epithelial and stromal cell types, which are of paramount importance in vivo. The behavior of endometrial cells in vitro depends on the source and in-vivo state of the endometrial cells used for the model, the purity of cell preparations, culture conditions, the nature of the ECM used in the model and their duration in culture. These models may be used to study physiological events at the cellular and molecular levels, enhance our knowledge of biochemical effects of steroids, growth factors, pharmacological agents and immunomodulatory agents on the cells, study embryo implantation, and assess endometriosis.

Immortalized endometrial cell lines have been developed and validated as more controlled experimental paradigms. Defined cellular components, maintenance of a differentiated state and preservation of in-vivo characteristics are essential. Immortalized endometrial cell lines serve as powerful tools to address mechanisms underlying growth, differentiation and specific gene expression in uterine epithelial and stromal cells.

Computer-generated mathematical models have been used to generate 3D reconstruction of histological parallel serial sections displaying microvascular and glandular structures in human endometrium, bridge the relationship between the observations in the clinic and underlying movements of the individual tumor cells, assess the efficacy of preoperative radiation treatment in reducing the visible size of endometrial tumors and for light dosimetry in photodynamic destruction of human endometrium. Recent demands from animal protectionists may be satisfied by human tissue and cell culture models and mathematical model for biological, pharmacological, and toxicological assays.

Ultimately, validation of any model system is of paramount importance. Models that do not recapitulate the in-vivo condition are invalid and often infect the literature with confusing and often conflicting data. Valid endometrial paradigms enhance our understanding of endometrial function and disease including various aspects of cell proliferation and differentiation, steroid hormone, growth factor and cytokine responsiveness and action, autocrine and paracrine communication within and between endometrial cells and with the embryo and interactions with the extracellular matrix, tumorigenesis, and the effects of various pharmacological, immunomodulatory, xenobiotic and gene therapy approaches on endometrial function at the molecular, cellular, and proteomic levels, most with a similar translational goal for therapeutic use.

REFERENCES

1. Denker HW. Endometrial receptivity: cell biological aspects of an unusual epithelium. A review. Ann Anat 1994; 176: 53–60.
2. de Ziegler D, Fanchin R, de Moustier B et al. The hormonal control of endometrial receptivity: estrogen (E2) and progesterone. J Reprod Immunol 1998; 39: 149–66.
3. Ghosh D, Sengupta J. Endocrine and paracrine correlates of endometrial receptivity to blastocyst implantation in the human. Indian J Physiol Pharmacol 2004; 48: 6–30.
4. Kodaman PH, Taylor HS. Hormonal regulation of implantation. Obstet Gynecol Clin North Am 2004; 31: 745–66.
5. Beier HM, Beier-Hellwig K. Molecular and cellular aspects of endometrial receptivity. Hum Reprod Update 1998; 4: 448–58.
6. Sharpe-Timms KL, Glasser SR. Models for the study of uterine receptivity for blastocyst implantation. Semin Reprod Endocrinol 1999; 17: 107–15.
7. Lessey BA. Endometrial receptivity and the window of implantation. Baillières Best Pract Res Clin Obstet Gynaecol 2000; 14: 775–88.
8. Simon C, Martin JC, Pellicer A. Paracrine regulators of implantation. Baillières Best Pract Res Clin Obstet Gynaecol 2000; 14: 815–26.
9. Paria BC, Reese J, Das SK et al. Deciphering the cross-talk of implantation: advances and challenges. Science 2002; 296: 2185–8.
10. Rosario G, Sachdeva G, Okulicz WC et al. Role of progesterone in structural and biochemical remodeling of endometrium. Front Biosci 2003; 8: s924–35.
11. Cavagna M, Mantese JC. Biomarkers of endometrial receptivity – a review. Placenta 2003; 24(Suppl B): S39–47.
12. Horcajadas JA, Riesewijk A, Dominguez F et al. Determinants of endometrial receptivity. Ann NY Acad Sci 2004; 1034: 166–75.
13. Arnold LL, Asher SM, Schruefer JJ et al. The nonsurgical diagnosis of adenomyosis. Obstet Gynecol 1995; 3: 461–5.
14. Togashi K, Nishimura K, Itoh K et al. Adenomyosis: diagnosis with MR imaging. Radiology 1988; 166: 111–14.
15. Bradley LD, Falcone T, Magen AB. Radiographic imaging techniques for the diagnosis of abnormal uterine bleeding. Obstet Gynecol Clin North Am 2000; 27: 245–76.
16. Kunz G, Beil D, Huppert P, Leyendecker G. Structural abnormalities of the uterine wall in women with endometriosis and infertility visualized by vaginal sonography and magnetic resonance imaging. Hum Reprod 2000; 15: 76–82.
17. Gerety E, Harris RD. Endometriosis: epidemiology, current pathophysiological concepts, and imaging considerations. Appl Radiol 2001: 11–18.
18. Moore CM, Janish C, Eddy CA et al. Cytogenetic and fertility studies of a rheboon, rhesus macaque (*Macaca mulatta*) × baboon (*Papio hamadryas*) cross: further support for a single karyotype nomenclature. Am J Phys Anthropol 1999; 110: 119–27.
19. Stouffer RL. Pre-ovulatory events in the rhesus monkey follicle during ovulation induction. Reprod Biomed Online 2002; 4(Suppl 3): 1–4.
20. Hewitson L, Schatten G. The use of primates as models for assisted reproduction. Reprod Biomed Online 2002; 5: 50–5.
21. Kubisch HM, Ratterree MS, Williams VM et al. Birth of rhesus macaque (*Macaca mulatta*) infants after in vitro fertilization and gestation in female rhesus or pigtailed (*Macaca nemestrina*) macaques. Comp Med 2005; 55: 129–35.
22. Brenner RM, Rudolph L, Matrisian L et al. Non-human primate models; artificial menstrual cycles, endometrial matrix metalloproteinases and s.c. endometrial grafts. Hum Reprod 1996; 11(Suppl 2): 150–64.
23. Qin L, Wang YL, Bai SX et al. Temporal and spatial expression of integrins and their extracellular matrix ligands at the maternal–fetal interface in the rhesus monkey during pregnancy. Biol Reprod 2003; 69: 563–71.
24. Wei P, Chen XL, Song XX et al. VEGF, bFGF, and their receptors in the endometrium of rhesus monkey during menstrual cycle and early pregnancy. Mol Reprod Dev 2004; 68: 456–62.
25. Sun T, Li SJ, Diao HL et al. Cyclooxygenases and prostaglandin E synthases in the endometrium of the rhesus monkey during the menstrual cycle. Reprod 2004; 127: 465–73.
26. Ace CI, Okulicz WC. Differential gene regulation by estrogen and progesterone in the primate endometrium. Mol Cell Endocrin 1995; 115: 95–103.
27. Brenner RM, Slayden OD. Steroid receptors in blood vessels of the rhesus macaque endometrium: a review. Arch Histol Cytol 2004; 67: 411–16.

28. Critchley HO, Brenner RM, Henderson TA et al. Estrogen receptor beta, but not estrogen receptor alpha, is present in the vascular endothelium of the human and nonhuman primate endometrium. J Clin Endocrinol Metab 2001; 86: 1370–8.

29. Goldsmith LT, Weiss G. Relaxin regulates endometrial structure and function in the rhesus monkey. Ann NY Acad Sci 2005; 1041: 110–17.

30. Golos TG. Pregnancy initiation in the rhesus macaque: towards functional manipulation of the maternal–fetal interface. Reprod Biol Endocrinol 2004; 2: 35.

31. Patton DL, Kidder GG, Sweeney YC et al. Effects of nonoxynol-9 on vaginal microflora and chlamydial infection in a monkey model. Sex Transm Dis 1996; 23: 461–4.

32. Patton DL, Sweeney YT, McKay TL et al. 0.25% chlorhexidine gluconate gel. A protective topical microbicide. Sex Transm Dis 1998; 25: 421–4.

33. Patton DL, Sweeney YT, Stamm WE. Significant reduction in inflammatory response in the macaque model of chlamydial pelvic inflammatory disease with azithromycin treatment. J Infect Dis 2005; 192: 129–35.

34. Trisomboon H, Malaivijitnond S, Watanabe G et al. Ovulation block by Pueraria mirifica: a study of its endocrinological effect in female monkeys. Endocrine 2005; 26: 33–9.

35. Fraser HM, Wilson H, Rudge JS et al. Single injections of vascular endothelial growth factor trap block ovulation in the macaque and produce a prolonged, dose-related suppression of ovarian function. J Clin Endocrinol Metab 2005; 90: 1114–22.

36. Siler-Khodr TM, Yu FQ, Wei P et al. Contraceptive action of a gonadotropin-releasing hormone II analog in the rhesus monkey. J Clin Endocrinol Metab 2004; 89: 4513–20.

37. Jensen JT, Rodriguez MI, Liechtenstein-Zabrak J et al. Transcervical polidocanol as a nonsurgical method of female sterilization: a pilot study. Contraception 2004; 70: 111–15.

38. Sengupta J, Dhawan L, Lalitkumar PGL et al. A multiparametric study of the action of mifepristone used in emergency contraception using the rhesus monkey as a primate model. Contraception 2003; 68: 453–69.

39. Yamamoto Y, Thau RB. Characterizations of anti-oLH beta antibodies acting as contraceptives in rhesus monkeys. II. In vivo neutralizing ability for gonadotropic hormones. J Reprod Immunol 1983; 5: 195–202.

40. Jainkittivong A, Langlais RP. Herpes B virus infection. Oral Surg Oral Med Oral Pathol Oral Radiol Endod 1998; 85: 399–403.

41. D'Hooghe TM, Nugent NP, Cuneo S et al. Recombinant human TNFRSF1A (r-hTBP1) inhibits the development of endometriosis in baboons: a prospective, randomized, placebo- and drug-controlled study. Biol Reprod 2006; 74: 131–6.

42. Fazleabas AT. A baboon model for inducing endometriosis. Methods Mol Med 2006; 121: 95–9.

43. Fazleabas AT. A baboon model for simulating pregnancy. Methods Mol Med 2006; 121: 101–10.

44. Fazleabas AT, Verhage HG. A simple technique for sampling the uterine cavity of the baboon. Theriogenology 1987; 27: 645–53.

45. Strakova Z, Srisuparp S, Fazleabas AT. Interleukin-1beta induces the expression of insulin-like growth factor binding protein-1 during decidualization in the primate. Endocrinology 2000; 141: 4664–70.

46. Strakova Z, Mavrogianis P, Meng X et al. In vivo infusion of interleukin-1beta and chorionic gonadotropin induces endometrial changes that mimic early pregnancy events in the baboon. Endocrinology 2005; 146: 4097–104.

47. Kim JJ, Jaffe RC, Fazleabas AT. Comparative studies on the in vitro decidualization process in the baboon (*Papio anubis*) and human. Biol Reprod 1998; 59: 160–8.

48. Kim JJ, Fazleabas AT. Uterine receptivity and implantation: the regulation and action of insulin-like growth factor binding protein-1 (IGFBP-1), HOXA10 and forkhead transcription factor-1 (FOXO-1) in the baboon endometrium. Reprod Biol Endocrinol 2004; 16: 2–34.

49. Srisuparp S, Strakova Z, Brudney A et al. Signal transduction pathways activated by chorionic gonadotropin in the primate endometrial epithelial cells. Biol Reprod 2003; 68: 457–64.

50. Jones CJ, Enders AC, Fazleabas AT. Early implantation events in the baboon (*Papio anubis*) with special reference to the establishment of anchoring villi. Placenta 2001; 22: 440–56.

51. Niklaus AL, Babischkin JS, Aberdeen GW et al. Expression of vascular endothelial growth/permeability factor by endometrial glandular epithelial and stromal cells in baboons during the menstrual cycle and after ovariectomy. Endocrinology 2002; 143: 4007–17.

52. D'Hooghe TM, Bambra CS, Cornillie FJ et al. Prevalence and laparoscopic appearance of spontaneous endometriosis in the baboon (*Papio anubis, Papio cynocephalus*). Biol Reprod 1991; 45: 411–16.

53. D'Hooghe TM, Bambra CS, Raeymaekers BM et al. Increased prevalence and recurrence of retrograde menstruation in baboons with spontaneous endometriosis. Hum Reprod 1996; 11: 2022–5.

54. D'Hooghe TM, Bambra CS, Raeymaekers BM et al. Intrapelvic injection of menstrual endometrium causes endometriosis in baboons (*Papio cynocephalus, Papio anubis*). Am J Obstet Gynecol 1995; 173: 125–34.

55. Fazleabas AT, Brudney A, Gurates B et al. A modified baboon model for endometriosis. Ann NY Acad Sci 2002; 955: 308–17.

56. Barrier BF, Bates GW, Leland MM et al. Efficacy of anti-tumor necrosis factor therapy in the treatment of spontaneous endometriosis in baboons. Fertil Steril 2004; 81(Suppl 1): 775–9.

57. D'Hooghe TM, Bambra CS, Suleman MA et al. Development of a model of retrograde menstruation in baboons (*Papio anubis*). Fertil Steril 1994; 62: 635–8.

58. D'Hooghe TM, Debrock S, Kyama CM et al. Baboon model for fundamental and preclinical research in endometriosis. Gynecol Obstet Invest 2004; 57: 43–6.

59. Coelho AM Jr, Carey KD. A social tethering system for nonhuman primates used in laboratory research. Lab Anim Sci 1990; 40: 388–94.

60. Seier JV, Chwalisz K, Louw J et al. Endometrial function in vervet monkeys (*Cercopithecus aethiops*): morphology, beta3 integrin and insulin-like growth factor binding protein-1 expression during the menstrual cycle and pregnancy in the normal and disrupted endometrium. J Med Primatol 2002; 31: 330–9.

61. Owiti GE, Cukierski M, Tarara RP et al. Early placentation in the African green monkey (*Cercopithecus aethiops*). Acta Anat (Basel) 1986; 127: 184–94.

62. Kudolo GB, Mbai FN, Eley RM. Reproduction in the vervet monkey (*Cercopithecus aethiops*): endometrial estrogen and progestin receptor dynamics during normal and prolonged menstrual cycles. J Endocrinol 1986; 110: 429–39.

63. Palmer AE, London WT, Sly DL et al. Spontaneous preeclamptic toxemia of pregnancy in the patas monkey (*Erythrocebus patas*). Lab Anim Sci 1979; 29: 102–6.

64. Gille JH, Moore DG, Sedgwick CJ. Placental infarction: a sign of pre-eclampsia in a patas monkey (*Erythrocebus patas*). Lab Anim Sci 1977; 27: 119–21.

65. Harding RD, Hulme MJ, Lunn SF et al. Plasma progesterone levels throughout the ovarian cycle of the common marmoset (*Callithrix jacchus*). J Med Primatol 1982; 11: 43–51.

66. Harlow CR, Gems S, Hodges JK et al. The relationship between plasma progesterone and the timing of ovulation

and early embryonic development in the marmoset monkey (*Callithrix jacchus*). J Zool Lond 1983; 201: 273–82.

67. Harlow CR, Hearn JP, Hodges JK. Ovulation in the marmoset monkey: endocrinology, prediction and detection. J Endocrinol 1984; 103: 17–24.

68. Rune GM, Leuchtenberg U, Schroter-Kermani C et al. Zonal differentiation of the marmoset (*Callithrix jacchus*) endometrium. J Anat 1992; 181: 301–12.

69. Kholkute SD, Katkam RR, Nandedkar TD et al. Leukaemia inhibitory factor in the endometrium of the common marmoset *Callithrix jacchus*: localization, expression and hormonal regulation. Mol Hum Reprod 2000; 6: 337–43.

70. Dalrymple A, Jabbour HN. Localization and signaling of the prolactin receptor in the uterus of the common marmoset monkey. J Clin Endocrinol Metab 2000; 85: 1711–18.

71. Einspanier A, Muller D, Lubberstedt J et al. Characterization of relaxin binding in the uterus of the marmoset monkey. Mol Hum Reprod 2001; 7: 963–70.

72. Kholkute SD, Nandedkar TD, Puri CP. Localization of estrogen and progesterone receptors in the endometrium of common marmosets *Callithrix jacchus*. Indian J Exp Biol 2000; 38: 425–31.

73. Rowe AJ, Wulff C, Fraser HM. Angiogenesis and microvascular development in the marmoset (*Callithrix jacchus*) endometrium during early pregnancy. Reproduction 2004; 128: 107–16.

74. Jones CPJ, Fazleabas AT, McGinlay PB et al. Cyclic modulation of epithelial glycosylation in human and baboon (*Papio anubis*) endometrium demonstrated by the binding of the agglutinin from Dolichos biflorus. Biol Reprod 1998; 58: 20–7.

75. Bany BM, Cross JC. Post-implantation mouse conceptuses produce paracrine signals that regulate the uterine endometrium undergoing decidualization. Dev Biol 2006; 294: 445–56.

76. Lee KY, DeMayo FJ. Animal models of implantation. Reproduction 2004; 128: 679–95.

77. Tranguch S, Daikoku T, Guo Y et al. Molecular complexity in establishing uterine receptivity and implantation. Cell Mol Life Sci 2005; 62: 1964–73.

78. Lubahn DB, Moyer JS, Golding TS et al. Alteration of reproductive function but not prenatal sexual development after insertional disruption of the mouse estrogen receptor gene. Proc Natl Acad Sci USA 1993; 90: 11162–6.

79. Krege JH, Hodgin JB, Couse JF et al. Generation and reproductive phenotypes of mice lacking estrogen receptor beta. Proc Natl Acad Sci USA 1998; 95: 15677–82.

80. Dupont S, Krust A, Gansmuller A et al. Effect of single and compound knockouts of estrogen receptors alpha (ERalpha) and beta (ERbeta) on mouse reproductive phenotypes. Development 2000; 127: 4277–91.

81. Cooke PS, Buchanan DL, Young P et al. Stromal estrogen receptors mediate mitogenic effects of estradiol on uterine epithelium. Proc Natl Acad Sci USA 1997; 94: 6535–40.

82. Fisher CR, Graves KH, Parlow AF et al. Characterization of mice deficient in aromatase (ArKO) because of targeted disruption of the cyp19 gene. Proc Natl Acad Sci USA 1998; 95: 6965–70.

83. Britt KL, Drummond AE, Cox VA et al. An age-related ovarian phenotype in mice with targeted disruption of the Cyp 19 (aromatase) gene. Endocrinology 2000; 141: 2614–23.

84. Lydon JP, DeMayo FJ, Funk CR et al. Mice lacking progesterone receptor exhibit pleiotropic reproductive abnormalities. Genes Dev 1995; 9: 2266–78.

85. Conneely OM, Mulac-Jericevic B, Lydon JP et al. Reproductive functions of the progesterone receptor isoforms: lessons from knock-out mice. Mol Cell Endocrinol 2001; 179: 97–103.

86. Onate SA, Tsai SY, Tsai MJ et al. Sequence and characterization of a coactivator for the steroid hormone receptor superfamily. Science 1995; 270: 1354–7.

87. Xu J, Qiu Y, DeMayo FJ, Tsai SY. Partial hormone resistance in mice with disruption of the steroid receptor coactivator-1(SRC-1) gene. Science 1998; 279: 1922–5.

88. Xu J, Liao L, Ning G et al. The steroid receptor coactivator SRC-3 (p/CIP/RAC3/AIB1/ACTR/TRAM-1) is required for normal growth, puberty, female reproductive function, and mammary gland development. Proc Natl Acad Sci USA 2000; 97: 6379–84.

89. Nagel SC, Hagelbarger JL, McDonnell DP. Development of an ER action indicator mouse for the study of estrogens, selective ER modulators (SERMs), and Xenobiotics. Endocrinology 2001; 142: 4721–8.

90. Ciana P, Di Luccio G, Belcredito S et al. Engineering of a mouse for the in vivo profiling of estrogen receptor activity. Mol Endocrinol 2001; 15: 1104–13.

91. Lemmen JG, Arends RJ, van Boxtel AL et al. Tissue- and time-dependent estrogen receptor activation in estrogen reporter mice. J Mol Endocrinol 2004; 32: 689–701.

92. Shang Y, Brown M. Molecular determinants for the tissue specificity of SERMs. Science 2002; 295: 2465–8.

93. Paech K, Webb P, Kuiper GG et al. Differential ligand activation of estrogen receptors ERalpha and ERbeta at AP1 sites. Science 1997; 277: 1508–10.

94. Lemmen JG, Arends RJ, van der Saag PT et al. In vivo imaging of activated estrogen receptors in utero by estrogens and bisphenol A. Environ Health Perspect 2004; 112: 1544–9.

95. Welshons WV, Nagel SC, Vom Saal FS. Large effects from small exposures. III. Endocrine mechanisms mediating effects of bisphenol A at levels of human exposure. Endocrinology 2006; 147(6 Suppl): S56–69.

96. Harris HA, Bruner-Tran KL, Zhang X et al. A selective estrogen receptor-beta agonist causes lesion regression in an experimentally induced model of endometriosis. Hum Reprod 2005; 20: 936–41.

97. Vernon MW, Wilson EA. Studies on the surgical induction of endometriosis in the rat. Fertil Steril 1985; 44: 684–94.

98. Cummings AM, Metcalf JL. Induction of endometriosis in mice: a new model sensitive to estrogen. Reprod Toxicol 1995; 9: 233–8.

99. Moon CE, Bertero MB, Curry TE et al. The presence of luteinized unruptured follicle syndrome (LUFS) and altered folliculogenesis in rats with surgically induced endometriosis. Am J Obstet Gynecol 1993; 169: 676–82.

100. Berkley KJ, Dmitrieva N, Curtis KS et al. Innervation of ectopic endometrium in a rat model of endometriosis. Proc Natl Acad Sci USA 2004; 101: 11094–8.

101. Cason AM, Samuelsen CL, Berkley KJ. Estrous changes in vaginal nociception in a rat model of endometriosis. Horm Behav 2003; 44: 123–31.

102. Sharpe KL, Bertero MC, Vernon MW. Follicular atresia and infertility in rats treated with a gonadotropin releasing hormone (GnRH) antagonist. Endocrinology 1990; 127: 25–31.

103. Sharpe-Timms KL, Zimmer RL, Jolliff WJ et al. Gonadotropin-releasing hormone agonist (GnRHa) therapy alters activity of plasminogen activators (PA), matrix metalloproteinases (MMP) and of their inhibitors (PAI and MMPI) in rat models for adhesion formation and endometriosis: potential GnRHa-regulated mechanisms reducing adhesion formation. Fertil Steril 1998; 69: 916–23.

104. Sharpe-Timms KL, Keisler LW, McIntush EW et al. Tissue inhibitor of metalloproteinase-1 (TIMP-1) concentrations are attenuated in peritoneal fluid and sera of women with endometriosis and restored in sera by gonadotropin-releasing hormone agonist (GnRHa) therapy. Fertil Steril 1998; 69: 1128–34.

105. Wright JA, Sharpe-Timms KL. Gonadotropin-releasing hormone agonist (GnRHa) therapy reduces postoperative adhesion formation and reformation following adhesiolysis in rat

models for adhesion formation and endometriosis. Fertil Steril 1995; 63: 1094–100.

106. Ozdemir I, Ustundag N, Guven A et al. Effect of clomiphene citrate on ovarian, endometrial, and cervical histologies in a rat model. Gynecol Obstet Invest 2005; 60: 181–5.

107. Qu F, Zhou J, Ma B. The effect of Chinese herbs on the cytokines of rats with endometriosis. J Alternative Complementary Med 2005; 11: 627–30.

108. Sharpe KL, Bertero MC, Vernon MW. Spontaneous and steroid-induced recurrence of endometriosis following suppression by a gonadotropin releasing hormone antagonist in the rat. Am J Obstet Gynecol 1991; 164: 187–94.

109. Sharpe KL, Zimmer RL, Griffin WT et al. Polypeptides synthesized and released by human endometriosis tissue differ from those of the uterine endometrium in culture. Fertil Steril 1993; 60: 839–51.

110. Sharpe KL, Vernon MW. Polypeptides synthesized and released by rat ectopic uterine implants differ from those of the uterus in culture. Biol Reprod 1993; 48: 1334–40.

111. Sharpe-Timms KL, Penney LL, Zimmer RL et al. Partial purification and amino acid sequence analysis of endometriosis protein-II (ENDO-II) reveals homology with tissue inhibitor of metalloproteinases-1 (TIMP-1). J Clin Endocrin Metab 1995; 80: 3784–7.

112. Sharpe-Timms KL, Piva M, Ricke EA et al. Endometriotic lesions synthesize and secrete a haptoglobin-like protein. Biol Reprod 1998; 58: 988–94.

113. Piva M, Sharpe-Timms KL. Peritoneal endometriotic lesions differentially express a haptoglobin-like gene. Mol Hum Reprod 1999; 5: 71–8.

114. Sharpe-Timms KL, Ricke EA, Piva M et al. Differential in vivo expression and localization of endometriosis protein-I (ENDO-I), a haptoglobin homologue, in endometrium and endometriotic lesions. Hum Reprod 2000; 15: 2180–5.

115. Cox KE, Piva M, Sharpe-Timms KL. Differential regulation of matrix metalloproteinase-3 gene expression in endometriotic lesions as compared to endometrium. Biol Reprod 2001; 65: 1297–303.

116. Sharpe-Timms KL, Zimmer RL, Ricke EA et al. Endometriotic haptoglobin binds peritoneal macrophages and alters their function in endometriosis. Fertil Steril 2002; 78: 810–19.

117. Piva MA, Moreno I, Sharpe-Timms KL. Glycosylation and over-expression of endometriosis-associated peritoneal haptoglobin. Glycoconj J 2003; 19: 33–41.

118. Gottschalk C, Malberg K, Arndt M et al. Matrix metalloproteinases and TACE play a role in the pathogenesis of endometriosis. Adv Exp Med Biol 2000; 477: 483–6.

119. Szamatowicz J, Laudanski P, Tomaszewska I. Matrix metalloproteinase-9 and tissue inhibitor of matrix metalloproteinase-1: a possible role in the pathogenesis of endometriosis. Hum Reprod 2002; 17: 284–8.

120. Osteen KG, Yeaman GR, Bruner-Tran KL. Matrix metalloproteinases and endometriosis. Semin Reprod Med 2003; 21: 155–64.

121. Uzan C, Cortez A, Dufournet C et al. Eutopic endometrium and peritoneal, ovarian and bowel endometriotic tissues express a different profile of matrix metalloproteinases-2, -3 and -11, and of tissue inhibitor metalloproteinases-1 and -2. Virchows Archiv 2004; 445: 603–9.

122. Laudanski P, Szamatowicz J, Ramel P. Matrix metalloproteinase-13 and membrane type-1 matrix metalloproteinase in peritoneal fluid of women with endometriosis. Gynecol Endocrinol 2005; 21: 106–10.

123. Osteen KG, Bruner-Tran KL, Eisenberg E. Reduced progesterone action during endometrial maturation: a potential risk factor for the development of endometriosis. Fertil Steril 2005; 83: 529–37.

124. Grummer R, Schwarzer F, Bainczyk K et al. Peritoneal endometriosis: validation of an in-vivo model. Hum Reprod 2001; 16: 1736–43.

125. Bruner-Tran KL, Webster-Clair D, Osteen KG. Experimental endometriosis: the nude mouse as a xenographic host. Ann NY Acad Sci 2002; 955: 328–39.

126. Bruner-Tran KL, Zhang Z, Eisenberg E et al. Down-regulation of endometrial matrix metalloproteinase-3 and -7 expression in vitro and therapeutic regression of experimental endometriosis in vivo by a novel non-steroidal progesterone receptor agonist, tanaproget. J Clin Endocrinol Metabol 2006; 91: 1554–60.

127. Somigliana E, Vigano P, Rossi G et al. Endometrial ability to implant in ectopic sites can be prevented by interleukin-12 in a murine model of endometriosis. Hum Reprod 1999; 14: 2944–50.

128. Somigliana E, Vigano P, Zingrillo B et al. Induction of endometriosis in the mouse inhibits spleen leukocyte function. Acta Obstet Gynecol Scand 2001; 80: 200–5.

129. Hirata T, Osuga Y, Yoshino O et al. Development of an experimental model of endometriosis using mice that ubiquitously express green fluorescent protein. Hum Reprod 2005; 20: 2092–6.

130. Okabe M, Ikawa M, Kominami K et al. 'Green mice' as a source of ubiquitous green cells. FEBS Lett 1997; 407: 313–19.

131. Fortin M, Lepine M, Page M et al. An improved mouse model for endometriosis allows noninvasive assessment of lesion implantation and development. Fertil Steril 2003; 80(Suppl 2): 832–8.

132. Defrere S, Van Langendonckt A, Ramos RG et al. Quantification of endometriotic lesions in a murine model by fluorimetric and morphometric analyses. Hum Reprod 2006; 21: 810–17.

133. Hull ML, Charnock-Jones DS, Chan CL et al. Antiangiogenic agents are effective inhibitors of endometriosis. J Clin Endocrinol Metabol 2003; 88: 2889–99.

134. Hull ML, Prentice A, Wang DY et al. Nimesulide, a COX-2 inhibitor, does not reduce lesion size or number in a nude mouse model of endometriosis. Hum Reprod 2005; 20: 350–8.

135. Nap AW, Griffioen AW, Dunselman GA et al. Antiangiogenesis therapy for endometriosis. J Clin Endocrinol Metabol 2004; 89: 1089–95.

136. Eggermont J, Donnez J, Casanas-Roux F et al. Time course of pelvic endometriotic lesion revascularization in a nude mouse model. Fertil Steril 2005; 84: 492–9.

137. Zaino RJ, Satyaswaroop PG, Mortel R. Histologic response of normal human endometrium to steroid hormones in athymic mice. Hum Pathol 1985; 16: 867–72.

138. Bruner-Tran KL, Rier SE, Eisenberg E et al. The potential role of environmental toxins in the pathophysiology of endometriosis. Gynecol Obstet Invest 1999; 48(Suppl 1): 45–56.

139. Satyaswaroop PG, Zaino RJ, Mortel R. Steroid receptors and human endometrial carcinoma: studies in a nude mouse model. Cancer Metastasis Rev 1987; 6: 223–41.

140. Zaino RJ, Satyaswaroop PG, Mortel R. Hormonal therapy of human endometrial adenocarcinoma in a nude mouse model. Cancer Res 1985; 45: 539–41.

141. Riondel J, Jacrot M, Picot F et al. Therapeutic response to taxol of six human tumors xenografted into nude mice. Cancer Chemother Pharmacol 1986; 17: 137–42.

142. Satyaswaroop PG. Development of a preclinical model for hormonal therapy of human endometrial carcinomas. Ann Med 1993; 25: 105–11.

143. Daftary GS, Taylor HS. Reproductive tract gene transfer. Fertil Steril 2003; 80: 475–84.

144. Kimura T, Nakamura H, Koyama S et al. In vivo gene transfer into the mouse uterus: a powerful tool for investigating implantation physiology. J Reprod Immunol 2005; 67: 13–20.

145. Charnock-Jones DS, Sharkey AM, Jaggers DC et al. In-vivo gene transfer to the uterine endometrium. Hum Reprod 1997; 12: 17–20.

146. Bagot CN, Troy PJ, Taylor HS. Alteration of maternal Hoxa10 expression by in vivo gene transfection affects implantation. Gene Ther 2000; 7: 1378–84.

147. Ding Y-Q, Zhu L-Z, Bagchi MK et al. Progesterone stimulates calcitonin gene expression in the uterus during implantation. Endocrinology 1994; 135: 2265–74.

148. Zhu L-J, Bagchi MK, Bagchi IC. Attenuation of calcitonin gene expression in pregnant rat uterus leads to a block in embryonic implantation. Endocrinology 1998; 139: 330–9.

149. Gui Y, Zhang J, Yuan L et al. Regulation of HOXA-10 and its expression in normal and abnormal endometrium. Mol Hum Reprod 1999; 5: 866–73.

150. Satokata I, Benson G, Maas R. Sexually dimorphic sterility phenotypes on Hoxa10 deficient mice. Nature 1995; 374: 46–63.

151. Eun Kwon H, Taylor HS. The role of HOX genes in human implantation Ann NY Acad Sci 2004; 1034: 1–18.

152. Taylor HS, Arici A, Olive D et al. HOXA10 is expressed in response to sex steroids at the time of implantation in the human endometrium. J Clin Invest 1998; 101: 1379–84.

153. Chau YM, Pando S, Taylor HS. HOXA11 silencing and endogenous HOXA11 antisense ribonucleic acid in the uterine endometrium. J Clin Endocrinol Metab 2002; 87: 2674–80.

154. Nakamura H, Kimura T, Ogita K et al. NF kappaB activation at implantation window of the mouse uterus. Am J Reprod Immunol 2004; 51: 16–21.

155. Page M, Tuckerman EM, Li T-C et al. Expression of nuclear factor kappa B components in human endometrium. J Reprod Immunol 2002; 54: 1–13.

156. Nakamura H, Kimura T, Ogita K et al. Alteration of the timing of implantation by in vivo gene transfer: delay of implantation by suppression of nuclear factor κB activity and partial rescue by leukemia inhibitory factor. Biochem Biophys Res Commun 2004; 321: 886–92.

157. Saeki Y, Matsumoto N, Nakano Y et al. Development and characterization of cationic liposomes conjugated with HVJ (Sendai virus): reciprocal effect of cationic lipid for in vitro and in vivo gene transfer. Hum Gene Ther 1997; 8: 1965–72.

158. Kaneda Y. New vector innovation for drug delivery: development of fusigenic non-viral particles. Curr Drug Targets 2003; 4: 599–602.

159. Kaneda Y, Nakajima T, Nishikawa T et al. Hemagglutinating virus of Japan (HVJ) envelope vector as a versatile gene delivery system. Mol Ther 2002; 6: 219–26.

160. Nakamura H, Kimura T, Ikegami H et al. Highly efficient and minimally invasive in-vivo gene transfer to the mouse uterus using haemagglutinating virus of Japan (HVJ) envelope vector. Mol Hum Reprod 2003; 9: 603–9.

161. Hsieh Y-Y, Lin C-S, Sun Y-L et al. In vivo gene transfer of leukemia inhibitory factor (LIF) into mouse endometrium. J Assist Reprod Genet 2002; 19: 79–83.

162. Saeki Y, Wataya-Kaneda M, Tanaka K et al. Sustained transgene expression in vitro and in vivo using an Epstein–Barr virus replicon vector system combined with HVJ-liposomes. Gene Ther 1998; 5: 1031–7.

163. Bulletti C, Jassoni VM, Lubicz L et al. Extracorporeal perfusion of the human uterus. Am J Obstet Gynecol 1986; 154: 683–8.

164. Bulletti C, Jassoni VM, Ciotti PM et al. Extraction of estrogens by human perfused uterus. Effect of membrane permeability and binding by serum proteins on differential influx into endometrium and myometrium. Am J Obstet Gynecol 1988; 159: 509–15.

165. Richter O, Wardelmann E, Dombrowski F et al. Extracorporeal perfusion of the human uterus as an experimental model in gynaecology and reproductive medicine. Hum Reprod 2000; 15: 1235–40.

166. Kaufman DG, Adeamec TA, Walton LA et al. Studies of human endometrium in organ culture. Methods Cell Biol 1980; 21β: 1–27.

167. Csermely T, Demers LM, Hughes EC. Organ culture of human endometrium. Effects of progesterone. Obstet Gynecol 1969; 34: 252–9.

168. Gurpide E, Welch M. Dynamics of uptake of estrogens and androgens by human endometrium. J Biol Chem 1969; 244: 5159–69.

169. Tseng L, Stolee A, Gurpide E. Quantitative studies on the uptake and metabolism of estrogens and progesterone by human endometrium. Endocrinology 1972; 90: 390–404.

170. Dudley DJ, Hatasaka HH, Branch DW et al. A human endometrial explant system: validation and potential applications. Am J Obstet Gynecol 1992; 167: 1774–80.

171. Stoklosowa S. Three dimensional tissue and organ models in vitro: their application in basic and practical research. Folia Histochem Cytobiol 2001; 39: 91–6.

172. Hohn HP, Winterhager E, Busch LC et al. Rabbit endometrium in organ culture: morphological evidence for progestational differentiation in vitro. Cell Tissue Res 1989; 257: 505–18.

173. Wild RA, Zhang RJ, Medders D. Whole endometrial fragments form characteristics of in vivo endometriosis in a mesothelial cell co-culture system: an in vitro model for the study of the histogenesis of endometriosis. J Soc Gynecol Invest 1994; 1: 65–8.

174. Tan Y, Tan D, He M et al. A model for implantation: coculture of blastocysts and uterine endometrium in mice. Biol Reprod 2005; 72: 556–61.

175. Negami AI, Tominaga T. Gland and epithelium formation in vitro from epithelial cells of the human endometrium. Hum Reprod 1989; 4: 620–4.

176. White TEK, DiSant'agnese PA, Miller RK. Human endometrial cells grown on an extracellular matrix form simple columnar epithelia and glands. In Vitro Cell Dev Biol 1990; 26: 636–42.

177. Branham WS, Lyn-Cook BD, Andrews A et al. Growth of neonatal rat uterine luminal epithelium on extracellular matrix. In Vitro Cell Dev Biol 1991; 27A: 442–6.

178. Martelli M, Campana A, Bischof P. Secretion of matrix metalloproteinases by human endometrial cells in vitro. J Reprod Fertil 1993; 98: 67–76.

179. Fleming H. Differentiation in human endometrial cells in monolayer culture: dependence on a factor in fetal bovine serum. J Cell Biochem 1995; 57: 262–70.

180. Fleming H. Structure and function of cultured endometrial epithelial cells. Semin Reprod Endocrinol 1999; 17: 93–106.

181. Irwin JC, Kirk D, King RJ et al. Hormonal regulation of human endometrial stromal cells in culture: an in vitro model for decidualization. Fertil Steril 1989; 52: 761–8.

182. Cunha GR, Bigsby RM, Cooke PS et al. Stromal–epithelial interactions in adult organs. Cell Differ 1985; 17: 137–48.

183. Bentin-Ley U, Pedersen B, Lindenberg S et al. Isolation and culture of human endometrial cells in a three-dimensional culture system. J Reprod Fertil 1994; 101: 327–32.

184. Osteen KG, Rodgers WH, Gaire M et al. Stromal–epithelial interaction mediates steroidal regulation of metalloproteinase expression in human endometrium. Proc Natl Acad Sci USA 1994; 91: 10129–33.

185. Bruner KL, Rodgers WH, Gold LI et al. Transforming growth factor beta mediates the progesterone suppression of an epithelial metalloproteinase by adjacent stroma in the human endometrium. Proc Natl Acad Sci USA 1995; 92: 7362–6.

186. Classen-Linke I, Kusche M, Knauthe R et al. Establishment of a human endometrial cell culture system and characterization of its polarized hormone responsive epithelial cells. Cell Tissue Res 1996; 287: 171–85.

187. Lockwood CJ, Schatz F. A biological model for the regulation of peri-implantational hemostasis and menstruation. J Soc Gynecol Invest 1996; 3: 159–65.

188. Yang H, Han S, Kim H et al. Expression of integrins, cyclooxygenases and matrix metalloproteinases in three-dimensional human endometrial cell culture system. Exp Mol Med 2002; 34: 75–82.

189. Hoegh AM, Islin H, Moller C et al. Identification of differences in gene expression in primary cell cultures of human endometrial epithelial cells and trophoblast cells following their interaction. J Reprod Immunol 2006; 70: 1–19.

190. Negami AI. [Implantation model in vitro]. Nippon Sanka Fujinka Gakkai Zasshi 1992; 44: 949–59. [in Japanese]

191. Sharpe KL, Zimmer RL, Khan RS et al. Proliferative and morphogenic changes induced by the co-culture of rat uterine and peritoneal cells: a cell culture model for endometriosis. Fertil Steril 1992; 58: 1220–9.

192. Fasciani A, Bocci G, Xu J et al. Three-dimensional in vitro culture of endometrial explants mimics the early stages of endometriosis. Fertil Steril 2003; 80: 1137–43.

193. Brosens JJ, Takeda S, Acevedo CH et al. Human endometrial fibroblasts immortalized by simian virus 40 large T antigen differentiate in response to a decidualization stimulus. Endocrinology 1996; 137: 2225–31.

194. Kyo S, Nakamura M, Kiyono T et al. Successful immortalization of endometrial glandular cells with normal structural and functional characteristics. Am J Pathol 2003; 163: 2259–69.

195. Krikun G, Mor G, Lockwood C. The immortalization of human endometrial cells. Methods Mol Med 2006; 121: 79–83.

196. Manconi F, Markham R, Cox G et al. Computer-generated, three-dimensional reconstruction of histological parallel serial sections displaying microvascular and glandular structures in human endometrium. Micron 2001; 32: 449–53.

197. Blumenson LE, Bross IDJ. Use of a mathematical model to bridge the clinic–laboratory gap: local spread of endometrial cancer J Theor Biol 1973; 38: 397–411.

198. Blumenson LE, Bross ID, Slack NH. Application of a mathematical model to a clinical study of the local spread of endometrial cancer. Cancer 1971; 28: 735–44.

199. Tromberg BJ, Svaasand LO, Fehr MK et al. A mathematical model for light dosimetry in photodynamic destruction of human endometrium. Phys Med Biol 1996; 41: 223–37.

38 Endometrial effects of hormonal contraception

Hilary OD Critchley and David T Baird

Synopsis

Background

- The world's increasing population will impact strongly on health and social well-being.
- Many women do not use contraception, particularly adolescents and those over 40 years old and in developing countries.
- In spite of the choice and variety of methods available, there is still need for contraceptive development.
- The ideal contraceptive should combine safety and efficacy with convenience and acceptability of use.
- In principle, a regimen that targeted the endometrium might specifically and selectively block implantation.
- In practice, most contraceptive regimens impact primarily on pituitary–hypothalamic function and thus affect the ovary, with some having an effect on the endometrium.

Basic Science

- The classical histological changes seen in the endometrial cycle result from the actions of estrogen followed by progesterone combined with estrogen.
- Complexity in tissue response arises from the interaction of various different steroids – endogenous hormones and their metabolites as well as analogues administered as part of a contraceptive regimen – with the different receptors present in endometrial cells, including ERα, ERβ, PR-A, PR-B, and AR.
- Route of administration – oral, intrauterine, or transdermal – is a further important variable influencing responses in the endometrium.
- Much remains to be learned about angiogenesis and vessel stability in endometrium exposed to contraceptive steroids.

Clinical

- Most emergency (single-dose) contraception affects ovulation.
- Prolonged use of the combined oral contraceptive (21/28 days) leads to an atrophic endometrium with a monthly withdrawal bleed followed by a brief regenerative phase.
- Progesterone-only contraception is safe and effective, but unscheduled or 'breakthrough' bleeding is a considerable inconvenience and deterrent to its use.
- It is hypothesized that the lack of exposure in most regimens to a period of unopposed estrogen (i.e. estrogen in the absence of progestin) accounts for most cases of irregular bleeding.
- Amenorrhea as a potential health benefit of endometrial contraception and remains a realistic challenge for future research and development.

INTRODUCTION

In spite of the significant advances in contraceptive practices over the past four decades, there remains a need for improved methods of contraception and greater choice of acceptable methods.[1] The oral contraceptive remains the most widely used method of contraception in developed countries (22 million users in five European countries).[2] Other important developments in contraception have been the reversible long-term progestogen-only methods that include depot injections, subdermal implants, and the intrauterine delivery route (levonorgestrel-releasing intrauterine system, LNG-IUS). Long-acting reversible contraceptives (LARCs) are among the most effective methods and there is less dependence on users' compliance and correct method of use.[3] Furthermore, LARCs are a cost-effective contraceptive option.[4] Other developments still based on the sex hormones that broaden the choice and the range of methods available are the delivery of constant low doses of both an estrogen and a progestogen either by a transdermal patch or vaginal ring. Over the next 50 years the world's population figures are predicted to rise from about 6057 million to 9322 million.[5] Much of this increase will be in developing countries and will have a major impact upon health and social well-being. Even in developed countries some women still fail to use contraception. In a recent report on contraceptive use in five European countries no method was being used by 23% of the study population.[2] Particularly at risk are adolescent girls and women over 40 years.[6] Thus, in spite of the choice and variety of methods, there is still need for contraceptive development. The ideal contraceptive should combine safety and efficacy with convenience and acceptability of use, and should also offer additional health benefits such as improved menstrual bleeding patterns.

The uterine endometrium plays a pivotal role in reproductive events. Its cycles of cellular proliferation and differentiation in response to the prevailing endocrine and paracrine environment, with regular menstrual bleeding, are the outward manifestation of cyclical ovarian function (see Chapter 5). In a developed society, the average woman will menstruate on some 400 occasions during her reproductive life span. In contrast, in a less well-developed society and prior to the availability of effective contraceptive methods, which have permitted women to regulate their own fertility, the majority of women will see few or no menstrual periods.[7] Consequently, novel and effective methods of endometrial contraception that have amenorrhea (no bleeding) as a potential health benefit (reduced menstrual blood loss; less anemia and maintenance of iron stores) may be attractive to many women.

Classic studies from Markee[8] and Corner and colleagues[9] established the role for ovarian steroids, estradiol and progesterone, in orchestrating the changes in endometrial structure and function over the menstrual cycle. Progesterone is essential for the establishment and maintenance of pregnancy following a period of exposure of the endometrium to estrogen. Unopposed estrogen during the follicular phase of the cycle promotes regeneration and proliferation. It is essential for the up-regulation of progesterone receptors (PRs), which permit the endometrium to respond to progesterone in the luteal phase. The sex steroids, acting through cognate receptors, initiate a cascade of gene and protein expression that is crucial for implantation. Novel molecular technologies, including microarray studies with detailed bioinformatics analysis techniques, have contributed to a valuable literature on gene profiles during the putative receptive phase of human endometrium[10–14] (see Chapter 14). Such knowledge is as important for fertility control (contraception) as it is for understanding how disturbances of endometrial structure and function may play a role in subfertility.

Here we consider the effects of contraceptive agents upon endometrial structure and function and describe the current literature on agents which may offer novel approaches for endometrial contraception.

ENDOMETRIAL RESPONSE TO EXOGENOUS SEX HORMONES (COMBINED ESTROGEN–PROGESTOGEN DELIVERY)

The administration of exogenous sex steroids will not necessarily result in histological features in the endometrium that resemble those characteristic of the normal menstrual cycle. It is the sequential exposure of the endometrium to the natural steroids estradiol and progesterone that leads to the characteristic morphological changes[15,16] (see Chapter 5). Estrogen exposure during the follicular phase is responsible for endometrial proliferation. Exposure to progesterone in the luteal phase results in secretory differentiation. Progesterone is antiestrogenic (see Chapter 9) and inhibits endometrial growth and glandular differentiation. It is the fall in circulating levels of estrogen and progesterone in the absence of conception that triggers the onset of menstruation.[17,18]

It is important to appreciate that most current methods of hormonal contraception lack a period of unopposed estrogen. The sole exception is the so-called sequential regimen of combined oral contraception which was introduced in an attempt to obtain better control of endometrial bleeding by simulating the natural ovarian cycle. However, it has largely been abandoned because of the relatively high failure rate. Exogenous administration of sex steroids, such as the combined oral contraceptive (COC) pill, will profoundly influence endometrial histology. The endometrial response to sex steroid exposure will reflect the prevailing endogenous sex hormone milieu plus the dose and formulation of steroid delivery, the route of delivery of the steroid, and the timing and duration of administration.

For example, estrogen delivery to a woman in the follicular phase will likely result in a prolonged proliferative phase, delayed or absent ovulation, and a short or absent secretory phase. In contrast, estrogen delivery during the luteal phase causes enhanced stromal edema, delayed stromal maturation, and incomplete secretory transformation of the glandular epithelium. These features are not dissimilar to those described in the context of deficiency of progesterone exposure in the luteal phase.[16,19,20]

Estrogens induce expression of both estrogen receptors (ERs) and PRs.[21,22] Progestogens only induce effects in the endometrium when the tissue has been previously exposed to estrogen and when PRs have been induced. The general response to progestogens includes inhibition of endometrial proliferation (antiestrogenic effect) and differentiation and maturation of epithelial and stromal cells.[23] The stage of the menstrual cycle at which progestogen exposure takes place will be a determinant of the resulting endometrial morphology. For example, when exposure to progestogen is in the early proliferative phase there is little evidence of stromal decidualization or spiral artery differentiation. Administration later in the proliferative phase, after a period of estrogen exposure, results in endometrial features of stromal pseudodecidualization with glands that are small and inactive. Exposure to longer-term progestogen therapy results in an atrophic endometrium where the stroma is compact, has small inactive glands, and spiral artery development is not present.[23] As discussed later, exposure to very high dosages of intrauterine progestogen will cause profound features of decidualization (see Chapter 24) and glandular atrophy.[24] The histological changes develop within 1 month after insertion and persist until the system is removed. Such marked morphological changes are not observed with systemic administration.

With prolonged use of combined oral contraception where estrogen (ethinyl estradiol) and progestogen are administered together for 21 out of 28 days each month, cyclic changes in endometrial histology will be superseded by an atrophic state.[23] Morphology reflects the specific formulation of steroids within the preparation. A withdrawal bleed is anticipated at the end of each 21-day period of combined hormone

exposure. This event is followed by a period of regeneration where the proliferation phase is brief due to the coincident inhibitory action of the constituent progestogen and, consequently, the endometrium remains shallow and inactive. Any secretory features evident resemble those of the early secretory phase. Thus, there is minimal spiral artery growth and differentiation, glandular secretory transformation, or pseudodecidualization.[23]

Prolonged exposure to COC preparations is associated with breakthrough bleeding (BTB), described by some as due to patchy necrosis.[25] The endometrial blood vessels are thin and dilated and a defect in vessel wall integrity is a likely contributing factor to unscheduled bleeding episodes. This is also the case with progestogen-only contraceptive (POC) preparations. In a recent study of endometrial microstructure in 37 women with 84 days consecutive administration of a combined ethinyl estradiol (30 µg)/levonorgestrel (150 µg) preparation, endometrial biopsy demonstrated in nearly two-thirds of users an inactive or atrophic endometrium.[26] Following withdrawal, there was a rapid reversion to normal cyclical histological features and no evidence of hyperplasia or other endometrial pathology. Thus, all regimens of hormonal contraception can result in an upset in the pattern of menstrual bleeding. This is not surprising because essentially none of them reproduce the sequence of priming with estrogen followed by estrogen and progestogen which occurs in the normal cycle. It is our contention that most of the irregular bleeding associated with hormonal contraception is due to the lack of an episode of unopposed estrogen.

ENDOMETRIUM IN EMERGENCY CONTRACEPTION

Large single doses of ethinyl estradiol and/or levonorgestrel as emergency contraceptives prevent pregnancy mostly by inhibiting or delaying ovulation.[27] The effects of these compounds on the endometrium when given after ovulation are minimal.

The effects of a single dose of a combined estrogen/progestogen preparation as used for emergency contraception have been described.[28] A delay in glandular maturation was reported. When two doses (100 µg ethinyl estradiol and 1 mg/dl norgestrel) were taken with a 12 hour separation at the time of anticipated ovulation, the result was desynchronization of the development of glandular and stromal cell compartments. There was a reported lag in glandular development.[25,29] Whether this

Table 38.1 Classification of progestogenic compounds

	First generation	Second generation	Third generation
Estranes	Norethindrone (norethisterone) Norethindrone acetate Ethynodiol diacetate		
Gonanes	Norgestrel	Levonorgestrel	Desogestrel Norgestimate Gestodene
Pregnanes	Medroxyprogesterone acetate Cyproterone acetate Dydrogesterone		
Others	Drospirenone		

Reproduced from Milling Smith and Critchley,[39] with kind permission of Springer Science and Business Media.

aberration in endometrial development and assumed disturbance of normal function explains the failure of conception when emergency contraception is taken has yet to be proven.

There are data demonstrating that the late follicular phase administration of the widely used emergency contraceptive levonorgestrel (LNG) alone (LNG 0.75 mg, two doses 12 hours apart) influences expression of endometrial secretory products later in the cycle.[30] The luteal phase secretory pattern of glycodelin in both serum and endometrium was reported as altered. Glycodelin-A is a progesterone-regulated product of luteal phase endometrium that is maximally expressed during the late luteal phase,[31] and reduced expression may be associated with perturbation of any immunosuppressive action this protein may exhibit.[32] No histological differences have been reported in ovulatory cycles among women who take LNG at mid cycle.[33]

Use of antiprogestogens has been explored for emergency contraception.[34,35] Treatment with mifepristone as a single dose ranging from 10 to 600 mg is a highly effective hormonal method of emergency contraception. Mifepristone inhibits ovulation or delays endometrial development if given before or after ovulation, respectively. Administration of a single dose of mifepristone in the early luteal phase (LH+2) has a marked effect on endometrial morphology.[36,37] Its mode of action is likely to be mainly impairment of ovarian function, either inhibiting or delaying the luteinizing hormone (LH) surge, but it may also inhibit implantation.[38]

POC METHODS AND ENDOMETRIAL RESPONSES TO PROGESTOGENS

Progestogens are defined as synthetic compounds that maintain a secretory endometrium. POCs are safe and effective. Minor molecular alterations to the structure of progesterone produce striking changes in pharmacological properties, including tissue availability, half-life, absorbance, and side effects. A variety of synthetic progestogens are utilized in contraceptive preparations (Table 38.1).[39] The gonanes and estranes[40] are structural classifications for derivatives of 19-nortestosterone. All estranes require conversion into norethindrone for biological activity. The gonanes include the common contraceptive progestogen levonorgestrel, as well as a more recent third-generation, less-androgenic progestogen, desogestrel. A third group of progestogens, pregnanes, originating from 17α-hydroxyprogesterone, includes cyproterone acetate and medroxyprogesterone acetate (MPA). A newer progestogen, drospirenone, is not derived from testosterone or progesterone but originates from spironolactone, a mineralocorticoid receptor antagonist. There are many forms of POCs available (Table 38.2),[39] utilizing variable delivery routes with differing doses and formulation of progestogen.

The contraceptive actions of POCs are consequent upon a number of mechanisms that reflect the contraceptive type and dosage. Contraceptive mechanisms include inhibition of ovulation, suppression of normal luteal activity, alterations to endometrial structure and function, and the production of hostile cervical mucus. Some POCs (e.g. Cerazette) contain a high enough dose of gestogen (75 µg desogestrel) to reliably inhibit ovulation. Ovulation usually occurs with other POCs – e.g. 0.350 mg norethisterone (Micronor, Janssen–Cilag; Noriday, Pharmacia) or 30 µg levonorgestrel (Microval, Wyeth; Norgeston, Schering) – all of which rely for their contraceptive efficacy on effects on cervical mucus and endometrium.

All POCs are associated with the side effect of unscheduled BTB. The amount and character of BTB varies with the method used, and many women report

Table 38.2 Commonly prescribed progestogen contraceptives

Delivery route	Contraceptive	Progestogen formulation	Dose
Oral (mini pills)	Second generation	Levonorgestrel	25 µg–75 µg/day
		Norethindrone	35 µg/day
	Third generation	Desogestrel	75 µg/day
Intramuscular injection	Depo-Provera	Depot MPA (DMPA)	150 mg/3 months
Subdermal implants	Norplant	Levonorgestrel	40–50 µg/day
	Implanon	3-keto desogestrel (etonogestrel)	67 µg/day
Intrauterine delivery system	Mirena (LNG-IUS)	Levonorgestrel	20 µg/day

Reproduced from Milling Smith and Critchley,[39] with kind permission of Springer Science and Business Media.

a reduction in troublesome BTB with time.[40] By way of example, BTB is present in up to 55% of women after 3 months' use of the LNG-IUS (levonorgestrel 20 µg daily)[41] and as many as half of women using Norplant request removal of the implant within the first year of use due to menstrual disturbances.[42]

The mechanisms of BTB with POCs have not been fully established. There are many lines of evidence to indicate the presence of superficial blood vessel fragility. Review of the published data also indicates that there are local changes in endometrial steroid response, cellular integrity, tissue perfusion, and aberration of locally produced angiogenic factors in the endometrium of women with a complaint of unscheduled BTB with progestogen-only contraception.[24,39] Thus far, there are no established long-term interventions available to reliably overcome unscheduled bleeding. This remains an area of endometrial physiology where a more detailed understanding of the mechanisms involved is needed.

The most striking endometrial response to exogenous progestogen is observed with the intrauterine delivery of levonorgestrel, which induces a rapid and dramatic transformation of the endometrium and is worthy of separate comment (Figure 38.1). Features are characterized by extensive decidualization of the stromal cells associated with a leukocyte infiltrate, atrophy of the glandular and surface epithelium, and alterations in the vasculature (suppression of spiral artery formation and presence of large distended vessels). There is a strong expression of local factors associated with decidualization, including prolactin and coincidental expression of the prolactin receptor in decidualized stromal cells, especially close to blood vessels. Other markers of decidualization, insulin-like growth factor binding protein 1 (IGFBP-1) and tissue factor (TF), are also strongly expressed in endometrium exposed to intrauterine LNG.[24,43,44]

The functional response of the endometrium to progestogen administration includes changes in sex

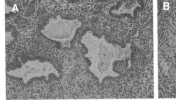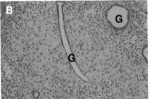

Figure 38.1 (A) Secretory phase endometrium illustrating large convoluted glands in an edematous stroma. Spiral artery differentiation is well developed. (B) Endometrium exposed to intrauterine delivery of levonorgestrel (LNG-IUS). The glands (G) are atrophic and the stroma decidualized. Spiral artery formation is suppressed.

steroid receptor expression, with down-regulation in both glandular and stromal cells. The consequence of a decrease in steroid receptor expression will influence the cascade of downstream molecular and cellular events. A summary of progesterone and progestogen effects on endometrial structure and function is presented in Table 38.3.[39]

The short-term administration of synthetic progestogens decreases the endometrial expression of the progesterone receptor.[45] Endometrium exposed to intrauterine delivery of 20 µg of levonorgestrel (LNG-IUS) responds with an initial down-regulation in both ER and PR.[46,47] Interestingly after 6–12 months' exposure to intrauterine LNG, an increase in the PR-A receptor relative to PR-B was reported.[46] In contrast, administration of subdermal levonorgestrel (Norplant) is associated with an increase or a persistence of endometrial PR expression. It is not known whether these increased/persistent PRs are functional.[48,49] Furthermore, studies on endometrial sex steroid receptor expression among Norplant users reported that although PR protein expression remains elevated, PR mRNA levels showed a decline within the glands and stroma. Among Norplant users, those women who reported amenorrhea demonstrated more PR mRNA in the stroma than women with unscheduled bleeding.[49] On the other hand, women using an intrauterine route of

Table 38.3 Summary of progesterone and progestogen effects on endometrial structure and function

Endometrial type	Estrogen receptor (ER)	Progesterone receptor (ER)	Vascular morphology	Vascular density	Structural integrity
Proliferative:					
Glands	Increased	Increased	No change	No change	No change
Stroma	Increased	Increased			
Secretory:					
Glands	Decreased	Decreased	No change	No change	No change
Stroma	Decreased	Persists (PR-A dominant)			
Levonorgestrel-releasing intrauterine system:					
Short term	Decreased	Decreased	Dilated thin walled	Increased	Decreased
Long term		Decreased (with increased PR-A:PR-B)			
Subdermal LNG (Norplant)		Increased protein Decreased mRNA	Dilated thin walled Fragile	Increased	Decreased
Medroxyprogesterone acetate		Decreased	Dilated thin walled	Decreased with high dose	
Northisterone				Decreased with high dose	
Etonogestrel (Implanon)				No change	Decreased

Reproduced from Milling Smith and Critchley,[39] with kind permission of Springer Science and Business Media. Empty cells indicate unknown findings.

LNG delivery (LNG-IUS) exhibited no difference in steroid receptor expression among those with unscheduled BTB compared to those without breakthrough bleeding. The significance of differential PR expression in the endometrium is yet to be determined. It is very important to recognize that differential PR expression in response to exposure to LNG is a result of local endometrial progestogen concentrations. The local endometrial LNG concentrations in women using an LNG-IUS are 1000-fold greater than serum concentrations or LNG levels among subdermal LNG (Norplant) users.[50] Local factors rather than systemic hormones are thus most likely to be implicated in the mechanisms responsible for the control of endometrial bleeding.

During the menstrual cycle, the androgen receptor (AR) is expressed predominantly in the endometrial stroma, and there is considerably higher intensity of AR immunostaining during the proliferative as compared to the secretory phase.[51] Administration of androgens/androgenic progestogens will suppress estrogen action in the endometrium, and this effect is most likely mediated by endometrial AR. The physiological roles, if any, for AR in the menstrual process and the regulation of AR expression are yet to be determined. LNG binds to the AR[52] and there is a significant decrease in AR expression in endometrium exposed to intrauterine LNG.[53]

EFFECTS OF POCS ON ENDOMETRIAL VASCULAR MORPHOLOGY AND FUNCTION

In the normal endometrium the microvasculature of capillaries and venous plexuses is distal to the spiral arterioles which are under the control of steroid hormones.[54] Human endometrial endothelial cells do not express PR or the classic ERα isoform, but do express the more recently identified ERβ isoform.[55] The mechanisms by which estrogens influence the microvasculature are, however, poorly understood.

POC use has been shown to result in changes to the endometrial vasculature, including superficial vascular dilatation, new vessel formation, altered microvessel density, and increased vascular fragility. Such modifications suggest that exogenous progestogen administration interferes with normal angiogenesis.

For example, large, thin-walled vessels are seen in the superficial endometrial stroma of women using the LNG-IUS. Despite the observations of abnormal vessel development as a result of long-term progestogen-only contraceptive use, the mechanism that causes aberrant angiogenesis and vascular fragility remains unknown.[56,57] Since progesterone receptors are prominent in perivascular cells but absent in the endothelium,[54,55,58] local LNG-induced effects on the endothelium may be indirectly mediated. A greater understanding of the changes in endometrial vessel morphology with exogenous progestogen administration will be important if the mechanisms of unscheduled BTB associated with POC are to be elucidated. There is also a need to consider the effects of the lack of exposure of the endometrium to unopposed estrogen.

In this context, it is notable that in reproductive tissues the local concentrations of sex steroids are modulated by hydroxysteroid dehydrogenase (HSDs) enzymes. The various HSDs are multigene families. The human 17βHSD family has at least six known members, each being a separate gene product from a different chromosome with distinct properties in terms of substrates and redox direction. The type 2 form (17βHSD-2) plays a major role in the inactivation of estradiol (E_2) to estrone (E_1). This 17βHSD-2 isoform is expressed in endometrial glandular epithelium and is up-regulated by progesterone. Its activity decreases when progesterone concentrations fall prior to menstruation or after antiprogestogen administration[59] and as a consequence the endometrium is exposed to a more 'estrogenic' environment.

In the first months of intrauterine exposure to LNG (LNG-IUS), 17βHSD-2 mRNA expression remains elevated, with a decline in expression by 6 months after insertion.[53] Therefore, as 17βHSD-2 converts estradiol (E_2) to the weaker estrogen estrone (E_1), the endometrial glands would be exposed to higher levels of E_1 and thus the endometrium may exhibit an intracellular 'estrogen deficiency'. This intracrine modulation of the local endometrial environment is at a time when unscheduled bleeding episodes are often reported. Furthermore, E_2-dependent products of the glands with paracrine actions within the endometrium would also be suppressed. Empirical approaches to managing unscheduled bleeding involve administration of exogenous estrogen or antiprogestins. In each case the concentration of estrogens in the endometrium will rise, either directly or by inhibition of 17βHSD type 2. In addition, antiprogestins up-regulate ER. It would be reasonable to hypothesize that unscheduled BTB episodes may at least in part be due to an intracellular estrogen deprivation that either directly or indirectly leads to vascular fragility.[53]

Over the course of the normal menstrual cycle, there is little change in blood vessel density.[60] Any effect of POCs on the endometrial vasculature reflects the dose, duration, and formulation of progestogen administered.

There is evidence that use of POCs results in disruption in normal endometrial vessel formation. Women using higher doses of injectable norethisterone, or MPA, exhibit a decrease in endometrial vessel density.[56] In contrast, administration of Norplant, the low-dose LNG implant, results in an increase in microvessel density.[60] Dilated superficial endometrial vessels have been identified by several groups in endometrium from women administered exogenous steroids.[61] There are many lines of evidence that the integrity and support of endometrial small vessels is altered by POCs, and in particular with subdermal implants such as Norplant. Exogenous progestogen administration may result in small vessels in the endometrium that are more fragile and prone to unscheduled bleeding.[61]

The newer subdermal implant Implanon delivers another progestogen, etonogestrel (3-keto-desogestrel). To date studies on the endometrial effects of Implanon have not shown any change in endothelial cell density.[62]

A reduction in vascular smooth muscle α-actin has been observed in the endometrium of women using subdermal LNG (Norplant).[63] In addition to the loss of structural support, alterations in basement membrane components may have effects on vessel formation and permeability. For example, basement membrane abnormalities could result in endothelial cell breakdown. However, no correlation was found between bleeding episodes and basement membrane components among women using Norplant POC.[64] Studies conducted on endometrial biopsies collected during the first month of Implanon use demonstrated a significant reduction in the number of vessels surrounded by the basement membrane components laminin, collagen IV, and heparan sulfate proteoglycan.[64] The published reports on changes in basement membrane components with subdermal LNG use are, however, inconsistent.[65,66] A decrease in basement membrane integrity could be caused by a decrease in production or an increase in extracellular proteolytic activity.[39] It remains to be established whether changes in vessel morphology are a consequence of aberrant angiogenesis, altered vascular perfusion, or a result of a direct effect on vessel structure and function by locally produced vasoactive mediators.[61]

Most studies report increases in angiogenic factors in the endometrium of women taking POCs. Although progesterone does not result in modifications in vascular endothelial growth factor (VEGF) expression, it has been reported to increase the angiogenic inhibitor thrombospondin 1 (TSP-1), whereas synthetic progestogens have minimal effect.[67] This may go some way to explain why, in contrast to the situation described with synthetic gestogens, aberrant angiogenesis is not normally seen in response to progesterone during the physiological menstrual cycle. More recently, studies in an endometrial epithelial cell-line (Ishikawa cells) have demonstrated that an antiprogestogen, mifepristone, inhibited the progesterone-induced increase in TSP-1 expression. The data from these studies have raised the hypothesis that the low rate of vaginal bleeding experienced by women exposed to mifepristone may be due to lack of stimulation of angiogenic factors.[68] A detailed review of endometrial angiogenesis appears in Chapter 7. POC use influences other angiogenic and angiostatic factors. The expression of angiopoietins (Ang-1 and Ang-2) is influenced by progestogen contraceptive administration and is associated with thrombin formation and tissue hypoxia. Unscheduled bleeding will result in thrombin formation within the endometrium. Thrombin has been reported to decrease Ang-1 protein and mRNA expression in human endometrial stromal cells but only minimally decrease Ang-2, in endometrial endothelial cells.[69] The consequence of a modification in local angiopoietin levels is a decrease in endothelial cell stability with an enhancement of further aberrant angiogenesis.

Tissue factor (TF) is an initiator of hemostasis, and levels of the protein are raised with intrauterine delivery of LNG, aiding thrombin formation.[44] However, levels of TF are initially decreased with subdermal delivery of LNG, rebounding to a persistently elevated level after 1 year of use.[70] One of the roles of thrombin is to raise levels of the proinflammatory and angiogenic factor, cytokine interleukin-8 (IL-8), the levels of which are usually decreased with decidualization. Hypoxia has also been demonstrated to cause an increase in IL-8.[44] These observations are important, as studies investigating uterine blood flow with subdermal LNG use have shown a significant decrease in endometrial perfusion.[71] Consequently, both the contraceptive LNG-IUS and LNG implant systems may lead to aberrant angiogenesis as a result of increasing TF levels and increased IL-8 levels secondary to both hypoxia and enhanced thrombin formation.[44]

EFFECTS OF POCS ON ENDOMETRIAL REMODELING ENZYMES

Progesterone has a regulatory effect on endometrial remodeling and specifically matrix metalloproteinase MMP activity[72] (see Chapter 23). Progesterone suppresses MMP activation, and withdrawal of progesterone results in an increase in MMP:TIMP (tissue inhibitor of metalloproteinase) ratio.[73] Progestin-only contraception is associated with a perimenstrual pattern of endometrial expression of MMPs and their

inhibitors. The use of subdermal LNG implants (Norplant) and Depo-Provera (DMPA; injectable MPA) have both been shown to cause expression of MMP and TIMP similar to that seen in shedding perimenstrual tissue. Progestogens can also influence expression of TIMPs, which may result in an increase in MMP activity. By way of example, use of DMPA led to a reduction in TIMP-1, -2, and -3 expression in endometrium but no correlation with endometrial bleeding patterns was recorded.[74–76]

Administration of high-dose progestogens is accompanied by an increase in endometrial leukocytes.[77,78] An elevated leukocyte infiltrate is observed early after insertion of an LNG-IUS and comprises mainly CD56+ uterine natural killer (uNK) cells and macrophages. Interestingly, strong VEGF immunoreactivity has been reported in macrophages in endometrium from women with an LNG-IUS.[62] In the atrophic endometrium from women using subdermal LNG (Norplant), increased numbers of macrophages (CD68+) correlate with abnormal endometrial bleeding.[79] The mechanisms that account for an increased leukocyte population have not yet been determined. Expression of the chemokine IL-8 is increased in endometrium after insertion of an LNG-IUS, with a decrease observed 6 months postinsertion. Another inflammatory mediator, cyclooxygenase 2 (COX-2), is similarly expressed in the early months after insertion of an LNG-IUS, an observation that contrasts with the initial suppression of prostaglandin dehydrogenase (PGDH) activity. These changes would result in a relatively high concentration of prostaglandins locally in the endometrium in the early months after insertion of an LNG-IUS.[43]

Activated mast cells in the endometrium have the potential to stimulate MMP production by endometrial stromal cells. MMP-1 expression was significantly greater in Norplant users compared with DMPA-exposed endometrium or menstrual phase control endometrial biopsies. Furthermore, activated mast cells, as detected by the presence of extracellular mast cell tryptase, predominated in the endometrium of Norplant users and were also seen with DMPA use in similar quantities to menstrual controls.[75] No correlation was made between MMP immunostaining patterns and the number of bleeding days reported by subjects. Data derived from endometrial biopsies collected from women using the contraceptive LNG-IUS demonstrated a significant increase in numbers of mast cells containing MMP-1 in women experiencing BTB compared to those with no reported bleeding problem.[80]

ENDOMETRIAL EFFECTS OF ANTIPROGESTOGENS AND POTENTIAL ROLE AS AN ESTROGEN-FREE CONCEPTION OPTION

Mifepristone is a synthetic C19 norsteroid and a potent progesterone antagonist.[81] The compound is best known for induction of abortion in early pregnancy. Its other potential uses include emergency contraception and even a 'once-a-month' contraceptive pill.[82] Continuous daily administration of doses between 2 and 10 mg suppresses ovulation, although some follicular activity may persist.[83–86] Contraceptive potential was demonstrated in a randomized double-blind trial where women were administered a low daily dose (2 or 5 mg mifepristone) for 120 days. Ninety percent were reported to be anovulatory and amenorrheic although their circulating estradiol levels fell within the mid-follicular phase range.[87]

Before the concept of daily administration of mifepristone can be advanced for estrogen-free contraception with the added health benefit of amenorrhea it will be necessary to demonstrate endometrial safety. To date, histological examination of endometrium exposed to low doses of mifepristone (2 and 5 mg) has revealed no evidence of hyperplastic, atypical, or malignant features.[88,89] Typical endometrial features with low-dose mifepristone exposure are inactive proliferative or cystic changes with a dense stroma (Figure 38.2). There is an accompanying decrease in markers of proliferation (mitotic index; Phospho-H3 mitosis marker[90] and Ki67 immunoreactivity). There is an increase in glandular androgen receptor expression and, with prolonged administration of up to 120 days, a down-regulation of the progesterone receptor.[89] Acute and short-term antiprogestogen administration is associated with an up-regulation of all three sex steroid receptors (ER, PR, and AR) in both glandular and stromal cell components of the endometrium[51,91] and inhibition of endometrial factors of potential importance for implantation.[38,91,92] There is evidence of inhibition of progesterone-dependent endometrial protein expression such as the enzymes PGDH and 17βHSD-2 and the protein glycodelin.[59,91,93] An increase in AR protein expression in mifepristone-exposed endometrium may result in an increased binding of androgens, which in turn may antagonize the effects of estrogen on endometrial growth. This curious up-regulation of the AR in both glandular and stromal cells following administration of antiprogestogen in human endometrium is also observed in the non-human primate endometrium.[51] Furthermore, in a non-human primate model, treatment with an antiandrogen flutamide has been shown to block the antiproliferative effect (endometrial thickness, stromal compaction, and mitotic index) of the progesterone receptor antagonist (ZK137316).[94,95]

This observation supports an hypothesis that the endometrial AR may be a critical component of the mechanism by which antiprogestogens suppress endometrial proliferation in the presence of circulating estrogens.[96]

Chronic antiprogestogen administration inhibits both endometrial secretion and proliferation (antiestrogen effects). This effect has been described as a 'functional non-competitive anti-estrogenic action' of an antiprogestin.[96–98] Since only the endometrial epithelium demonstrates this phenomenon, it has more recently been termed an 'endometrial anti-proliferative effect' of antiprogestogens.[96]

CONCLUDING COMMENTS

Current methods of hormonal contraception are highly effective if used consistently and are safe in the majority of women. Epidemiological studies have demonstrated that they convey many long-term health benefits such as a reduction in the incidence of endometrial and ovarian cancer. However, some women fail to use the methods consistently because of minor side effects such as breast tenderness and particularly breakthrough bleeding. This latter side effect is the commonest reason why women discontinue contraceptive methods, particularly POCs. Regular monthly withdrawal bleeding is much more predicable and lighter in women using COCs and is one of the reasons for their widespread popularity. However, estrogen-containing contraceptives are contraindicated in older women who smoke because of the increased risk of myocardial infarction and venous thromboembolism. Moreover, their use is associated with a small but significant risk in developing breast cancer.

Thus, there remains a need for improved methods of contraception and greater choice of acceptable methods. Important non-contraceptive health benefits such as reduced and regular menstrual blood loss, fewer painful periods, less anemia, and maintenance of iron stores are important in order to improve quality of life for women.[99] Any novel contraceptive developments must take account of these issues. Given the pivotal role of progesterone in the establishment of pregnancy, compounds that interrupt its action will have major effects on reproductive function. There are preparations available that have the potential to meet

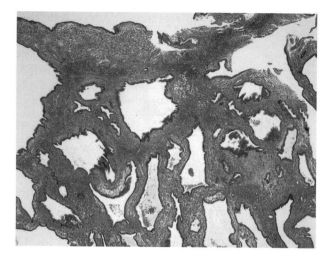

Figure 38.2 Photomicrograph showing the features of cystic glandular dilatation and compact cellular stroma obtained from a patient receiving 5 mg of mifepristone daily for 24 weeks.[100]

this ideal, if clinical researchers are given the opportunity to take forward development.

ACKNOWLEDGMENTS

The authors would like to thank Mrs Meg Anderson for her secretarial assistance. We are grateful to Dr ARW Williams for provision of the histological image of antiprogestogen-exposed endometrium, and to Mr Ted Pinner and Ms Corrine Macleod for assistance with preparation of figures.

REFERENCES

1. Baird DT, Glasier AF. Science, medicine and the future: contraception. BMJ 1999; 319: 969–72.
2. Skouby SO. Contraceptive use and behaviour in the 21st century: a comprehensive study across five European countries. Eur J Contracept Reprod Health Care 2004; 9: 57–68.
3. Peterson HB, Curtis KM. Long acting methods of contraception. New Engl J Med 2005; 353: 2169–75.
4. Mavranezouli I, Wilkinson C. Long-acting reversible contraceptives: not only effective, but also a cost-effective option for the National Health Service. J Fam Plann Reprod Health Care 2006; 32: 3–5.
5. United Nations. World Population Prospects: The 2000 Revision. New York: United Nations, 1999.
6. Oddens BJ, Visser AP, Vemer HM et al. Contraceptive use and attitudes in Great Britain. Contraception 1994; 49: 73–86.
7. Short RV. Oestrous and menstrual cycles. In: Austin CR, Short RV, eds. Hormonal Control of Reproduction. Cambridge: Cambridge University Press, 1984: 115–52.
8. Markee JE. Menstruation in intraocular endometrial transplants in the Rhesus monkey. Contr Embryol Carnegie Instn 1940; 177: 211–308.
9. Corner GW, Allen WM. Physiology of the corpus luteum II. Production of a special uterine reaction (progestational proliferation) by extracts of the corpus luteum. Am J Physiol 1929; 88: 326–39.
10. Kao LC, Tulac S, Lobo S et al. Global gene profiling in human endometrium during window of implantation. Endocrinology 2002; 143: 2119–38.
11. Talbi S, Hamilton AE, Vo KC et al. Molecular phenotyping of human endometrium distinguishes menstrual cycle phases and underlying biological processes in normo-ovulatory women. Endocrinology 2006; 147: 1097–121.
12. Riesewijk A, Martin J, van Os R et al. Gene expression in profiling of human endometrial receptivity on days LH+2 versus LH+7 by microarray technology. Mol Hum Reprod 2003; 9: 253–64.
13. Borthwick JM, Charnock-Jones DS, Tom BD et al. Determination of the transcript profile of human endometrium. Mol Hum Reprod 2003; 9: 19–33.
14. Ponnampalam AP, Weston GC, Trajstam AC et al. Molecular classification of human endometrial cycle stages by transcriptional profiling. Mol Hum Reprod 2004; 10: 879–93.
15. Noyes RW, Hertig AT, Rock J. Dating the endometrial biopsy. Fertil Steril 1950; 1: 3–25.
16. Buckley CH, Fox H. The normal endometrium as seen in biopsy material. In: Buckley CH, ed. Biopsy Pathology of the Endometrium. London: Chapman and Hall, 1989: 30–47.
17. Critchley HOD, Kelly RW, Brenner RM et al. Antiprogestins as a model for progesterone withdrawal. Steroids 2003; 68: 1061–8.
18. Jabbour HN, Kelly RW, Fraser H et al. Endocrine regulation of menstruation. Endocr Rev 2006; 27: 17–46.
19. Dallenbach-Hellweg G. Histopathology of the Endometrium, 3rd edn. Berlin: Springer-Verlag, 1981: 126–256.
20. Egger H, Kinderman G. Effects of high oestrogen doses on the endometrium. In: Dallenbach-Hellweg G, ed. Functional Morphologic Changes in Female Sex Organs Induced by Endogenous Hormones. Berlin: Springer-Verlag, 1980: 51–3.
21. Garcia E, Bouchard P, De Brux J et al. Use of immunocytochemistry of progesterone and estrogen receptors for endometrial dating. J Clin Endocrinol Metab 1988; 67: 80–7.
22. Lessey BA, Killam AP, Metzer DA et al. Immunohistochemical analysis of human uterine estrogen and progesterone receptors throughout the menstrual cycle. J Clin Endocrinol Metab 1988; 67: 334–40.
23. Buckley CH, Fox H. The effect of therapeutic and contraceptive hormones on the endometrium. In: Buckley CH, ed. Biopsy Pathology of the Endometrium. London: Chapman and Hall, 1989: 68–92.
24. Critchley HOD. Endometrial effects of progestogens. Gynaecol Forum 2003; 8: 6–10.
25. Okon MA, Li TC, Dockery P. Contraceptive steroids and endometrial morphology. In: Cameron IT, Fraser IS, Smith SK, eds. Clinical Disorders of the Endometrium and Menstrual Cycle. Oxford: Oxford University Press, 1998: 375–89.
26. Anderson FD, Hait H, Hsiu J et al. Endometrial microstructure after long-term use of a 91-day extended-cycle oral contraceptive regimen. Contraception 2005; 71: 55–9.
27. Croxatto HB Fuentealba B, Brache V et al. Effects of the Yuzpe regimen, given during the follicular phase, on ovarian function. Contraception 2002; 65: 121–8.
28. Yuzpe AA, Thurlow HJ, Ramzy I et al. Post coital contraception – a pilot study. J Reprod Med 1974; 13: 53–61.
29. Ling WY, Robichaud A, Zayid I et al. Mode of action of DL-norgestrel and ethinylestradiol combination in postcoital contraception. Fertil Steril 1979; 32: 297–302.
30. Durand M, Seppala M, Cravioto MC et al. Late follicular phase administration of levonorgestrel as an emergency contraceptive changes the secretory pattern of glycodelin in

serum and endometrium during the luteal phase of the menstrual cycle. Contraception 2005; 71: 451–7.

31. Julkunen M, Koistinen R, Sjoberg J et al. Secretory endometrium synthesized placental protein 14. Endocrinology 1986; 118: 1782–6.

32. Seppala M, Taylor RN, Koistinen H et al. Glycodelin: a major lipocalin protein of the reproductive axis with diverse actions in cell recognition and differentiation. Endocr Rev 2002; 23: 401–30.

33. Durand M, Cravioto MC, Raymond EG et al. On the mechanism of action of short-term levonorgestrel administration in emergency contraception. Contraception 2001; 64: 227–34.

34. Glasier A, Thong KJ, Mackie M et al. Mifepristone (RU486) compared with high-dose estrogen and progestogen for emergency postcoital contraception. N Engl J Med 1992; 327: 1041–4.

35. Webb AM, Russell J, Elstein M. Comparison of Yuzpe regimen, danazol, and mifepristone (RU486) in oral postcoital contraception. BMJ 1992; 305: 927–31.

36. Gemzell-Danielsson K, Marions L, Bygdeman M. Effects of mifepristone on endometrial receptivity. Steroids 2003; 68: 1069–75.

37. Cameron ST, Glasier AF, Narvekar N et al. Effects of onapristone on postmenopausal endometrium. Steroids 2003; 68: 1053–9.

38. Gemzell-Danielsson K, Mandl I, Marions L. Mechanisms of action of mifepristone when used for emergency contraception. Contraception 2003; 68: 471–6.

39. Milling Smith OP, Critchley HO. Progestogen only contraception and endometrial breakthrough bleeding. Angiogenesis 2005; 8: 117–26.

40. Collins J, Crosignani PG. Hormonal contraception without estrogens. Hum Reprod Update 2003; 9: 373–86.

41. Irvine GA, Campbell-Brown MB, Lumsden MA et al. Randomised comparative trial of the levonorgestrel intrauterine system and norethisterone for treatment of idiopathic menorrhagia. Br J Obstet Gynaecol 1998; 105: 592–8.

42. Peers T, Stevens JE, Graham J et al. Norplant implants in the UK: first year continuation and removals. Contraception 1996; 53: 345–51.

43. Jones RL, Critchley HOD. Morphological and functional changes in human endometrium following intrauterine levonorgestrel delivery. Hum Reprod 2000; 15: 162–72.

44. Lockwood CJ, Kumar P, Krikun G et al. Effects of thrombin, hypoxia, and steroids on interleukin-8 expression in decidualized human endometrial stromal cells: implications for long-term progestin-only contraceptive-induced bleeding. J Clin Endocrinol Metab 2004; 89: 1467–75.

45. Lane G KR, Whitehead M. The effects of oestrogen and progestogens on endometrial biochemistry. In: Studd JWW, Whitehead MI, eds. The Menopause. Oxford: Blackwell; 1988: 213–26.

46. Critchley HO, Wang H, Kelly RW et al. Progestin receptor isoforms and prostaglandin dehydrogenase in the endometrium of women using a levonorgestrel-releasing intrauterine system. Hum Reprod 1998; 13: 1210–17.

47. Hurskainen R, Salmi A, Paavonen J et al. Expression of sex steroid receptors and Ki-67 in the endometria of menorrhagic women: effects of intrauterine levonorgestrel. Mol Hum Reprod 2000; 6: 1013–18.

48. Critchley HO, Bailey DA, Au CL et al. Immunohistochemical sex steroid receptor distribution in endometrium from long-term subdermal levonorgestrel users and during the normal menstrual cycle. Hum Reprod 1993; 8: 1632–9.

49. Lau TM, Witjaksono J, Affandi B et al. Expression of progesterone receptor mRNA in the endometrium during the normal menstrual cycle and in Norplant users. Hum Reprod 1996; 11: 2629–34.

50. Pekonen F, Nyman T, Lahteenmaki P et al. Intrauterine progestin induces continuous insulin-like growth factor-binding protein-1 production in the human endometrium. J Clin Endocrinol Metab 1992; 75: 660–4.

51. Slayden OD, Nayak NR, Burton KA et al. Progesterone antagonists increase androgen receptor expression in the rhesus macaque and human endometrium. J Clin Endocrinol Metab 2001; 86: 2668–79.

52. Kloosterboer HJ, Vonk-Noordgraaf CA, Turpijn EW Selectivity in progesterone and androgen receptor binding of progestogens used in oral contraceptives. Contraception 1988; 38: 325–32.

53. Burton KA, Henderson TA, Hiller SG et al. Local levonorgestrel regulation of androgen receptor and 17beta-hydroxysteroid dehydrogenase type 2 expression in human endometrium. Hum Reprod 2003; 18: 2610–17.

54. Perrot-Applanat M, Deng M, Fernandez H et al. Immunohistochemical localisation of estradiol and progesterone receptors in human uterus throughout pregnancy: expression in endometrial blood vessels. J Clin Endocrinol Metab 1994; 78: 216–24.

55. Critchley HO, Brenner RM, Henderson TA et al. Estrogen receptor beta, but not estrogen receptor alpha, is present in the vascular endothelium of the human and nonhuman primate endometrium. J Clin Endocrinol Metab 2001; 86: 1370–8.

56. Song JY, Markham R, Russell P et al. The effect of high-dose medium- and long-term progestogen exposure on endometrial vessels. Hum Reprod 1995; 10: 797–800.

57. McGavigan CJ, Dockery P, Metaxa-Mariatou V et al. Hormonally mediated disturbance of angiogenesis in the human endometrium after exposure to intrauterine levonorgestrel. Hum Reprod 2003; 18: 77–84.

58. Leece G, Meduri G, Ancelin M et al. Presence of estrogen receptor β in the human endometrium through the cycle: expression in glandular, stromal and vascular cells. J Clin Endocrinol Metab 2001; 86: 1379–86.

59. Maentausta O, Svalander P, Danielsson KG et al. The effects of an antiprogestin, mifepristone, and an antiestrogen, tamoxifen, on endometrial 17b-hydroxysteroid dehydrogenase and progestin and estrogen receptors during the luteal phase of the menstrual cycle: an immunohistochemical study. J Clin Endocrinol Metab 1993; 77: 913–18.

60. Rogers PA, Au CL, Affandi B. Endometrial microvascular density during the normal menstrual cycle and following exposure to long-term levonorgestrel. Hum Reprod 1993; 8(9): 1396–404.

61. Hickey M, Fraser IS. The structure of endometrial microvessels. Hum Reprod 2000; 15(Suppl 3): 57–66.

62. Charnock-Jones DS, Macpherson AM, Archer DF et al. The effect of progestins on vascular endothelial growth factor, oestrogen receptor and progesterone receptor immunoreactivity and endothelial cell density in human endometrium. Hum Reprod 2000; 15(Suppl 3): 85–95.

63. Rogers PA, Plunkett D, Affandi B. Perivascular smooth muscle alpha-actin is reduced in the endometrium of women with progestin-only contraceptive breakthrough bleeding. Hum Reprod 2000; 15(Suppl 3): 78–84.

64. Hickey M, Simbar M, Markham R et al. Changes in vascular basement membrane in the endometrium of Norplant users. Hum Reprod 1999; 14: 716–21.

65. Palmer JA, Lau TM, Hickey M et al. Immunohistochemical study of endometrial microvascular basement membrane components in women using Norplant. Hum Reprod 1996; 11: 2142–50.

66. Kelly FD, Tawia SA, Rogers PA. Immunohistochemical characterization of human endometrial microvascular basement membrane components during the normal menstrual cycle. Hum Reprod 1995; 10: 268–76.

67. Mirkin S, Navarro F, Archer DF. Hormone therapy and endometrial angiogenesis. Climacteric 2003; 6: 273–7.

68. Mirkin S, Archer DF. Effects of mifepristone on vascular endothelial growth factor and thrombospondin-1 mRNA in Ishikawa cells; implication for the endometrial effects of mifepristone. Contraception 2004; 70: 327–33.

69. Krikun G, Critchley H, Schatz F et al. Abnormal uterine bleeding during progestin-only contraception may result from free radical-induced alterations in angiopoietin expression. Am J Pathol 2002; 161: 979–86.

70. Runic R, Schatz F, Wan L et al. Effects of norplant on endometrial tissue factor expression and blood vessel structure. J Clin Endocrinol Metab 2000; 85: 3853–9.

71. Hickey M, Carati C, Manconi F et al. The measurement of endometrial perfusion in norplant users: a pilot study. Hum Reprod 2000; 15: 1086–91.

72. Salamonsen LA, Zhang J, Hampton A et al. Regulation of matrix metalloproteinases in human endometrium. Hum Reprod 2000, 15(Suppl 3): 112–19.

73. Salamonsen LA, Butt AR, Hammond FR et al. Production of endometrial matrix metalloproteinases, but not their tissue inhibitors, is modulated by progesterone withdrawal in an in vitro model for menstruation. J Clin Endocrinol Metab 1997; 82: 1409–15.

74. Zhang J, Nie G, Jian W et al. Mast cell regulation of human endometrial matrix metalloproteinases: a mechanism underlying menstruation. Biol Reprod 1998; 59: 693–703.

75. Vincent AJ, Zhang J, Ostor A et al. Matrix metalloproteinase-1 and -3 and mast cells are present in the endometrium of women using progestin-only contraceptives. Hum Reprod 2000; 15: 123–30.

76. Vincent AJ, Zhang J, Ostor A et al. Decreased tissue inhibitor of metalloproteinase in the endometrium of women using depot medroxyprogesterone acetate: a role for altered endometrial matrix metalloproteinase/tissue inhibitor of metalloproteinase balance in the pathogenesis of abnormal uterine bleeding? Hum Reprod 2002; 17: 189–98.

77. Song JY, Russell P, Markham R et al. Effects of high dose progestogens on white cells and necrosis in human endometrium. Hum Reprod 1996; 11: 1713–18.

78. Critchley HO, Wang H, Jones RL et al. Morphological and functional features of endometrial decidualization following long-term intrauterine levonorgestrel delivery. Hum Reprod 1998; 13: 1218–24.

79. Clark DA, Wang S, Rogers P et al. Endometrial lymphomyeloid cells in abnormal uterine bleeding due to levonorgestrel (Norplant). Hum Reprod 1996; 11: 1438–44.

80. Milne SA, Rakhyoot A, Drudy TA et al. Co-localization of matrix metalloproteinase-1 and mast cell tryptase in the human uterus. Mol Hum Reprod 2001; 7: 559–65.

81. Ulmann A. The development of mifepristone: a pharmaceutical drama in three acts. J Am Med Women's Assoc 2000; 55(Suppl 3): 117–20.

82. Baird DT. Antigestogens: the holy grail of contraception. Reprod Fertil Dev 2001; 13: 1–6.

83. Ledger WL, Sweeting VM, Hillier H et al. Inhibition of ovulation by low dose mifepristone (RU486). Hum Reprod 1992; 7: 945–50.

84. Croxatto HB, Salvatierra AM, Croxatto HD et al. Effects of continuous treatment with low dose mifepristone throughout one menstrual cycle. Hum Reprod 1993; 8: 201–7.

85. Cameron ST, Thong KJ, Baird DT. Effect of daily low dose mifepristone on the ovarian cycle and on the dynamics of follicle growth. Clin Endocrinol (Oxf) 1995; 43: 407–14.

86. Cameron ST, Critchley HOD, Thong KJ et al. Effects of daily low dose mifepristone on endometrial maturation and proliferation. Hum Reprod 1986; 11: 2518–26.

87. Brown A, Cheng L, Lin S et al. Daily low dose mifepristone has contraceptive potential by suppressing ovulation and menstruation: a double blind randomised control trial of 2mg and 5mg per day for 120 days. J Clin Endocrinol Metab 2002; 87: 63–70.

88. Baird DT, Brown A, Critchley HOD et al. Effect of long-term treatment with low dose mifepristone on the endometrium Hum Reprod 2003; 18: 61–8.

89. Narvekar N, Cameron S, Critchley HOD et al. Low dose mifepristone inhibits endometrial proliferation and up-regulates androgen receptor J Clin Endocrinol Metab 2004; 89: 2491–7.

90. Brenner RM, Slayden OD, Rodgers WH et al. Immunocytochemical assessment of mitotic activity with an antibody to phosphorylated histone H3 in the macaque and human endometrium. Hum Reprod 2003; 18: 1185–93.

91. Cameron ST, Critchley HOD, Buckley CH et al. Effect of two antiprogestins (mifepristone and onapristone) on endometrial factors of potential importance for implantation. Fertil Steril 1997; 67: 1046–53.

92. Ghosh D, Kumar PG, Sengupta J. Effect of early luteal phase administration of mifepristone (RU486) on leukaemia inhibitory factor, transforming growth factor beta and vascular endothelial growth factor in the implantation stage endometrium of the rhesus monkey. J Endocrinol 1998; 157: 115–25.

93. Lalitkumar PG, Sengupta J, Karande AA et al. Placental protein 14 in endometrium during the menstrual cycle and effect of early luteal phase mifepristone administration on its expression in implantation stage endometrium in the rhesus monkey. Hum Reprod 1998; 13: 3478–86.

94. Brenner R, Slayden OD, Critchley HOD. Anti-proliferative effects of progesterone antagonists in the primate endometrium: a potential role for the androgen receptor. Reproduction 2002; 124: 167–72.

95. Slayden OD, Brenner RM. Flutamide counteracts the antiproliferative effects of antiprogestins in the primate endometrium. J Clin Endocrinol Metab 2003; 88: 946–9.

96. Brenner R, Slayden OD, Nayak NR et al. A role for the androgen receptor in the endometrial antiproliferative effects of progesterone antagonists. Steroids 2003; 68: 1033–9.

97. Wolf JP, Hsiu JG, Anderson TL et al. Noncompetitive antiestrogenic effect of RU486 in blocking the estrogen-stimulated luteinizing surge and the proliferative action of estradiol on endometrium in castrate monkeys. Fertil Steril 1989; 52: 1055–60.

98. Hodgen GD, van Uem JF, Chillik CF et al. Non-competitive antioestrogenic activity of progesterone antagonists in primate models. Hum Reprod 1994; 9: 77–81.

99. The ESHRE Capri Workshop Group. Noncontraceptive health benefits of combined oral contraception. Hum Reprod Update 2005; 11: 513–25.

100. Lakha F, Ho PC, van der Spuy Z et al. A novel estrogen-free oral contraceptive pill for women: multicenter double blind randomised control trial of mifepristone and levonorgestrel. Hum Reprod 2007; 22: 2428–36.

39 Endometiral effects of selective progesterone receptor modulators

Kristof Chwalisz, Alistair Williams, and Robert Brenner

INTRODUCTION

Since the isolation of progesterone in 1934,[1,2] the primary natural ligand of the progesterone receptor (PR), many steroidal and non-steroidal compounds have been synthesized, which exhibit a high binding affinity to PR and specific effects in progesterone target tissues. Three classes of compounds belong to the PR ligand family: PR agonist (progestins), PR antagonists (PRAs, antiprogestins, also known as progesterone antagonists), and selective progesterone receptor modulators (SPRMs). In this review, to avoid confusion with the PR-A isoform (PR-A), we use the abbreviation PA to mean PR antagonists.

SPRMs, which have partial or mixed progesterone agonist/antagonist activities, may exhibit tissue-specific effects. Because of these properties, SPRMs have the potential to provide the beneficial effects of progestins and PAs while avoiding their drawbacks. The 11β-benzaldoxime-substituted estratrienes (J compounds; Figure 39.1), are the best-known steroidal SPRMs.[3,4] Asoprisnil (J867), which belongs to this group, is the first SPRM that has reached clinical development for the treatment of women with symptomatic uterine leiomyomata and endometriosis. More recently, several non-steroidal SPRMs, e.g. benzimidazole-2-thione analogues,[5] 5-benzylidene-1,2-dihydrochromeno[3,4-f]quinolines,[6] and new steroidal SPRMs related to dexamethasone (dexamethasonemesylate and dexamethasoneoxetanone)[7] have been described. Since these compounds are still in the early stage of development, little information about their effects in vivo is currently available.

Progesterone plays a crucial role in controlling the key reproductive functions in females, including ovulation, implantation, pregnancy maintenance, and parturition. These functions of progesterone are mediated by PR, which is expressed in at least two isoforms, PR-A and PR-B. PR is present in various tissues in the body, predominantly in the reproductive tract. Pharmacological studies with PAs and SPRMs show

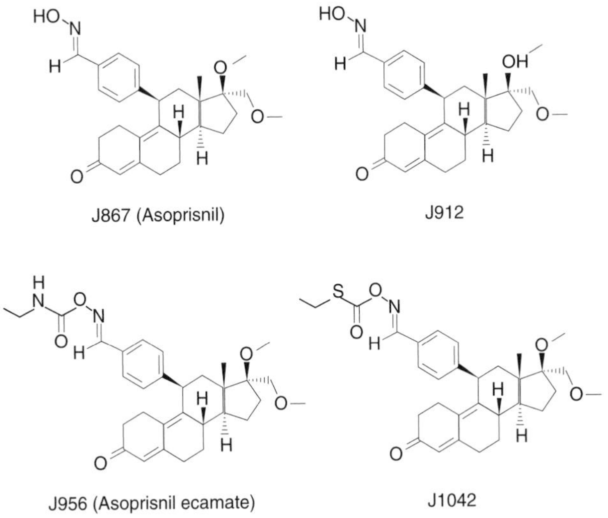

Figure 39.1 Chemical structures of major 11β-benzaldoxime substituted SPRMs.

that the endometrium of non-human primates and humans is the most sensitive tissue in the body to PR ligands. The endometrial effects of compounds belonging to these classes, e.g. suppression of uterine bleeding[8] or changes in endometrial morphology and marker proteins,[9–11] can be observed at doses that have no effects on ovulation or morphology of non-endometrial tissues of the reproductive tract. The endometrial effects of SPRMs have been extensively studied in non-human primates and more recently in humans. The characterization of these effects using morphological, cellular, and molecular criteria is not only important for the understanding of the mechanism of amenorrhea and the endometrial antiproliferative effect but also is crucial for the assessment of endometrial safety during the clinical development of SPRMs. In this chapter, we review the effects of SPRMs on the endometrium of non-human primates and women. In addition, we describe the rationale for the use of SPRMs in the treatment of women with various gynecological disorders, including uterine leiomyomata, endometriosis, and abnormal uterine bleeding.

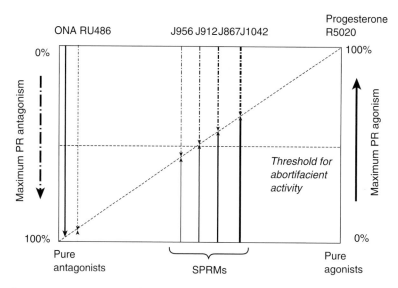

Figure 39.2   Spectrum of progesterone agonist and antagonist activities of major 11β-benzoxime-substituted SPRMs and PAs. The figure is based on studies in rabbits (McPhail test) and guinea pigs (luteolysis inhibition assay, induction of labor). ONA, onapristone; RU486, mifepristone; R5020, pure progestin promegestone; J867, asoprisnil; PR, progesterone receptor. (Reproduced form Schubert et al,[4] with permission.)

DEFINITION AND BIOLOGICAL PROPERTIES OF SPRMs

SPRMs can be defined by both functional and molecular criteria. Using the functional criteria, SPRMs are defined as PR ligands that exert clinically relevant tissue-selective progesterone agonist, antagonist, partial, or mixed agonist/antagonist effects on various progesterone target tissues in an in-vivo situation depending on the biological action studied.[12] This definition, particularly the presence of tissue-selective effects, is based on biological actions in animals and women, analogous to other selective steroid receptor modulators, such as selective estrogen receptor modulators (SERMs), or selective androgen receptor modulators (SARMs), and is consistent with the steroid receptor modulator (SRM) definition proposed by Smith and O'Malley.[13] The term partial PR agonist or antagonist means that a given compound possesses some agonist or antagonist activity in pharmacological bioassays, e.g. transactivation assays in cell lines or in-vivo bioassays, but not to the extent of pure agonists or antagonists. Partial PR agonists or antagonists usually reach a plateau in their dose–response curves that is below the plateau of full agonists or antagonists. Compounds with mixed PR agonist/antagonist activities may induce agonist effects in one tissue and antagonist effects in other tissues. Based on the data from animal studies generated during this program, it was possible to rank the new SPRMs and the reference compounds according to the ratio of their PR agonist and antagonist activities

(Figure 39.2). During the drug discovery program, the classical McPhail assay in intact, immature, estrogen-primed rabbits was used for the assessment of progesterone agonist and antagonist activities of J-compounds at the endometrial level.[4] Asoprisnil elevated McPhail scores in a dose-dependent manner; however, the agonist effects never reached the maximum response of progesterone. When assessed as a PR antagonist, asoprisnil and other J compounds showed only partial antagonist effects and none of the compounds reached the inhibition level achieved with mifepristone (RU486), which showed no agonist activity in this test. The pharmacological studies in animals also suggest that there is an inverse relationship between the amount of partial agonist activity, as assessed with the McPhail bioassay, and the effects on pregnancy. The 11β-benzaldoxime SPRMs with high progesterone agonist activity had low abortifacient activity and a high ability to suppress estrogen effects in the uterus.[4] In contrast, the PAs (e.g. onapristone or mifepristone) lacked tissue selectivity and were very effective in blocking the functions of progesterone during all stages of pregnancy. Table 39.1 presents the key pharmacological properties of PR agonists, PAs, and SPRMs.

Asoprisnil was selected for further development based on its pronounced PR agonist activity, endometrial antiproliferative effects in non-human primates, and marginal labor-inducing activity.[4] More recently, the tissue-selective effects of asoprisnil were confirmed in women. The results of early clinical trials showed that asoprisnil controls uterine bleeding irrespective of

Table 39.1 Key pharmacological properties of PR ligands

Model	Agonists	SPRMs	Antagonists
McPhail test[a]	Agonist	Partial and mixed agonists/antagonists	Antagonists
Abortifacient activity[b]	Absent	Marginal or absent	High
Cervical ripening[b]	Absent	Low or absent	High
Antiovulatory activity[c]	High	Inconsistent effects, dose-independent	High
Endometrial effect[c]	Secretory transformation	SPRM effect (non-physiological secretory patterns)	'Inactive non-secretory pattern'
Uterine bleeding[c]	Breakthrough bleeding and spotting	Amenorrhea via an endometrial effect	Amenorrhea due to anovulation

[a]Rabbits. [b]Guinea pigs. [c]Humans.

the effects on luteinization,[8] and reduces leiomyoma volume in the presence of follicular phase estrogen concentrations.[12]

The molecular definition of SPRMs is based on the ability of a liganded PR to interact with coregulators.[13] Coregulators (coactivators and corepressors) are nuclear proteins that form multiple complexes with nuclear receptors and modulate their transcriptional activity.[14–17] Coactivators enhance transcriptional activity of nuclear receptors, whereas corepressors elicit inhibitory effects on nuclear receptors. The relative balance of coactivator and corepressor expression within a given target cell determines the relative agonist vs antagonist activity of selective receptor modulators (SRMs).[13] This model was originally developed to explain the molecular mechanism of action of SERMs such as tamoxifen and raloxifene,[18] but seems to be valid for all known SRMs, including SPRMs, SARMs, and selective glucocorticoid receptor modulators (SGRMs). Pure PR antagonists such as onapristone, mifepristone, and CDB-2914 either favor interaction of PR with corepressors or inhibit interactions with coactivators, whereas pure PR agonists promote the interaction of the nuclear receptor with coactivators.[19,20] Finally, SPRMs induce an intermediate state of interaction between nuclear receptors and coactivators.[13,19,21] Since the availability of both coactivators and corepressors is dependent on tissue and hormonal milieu, the cell type- and promoter-specific differences in coregulator recruitment determine the tissue selectivity of SPRMs.[12,13] More recent molecular studies show that asoprisnil-liganded PR promotes the recruitment of the coactivator SRC-1 in an in-vitro model,[22] which could explain the partial agonist effects observed in animal models and humans. The PR specificity, i.e. the absence of a pharmacologically relevant binding to other steroid receptors (such as GR, AR, or estrogen receptor [ER]), is not included in the definition of an SPRM.[12] Figure 39.3 presents the molecular mechanism of action of SPRMs.

EFFECTS OF SPRMs ON THE NON-HUMAN PRIMATE ENDOMETRIUM

The endometrium of menstruating (Old World) non-human primates seems to share a lot of similarities with the human endometrium in terms of hormonal regulation of cell proliferation and differentiation, menstrual cyclicity, and molecular mechanisms of menstruation and tissue repair.[23] In non-human primates and women, estrogen is the primary mitogen in the endometrium. Progesterone and synthetic progestins oppose the effects of estrogen on the endometrial epithelium, and thereby protect the endometrium from the development of hyperplasia. The antiproliferative action of progesterone on the primate endometrial epithelium involves multiple mechanisms, including down-regulation of ER, induction of 17β-hydroxysteroid dehydrogenase (17βHSD) type 2 that catalyzes the conversion of estradiol to the less active estrone, inhibition of estrogen-induced protooncogenes (cjun, cfos), and regulation of cyclins.[24]

Endometrial antiproliferative effect in non-human primates

Keeping in mind the inhibitory effects of progesterone on endometrial proliferation, the observation made by Hodgen's group of 'antiestrogenic' effects of mifepristone on the macaque endometrium[25] was unexpected and surprising. This effect was originally described as a 'non-competitive antiestrogenic effect' since mifepristone does not bind to ER. The endometrial effects of various PAs were studied in more detail by Brenner and colleagues.[11,26–28] Since this phenomenon does not occur in all species,[29] or in other regions of the primate reproductive tract, it is best referred to as an 'endometrial antiproliferative effect'.[26]

Asoprisnil and structurally-related SPRMs also showed endometrial antiproliferative effects in cynomolgus

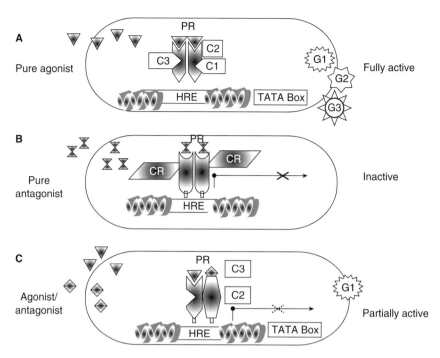

Figure 39.3 Hypothetical representation of the potential agonistic and antagonistic activities of SPRMs. (**A**) 'Pure' agonist ligands bind to the progesterone receptor (PR), inducing dimerization and conformational changes, which promote recruitment of coactivators (C1, C2, C3). The ligand–receptor complex, bound to the response element (HRE) of the promoter region of the target genes, will induce transactivation of progesterone responsive genes (G1, G2, G3). (**B**) The 'Pure' antagonist activity, in the presence or absence of progesterone, induces conformational changes that inactivate the AF-2 domain in the carboxyl terminal tail of the PR, thus preventing the receptor–ligand DNA complex from interacting with coactivators and will promote recruitment of corepressors (CR). (**C**) The partial agonist/antagonist activity of SPRM ligands may be explained by the induction of an intermediate conformation of PR, thus allowing its interaction (i) with both coactivators and corepressors, or (ii) with selected coactivators. The relative balance of coactivators and corepressors within a given cell will determine the relative agonist vs antagonist activity of an SPRM. An alternative possibility of partial agonist and antagonist activity in the presence of progesterone may be explained by binding of the SPRM to the PR followed by heterodimerization with progesterone bound to PR. The heterodimers will be less effective at binding to the HRE and activating gene transcription. (Reproduced from Chwalisz et al[12] and DeManno et al[30] with permission.)

monkeys.[24] In fact, studies in non-human primates played an important role in the discovery and conceptualization of SPRMs.[4] The antiproliferative effect of asoprisnil was confirmed in chronic toxicological studies conducted in intact cynomolgus macaques. These studies, which were of 39-week duration and employed various doses of asoprisnil (20, 60, 160, and 480 mg/kg/day), consistently showed endometrial atrophy (thinning) accompanied by a trend towards more compact stromal appearance and underdeveloped endometrial glands without signs of any secretory activity.[30] These effects occurred at all asoprisnil doses.

The effects of asoprisnil on endometrial morphology were evaluated in cynomolgus monkeys treated with lower doses of asoprisnil for a shorter period of time.[31,32] The monkeys were treated orally for 90 days with either asoprisnil (10, 30, and 90 mg/kg) or a placebo. The entire reproductive tract was removed from each animal and assessed for general histological changes, including spiral artery development, endometrial thickness, and stromal compaction. The effects on the proliferative

state were quantified by assessing two markers of proliferation – a cell-cycle non-specific marker Ki-67 and phosphorylated histone 3 (Phospho-H3), a cell-cycle specific marker that is expressed only in mitotic chromosomes and provides a direct indication of mitotic activity.[33] This study showed that all doses of asoprisnil significantly suppressed the proliferation markers Ki-67 and Phospho-H3 in the endometrial glands, and the two higher doses caused significant shrinkage in endometrial thickness without inducing progestational effects such as glandular sacculation and secretion (Figure 39.4). As in previous toxicological studies, there was a trend in stromal compaction, but no evidence of spiral artery degeneration. These effects occurred in the presence of physiologically adequate estrogen concentrations, as evidenced by estrogenic effects on the vagina, which was in an estrogenized state (assessed by a degree of cornification) in all asoprisnil-treated animals.

In summary, these studies showed that asoprisnil exhibits an endometrial antiproliferative effect in macaques, but, unlike a PA, does not induce spiral

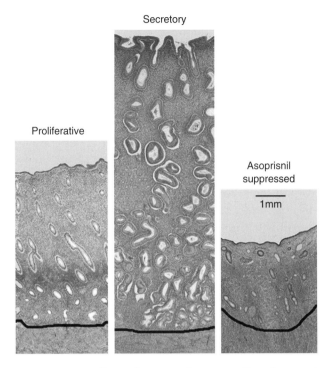

Secretory

Proliferative

Asoprisnil
suppressed

1mm

Figure 39.4 Effect of asoprisnil on overall endometrial histology of intact cynomolgus macaques. Photomicrographic comparison of endometrial histology of typical control animals (proliferative and secretory phases) vs asoprisnil-treated (90 mg/kg) animals. Original magnification ~ 4×. (Reproduced from Chwalisz et al[32] with permission. See also color plate section.)

artery degeneration and has only moderate effects on stromal compaction.

EFFECTS OF SPRMs ON THE HUMAN ENDOMETRIUM

To our knowledge, only two SPRMs, asoprisnil and J956, have been evaluated to date in humans regarding endometrial effects. Some asoprisnil studies have been published as full reports,[8] or in abstract form.[34–36] Phase 1 human studies have already revealed that these compounds induce distinctive effects on endometrial function and morphology that have not been described with any pharmacological agent before – (1) suppression of uterine bleeding via an endometrial effect and (2) unique endometrial morphology ('non-physiological secretory patterns' or 'SPRM endometrial effect') that seems to reflect the mixed progesterone agonist/antagonist properties of these compounds.[8]

Effects on uterine bleeding

The effects of asoprisnil on bleeding patterns are dependent on the dose. At lower doses (< 10 mg 1day),

a reduction in the intensity and duration of menstrual bleeding in the presence of normal menstrual cyclicity was generally observed. At higher doses (≥ 10 mg/day), suppression of uterine bleeding (defined as no bleeding requiring sanitary protection) and amenorrhea (no bleeding or spotting) occurred in the majority of women treated with asoprisnil. The effects of asoprisnil on uterine bleeding were rapid, and had already occurred during the first month of treatment. In addition, the troublesome breakthrough bleeding and spotting commonly observed during continuous progestin treatment[37] were rarely observed in women treated with asoprisnil.

The effects of asoprisnil on ovarian and menstrual cycle were studied in healthy volunteers in a phase 1 setting.[8] In this double-blind, dose-escalation study, 60 regularly cycling premenopausal women were treated with asoprisnil (dose range 5–100 mg/day) for a 28-day duration, beginning during the first 4 days of the menstrual cycle. Asoprisnil consistently prolonged the menstrual cycle at doses of ≥ 10 mg/day after treatment for 28 days. However, the effects on luteal phase progesterone, indicative of luteinization, were inconsistent and lacked dose dependency. Asoprisnil suppressed periovulatory serum estradiol concentrations, but not below those seen during the follicular phase. This study provided the first evidence that asoprisnil may control uterine bleeding predominantly via an endometrial effect.

The effects of asoprisnil on uterine bleeding were also studied in 129 patients with leiomyomata.[35] In this multicenter, randomized, double-blind, placebo-controlled, phase 2 study, asoprisnil (5 mg, 10 mg, and 25 mg) or a placebo was administered orally once daily for 12 weeks, beginning during the first 4 days of the menstrual cycle. Uterine bleeding was assessed by the patients using a daily bleeding diary, and a monthly 5-point score (0 = none, 1 = spotting [no protection or only requiring use of a panty shield], 2 = light bleeding [1–2 tampons or pads], 3 = medium bleeding [3–4 tampons or pads], or 4 = heavy bleeding [more than 4 tampons or pads]) to assess heavy uterine bleeding (self-reported menorrhagia). Daily bleeding diaries showed a dose-dependent suppression of uterine bleeding reflected in a significant reduction in average monthly spotting and bleeding scores (15.6 for placebo vs 7.3, 4.7, and 1.3 for asoprisnil 5, 10, and 25 mg, respectively; $p < 0.001$). Subjects with self-reported heavy uterine bleeding at baseline (76%) showed a decrease in menorrhagia scores after only 1 month of treatment. Asoprisnil dose-dependently suppressed uterine bleeding throughout treatment, with rates of 28%, 64%, and 83% for the 5, 10, and 25 mg doses, respectively, compared with 0% in the placebo group. This study showed that asoprisnil also controls heavy uterine bleeding associated with leiomyomata.

Suppression of uterine bleeding, via an endometrial effect, is a surprising finding that has not been previously described. All known pharmacological agents, including continuous oral contraceptives or depot-progestins,[38] gonadotropin-releasing hormone (GnRH) agonists,[39] and mifepristone[40–42] produce amenorrhea via anovulation. Continuous administration of the PA mifepristone induces anovulation and amenorrhea at daily doses of 2 mg and 5 mg,[40] and more consistently at higher doses of 50 or 100 mg/day.[41]

The asoprisnil effects on uterine bleeding were accompanied by a reduction in leiomyoma volume and improvement in pressure-related symptoms (pelvic pressure and bloating). Median percent decrease from baseline in leiomyoma volume was statistically significant at 25 mg compared with placebo after 4 and 8 weeks of treatment; by week 12, leiomyoma volume was reduced by 36%. There was a significant reduction in bloating with the two highest doses and in pelvic pressure at 25 mg by week 12.

Asoprisnil also showed efficacy in suppressing endometriosis-associated pain symptoms in a randomized, placebo-controlled phase 2 study.[43] Asoprisnil (5 mg, 10 mg, and 25 mg, or placebo) was administered orally once daily for 12 weeks, beginning during the first 4 days of the menstrual cycle. The effect of asoprisnil on daily pain was measured in subject diaries using a 4-point grading scale (0 = none, 1 = mild, 2 = moderate, 3 = severe) for three categories of pain (non-menstrual pelvic pain, dysmenorrhea, and dyspareunia). An additional assessment of pain was made during monthly visits using a modified Biberoglu and Behrman 4-point pain scale. All three asoprisnil doses significantly ($p < 0.05$) reduced the average daily combined non-menstrual pelvic pain/dysmenorrhea scores at all treatment months compared with placebo, showing a mean reduction in pain score of approximately 0.5 compared with a decrease of less than 0.1 with placebo, with similar reductions for each of the active groups. Similar results were observed for non-menstrual pelvic pain and dysmenorrhea when analyzed separately using daily diaries or monthly assessment during visits. The exact mechanism of endometriosis-associated pain suppression by asoprisnil is still unknown. However, animal studies with various SPRMs and PAs suggest that these compounds suppress the production of uterine prostaglandins in a tissue-specific manner.[3]

Effects on endometrial morphology and proliferation markers

During early clinical studies with asoprisnil and J956, it became apparent that SPRMs induce unique morphological effects on the endometrium that cannot be assessed using the conventional criteria of Noyes,[44] due to the asynchronous appearance of endometrial glands and stroma. These effects were characterized by a combination of morphological features affecting the glands, stroma, and vessels, which are described below in more detail. A new classification system was therefore established by a group of expert gynecological pathologists from various academic institutions and a central reading laboratory, who have been involved in all asoprisnil trials.[8] This system is based on conventional criteria, as described in *Blaustein's Pathology of the Female Genital Tract*,[45] but includes a new category, 'non-physiologic secretory patterns', consisting of two subcategories: (i) 'non-physiologic secretory effect', and (ii) 'secretory pattern mixed type'. The first subcategory is characterized by weak secretory effects on the endometrial glands without any mitotic figures, and variable effects on endometrial stroma ranging from stromal compaction to focal predecidual changes. The second subcategory, 'secretory pattern, mixed type', differs from the first subcategory by the presence of isolated mitotic figures in endometrial glands. It should be noted that none of the characteristic features of endometrial glands, stroma, and vessels were on their own specific for the SPRMs (asoprisnil and J956); however, the occurrence of several features together allowed designation of the endometrium as showing 'non-physiologic secretory patterns'. We also realized that some of these features change during longer treatment duration. Therefore, we prefer using a broader term, 'SPRM endometrial effect', which better describes the morphological syndrome induced in the endometrium during treatment with SPRMs. The following paragraphs summarize the endometrial morphology that was observed after asoprisnil treatment for 28 days and 3 months.

After short-term treatment for 28 days, the 'SPRM endometrial effect' was already recognizable in about half of the women treated with various doses of asoprisnil.[8] These effects, which were quite discrete, were characterized by the presence of weakly secretory glands lined by inactive epithelium and variable effects on the stroma, which showed a tendency towards compaction. In addition, clusters of unusually thick-walled arterial vessels were occasionally observed.

After longer (>1 month) treatment, these effects became more consistent and frequent, particularly the

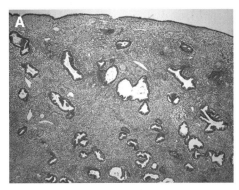
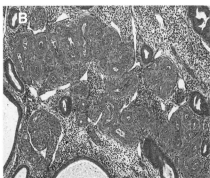

Figure 39.5   The 'SPRM endometrial effects' of asoprisnil after treatment for 3 months. (**A**) Representative full-thickness section of the endometrium from a hysterectomy specimen of a patient with symptomatic leiomyomata. Glands show a sinuous or serpentine profile, similar to the architecture of glands seen in the midsecretory phase of the menstrual cycle, with focal mild cystic dilatation. The stroma is compact, but non-decidualized. (**B**) Thick-walled muscularized vessel in endometrial stroma. (See also color plate section.)

changes in the arterial vessel wall. A detailed evaluation of the endometrial effects induced with asoprisnil after a 3-month treatment was conducted in patients with symptomatic leiomyomata awaiting hysterectomy.[36] This evaluation was based on the full-thickness endometrial samples obtained from hysterectomy specimens. In this double-blind, randomized, placebo-controlled study, 33 patients were treated with asoprisnil (10 mg or 25 mg/day) or a placebo. The non-specific proliferation marker Ki-67 and the mitosis-specific proliferation marker Phospho-H3 were assessed by immunohistochemistry in paraffin sections of endometrial samples. The numbers of glandular and stromal cells stained with Phospho-H3 in the endometrium were counted and expressed with respect to a measured area of the endometrium (mm²). Ki-67 was assessed in the endometrium using stereological methods.[36] The 'non-physiologic secretory pattern' was evident in the majority of endometrial samples from subjects treated with asoprisnil.[36] The endometrial glands showed mild tortuosity similar to the architecture of the secretory phase, but with a rarity of secretory activity or cytoplasmic vacuolation (Figure 39.5A). In addition, the endometrial glands frequently showed cystic dilatation; however, although nuclear stratification was present, there was a paucity of mitotic activity. There was, however, no evidence of hyperplastic changes in the glands, and no cytological atypia was seen to indicate any premalignant changes. A possible dose-dependent decrease in the numbers of mitotic figures in the endometrial glands was observed in asoprisnil-treated patients, and no glandular mitoses were identified in any of the endometrial samples from subjects taking 25 mg. With asoprisnil treatment, the endometrial stroma showed increasing compactness without decidual change, but the most characteristic stromal effect involved the vessels. After 3 months of asoprisnil treatment, the endometrium showed the formation of

unusual thick-walled muscular spiral arterioles and prominent aggregations of vessels in the stroma (Figure 39.5B). This effect was specific to the endometrium, since no changes in arterial vessels were found in non-endometrial tissues of the reproductive tract. Low Ki-67 and Phospho-H3 immunostaining was found in the endometrial glandular and stromal cells in both of the asoprisnil groups and in the secretory phase placebo group. Asoprisnil suppressed the expression of Ki-67 in endometrial stromal cells significantly below the level found in the stromal cells of the secretory phase placebo group.[36] There was a similar trend in Phospho-H3 expression, but this effect was not statistically significant. This suggests that the stromal cells may be more sensitive than the glandular cells to suppression by asoprisnil, as the proliferation markers Ki-67 and Phospho H3 in the glandular cells, already very low in the secretory phase, were not further suppressed by asoprisnil. In summary, this study confirmed both the presence of 'SPRM endometrial effect' as well as an antiproliferative effect on the endometrium in women after a 3-month asoprisnil treatment, based on the evaluation of full-thickness endometrial biopsies. In addition, the results of this study provided further evidence for the effects of asoprisnil on the endometrial arterial vasculature.

Endometrial differences between SPRMs and PAs

There are some morphological similarities between the endometrial effects of SPRMs and those of the PA mifepristone, but there are also significant differences. Cystic glandular dilatation with inactive epithelial appearances is common to both, and there is an antiproliferative effect.[46,47] However, no specific vascular changes have been identified in the stroma of a mifepristone-treated endometrium, and glands show a less tortuous morphology, generally showing simple tubular appearances or cystic dilatation. This suggests a pure antagonist effect of mifepristone on PR, whereas, with asoprisnil, the gland tortuosity probably reflects a partial agonist effect in addition to antagonist action.

Differences between the effects of PAs and SPRMs on human and non-human primate endometrium

Our studies also revealed some differences between the non-human primate models and women with respect to the endometrial effects of SPRMs and PAs. In both intact cycling, and ovariectomized estrogen-substituted macaques, a profound endometrial atrophy, associated with a dramatic reduction in endometrial thickness, was generally observed after treatment with SPRMs and some PAs, including mifepristone.[24] Although human studies with asoprisnil and mifepristone clearly showed an antiproliferative endometrial effect, such a profound endometrial atrophy was not observed. In cynomolgus macaques, neither secretory changes in endometrial glands, nor formation of thick-walled endometrial spiral arteries, were observed after asoprisnil treatment, indicating some important differences in the steroid receptor pharmacology of the monkey and human endometrium. The reason for these differences is unclear, but possibly the balance between agonist and antagonist effects of asoprisnil on the endometrium is shifted towards the agonist side in women, perhaps due to species differences in metabolic end products. Our studies with asoprisnil and previous experience with PAs suggest that the macaque endometrium is also more sensitive to PR ligands than the human endometrium, which could explain the stronger antagonistic effects of SPRMs and PAs in these animals.

SUMMARY AND CLINICAL OUTLOOK

In summary, studies in non-human primates and women demonstrated that 11β-benzaldoxime-substituted SPRMs control uterine bleeding and exhibit antiproliferative effects on the endometrium in the presence of follicular phase estradiol concentrations, as evidenced by a suppression of mitotic counts and a decrease in proliferation markers. Importantly, there is growing evidence that these results are predominantly due to an endometrial effect of these compounds. Clinical trials with this category of SPRMs revealed that this treatment leads to the development of unique histological appearances in the endometrium, termed 'SPRM endometrial

effect'. This histomorphological syndrome is characterized by the presence of endometrial glands showing tortuosity similar to the architecture of the secretory phase, separated by compacted stroma populated with thick-walled muscular arterial vessels.

Although the mechanism of asoprisnil-induced amenorrhea is still not completely understood, the current evidence suggests that asoprisnil may have an inhibitory effects on the function of spiral arteries. The most striking effect of asoprisnil on the human endometrium is the formation of thick-walled spiral arterioles, which appear to be specific to endometrial tissue. Interestingly, these effects clearly differ from those commonly observed in women using long-acting progestins or levonorgestrel-containing intrauterine systems that are associated with the formation of 'thin-walled' microvessels that are very fragile and frequently lead to breakthrough bleeding.[48-50] Although the molecular mechanisms of asoprisnil-induced amenorrhea remain unknown, the effects of asoprisnil on endometrial vessel morphology may explain, at least in part, the endometrial vessel's stability in asoprisnil-treated women.

Asoprisnil and other structurally related SPRMs exhibit an antiproliferative effect on the endometrium of non-human primates and women, as evidenced by low mitotic activity and a low level of proliferation markers in endometrial glands and stroma.[24,32,36] The mechanism of this effect remains unknown. Based on experiments conducted in cynomolgus macaques, we previously proposed that the endometrial antiproliferative effect of SPRMs and PAs might be due to the inhibition of angiogenesis.[24] However, studies with asoprisnil in women, as previously discussed, do not seem to support this hypothesis. More recently, the role of endometrial AR has been emphasized as a potential mechanism of the endometrial antiproliferative effects of PAs.[26,51-53] Androgens are known to inhibit estrogen effects in the primate endometrium.[53] The AR hypothesis was proposed based on the observation of greatly enhanced expression of AR in the endometrial glands of macaques treated with various PAs and in women treated with mifepristone.[51] Since up-regulation of AR was observed in the endometrial stroma of cynomolgus macaques treated with asoprisnil, its antiproliferative effect on the endometrial glandular epithelium might be mediated, at least in part, by AR-mediated stromal growth factors.[31] In addition, asoprisnil has weak androgenic properties, which may play a role in this respect.[30]

The 'SPRM endometrial effect' seems to reflect the non-physiological effects of compounds with mixed progesterone agonist/antagonist activities on endometrial glands and stroma. The clinical significance of these changes remains unknown. Although the glandular architectural features are not consistent with hyperplasia, the 'SPRM endometrial effect', which is unfamiliar to histopathologists, may lead to misdiagnoses of endometrial hyperplasia due to the presence of dilated glands. In addition, the thick-walled arterioles seen in Pipelle biopsies share similarities with 'feeder' vessels of endometrial polyps. It is important, therefore, that histopathologists examining endometrial biopsy specimens from SPRM-treated patients need to be aware of the unique 'SPRM endometrial effects', which do not easily fit with the current lexicon of histological diagnoses, to avoid misclassifying these appearances as simple hyperplasia or polyps. An expert meeting, convened by National Institutes of Health in April 2006 to discuss endometrial changes induced by SPRMs and PAs concluded that the descriptions of endometrial changes induced by these compounds do not fit current dictionaries, and new diagnostic categories need to be developed (Progesterone Receptor Modulators and the Endometrium – Changes and Consequences. April 7–8, 2006. Bethesda, MD, USA).

SPRMs have the potential to treat various gynecological disorders, particularly symptomatic leiomyomata, endometriosis, and treatment-resistant heavy uterine bleeding, without inducing estrogen deprivation.[12] Clinical studies with asoprisnil demonstrated that this SPRM effectively controls leiomyoma-associated symptoms, including heavy uterine bleeding and pressure-related symptoms, and reduces leiomyoma volume.[34] Furthermore, studies with asoprisnil showed its efficacy in controlling pain symptoms associated with endometriosis.[43] Further studies, in a larger study population, are needed to determine the optimal treatment regimens with asoprisnil or other SPRMs regarding both safety and efficacy outcomes.

ACKNOWLEDGMENT

We thank Gretchen Bodum for editing the manuscript.

REFERENCES

1. Allen WM, Wintersteiner O. Crystalline progesterone. Science 1934; 80: 190–1.
2. Butenandt A, Westphal U, Hohlweg W. [Uber das Hormon des corpus luteum]. Hopper-Seyler's Z Physiol Chem 1934; 227: 84–98. [in German]
3. Elger W, Bartley J, Schneider et al. Endocrine pharmacological characterization of progesterone antagonists and progesterone receptor modulators with respect to PR-agonistic and antagonistic activity. Steroids 2000; 65: 713–23.
4. Schubert G, Elger W, Kaufmann G et al. Discovery, chemistry, and reproductive pharmacology of asoprisnil and related 11beta-benzaldoxime substituted selective progesterone receptor modulators (SPRMs). Semin Reprod Med 2005; 23: 58–73.
5. Dong Y, Roberge JY, Wang Z et al. Characterization of a new class of selective nonsteroidal progesterone receptor agonists. Steroids 2004; 69: 201–17.
6. Zhi L, Tegley CM, Pio B et al. 5-benzylidene-1,2-dihydrochromeno[3,4-f]quinolines as selective progesterone receptor modulators. J Med Chem 2003; 46: 4104–12.
7. Giannoukos G, Szapary D, Smith CL, et al. New antiprogestins with partial agonist activity: potential selective progesterone receptor modulators (SPRMs) and probes for receptor- and coregulator-induced changes in progesterone receptor induction properties. Mol Endocrinol 2001; 15: 255–70.
8. Chwalisz K, Elger W, Stickler T et al. The effects of 1-month administration of asoprisnil (J867), a selective progesterone receptor modulator, in healthy premenopausal women. Hum Reprod 2005; 20: 1090–9.
9. Ishwad PC, Katkam RR, Hinduja IN et al. Treatment with a progesterone antagonist ZK 98.299 delays endometrial development without blocking ovulation in bonnet monkeys. Contraception 1993; 48: 57–70.
10. Katkam RR, Gopalkrishnan K, Chwalisz K et al. Onapristone (ZK 98.299): a potential antiprogestin for endometrial contraception. Am J Obstet Gynecol 1995; 173: 779–87.
11. Slayden OD, Zelinski-Wooten MB, Chwalisz K et al. Chronic treatment of cycling rhesus monkeys with low doses of the antiprogestin ZK 137 316: morphometric assessment of the uterus and oviduct. Hum Reprod 1998; 13: 269–77.
12. Chwalisz K, Perez MC, DeManno D et al. Selective progesterone receptor modulator development and use in the treatment of leiomyomata and endometriosis [published erratum appears in Endocr Rev 2005; 26: 703]. Endocr Rev 2005; 26: 423–38.
13. Smith CL, O'Malley BW. Coregulator function: a key to understanding tissue specificity of selective receptor modulators. Endocr Rev 2004; 25: 45–71.
14. Horwitz KB, Jackson TA, Bain DL et al. Nuclear receptor coactivators and corepressors. Mol Endocrinol 1996; 10: 1167–77.
15. Hull ML, Prentice A, Wang DY et al. Nimesulide, a COX-2 inhibitor, does not reduce lesion size or number in a nude mouse model of endometriosis. Hum Reprod 2004; 20: 665.
16. Chen JD, Evans RM. A transcriptional co-repressor that interacts with nuclear hormone receptors. Nature. 1995; 377: 454–47.
17. Onate SA, Tsai SY, Tsai MJ, O'Malley BW. Sequence and characterization of a coactivator for the steroid hormone receptor superfamily. Science 1995; 270: 1354–7.
18. McDonnell DP. The molecular pharmacology of SERMs. Trends Endocrinol Metab 1999; 10: 301–11.
19. Jackson TA, Richer JK, Bain DL et al. The partial agonist activity of antagonist-occupied steroid receptors is controlled by a novel hinge domain-binding coactivator L7/SPA and the corepressors N-CoR or SMRT. Mol Endocrinol 1997; 11: 693–705.
20. Wagner BL, Norris JD, Knotts TA et al. The nuclear corepressors NCoR and SMRT are key regulators of both ligand- and 8-bromo-cyclic AMP-dependent transcriptional activity of the human progesterone receptor. Mol Cell Biol 1998; 18: 1369–78.
21. Wagner BL, Pollio G, Leonhardt S et al. 16 alpha-substituted analogs of the antiprogestin RU486 induce a unique conformation in the human progesterone receptor resulting in mixed agonist activity. Proc Natl Acad Sci USA 1996; 93: 8739–44.
22. Melvin V, Perez M, Chwalisz K, Edwards D. Mechanism of action of the selective progesterone receptor modulator asoprisnil. Endocrine Society's 87th Annual Meeting, 2005: 613.

23. Brenner RM, Nayak NR, Slayden OD et al. Premenstrual and menstrual changes in the macaque and human endometrium: relevance to endometriosis. Ann NY Acad Sci 2002; 955: 60–74; discussion 86–68, 396–406.

24. Chwalisz K, Brenner RM, Fuhrmann UU et al. Antiproliferative effects of progesterone antagonists and progesterone receptor modulators on the endometrium. Steroids 2000; 65: 741–51.

25. Wolf JP, Hsiu JG, Anderson TL et al. Noncompetitive antiestrogenic effect of RU 486 in blocking the estrogen-stimulated luteinizing hormone surge and the proliferative action of estradiol on endometrium in castrate monkeys. Fertil Steril 1989; 52: 1055–60.

26. Brenner RM, Slayden OD, Critchley HO. Anti-proliferative effects of progesterone antagonists in the primate endometrium: a potential role for the androgen receptor. Reproduction 2002; 124: 167–72.

27. Slayden OD, Hirst JJ, Brenner RM. Estrogen action in the reproductive tract of rhesus monkeys during antiprogestin treatment. Endocrinology 1993; 132: 1845–56.

28. Slayden OD, Brenner RM. RU 486 action after estrogen priming in the endometrium and oviducts of rhesus monkeys (*Macaca mulatta*). J Clin Endocrinol Metab 1994; 78: 440–8.

29. Chwalisz K, Stockemann K, Fritzemeier KH, Fuhrmann U. Modulation of oestrogenic effects by progesterone antagonists in the rat uterus. Hum Reprod Update 1998; 4: 570–83.

30. DeManno D, Elger W, Garg R et al. Asoprisnil (J867): a selective progesterone receptor modulator for gynecological therapy. Steroids 2003; 68: 1019–32.

31. Brenner RM, Slayden OD, Garg R, Chwalisz K. Asoprisnil suppresses endometrial proliferation in cynomolgus macaques. J Soc Gynecol Invest 2005; 12(Suppl): 208A.

32. Chwalisz K, Garg R, Brener R et al. Role of nonhuman primate models in the discovery and clinical development of selective progesterone receptor modulators (SPRMs). Reprod Biol Endocrinol 2006; 4(Suppl 1): S8.

33. Brenner RM, Slayden OD, Rodgers WH et al. Immunocytochemical assessment of mitotic activity with an antibody to phosphorylated histone H3 in the macaque and human endometrium. Hum Reprod 2003; 18: 1185–93.

34. Chwalisz K, Parker RL, Williamson S et al. Treatment of uterine leiomyomas with the novel selective progesterone receptor modulator (SPRM) J867. J Soc Gynecol Investig 2003; 10(Suppl 2): 636.

35. Chwalisz K, Larsen L, McCrary K, Edmonds A. Effects of the novel selective progesterone receptor modulator (SPRM) asoprisnil on bleeding patterns in subjects with leiomyomata. J Soc Gynecol Invest 2004; 11(Suppl 2): 320–1A.

36. Williams AR, Critchley HO, Osei J, et al. The selective progesterone receptor modulator asoprisnil inhibits glandular proliferation and induces consistent morphological effects in human endometrium. J Soc Gynecol Investig 2006; 13(Suppl 2): 261–2A.

37. Fraser IS, Weisberg E, Minehan E, Johansson ED. A detailed analysis of menstrual blood loss in women using Norplant and Nestorone progestogen-only contraceptive implants or vaginal rings. Contraception 2000; 61: 241–51.

38. Lobo RA, Stanczyk FZ. New knowledge in the physiology of hormonal contraceptives. Am J Obstet Gynecol 1994; 170: 1499–507.

39. Conn PM, Crowley WF Jr. Gonadotropin-releasing hormone and its analogues. N Engl J Med 1991; 324: 93–103.

40. Brown A, Cheng L, Lin S, Baird DT. Daily low-dose mifepristone has contraceptive potential by suppressing ovulation and menstruation: a double-blind randomized control trial of 2 and 5 mg per day for 120 days. J Clin Endocrinol Metab 2002; 87: 63–70.

41. Kettel LM, Murphy AA, Morales AJ, Yen SS. Clinical efficacy of the antiprogesterone RU486 in the treatment of endometriosis and uterine fibroids. Hum Reprod 1994; 9(Suppl 1): 116–20.

42. Croxatto HB, Kovacs L, Massai R et al. Effects of long-term low-dose mifepristone on reproductive function in women. Hum Reprod 1998; 13: 793–8.

43. Chwalisz K, Mattia-Goldberg C, Lee M et al. Treatment of endometriosis with the novel selective progesterone receptor modulator (SPRM) asoprisnil. Fertil Steril 2004; 82(Suppl 2): S83–4.

44. Noyes R, Hertig AT, Rock J. Dating the endometrial biopsy. Fertil Steril 1950; 1: 3–25.

45. Mutter G, Ferenczy A. Anatomy and histology of the uterine corpus. In: Kurman R, ed. Blaustein's Pathology of the Female Genital Tract. New York: Springer-Verlag, 2002: 383–419.

46. Baird DT, Brown A, Critchley HO et al. Effect of long-term treatment with low-dose mifepristone on the endometrium. Hum Reprod 2003; 18: 61–8.

47. Narvekar N, Cameron S, Critchley HO et al. Low-dose mifepristone inhibits endometrial proliferation and up-regulates androgen receptor. J Clin Endocrinol Metab 2004; 89: 2491–7.

48. Hickey M, Dwarte D, Fraser IS. Superficial endometrial vascular fragility in Norplant users and in women with ovulatory dysfunctional uterine bleeding. Hum Reprod 2000; 15: 1509–14.

49. Hickey M, Fraser IS. The structure of endometrial microvessels. Hum Reprod 2000; 15 (Suppl 3): 57–66.

50. Simbar M, Manconi F, Markham R et al. A three-dimensional study of endometrial microvessels in women using the contraceptive subdermal levonorgestrel implant system, Norplant. Micron 2004; 35: 589–95.

51. Slayden OD, Nayak NR, Burton KA et al. Progesterone antagonists increase androgen receptor expression in the rhesus macaque and human endometrium. J Clin Endocrinol Metab 2001; 86: 2668–79.

52. Brenner RM, Slayden OD, Nayak NR et al. A role for the androgen receptor in the endometrial antiproliferative effects of progesterone antagonists. Steroids 2003; 68: 1033–9.

53. Brenner RM, Slayden OD. Progesterone receptor antagonists and the endometrial antiproliferative effect. Semin Reprod Med 2005; 23: 74–81.

40   In-utero gene transfer: promises and problems

Gaurang S Daftary and Hugh S Taylor

Synopsis

In utero gene transfer is one of several potential, advanced medical therapies for endometrial disorders. Several issues are important for success of this experimental technique to treat endometrial disorders related to implantation failure, endometrial hyperlasia and neoplasia, abnormal endometrial bleeding, and applications to contragestation.:

Clinical

- type of gene transfer vector
- route of administration
- timing in the cycle
- targets of interest

ABSTRACT

The rapidly evolving field of genomics and the resources provided by the Human Genome Project have generated great enthusiasm for translating these advances into clinically realizable gains. Gene therapy has been exploited as a novel modality to treat recalcitrant and conventionally untreatable diseases, ranging from inherited disorders such as cystic fibrosis to cancer. Additionally, gene therapy provides a more physiological ability to affect disease and has expanded the spectrum of current therapeutics. In most cases gene therapy application is specific and minimally invasive compared to alternatives using conventional therapy. Concomitant with the developments in genomics are significant advances in biomedical research. This has resulted in the development of a diverse range of gene delivery vehicles, capable of efficiently and specifically transferring therapeutic genes to their respective target tissues. Uterine transfection in animal models appears to be safe, efficient, and reproducible and, in preliminary trials, gene therapy has proven efficacious. The human uterus has also proven to be amenable to efficient gene transfection. Gene therapy to the human uterus is likely to expand the spectrum of therapeutics to disorders that are incompletely understood and therefore inadequately treated by conventional means such as embryo implantation defects and habitual abortion. Advances in therapeutic capability may alter the way in which uterine neoplasia, functional bleeding, and contraception are treated as well. Every new advance is accompanied by adverse reactions that are either predictable or unforeseen and need to be considered prior to the incorporation of this novel advance in translational medicine.

INTRODUCTION

Gene therapy is defined as any therapeutic procedure in which genes are pharmacologically introduced into human somatic cells, resulting in a desired therapeutic effect. Recent advances in genome research, such as the Human Genome Project, have led to greater understanding of the molecular defects underlying many diseases. The rapidly evolving field of translational research has resulted in the development of novel therapeutic approaches. One such application is the development of gene therapy. Gene therapy may be administered either directly to the target cells (in-vivo gene therapy) or, alternatively, target cells may be extracted from the organism and grown as explants which are then modified ex vivo by gene therapy, prior to reimplantation into the host organism.

Gene replacement was initially attempted in the treatment of inherited single gene disorders where no satisfactory conventional treatments exist. These conditions typically resulting from mutant alleles giving rise to genetic deficiencies. The first published report of successful gene therapy was for a rare metabolic disorder, severe combined immune deficiency (SCID), that results from congenital adenine deaminase deficiency (ADA).[1] This rare enzyme deficiency precludes lymphocytes from synthesizing antibodies to common viral antigens and results in morbidity and early mortality from common respiratory and gastrointestinal infections. The administration of ex-vivo genetically altered lymphocytes to patients with this disorder resulted in normalization of the T-lymphocyte count and ADA level, resulting in immunological competence. Likewise, insertion of a normal CFTR (cystic fibrosis transmembrane receptor) allele has been attempted with variable success in patients with cystic fibrosis.[2] Other single gene disorders where gene therapy has been attempted include α_1-antitrypsin deficiency, β-thalassemia, hemophilia A, and hemophilia B. There are currently over 4000 known single gene disorders and not all of them are amenable to gene replacement. For example, in the case of sickle cell anemia, the disease involves the production of an abnormal hemoglobin, HgS. Successful gene therapy for this disorder would therefore require not only the production of adequate amounts of normal hemoglobin but also suppression of HgS.

Novel therapeutic strategies such as gene therapy are being increasingly developed for the treatment of cancer. This is because conventional chemotherapy and radiation are often not able to cure the disease and are associated with multiple adverse effects. Increased understanding of the mechanisms leading to tumor growth has revealed multiple potential mechanisms by which gene therapy could be employed in the treatment of cancer. The basis for gene therapy in cancer stems from the development of transgenes, consisting of a cancer-specific promoter with a gene that has antitumor activity. Selective and robust expression of the antitumor effective gene within cancer cells maximizes efficacy while concomitantly minimizing damage to surrounding normal tissues. A number of cancer-specific promoters have been reported, such as probasin, human telomerase reverse transcriptase, surviving, ceruloplasmin, and HER-2. As a group, these are usually promoters of growth-promoting transcription factors that are expressed at higher levels in rapidly prolific neoplastic cells. Alternatively, antitumor genes are either proapoptotic, such as p53, E1A, BAX, FasL, or suicide genes.[3] Suicide genes are non-mammalian enzymes such as *HSV-TK* and *CDA* that convert non-toxic prodrugs such as ganciclovir and 5-fluorouracil to toxic metabolites, thereby effecting cell death.[4] Inhibition of angiogenesis may be yet another mechanism to arrest the growth of tumors.[5] Yet another approach to cancer-targeted gene therapy is through increased antitumor immunity, which can be achieved through immunization with genetically programmed cells such as melanoma cells capable of enhanced granulocyte–macrophage colony-stimulating factor (GM-CSF) secretion.[6] In the future, gene therapy-mediated immune modulation is likely to target tumor-specific antigens and immune cells capable of mounting an antitumor immune response.[7] Immune modulation through gene therapy has also been attempted to enhance host immunity in infections such as human immunodeficiency virus (HIV).[8]

Another area where gene therapy has great potential is the cardiovascular system. The administration of fibroblast growth factor 4 (FGF-4) and vascular endothelial growth factor (VEGF) has been shown in animals and humans to induce angiogenesis in a previously infarcted region in both the myocardium and in peripheral vascular disease.[9,10] Gene therapy is likely to have a major impact in this field not only because of the high incidence of coronary artery disease but also because of the ease of administration of gene therapy into the vasculature, resulting in high tissue-specific levels with minimal side effects due to non-specific transfection.

Given the advances in genomics and the preliminary success achieved when this knowledge has been translated into therapeutics, it is logical to extend this capability to the treatment of gynecological disorders. In this chapter, we consider potential indications of in-utero gene transfer. We further consider various methods for achieving gene transfer, their advantages and disadvantages, followed by applicability to the female reproductive tract. Finally, potential complications that could arise from such therapy are considered.

IN-UTERO GENE THERAPY: PROMISES

Gene therapy may be potentially applied to rectify a wide spectrum of molecular defects resulting from genomic errors. Molecular defects have been implicated in the pathogenesis of such uterine disorders as implantation defects, recurrent pregnancy loss, and cancer. Gene therapy to the female reproductive tract offers a novel, specific, and relatively non-invasive therapeutic approach to treat the molecular defects underlying these conditions. It is therefore likely to find wide applicability in gynecology.

A number of potential indications for gene transfer to the human female reproductive tract exist and may be amenable to genetic alteration. Implantation defects contribute to infertility and abortion. Such defects may coexist with other reproductive tract diseases such as endometriosis, hydrosalpinx, and polycystic ovary syndrome (PCOS) or may uniquely be the only underlying factor in patients with otherwise unexplained infertility or habitual abortion. Recent evidence has demonstrated the necessity of the homeobox genes Hoxa10 and Hoxa11 as well as the cytokine leukemia inhibitory factor (LIF) for embryo implantation.[11–13] Altered expression levels of the homeobox genes have been associated with human implantation defects.[14,15] As discussed later, implantation rates may be genetically augmented or diminished in the animal model through altered expression of these genes.[16] The possibility of altering implantation can be therapeutically used to either augment implantation rates, especially in conjunction with artificial reproductive technology, or to prevent implantation as a contraceptive.

Gene therapy is also likely to have a major impact in the treatment of uterine neoplasia. Uterine leiomyomas are common tumors seen in up to 77% of women.[17] These tumors are a frequent cause of morbidity such as abnormal uterine bleeding, pelvic pain, urinary and intestinal symptoms, and infertility. Fibroid uterus is currently the most common indication for hysterectomy. Whereas conventional methods of surgical treatment are usually effective, they result in significant morbidity. Furthermore, due to the recurrent nature of these tumors, conservative surgical procedures are often unable to effect a lasting cure, requiring repeated procedures or hysterectomy. A leiomyoma develops due to abnormal clonal proliferation of uterine myocytes. By genetically altering the rate of growth or by promoting apoptosis of the dysregulated myocytes in a fibroid by selective expression of antitumor genes as discussed above, it may be possible to easily, specifically, and repeatedly treat uterine fibroids without the need for surgical intervention. Endometrial cancer, the most common female genital tract malignancy, may also be amenable to targeted intervention at the molecular level using gene therapy. Either expression of tumor suppressor genes, genes inducing apoptosis such as p53, or suicide genes such as viral thymidine kinase in conjunction with chemotherapeutic agents, may be used for this purpose.

Novel approaches to treat dysfunctional bleeding may involve gene therapy to the vasculature, as is currently being investigated for use in cardiovascular disease. These may involve the use of antisense to VEGF or FGF to prevent neovascularization or treatment of vascular adventitia to regulate vascular remodeling.[18]

The adult human uterus can be transfected easily and with high efficiency.[19,20] High levels of gene expression can be achieved by this method. Given the technology, rapid advances in genomics, and knowledge of disease causality, gene therapy of female reproductive disorders is a logical advance in gynecological therapeutics.

In addition to administering gene therapy to the uterus for treatment of various uterine diseases, there are newly emergent applications for in-utero fetal gene therapy. As discussed later, multiple fetal sites for administration of gene therapy are readily accessible via ultrasound guidance. Early gene therapy to the fetus permits a potential cure for many currently incurable inherited diseases such as cystic fibrosis and sickle cell anemia, whose genetic basis has been well characterized.

ADMINISTRATION OF GENE THERAPY

Prior to considering the applicability of in-utero gene therapy, it is essential to briefly recapitulate the physiology of gene expression and thereby identify likely barriers to therapy using transgenes. In order to be expressed, a gene is initially transcribed into heteronuclear RNA (hnRNA), which is then spliced within the nucleus into mature messenger RNA (mRNA). Transcription requires that RNA polymerases bind to the gene promoter, which is a DNA sequence located 5′ of the transcription start site of most genes. In turn, the RNA polymerase recruits a number of regulatory proteins, including general transcription factors. Such binding either causes activation of RNA polymerase, resulting in gene transcription, or repression of RNA polymerase, resulting in inhibition of transcription. Gene expression levels therefore correspond to the relative state of activating and inhibitory influences and affect transcription through RNA polymerase. Mature mRNA is translated in the ribosomes into protein. The protein, in turn, is the functional effector of the gene.

In general, gene therapy aims to correct the underlying genetic defect through either gene repair, gene inhibition, or gene addition. With current technology, it is extremely difficult to achieve gene repair – involving excision of a gene segment containing an offending deletion, insertion, or inversion, followed by replacement by a corresponding but normal gene segment. However, silencing the expression of an abnormal gene through the use of antisense nucleotides or RNA interference (RNAi), or addition of multiple copies of a normal gene in a cell that is deficient for the gene, are the current focus of contemporary gene therapy trials. In vivo, diverse physiological processes are regulated by proteins functioning either intracellularly (e.g. transcription factors, enzymes, cytoskeletal proteins) or on the cell surface (e.g. follicle-stimulating hormone [FSH], luteinizing hormone [LH], and other peptide hormones). Whereas systemic administration of a cell-surface acting protein is facile, low rates of intracellular protein uptake limit the ability to treat diseases requiring intracellular protein. High intracellular protein expression can, however, be achieved with gene therapy by utilizing the intrinsic protein synthetic machinery in target cells. Synthesis of DNA for commercial use is relatively easy and inexpensive compared to manufacture of proteins. In addition, many proteins are immunogenic and therefore systemic administration is likely to invoke inflammatory reactions; this could result in degradation of the protein as well as put the patient at risk for potentially life-threatening complications. Finally, long-term stable transfection of the therapeutic transgene into the defective host cell genome may potentially effect a cure.

As DNA provides only the framework for synthesis of the actual effector protein, it is necessary to deliver the DNA into the target cell nucleus, where it can be processed. The process of gene administration to a cell or organ in most cases requires the use of a vector. A vector may be defined as a vehicle that permits passage of the transfected gene into the nucleus of the cell. Vectors may be classified into two categories – viral or non-viral. The gene of interest is inserted into either viral DNA or RNA or into plasmid DNA in series with a heterologous promoter that can drive gene expression in the target cell using host cell RNA polymerase and transcription factors. The nucleic acid component, comprising the gene of interest together with its flanking regulatory DNA sequence, is known as the 'expression cassette'. Key structural elements of vectors are a surface element that recognizes the target cell surface and elements that mediate internalization and transport to the nucleus. A vector differs from a drug in that it consists of a constellation of assembled components, each of which is uniquely engineered to improve overall vector performance.

To attain the desired therapeutic effect, the vector carrying the therapeutic gene must successfully target the tissue where gene expression is desired. On reaching the target tissue, the target gene must successfully traffic through the cytosol. Once in the nucleus, the expression of the gene should occur in a manner that closely resembles physiological gene expression. Most importantly, the therapeutic protein produced must have biological activity in vivo. Additionally, neither the vector nor the gene product should have toxic effects on the host. No single vector meets all these requirements, such that it may be used to administer gene therapy in all settings. The optimal gene delivery method varies by indication and depends on the type of disorder, the target tissue to be transfected, and the desired duration of transgene expression (transient or permanent).

Viruses efficiently deliver their nucleic acid into mammalian cells as an essential and critical part of their life cycle. Their ability to deliver genes into target cells has been honed through evolution. Consequently, viruses were the first choice as vehicles for gene transfer, because they efficiently recognize and enter cells, traffic through the cytosol, reach the nucleus, and express their genes. The process of introduction and expression of a therapeutic transgene in somatic cells using a viral vector is known as transduction. In order for a virus to function solely as a gene transduction vehicle and at the same time not induce disease or tissue damage, its ability to replicate in the host has to be prevented.[21] This is achieved by deleting genes necessary for viral replication and substituting the therapeutic transgene in the viral genome instead. Recombinant viruses are initially synthesized as infectious particles by a specialized packaging cell line.[22] These specialized packaging cells have been previously transfected with viral genes necessary for replication. Assembly of the viral capsid with altered viral genomic DNA in the packaging cell line results in the synthesis of recombinant viruses that are only capable of infecting target cells at initial contact. Being unable to replicate, they successfully transduce target organ cells with the gene of interest but are unable to cause infectious disease. Alternatively, the viral genomic packaging signal sequences, which direct newly synthesized viral genome to newly synthesized viral particles in the infected cell, may be deleted and appended to a therapeutic transgene. New viral particles synthesized by the expressed viral genes incorporate only the transgene, due to its association with the signal sequence. The viral progeny therefore function solely as vectors. Several different viruses have been used in clinical trials of gene therapy.[2,23] The most commonly used are retroviruses and adenoviruses. Other viruses under development as vectors include the adeno-associated virus (AAV), lentivirus, and herpes simplex virus (HSV).

Some of the initial trials involving viral vectors used retroviruses. Retroviral vectors are derived from C-type retroviruses such as the murine leukemia virus or lentiviruses such as human or feline immunodeficiency viruses. Retroviruses are RNA viruses. Once in the nucleus, activation of the enzyme reverse transcriptase encoded by the viral gene *pol* leads to viral DNA synthesis. The viral DNA contains long terminal repeat sequences that enable stable integration into the host cell genome. By deleting the gene ψ, necessary for viral encapsidation (and thus infectivity), it is possible to use these viruses as vehicles for long-term genetic transduction of target cells.

Retroviruses have a high gene transfer efficiency and stable chromosome integration allowing for long-term gene expression.[24] However, retroviruses can only transduce actively dividing cells. Additionally, inability to transduce cells with large DNA inserts (> 10 kb) is also a major limiting factor for use of this method.[25,26] The integration of the viral genome into the host cell genome is mediated by viral integrase and occurs at random locations, often at a different chromosomal site in each transduced cell, preferring actively transcribed sites.[27] Potential complications due to random integration of the DNA insert into the host cell genome have been reported.[28] These include insertional mutagenesis from disruption of essential host cell genes. Disruption of a tumor suppressor gene or activation of an oncogene could result in malignant transformation. This was seen clinically in two X-linked SCID patients that received gene therapy. Both patients developed leukemia and demonstrated genomic integration in close proximity to the LMO2 oncogene.[29] In other cases, diminished transgene expression may be due to transcriptional repression

from interruption of host gene regulatory regions or binding of inhibitory transcription factors to viral enhancer elements or epigenetic modification such as methylation or acetylation. Finally, provirus deletion during DNA repair or death of the infected target cell could terminate entirely the therapeutic benefit gained from the original gene therapy.

The natural tropism of the replication defective recombinant adenovirus initially prompted its use in the respiratory tract to treat cystic fibrosis.[2] It was subsequently found to be very effective at transducing a wide variety of cells and achieving high levels of transgene expression.[30] Unlike retroviruses, these viruses do not integrate into the host chromosomes. Instead, they express the transgene from an extrachromosomal location (episome). Transgene expression with these vectors is therefore transient in duration. Although there is no risk of insertional mutagenesis, potential complications from lack of tissue selectivity and immunogenicity have been reported.[31–33] Modifications to the adenovirus genome therefore are aimed at producing vectors that are less immunogenic to the host and less likely to cause disease.[34]

Advances in the development of viral vectors have led to the use of novel viruses such as the AAV, a non-pathogenic, defective, DNA parvovirus.[28] The viral genome integrates with that of the host cell potentially enabling stable long-term transduction.[35] The risk for insertional mutagenesis is, however, lower than that observed with retroviruses. Trials with other viral vectors such as lentiviruses and HSV are also in progress.[36,37]

Non-viral mechanisms of direct gene transfer involve such physical methods as direct injection, particle-mediated bombardment (gene gun) electroporation, and the related technique of ultrasonoporation. In addition, nucleic acids may also be combined with cationic lipids and transferred by a process known as lipofection. The process of introducing genetic material (DNA or RNA) into a target cell by non-viral mechanisms is known as transfection. The efficiency of gene transfer using these methods is in general diminished compared to that obtained with viral vectors. Additionally, lack of integration of the transfected gene into the target cell genome results in only transient gene expression. However, gene transfection by non-viral mechanisms is safer, easier, and less expensive to administer than using viral vectors and additionally enables transfer of larger DNA fragments to target cells. These advantages offer scope for large-scale clinical application.

Direct DNA injection involves microinjection of DNA into the target cell. In vivo, this method has been utilized therapeutically to transfect striated muscle in α_1-antitrypsin deficiency.[38] Due to the small number of cells that are successfully transfected, this method is better suited for ex-vivo transfection of single cells, such as producing transgenic organisms.[39] Another application of this technique is for genetic vaccination, where bacterial, viral, or tumor antigens may be expressed in host tissues and thereby invoke either a protective or therapeutic immune response.[40]

Particle-mediated gene delivery is a physical method that involves coating 1–3 μm inert particles with plasmid DNA, which are then transferred by either an electric discharge or gas pulse device.[41,42] The driving force generated enables the particles to penetrate the cell membrane. Transferred DNA is present in the nucleus as episomes and transfection is transient. In contrast to viral transduction, this method enables transfer of large amounts of DNA such as cosmids and artificial chromosomes. The physical nature of transfer precludes development of cytopathic immune responses, as seen with the use of viruses.[43] The skin is the most accessible site for in-vivo gene transfer and trials have focused on DNA immunization.[44] However, as with direct DNA injection, the ability to transfect organs in deeper locations is limited. Electroporation is another physical method of transfection that exposes cells to high voltage in the presence of DNA. The applied electrical force results in transient formation of hydrophilic pores in the cell membrane, thereby allowing the cell to take up DNA. Electroporation is useful in in-vitro and ex-vivo cellular gene transfer.[45,46] The technique is easy to perform, achieving rapid, efficient, and highly reproducible transfer of even large DNA inserts such as cosmids and artificial chromosomes.[47,48] In a related technique known as ultrasonoporation, DNA is incorporated into microbubbles, which are then burst in the vicinity of target cells, by the application of high-frequency ultrasound.[49] As with other physical methods of DNA transfer, the ability to transfect deeper tissues or whole organs is limited with electroporation.

Gene transfer using cationic liposomes is referred to as lipofection, and the complex comprising liposome and nucleic acid is termed 'lipoplex'.[50,51] Cationic lipids are fatty acids with a hydrophilic head and hydrophobic tail. Most cationic lipids used for gene transfer are cationic amphiphiles such as Lipofectamine (composed of a non-bilayer forming cationic lipid DOSPA [2,3-dioleyloxy-N-[2(sperminecarboxamido)ethyl]-N-N-dimethyl-1-propanaminium trifluoroacetate] and neutral helper lipid DOPE [dioleoyl phosphatidyl ethanolamine]. The positively charged lipid molecules in a lipoplex complex electrostatically with anionic nucleic acids (negative charge conferred by phosphate groups). Hydrophobic interactions result in condensation of the complex and encapsulation of the nucleic acid by the lipid. The lipoplex is taken up by the cell by either endocytosis, phagocytosis, or direct fusion with the cell membrane, depending on the cell type.[50] As discussed earlier, the efficiency of gene transfection depends on the ability of sufficient lipid–DNA complexes to resist lysosomal degradation and thereby deliver DNA for nuclear uptake. Compared to transfection using viral vectors, lipofection has low transfection efficiency. Advantages of lipofection include ease of performance, safety, and applicability to a wide range of host cell types. Modification in liposome composition such as addition of an SV40 nuclear localization peptide has improved gene transfer efficiency.[52] In order to ensure more reliable gene delivery to a target cell, a cell receptor-specific ligand (e.g. transferrin) may be included in the liposome–DNA complex. The resultant complex is known as a polyplex.[53] The ligand–receptor interaction further augments internalization by target cells, thereby improving selectivity and efficiency of gene expression. Other modifications include the incorporation of several functional domains specific for cytosol trafficking or endosomal destabilization in the plasmid used for lipofection so as to mimic viral infection and thereby achieve high transfection efficiency.[54,55]

While transfection and transduction have largely been used to introduce novel therapeutic transgenes into target cells lacking their expression, we will now consider methods that may be used to silence abnormal endogenous gene expression. Single-stranded DNA in cell-free systems has been shown to inhibit mRNA translation. This observation has resulted in the development of techniques that utilize exogenous nucleic acids to inhibit in-vivo gene expression.[56,57] Natural antisense RNA molecules have been described with the ability to influence gene expression.[58,59] Nucleic acid therapeutic technology uses two major approaches to modulate gene expression: anti-DNA or anti-mRNA.[60]

Anti-DNA (Anti-gene) approaches target genes by triple-helix-forming oligodeoxynucleotides (TFOs).[61,62] TFOs are typically 10–30 nucleotides in length and bind in the major groove of DNA to sequences that consist of runs of purines on one DNA strand and of pyrimidines on the complementary strand. This stringent requirement limits the potential for generalized application. TFOs alter gene expression by multiple mechanisms. These include inhibition of transcription, mutagenesis at the binding site, or by inducing homologous recombination. Additionally, an artificially tethered mutagen may also be delivered to the DNA via the TFO, thereby altering target gene expression.[62] Through mutagenesis and recombination, induction of long-term or heritable therapeutic alterations may be possible.

mRNA is susceptible to therapeutic manipulation either during transcription, transport from the nucleus, or during translation.[60] Numerous anti-mRNA approaches are therefore in current development. Antisense strategy constitutes the delivery of reverse complementary oligonucleotides (antisense) to a cell expressing the gene of interest.[63,64] Stable duplex complexes comprising mRNA-antisense are formed as a result. This could either interfere with splicing of hnRNA into mature mRNA or block translation.[65,66] The antisense nucleotide may in some cases promote degradation of bound mRNA by further allowing binding of endogenous nucleases such as RNase H.[67] Alternatively, intrinsic enzymatic activity can be artificially engineered into the antisense oligonucleotide itself (ribozyme). Ribozymes are composed of a catalytic motif surrounded by flanking nucleotides that bind target mRNA, enabling its degradation.[68] One such ribozyme, the hammerhead, employs divalent cations such as Mg^{2+} to accomplish RNA degradation.[69]

Another novel approach for targeting mRNA is post-transcriptional gene silencing or RNAi.[70-72] This approach is based on target mRNA degradation in the presence of intracellular double-stranded RNA (dsRNA). This results in post-transcriptional silencing of the target gene. Specific triggering dsRNA oligonucleotides are taken up by target cells and processed into multiple 21–25 base pair fragments known as small interfering RNA (siRNA) by the RNase III-like enzyme Dicer. The siRNA are then incorporated into a multiunit enzymatic complex known as RISC (RNA-induced silencing complex). The component siRNA directs the RISC complex to specific homologous target mRNA. The mRNA then undergoes enzymatic hydrolysis, thereby silencing the expression of the encoded target gene. Successful use of RNAi in mammalian cells indicates potential applicability in future gene therapy application.[73,74] In general, gene silencing through methods that involve the use of ribozymes or siRNA is more efficient than antisense methods. This is because, in addition to preventing mRNA expression, these methods utilize catalytic enzymes that lyse the target mRNA.

In summarizing the different methods of gene delivery described so far, the only method that results in stable, long-term gene expression is retroviral transduction. Potential complications of this method are insertional mutagenesis and generation of replication-competent retroviruses. Two novel agents, mammalian artificial chromosomes and Epstein–Barr virus-based vectors, are being investigated as agents with potential for long-term transfection. As these agents do not integrate with the host cell chromosomes, they lack the risks incurred with the use of retroviruses.[75-77]

APPLICATION OF IN-UTERO GENE TRANSFER

Prior to developing in-utero gene therapy protocols, it is first necessary to determine if the uterus itself is amenable to gene transfer. Several studies have shown high uterine transfection efficiency not only in animal models but also in human endometrial cells as well as ex vivo in the intact human uterus. Uterine gene transfer has been successfully achieved using both non-viral and viral vectors. Not only has the uterus been successfully transfected but also therapeutic consequences of such gene transfer have been obtained in the murine model.

Initial studies were performed to determine the feasibility of gene transfer to endometrial cells. Primary epithelial cells isolated from endometrial biopsies were transfected using liposome (Lipofectamine) and a plasmid-expressing firefly luciferase. A 5000-fold increase in luciferase expression ($p < 0.001$) was seen in cells transfected with luciferase compared to controls transfected with the carrier empty vector pcDNA.[78] Ishikawa cells are a well-differentiated endometrial adenocarcinoma cell line known to express estrogen and progesterone receptors;[79,80] they serve as a model of endometrial epithelial cells. As with primary endometrial epithelial cells, Ishikawa cells were also successfully transfected with the bacterial gene Lac-Z using a lipoplex consisting of Lipofectamine 20 µg/ml and 4 µg/ml DNA (pcDNA3.1/LacZ).[16] Nearly 80% of cells expressed at least moderate β-galactosidase staining (by immunohistochemistry using a β-gal solution [Boehringer Mannheim, Indianapolis, IN]), indicative of a high gene transfer efficiency. Efficient and reproducible in-vitro gene transfer to human endometrial cells offers the potential for in-vivo applicability of uterine gene therapy.

Successful non-viral vector-mediated uterine transfection has been achieved by liposome-mediated methods.[16,78,81,82] The efficiency of transfection depends on the stage of the murine estrus cycle.[83] Highest transfection efficiency was achieved in uteri during the

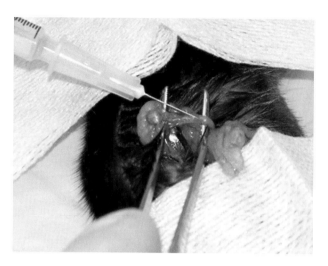

Figure 40.1 In-vivo intrauterine lipofection. Liposome-mediated in-vivo uterine transfection was performed by direct intraluminal uterine injection. An incision was made on the dorsal aspect on each side of the midline in the lumbar region to expose the ovary and the ovarian end of each uterine horn. One hundred microliters of diluted lipoplex were then injected into the uterine lumen at the ovarian end of each horn.

metestrus phase and pseudopregnancy. Furthermore, transgene expression was observed for up to 7 days after transfection. Liposome transfection is accomplished transluminally (Figure 40.1). It is therefore not surprising that the efficiency of transfection is most efficient in the luminal epithelium, the tissue adjacent to the lumen, compared to deeper tissues. This was corroborated by transfection of the murine uterus, using a lipoplex composed of the plasmid pcDNA3.1 containing the bacterial gene Lac-Z and liposome (Lipofectamine).[78] Mouse uteri were transfected on day 2 of pseudopregnancy. On day 4, the uteri were harvested and evaluated by immunohistochemistry for β-galactosidase expression. β-galactosidase was predominantly expressed by endometrial glandular epithelium and to a lesser extent by luminal epithelium. Analysis of other abdominal organs did not reveal β-galactosidase expression, suggestive of localized uterine transfection.

Uterine gene transfer using viral mechanisms has also been successfully employed in the animal model.[84,85] In the first such experiment, the viral envelope from the hemagglutinating virus of Japan (HVJ) was used successfully to transfect the murine uterus in vivo.[85] Transfection of the murine uterus using the HVJ envelope vector was performed using a construct expressing the luciferase gene on day 1.5 postcoitum. The construct was composed of cDNA of the reporter gene luciferase encased in the HVJ envelope. Compared

to controls treated by cationic liposome-mediated transfection, uteri treated with the HVJ viral envelope expressed higher luciferase levels.[85] Transfected gene expression was evident up to 3 days after treatment. No difference was noted in the rate or duration of pregnancy in treated mice. Furthermore, neither the litter size nor the birth weight or newborn anthropometric indices differed from those in untreated mice. Viral envelope vector-mediated uterine transfection seems to drive high levels of transgene expression over a limited duration of time and in preliminary experiments appears not to have significant deleterious effects. This method is based on the potent cell-fusion property of the HVJ viral envelope, additionally utilizing its intrinsic ability to efficiently enter the intracellular compartment, resulting in enhanced rates of gene transfer compared to liposomes. It differs from viral vector-mediated gene transduction in that the envelope serves only as a carrier, negotiating the cell membrane. Unlike transduction, where a viral genome-incorporated therapeutic transgene either integrates into the host cell genome, or is expressed from an episomal location, the viral envelope-transported transgene is subject to inactivation inside the cell, as would be the case with gene transfer using non-viral mechanisms.

Recently, uterine transduction has been successfully employed using a replication incompetent adenovirus vector carrying a dominant negative estrogen receptor (DN-ER) transgene, resulting in increased apoptosis and decreased cell proliferation in leiomyoma cell lines.[84] When these transduced leiomyoma cells were injected into nude mice, they were found to induce significantly smaller-sized fibroids, compared to those in controls injected with leiomyoma cells transduced ex vivo by an adenovirus vector carrying the LacZ gene. Furthermore, direct intratumor administration of the adenovirus carrying the DN-ER transgene inhibited the growth of the treated fibroid.[84] Fibroids are estrogen-dependent tumors; based on this physiological property, this gene therapy protocol inhibits trophic hormone-mediated tumor growth, constituting a novel approach to therapy.

Not only has the uterus proved amenable to efficient transfection using viral as well as non-viral vectors but also the prospect of therapeutic intervention in the uterus using gene therapy seems feasible. In all of the above experiments, uterine transfection was performed in the immediate postcoitum period with high transfection efficiency. To determine if genetic modification at this time impacts embryo implantation, uterine transfection with constructs that resulted in altered levels of expression of specific implantation-associated genes were performed. Altering the expression of the homeobox gene Hoxa10 in the murine uterus has been shown to impact implantation rates.[16] Homeobox genes are necessary for development, conferring tissue identity. They are transcription factors that function by activation or repression of downstream target genes.[86,87] In the murine reproductive tract, genes of the Hoxa cluster (a9, a10, a11, and a13) are necessary for differentiation of the Müllerian duct into adult reproductive structures.[88,89] The human orthologues of these murine homeotic genes (HOXA9, A10, A11, and A11) demonstrate a conserved spatial expression pattern in the adult human reproductive tract.[89] Although necessary for developmental specification within the reproductive tract, persistent Hoxa10 expression has been demonstrated in adult murine endometrium.[13,16,89,90] Female Hoxa10(−/−) mice, lacking adult endometrial Hoxa10 expression, demonstrate uterine factor infertility due to preimplantation and implantation defects.[13] Implantation site defects frequently consist of hemorrhage within the site itself, as well as in the adjacent uterine lumen. Also observed are small implantation sites with disorganized embryos and empty decidua suggestive of early degeneration of a postimplantation embryo. Furthermore, the size of the decidual swellings is reduced compared to wild-type uteri.[91] These implantation defects are implicit to Hoxa10(−/−) females, irrespective of paternal genotype. Similarly, implantation defects with deficient endometrial stromal, glandular, and decidual cell development in early gestation are also seen in Hoxa11(−/−) female mice.[92] In humans, reproductive tract diseases associated with diminished implantation such as endometriosis, hydrosalpinx, and PCOS have diminished endometrial HOXA10 expression levels.[14,15,93]

As discussed above, a functional consequence of aberrant adult endometrial Hoxa10 expression is evident as defective implantation, seen in Hoxa10(−/−) mice. Mice with a targeted disruption of the Hoxa10 gene are infertile due to defective embryo implantation.[13] When transferred into the uteri of Hoxa10(−/−) mice, neither their own embryos nor embryos from wild-type mice exhibit implantation. However, embryos from Hoxa10(−/−) mice implant normally when transferred to the uteri of wild-type pseudopregnant mice.[91]

The adult expression of developmental genes such as Hoxa10 and Hoxa11 probably preserves developmental plasticity, allowing tissue remodeling to occur during each reproductive cycle and pregnancy. Endometrial Hoxa10 expression reaches high levels in the latter half of the reproductive cycle, coincident with development of embryo receptivity. It is therefore likely that dynamic Hoxa10 expression in the adult endometrium is necessary for embryo implantation. This is evidenced in experiments where murine uteri are transfected with constructs that alter Hoxa10 expression levels such as Hoxa10 antisense (to block Hoxa10 expression) or pcDNA3.1/HOXA10 (a construct which constitutively expresses HOXA10). Whereas, the Hoxa10 antisense used a 30 bp phosphothiorate modified deoxyribonucleotide complimentary to the translation start site of HOXA10, the HOXA10 overexpression vector consists of the pcDNA3.1(+) plasmid (Invitrogen) carrying full-length HOXA10 cDNA.

In these experiments, nulliparous reproductive-aged mice were mated. Liposome-1 mediated in-vivo uterine transfection was performed by direct intrauterine injection on day 1 of pregnancy. Briefly, after making a midline abdominal incision, each uterine horn was exposed and injected with 100 µl lipoplex per horn. The lipoplex is composed of 16 µg/ml DNA (antisense or pcDNA3.1/HOXA10) and 40 µg/ml liposome (Lipofectamine – Gibco BRL, Gaithersburg, MD) in phosphate buffered saline (1X PBS). Pregnant mice were either euthanized on day 9 of pregnancy and the number of implantation sites determined or allowed to continue to term and litter size determined on the day of parturition. Whereas murine uteri transfected with Hoxa10 antisense demonstrated a decreased number of implantation sites (6.5 compared to 13.3 in controls; $p < 0.00002$), overexpression of Hoxa10 resulted in a consistently large litter size with low variability (Figure 40.2). The litter size in pcDNA3.1/HOXA10-treated mice was 11–14 pups compared to 0–13 pups per litter in controls ($p < 0.024$).

The absence of Hoxa10 expression, as demonstrated in Hoxa10(−/−) mice, results in implantation failure.[13] This may be due to absence of Hoxa10 during uterine development and/or abrogation of dynamic sex steroid-driven endometrial Hoxa10 expression in the adult. Treatment of the adult endometrium with Hoxa10 antisense adversely impacts implantation, indicating the necessary role of dynamic, adult endometrial Hoxa10 expression, in the development of embryo receptivity.[16] Endometrial receptivity can therefore be genetically enhanced to improve implantation rates (by augmenting Hoxa10 expression).[16] This therapeutic capability is likely to bring new hope in patients with such diseases as hydrosalpinx, endometriosis, and PCOS associated with diminished endometrial HOXA10 expression and infertility.[14,15,93] In these

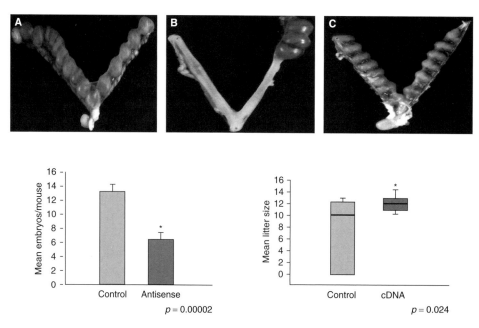

Figure 40.2 Variation in implantation rates following in-vivo altered endometrial HOXA10 expression levels using liposome-mediated gene transfection. Using HOXA10 antisense, embryo implantation rates were significantly diminished ($p=0.00002$) in antisense-treated mice compared to controls treated with a similar-sized inactive missense oligonucleotide. Compare control-treated mice shown in (**A**) with antisense-treated mice shown in (**B**). The average number of implantation sites was 13.3 in mice transfected with a control missense oligonucleotide and 6.5 in mice transfected with the Hoxa10 antisense oligonucleotide. (**C**) In contrast, this image demonstrates augmented endometrial HOXA10 expression levels using a construct (pcDNA3.1/HOXA10) that constitutively expresses the gene. This treatment resulted in consistently high litter sizes compared to controls treated with the empty vector pcDNA3.1(+). In the pcDNA3.1/HOXA10 group, mice gave birth to between 11 and 14 pups compared to litter sizes ranging from 0 to 13 in the control group. Statistical significance determined using a two-tailed unpaired t test ($p=0.024$).

patients, gene therapy may be successfully combined with assisted reproductive technology to further augment success rates for achieving pregnancy.

Implantation is also affected by the endometrial expression levels of the peptide hormone calcitonin. Calcitonin is expressed by endometrial glandular epithelium, where it is regulated by progesterone. Peak levels of expression are seen on days 3–5 of pregnancy, just prior to blastocyst implantation.[94,95] On day 6, after implantation, calcitonin is no longer expressed by this tissue. Diminished endometrial calcitonin expression attenuates implantation rates.[96] The temporal expression pattern of this molecule during the peri-implantation period suggests a role in embryo implantation. This was evidenced when pregnant rats were administered intrauterine antisense calcitonin in a lipoplex composed of calcitonin antisense and liposome DOTAP (N-[1-(2,3-dioleoyloxy)propyl]-N,N,N-trimethylammonium methyl sulfate; Boehringer Mannheim, Indianapolis, IN) on day 2 of pregnancy. Antisense calcitonin is composed of an oligonucleotide designed against exon IV of the calcitonin gene.[96] On day 9 of pregnancy, in comparison to controls treated with either saline or sense oligonucleotide, the number of implanted embryos in the uteri of antisense calcitonin-treated animals is reduced by 50–80% in most animals.

In addition to facile, efficient, and reproducible transfection of murine uteri, it is also possible to successfully and efficiently transfect the human uterus. This was demonstrated when intact uteri from two women undergoing hysterectomy were transfected with the bacterial gene Lac-Z.[19] On removal of the uteri, a lipoplex consisting of pcDNA3.1/LacZ (16 μg/ml) and Lipofectamine (40 μg/ml) in 1X PBS (total volume of 1 ml) was administered transcervically into the uterine cavity using an intrauterine insemination catheter (Wallach Surgical Devices, Orange, CT). The uteri were then immersed in minimum essential medium on ice for 4 hours. Uterine sections were evaluated by immunohistochemistry for β-galactosidase expression. Using this technique of gene transfer, high levels of expression of β-galactosidase were obtained in the endometrium. Expression was most abundant in the endometrial epithelium, where most cells stained for β-galactosidase. Intense staining was observed in 50% of endometrial epithelial cells, 25% of endometrial stromal cells, and 15% of superficial myometrial cells. Intensity of β-galactosidase expression decreased with increasing distance from the endometrial–myometrial junction. No β-galactosidase expression was evident beyond 1.75 cm from the endometrial–myometrial junction. In this study, no β-galactosidase expression was observed in either subserosal myometrium or blood vessels, indicative of localized uterine transfection. It is therefore evident that gene therapy to the human uterus is technically feasible. Given the potential indications for uterine gene therapy, it is likely to significantly impact the practice of gynecology.

An emerging area of gene therapy is in-utero administration of gene therapy to the developing fetus.[97] Such an approach has several advantages. Administering gene therapy early in gestation, at a preimmune stage of development, may preclude the development of an immune response to the vector, particularly a viral vector, thereby maximizing the efficacy of transduction. Another possible advantage from evading the immune response relates to avoidance of immune recognition and therefore disposal of the essential therapeutic transgene protein product that is necessary for the organism. In-utero fetal gene therapy would permit treatment of a disease prior to its onset. This is particularly relevant for diseases that have early-onset degenerative effects resulting in irreversible pathological damage such as phenylketonuria and cystic fibrosis. By targeting a relatively small overall number of cells in the organism in contrast to the fully developed adult, the efficiency of transfection, and the ability to transfect stem cells in the expectation of effecting lasting cures, is greater with fetal gene therapy. As the fetal liver is the major hematopoietic organ in early gestation, stem cell-targeted gene therapy to such an organism is greatly facilitated.[97] Furthermore, the tremendous synthetic capacity of hepatocytes ensures expression of a systemically required transgenic protein such as clotting factors VIII and IX in hemophilia. The fetal liver is amenable to ultrasound-guided direct and intraumbilical vein-mediated gene transfer.[98]

IN-UTERO THERAPY: PROBLEMS

One of the primary hurdles encountered with in-vivo gene transfer is achieving reliable levels of transgene expression in target tissues. This has necessitated development of diverse approaches designed to facilitate transfer of various types and sizes of nucleic acid inserts into cells with varying uptake specificity.

In general, viral vectors transduce target tissues more efficiently than transfection using non-viral vectors. However, viral vectors have the potential to spread beyond the target organ. This can lead to generalized viral replication and disease.

This is particularly important for the reproductive tract, where viral immunogenicity could invoke inflammatory reactions in the endometrium. Such iatrogenic endometrial inflammation may actually diminish implantation rates rather than augment them therapeutically. Furthermore, the inflammatory endometrial environment may be harmful for the early-developing conceptus, resulting in increased rates of abortion. Another concern with the use of viral vectors, especially retroviral vectors, is the potential for insertional mutagenesis due to their ability to integrate into the host cell chromosome. As discussed earlier, this has already been shown to result in the development of cancer in previous recipients of gene therapy due to non-random insertion of viral nucleic acids into the host cell genome. Current research is focused on the development of expression cassettes that target non-coding regions of the genome for insertion. With uterine gene therapy in particular, there remains a risk of persistent endometrial viral colonization that is capable of transplacental transfer to a developing fetus. Such a possibility may have serious consequences such as teratogenicity from infection of various fetal somatic tissues. Cytomegalovirus (CMV) is a potent viral teratogen that is capable of inducing profound anomalies in the developing offspring. Another potential complication could arise from viral infection of the fetal germ line. Due to a paucity of total cell number, the early-developing conceptus has a high ratio of germ cells to somatic cells and may be at very high risk for germ line infection, the effects of which could affect subsequent generations. The societal impact of such an adverse event is a cause of grave concern.

Liposome-mediated gene transfer to the human female reproductive tract appeared not to spread beyond the uterus, as evidenced by lack of β-galactosidase expression in deep subserosal myometrium and blood vessels.[19] Although less efficient than viral gene transfer methods, lipofection appears to be an effective and safe means of gene delivery to the female reproductive tract.

CONCLUSION

Prior to the addition of in-utero gene therapy to the therapeutic armamentarium, it is first necessary to develop specific indications and protocols for such administration. Concomitantly, it is necessary to monitor the safety of in-utero administered gene therapy. In a recent phase 1 clinical trial, patients with advanced breast or ovarian cancer were treated with intracavitary (thoracic and peritoneal, respectively) gene therapy.[99] In this toxicity determination trial, intracavitary EIA (an adenovirus gene associated with down-regulation of the HER-2/neu oncogene and apoptosis) was administered in combination with the liposome. Tumor cells expressing the transfected gene E1A simultaneously also demonstrated diminished HER-2/neu expression as well as enhanced apoptosis. Transfer of genes with tumor suppressive effects is a novel therapeutic strategy for patients with advanced cancer. Although not administered directly into the reproductive tract, this trial determines that it is possible to effect genetic modification as a therapeutic modality for reproductive tract diseases.

The ease of transfection of the human uterus makes it likely to be adapted for use in an outpatient setting.[19] Additionally, transgene expression with this technique is efficient, rapid, and reproducible and in the animal model lipofection has been successfully exploited to achieve therapeutic gains.[16,96] Transcervical gene therapy to the human uterus is unlikely to cause significant patient discomfort beyond that experienced at the time of intrauterine insemination, as the equipment used for gene transfer is the same. Efficient uterine gene transfection further enhances the potential of reproductive tract gene therapy.

REFERENCES

1. Blaese RM, Culver KW, Miller AD et al. T lymphocyte-directed gene therapy for ADA- SCID: initial trial results after 4 years. Science 1995; 270(5235): 475–80.
2. Knowles MR, Hohneker KW, Zhou Z et al. A controlled study of adenoviral-vector-mediated gene transfer in the nasal epithelium of patients with cystic fibrosis. N Engl J Med 1995; 333(13): 823–31.
3. Drozdzik M, Qian C, Lasarte JJ et al. Antitumor effect of allogenic fibroblasts engineered to express Fas ligand (FasL). Gene Ther 1998; 5(12): 1622–30.
4. Palu G, Cavaggioni A, Calvi P et al. Gene therapy of glioblastoma multiforme via combined expression of suicide and cytokine genes: a pilot study in humans. Gene Ther 1999; 6(3): 330–7.
5. O'Reilly MS, Holmgren L, Shing Y et al. Angiostatin: a novel angiogenesis inhibitor that mediates the suppression of metastases by a Lewis lung carcinoma. Cell 1994; 79(2): 315–28.
6. Soiffer R, Lynch T, Mihm M et al. Vaccination with irradiated autologous melanoma cells engineered to secrete human granulocyte–macrophage colony-stimulating factor generates potent antitumor immunity in patients with metastatic melanoma. Proc Natl Acad Sci USA 1998; 95(22): 13141–6.
7. Huang AY, Golumbek P, Ahmadzadeh M et al. Role of bone marrow-derived cells in presenting MHC class I-restricted tumor antigens. Science 1994; 264(5161): 961–5.
8. Wong-Staal F, Poeschla EM, Looney DJ. A controlled, Phase 1 clinical trial to evaluate the safety and effects in HIV-1 infected humans of autologous lymphocytes transduced with a ribozyme that cleaves HIV-1 RNA. Hum Gene Ther 1998; 9(16): 2407–25.
9. Giordano FJ, Ping P, McKirnan MD et al. Intracoronary gene transfer of fibroblast growth factor-5 increases blood flow and contractile function in an ischemic region of the heart. Nat Med 1996; 2(5): 534–9.
10. Laitinen M, Hartikainen J, Hiltunen MO et al. Catheter-mediated vascular endothelial growth factor gene transfer to human coronary arteries after angioplasty. Hum Gene Ther 2000; 11(2): 263–70.
11. Stewart CL, Kaspar P, Brunet LJ et al. Blastocyst implantation depends on maternal expression of leukaemia inhibitory factor. Nature 1992; 359(6390): 76–9.
12. Hsieh-Li HM, Witte DP, Weinstein M et al. Hoxa 11 structure, extensive antisense transcription, and function in male and female fertility. Development 1995; 121(5): 1373–85.
13. Satokata I, Benson G, Maas R. Sexually dimorphic sterility phenotypes in Hoxa10-deficient mice. Nature 1995; 374(6521): 460–3.
14. Cermik D, Selam B, Taylor HS. Regulation of HOXA-10 expression by testosterone in vitro and in the endometrium of patients with polycystic ovary syndrome. J Clin Endocrinol Metab 2003; 88(1): 238–43.
15. Daftary GS, Taylor HS. Hydrosalpinx fluid diminishes endometrial cell HOXA10 expression. Fertil Steril 2002; 78(3): 577–80.
16. Bagot CN, Troy PJ, Taylor HS. Alteration of maternal Hoxa10 expression by in vivo gene transfection affects implantation. Gene Ther 2000; 7(16): 1378–84.
17. Cramer SF, Patel A. The frequency of uterine leiomyomas. Am J Clin Pathol 1990; 94(4): 435–8.
18. Hiltunen MO, Turunen MP, Turunen AM et al. Biodistribution of adenoviral vector to nontarget tissues after local in vivo gene transfer to arterial wall using intravascular and periadventitial gene delivery methods. FASEB J 2000; 14(14): 2230–6.
19. Daftary GS, Taylor HS. Efficient liposome-mediated gene transfection and expression in the intact human uterus. Hum Gene Ther 2001; 12(17): 2121–7.
20. Daftary GS, Taylor HS. Reproductive tract gene transfer. Fertil Steril 2003; 80(3): 475–84.
21. Perkins AS, Kirschmeier PT, Gattoni-Celli S, Weinstein IB. Design of a retrovirus-derived vector for expression and transduction of exogenous genes in mammalian cells. Mol Cell Biol 1983; 3(6): 1123–32.
22. Miller AD. Retroviral vectors. Curr Top Microbiol Immunol 1992; 158: 1–24.
23. Anderson WF. Human gene therapy. Nature 1998; 392(6679 Suppl): 25–30.
24. Boris-Lawrie K, Temin HM. The retroviral vector. Replication cycle and safety considerations for retrovirus-mediated gene therapy. Ann NY Acad Sci 1994; 716: 59–70; discussion 71.
25. Miller DG, Adam MA, Miller AD. Gene transfer by retrovirus vectors occurs only in cells that are actively replicating at the time of infection. Mol Cell Biol 1990; 10(8): 4239–42.
26. Challita PM, Kohn DB. Lack of expression from a retroviral vector after transduction of murine hematopoietic stem cells is associated with methylation in vivo. Proc Natl Acad Sci USA 1994; 91(7): 2567–71.
27. Laufs S, Gentner B, Nagy KZ et al. Retroviral vector integration occurs in preferred genomic targets of human bone marrow-repopulating cells. Blood 2003; 101(6): 2191–8.
28. Smith KT, Shepherd AJ, Boyd JE, Lees GM. Gene delivery systems for use in gene therapy: an overview of quality assurance and safety issues. Gene Ther 1996; 3(3): 190–200.
29. Hacein-Bey-Abina S, Von Kalle C, Schmidt M et al. LMO2-associated clonal T cell proliferation in two patients after gene therapy for SCID-X1. Science 2003; 302(5644): 415–19.

30. Neering SJ, Hardy SF, Minamoto D et al. Transduction of primitive human hematopoietic cells with recombinant adenovirus vectors. Blood 1996; 88(4): 1147–55.

31. Wickham TJ, Mathias P, Cheresh DA, Nemerow GR. Integrins alpha v beta 3 and alpha v beta 5 promote adenovirus internalization but not virus attachment. Cell 1993; 73(2): 309–19.

32. Lehrman S. Virus treatment questioned after gene therapy death. Nature 1999; 401(6753): 517–18.

33. Marshall E. Gene therapy death prompts review of adenovirus vector. Science 1999; 286(5448): 2244–5.

34. Wang Q, Finer MH. Second-generation adenovirus vectors. Nat Med 1996; 2(6): 714–16.

35. Snyder RO, Spratt SK, Lagarde C et al. Efficient and stable adeno-associated virus-mediated transduction in the skeletal muscle of adult immunocompetent mice. Hum Gene Ther 1997; 8(16): 1891–900.

36. Poeschla E, Corbeau P, Wong-Staal F. Development of HIV vectors for anti-HIV gene therapy. Proc Natl Acad Sci USA 1996; 93(21): 11395–9.

37. Todo T, Rabkin SD, Sundaresan P et al. Systemic antitumor immunity in experimental brain tumor therapy using a multi-mutated, replication-competent herpes simplex virus. Hum Gene Ther 1999; 10(17): 2741–55.

38. Zhang G, Song YK, Liu D. Long-term expression of human alpha1-antitrypsin gene in mouse liver achieved by intravenous administration of plasmid DNA using a hydrodynamics-based procedure. Gene Ther 2000; 7(15): 1344–9.

39. Anderson WF, Killos L, Sanders-Haigh L, Kretschmer PJ, Diacumakos EG. Replication and expression of thymidine kinase and human globin genes microinjected into mouse fibroblasts. Proc Natl Acad Sci USA 1980; 77(9): 5399–403.

40. Timmerman JM, Singh G, Hermanson G et al. Immunogenicity of a plasmid DNA vaccine encoding chimeric idiotype in patients with B-cell lymphoma. Cancer Res 2002; 62(20): 5845–52.

41. Yang NS, Sun WH. Gene gun and other non-viral approaches for cancer gene therapy. Nat Med 1995; 1(5): 481–3.

42. Yang NS, Burkholder J, Roberts B et al. In vivo and in vitro gene transfer to mammalian somatic cells by particle bombardment. Proc Natl Acad Sci USA 1990; 87(24): 9568–72.

43. Yang NS, Sun WH, McCabe D. Developing particle-mediated gene-transfer technology for research into gene therapy of cancer. Mol Med Today 1996; 2(11): 476–81.

44. Cheng L, Ziegelhoffer PR, Yang NS. In vivo promoter activity and transgene expression in mammalian somatic tissues evaluated by using particle bombardment. Proc Natl Acad Sci USA 1993; 90(10): 4455–9.

45. Toneguzzo F, Keating A. Stable expression of selectable genes introduced into human hematopoietic stem cells by electric field-mediated DNA transfer. Proc Natl Acad Sci USA 1986; 83(10): 3496–9.

46. Van Tendeloo VF, Willems R, Ponsaerts P et al. High-level transgene expression in primary human T lymphocytes and adult bone marrow CD34+ cells via electroporation-mediated gene delivery. Gene Ther 2000; 7(16): 1431–7.

47. Potter H, Weir L, Leder P. Enhancer-dependent expression of human kappa immunoglobulin genes introduced into mouse pre-B lymphocytes by electroporation. Proc Natl Acad Sci USA 1984; 81(22): 7161–5.

48. Weaver JC. Electroporation theory. Concepts and mechanisms. Methods Mol Biol 1995; 55: 3–28.

49. Miller DL, Pislaru SV, Greenleaf JE. Sonoporation: mechanical DNA delivery by ultrasonic cavitation. Somat Cell Mol Genet 2002; 27(1–6): 115–34.

50. Felgner PL, Gadek TR, Holm M et al. Lipofection: a highly efficient, lipid-mediated DNA-transfection procedure. Proc Natl Acad Sci USA 1987; 84(21): 7413–17.

51. Felgner PL, Barenholz Y, Behr JP et al. Nomenclature for synthetic gene delivery systems. Hum Gene Ther 1997; 8(5): 511–12.

52. Branden LJ, Mohamed AJ, Smith CI. A peptide nucleic acid-nuclear localization signal fusion that mediates nuclear transport of DNA. Nat Biotechnol 1999; 17(8): 784–7.

53. Cotten M, Langle-Rouault F, Kirlappos H et al. Transferrin-polycation-mediated introduction of DNA into human leukemic cells: stimulation by agents that affect the survival of transfected DNA or modulate transferrin receptor levels. Proc Natl Acad Sci USA 1990; 87(11): 4033–7.

54. Wagner E, Plank C, Zatloukal K et al. Influenza virus hemagglutinin HA-2 N-terminal fusogenic peptides augment gene transfer by transferrin–polylysine–DNA complexes: toward a synthetic virus-like gene-transfer vehicle. Proc Natl Acad Sci USA 1992; 89(17): 7934–8.

55. Wagner E, Zatloukal K, Cotten M et al. Coupling of adenovirus to transferrin–polylysine/DNA complexes greatly enhances receptor-mediated gene delivery and expression of transfected genes. Proc Natl Acad Sci USA 1992; 89(13): 6099–103.

56. Paterson BM, Roberts BE, Kuff EL. Structural gene identification and mapping by DNA–mRNA hybrid-arrested cell-free translation. Proc Natl Acad Sci USA 1977; 74(10): 4370–4.

57. Stephenson ML, Zamecnik PC. Inhibition of Rous sarcoma viral RNA translation by a specific oligodeoxyribonucleotide. Proc Natl Acad Sci USA 1978; 75(1): 285–8.

58. Simons RW, Kleckner N. Translational control of IS10 transposition. Cell 1983; 34(2): 683–91.

59. Chau YM, Pando S, Taylor HS. HOXA11 silencing and endogenous HOXA11 antisense ribonucleic acid in the uterine endometrium. J Clin Endocrinol Metab 2002; 87(6): 2674–80.

60. Opalinska JB, Gewirtz AM. Nucleic-acid therapeutics: basic principles and recent applications. Nat Rev Drug Discov 2002; 1(7): 503–14.

61. Stasiak A. Getting down to the core of homologous recombination. Science 1996; 272(5263): 828–9.

62. Knauert MP, Glazer PM. Triplex forming oligonucleotides: sequence-specific tools for gene targeting. Hum Mol Genet 2001; 10(20): 2243–51.

63. Gewirtz AM, Sokol DL, Ratajczak MZ. Nucleic acid therapeutics: state of the art and future prospects. Blood 1998; 92(3): 712–36.

64. Stein CA. How to design an antisense oligodeoxynucleotide experiment: a consensus approach. Antisense Nucleic Acid Drug Dev 1998; 8(2): 129–32.

65. Dominski Z, Kole R. Identification and characterization by antisense oligonucleotides of exon and intron sequences required for splicing. Mol Cell Biol 1994; 14(11): 7445–54.

66. Summerton J, Weller D. Morpholino antisense oligomers: design, preparation, and properties. Antisense Nucleic Acid Drug Dev 1997; 7(3): 187–95.

67. Crooke ST. Molecular mechanisms of antisense drugs: RNase H. Antisense Nucleic Acid Drug Dev 1998; 8(2): 133–4.

68. Usman N, Blatt LM. Nuclease-resistant synthetic ribozymes: developing a new class of therapeutics. J Clin Invest 2000; 106(10): 1197–202.

69. Eckstein F. The hammerhead ribozyme. Biochem Soc Trans 1996; 24(3): 601–4.

70. Nishikura K. A short primer on RNAi: RNA-directed RNA polymerase acts as a key catalyst. Cell 2001; 107(4): 415–18.

71. Elbashir SM, Lendeckel W, Tuschl T. RNA interference is mediated by 21- and 22-nucleotide RNAs. Genes Dev 2001; 15(2): 188–200.

72. Tuschl T. Expanding small RNA interference. Nat Biotechnol 2002; 20(5): 446–8.

73. Elbashir SM, Harborth J, Lendeckel W et al. Duplexes of 21-nucleotide RNAs mediate RNA interference in cultured mammalian cells. Nature 2001; 411(6836): 494–8.

74. Yu JY, DeRuiter SL, Turner DL. RNA interference by expression of short-interfering RNAs and hairpin RNAs in mammalian cells. Proc Natl Acad Sci USA 2002; 99(9): 6047–52.

75. Calos MP. The potential of extrachromosomal replicating vectors for gene therapy. Trends Genet 1996; 12(11): 463–6.

76. Wohlgemuth JG, Kang SH, Bulboaca GH et al. Long-term gene expression from autonomously replicating vectors in mammalian cells. Gene Ther 1996; 3(6): 503–12.

77. Harrington JJ, Van Bokkelen G, Mays RW et al. Formation of de novo centromeres and construction of first-generation human artificial microchromosomes. Nat Genet 1997; 15(4): 345–55.

78. Charnock-Jones DS, Sharkey AM, Jaggers DC et al. In-vivo gene transfer to the uterine endometrium. Hum Reprod 1997; 12(1): 17–20.

79. Nishida M, Kasahara K, Kaneko M et al. [Establishment of a new human endometrial adenocarcinoma cell line, Ishikawa cells, containing estrogen and progesterone receptors]. Nippon Sanka Fujinka Gakkai Zasshi 1985; 37(7): 1103–11. [in Japanese]

80. Lessey BA, Ilesanmi AO, Castelbaum AJ et al. Characterization of the functional progesterone receptor in an endometrial adenocarcinoma cell line (Ishikawa): progesterone-induced expression of the alpha1 integrin. J Steroid Biochem Mol Biol 1996; 59(1): 31–9.

81. Bagot CN, Kliman HJ, Taylor HS. Maternal Hoxa10 is required for pinopod formation in the development of mouse uterine receptivity to embryo implantation. Dev Dyn 2001; 222(3): 538–44.

82. Daftary GS, Taylor HS. Pleiotropic effects of Hoxa 10 on the functional development of peri-implantation endometrium. Mol Reprod Dev. 2004; 67(1): 8–14.

83. Relloso M, Esponda P. In-vivo transfection of the female reproductive tract epithelium. Mol Hum Reprod 2000; 6(12): 1099–105.

84. Al-Hendy A, Lee EJ, Wang HQ, Copland JA. Gene therapy of uterine leiomyomas: adenovirus-mediated expression of dominant negative estrogen receptor inhibits tumor growth in nude mice. Am J Obstet Gynecol 2004; 191(5): 1621–31.

85. Nakamura H, Kimura T, Ikegami H et al. Highly efficient and minimally invasive in-vivo gene transfer to the mouse uterus using haemagglutinating virus of Japan (HVJ) envelope vector. Mol Hum Reprod 2003; 9(10): 603–9.

86. Krumlauf R. Hox genes in vertebrate development. Cell 1994; 78(2): 191–201.

87. McGinnis W, Krumlauf R. Homeobox genes and axial patterning. Cell 1992; 68(2): 283–302.

88. Block K, Kardana A, Igarashi P, Taylor HS. In utero diethylstilbestrol (DES) exposure alters Hox gene expression in the developing Müllerian system. FASEB J 2000; 14(9): 1101–8.

89. Taylor HS, Vanden Heuvel GB, Igarashi P. A conserved Hox axis in the mouse and human female reproductive system: late establishment and persistent adult expression of the Hoxa cluster genes. Biol Reprod 1997; 57(6): 1338–45.

90. Taylor HS, Arici A, Olive D, Igarashi P. HOXA10 is expressed in response to sex steroids at the time of implantation in the human endometrium. J Clin Invest 1998; 101(7): 1379–84.

91. Benson GV, Lim H, Paria BC et al. Mechanisms of reduced fertility in Hoxa-10 mutant mice: uterine homeosis and loss of maternal Hoxa-10 expression. Development 1996; 122(9): 2687–96.

92. Gendron RL, Paradis H, Hsieh-Li HM et al. Abnormal uterine stromal and glandular function associated with maternal reproductive defects in Hoxa-11 null mice. Biol Reprod 1997; 56(5): 1097–105.

93. Taylor HS, Bagot C, Kardana A et al. HOX gene expression is altered in the endometrium of women with endometriosis. Hum Reprod 1999; 14(5): 1328–31.

94. Ding YQ, Bagchi MK, Bardin CW, Bagchi IC. Calcitonin gene expression in the rat uterus during pregnancy. Recent Prog Horm Res 1995; 50: 373–8.

95. Ding YQ, Zhu LJ, Bagchi MK, Bagchi IC. Progesterone stimulates calcitonin gene expression in the uterus during implantation. Endocrinology 1994; 135(5): 2265–74.

96. Zhu LJ, Bagchi MK, Bagchi IC. Attenuation of calcitonin gene expression in pregnant rat uterus leads to a block in embryonic implantation. Endocrinology 1998; 139(1): 330–9.

97. Waddington SN, Kramer MG, Hernandez-Alcoceba R et al. In utero gene therapy: current challenges and perspectives. Mol Ther 2005; 11(5): 661–76.

98. Song S, Embury J, Laipis PJ et al. Stable therapeutic serum levels of human alpha-1 antitrypsin (AAT) after portal vein injection of recombinant adeno-associated virus (rAAV) vectors. Gene Ther 2001; 8(17): 1299–306.

99. Hortobagyi GN, Ueno NT, Xia W et al. Cationic liposome-mediated E1A gene transfer to human breast and ovarian cancer cells and its biologic effects: a phase I clinical trial. J Clin Oncol 2001; 19(14): 3422–33.

41 Gamete quality and assisted reproductive technologies

Catherine MH Combelles and Catherine Racowsky

INTRODUCTION

Among the 15% of couples reported to receive infertility services in the USA, over 100 000 assisted reproductive technologies (ART) treatment cycles are reported each year.[1] The field of ART comprises treatment strategies during which the egg (oocyte) and sperm are manipulated outside of the body. With the first successful birth in 1978 in the UK, in-vitro fertilization (IVF) represents the oldest ART technique.[2] Following rapid demands and advances in the field, ART treatment now includes a number of related procedures, among which are gamete intrafallopian tube transfer (GIFT), zygote intrafallopian tube transfer (ZIFT), and intracytoplasmic sperm injection (ICSI). Since 1991, ICSI has been used to microinject a single spermatozoon directly into the cytoplasm of a mature oocyte.[3] IVF and ICSI are most commonly employed, accounting in the USA for about 43% and 56% of reported ART cycles, respectively.[1] Beyond these treatment strategies (IVF, ICSI, GIFT, ZIFT), additional laboratory manipulations may be performed, including embryo cryopreservation, preimplantation genetic diagnosis (PGD), assisted hatching (AH), and extended embryo culture to the blastocyst stage.[4,5]

Regardless of which ART procedure is performed, they all entail the following sequential steps: patient preparation for gamete retrieval, gamete isolation and preparation, fertilization and embryo culture in the laboratory, followed by embryo transfer back to the woman's uterus. While each step in an ART cycle is subject to cancellation or to varying degrees of success, it has become increasingly clear that the gametes are a limiting factor in final reproductive outcome. It is true that in certain instances of gonad failure, gametes may represent a limiting resource in the laboratory; however, it is quality, rather than quantity, of gametes that most significantly impacts the overall influence of the gametes on cycle outcome.

In this chapter, we examine the issue of gamete quality, beginning with the means by which 'quality' may be defined and the importance of good gametes in the ART laboratory. Methods to evaluate gamete quality will be presented along with factors underlying superior vs inferior quality gametes. In this respect, we address potential variables that may influence gamete quality, not only in the laboratory but also within the human body. We highlight how current knowledge is being applied in attempts to maximize gamete quality during ART treatment. In addition, we identify areas that will benefit from improvement and in which great strides should be made.

GAMETE QUALITY AND ITS IMPORTANCE IN ART

In the early stages of ART when only one or perhaps two oocytes were retrieved without gonadotropin stimulation,[2,6] the number of available oocytes severely restricted success rates; consequently, the focus was placed on introducing[7,8] and then improving[9–11] ovarian stimulation regimens. More recently, limitations imposed by either the absence, or a very low number, of sperm in the ejaculate have been addressed by introduction of epididymal aspiration and/or testicular biopsy.[12] Today, within the biological constraints imposed by ovarian and testicular function, most of the limitations associated with gamete quantity have been overcome. Now at the forefront of gamete biology in ART is no longer a need for additional gametes, but rather a more recently appreciated and essential focus on the quality of gametes.

Gametes are often described by their quality, a characteristic that remains ill-defined in both ovarian and testicular biology. On a superficial level, gamete quality can be described as the ability of spermatozoa and oocytes to support fertilization and subsequent embryonic development to term. Less generally, gamete quality may in turn refer to the ability of a gamete to complete a specific event, itself known to be required for a conceptus to develop to term into a healthy child. Based on the complex development of gametes, it is thus critical to understand the molecular and cellular mechanisms that underlie normal gamete function; some of these mechanisms are presented in the 'Biological significance of gamete quality' section.

Gametes vary considerably in their quality, as illustrated by the range of reproductive successes. As a matter of fact, most human conceptions fail to develop to term, with only about 40% of fertilized zygotes estimated to result in the birth of healthy term fetuses in the USA.[13] While the origins of such poor developmental potential are likely to vary and be multiple, many failures can be traced back to gametes and their quality. Indeed, compromised gamete quality affects several reproductive parameters, including embryo development, implantation, fetal development, maintenance of pregnancy, and live birth. It is clear that gamete quality impacts not only natural but also assisted conceptions during ART treatment. Interestingly, the normal fecundity rate, as measured by the probability of achieving a live birth within a single month, is only about 20–25%, thereby not substantially deviating from the overall live birth rate of 28% per cycle in the USA infertility population following ART treatment.[1,14] Since ART bypasses some of the significant hurdles during development, there remains the opportunity for improvement in ART outcome. Indeed, our ability to understand, diagnose, and optimize gamete quality is likely to ensure such increased success rates in a greater number of patients adopting assisted conception technologies.

A well-accepted measure of reproductive success has been live birth rates; however, it has become increasingly clear that outcomes should also include additional assessments. Indeed, defects may not become apparent until later adulthood, albeit their origins possibly occurring during some of the earliest developmental periods. The Barker hypothesis or Fetal Origins of Adult Disease postulates that certain chronic adult diseases (such as coronary heart diseases, strokes, and diabetes) originate during fetal life.[15,16] The hypothesis has received significant support from not only epidemiological data in humans but also basic science studies in animals.[17,18] Furthermore, evidence is emerging that conditions around the time of conception may impact later development and adult health.[19-21] Given the current controversies with respect to the safety of ART, long-term and appropriately designed surveillance studies are necessary;[22,23] these will continue to augment our knowledge of potential effects of ART treatment on the overall health of its resulting offspring. In this effort, the potential contribution of gamete quality to detrimental effects will also need to be identified, in turn necessitating our ability to understand and assess gamete quality.

BIOLOGICAL SIGNIFICANCE OF GAMETE QUALITY

In this section, we define some of the key aspects of gamete functions that are believed to contribute to embryo quality and perhaps even to its complete development to term (Table 41.1).

Male gamete

Fertilization and egg activation

A good-quality sperm is one that possesses fertilizing and egg-activating abilities. Fertilization is clearly a process entailing a complex set of multiple events, among which are:

- penetration of the cumulus cell layer surrounding the oocyte
- recognition of, binding to, and penetration of the zona pellucida
- fusion of sperm and oocyte membranes
- egg activation events
- and formation, migration, and fusion of the pronuclei.[24,25]

Egg activation involves a complex sequence of events, among which are re-entry into the meiotic cell cycle, transition into mitosis, release of cortical granules, and recruitment of maternal transcripts.[26,27] Proper activation of these events is dependent on a series of characteristic calcium oscillations, which further influence normal patterns of embryonic development.[26,28] Although the oocyte becomes equipped with the ability to undergo egg activation during oogenesis (see below), the process is not initiated until sperm entry. More precisely, cytosolic rises in calcium are triggered and modulated by the so-called sperm factor, the exact composition of which remains undefined.[26] A current model proposes the involvement of a sperm-specific novel phospholipase C (PLC) ζ in the release of calcium from intracellular stores in the oocyte and the triggering of signaling cascades and egg activation at large.[29,30] While much of this work has focused on animal models, recent work also supports the role of PLCζ in triggering calcium oscillations and egg activation events in human oocytes.[31] In addition, the importance of calcium transients has been reported in human oocytes undergoing ICSI, despite circumvention of many of the sperm–egg binding and membrane fusion events.[32,33] The potential differences in egg activation and fertilization between oocytes inseminated by conventional IVF and ICSI

Table 41.1   Determinants of gamete quality together with some of their known or proposed biological significance(s)

Determinants[a]	Biological significance(s)
Sperm	
Activation and hyperactivation	Motility necessary for gamete transport and fertilizing ability (penetration of cumulus and egg layers)
Morphology	Normal morphology is not essential for gamete transport but perhaps indicates chromosomal abnormalities
Meiotic segregation	Meiotic arrests, structural chromosome reorganizations, aneuploidy or diploidy all result in failed or abnormal embryonic development
DNA strand integrity	DNA strand breaks may reflect apoptotic spermatozoa
Chromatin packing	Histone-to-protamine substitution provides protection from DNA damage
Gene imprinting	Paternal contribution of gene activities
Centriole	Fertilization and formation of normal spindles during early cleavage divisions
Non-nuclear determinants:	
• Mitochondrial reduction	• For contribution of mitochondria solely from the egg
• Biochemical modifications of the plasma membrane	• Adequate recognition of the egg, binding to its layers, and fusion of membranes
Sperm factor	Ability to elicit calcium oscillations during egg activation
Oocyte	
Cytoplasmic maturation:	Meiotic competence and ability to support fertilization and early embryonic development
• Organelles	
• Molecular stores	
• Polarity	
• Ca^{2+} transients activity	
• Sperm nucleus remodeling activity	
• Cumulus cells	
Zona pellucida	Ovarian folliculogenesis, oogenesis, fertilization, and early embryonic development
Chromosomal segregation	Meiotic errors result in embryo/fetal inviability and pregnancy loss
Chromatin remodeling and gene imprinting patterns	Transcriptional activation and repression

[a]Collectively, these determinants permit an oocyte and sperm to support fertilization and embryonic development to term (references cited in 'Biological significance of gamete quality' section of the text)

remain contentious and are the subject of intense investigation.[27,32,34] Most recently, concern was documented in the mouse with the non-physiological presence of the sperm acrosome in the egg cytoplasm post-ICSI.[35]

In the context of gamete quality and ART, the question is whether oocytes and spermatozoa from infertility patients possess all of the factors required to complete what appears to be a complex and carefully regulated program of egg activation. Moreover, with ART techniques such as ICSI that bypass normal cell–cell recognition and membrane fusion, additional knowledge is warranted as to the relative contributions of gamete quality and fertilization outcome in such circumstances. Undoubtedly, fertilization and egg activation are extremely intricate processes. With potential errors existing at any of its multiple events, fertilization represents a risky business that ultimately relies on good gamete quality.

Sperm motility

Good sperm motility typically reflects normal male fertility. While poorly motile or immotile sperm are unequivocally characteristic of infertile or sterile individuals, underlying causes for variations in sperm motility remain ill-defined.[36,37] Understanding the precise mechanisms of sperm motility may permit targeted treatment, thereby improving sperm quality in ART without having to rely on techniques such as ICSI that abolish the requirement for sperm motility altogether. In vivo, sperm motility is vital to the rendezvous of gametes and the completion of fertilization in the oviduct. In addition, there are two forms of physiological motility, both of which appear to be required for fertilization in several species: one is activated motility, as present in freshly ejaculated sperm; the other is referred to as hyperactivated motility, which is acquired in the female reproductive tract.[25,37,38] Clinically, it is activated motility that is typically assessed, with very little being known about the control and measures of hyperactivation in sperm in vitro.[38,39] Multiple cellular and molecular components provide sperm with the ability to swim; for instance, a flagellum with its axonemal core and associated mitochondrial and fibrous sheaths together ensure the continued movement of sperm, necessary energy sources, and proper support.[37] Studies have begun to highlight the multiple aspects of sperm motility that are subject to failure. Defects in flagellar ultrastructure, axonemal proteins, metabolism, calcium signaling, protein phosphorylation, and other regulatory pathways are all potential candidates for cases of suboptimal sperm motility, and thus sperm quality, in ART.[36] However, despite ongoing strides in our knowledge of sperm motility, minimal translation from the bench to ART has occurred to date.

Sperm morphology

A mature spermatozoon can be characterized based on gross external morphology of each of its three main structural elements: i.e. the head, the midpiece, and the tail. Not only have the dimensions and proportions been considered but also the overall shape of the sperm.[40,41] Significant differences in parameters of sperm morphology exist among male gametes of a single species and even when comparing individual sperm within a given semen specimen. The exact biological significance that such variation represents remains to be established; interestingly, aberrant sperm morphologies do not preclude gamete transport to its destination. Thus, although a potential relationship between abnormalities in sperm morphology and chromosome complements is conceivable, conclusive evidence is absent in the human. In the mouse, a moderate correlation exists between atypical sperm forms and reduced sperm quality.[42,43] However, mouse sperm with highly anomalous external appearances can still fertilize and support full development to term.[44] Given the lack of robust evidence for the functional significance of sperm morphology, much remains uncertain as to its utility in the ART laboratory (see 'Assessment of gamete quality in ART' section).

Sperm nuclear determinants

The sperm contributes half of the genome to the newly created conceptus, and it does so in a very specialized manner. Indeed, the sperm nucleus becomes highly modified to accommodate its journey through the male and female reproductive tracts and the final delivery of intact DNA to the oocyte at fertilization. However, inaccuracies may occur at several steps in the nuclear differentiation process of spermatozoa, and the types of nuclear defects include various gross chromosome meiotic errors, Y microdeletions (see 'Factors influencing gamete quality in ART' section), epigenetic anomalies, and DNA damage. In this section, we present some of the unique characteristics of sperm nuclei and relevant evidence for specific defects known to influence gamete quality and thus ART outcome.

Meiosis is a complex cell division process prone to errors, thereby leading to aneuploidy (abnormal chromosome numbers) or diploidy (no reductive chromosome division). While greater detail on the relevance of aneuploidy in ART is presented in the next section on oocytes, we focus on sperm aneuploidy here. Male gametes display meiotic anomalies that may result in meiotic arrests (from sex chromosome aneuploidies) or abnormal meiotic configurations (due to structural chromosome reorganizations);[45] as a result, chromosomally imbalanced sperm are formed, at rates between 1 and 8% depending on patient populations and meiotic anomalies under study.[46-49] Any interference in the normal male meiotic process may result in aneuploid spermatozoa that will then affect normal restoration of diploidy at fertilization and subsequent embryonic development. In addition, diploid spermatozoa frequently occur in infertile males, and thus contribute to a significant proportion of sperm anomalies in ART.[48] Although the mechanisms underlying the production of diploid spermatozoa remain poorly defined, a meiotically unreduced spermatozoon results in triploidy following fertilization, and thus abortive embryos. With some infertile men exhibiting chromosomal anomalies in strictly meiotic cells, and not in somatic cells as detected by routine karyotypes, the clinical relevance of male meiotic disorders is of utmost importance in ART.[50]

Sperm cells may possess nuclear abnormalities such as breaks in their DNA strands. While a correlation has been established in animal studies between nuclear DNA anomalies and diminished reproductive outcome, how DNA strand breaks may impact human ART success has not been clearly defined to date.[51,52] Sperm DNA anomalies may originate during spermatogenesis in the testes. Indeed, complex events define sperm development, with extensive cell division (by mitosis and meiosis), cell differentiation, and cell death. Sperm cell death, by a programmed mechanism of apoptosis, occurs normally as a way to ensure the development of an appropriate number and quality of spermatozoa.[53] DNA breaks may be indicative of apoptosis in spermatozoa, or other errors during the differentiation process, including problems in chromatin packaging during the histone to protamine substitution.[52] During spermiogenesis, 85% of the classical histones are exchanged with sperm-specific protamine proteins;[54] the latter set of proteins permits an extreme state of chromatin packing and increased protection from DNA damage.[55] This exchange is central to normal sperm function, notably during the posttesticular life of these highly specialized cells; indeed, spermatozoa spend a great deal of time as single entities, without the protection that surrounding somatic cells (such as Sertoli cells) normally afford them in the testis. Given the susceptibility of sperm to DNA damage, whether of exogenous or endogenous origins, proper DNA packaging appears fundamental for normal sperm function.

Another emerging role of sperm is the particular gene imprinting pattern with which it provides the mature egg and newly created embryo. Indeed, epigenetic processes of global chromatin alterations are pivotal and allow specific patterns of gene expression and silencing.[56] It must be emphasized that while DNA methylation represents the best understood mode by which gene activity is epigenetically modified, histone modifications are also involved in the genetic imprinting of gametes. A number of genes are known to become imprinted, and patterns differ between the DNA of male or female origin. As a result, contributions from both maternal and paternal imprints appear to be required for the normal development of a conceptus; any abnormalities give rise to adult imprinting disorders (e.g. Beckwith–Wiedemann and Angelman syndromes) or other growth and developmental defects in utero (e.g. large offspring syndrome).[57,58]

Spermatogenesis and oogenesis are critical periods during development when patterns of gene imprints are first established in gametes.[59,60] In the female, gene imprinting occurs in preovulatory follicles before resumption of meiosis and patterns are maintained through oocyte maturation, fertilization, and embryonic development. In the male, gene imprinting takes place before and during postmeiotic maturation of round spermatids into mature sperm as chromatin becomes compacted. Maintenance of imprinting patterns must also occur through fertilization and postfertilization events. Subsequently, specific timing of maternal and paternal imprint initiation, loss, or maintenance occurs during early embryogenesis.[59,60]

Interestingly, altered genetic imprints have been documented in spermatozoa in distinct cases of failed spermatogenesis, thereby supporting the significance of epigenetic factors in sperm quality.[61,62]

Sperm non-nuclear determinants

It is essential to emphasize that not only sperm nuclear but also non-nuclear determinants are likely to underlie reproductive success. With the extreme reduction in cytoplasmic components that is characteristic of mature spermatozoa, the relative involvement of nonnuclear sperm factors to successful fertilization and embryo development has not received as much attention as the sperm genome. Indeed, while the sperm has become highly specialized to provide the newly fertilized egg with the paternal genome, it also appears to contribute in other ways, notably with respect to centrosomes. With an absence of centrioles in mature mammalian oocytes, the sperm contributes its centriole to the newly fertilized zygote.[63] Importantly, variations in centrosomal elements in spermatozoa of suboptimal quality underlie cases of fertilization failure and poor reproductive outcome.[64,65] Similarly, sperm defects may lead to the non-elimination of paternal mitochondria at fertilization and, consequently, disrupted embryogenesis.[66] Another nonnuclear determinant of optimal sperm quality may also lie in the sperm factor and its ability to trigger and sustain egg activation events; such a possibility merits further investigation. During spermiogenesis, there are other specializations that occur in the non-nuclear compartments of the sperm.[67] For example, the biochemical composition of the plasma membrane becomes modified. Also, cellular components must be placed in the right place to achieve their normal functions; for example, the acrosome and receptors for oocytes must be located in the head and equatorial regions, respectively. Unquestionably, whether it be at the nuclear or non-nuclear levels, a spermatozoon must become equipped with a broad set of factors and specializations so that it functions properly and supports subsequent embryonic development.

Female gamete

Meiotic and developmental competencies

At the outset, it must be mentioned that oogenesis is a remarkably complex process that entails a protracted growth phase that is coordinated with follicular development, followed by oocyte maturation, a time during which the oocyte resumes and completes meiosis-I before arrest at metaphase of meiosis-II. It is at this arrested stage of metaphase-II that mature oocytes are retrieved for ART treatment. Oocytes can be described by at least two competencies that are acquired sequentially: meiotic competence refers to the ability of oocytes to resume and complete meiosis (and thus undergo the process of oocyte maturation); developmental competence refers to an oocyte that can be fertilized and support development to term. Clearly, both aptitudes are required and represent hallmarks of oocyte quality. Indeed, metaphase-II oocytes that do not properly complete maturation of both the nucleus and cytoplasm are developmentally compromised.[68–70] In addition, each competency comprises a multitude of modifications, which occur or may fail at discrete and possibly even independent times.

Oocyte cytoplasmic compartment

Various lines of experimental evidence have lent credence to the establishment of the cytoplasm as a key determinant of oocyte quality.[70,71] Cytoplasmic maturation, and thus cytoplasmic quality, entails a wide array of cell functions and characteristics, including both biochemical and structural properties. Examples of these include modifications in oocyte metabolism, cytoskeletal organization, and determinants of calcium transients, all of which in turn impact nuclear events more immediately, and early embryonic development more distantly.

A considerable number of organelles and molecules are produced and stockpiled during oogenesis, although the precise nature of only relatively few has been defined.[72] This accumulation occurs in preparation for (1) the completion of meiosis and fertilization, (2) bursts in metabolic activity and protein synthesis at fertilization, and (3) the support of early embryonic cleavages until the time of zygotic genome activation when the preimplantation embryo begins synthesizing its own gene transcripts for the first time. It is hardly debatable that embryogenesis is rooted in oogenesis, a theme that appears relevant across multiple animal models.[73] What structural and chemical complements provide an oocyte with optimal meiotic and developmental potential represents a relatively unexplored area of study in human ART. Lastly, not only should an oocyte accumulate proper components but also it must segregate them properly during the unique process of asymmetric cytokinesis. An active and promising area of study in mammalian oogenesis concerns defining the role of the cytoskeleton in spatially and temporally regulating the segregation of cellular and molecular components.[70,74] While oocytes exhibit polarization, the exact clinical significance remains debatable.[75–77] Of interest is evidence for an association between the alignment of the pronuclei with respect to the first polar body and developmental competency of resulting embryos.[78,79]

There are several examples of specific activities that the oocyte must acquire during its development. As discussed above, oocytes must be able to generate and sustain calcium oscillations to ensure normal egg activation at fertilization.[80] Among many other processes, this is an example of an ability that is acquired during oocyte development and more precisely later during oocyte maturation.[81] Similarly, sperm chromatin needs to be extensively reconfigured at fertilization, and oocytes exhibit a temporal window during which they display such chromatin-remodeling activity.[82] The cytoplasm of the oocyte must also provide a chemically reducing environment to allow for the decondensation of the sperm nucleus and normal formation of the male pronucleus.[63] Thus, a number of postfertilization events are dependent on the quality of oocyte maturation. It is also important to note that the oocyte and its surrounding cumulus cells together are required for the normal function of both cell compartments during oogenesis[83–85] and even fertilization.[86] Lastly, the outer extracellular matrix of the oocyte, the zona pellucida, is also at the forefront of oocyte quality; indeed, it plays a significant role all the way from follicular to early embryonic development and variants in its organization underlie impaired fertility in animal models, and possibly also in the human.[87,88]

Oocyte nuclear compartment

Abnormalities in chromosome segregation, resulting in aneuploidy, are of central concern in human reproduction; such abnormalities constitute a leading cause of pregnancy loss following both natural conception and assisted reproduction.[49,84] The incidence of aneuploidy is age-related and also varies according to the developmental stage examined; in ART, early preimplantation human embryos display aneuploidy at an incidence as high as 60%.[90–92] The majority of chromosomal abnormalities are not compatible with embryo or fetal viability, thus influencing reproductive outcomes. Since errors in chromosome numbers in the embryo may arise from meiotic and/or mitotic chromosome malsegregations, cytogenetic analysis of human gametes has provided further insights into the origins of aneuploidy in humans. While the paternal origin of chromosome errors cannot be ignored (as discussed above), oocytes are particularly prone to errors.

Indeed, a wide range of oocytes (from 20 up to 60%) display missing or additional chromosomes in studies analyzing a very large number of oocytes, using both traditional and novel cytogenetic techniques.[49,93–95] Importantly, whether this rate is representative of oocytes normally developing in vivo remains to be demonstrated conclusively, although analysis of oocytes from unstimulated ovaries suggests that this may be the case.[96] However, efforts should be placed on applying the currently broad set of karyotyping tools such as spectral karyotype (SKY) imaging[97,98] and complete genomic hybridization (CGH)[99] to non-preselected oocytes from the fertile population.[49,100]

Regarding the mechanisms underlying human aneuploidies, most errors have been attributed to malsegregation during the first meiotic division of the oocyte.[49,89] The reasons for such high error rates represent an active area of study, and the unique timing of female meiosis and oocyte development in the ovary has been considered. In addition, oocytes are believed to be permissive in their cell cycle checkpoints, as they will progress through oogenesis despite fundamental meiotic errors;[101] this may in turn account for the heightened susceptibility to aneuploidy of human oocytes.[102] Regardless, advanced maternal age is the most widely recognized factor predisposing gametes to increased aneuploidy risks.[103] In addition, external agents, such as toxins, are under intense current investigation in this regard.[104]

Proper patterns of gene imprinting are also established during oocyte development[105] and, as mentioned above for spermatozoa, these epigenetic modifications have an essential role in later embryonic development. On a more global note, chromatin remodeling also has a central impact on oocyte competence. Recent analytical tools in gene expression are beginning to identify changes in transcript levels that occur at key transition stages during oocyte development in several animal models.[106–108] Upon completion, these studies will allow the exact patterns of transcriptional activity and repression to be determined during oocyte development. Also, whether these changes in gene activity represent underpinnings of subsequent oocyte quality will warrant additional examination. Current evidence, in the mouse, indicates that oocytes undergo global transcriptional repression during later phases of oogenesis at a time when chromatin condensation occurs.[109] Studies exploring the conservation of such mechanisms to human oocyte development have been limited to date[110] and merit further consideration.

PREDICTION OF GAMETE QUALITY IN ART

The possibility that gamete quality may be predicted upon initial examination is certainly attractive in the treatment of infertility by ART. Indeed, if one could reliably predict the probability of the available oocytes and sperm to support full development, patient counseling and management would be more effective. Furthermore, test(s) of gamete quality could be of invaluable prognostic value: cases of very poor predictive quality would probably indicate use of gamete donation; in less severe cases, one might be able to tailor treatment strategy appropriately. In addition, predicting gamete quality would certify that gametes are and remain of optimal quality at all steps; this would not only ensure successful treatment but also control for proper medical and laboratory protocols. With only good-quality gametes selected, then embryos of the best developmental potential would be consistently available, thereby allowing the transfer of fewer embryos. As a result, widespread use of single embryo transfers may become a reality across most patient groups. Our ability to predict gamete quality will thus overcome the currently low implantation rates and overall improve ART outcome.

ASSESSMENT OF GAMETE QUALITY IN ART

With growing demands for ART, significant advents have been made in developing tools used in evaluating oocyte and sperm quality. A summary of approaches commonly used in a contemporary ART laboratory are presented in this section (Figure 41.1).

Male gamete

Routine semen analysis

Conventionally, a male gamete has been assessed based on the patient's semen analysis with qualitative and semiquantitative methods according to criteria published by the World Health Organization.[40] Such semen analyses include not only assessment of the volume and other properties of the ejaculate including viscosity and presence of leukocytes but also the number, motility, and morphology of spermatozoa. Importantly, a patient's overall sperm quality should be based on more than one ejaculate due to common variability in results from sample to sample. Indeed, it is characteristic for human semen to display a great

Sperm	Oocyte

➢ Routine semen analysis
  • Volume, viscosity of semen
  • Presence of leukocytes
  • Number, motility, morphology of spermatozoa
➢ Functional analysis
  • Ability to penetrate the zona pellucida
➢ Nuclear assessment
  • Integrity of DNA
  • Analysis of chromosomes
	➢ Morphological grading of cumulus–oocyte complex
	  • Expansion
	  • Organization of cumulus cell layers
	➢ Morphology of cellular elements (visible in ICSI cases)
	  • Characteristics of the cytoplasm
	  • Structural analysis of the zona pellucida
	  • Imaging of the meiotic spindle
	  • Features of the first polar body
	➢ Nuclear assessment
	  • Analysis of chromosomes
	➢ Indirect predictors
	  • Content of follicular fluid
	  • Properties (viability, growth, expression profiles) of granulosa cells
	➢ Subsequent measures on the resulting embryo
	  • Morphology (cell number, symmetry, fragmentation)
	  • Metabolic profiling
	  • Secretome

Figure 41.1   Summary of potential approaches used to assess gamete quality in the contemporary ART laboratory. (References cited in 'Assessment of gamete quality in ART' section.)

deal of heterogeneity, including grossly abnormal sperm, that far exceeds that from ejaculates of other species. Nonetheless, the utility of standard semen parameters in predicting sperm normal function remains questionable.[111,112] First, these criteria are not robust predictors of fertility potential and, secondly, limitations prevail in the ability of current laboratory practices to employ these analyses reliably. Abnormal semen parameters, such as sperm morphologies below reference values by the WHO, fail to preclude fertilization success during ART. Clearly, more information is needed on the biological significance of irregular sperm morphology; also, the possibility of a correlation with more subtle developmental defects later into fetal life remains to be considered. Lastly, with respect to implementation of universal WHO standards to semen analysis in the ART laboratory, too much technical bias exists in this relatively subjective approach, even when using computer-assisted semen analyzers.[113,114] Nonetheless, the use of standard semen analysis remains an invaluable diagnostic tool that deserves supplementation with additional, and perhaps more reliable, measures of sperm quality.

Functional analysis

As alternative strategies, functional tests have been considered.[115] One example is the sperm penetration assay, which directly assesses the ability of sperm to initiate the early events during fertilization, and more precisely the penetration of the oocyte's zona pellucida. However, such tests are expensive, time-consuming, and generally not amenable to routine use in the ART laboratory. Perhaps with time, significant technological advances will allow the incorporation of functional sperm assays in ART. This remains an attractive approach, as ultimately only normal function may reliably predict superior sperm quality.

Nuclear assessment

Tests of sperm quality are currently being used by several laboratories to assess the nuclear integrity of the sperm. Such tests are of particular relevance given that sperm nuclear abnormalities exist and account for a large proportion of male infertility.[52] Also, because of the potential risks of creating embryos from ICSI using abnormal sperm that have not been selected physiologically at the level of the corona and zona pellucida, significant efforts have been placed in the last few years on developing methods to evaluate sperm DNA damage.

The phenomenon of DNA strand breaks has been described in a significant proportion of men undergoing ICSI treatment with poor semen parameters.[51,52] Therefore, some of the most recent efforts in developing optimal laboratory techniques for sperm evaluation relate to assessment of DNA integrity. An early test utilized a TUNEL technique (or terminal deoxynucleotidyl transferase-mediated dUTP nick-end labeling) that labels DNA breaks without quantifying them. In an effort to quantify nuclear integrity, a Sperm Chromatin Structure Assay (SCSA) has been developed. The SCSA is based on a flow-cytometric measurement of the proportion of fragmented DNA in an ejaculate sample.[116]

A growing body of studies has focused on defining the precise relationships between DNA fragmentation and ART outcomes.[117] Yet, several conflicting findings exist regarding the relationship between DNA damage and sperm quality.[117–120] Currently, further data must be acquired with respect to who may benefit from using SCSA before it becomes a routine ART assessment of gamete quality for clinical diagnosis; thus, guidelines remain to be established. Indeed, with several studies demonstrating that damaged DNA does not preclude spermatozoa from supporting complete embryonic development, the predictive value of sperm DNA integrity lacks conclusive findings. Possible limitations may reside in the inability of SCSA to distinguish between DNA breaks on the one hand, and chromatin packaging errors, on the other. Given the vital role of protamines in sperm chromatin packing and function, protamine deficiencies have been measured, related to DNA damage, and negatively correlated with fertilization rates after ICSI.[121] However, no link has been found between sperm protamine deficiency and embryo quality.[119,121] Under more recent consideration is the potential development of a magnetic cell sorting test to select non-apoptotic sperm, an interesting novel approach given that apoptotic spermatozoa are present in ejaculates.[122] However, further validation is needed to clarify any benefit of selecting non-apoptotic sperm for enhanced ART outcome.

It is clear from the above discussion, that much research in clinical andrology has been undertaken during the last few years, with the development and testing of a multitude of tests of sperm chromatin structure. All of these continue to be under intense investigation, in search of validation between a given test and markers of sperm quality together with a defined relationship to fertility. Overall, continued large-scale, prospective, and standardized trials are needed to ascertain the predictive value of sperm DNA integrity assays in ART. Furthermore, one cannot rule out the possibility that sperm DNA damage impairs fetal or neonatal development, rather than the early endpoints studied to date. Indeed, a possibility meriting further investigation is that despite an ability to support a pregnancy, sperm with DNA damage may be associated with subtle defects that are either very rare or distant in the health of the resultant child.[123]

Chromosomal anomalies occur at an elevated incidence in infertile males.[45,48,124] In selected patient populations, meiotic disorders can be identified using sperm chromosome analyses by fluorescence in-situ hybridization (FISH); such information may permit the establishment of ART prognosis and also the recommendation for PGD in certain cases. One pitfall with this approach is that while it guides treatment options, it fails to select good-quality sperm non-invasively. Therefore, there is a continued need for improvements in our ability to diagnose and predict sperm quality. Much progress awaits clinical andrology, specifically with regard to selection against the large numbers of abnormal sperm typically present during ART treatment. Furthermore, it is likely that no single sperm parameter will be used alone, but rather that a combinatorial approach will be adopted.

Female gamete

Simplicity defines neither oocyte quality nor embryo quality. This is true not only at the cellular level (as presented in the 'Biological significance of gamete quality' section) but also on a practical level with respect to assessment. Nevertheless, much can be learned from the evaluation of embryo quality. Once reliable tools exist to predict embryo viability, these can, in turn, be used in studies aimed at predicting and improving oocyte quality. Indeed, this will permit a wide range of investigations that are not currently possible since an oocyte can only be confirmed as having good quality upon its subsequent development to term into a healthy fetus. Such a paradigm clearly represents considerable restrictions in clinical ART.

Morphological and non-invasive evaluation

Since the inception of ART, attention has focused on the morphological evaluation of human embryos using a multitude of parameters, each of which has been considered for direct links with reproductive success.[125,126] No consensus yet exists on the robustness by which morphological assessment indeed predicts embryo quality; however, it still remains the single most frequently used tool to select embryos of presumably highest developmental potential in ART. Conventional criteria used for embryo morphological assessment include cell number, symmetry, and fragmentation of blastomeres. Attempts also exist to develop morphological parameters to assess oocyte quality, again targeting many of the structural elements of oocytes.[127,128]

Morphological evaluation of the human oocyte is often limited to characteristics of the intact cumulus–oocyte complex immediately after retrieval from the patient. Cumulus grading has been based on overall dimensions, degree of expansion, and homogeneity of cumulus cell layers around the oocyte.[129–131] While lower grade cumulus–oocyte complexes, which are grossly disorganized, often correlate with compromised oocyte quality, the wide range of even intact complexes largely fails to predict later gamete quality. Such a theme when using morphological predictors of gamete or embryo quality is rather common in ART, with clear deviations from the norm indicative of poor outcome while cells with apparently regular morphology still display a wider range of developmental potential. Clearly, difficulty remains regarding the morphological determination of oocyte quality.

In contrast to morphological evaluation for assessment of oocyte quality, biochemical approaches have been used to identify markers in follicular fluid or isolated granulosa or cumulus.[128,132,133] Preliminary evidence also suggests the potential utility of the degree of perifollicular vascularity as a predictor of oocyte quality.[134,135] Here again, however, technical drawbacks and inconsistencies in findings have hindered significant progress along these lines of research.

A more thorough evaluation of oocyte morphology is possible once cumulus cells are removed. However, this approach is strictly limited to one type of ART cycle, which utilizes ICSI, in which a sperm is injected into a denuded oocyte. Several oocyte morphological parameters have been considered, including characteristics of the cytoplasm, structural analysis of the zona pellucida, imaging of the meiotic spindle, and morphology of the first polar body.[128] A relationship between polar body features (size, fragmentation, surface smoothness) and oocyte quality remains tentative and deserves more experimental data for support.[136] In the last few years, developments in optical systems for polarized light microscopy have made possible the analysis of spindle architecture using the Polscope.[137] This instrument permits the non-invasive measurement of microtubule density, and thus visualization of spindle structure.[138]

Evidence continues to accumulate regarding the clinical use and relevance of the Polscope as a measure of oocyte quality and subsequent formation of euploid embryos. Collectively, these data support the putative utility of the Polscope as a predictor of oocyte quality, but not without some conflicting results.[136,138] Animal studies point to the complexity of spindle structures under various situations;[139–141] thus, the assessment of finer details of meiotic spindles in human oocytes may not be identifiable using the Polscope. Nonetheless, the instrument is considered to have potential use as a quality control tool to prevent physical damage to the meiotic spindle when performing ICSI.[139] Its use has

also been extended to evaluating the organization of the zona pellucida.[142,143] The multilaminar arrangement of the zona pellucida becomes apparent with Polscope microscopy and, thus far, initial studies have related variations in zona structure to gamete quality and ultimately pregnancy outcome.[144,145]

Overall, with limitations regarding the significance and predictive value of oocyte morphology, alternative criteria need to be considered. Besides, in view of the critical role of cumulus cells in supporting oocyte function, tests relying on oocytes free of cumulus cells will neither be applicable to, nor recommended for, conventional IVF cycles, even upon successful optimization. As is the case for sperm analysis, the exact nature of the correlation between oocyte morphology and viability still awaits further understanding. For example, the significance of oocyte cytoplasmic granularity, oocyte shape, and membrane irregularities are not known. Extensive studies should be conducted with animal oocytes, for which availability is not restrictive and the range of possible manipulations is non-limiting. Notably, animal studies have increasingly focused on the assessment of relative transcript abundance between gametes and embryos at different developmental stages.[107,146] With modern advents in broad-scale gene expression profiling, a new field of embryogenomics is emerging, promising to contribute significantly to our basic understanding and management of gamete quality in ART. Innovative strategies in the non-invasive evaluation of molecular aspects of gamete and embryo function may also prove applicable to clinical ART in the future.[147] Also, a proteomic approach may prove instrumental in establishing patterns of protein expression in good-quality gametes, as such a strategy begins to be employed in embryos.[128,148] Ideally, a secreted protein profile (or secretome) of embryos and possibly even of cumulus–oocyte complexes will allow the non-invasive, routine, and reliable prediction of positive reproductive outcome. Lastly, focusing on the health of gametes, and particularly oocytes, metabolic output or nutrient consumption may be assessed non-invasively, as has been investigated in human embryos.[149–153] Clearly, the time has come for the general application of non-invasive markers to the assessment of gamete quality in ART, pending further technological advances and experimental support.[154]

Nuclear assessment

On an increasingly routine level, embryos are assessed for their chromosomal normalcy based on chromosomal analysis. In conjunction with PGD, a broad range of cytogenetic techniques is used in genetic screens of cleavage-stage human embryos in selected patients. For instance, in patients of advanced maternal age for whom embryo morphological analysis does not accurately predict developmental potential, PGD may provide an efficacious treatment strategy provided sufficient available embryos can be biopsied.[91] Similarly, individual oocytes may be evaluated by polar body aneuploidy screening.[95] When performed on the polar bodies resulting from the two meiotic divisions, the use of FISH analysis has provided a certain degree of predictive value for aneuploidy occurrence.[155,156] Then again, just as the use of PGD on embryos remains controversial as an effective screening tool for aneuploidy, further testing and improvement merit attention with respect to the cytogenetic analysis of polar bodies.[157] Intrinsic limitations for polar body analysis lie in the quality of chromosome spreads and the natural fragmentation and degeneration of polar bodies.

In contrast to the currently limited value of oocyte assessment, the efficacy of embryo grading has undergone considerable improvement and optimization since its initial implementation in the ART laboratory. Notably, cumulative scoring has been developed over two decades of extensive research and it entails successive morphological embryo grading from egg retrieval to embryo transfer. The incorporation of several parameters into a single predictive score of embryo quality currently appears to be of clinical value, with a significant improvement in success rates.[158–161] Following their development and proven utility, it is thus conceivable that markers of oocyte and sperm quality also become integrated into a cumulative scoring system.

In conclusion, a great deal of effort is currently centered around developing assays that will allow the assessment of gamete quality without interfering with its normal development. It is also of utmost importance that non-invasive assays are quantitative, given that consistency is a clear limitation in ART for any assays that rely on a qualitative form of assessment. A critical need exists to develop tests for the normal nuclear and cytoplasmic function of gametes, including assaying for chromosomal normalcy as well as recently identified genetic and epigenetic parameters.

FACTORS INFLUENCING GAMETE QUALITY IN ART

With the complexity of gamete development, it is not surprising that a multitude of factors may undermine gamete quality and normal function. These factors may be considered in two general classes: those relating to the laboratory environment, and those exerting an effect in the body prior to gamete retrieval. In addition, it is important to note that genetic and epigenetic parameters also exert their impact on gamete quality. While the nature of interplays among all sources of factors remains uncertain, it is conceivable that, for example, genetic and exogenous factors themselves predispose gametes to epigenetic modifications. In this section, we summarize key factors and conditions suggested to influence gamete quality (Figure 41.2).

In the laboratory

The isolation, preparation, and culture of gametes in the laboratory (singly or together) undoubtedly expose these cells to hazards not normally encountered in the male or female reproductive tracts. Notably, gametes may be unable to sustain normal cell structure and function in this artificial environment. Furthermore, one must ask what constitutes the 'normal environment' and the 'normal responses' of the gametes to this environment; alas, much remains unknown in these realms. For example, the percent oxygen that prevails in the ovary during follicular development, in the Fallopian tube after ovulation, and in the uterine environment during the peri-implantation period, is of pivotal relevance when attempting to mirror physiological conditions ex vivo. In this respect, controversy still exists as to the nature of influences, positive or negative, of elevated oxygen tension on human gamete function.[162–164] Nonetheless, sperm, oocytes, and resulting embryos are all subject to oxidative stress when manipulated and cultured ex vivo. Substantial levels of reactive oxygen species (ROS) are present during ART treatment, and thus a rising concern exists regarding the overall role of oxidative stress in ART.[165,166] For instance, high levels of ROS may lead to an increased incidence of DNA strand breaks in spermatozoa, in turn reducing overall reproductive outcome.[167] Strategies under investigation to overcome oxidative stress have been to reduce the incubation time between sperm and oocytes at fertilization as well as to use lowered concentrations of sperm.[168] Indisputably, multiple approaches will be necessary to overcome oxidative stress in gametes during ART.

Studies in domestic animals support the central role of the oocyte in determining its later ability to develop into a blastocyst; however, the quality of the resulting blastocyst appears to be largely influenced by the culture environment.[146,169] Based on animal studies, experimental evidence has accumulated on significant

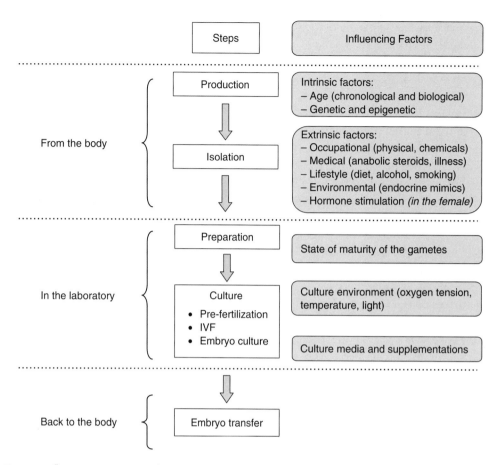

Figure 41.2   Factors influencing gamete quality at each step in ART, from the origin of gametes in the body ('produced' step) to the artificial conditions of the laboratory ('culture' step). (References cited in 'Factors influencing gamete quality in ART' section.)

disparities in the quality of oocytes and embryos that developed in vitro when compared to in vivo.[71,170–172] Among the multiple parameters, the relative abundance of transcripts has been shown to be discrepant.[173] Interestingly, many transcripts that are related to developmental competence are detected at different levels depending on the milieu in which oogenesis and oocyte maturation occur. Continued comparison between in-vitro and in-vivo produced gametes and embryos is necessary before we can truly model ART techniques to replicate in-vivo processes.

It is indisputable that human gametes are extremely sensitive to their environment. Thus, every attempt is typically made during ART manipulation ex vivo to mirror known conditions in vivo. For example, temperature fluctuations are known to impair the oocyte cytoskeleton.[139,174] The meiotic spindle is particularly prone to damage, thereby possibly underlying chromosomal abnormalities and the impaired segregation of subcellular components in resultant embryos. Given that damage may not always be reversible and oocyte function may proceed despite severe deficiencies, a critical need arises to control all potential insults

during oocyte retrieval and subsequent manipulation. The use of non-invasive imaging technology, such as the Polscope discussed above, may allow improved quality control and minimize potential deviations from normal spindle characteristics.

Recent studies using animal models have highlighted potential dangers resulting from apparently benign manipulations often performed in the ART laboratory. For example, simply culturing mouse embryos in vitro caused altered gene expression,[175,176] and different culture media altered patterns of genomic imprinting.[177] With the considerable expansion of commercially available media, an increasing number of studies have compared embryo quality among different culture conditions.[178–180] Moreover, a recent study has revealed an association between the type of culture medium used to culture human embryos from day 1 to day 3, and the level of human chorionic gonadotropin (hCG) in maternal serum early in pregnancy.[181] For a varied set of studied markers, all reports to date point towards the critical influence of a suboptimal culture environment on embryo quality, and thus conceivably gamete function and ART outcome.

With respect to culture medium supplementation, and most particularly sources of exogenous energy sources, the use of serum is no longer employed in ART. Rather, defined and purified protein preparations are used in order not only to alleviate putative defects from pathogenic contaminants but also to minimize growth defects. Indeed, fetal and placental growth abnormalities have been identified in animal studies and attributed to the serum components in culture media.[182] Although much effort has centered on the influence of embryo culture media on gene expression, particularly when using extended culture to the blastocyst stage, the effect does not appear restricted to prolonged culture duration. Indeed, relatively short cultures (of approximately 1 day) alter normal patterns of gene expression in animal models.[169] However, these studies have focused on the early embryo, and the relevance of timing and characteristics between the culture environment and quality remains to be determined for gametes. Further research is clearly required to investigate the influence of media compositions in sustaining normal gene expression in human gametes and embryos. Meiotic errors should also be considered when evaluating culture conditions, during either in-vitro fertilization or in-vitro maturation, since elevated aneuploidy error rates have been associated with the use of these in-vitro techniques in human and animal models.[96,183,184] Most recently, variants in components of IVF media were shown to influence subsequent epigenetic marks, and more precisely levels of genomic cytosine methylation, in bovine fetuses.[185]

The use of immature gametes represents an additional challenge in ART. Examples include the use of prophase-I arrested oocytes that have not yet completed oocyte maturation and spermatogenic cells such as testicular round spermatids. Despite intense attention, in-vitro maturation of human oocytes remains an experimental procedure that awaits significant improvements.[186] Indeed, a major constraint lies in the inability to emulate in-vivo conditions for the maturation of human oocytes in the laboratory.[187] Similarly for prespermatozoon cells, concern prevails as to the normalcy of immature gametes and our current inability to sustain their development in vitro.[34] Notably, compromised patterns of gene imprinting associated with the in-vitro handling of immature gametes may be inconsistent with their safe and routine use in present-day ART.

In conclusion, suboptimal conditions in the laboratory are particularly detrimental to gamete quality, even when exposure is for a very limited time interval. Optimal quality of gametes in the ART laboratory may be achieved by (1) optimizing the protocols associated with isolation, (2) maintaining the quality of gametes at the time of isolation and during preparation, and (3) reducing potential sources of factors that may reduce gamete quality during culture.

In the body

Of relevance is also our ability to understand the origins of varying gamete quality in the body; indeed, such knowledge of the basic factors influencing sperm and oocyte quality will permit not only the identification of any abnormalities but also the optimization of ART. Animal studies have also emphasized the importance of oocyte origin in determining blastocyst yield; this is in contrast to postfertilization culture conditions that have been associated with blastocyst quality and subsequent development of a healthy offspring.[169] It is without doubt then that all aspects of gamete and embryo quality ought to be considered in ART, including both the culture conditions and the physiological environment provided within the body. One evident determinant of gamete quality is age of the individual, regardless of the sex; indeed, advanced age is associated with gametes of severely diminished quality, not only in the female but also in the male.[188] While the focus has historically been placed on the woman, and her fertility and quality of her oocytes, it has become increasingly clear that male infertility accounts for a significant percentage (up to 40%) of infertility diagnoses among all ART cycles.[1]

Besides age, sperm quality appears to be influenced by a wide array of compounds and conditions. The vast majority of studies have examined potential relationships between changes in the environment and reproductive health, including subfertility and infertility in not only humans but also wildlife and experimental animals. This increased research attention contributes to an understanding of the etiology of infertility and predictors of ART outcome. Focusing more specifically on gamete quality, several studies have supported the hypothesis that environmental influences may impair normal sperm development.[189] More precisely, influences may be classified under one of several broad categories: environmental, occupational, medical, and lifestyle.[189,190] Occupational exposures that may impair reproductive function include the physical, psychosocial (stress), and chemical environments (solvents, metals, agriculture). To date, studies have failed to establish conclusively that common occupational insults directly lead to adverse IVF outcomes.[191] Uptake of anabolic steroids is known to affect sperm production, with limited recovery after interrupting steroid use.[192] Other sources of chemical exposures arise from lifestyle choices, including diet, alcohol, caffeine, or smoking.[193] For instance, obesity correlates with diminished sperm quality. From studies to date, the effects of caffeine and alcohol consumption remain undefined. In contrast, a more robust relationship exists between smoking, notably nicotine exposure, and reduced reproductive function. While the exact mechanisms of action of smoking remain to be identified, an impaired ability of sperm to fertilize and more precisely bind to the oocyte's zona pellucida has been implicated.[191] A last potential origin of chemicals is from inadvertent exposures to toxin-containing air, water, and food; among such pollutants are a wide variety of endocrine-disrupting chemicals. These compounds present a serious public health concern noteworthy of heightened scrutiny. Indeed, given their ability to mimic natural hormones, notably estrogen, their aptitude to interfere with normal gamete development is not surprising. Although controversy remains regarding the exact links between fertility and endocrine-disrupting chemicals, animal studies have provided invaluable evidence for deleterious effects on sperm and oocyte characteristics.[194,195] All of the insight gained from animal models has greatly advanced our understanding of the 'whether, which, how, and when' environmental contaminants affect gamete quality.

It is undeniable that at multiple times in their life history, spermatozoa appear vulnerable to a number of toxic environmental substances such as pesticides, herbicides, and industrial agents. Yet, a great deal of uncertainty remains regarding such relevance to ART mainly due to some of the inherent limitations in study designs employed to date. Indeed, numerous problems arise in interpreting exposure studies. While many of the early human studies have been population-based and provided correlative evidence, more recent advances in available tools and an improved understanding of normal sperm function have opened new and promising avenues of research in this field. For example, sperm DNA damage may constitute a better bioassay to test a wide range of compounds; however, as outlined in the above section, a reliable test will first need to be implemented. Indeed, sensitive, reliable, and routine screening tools need to be used in future studies aimed at defining parameters affecting gamete quality. It is also important to note that studies focusing on specific external influences are likely to be confounded by a complex set of other factors, intrinsic in nature, that also affect spermatogenesis, whether these be genetic or developmental features. Also, conditions

disrupting normal temperature regulation in the testes and illnesses causing infection may also, in turn, influence sperm quality through damage to the DNA.[196] It is likely that prior gamete exposures to compounds may confound our ability to discern among other causes underlying any specific defect.

The precise influence of environmental threats on the quality of oocytes in situ remains uncertain, this being due either to a lack of studies or to inconclusive or even conflicting results. Among the range of factors suspected to undermine oocyte quality in vivo are alcohol consumption, smoking, and diet, all of which have received significant attention in recent decades.[193] As mentioned above, one of the most studied etiological factors for the precipitous drop in oocyte quality during a woman's life is her age.[188] Indeed, oocyte quality rapidly declines during the normal process of reproductive aging at menopause. Nonetheless, a distinction must be made between chronological and biological aging as both processes take place in women and are associated with compromised oocyte quality. Indeed, a fall in ovarian reserve often precedes a woman's menopausal clock. Thus, many women undergoing ART exhibit a progressive reduction in oocyte quality that could be managed better if predicted more accurately.[197,198] Clearly, the field of ART needs to be able to rely on markers of ovarian reserve that will account not only for the quantity but also the quality of oocytes that a woman possesses.

The current paucity of, and inconsistency among data on potential reproductive hazards, precludes the establishment of definitive links between specific insults and gamete quality. But undoubtedly, both men and women face such risks to their fertility; thus, as further studies unravel the exact mechanisms by which gametes are affected, we will be better positioned to control such external factors, and prevent any potential decline in gamete quality and related decrease in ART success.

Another unique aspect of ART treatment is the routine use of ovarian hormone stimulation. Since such external hormonal manipulations salvage follicles that would otherwise undergo atresia, it is not surprising that there is typically considerable heterogeneity in the cohort of oocytes retrieved. Moreover, such exogenous hormone stimulation has been shown, at least in animal models, to modify the follicular environment that, in turn, affects oocyte quality.[107,199] However, there is a paucity of evidence directly demonstrating the effects of specific stimulation protocols used in ART on oocyte quality. The types of ART stimulation protocols are multiple, and considerable variations exist in responses among individuals. Specific stimulation regimens influence embryo quality and cycle outcome differently.[9,200,201] However, the underlying mechanisms by which various stimulations affect oocyte quality within the ovary and after retrieval remain to be defined. Recent reports have proposed a correlation between ovarian stimulation and imprinting modifications.[57] Oocytes normally acquire unique patterns of imprints during the growth and maturation phases of oogenesis at a time when hormones and paracrine factors are largely influencing the ovarian follicle and oocyte. Clearly, under the influence of exogenous and non-physiological levels of gonadotropins and steroids, processes naturally under the control of hormones may be incorrectly regulated and at a risk of not proceeding accurately. Along this same line of reasoning, whether ovarian stimulation results in an increased incidence of aneuploidy merits additional scrutiny;[91,92] of relevance are studies in mice with oocyte growth defects that show a greater risk of chromosomal non-disjunction.[202] Thus, it is conceivable that by modifying the normal balance of oocyte growth during folliculogenesis, hormone supplementation impairs oocyte quality at the level of chromosomal segregation during meiosis. This hypothesis deserves careful further testing, with assessments of a broad array of nuclear and cytoplasmic determinants of oocyte quality being made.

Dramatic advances in genetics have permitted the creation and phenotypic characterization of a large number of mouse knockouts for genes related to mammalian fertility. Such genetic models have provided tremendous insight into not only the genetic basis of infertility but also the identification and characterization of molecules involved in normal sperm and oocyte function.[203–205] In addition, during the last decade, great strides have been made towards genetically testing severe clinical cases of male infertility, including azoospermia, in which there is a complete absence of sperm in semen. As a result, the genetic basis of some forms of previously classified 'idiopathic' male infertility has been unraveled with notably the identification of DAZ, the deleted in azoospermia gene.[45,206] With the discovery of additional genes, DAZ has been renamed AZFc, representing one of several AZF or azoospermia factor genes.[62] With a 47,XXY karyotype, Klinefelter's syndrome represents the most frequent genetic cause of male infertility, trailed by Y chromosome microdeletions, as first discovered in the 1970s. Since then, a multitude of loci not only have been identified on deleted regions of the Y chromosome, named AZFa-d, but also linked with non-obstructive severe oligozoospermia or azoospermia.[62,207–209] Not surprisingly, the genes associated with Y chromosome deletions play a role in spermatogenesis, such as in Sertoli cell numbers and function, meiotic progression, or even in postmeiotic differentiation. Clinically, the range of phenotypes resulting from AZF deletions varies significantly, an expected phenomenon given the large number of genes lying in these chromosomal regions.[206] During ART, men with Y chromosome deletions can father children using ISCI; interestingly, although they have reduced fertilization rates, pregnancy rates are comparable to control groups.[210,211] Regarding testing for microdeletions, molecular diagnostic tools exist and are offered to patients considering ART treatment in Europe.[212] Overall, our current understanding of the genetic basis of human infertility is minimal and restricted to just a few genes. Efforts in identifying genetic causes in both males and females are ongoing and, clearly, knowledge gained from mouse infertility mutants will likely prove instrumental to such endeavor.

In summary, given the influence of both the origin of gametes, and the culture environment on embryo quality, optimization efforts should focus on all potential variables affecting gamete quality. In addition, it is likely that the numerous factors believed to influence gamete quality independently also interact with each other either in an additive or synergistic manner, thereby obscuring and possibly confounding analysis. Thus, increased care must be taken in ART data analyses in order to avoid any potential bias in interpretation.

CONCLUSION

In the present chapter, we have summarized some of the past and current work pertinent to gamete quality, along with current challenges in this rapidly evolving technological field of ART. Among some of the significant advents in ART, ICSI has permitted the treatment of patients with severe gamete defects, notably in cases with highly abnormal sperm. However, much remains to be unraveled for what is likely to be a spectrum of infertility or subfertility disorders that are multifactorial or multigenic in origin. An enhanced and detailed understanding of basic gamete development will not only assist a broader population of patients than in the present but also optimize overall success outcomes for all.

Clearly, factors underlying human fertility are complex, and efforts will continue to be placed on improving patient-tailored approaches to diagnosis and treatment. Indeed, there is a pressing need for advances in our ability to predict, measure, and maintain optimal sperm and oocyte function. Continued work using animal models and their careful application to human studies promise to provide an ever-refined outlook on the essential impact of gamete quality in assisted conception. Future research should focus on identifying all relevant conditions or factors affecting gamete quality in ART. Additionally, in light of the vulnerability of non-human gametes to altered gene expression and epigenetic modifications, the exact influences of culture media on human gametes must be assessed during all routine procedures employed in the ART laboratory. Studies that deserve immediate attention should hence focus on possible detrimental effects that current culture conditions may cause to gametes. Novel techniques must be continually and carefully implemented with combined approaches, such as morphological and non-invasive bioassays, likely to prove most successful. It is an exciting time in ART as multiple prospects for improved production, isolation, preparation, and use of optimal quality gametes are on the horizon. Indisputably, oocyte quality persists at the forefront of success during ART; however, the importance of superior sperm characteristics has gained novel appreciation, in need of further scrutiny. Advances in basic gamete biology, together with continued implementation and analysis of ART protocols, promise to result in much-awaited breakthroughs, and ultimately clinical efficiency and safety.

REFERENCES

1. CDC, Center for Disease Control and Prevention. 2003 Assisted reproductive technology success rates. National summary and fertility clinic reports. Atlanta, GA, USA, 2005.
2. Steptoe PC, Edwards RG. Birth after the reimplantation of a human embryo. Lancet 1978; 2: 366.
3. Palermo G, Joris H, Devroey P, Van Steirteghem AC. Pregnancies after intracytoplasmic injection of single spermatozoon into an oocyte. Lancet 1992; 340: 17–18.
4. Da Motta EL, Serafini P. The treatment of infertility and its historical context. Reprod Biomed Online 2002; 5: 65–77.
5. Hardy K, Wright C, Rice S et al. Future developments in assisted reproduction in humans. Reproduction 2002; 123: 171–83.
6. Edwards RG, Steptoe PC, Purdy JM. Establishing full-term human pregnancies using cleaving embryos grown in vitro. Br J Obstet Gynaecol 1980; 87: 737–56.
7. Edwards RG, Steptoe PC. Current status of in-vitro fertilisation and implantation of human embryos. Lancet 1983; 2: 1265–9.
8. Steptoe PC, Edwards RG, Walters DE. Observations on 767 clinical pregnancies and 500 births after human in-vitro fertilization. Hum Reprod 1986; 1: 89–94.
9. Diedrich K, Felberbaum R. New approaches to ovarian stimulation. Hum Reprod 1998; 13(Suppl 3): 1–13; discussion 14–17.
10. Lunenfeld B. Development of gonadotrophins for clinical use. Reprod Biomed Online 2002; 4(Suppl 1): 11–17.
11. Macklon NS, Stouffer RL, Giudice LC, Fauser BC. The science behind 25 years of ovarian stimulation for IVF. Endocr Rev 2006; 27: 170–207.
12. Safran A, Reubinoff BE, Porat-Katz A et al. Assisted reproduction for the treatment of azoospermia. Hum Reprod 1998; 13(Suppl 4): 47–60.
13. Jones RE, Lopez KH. Pregnancy. In: Human Reproductive Biology, 3rd edn. Elsevier: Academic Press, 2006: 253–97.
14. Hamilton BE, Martin JA, Ventura SJ et al. Births: preliminary data for 2004. Natl Vital Stat Rep 2005; 54: 1–17.
15. Godfrey KM, Barker DJ. Fetal programming and adult health. Public Health Nutr 2001; 4: 611–24.
16. Hales CN, Barker DJ. The thrifty phenotype hypothesis. Br Med Bull 2001; 60: 5–20.
17. Langley-Evans SC, Langley-Evans AJ, Marchand MC. Nutritional programming of blood pressure and renal morphology. Arch Physiol Biochem 2003; 111: 8–16.
18. Langley-Evans SC. Developmental programming of health and disease. Proc Nutr Soc 2006; 65: 97–105.
19. Kwong WY, Wild AE, Roberts P et al. Maternal undernutrition during the preimplantation period of rat development causes blastocyst abnormalities and programming of postnatal hypertension. Development 2000; 127: 4195–202.
20. Bloomfield FH, Oliver MH, Hawkins P et al. A periconceptional nutritional origin for noninfectious preterm birth. Science 2003; 300: 606.
21. Bloomfield FH, Oliver MH, Hawkins P et al. Periconceptional undernutrition in sheep accelerates maturation of the fetal hypothalamic–pituitary–adrenal axis in late gestation. Endocrinology 2004; 145: 4278–85.
22. Bower C, Hansen M. Assisted reproductive technologies and birth outcomes: overview of recent systematic reviews. Reprod Fertil Dev 2005; 17: 329–33.
23. Wright VC, Schieve LA, Reynolds MA, Jeng G. Assisted reproductive technology surveillance – United States, 2002. MMWR Surveill Summ 2005; 54: 1–24.
24. Wassarman PM, Jovine L, Litscher ES. A profile of fertilization in mammals. Nat Cell Biol 2001; 3: E59–64.
25. Evans JP, Florman HM. The state of the union: the cell biology of fertilization. Nat Cell Biol 2002; 4(Suppl): s57–63.
26. Fissore RA, Kurokawa M, Knott J et al. Mechanisms underlying oocyte activation and postovulatory ageing. Reproduction 2002; 124: 745–54.
27. Williams CJ. Signalling mechanisms of mammalian oocyte activation. Hum Reprod Update 2002; 8: 313–21.
28. Ducibella T, Huneau D, Angelichio E et al. Egg-to-embryo transition is driven by differential responses to Ca^{2+} oscillation number. Dev Biol 2002; 250: 280–91.
29. Swann K, Larman MG, Saunders CM, Lai FA. The cytosolic sperm factor that triggers Ca^{2+} oscillations and egg activation in mammals is a novel phospholipase C: PLCzeta. Reproduction 2004; 127: 431–9.
30. Kurokawa M, Sato K, Wu H et al. Functional, biochemical, and chromatographic characterization of the complete $[Ca^{2+}]i$ oscillation-inducing activity of porcine sperm. Dev Biol 2005; 285: 376–92.
31. Rogers NT, Hobson E, Pickering S et al. Phospholipase Czeta causes Ca^{2+} oscillations and parthenogenetic activation of human oocytes. Reproduction 2004; 128: 697–702.
32. Ludwig M, Schroder AK, Diedrich K. Impact of intracytoplasmic sperm injection on the activation and fertilization process of oocytes. Reprod Biomed Online 2001; 3: 230–40.
33. Kurokawa M, Fissore RA. ICSI-generated mouse zygotes exhibit altered calcium oscillations, inositol 1,4,5-trisphosphate receptor-1 down-regulation, and embryo development. Mol Hum Reprod 2003; 9: 523–33.

34. Yanagimachi R. Intracytoplasmic injection of spermatozoa and spermatogenic cells: its biology and applications in humans and animals. Reprod Biomed Online 2005; 10: 247–88.

35. Morozumi K, Yanagimachi R. Incorporation of the acrosome into the oocyte during intracytoplasmic sperm injection could be potentially hazardous to embryo development. Proc Natl Acad Sci USA 2005; 102: 14209–14.

36. Turner RM. Tales from the tail: what do we really know about sperm motility? J Androl 2003; 24: 790–803.

37. Turner RM. Moving to the beat: a review of mammalian sperm motility regulation. Reprod Fertil Dev 2006; 18: 25–38.

38. Suarez SS, Pacey AA. Sperm transport in the female reproductive tract. Hum Reprod Update 2006; 12: 23–37.

39. De Jonge C. Biological basis for human capacitation. Hum Reprod Update 2005; 11: 205–14.

40. World Health Organization. WHO laboratory manual for the examination of human semen and sperm-cervical mucus interaction. Cambridge, UK: Cambridge University Press, 1999.

41. Sun F, Ko E, Martin RH. Is there a relationship between sperm chromosome abnormalities and sperm morphology? Reprod Biol Endocrinol 2006; 4: 1.

42. Kishikawa H, Tateno H, Yanagimachi R. Chromosome analysis of BALB/c mouse spermatozoa with normal and abnormal head morphology. Biol Reprod 1999; 61: 809–12.

43. Pyle A, Handel MA. Meiosis in male PL/J mice: a genetic model for gametic aneuploidy. Mol Reprod Dev 2003; 64: 471–81.

44. Burruel VR, Yanagimachi R, Whitten WK. Normal mice develop from oocytes injected with spermatozoa with grossly misshapen heads. Biol Reprod 1996; 55: 709–14.

45. Griffin DK, Finch KA. The genetic and cytogenetic basis of male infertility. Hum Fertil (Camb) 2005; 8: 19–26.

46. Jacobs PA. The chromosome complement of human gametes. Oxf Rev Reprod Biol 1992; 14: 47–72.

47. Hassold TJ. Nondisjunction in the human male. Curr Top Dev Biol 1998; 37: 383–406.

48. Egozcue S, Blanco J, Vendrell JM et al. Human male infertility: chromosome anomalies, meiotic disorders, abnormal spermatozoa and recurrent abortion. Hum Reprod Update 2000; 6: 93–105.

49. Hassold T, Hunt P. To err (meiotically) is human: the genesis of human aneuploidy. Nat Rev Genet 2001; 2: 280–91.

50. Egozcue J, Sarrate Z, Codina-Pascual M et al. Meiotic abnormalities in infertile males. Cytogenet Genome Res 2005; 111: 337–42.

51. Irvine DS, Twigg JP, Gordon EL et al. DNA integrity in human spermatozoa: relationships with semen quality. J Androl 2000; 21: 33–44.

52. Spano M, Seli E, Bizzaro D et al. The significance of sperm nuclear DNA strand breaks on reproductive outcome. Curr Opin Obstet Gynecol 2005; 17: 255–60.

53. Blanco-Rodriguez J. A matter of death and life: the significance of germ cell death during spermatogenesis. Int J Androl 1998; 21: 236–48.

54. Ward WS, Coffey DS. DNA packaging and organization in mammalian spermatozoa: comparison with somatic cells. Biol Reprod 1991; 44: 569–74.

55. Braun RE. Packaging paternal chromosomes with protamine. Nat Genet 2001; 28: 10–12.

56. Jaenisch R, Bird A. Epigenetic regulation of gene expression: how the genome integrates intrinsic and environmental signals. Nat Genet 2003; 33(Suppl): 245–54.

57. Horsthemke B, Ludwig M. Assisted reproduction: the epigenetic perspective. Hum Reprod Update 2005; 11: 473–82.

58. Thompson JR, Williams CJ. Genomic imprinting and assisted reproductive technology: connections and potential risks. Semin Reprod Med 2005; 23: 285–95.

59. Lucifero D, Mann MR, Bartolomei MS, Trasler JM. Gene-specific timing and epigenetic memory in oocyte imprinting. Hum Mol Genet 2004; 13: 839–49.

60. Allegrucci C, Thurston A, Lucas E, Young L. Epigenetics and the germline. Reproduction 2005; 129: 137–49.

61. Marques CJ, Carvalho F, Sousa M, Barros A. Genomic imprinting in disruptive spermatogenesis. Lancet 2004; 363: 1700–2.

62. Seli E, Sakkas D. Spermatozoal nuclear determinants of reproductive outcome: implications for ART. Hum Reprod Update 2005; 11: 337–49.

63. Sutovsky P, Schatten G. Paternal contributions to the mammalian zygote: fertilization after sperm-egg fusion. Int Rev Cytol 2000; 195: 1–65.

64. Navara CS, First NL, Schatten G. Phenotypic variations among paternal centrosomes expressed within the zygote as disparate microtubule lengths and sperm aster organization: correlations between centrosome activity and developmental success. Proc Natl Acad Sci USA 1996; 93: 5384–8.

65. Terada Y. Human sperm centrosomal function during fertilization, a novel assessment for male sterility. Hum Cell 2004; 17: 181–6.

66. St John JC, Lloyd R, El Shourbagy S. The potential risks of abnormal transmission of mtDNA through assisted reproductive technologies. Reprod Biomed Online 2004; 8: 34–44.

67. Tanaka H, Baba T. Gene expression in spermiogenesis. Cell Mol Life Sci 2005; 62: 344–54.

68. Eppig JJ. Coordination of nuclear and cytoplasmic oocyte maturation in eutherian mammals. Reprod Fertil Dev 1996; 8: 485–9.

69. Fulka J Jr, First NL, Moor RM. Nuclear and cytoplasmic determinants involved in the regulation of mammalian oocyte maturation. Mol Hum Reprod 1998; 4: 41–9.

70. Albertini DF, Sanfins A, Combelles CM. Origins and manifestations of oocyte maturation competencies. Reprod Biomed Online 2003; 6: 410–15.

71. Moor RM, Dai Y, Lee C, Fulka J Jr. Oocyte maturation and embryonic failure. Hum Reprod Update 1998; 4: 223–36.

72. Picton H, Briggs D, Gosden R. The molecular basis of oocyte growth and development. Mol Cell Endocrinol 1998; 145: 27–37.

73. Gosden RG. Oogenesis as a foundation for embryogenesis. Mol Cell Endocrinol 2002; 186: 149–53.

74. Brunet S, Maro B. Cytoskeleton and cell cycle control during meiotic maturation of the mouse oocyte: integrating time and space. Reproduction 2005; 130: 801–11.

75. Edwards RG, Beard HK. Oocyte polarity and cell determination in early mammalian embryos. Mol Hum Reprod 1997; 3: 863–905.

76. Gardner RL. Polarity in early mammalian development. Curr Opin Genet Dev 1999; 9: 417–21.

77. Plancha CE, Sanfins A, Rodrigues P, Albertini D. Cell polarity during folliculogenesis and oogenesis. Reprod Biomed Online 2005; 10: 478–84.

78. Scott L. The biological basis of non-invasive strategies for selection of human oocytes and embryos. Hum Reprod Update 2003; 9: 237–49.

79. Scott L. Pronuclear scoring as a predictor of embryo development. Reprod Biomed Online 2003; 6: 201–14.

80. Abbott AL, Ducibella T. Calcium and the control of mammalian cortical granule exocytosis. Front Biosci 2001; 6: D792–806.

81. Cheung A, Swann K, Carroll J. The ability to generate normal Ca^{2+} transients in response to spermatozoa develops during the final stages of oocyte growth and maturation. Hum Reprod 2000; 15: 1389–95.

82. McLay DW, Clarke HJ. Remodelling the paternal chromatin at fertilization in mammals. Reproduction 2003; 125: 625–33.

83. Eppig JJ. Intercommunication between mammalian oocytes and companion somatic cells. Bioessays 1991; 13: 569–74.

84. Albertini DF, Combelles CM, Benecchi E, Carabatsos MJ. Cellular basis for paracrine regulation of ovarian follicle development. Reproduction 2001; 121: 647–53.

85. Eppig JJ. Oocyte control of ovarian follicular development and function in mammals. Reproduction 2001; 122: 829–38.

86. Tanghe S, Van Soom A, Nauwynck H et al. Minireview: functions of the cumulus oophorus during oocyte maturation, ovulation, and fertilization. Mol Reprod Dev 2002; 61: 414–24.

87. Rankin T, Soyal S, Dean J. The mouse zona pellucida: folliculogenesis, fertility and pre-implantation development. Mol Cell Endocrinol 2000; 163: 21–5.

88. Conner SJ, Lefievre L, Hughes DC, Barratt CL. Cracking the egg: increased complexity in the zona pellucida. Hum Reprod 2005; 20: 1148–52.

89. Nicolaidis P, Petersen MB. Origin and mechanisms of nondisjunction in human autosomal trisomies. Hum Reprod 1998; 13: 313–19.

90. Márquez C, Sandalinas M, Bahce M et al. Chromosome abnormalities in 1255 cleavage-stage human embryos. Reprod Biomed Online 2000; 1: 17–26.

91. Munné S. Chromosome abnormalities and their relationship to morphology and development of human embryos. Reprod Biomed Online 2006; 12: 234–53.

92. Munné S, Ary J, Zouves C et al. Wide range of chromosome abnormalities in the embryos of young egg donors. Reprod Biomed Online 2006; 12: 340–6.

93. Márquez C, Cohen J, Munné S. Chromosome identification in human oocytes and polar bodies by spectral karyotyping. Cytogenet Cell Genet 1998; 81: 254–8.

94. Kuliev A, Cieslak J, Verlinsky Y. Frequency and distribution of chromosome abnormalities in human oocytes. Cytogenet Genome Res 2005; 111: 193–8.

95. Pellestor F, Anahory T, Hamamah S. The chromosomal analysis of human oocytes. An overview of established procedures. Hum Reprod Update 2005; 11: 15–32.

96. Volarcik K, Sheean L, Goldfarb J et al. The meiotic competence of in-vitro matured human oocytes is influenced by donor age: evidence that folliculogenesis is compromised in the reproductively aged ovary. Hum Reprod 1998; 13: 154–60.

97. Fung J, Weier HU, Goldberg JD, Pedersen RA. Multilocus genetic analysis of single interphase cells by spectral imaging. Hum Genet 2000; 107: 615–22.

98. Weier HU, Weier JF, Renom MO et al. Fluorescence in situ hybridization and spectral imaging analysis of human oocytes and first polar bodies. J Histochem Cytochem 2005; 53: 269–72.

99. Wilton, L. Preimplantation genetic diagnosis and chromosome analysis of blastomeres using comparative genomic hybridization. Hum Reprod Update 2005; 11: 33–41.

100. Pellestor F, Andreo B, Anahory T, Hamamah S. The occurrence of aneuploidy in human: lessons from the cytogenetic studies of human oocytes. Eur J Med Genet 2006; 49: 103–16.

101. LeMaire-Adkins R, Radke K, Hunt PA. Lack of checkpoint control at the metaphase/anaphase transition: a mechanism of meiotic nondisjunction in mammalian females. J Cell Biol 197; 139: 1611–19.

102. Hunt PA, Hassold TJ. Sex matters in meiosis. Science 2002; 296: 2181–3.

103. Pellestor F, Anahory T, Hamamah S. Effect of maternal age on the frequency of cytogenetic abnormalities in human oocytes. Cytogenet Genome Res 2005; 111: 206–12.

104. Handel MA, Sun F. Regulation of meiotic cell divisions and determination of gamete quality: impact of reproductive toxins. Semin Reprod Med 2005; 23: 213–21.

105. Bao S, Obata Y, Carroll J et al. Epigenetic modifications necessary for normal development are established during oocyte growth in mice. Biol Reprod 2000; 62: 616–21.

106. Goto T, Jones GM, Lolatgis N et al. Identification and characterisation of known and novel transcripts expressed during the final stages of human oocyte maturation. Mol Reprod Dev 2002; 62: 13–28.

107. Pan H, O'Brien MJ, Wigglesworth K et al. Transcript profiling during mouse oocyte development and the effect of gonadotropin priming and development in vitro. Dev Biol 2005; 286: 493–506.

108. Zeng F, Schultz RM. RNA transcript profiling during zygotic gene activation in the preimplantation mouse embryo. Dev Biol 2005; 283: 40–57.

109. De La Fuente R, Viveiros MM, Burns KH et al. Major chromatin remodeling in the germinal vesicle (GV) of mammalian oocytes is dispensable for global transcriptional silencing but required for centromeric heterochromatin function. Dev Biol 2004; 275: 447–58.

110. Combelles CM, Cekleniak NA, Racowsky C, Albertini DF. Assessment of nuclear and cytoplasmic maturation in in-vitro matured human oocytes. Hum Reprod 2002; 17: 1006–16.

111. Eggert-Kruse W, Schwarz H, Rohr G et al. Sperm morphology assessment using strict criteria and male fertility under in-vivo conditions of conception. Hum Reprod 1996; 11: 139–46.

112. Keel BA. How reliable are results from the semen analysis? Fertil Steril 2004; 82: 41–4.

113. Jequier AM. Clinical andrology – still a major problem in the treatment of infertility. Hum Reprod 2004; 19: 1245–9.

114. Graves JE, Higdon HL, 3rd, Boone WR, Blackhurst DW. Developing techniques for determining sperm morphology in today's andrology laboratory. J Assist Reprod Genet 2005; 22: 219–25.

115. Weber RF, Dohle GR, Romijn JC. Clinical laboratory evaluation of male subfertility. Adv Clin Chem 2005; 40: 317–64.

116. Evenson DP, Larson KL, Jost LK. Sperm chromatin structure assay: its clinical use for detecting sperm DNA fragmentation in male infertility and comparisons with other techniques. J Androl 2002; 23: 25–43.

117. Agarwal A, Said TM. Role of sperm chromatin abnormalities and DNA damage in male infertility. Hum Reprod Update 2003; 9: 331–45.

118. Morris ID, Ilott S, Dixon L, Brison DR. The spectrum of DNA damage in human sperm assessed by single cell gel electrophoresis (Comet assay) and its relationship to fertilization and embryo development. Hum Reprod 2002; 17: 990–8.

119. Benchaib M, Braun V, Lornage J et al. Sperm DNA fragmentation decreases the pregnancy rate in an assisted reproductive technique. Hum Reprod 2003; 18: 1023–8.

120. Giwercman A, Richthoff J, Hjollund H et al. Correlation between sperm motility and sperm chromatin structure assay parameters. Fertil Steril 2003; 80: 1404–12.

121. Nasr-Esfahani MH, Salehi M, Razavi S et al. Effect of sperm DNA damage and sperm protamine deficiency on fertilization and embryo development post-ICSI. Reprod Biomed Online 2005; 11: 198–205.

122. Said T, Agarwal A, Grunewald S et al. Selection of nonapoptotic spermatozoa as a new tool for enhancing assisted reproduction outcomes: an in vitro model. Biol Reprod 2006; 74: 530–7.

123. Aitken RJ, Sawyer D. The human spermatozoon – not waving but drowning. Adv Exp Med Biol 2003; 518: 85–98.

124. Egozcue J, Blanco J, Anton E et al. Genetic analysis of sperm and implications of severe male infertility – a review. Placenta 2003; 24(Suppl B): S62–5.

125. Racowsky C, Combelles CM, Nureddin A et al. Day 3 and day 5 morphological predictors of embryo viability. Reprod Biomed Online 2003; 6: 323–31.

126. Van Soom A, Mateusen B, Leroy J, De Kruif A. Assessment of mammalian embryo quality: what can we learn from embryo morphology? Reprod Biomed Online 2003; 7: 664–70.

127. Coticchio G, Sereni E, Serrao L et al. What criteria for the definition of oocyte quality? Ann NY Acad Sci 2004; 1034: 132–44.

128. Combelles CM, Racowsky C. Assessment and optimization of oocyte quality during assisted reproductive technology treatment. Semin Reprod Med 2005; 23: 277–84.

129. Veeck LL, Wortham JW Jr, Witmyer J et al. Maturation and fertilization of morphologically immature human oocytes in a program of in vitro fertilization. Fertil Steril 1983; 39: 594–602.

130. Gregory L, Booth AD, Wells C, Walker SM. A study of the cumulus–corona cell complex in in-vitro fertilization and embryo transfer; a prognostic indicator of the failure of implantation. Hum Reprod 1994; 9: 1308–17.

131. Lin YC, Chang SY, Lan KC et al. Human oocyte maturity in vivo determines the outcome of blastocyst development in vitro. J Assist Reprod Genet 2003; 20: 506–12.

132. Enien WM, Chantler E, Seif MW, Elstein M. Human ovarian granulosa cells and follicular fluid indices: the relationship to oocyte maturity and fertilization in vitro. Hum Reprod 1988; 13: 1303–6.

133. Saith RR, Srinivasan A, Michie D, Sargent IL. Relationships between the developmental potential of human in-vitro fertilization embryos and features describing the embryo, oocyte and follicle. Hum Reprod Update 1998; 4: 121–34.

134. Van Blerkom J. Can the developmental competence of early human embryos be predicted effectively in the clinical IVF laboratory? Hum Reprod 1997; 12: 1610–14.

135. Borini A, Tallarini A, Maccolini A et al. Perifollicular vascularity monitoring and scoring: a clinical tool for selecting the best oocyte. Eur J Obstet Gynecol Reprod Biol 2004; 115(Suppl 1): S102–5.

136. De Santis L, Cino I, Rabellotti E et al. Polar body morphology and spindle imaging as predictors of oocyte quality. Reprod Biomed Online 2005; 11: 36–42.

137. Oldenbourg R. Polarized light microscopy of spindles. Methods Cell Biol 1999; 61: 175–208.

138. Keefe D, Liu L, Wang W, Silva C. Imaging meiotic spindles by polarization light microscopy: principles and applications to IVF. Reprod Biomed Online 2003; 7: 24–9.

139. Eichenlaub-Ritter U, Shen Y, Tinneberg HR. Manipulation of the oocyte: possible damage to the spindle apparatus. Reprod Biomed Online 2002; 5: 117–24.

140. Sanfins A, Lee GY, Plancha CE et al. Distinctions in meiotic spindle structure and assembly during in vitro and in vivo maturation of mouse oocytes. Biol Reprod 2003; 69: 2059–67.

141. Ibañez E, Sanfins A, Combelles CM et al. Genetic strain variations in the metaphase-II phenotype of mouse oocytes matured in vivo or in vitro. Reproduction 2005; 130: 845–55.

142. Keefe D, Tran P, Pellegrini C, Oldenbourg R. Polarized light microscopy and digital image processing identify a multilaminar structure of the hamster zona pellucida. Hum Reprod 1997; 12: 1250–2.

143. Pelletier C, Keefe DL, Trimarchi JR. Noninvasive polarized light microscopy quantitatively distinguishes the multilaminar structure of the zona pellucida of living human eggs and embryos. Fertil Steril 2004; 81(Suppl 1): 850–6.

144. Gabrielsen A, Lindenberg S, Petersen K. The impact of the zona pellucida thickness variation of human embryos on pregnancy outcome in relation to suboptimal embryo development. A prospective randomized controlled study. Hum Reprod 2001; 16: 2166–70.

145. Shen Y, Stalf T, Mehnert C et al. High magnitude of light retardation by the zona pellucida is associated with conception cycles. Hum Reprod 2005; 20: 1596–606.

146. Corcoran D, Fair T, Lonergan P. Predicting embryo quality: mRNA expression and the preimplantation embryo. Reprod Biomed Online 2005; 11: 340–8.

147. Yamagata K, Yamazaki T, Yamashita M et al. Noninvasive visualization of molecular events in the mammalian zygote. Genesis 2005; 43: 71–9.

148. Krussel JS, Huang HY, Hirchenhain J et al. Is there a place for biochemical embryonic preimplantational screening? J Reprod Fertil Suppl 2000; 55: 147–59.

149. Gardner DK, Lane M, Stevens J, Schoolcraft WB. Noninvasive assessment of human embryo nutrient consumption as a measure of developmental potential. Fertil Steril 2001; 76: 1175–80.

150. Houghton FD, Hawkhead JA, Humpherson PG et al. Noninvasive amino acid turnover predicts human embryo developmental capacity. Hum Reprod 2002; 17: 999–1005.

151. Brison DR, Houghton FD, Falconer D et al. Identification of viable embryos in IVF by non-invasive measurement of amino acid turnover. Hum Reprod 2004; 19: 2319–24.

152. Houghton FD, Leese HJ. Metabolism and developmental competence of the preimplantation embryo. Eur J Obstet Gynecol Reprod Biol 2004; 115(Suppl 1): S92–6.

153. Preis KA, Seidel G Jr, Gardner DK. Metabolic markers of developmental competence for in vitro-matured mouse oocytes. Reproduction 2005; 130: 475–83.

154. Sakkas D, Gardner DK. Noninvasive methods to assess embryo quality. Curr Opin Obstet Gynecol 2005; 17: 283–8.

155. Verlinsky Y, Cieslak J, Ivakhnenko V et al. Prevention of age-related aneuploidies by polar body testing of oocytes. J Assist Reprod Genet 1999; 16: 165–9.

156. Kuliev A, Cieslak J, Ilkevitch Y, Verlinsky Y. Chromosomal abnormalities in a series of 6,733 human oocytes in preimplantation diagnosis for age-related aneuploidies. Reprod Biomed Online 2003; 6: 54–9.

157. Shahine LK, Cedars MI. Preimplantation genetic diagnosis does not increase pregnancy rates in patients at risk for aneuploidy. Fertil Steril 2006; 85: 51–6.

158. De Placido G, Wilding M, Strina I et al. High outcome predictability after IVF using a combined score for zygote and embryo morphology and growth rate. Hum Reprod 2002; 17: 2402–9.

159. Rienzi L, Ubaldi F, Iacobelli M et al. Day 3 embryo transfer with combined evaluation at the pronuclear and cleavage stages compares favourably with day 5 blastocyst transfer. Hum Reprod 2002; 17: 1852–5.

160. Fisch JD, Sher G, Adamowicz M, Keskintepe L. The graduated embryo score predicts the outcome of assisted reproductive technologies better than a single day 3 evaluation and achieves results associated with blastocyst transfer from day 3 embryo transfer. Fertil Steril 2003; 80: 1352–8.

161. Ciray HN, Karagenc L, Ulug U et al. Early cleavage morphology affects the quality and implantation potential of day 3 embryos. Fertil Steril 2006; 85: 358–65.

162. Dumoulin JC, Meijers CJ, Bras M et al. Effect of oxygen concentration on human in-vitro fertilization and embryo culture. Hum Reprod 1999; 14: 465–9.

163. Catt JW, Henman M. Toxic effects of oxygen on human embryo development. Hum Reprod 2000; 15(Suppl 2): 199–206.

164. Bahceci M, Ciray HN, Karagenc L et al. Effect of oxygen concentration during the incubation of embryos of women undergoing ICSI and embryo transfer: a prospective randomized study. Reprod Biomed Online 2005; 11: 438–43.

165. Agarwal A, Gupta S, Sharma R. Oxidative stress and its implications in female infertility – a clinician's perspective. Reprod Biomed Online 2005; 11: 641–50.

166. Agarwal A, Gupta S, Sharma RK. Role of oxidative stress in female reproduction. Reprod Biol Endocrinol 2005; 3: 28.

167. Aitken RJ, Baker MA, Sawyer D. Oxidative stress in the male germ line and its role in the aetiology of male infertility and genetic disease. Reprod Biomed Online 2003; 7: 65–70.

168. Dirnfeld M, Bider D, Koifman M et al. Shortened exposure of oocytes to spermatozoa improves in-vitro fertilization outcome: a prospective, randomized, controlled study. Hum Reprod 1999; 14: 2562–4.

169. Lonergan P, Rizos D, Gutierrez-Adan A et al. Effect of culture environment on embryo quality and gene expression – experience from animal studies. Reprod Biomed Online 2003; 7: 657–63.

170. Mermillod P, Oussaid B, Cognie Y. Aspects of follicular and oocyte maturation that affect the developmental potential of embryos. J Reprod Fertil Suppl 1999; 54: 449–60.

171. Moor R, Dai Y. Maturation of pig oocytes in vivo and in vitro. Reprod Suppl 2001; 58: 91–104.

172. Sutton ML, Gilchrist RB, Thompson JG. Effects of in-vivo and in-vitro environments on the metabolism of the cumulus–oocyte complex and its influence on oocyte developmental capacity. Hum Reprod Update 2003; 9: 35–48.

173. Watson AJ, De Sousa P, Caveney A et al. Impact of bovine oocyte maturation media on oocyte transcript levels, blastocyst development, cell number, and apoptosis. Biol Reprod 2000; 62: 355–64.

174. Pickering SJ, Braude PR, Johnson MH et al. Transient cooling to room temperature can cause irreversible disruption of the meiotic spindle in the human oocyte. Fertil Steril 1990; 54: 102–8.

175. Ho Y, Wigglesworth K, Eppig JJ, Schultz RM. Preimplantation development of mouse embryos in KSOM: augmentation by amino acids and analysis of gene expression. Mol Reprod Dev 1995; 41: 232–8.

176. Rinaudo P, Schultz RM. Effects of embryo culture on global pattern of gene expression in preimplantation mouse embryos. Reproduction 2004; 128: 301–11.

177. Doherty AS, Mann MR, Tremblay KD et al. Differential effects of culture on imprinted H19 expression in the preimplantation mouse embryo. Biol Reprod 2000; 62: 1526–35.

178. Biggers JD. Thoughts on embryo culture conditions. Reprod Biomed Online 2002; 4(Suppl 1): 30–8.

179. Biggers JD, Racowsky C. The development of fertilized human ova to the blastocyst stage in KSOM(AA) medium: is a two-step protocol necessary? Reprod Biomed Online 2002; 5: 133–40.

180. Summers MC, Biggers JD. Chemically defined media and the culture of mammalian preimplantation embryos: historical perspective and current issues. Hum Reprod Update 2003; 9: 557–82.

181. Orasanu B, Jackson KV, Hornstein MD, Racowsky C. Effects of culture medium on hCG levels and their value in predicting successful IVF outcome. Reprod BioMed Online 2006; 12: 590–8.

182. Khosla S, Dean W, Reik W, Feil R. Culture of preimplantation embryos and its long-term effects on gene expression and phenotype. Hum Reprod Update 2001; 7: 419–27.

183. Nogueira D, Staessen C, Van de Velde H, Van Steirteghem A. Nuclear status and cytogenetics of embryos derived from in vitro-matured oocytes. Fertil Steril 2000; 74: 295–8.

184. Bean CJ, Hassold TJ, Judis L, Hunt PA. Fertilization in vitro increases non-disjunction during early cleavage divisions in a mouse model system. Hum Reprod 2002; 17: 2362–7.

185. Hiendleder S, Wirtz M, Mund C. Tissue-specific effects of in vitro fertilization procedures on genomic cytosine methylation levels in overgrown and normal sized bovine fetuses. Biol Reprod 2006; 75: 17–23.

186. Rao GD, Tan SL. In vitro maturation of oocytes. Semin Reprod Med 2005; 23: 242–7.

187. Combelles CM, Fissore RA, Albertini DF, Racowsky C. In vitro maturation of human oocytes and cumulus cells using a co-culture three-dimensional collagen gel system. Hum Reprod 2005; 20: 1349–58.

188. Baird DT, Collins J, Egozcue J et al. Fertility and ageing. Hum Reprod Update 2005; 11: 261–76.

189. Aitken RJ, Koopman P, Lewis SE. Seeds of concern. Nature 2004; 432: 48–52.

190. Hampton T. Researchers discover a range of factors undermine sperm quality, male fertility. JAMA 2005; 294: 2829–31.

191. Younglai EV, Holloway AC, Foster WG. Environmental and occupational factors affecting fertility and IVF success. Hum Reprod Update 2005; 11: 43–57.

192. Lombardo F, Sgro P, Salacone P et al. Androgens and fertility. J Endocrinol Invest 2005; 28: 51–5.

193. Klonoff-Cohen H. Female and male lifestyle habits and IVF: what is known and unknown. Hum Reprod Update 2005; 11: 179–203.

194. Pocar P, Brevini TA, Fischer B, Gandolfi F. The impact of endocrine disruptors on oocyte competence. Reproduction 2003; 125: 313–25.

195. Safe S. Endocrine disruptors and human health: is there a problem. Toxicology 2004; 205: 3–10.

196. Sharma RK, Said T, Agarwal A. Sperm DNA damage and its clinical relevance in assessing reproductive outcome. Asian J Androl 2004; 6: 139–48.

197. te Velde ER, Scheffer GJ, Dorland M et al. Developmental and endocrine aspects of normal ovarian aging. Mol Cell Endocrinol 1998; 145: 67–73.

198. Macklon NS, Fauser BC. Ovarian reserve. Semin Reprod Med 2005; 23: 248–56.

199. Blondin P, Bousquet D, Twagiramungu H et al. Manipulation of follicular development to produce developmentally competent bovine oocytes. Biol Reprod 2002; 66: 38–43.

200. Fauser BC, Bouchard P, Coelingh Bennink HJ. Alternative approaches in IVF. Hum Reprod Update 2002; 8: 1–9.

201. Racowsky C, Orasanu B, Hinrichsen MJ, Ginsburg ES. Embryo quality based on ovulation induction: defining the differences. Reprod Biomed Online 2005; 11: 22–5.

202. Hodges CA, Ilagan A, Jennings D et al. Experimental evidence that changes in oocyte growth influence meiotic chromosome segregation. Hum Reprod 2002; 17: 1171–80.

203. Matzuk MM, Lamb DJ. Genetic dissection of mammalian fertility pathways. Nat Cell Biol 2002; 4(Suppl): s41–9.

204. Shah K, Sivapalan G, Gibbons N et al. The genetic basis of infertility. Reproduction 2003; 126: 13–25.

205. Roy A, Matzuk MM. Deconstructing mammalian reproduction: using knockouts to define fertility pathways. Reproduction 2006; 131: 207–19.

206. Diemer T, Desjardins C. Developmental and genetic disorders in spermatogenesis. Hum Reprod Update 1999; 5: 120–40.

207. Reijo R, Alagappan RK, Patrizio P, Page DC. Severe oligozoospermia resulting from deletions of azoospermia factor gene on Y chromosome. Lancet 1996; 347: 1290–3.

208. Vogt PH, Edelmann A, Kirsch S et al. Human Y chromosome azoospermia factors (AZF) mapped to different subregions in Yq11. Hum Mol Genet 1996; 5: 933–43.

209. Vogt PH. Azoospermia factor (AZF) in Yq11: towards a molecular understanding of its function for human male fertility and spermatogenesis. Reprod Biomed Online 2005; 10: 81–93.

210. Oates RD, Silber S, Brown LG, Page DC. Clinical characterization of 42 oligospermic or azoospermic men with microdeletion of the AZFc region of the Y chromosome, and of 18 children conceived via ICSI. Hum Reprod 2002; 17: 2813–24.

211. Choi JM, Chung P, Veeck L et al. AZF microdeletions of the Y chromosome and in vitro fertilization outcome. Fertil Steril 2004; 81: 337–41.

212. Simoni M, Bakker E, Krausz C. EAA/EMQN best practice guidelines for molecular diagnosis of y-chromosomal microdeletions. State of the art 2004. Int J Androl 2004; 27: 240–9.

42 Unanswered questions and proposed solutions in assisted reproductive technologies

Jose M Navarro, Hey-Joo Kang, Glenn L Schattman, and Zev Rosenwaks

INTRODUCTION

The worldwide application and success of assisted reproductive technology (ART) has advanced our knowledge about the complex nature of the human endometrium as it prepares for implantation. Prior to the first live birth from in-vitro fertilization (IVF) in 1978,[1] the efficiency of human implantation was unknown. Since that time, we have come to appreciate that many apparently 'normal' embryos do not, in fact, implant. These observations have led to intensive research directed at identifying the rate-limiting steps of implantation.

Embryo implantation is a complex process that involves dynamic interactions between the embryo and the endometrium. The induction of a receptive endometrium requires exposure to adequate temporal secretions of follicular and early secretory phase ovarian hormones. Consequent to exposure to ovarian hormones, the endometrium undergoes structural and biochemical transformations necessary to create an environment conducive to blastocyst implantation.[2]

For successful implantation to occur, the endometrium and the fertilized ovum must undergo exquisitely synchronized developmental changes. In the context of ART, failure to adequately control synchronization between the temporal events of embryo development and the proper progression of endometrial maturation may lead to implantation failure. As the molecular mechanisms controlling these changes are not yet fully elucidated, we must rely on clinical paradigms – such as the egg donation model – to define the tolerance of dyssynchrony. The list of identified factors that may be involved in endometrial implantation is constantly expanding and includes hormones, growth factors, and cell adhesion molecules, all acting in concert to make the endometrium receptive to trophoblast invasion. The average implantation rate for a day 3 embryo is approximately 15%, although in young women (younger than 34 years old)

it may be as high as 30–35%.[3] The relatively low efficiency of implantation in IVF has led to a number of studies focusing on key areas such as (1) optimal secretory phase endometrium composition, (2) the importance of endometrial thickness, and (3) the role of cytokines, integrins, and steroid receptor activity. Recognition of reliable histological and biochemical markers may enable us to improve uterine receptivity and increase implantation rates of human embryos.

THE LUTEAL PHASE DEFECT: DOES IT AFFECT IMPLANTATION SUCCESS?

Definitions and general concepts

The luteal phase defect (LPD), a condition associated with inadequate endometrial development, was initially described in 1949 by Jones et al.[4] The most direct cause of an LPD is inadequate progesterone secretion by the corpus luteum, although it can also occur if progesterone is secreted for a relatively short period (< 10 days) during the luteal phase. Rarely, an inadequate endometrial response to normal physiological levels of progesterone can also manifest as LPD.

The question of what causes luteal cells to secrete inadequate amounts of progesterone is difficult to answer. The primary steroidogenic cells of the corpus luteum are large luteal cells originating from follicular granulosa cells. These cells produce estrogens and progesterone as well as peptides which act in an autocrine and paracrine fashion. Equally important are small luteal cells derived from follicular theca cells which are responsive to luteinizing hormone (LH) pulses and also secrete estrogens and progesterone.[5] Therefore, any factors that disturb ovulatory function will influence the efficient development and luteinization of granulosa and theca cells destined to secrete progesterone, resulting in a luteal phase defect.

Inadequate pituitary LH pulsatility, inadequate follicle-stimulating hormone (FSH) stimulation in the follicular phase which typically promotes LH receptor expression on granulosa cells during the periovulatory period, or aberrant pulsatility of gonadotropin-releasing hormone (GnRH), have all been proposed as possible mechanisms which can result in LPD. Other less likely causes include decreased responsiveness of the endometrium to progesterone or elevated prolactin levels.

Whereas the underlying pathophysiology leading to LPD is complex, the endpoint seems to be a deficiency in progesterone production. This manifests in poor endometrial development that can result in either the absence of implantation or abnormal early implantation. As luteal progesterone is routinely administered following IVF procedures, any coincident progesterone insufficiency may be overcome with contemporary protocols utilizing progesterone supplementation.

Diagnosis of LPD

There are two methods used to diagnose LPD. Traditionally, two endometrial biopsies performed in consecutive cycles in the mid to late secretory phase which show a lag in histological development of greater than 2 days of that expected for the 'actual' postovulatory day (based either on an LH surge or the subsequent menstrual day) is diagnostic of LPD. The histological criteria are based upon the original study by Noyes and co-workers.[6] The second method by which to diagnose LPD is measurement of serum progesterone levels. The hallmark of normal corpus luteum function is adequate progesterone secretion within 3–4 days following the LH surge (>2.5 ng/ml). A single mid luteal progesterone measurement of <10 ng/ml is considered abnormal; however, because progesterone is secreted in a pulsatile manner a single measurement may not be representative and could lead to a false-positive diagnosis in 15% of cases.[3] The solution to this dilemma is to measure serial progesterone levels on luteal days 5, 7, and 9 following the LH surge. A single value >10 ng/ml or a sum of three values >30 ng/ml is reflective of an adequate luteal phase.[7]

Clinical issues associated with LPD

The incidence of LPD may be as high as 3–10% in the general population and in 25% of women with recurrent pregnancy failure (≥3 first trimester losses).[8] While the majority of early pregnancy losses are chromosomal in nature, in some instances the losses may be associated with poor endometrial development from a luteal phase defect. However, studies of couples with recurrent pregnancy losses who were treated with progesterone have failed to conclusively show any benefit in outcome.[9]

The question remains as to whether LPD is a valid cause of infertility and if the endometrial biopsy is a valid method to diagnose it. Serial endometrial biopsies in parous women show equivalent rates of LPD compared to the infertile population.[10] In addition, a recent study by Coutifaris et al[11] evaluated 847 female volunteers. Endometrial biopsies were performed on days 21–22 and 26–27 in fertile and non-fertile couples. Out-of-phase biopsies sampled in the mid luteal phase in fertile and non-fertile women were found in 49.4% vs 43.2% of couples, respectively. Thus, in these studies an endometrial biopsy failed to discriminate between fertile and non-fertile groups, raising the question of the usefulness of endometrial biopsies in the initial evaluation of the infertile couple.

Overcoming LPD in ART

Controlled ovarian hyperstimulation (COH) with gonadotropins is designed to effect synchronous multifollicular recruitment in an effort to harvest several mature oocytes in a single cycle. Pituitary downregulation with GnRH analogues serves to suppress endogenous FSH and LH secretion, resulting in better control of ovarian stimulation cycles. Not infrequently, these protocols are associated with a consequent short or inadequate luteal phase. One solution for replacing pituitary support of the corpora lutea in this context is to use supplemental human chorionic gonadotropin (hCG). A meta-analysis revealed improved pregnancy rates with supplemental hCG[12] but this was associated with an unacceptably high rate (>5%) of ovarian hyperstimulation syndrome (OHSS). This complication can be reduced by using progesterone for luteal support soon after oocyte retrieval. Supplemental luteal phase progesterone has been shown to increase pregnancy rates in ART cycles in several studies.[13] In a meta-analysis by Pritts and Atwood, intramuscular progesterone in oil was shown to be superior with regard to implantation and pregnancy rates when compared to vaginal progesterone.[13]

Based on the above observations, it seems that the significance of the luteal phase defect as a major cause of infertility has been brought into question. It is possible that its very definition – both by histological criteria (2 days of developmental lag) and progesterone production – may be faulty. It is our experience that a developmental lag of >4–5 days is most often associated with pregnancy losses and/or infertility.

Nevertheless, the data from ART provide compelling evidence that adequate progesterone exposure following exogenous stimulation is necessary for both early implantation and early pregnancy maintenance. Thus, adequate progesterone supplementation should be administered, such that cycles associated with either short luteal phases or inadequate progesterone production can be rescued.

ART, ENDOMETRIAL THICKNESS, AND EMBRYO IMPLANTATION

Much of our knowledge about preparing the endometrium for implantation comes from our experience with oocyte donation. Recipients of donor ova undergo programmed cycles that are designed to mimic the natural cycle. Briefly, endometrial development is accomplished by exposure to exogenous estrogens and progesterone. Estrogens can be delivered orally, intramuscularly, or by the application of estradiol patches in a controlled and monitored fashion, followed by intramuscular or intravaginal progesterone to effect endometrial secretory changes.

The first successful birth following oocyte donation was reported in 1984 in an ovarian failure patient.[14] Thousands of babies have been born with this treatment approach in the past two decades. The success of ovum donation programs highlights the importance of creating an adequate hormonal environment in preparation for implantation.

ART has provided the opportunity to study the impact of endometrial thickness on implantation and pregnancy rates. Sequential transvaginal ultrasound assessments allow the clinician to monitor follicular development as well as permit the tracking of endometrial thickness and architecture. The measurement of the endometrial lining on the day of ovulation trigger is the most common reference point from which to study its impact on IVF outcomes.

The thin endometrium

To date, there have been over 40 clinical studies addressing the question of endometrial thickness and its impact on pregnancy rates in IVF. Most agree with the clinical observation that a thin endometrial lining (<7 mm) is a negative predictive factor for pregnancy outcome.

Furthermore, a profoundly thin lining of <5 mm should be evaluated by hysterosalpingography or by saline infusion sonogram to check for evidence of intrauterine synechiae (Asherman's syndrome). Asherman's syndrome is an uncommon condition, but when diagnosed can contribute significantly to subfertility. Hysteroscopic resection of intrauterine adhesions is the treatment of choice and can improve pregnancy outcome.[15] Direct lysis of adhesions by cutting, cautery, or laser yields better results than the traditional dilatation and curettage.[16]

Upon exclusion of synechiae as a cause of a thin endometrium and documentation of normal hormonal responsiveness of the endometrium on biopsy, several approaches can be applied to enhance endometrial thickness. Options include vaginal/oral estrogen supplementation or vaginal/oral sildenafil 25–50 mg every other day in the follicular phase. Sildenafil (Viagra) is a type 5-phosphodiesterase inhibitor that augments the vasodilatory effects of nitric oxide on vascular smooth muscle by preventing the degradation of cyclic guanyl monophosphate.[17] Despite the fact that both treatment modalities have shown improvements in endometrial thickness, the efficacy of either method in improving pregnancy rates has not been established.[16–17]

Most studies in ART patients have supported the finding that pregnancy is less likely to occur in cycles associated with an endometrial thickness of <7–8 mm.[18] Although attempts to improve a thin endometrium should always be made, the patient should be reassured that a thin endometrium does not preclude the establishment of a successful pregnancy. In fact, there have been several reports of pregnancies occurring when endometrial thickness was <5 mm. In a study reported in 1995 endometrial thickness was prospectively evaluated the endometrial thickness in 516 IVF cycles with embryo transfer.[20] In this series, 12 patients had an endometrial thickness of 6 mm, among which the clinical and ongoing pregnancy rates were 30% and 20%, respectively. This finding supports the hypothesis that pregnancy rates following ART procedures are influenced only marginally by the degree of endometrial thickness. Therefore, the finding of a thin endometrium should hardly ever be used as the sole reason for cycle cancellation.

The thick endometrium

The endometrium proliferates in response to rising estrogen levels from the maturing follicle.[5] In ART, the simultaneous recruitment of multiple follicles produces supraphysiological estrogen levels. This can potentially lead to the development of an endometrial lining that is greater than one would achieve in a natural cycle. Assuming that any intrauterine pathology such as an endometrial polyp or myoma has been eliminated in the initial evaluation of the infertile couple, this begs the question of whether there exists an upper limit of endometrial thickness necessary for implantation success.

A lining that measures > 14 mm is generally considered to be a thick endometrium. Although there have been two small studies reporting adverse pregnancy outcomes in ART cycles associated with thick endometrial linings,[20–21] the majority of clinical trials have found that having an excessively thick endometrial lining has no impact on ART success.[13] There is also little evidence to support any particular advantage when the endometrium is > 14 mm in thickness.

The architecture of an endometrial lining is also of significance. As the endometrial cavity is a potential space, the classic trilaminar appearance by ultrasound reflects the outer borders of the endometrium, with the sonolucent center line representing the apposition of the anterior and posterior walls. The absence of this trilaminar pattern in the follicular phase should alert the physician to the possibility of premature progesterone exposure or intrauterine pathology.

In conclusion, there appears to be no absolute endometrial thickness which precludes implantation; the decision to proceed with artificial insemination or embryo transfer should not be exclusively based on the measured endometrial thickness. Rather, the decision to proceed should be individualized to the patient's clinical history, response to treatment, and likelihood of treatment success.

Non-invasive methods to evaluate the endometrium

Two-dimensional (2D) ultrasound has proven its utility in gynecology. It has become the most widely accepted modality to evaluate the female reproductive system. 2D ultrasound permits the clinician to detect the presence of intrauterine pathology as well as the thickness and architecture of the endometrium. However, the accuracy of 2D vaginal ultrasound in endometrial assessment is observer- and technique-dependent, and there are many confounding factors which may contribute to the inter-observer variability.

Three-dimensional (3D) ultrasound measurement of endometrial volume appears to be a promising technique. Complete endometrial volume estimation has been suggested to improve the sensitivity, specificity, and reproducibility compared with conventional 2D

endometrial evaluation. The usefulness of 3D ultrasound has been confirmed by the observed correlation between endometrial volume and implantation rates.[23] In addition, the predictive value of 3D ultrasonographic measurement of endometrial volume and/or thickness may prove to be better than the value of 2D measurements,[24] although this finding has yet to be confirmed. It has been suggested that magnetic resonance imaging (MRI) could also be a reliable endometrial measurement technique,[24] although the high cost limits its applicability for routine use.

Uterine and utero-ovarian blood flow – expressed as the pulsatility or resistance index as well as the endometrial or subendometrial blood flow distribution pattern – assessed by transvaginal color Doppler have both been proposed as predictors of implantation success.[25] However, the cost-effectiveness of these methods, as well as the confirmation of their predictive value, must be established before they can be generally applied in clinical practice.

STEROID RECEPTORS AND PHARMACOLOGY IN ART

Clomiphene citrate

Clomiphene citrate (CC) is a non-steroidal compound structurally similar to tamoxifen and diethylstilbestrol. It is a mixed estrogen agonist/antagonist that can bind to the nuclear estrogen receptor (ER) for long periods of time, thereby inhibiting the process of ER replenishment. Clomiphene's action at the hypothalamus results in a perceived lower estradiol milieu, resulting in an increased GnRH pulsatility and amplitude, and thus culminating in a rise in gonadotropin release and multiple follicular development.[26]

Clomiphene citrate acts as an estrogen antagonist at the level of the endometrium and cervix in premenopausal women. The endometrium of women treated with CC is notably thinner, as evidenced by ultrasound assessment in the late follicular phase. Endometrial biopsies performed 7 days after ovulation in regularly cycling women followed by CC-treated cycles have shown a notable decrease in the density of glandular cells in the CC-treated samples. There is also a concomitant increase in the number of vacuolated cells.[26] Studies have also suggested a decrease in ER expression during the late follicular phase in CC-treated cycles. The addition of human menopausal gonadotropin (hMG) to CC treatment can restore endometrial histology,[27,28] an effect attributed to higher levels of estradiol resulting from hMG ovarian stimulation compared with CC alone. Clomiphene citrate also decreases the quality of cervical mucus, an effect largely overcome by intrauterine insemination.

Gonadotropins

The endometrium in ART is an endocrinologically altered environment due to the effect of gonadotropin therapy causing supraphysiologic hormone levels. Studies comparing the endometrium following exposure to exogenous gonadotropins with natural cycles have shown premature secretory changes in the postovulatory and early luteal phase, followed by dyssynchronous glandular and stromal differentiation in the mid luteal phase. A modified endometrial steroid receptor regulation and premature expression of pinopodes and integrins are in line with the observation of precocious luteal transformation following ovarian stimulation, although its clinical relevance is unclear.[29]

There is a potentially adverse effect of supraphysiological estradiol (E_2) levels on the endometrium. It has been proposed that high estrogen levels may inhibit embryo implantation during COH. Although some studies have not found any adverse effect of estradiol on endometrial receptivity, others have reported decreased implantation rates when the endometrium was exposed to supraphysiological levels of estradiol.[28–29] The high rates of embryo implantation in donor oocyte recipients supports the theory that altered endometrial receptivity in IVF-stimulated cycles may affect embryo implantation, as estradiol levels in donor oocyte recipients are similar to natural cycles. To this end, Levi et al[30] studied endometrial receptivity and embryo implantation by comparing IVF patients with supraphysiological E_2 levels with oocyte donor recipients. Both groups were similar with regards to stimulation protocol, ovarian responses, embryo quality, and the number of embyos transferred. In this study, controlled ovarian stimulation did not affect endometrial receptivity or the probability of pregnancy.

The impact of elevated estradiol levels on IVF implantation efficiency is controversial. Several clinical trials and meta-analyses have compared various ART protocols utilizing hMG, urinary FSH (uFSH), or recombinant FSH (rFSH). Compelling evidence for the superiority of any one of the gonadotropin preparations currently in use is lacking.[29–32] In some studies, IVF stimulation protocols using the step-down approach improved pregnancy rates.[33] The authors implied that such protocols, by virtue of their 'lower'

estradiol levels, may lead to improved implantation efficiency. However, it is difficult to determine whether their results were secondary to improved oocyte quality or endometrial receptivity. In addition to secretory changes, ovarian stimulation for IVF alters receptor kinetics in the follicular phase. Prolongation of the follicular phase is associated with a decreased probability of pregnancy because of advanced secretory changes in the endometrium.[34]

Endometrial biopsies of donors present a unique opportunity to study steroid receptor expression in the secretory phase following gonadotropin administration and how this may relate to implantation. In the natural cycle of fertile women, immunohistochemical studies for steroid receptors show the tissue stains similarly for ERs and progesterone receptors (PRs) in the late proliferative phase until the time of ovulation, when there is an abrupt decline in stromal ER staining. However, in COH donor cycles there is a decline in ER staining, beginning 2 days earlier than in natural cycles. The same pattern exists with PR, where immunohistochemical staining declines in the late secretory phase of COH cycles 2 days earlier than in the natural cycle.[34]

The clinical relevance of endometrial advancement caused by COH is evidenced by autologous frozen embryo cycles. In an effort to decrease the risk of multiple gestations, excess embryos produced in a fresh IVF cycle may be cryopreserved for use in a future cycle. When thawed day 6 blastocysts are transferred on an endometrial cycle day equivalent to day 5 after ovulation, pregnancy rates are higher than transfer of a day 6 embryo 1 day later.[35,36] This evidence supports the notion that if the embryo is transferred following closure of the implantation window, pregnancy is less likely to occur.

In summary, it is widely accepted that COH advances endometrial maturation compared to the natural cycle. This effect is probably the result of higher estrogen and progesterone levels reached earlier in COH cycles compared to the serum levels found in naturally cycling women. Earlier and higher progesterone concentrations in COH cycles may result in advancement of endometrial maturation – an earlier closure of the implantation window.[37] This highlights the significance of embryo–endometrial synchrony and the critical importance of performing embryo transfers during the brief period of endometrial receptivity.

STEROID RECEPTORS

The progesterone receptors expressed in the human endometrium exist in two forms, progesterone receptor

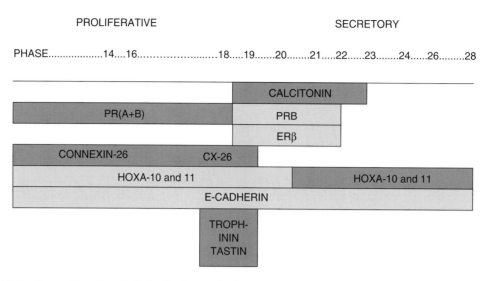

Figure 42.1   Molecular profile of epithelial cells during the human menstrual cycle.

A (PR-A) and progesterone receptor B (PR-B). These steroid receptors show maximal expression at ovulation, with a gradual decrease during the first half of the luteal phase and becoming barely detectable after day 20 of the menstrual cycle.[38] Although progesterone regulates many of the genes responsible for implantation, the virtual absence of PR in endometrial epithelial cells has proven difficult to explain. Recently, the two isoforms were shown to be co-expressed in epithelial cells at highly variable levels during the cycle and on different cell types. During the first half of the luteal phase, expression of both PR-A and PR-B decreases. In the middle of the luteal phase, the expression of PR-B becomes predominant in the vast majority of epithelial cells, a phenomenon that coincides with the second estradiol peak. At the end of the luteal phase, global PR expression is extremely low, but background PR-B staining is still visible.[39] PR-B is by far the stronger transcription activator of the two isoforms and is probably responsible for the regulation of global gene expression. The PR-A/PR-B ratio in each cell is the determinant of its final effect on the endometrium.

There are also two estrogen receptor isoforms, ERα and ERβ, and both are expressed in the human endometrium. They structurally differ in that ERα receptor contains a transcription activator function (TAF-1) in the regulatory domain that can activate gene transcription independent of hormone binding. The ERα isoform is the predominant isoform during the entire menstrual cycle, while ERβ is expressed mostly in the glandular epithelium at the time of implantation. Each endometrial cell can potentially express the four receptor isoforms: these vary in amounts during the cycle and also interact and share co-activators/co-repressors within the same cell.[40] The molecular profile of epithelial cells during the human menstrual cycle is summarized in Figure 42.1.

Pinopode formation in ART

At the time of implantation, the apical membrane of the epithelial cells lining the uterine cavity lose their microvilli and develop large and smooth membrane projections.[41] Due to their pinocytotic function, these projections were named pinopodes. In an idealized 28-day cycle, the pinopodes appear on day 20 of the menstrual cycle in humans and have been proposed to mark the opening of the implantation window. This dramatic morphological transformation of the surface epithelial apical membranes is known to have a relatively brief life span. It does not exceed 48 hours in the human menstrual cycle and is fully developed for only 24 hours. Their appearance is under the control of progesterone and can vary for up to 3 days in the human menstrual cycle.[42]

During IVF stimulation, the temporal appearance of pinopodes demonstrates greater variation compared to that of natural cycles. Endometrial biopsies of ovum donors following COH using a scanning electron microscope demonstrate the presence of pinopodes as early as cycle day 18 and extending to cycle day 22, compared to non-stimulated controls where pinopode expression is observed on cycle days 20–22.[20] Since most studies suggest that the window of transfer for 3-day-old embryos is between days 17 and 19, considering that another 2–3 days of intrauterine growth is necessary to reach the blastocyst stage, one can extrapolate that the window of implantation for blastocysts is day 21 or 22. However, most of these data are purely descriptive and the functional significance of this model in the human is still highly speculative.

Observations of pinopode expression in women who receive donor oocytes are in agreement with our current understanding of the window of implantation. With uniform and controlled estrogen and progesterone replacement designed to mimic the natural cycle, the transfer of 3-day-old embryos between cycle days 16–19 optimized implantation and pregnancy rates.[43] Embryo transfer performed prior to cycle day 16 or beyond cycle day 20 failed to achieve a pregnancy. Given that the time period of endometrial receptivity is narrow, the embryo must be in place during this critical period of receptivity for successful implantation to occur.

DETERMINANTS OF ENDOMETRIAL RECEPTIVITY

The sex steroids (estrogen and progesterone) are critical for both the proliferation and differentiation of the endometrium, such that it can undergo its specialized functions which facilitate implantation. As the endometrium prepares for implantation, the glands exhibit subnuclear vacuoles that migrate toward the luminal surface, resulting in functional secretory glands. As the glands and spiral arterioles progressively become more tortuous, the stroma becomes increasingly edematous and decidualization – the differentiation of the fibroblast-like stromal cells into large polypoid decidual cells destined to form the maternal component of the placenta – occurs. The concomitant increase in vascular permeability also allows the infiltration of inflammatory cells and cytokines. This coordinated series of events culminates in the creation of a receptive endometrium with a 'window of implantation' presumed to occur between cycle days 19 and 21.[41–43] Although the importance of estrogen and progesterone in creating this receptive state is undisputed, they must act through various transcription factors, steroid receptors, cytokines, and cofactors to achieve endometrial cell differentiation.

Homeobox gene

Homeobox genes were first identified in *Drosophila melanogaster* and have subsequently been identified in many other species. A particular subgroup of homeobox genes in humans is called the HOX genes. These are four special clusters of genes located on chromosomes 2, 7, 12, and 17. Each HOX gene contains a highly conserved 183 base pair sequence known as the homeobox that encodes a 61 amino acid domain. This 61 amino acid domain is referred to as the homeodomain and acts as a transcriptional regulator by binding to DNA at the promoter region of a target gene.[44]

The HOX genes are responsible for the differentiation of the Müllerian ducts. The location of each HOX gene, starting at the 3' position, determines which Müllerian structure is formed at the most anterior position in the body. For instance, HOXA-9 is located at the 3' end and is expressed in areas destined to become the Fallopian tube, whereas HOXA-10 is expressed in the developing uterus, HOXA-11 in the lower uterine segment, and HOXA-13 (located closest to the 5' end) is expressed in the upper vagina. Following the completion of embryogenesis, most tissues do not continue to express HOX genes; however, the endometrium is one of the few tissues in the adult that does.

Evidence supporting the importance of HOX genes in implantation comes from experiments showing complete failure of implantation in mice with homologous mutations in either the Hoxa-10 or Hoxa-11 gene. When embryos from the Hoxa-deficient mice were transferred into wild-type mice, implantation was successful.[46] Several molecular defects have also been identified in the endometrium of these HOXA-10 null mice. For instance, the endometrial response to sex steroids is abnormal[49] and a similar infertile phenotype was observed in the HOXA-11 knockout mice.[50]

These results have prompted researchers to study the expression of these two genes in the adult human endometrium. They are expressed in the surface epithelium and in the stromal cells in a cyclic manner. HOXA-10 predominates in the epithelial cells, while HOXA-11 is mostly expressed in the stroma.[51] Expression is low in the follicular and early luteal phases, but rises to maximum during the mid luteal phase, persisting until menstruation; both estradiol and progesterone have been shown to up-regulate the expression of both Hoxa-10 and Hoxa-11.[49]

The HOX genes are essential determinants of uterine embryogenesis, menstrual remodeling, and implantation success. They appear to control the remodeling and proper differentiation of the endometrial lining during each menstrual cycle and pregnancy (Table 42.1). The target genes of these HOX clusters have not yet been identified, but it is interesting to note that the promoter regions of genes for some adhesion molecules contain sequences capable of binding to the homeodomain.[52] HOX genes also govern uterine morphogenesis, finely

Table 42.1   Expression of the Hoxa/HOXA genes in the genital tract

Organ	Rodent embryo	Adult mouse	Adult human
Fallopian tubes	HOXA 9, 10, 11, 13	9	9
Uterus	HOXA 9, 10, 11, 13	10,11	10,11
Cervix	HOXA 9, 10, 11, 13	11,13	11,13
Vagina	HOXA 9, 10, 11, 13	13	13

Adapted from ref 74.

determining tissue identity in space and function. Many groups have compared the epithelial morphological changes observed during the receptivity acquisition to the epithelial–mesenchymal transformation described during embryogenesis.[52] It is also interesting to note that mice deficient in HOXA-11 gene have greatly diminished levels of leukemia inhibitory factor (LIF).[53] Although much has been discovered about the HOX genes and their important role in endometrial differentiation, the full extent of their role in endometrial receptivity and implantation has yet to be elucidated.

Proteins involved in endometrial receptivity

Cytokines

Cytokines are multifunctional glycoproteins that mediate intercellular communication by binding to specific receptors on the surface of target cells. They were originally thought to be produced exclusively by the hematopoietic system, but it is now known that cytokines are produced by and act upon other cell types and tissues. In the uterus, colony-stimulating factor-1 (CSF-1) was the first cytokine identified as being a product of uterine epithelial cells rather than invading leukocytes.[54] It is now known that several cytokines are produced by endometrial stromal, epithelial, and decidual cells. There is significant redundancy in the actions of cytokines, with several different cytokines exerting overlapping functions. This makes it difficult to identify individual cytokines that may be crucial for successful implantation, and whose production is affected by the hormonal manipulation of ART.

The sex steroids induce the expression of cytokines interleukin-1 (IL-1) and LIF. These are two of the many cytokines considered part of the apposition and adhesion steps of blastocyst implantation. LIF was originally discovered to induce macrophage differentiation of the myeloid leukemic cell line M1. In the endometrium, it has demonstrated effects on proliferation, differentiation, and cell survival, which are all essential to blastocyst implantation and survival. LIF is a cytokine expressed in the uterine endometrial glands on cycle days 18–28 in the postovulatory phase of a 28-day cycle.[55] The expression of LIF appears to be under maternal control as its expression is paralleled in pseudopregnant mice. Further evidence to support the maternal control of LIF expression rather than blastocyst control is that peak expression of LIF mirrors peak estradiol concentration and always precedes implantation of the blastocyst.[56]

The importance of LIF is evidenced by murine experiments where females lacking a functional LIF gene are fertile but their blastocysts fail to implant. However, the same blastocysts from LIF-deficient mice are viable when transferred to a wild-type recipient.[55] Subsequent studies suggesting the importance of LIF in implantation success have led to commercially available supplementation of this and other cytokines in ART media. However, there have not been controlled studies showing any improvement in ART success, perhaps because LIF acts in both an autocrine and paracrine manner to exert local effects.

There are several other cytokines expressed by endometrial cells and their surrounding lymphocytes during the peri-implantation period. Interleukin-11 (IL-11) is a growth factor with pleiotropic actions. IL-11 mRNA is maximal in the pregnant uterus at the time of decidualization, and mice lacking IL-11 receptors have impaired fertility with smaller litter sizes.[57] The importance of IL-1 is more controversial, but in-vitro studies reveal that IL-1 is detected in embryo culture conditions only in the presence of endometrial cofactors. CSF-1 is a glycoprotein that modulates proliferation, differentiation, and survival, with markedly increased expression in the luminal and glandular epithelium during pregnancy.[56] A detailed description of all cytokines expressed in the peri-implantation period is beyond the scope of this chapter; however, the importance of cytokines in successful blastocyst implantation should be underscored.

Integrins

Integrins are a class of cell adhesion molecules that interact with extracellular matrix ligands, matrix metalloproteinases (MMPs), and other cell adhesion molecules to exert their physiological effect. Beyond their known function of cell-to-cell adhesion and as receptors for various ligands involved in implantation, their detailed role is not currently known. More than 20 heterodimers have been identified to date. Many have been found to have roles in the landmark events of reproduction, from fertilization to birth.[58] In the endometrium, some integrins are constitutively expressed while others are steroid-regulated and thus vary during the menstrual cycle.

The most studied integrin is $\alpha_v\beta_3$, which is found on the apical epithelial surface of both the luminal endometrium and the embryo during the window of implantation. The ligand of the $\alpha_v\beta_3$ integrin is osteoponin, and the function of this receptor–ligand product is to facilitate attachment of the embryo to the apical surface of the epithelium prior to invasion. The expression of the $\alpha_v\beta_3$ integrin, together with pinopode formation, is considered by many to be the hallmark for the brief period of endometrial receptivity.

Trophinin, tastin, and bystin

The identification of these three molecules has been a very interesting development in implantation physiology. Their isolation resulted from the systematic screening of a cDNA library that searched for molecules able to confer an adhesive phenotype to human endometrial and trophoblastic cells. Trophinin resembles an adhesion molecule with a large membrane domain exposed to the extracellular milieu and a cytoplasmic domain containing phosphorylation sites. Tastin is a completely intracellular molecule interacting with trophinin to produce an adhesive phenotype to the endometrial epithelial cells. When they are incorporated together into the cell, the trophinin molecules cluster in multivalent adhesion sites at the membrane surface. When incorporated alone, the trophinin molecules are scattered all along the cell membrane and tastin molecules show a diffuse distribution in the cytoplasm.[59]

Trophinin and tastin have been isolated in the human endometrial cells between days 16 and 17 of the menstrual cycle. Trophinin, however, is not secreted into the uterine cavity until day 20 of the menstrual cycle.[60] Trophinin molecules have also been isolated in human syncytiotrophoblast, thus acting as a potential adhesion factor to the placenta.

A third molecule was identified as forming a molecular bridge between trophinin and tastin. This molecule is the human homologue of the *Drosophila* gene *bys*, named bystin. Trophinin, tastin, and bystin are expressed at the uteroplacental interface and appear at about the 6th week of pregnancy and disappear after week 10.[61,62] This model, comprising a membrane adhesion molecule and two cytoplasmic molecules, realizes the typical complex for in-and-out adhesive communication. It is very finely regulated during the

menstrual cycle to form clustered adhesion sites at the surface of the epithelial cell and has phosphorylation sites that are potentially able to transmit intracellular messages. This very sophisticated model also suggests that the integrin story in the human endometrium at the time of implantation is still incomplete, since the intracellular mechanisms associated with the appearance of these molecules are not fully understood.

Matrix metalloproteinases

After the embryo adheres to the endometrium, it must then invade the basement membrane to establish a connection to the maternal circulation. Matrix metalloproteinases are a group of proteolytic enzymes that degrade the basement membrane and the extracellular matrix. Through this mechanism, MMPs facilitate trophoblast invasion of the endometrium.[63] The MMPs are regulated locally by tissue inhibitors of metalloproteinases (TIMPs)[64] to limit the degree of trophoblastic invasion.

The cell-polarity/adhesive-phenotype model

Epithelial cells in the endometrium are typically polarized in the manner of a simple epithelium. The cells are cylindrically shaped with basal nucleus and apical organelles. Microvilli are located at the apex, tight and gap junctions are distributed at the apicolateral side of the membrane, adherens junctions are distributed at the basolateral side of the cell, and actin filaments are located along the lateral walls. With the acquisition of an adhesive phenotype coinciding with the appearance of the pinopodes, the morphology and polarity of the cells change dramatically. The epithelial cell typically becomes round, the tight junctions disappear, the molecular complexes forming the adherens junctions are dissociated, and the actin filaments are diffusely distributed in the cell. These morphological and cellular changes resemble the malignant transformation of epithelial cells. Therefore, the genes determining the malignant transformation of an epithelial cell could very well be essential for the acquisition of endometrial receptivity. For example, the apoptosis gene Bcl-2 is expressed in a cyclical manner in human endometrium, suggesting a hormonal regulation in secretory endometrial remodeling.[65]

IMPROVING ENDOMETRIAL RECEPTIVITY

Failure to conceive with IVF has been attributed in some cases to poor endometrial development. Endometrial growth is thought to depend on uterine artery blood flow. Nitric oxide relaxes vascular smooth muscle through a cGMP-mediated pathway and nitric oxide isoforms have been identified in the uterus. Sildenafil citrate, a type 5-specific phosphodiesterase inhibitor, augments the vasodilatory effects of nitric oxide by preventing the degradation of cGMP. However, reports of pregnancy rates in women with a history of poor endometrial development treated with sildefanil citrate have been mixed.

A preliminary report showed that the combination of sildenafil citrate and estradiol valerate improved blood flow and endometrial thickness in all patients studied.[66] In addition, the effect of vaginally administered sildenafil has been evaluated in a retrospective cohort analysis of infertile women with poor endometrial development.[67,68] Vaginal administration of sildenafil citrate enhanced endometrial development in 70% of the patients studied, and high implantation and ongoing pregnancy rates were achieved in a cohort with a poor prognosis for success. Lastly, Check et al[68] studied women failing to attain an 8 mm endometrial thickness treated with sildenafil or vaginal estradiol therapy. In this cohort, neither sildenafil nor vaginal estradiol improved endometrial thickness.

Estradiol supplementation at different doses from the early proliferative phase to the late secretory phase has been proposed to improve the chances of conception.[69] It has also been suggested that the transdermal administration of estradiol with ovarian stimulation could improve the endometrial development; however, evidence that these improve endometrial development (thickness and pattern) have been inconsistent.[69,70]

Success after IVF is dependent upon many factors, many of which depend not only on the patient but also on the skills of the treating physician.[72] The embryo transfer technique is the final 'physician-guided' step in IVF. After transfer, success of IVF relies on the ability of the embryo to develop and implant. Variables such as the presence of hydrosalpinges, age, or uterine anomalies will independently affect the chance for conception with IVF. Consistent criteria for grading embryo transfers are lacking.

Additional variables that may be assessed include transfer catheter type, difficulty of transfer, presence of mucus and/or blood, and retained embryos. Recently, a systematic review and meta-analysis showed that using a soft embryo catheter for embryo transfer resulted in a significantly higher pregnancy rate compared to stiff catheters.[72] They suggested that better implantation rates are due to less trauma caused to the endometrium by the soft catheter. Conversely, there have been several groups that have explored the possibility that local injury of the endometrium increases the incidence of implantation. In a prospective study of 134 IVF patients, embryo transfer was preceded by repeated endometrial biopsies resulting in a doubling of the live birth rate.[74]

CONCLUSION

Assisted reproductive technologies have allowed a more precise study of the embryo–endometrium interaction during the window of implantation. The development and differentiation of the endometrium is closely regulated by complex mechanisms, many of which are not yet fully understood. The importance of evolving concepts such as homeobox genes, adhesion molecules, cytokines, and steroid receptor function highlight the multifaceted nature of implantation.

The individual roles the endometrium and the embryo play with regard to implantation remain controversial. There is increasing doubt about the clinical value of assessing the receptiveness of the endometrium with a single marker, as the development and differentiation of the endometrium are closely regulated by complex mechanisms that are not well understood. The clinician's task should therefore be to focus on improving follicular stimulation and embryo culture conditions as well as the uterine environment. The cost and difficulty in studying embryo implantation in primates have limited clinical experiments primarily to the rodent model. Extrapolation to the human must be made with caution, as many differences exist between the two species.

Ideally, if a universal, non-invasive secretory marker of endometrial receptivity could be identified this would enhance the clinician's ability to both evaluate and optimize the endometrial environment. Analysis of endometrial protein expression patterns obtained from uterine flushings may offer a relatively non-invasive means of assessing endometrial receptivity during fertility treatment cycles. Future directions aimed at improving endometrial receptivity include analysis of comparative genomic hybridization in blastocysts and endometrial cells as well as the search for genetic determinants of endometrial receptivity.

REFERENCES

1. Steptoe PC, Edwards RG. Birth after the reimplantation of a human embryo. Lancet 1976; 2(8085): 366.
2. Psychoyos A. Uterine receptivity for nidation. Ann NY Acad Sci 1986; 476: 36–42.
3. Spandorfer SD, Chung PH, Kligman I et al. An analysis of the effect of age on implantation rates. J Assist Reprod Genet 2000; 17: 303–6.

4. Jones GES. Some newer aspects of the mangement of infertility. JAMA 1949; 141: 1123–9.

5. Bukulmez O, Arici A. Luteal phase defect: myth or reality. Obstet Gynecol Clin North Am 2004; 31: 727–44.

6. Noyes RW, Hertig MD, Rock MD. Dating of the endometrial biopsy. Fertil Steril 1950; 1: 3–25.

7. Speroff L, Fritz MC. Assisted reproductive technologies. Clinical Gynecologic Endocrinology and Infertility, 6 edn. Baltimore: Lippincott, Williams & Wilkins, 2005: 1013–15.

8. Ginsberg KA. Luteal phase defect. Etiology, diagnosis, and management. Endocrinol Metab Clin North Am 1992; 21(1): 85–104.

9. Coulam CB, Stern JJ. Endocrine factors associated with recurrent spontaneous abortion. Clin Obstet Gynecol 1994; 37: 730–44.

10. Davis OK, Berkeley AS, Naus GJ. The incidence of luteal phase defect in normal, fertile women, determined by serial endometrial biopsies. Fertil Steril 1989; 51: 582–6.

11. Coutifaris C, Myers E, Guzick D et al. Histologic dating of timed endometrial biopsy tissue is not related to fertility status. Fertil Steril 2004; 82: 1264–72.

12. Soliman S, Daya S, Collins J, Hughes EG. The role of luteal phase support in infertility treatment: a meta-analysis of randomized trials. Fertil Steril 1994; 61: 1068–76.

13. Pritts EA, Atwood AK. Luteal phase support in infertility treatment: a meta-analysis of the randomized trials. Hum Reprod 2002; 17(9): 2287–99.

14. Lutjen P, Trounson A, Leeton J et al. The establishment and maintenance of pregnancy using in-vitro fertilization and embryo donation in a patient with primary ovarian failure. Nature 1984; 307: 174–5.

15. Valle RF, Sciarra JJ. Intrauterine adhesions: hysteroscopic diagnosis, classification, treatment, and reproductive outcome. Am J Obstet Gynecol 1988; 158: 1459–70.

16. Fanchin R, Righini C, Schonauer LM et al. Vaginal versus oral E_2 administration: effects on endometrial thickness, uterine perfusion, and contractility. Fertil Steril 2001; 76: 994–8.

17. Palmer MJ, Bell AS, Fox DN et al. Design of second generation phosphodiesterase 5 inhibitors. Curr Top Med Chem 2007; 7(4): 433–54.

18. Richter K, Bugge K, Bromer J. Relationship between endometrial thickness and embryo implantation, based on 1,294 cycles of in vitro fertilization with transfer of two blastocyst-stage embryos. Fertil Steril 2007; 87(1): 53–9.

19. Noyes N, Liu HC, Sultan K et al. Endometrial thickness appears to be a significant factor in embryo implantation in in-vitro fertilization. Hum Reprod 1995; 10: 919–22.

20. Dickey RP, Olar TT, Curole DN et al. Endometrial pattern and thickness associated with pregnancy outcome after assisted reproduction technologies. Hum Reprod 1992; 7: 418–21.

21. Rinaldi L, Lisi F, Floccari A et al. Endometrial thickness as a predictor of pregnancy after in vitro fertilization but not after intracytoplasmic sperm injection. Hum Reprod 1996; 11: 1538–41.

22. Raga F, Bonilla-Musoles F, Casan EM et al. Assessment of endometrial volume by three-dimensional ultrasound prior to embryo transfer: clues to endometrial receptivity. Hum Reprod 1999; 14: 2851–4.

23. Yaman C, Ebner T, Sommergruber M, et al. Role of three-dimensional ultrasonographic measurement of endometrium volume as a predictor of pregnancy outcome in an IVF-ET program: a preliminary study. Fertil Steril 2000, 74: 797–801.

24. Turnbull LW, Rice CF, Horsman A et al. Magnetic resonance imaging and transvaginal ultrasound of the uterus prior to embryo transfer. Hum Reprod 1994; 9: 2438–43.

25. Maugey-Laulom B, Commenges-Ducos M, Jullien V et al. Endometrial vascularity and ongoing pregnancy after IVF. Eur J Obstet Gynecol Reprod Biol 2002; 04: 137–43.

26. Sereepapong W, Suwajanakorn S, Triratanachat S et al. Effect of clomiphene citrate on the endometrium of regularly cycling women. Fertil Steril 2000; 73(2): 287–91.

27. Graf MJ, Reyniak JV, Battle-Mutter P. Histologic evaluation of the luteal phase in women following follicle aspiration for oocyte retrieval. Fertil Steril 1988; 49: 616.

28. Bourgain C, Devroey P. The endometrium in stimulated cycles for IVF. Hum Reprod Update 2003; 9(6): 512–22.

29. Levi AJ, Drews MR, Bergh PA et al. Controlled ovarian hyperstimulation does not adversely affect endometrial receptivity in in vitro fertilization cycles. Fertil Steril 2001; 76: 640–4.

30. Collins JL. A turbulent arena. Fertil Steril 2003; 80: 1117.

31. van Wely M, Westergaard LG, Bossuyt PM, van der Veen F. Human menopausal gonadotropin and recombinant follicle-stimulating hormone for controlled ovarian hyperstimulation in assisted reproductive cycles: a meta-analysis. Fertil Steril 2003; 80: 1121.

32. Simon C, Cano, Valbuena D et al. Clinical evidence for a detrimental effect in uterine receptivity of high serum oestradiol concentrations in high and normal responder patients. Hum Reprod 1995; 10: 2432–7.

33. Kolibianakis EM. Optimizing ovarian stimulation for IVF using GnRH antagonists. J Gynecol Obstet Biol Reprod 2004; 33: 3S42–5.

34. Develioglu O, Hsiu J, Nikas G et al. Endometrial estrogen and progesterone receptor and pinopode expression in stimulated cycles of donor oocytes. Fertil Steril 1999; 71: 1040–7.

35. Veeck L, Bodine R, Clarke R. High pregnancy rates can be achieved after freezing and thawing human blastocysts. Fert Steril 2004; 82: 1418–27.

36. Shapiro BS, Daneshmand ST, Garner FC et al. Comparing day 5 and day 6 blastocyst transfers in fresh autologous, frozen autologous, and fresh oocyte donor cycles. Fertil Steril 2006; 86(S1): S6.

37. Propst AM, Hill JA, Ginsberg ES et al. A randomized study comparing Crinone 8% and intramuscular progesterone supplementation in in vitro fertilization–embryo transfer cycles. Fertil Steril 2001; 76: 1144–9.

38. Garcia E, Bouchard P, Brux JD et al. Use of immunohistochemistry of progesterone and estrogen receptors for endometrial dating. J Clin Endocrinol Metab 1988; 67: 80–7.

39. Mote PA, Balleine RL, McGowan EM, Clarke CL. Colocalization of progesterone receptors A and B by dual immunofluorescent histochemistry in human endometrium during the menstrual cycle. J Clin Endocrinol Metab 1999; 84: 2963–71.

40. Matsuzaki S, Fukaya T, Suzuki T et al. Oestrogen receptor alpha and beta mRNA expression in human endometrium throughout the menstrual cycle. Mol Hum Reprod 1999; 5: 559–64.

41. Psychoyos A, Mandon P [Study of the surface of the uterine epithelium by scanning electron microscopy. Observations in the rat at the 4th and 5th day of pregnancy. CR Acad Sci Hebd Seances Acad Sci D 1971; 272: 2723–9. [in French]

42. Nikas G, Psychoyos A. Uterine pinopodes in peri-implantation human endometrium. Clinical relevance. Ann NY Acad Sci 1997; 816: 129–42.

43. Navot D, Scott RT, Droesch K et al. The window of embryo transfer and the efficiency of human conception in vitro. Fertil Steril 1991; 55: 114–18.

44. Daftary G, Taylor H. Implantation in the human: the role of HOX genes. Semin Reprod Med 2000; 18(3): 311–20.

45. McGinnis W, Krumlauf R. Homeobox genes and axial patterning. Cell 1992; 68: 283–302.

46. Satokata I, Benson G, Maas R. Sexually dimorphic sterility phenotypes in Hoxa-10 deficient mice. Nature 1995; 374: 460–3.

47. Hsieh L, Witte DP, Weinstein M et al. Hoxa11 structure, extensive antisense transcription, and function in male and female infertility. Development 1995; 121: 1373–85.

48. Lim H, Ma L, Ma W-g et al. Hoxa-10 regulates uterine stromal cell responsiveness to progesterone during implantation and decidualization in the mouse. Mol Endocrinol 1999; 13: 1005–16.

49. Taylor HS, Igarashi P, Olive DL, Arici A. Sex steroids mediate HOXA 11 expression in the human peri-implantation endometrium. J Clin Endocrinol Metab 1999; 84: 1129–35.

50. Taylor HS, Arici A, Olive D, Igarashi P. HOXA10 is expressed in response to sex steroids at the time of implantation in the human endometrium. J Clin Invest 1998; 101: 1379–84.

51. Goomer RS, Holst BD, Wood IC et al. Regulation in vitro of L-CAM enhancer by homeobox genes HoxD9 and HNF-1. Proc Natl Acad Sci USA 1994; 91: 7985–9.

52. Denker H-W. Implantation: a cell biological paradox. J Exp Zool 1993; 266: 541–58.

53. Gendron RL, Paradis H, Hsieh-Li HM et al. Abnormal uterine stromal and glandular function associated with maternal reproductive defects in Hoxa-11 null mice. Biol Reprod 1997; 56: 1097–105.

54. Arceci RJ, Shanahan F, Stanley ER, Pollard JW. Temporal expression and location of colony-stimulating factor-1 (CSF-1) and its receptor in the female reproductive tract are consistent with CSF-1-regulated placental development. Proc Natl Acad Sci USA 1989; 86: 8818–22.

55. Stewart C, Kaspar P, Brunet L et al. Blastocyst implantation depends on maternal expression of leukaemia inhibitory factor. Nature 1992; 359: 76–9.

56. Salamonsen L, Dimitriadis E, Robb L. Cytokines in implantation. Semin Reprod Med 2000; 18: 299–310.

57. Robb L, Li R, Hartley L. Infertility in female mice lacking the receptor for interleukin 11 is due to a defective uterine response to implantation. Nat Med 1998; 4: 303–8.

58. Lessey BA, Damjanovich L, Coutifaris C et al. Integrin adhesion molecules in the human endometrium. Correlation with the normal and abnormal menstrual cycle. J Clin Invest 1992; 90: 188–95.

59. Fukuda MN, Sato T, Nakayama J et al. Trophinin and tastin, a novel cell adhesion molecule complex with potential involvement in embryo implantation. Genes Dev 1995; 9: 1199–210.

60. Suzuki N, Nakayama J, Shih I-M et al. Expression of trophinin, tastin, and bystin by trophoblast and endometrial cells in human placenta. Biol Reprod 1999; 60: 621–7.

61. Suzuki N, Zara J, Sato T et al. A cytoplasmic protein, bystin, interacts with trophinin, tastin, and cytokeratin and may be involved in trophinin-mediated cell adhesion between trophoblast and endometrial epithelial cells. Proc Nat Acad Sci USA 1998; 95: 5027–32.

62. Cross JC, Werb Z, Fisher SJ. Implantation and the placenta: key pieces of the development puzzle. Science 1994; 266(5190): 1508–18.

63. Woessner JF. Matrix metalloproteinases and their inhibitors in connective tissue remodeling. FASEB J 1991; 5(8): 2145–54.

64. Zhang J, Salamonsen LA. Tissue inhibitor of metalloproteinases (TIMP)-1, -2 and -3 in human endometrium during the menstrual cycle. Mol Hum Reprod 1997; 3(9): 735–41.

65. Gompel A, Sabourin J, Martin A et al. Bcl-2 expression in normal endometrium during the menstrual cycle. Am J Pathol 1994; 144: 1195–202.

66. Sher G, Fish JD. Vaginal sildenafil (Viagra): a preliminary report of a novel method to improve uterine artery blood flow and endometrial development in patients undergoing IVF. Hum Reprod 2000; 15: 806–9.

67. Sher G, Fish JD. Effect of vaginal sildenafil on the outcome of in vitro fertilization (IVF) after multiple IVF failures attributed to poor endometrial development. Fertil Steril 2002; 78: 1073–6.

68. Check JH, Graziano V, Lee G et al. Neither sildafenil nor vaginal estradiol improves endometrial thickness in women with thin endometria after taking estradiol in graduating doses. Clin Exp Obstet Gynecol 2004; 31: 99–102.

69. Jung H, Roth HK. The effects of E_2 supplementation from the early proliferative phase to the late secretory phase of the endometrium in HMG-stimulated IVF-ET. J Assist Reprod Genet 2000; 17: 28–33.

70. Shimoya K, Tomiyama T, Hashimoto K et al. Endometrial development was improved by transdermal estradiol in patients treated with clomiphene citrate. Gynecol Obstet Invest 1999; 47: 251–4.

71. Spandorfer SD, Goldstein J et al. Difficult embryo transfer has a negative impact on the outcome of in vitro fertilization. Fertil Steril 2003; 79: 654–5.

72. Abou-Setta AM, Al-Inany HG, Mansour RT et al. Soft versus firm embryo transfer catheters for assited reproduction: a systematic review and meta-analysis. Hum Reprod 2005; 20: 3114–21.

73. Barash A, Dekel N, Fieldust S et al. Local injury to the endometrium doubles the incidence of successful pregnancies in patients undergoing in vitro fertilization. Fertil Steril 2003; 79: 1317–22.

74. Taylor HS, Vanden Heuv el GB, Igarashi P. A conserved Hox axis in the human female reproductive system: late establishment persistent adult expression of the Hoxa cluster genes. Biol Reprod 1997; 57(6): 1338–45.

43 Clinical relevance of endometrial assessment

Aimee Seungdamrong and Peter G McGovern

Synopsis

The selective estrogen receptor modulator (SERM), clomiphene citrate (CC), has been used for decades to induce ovulation in anovulatory women desiring pregnancy and as a treatment for ovulatory women with infertility. Due to its estrogenic/anti-estrogenic effects, it has, in some women, adverse effects on endometrial thickness and pattern observed by ultrasound. Lower limits of endometrial thickness are difficult to define with regard to a "cut off" below which no pregnancy can occur. However, endometrial patterns of a trilaminar type are good predictors of endometrial development and pregnancy.

Clinical

- CC has effects on a variety of endometrial "biomarkers" of uterine receptivity, but the results have been inconclusive with regard to predictors of endometrial receptivity and pregnancy establishment and maintenance.
- In addition to CC, gonadotropins are commonly used for fertility therapy. This treatment modality results in changes in histology (advancement of the endometrium), decreased pinopodes, and changes in molecular markers of receptivity. These may contribute to the decreased implantation rates in women undergoing these therapies for infertility compared to fertile controls.
- Gonadotropin therapy increases pregnancy rates, thickens endometrium, and also decreases miscarriage rates in select populations.
- However, endometrial dyssynchrony - whether delayed or accelerated development) can occur with gonadotropin therapies and may compromise the conception potential of a given cycle.

EFFECTS OF CLOMIPHENE CITRATE ON THE ENDOMETRIUM

INTRODUCTION

Clomiphene citrate (CC) is a non-steroidal selective estrogen receptor modulator (SERM) that consists of two stereoisomers which have tissue-specific estrogen agonist and antagonist actions. It is widely used to stimulate ovulation by interfering with the estrogen negative feedback mechanism on the pituitary gland. While its antagonism of estrogen action at the level of the hypothalamus and pituitary results in elevated follicle-stimulating hormone (FSH) levels and therefore stimulates follicle development in the ovary, it also acts as an estrogen antagonist in the endometrium, where it may have negative effects upon endometrial development, receptivity to embryo implantation, and pregnancy. The potential clinical effect is an increase in pregnancy rate, but a smaller increase than that which would be predicted by the magnitude of the increase in the number of follicles which reach ovulation.[1–3] Investigators have used a variety of diagnostic methods to attempt to better study the effects of clomiphene citrate upon the endometrium, although it is important to remember that the only important outcome of interest is successful pregnancy.

INDIRECT (ULTRASOUND) ASSESSMENT OF ENDOMETRIAL CHANGES AFTER CLOMIPHENE CITRATE

One theory is that clomiphene citrate decreases the amount of endometrial proliferation compared to natural cycles, as evidenced by decreased endometrial thickness seen on transvaginal ultrasound. Studies in infertile women have often shown that CC decreases endometrial thickness when compared with spontaneous cycles. It is also decreased when compared to fertile controls.[4] This antagonism may result in fewer conceptions or an increase in very early abortions.[5] Ultrasound evaluation of the endometrium is readily accessible during routine monitoring for ovarian stimulation cycles using CC. However, the predictive value of the measurement of endometrial thickness or pattern on pregnancy outcome is still unclear.

Endometrial thickness

A large number of retrospective analyses have attempted to show that endometrial thickness is a good predictor of normal endometrial development. While many have shown that the endometrium is usually thicker in pregnant vs non-pregnant cycles, results have been inconsistent and the majority of investigators have noted that they cannot develop an endometrial thickness below which no successful pregnancies occur. Thus, there is no useful cutoff below which treatment cycles should be cancelled. It is sometimes thought that the greater the thickness of the endometrium, the better the pregnancy rate will be. Kolibianakis et al attempted to correlate endometrial thickness in clomiphene citrate cycles on the day of human chorionic gonadotropin (hCG) administration with ongoing pregnancy rates. While the number of follicles and estradiol level on the day of ovulation were significantly higher in the pregnant vs non-pregnant group, no relationship was seen between endometrial thickness and subsequent pregnancy.[6] Nakamura et al studied endometrial thickness in control vs clomiphene citrate cycles in an infertility population. Mid secretory and late luteal endometrial thickness in the clomiphene citrate cycles were thinner than in the control cycles (7.6±1.4 mm vs 8.5±1.7 mm). Furthermore, while the endometrial thickness in the control cycles correlated well with estradiol levels 1–3 days before ovulation, this relationship was not seen in the clomiphene citrate cycles.[7] This discrepancy between endometrial thickness and estrogen levels may be secondary to estrogen receptor (ER) blockage by clomiphene citrate.

Thus, while most studies note a reduced endometrial thickness after clomiphene citrate administration, the effect of this upon the most important outcome measure, pregnancy, remains unclear.

Endometrial pattern

The biochemical changes resulting in different sonographic densities and/or patterns have never been elucidated. Despite this, a trilaminar appearance of the endometrial stripe has been suggested as a better predictor of good endometrial development and pregnancy as compared to the homogeneous pattern. In a population of infertility patients, endometrial pattern was measured with transvaginal ultrasound at two time points: 1–3 days before ovulation and 6–8 days afterwards. A natural control cycle followed by a clomiphene citrate cycle was observed in all patients. The more favorable trilaminar endometrial pattern was seen more often in the control cycles than in the clomiphene citrate cycles. In cycles that resulted in pregnancy, a favorable pattern was seen more often than in non-pregnant cycles (72% vs 39% respectively).[7]

Similar results were seen when clomiphene citrate and gonadotropins were used in combination. Endometrial appearance after stimulation with 50–100 mg of clomiphene citrate followed by three doses of gonadotropins produced both trilaminar and homogeneous endometrial patterns in patients attempting to achieve pregnancy. In those patients that achieved pregnancy, 87% had a trilaminar-appearing endometrium compared to 57% of the patients that did not become pregnant. Although this difference was evaluated retrospectively, it was statistically significant. Despite the difference in pattern, the mean endometrial thickness did not differ significantly between the pregnant and non-pregnant groups (12.1 vs 11.0, respectively).[8] A prospective study by Hock et al looked at pregnancy rates when patients were separated by the sonographic appearance of the endometrial lining. Patients received CC followed by gonadotropins and endometrial thickness and pattern were evaluated on the day of hCG administration. In the group with a trilaminar appearance, a pregnancy rate of 21% was seen. In the homogeneous endometrium group, a pregnancy rate of 8% was seen ($p < 0.02$). This difference was statistically significant.[9] In this study, only endometrial pattern, and not endometrial thickness, was important as a predictor of pregnancy. While these studies suggest that a trilaminar endometrial pattern on ultrasound is favorable for pregnancy, the less favorable homogeneous pattern can still result in successful pregnancies. There have been no studies to attempt to discover potential mechanisms through which one might assist the conversion from the less to more favorable pattern. Thus, the practical value of assessing endometrial pattern is questionable.

DIRECT ASSESSMENT OF ENDOMETRIAL CHANGES AFTER CLOMIPHENE CITRATE

A more direct approach to evaluation of endometrial function is through endometrial biopsy and histological or molecular evaluation of the sample.

Histological evaluation of endometrial dating

Evaluation of the endometrium by light microscopic features of hematoxylin and eosin (H&E)-stained

endometrial biopsies is used to measure the maturity and development of the endometrium. The histological appearance of the endometrium changes throughout the menstrual cycle. In the luteal phase, epithelial proliferation stops and the endometrial glands increase secretory output. The endometrium reorganizes itself into a three-layered structure which then acquires stromal edema. Around the 'window of implantation', days 21–22 of the cycle, multiple cytokines, adhesion molecules, and cell signaling molecules are modified to allow the embryo to adhere to and implant within the uterine lining.[10] Endometrial evaluation has classically been performed by histological evaluation of leukocytic infiltration, stromal mitoses, pseudodecidual reaction, stromal edema, basal vacuolation, pseudostratification of nuclei, and gland mitoses. These markers have been used to assign a day of development to the endometrium.[11] This allows a measure of the maturity of the endometrium based on standardized criteria.[11] When the day of endometrial histology is more than 2 days behind the cycle day based upon the day of ovulation (e.g. histological day 22 on cycle day 26 or 12 days post-LH [luteinizing hormone] surge), then the endometrium is termed 'out-of-phase'. Such out-of-phase endometria are supposed to result in fewer pregnancies and more miscarriages because the dyssynchrony between embryo stage and endometrial development makes proper implantation more difficult.

Abnormalities of glandular development could account for the lower than expected pregnancy rates seen in CC cycles.[12] It is thought that clomiphene citrate may delay endometrial maturation and result in more out-of-phase endometria than seen in normal controls. Sereepapong et al examined the ultrasound findings and endometrial biopsies of 30 normo-ovulatory women in the mid luteal phase both in control cycles and after 200 mg of CC on days 3–7 of the menstrual cycle. Histological dating and ultrasound findings were similar in the CC-treated cycles compared to the control cycles in the same volunteers. However, in the CC group, the number of endometrial glands per square millimeter was decreased while the number of vacuolated cells per 1000 glandular cells was higher.[12] Palomino et al compared 13 CC-treated women to 18 natural cycle controls, all healthy volunteers. Based on Noyes' criteria, the CC-treated group had a significantly higher percentage of endometrial biopsies that were out of phase than the natural cycle group (38.4% vs 16.6%). Therefore, CC increased the percentage of out-of-phase endometrium.[13] Bonhoff et al examined endometrial biopsies from normal ovulatory women in the luteal phase and compared them to CC-treated patients. Patients treated with clomiphene citrate had decreased density of endometrial glands in the early luteal phase as

well as decreased glandular height compared to controls.[14] While much of this work has been performed in healthy ovulatory volunteers, who may have different responses to clomiphene citrate than infertile anovulatory women, they do support the hypothesis that clomiphene citrate alters endometrial development in comparison to natural cycles.

Molecular markers of endometrial receptivity

The last decade has seen an explosion in attempts to use molecular biology techniques for the evaluation of endometrial function. Most investigations have focused their attention on the presumed window of implantation in the mid luteal phase (cycle days 19–23). Multiple cytokines and proteins have been examined during the mid luteal phase/early implantation phase of the endometrium. The most studied markers to date have been integrins, leukemia inhibitory factor (LIF), E-cadherin, and oxytocin receptor.

Integrins are expressed in epithelial endometrium in peak amounts during the implantation period and are therefore potential biomarkers for uterine receptivity. Lack of integrins can be a cause for infertility.[10] In luteal phase deficiency, the progesterone receptor is inadequately down-regulated and integrin expression remains low. Clomiphene citrate acts as an antiestrogen in the endometrium and may interfere with integrin expression. Palomino et al investigated this hypothesis in 13 CC-treated women compared to 18 natural cycle controls. After evaluating endometrial samples for histological dating, they found that β_3 integrin levels detected by immunohistochemistry in out-of-phase samples of both groups were significantly lower compared to the in-phase samples of the same group. In the natural cycle, β_3 integrin levels from both the in-phase and out-of-phase endometrium were higher than in the similarly scored endometrium of CC cycles. Therefore, CC decreases the amount of β_3 integrin in both in-phase and out-of-phase endometrium.[13] Lacin et al studied the production of β_1, β_3, α_v integrins in the implantation window in patients with unexplained infertility who were given clomiphene citrate. Endometrial biopsies were done in patients on the 7th or 8th day after ovulation in a natural cycle and in a CC cycle. Integrin expression was evaluated by immunohistochemistry and the biopsies of the natural cycle were compared to the CC cycles. No difference was seen between the CC and natural cycles in these patients.[4]

Leukemia inhibitory factor is a glycoprotein cytokine that is shown in knockout experiments to be critical for implantation in the mouse. It is most abundant in secretory phase endometrium. Kuscu et al studied the levels of LIF in 11 women with unexplained infertility. When endometrial biopsies in natural cycles were compared with CC cycles in the same patients, no difference was seen in LIF levels between the natural cycles, and the CC-treated cycles.[15]

E-cadherin is a cell adhesion molecule that may play a role in increasing the adhesion of the embryo to the endometrium during implantation. It is expressed continuously throughout the menstrual cycle but the mRNA for E-cadherin is elevated during the luteal phase. Progesterone may induce this gene expression. Dawood et al examined the protein and mRNA levels of E-cadherin in mid luteal endometrial biopsy specimens of normal and CC-treated cycles. Despite elevated luteal phase progesterone levels in the CC-treated cycles, they found similar levels of E-cadherin mRNA expression in both groups. E-cadherin protein levels were elevated in CC-treated cycles, but not significantly.[16]

Dawood et al[17] also examined the levels of mRNA and protein of the oxytocin receptor in the same group of patients. In the control cycles, patients had higher levels of oxytocin receptor protein compared to the CC-treated cycles. However, mRNA levels were not significantly different between the two groups.

Work in this area continues. Studies to date have been inconclusive, possibly due to significant individual and temporal variation in endometrial function, along with the technical difficulties of performing molecular analyses upon samples containing differing proportions of glandular vs stromal cells. While these molecular markers have not provided conclusive evidence for the type of change effected by CC upon the endometrium, they do serve to illustrate that CC-treated endometrium may be different from natural cycle endometrium.[17]

CLINICAL MANAGEMENT OF THE ENDOMETRIUM AFTER CLOMIPHENE CITRATE

Timing of clomiphene citrate administration

Clomiphene citrate may be started at different days of the menstrual cycle. Starting too late in the cycle of an ovulatory woman would prevent the support of multiple follicles, as dominant follicle selection may have already occurred, but might be advantageous if it allowed a longer period of estrogen stimulation of endometrial development before exposure to the estrogen antagonist. In order to evaluate this issue, the timing of clomiphene citrate start day upon endometrial development has been studied. Triwitayakorn et al evaluated endometrial thickness and appearance using transvaginal ultrasound 7 days after

ovulation in healthy ovulatory volunteers treated with different clomiphene citrate regimens. No difference was found in endometrial thickness after administration of clomiphene citrate on days 1–5 of the menstrual cycle compared to administration on days 5–9. This was despite the fact that the second group had higher estradiol levels on the day of ovulation. Furthermore, no difference between dating or morphometric appearance was seen in mid luteal endometrial biopsies of either group.[18] Cheung et al also investigated different clomiphene citrate regimens in healthy ovulatory volunteers. They too found no change in mid-luteal endometrial thickness between groups taking CC on either days 2–6 of the menstrual cycle or on days 5–9.[19] Thus, the timing of clomiphene citrate administration seems to have no significant effect upon endometrial development.

Clomiphene citrate dose

Higher clomiphene citrate doses have been suspected as being more adverse for endometrial development. Investigators have therefore tried to confirm a dose–response relationship between clomiphene citrate dose and poor endometrial development. In a study looking at the relationship between increased patient weight and the dose of clomiphene citrate in the cycle of pregnancy success, an evaluation of the effects of clomiphene citrate on endometrial thickness was included. With increases in clomiphene citrate from 25 mg to >150 mg, no change in endometrial thickness on the day of hCG administration was seen.[20] In general, the literature has not supported a clear dose–response relationship between CC dose and adverse endometrial effects.

Clomiphene citrate with estrogen add-back therapy

To alleviate the negative effects of clomiphene citrate on the endometrium, investigators have attempted the addition of exogenous estrogen during or immediately after clomiphene citrate administration. Although this approach may result in a thicker endometrium, there is a theoretical risk that estrogen administration may interfere with the hypothalamic–pituitary negative feedback mechanisms which should be inhibited by CC, which may therefore inhibit the pituitary FSH response to CC. There have been no studies to look at this issue to date. A number of trials have been successful in increasing endometrial thickness at either time of hCG administration or in the mid luteal phase with the use of estrogen. Eleven oligo-ovulatory or anovulatory patients with no other medical or gynecological problems were given 100 mg of clomiphene citrate for days 5–9 of their menstrual cycle with or without 4 mg of transdermal estrogen from day 8 until the day of ovulation. Patients with the additional estrogen treatment had a significantly thicker endometrial lining around the time of ovulation.[21] Unfer and colleagues used healthy ovulatory patients to examine the effects of estradiol addition to clomiphene citrate on the endometrium without a background of infertility. They randomized patients into three arms: clomiphene citrate alone, clomiphene citrate plus 5 µg of ethinyl estradiol (EF), and clomiphene citrate + 2 µg of ethinyl estradiol. They found that addition of ethinyl estradiol increased the endometrial thickness when measured 7 days after ovulation. Furthermore, the percentage of endometrial biopsies that were in phase was increased with addition of ethinyl estradiol. Both of these differences were statistically significant but there was no difference between the two doses of ethinyl estradiol.[22] A randomized clinical trial of 64 women with infertility and oligo/amenorrhea treated subjects with either CC alone or CC followed by ethinyl estradiol. They showed that the addition of estrogen increased endometrial thickness when measured on the day of hCG administration. They also found that the miscarriage rate was lower (6.25% vs 18.75%) and the ongoing pregnancy rate higher (37.5% vs 6.25%) in the CC + EE group compared to the placebo group. There were no statistically significant differences in serum levels of LH, FSH, or E_2 levels between the groups.[23] Despite improvements in endometrial thickness, concerns about reducing the response to CC, along with inconclusive effects upon pregnancy rates, have led most authorities to recommend estrogen add-back only in cases where a thin endometrium is seen after CC.

Phytoestrogens

Phytoestrogens (PEs) are compounds found in plants and fungi with estrogenic activity that may have a higher affinity than CC for estrogen receptor-β (ERβ). This may help to decrease some of CC's antagonistic effects on the endometrium.[24] Phytoestrogens were administered in conjunction with clomiphene citrate in a randomized trial of 134 women with infertility. These women had oligomenorrhea but positive progesterone challenge tests and were randomized to either CC for 5 days or CC for 5 days + 1500 mg of phytoestrogens for 10 days starting on the same day as the CC. The phytoestrogens consisted of the soy isoflavones genistein, daidzein, and glycitein. Endometrial thicknesses were measured on the day of hCG administration and were found to be thicker in the patients treated with CC and PE. Furthermore, the pregnancy rate was higher in the group treated with CC + PE and the miscarriage rate was lower.[25] This effect may have

been modulated by PE activation of ERβ and an increase in the progesterone receptor. This may have then improved the endometrial quality during the luteal phase.[24]

Potential disadvantages of using botanical preparations include: lack of standardization, resulting in significant variability of content and efficacy from batch to batch; lack of quality control and regulation, resulting in possible contamination or adulteration; and possible errors in compounding.[26] Without any reason to expect better results from phytoestrogens as compared to standard pharmaceutical estrogen preparations, there seems to be little rationale for their use at this time.

Overall, estrogen supplementation during or just after ovarian stimulation with clomiphene citrate has been shown to improve endometrial thickness and increase the percentage of in-phase endometrial biopsies, but the ability of these changes to increase the occurrence of successful pregnancy has yet to be demonstrated conclusively.

EFFECTS OF GONADOTROPINS ON THE ENDOMETRIUM

Gonadotropins are glycoprotein hormones consisting of two polypeptide subunits (α and β) of which the α subunit is identical in the hormones FSH, LH, hCG, and thyroid-stimulating hormone (TSH). However, TSH is not active on the reproductive organs. The β subunit of each hormone confers its identity and therefore bioactive specificity. The α subunit gene is expressed in the pituitary and the placenta. LH and hCG β subunits are similar and have cross-actions on the LH receptor. LH and FSH are secreted by the gonadotrope cells in the anterior lobe of the pituitary. They are under regulation by pulsatile gonadotropin-releasing hormone (GnRH) secretion by the hypothalamus. Exogenous gonadotropin stimulation with both human menopausal gonadotropins and, more recently, recombinant FSH has been used as a treatment for poor endometrial development in women with recurrent pregnancy loss, infertility associated with a luteal phase defect, poor ovarian function, as well as unexplained infertility. For in-vitro fertilization cycles, FSH and LH are often used in conjunction with a GnRH agonist or antagonist as well as hCG. There have been concerns raised, however, that the multiple follicles produced may result in supraphysiological levels of estrogen and accelerated endometrial development, resulting in increased dyssynchrony between endometrial and embryo development. This may vary significantly from study to study and from person to person, depending upon the degree of ovarian stimulation and an individual's response. A woman who develops eight follicles and an estradiol level of 1500 pg/ml after 5 days of gonadotropin stimulation may have very different endometrial effects as compared to a woman who responds with three follicles and an estradiol level of 600 pg/ml after 9 days of gonadotropin stimulation. Thus, studies utilizing more aggressive gonadotropin stimulation or those with a population enriched with more responsive subjects may find more problems with accelerated endometrial development as compared to studies in which the population had lower responders and a less-aggressive ovarian stimulation regimen.

INDIRECT (ULTRASOUND) ASSESSMENT OF ENDOMETRIAL CHANGES AFTER GONADOTROPINS

Endometrial thickness and pattern

As with clomiphene citrate, ultrasound evaluation of the endometrium has been used during monitoring of stimulation cycles with gonadotropins. Many groups have attempted to correlate endometrial thickness and/or pattern with pregnancy outcome. Leibovitz and colleagues sonographically evaluated the endometrium of in-vitro fertilization (IVF) patients throughout their stimulation cycles and showed a statistically significant increase in endometrial thickness in pregnant compared to non-pregnant patients in the late luteal phase of the cycle. However, no difference in endometrial thickness was seen between pregnant and non-pregnant IVF patients at time points before oocyte retrieval or in the early to mid luteal phase.[27] Oliveira et al also analyzed the value of endometrial thickness and pattern inpredicting pregnancy status. IVF patients were separated into two groups based on sonographic appearance of the endometrium on the day of hCG administration. When the trilaminar endometrial pattern group was compared to the homogeneous endometrial pattern group, there was no difference in clinical pregnancy rates. However, within the trilaminar group, the endometrial thickness in pregnancy cycles was significantly greater than in the non-pregnant cycles. When endometrial pattern was disregarded, however, the endometrial thickness was not significantly different between the pregnant and non-pregnant groups.[28]

Bohrer et al performed a prospective study in patients undergoing gonadotropin–IUI (intrauterine insemination) stimulation cycles. In patients with trilaminar endometrial patterns, the endometrial thickness on the day of hCG administration was found to be greater than in patients with a homogeneous pattern. The patients with a trilaminar endometrium had a higher percentage of pregnancies.[29] In women treated with human menopausal gonadotropins alone, the endometrial thickness of conception vs non-conception cycles was compared. There were no significant differences between the two groups (11.9 mm vs 11.2 mm, respectively).[30]

In conclusion, ultrasound evaluation of endometrial thickness and pattern remains a less than perfect marker of endometrial development in ovarian stimulation cycles, due to the unclear relationship between these measures and successful pregnancy.

DIRECT ASSESSMENT OF ENDOMETRIAL CHANGES AFTER GONADOTROPIN STIMULATION

Histology for endometrial dating

As with clomiphene citrate, endometrial dating by comparison of endometrial biopsies has been used to evaluate the effects of gonadotropins on the endometrium. Simon et al performed a comprehensive comparison of the changes in the endometrium of oocyte donors in natural cycles and in gonadotropin stimulation cycles combined with one of two different dose regimens of GnRH antagonist or a standard GnRH agonist long protocol. Endometrial dating on biopsy in the early and mid luteal phase followed the pattern of the natural cycle for both antagonist protocols but the GnRH agonist group more frequently demonstrated delayed development.[31]

Electron microscopy

Pinopodes are large, smooth membrane projections that develop on the apical membranes of endometrial epithelial cells. They are thought to be markers of endometrial receptivity since they only appear during the implantation window in normal endometrium. Pinopode formation and regression is accelerated in controlled ovarian hyperstimulation (COH) cycles compared to natural cycles.[32,33] Electron microscopy is expensive and not readily available and therefore light microscopy with routine histological samples has been used to evaluate the endometrium for pinopodes.[34] Simon et al performed a comprehensive comparison of endometrial changes in oocyte donors in natural cycles, and in stimulation cycles using one of two different dose regimens of GnRH antagonist or a standard long GnRH agonist protocol. Endometrial samples in this study were evaluated on day 2 after LH surge or hCG administration. No pinopodes were seen in any of the groups. On day 7 after LH surge or hCG administration, around 6% of the endometrial samples showed evidence of pinopodes for the natural and antagonist cycles, whereas the long agonist cycle patients revealed pinopodes in only 2.6% of samples.[31]

Pathological examination of the luteal phase endometrium by light microscopy and electron microscopy is not useful during a treatment cycle as interruption of a pregnancy could occur with sampling of the endometrium. Thus, the studied cycle is never the actual cycle of conception. Due to intercycle variability, this inability to directly evaluate the endometrium in the cycle of interest adds a layer of complexity and confusion to these types of analyses. Furthermore, while pinopodes are potential markers for endometrial receptivity, they appear at variable times and are not consistent from cycle to cycle.[35]

Effect of gonadotropins on molecular markers of endometrial receptivity

Since estrogen receptor decline is a normal occurrence in the late luteal and early pregnancy endometrium, Ohno and Fujimoto looked at the presence of estrogen and progesterone receptors in the endometrium of both natural and stimulated cycles. There was no difference in endometrial patterns between non-pregnant and pregnant cycles, or between natural and gonadotropin cycles. With increased serum estrogen levels in gonadotropin cycles, they noted a decrease in enzyme immunoassay measured estrogen receptor content in the endometrium collected through endometrial biopsy but no change in the progesterone receptor levels. This trend was not statistically significant.[36]

Simon et al performed a comprehensive comparison of the changes in the endometrium of oocyte donors in natural cycles and in stimulation cycles using a GnRH antagonist or a standard GnRH agonist long protocol. Estrogen and progesterone receptor expression followed the pattern seen in the natural cycles, with no significant differences among the natural and treatment groups. Endometrial samples in this study were evaluated on day 2 after LH surge or hCG administration. Gene expression profiling also examined the difference among these four groups. The authors concluded that the GnRH antagonist group showed patterns of expression of implantation genes more similar to the natural cycles than the agonist group. As these patients were oocyte donors, pregnancy data for the endometrium evaluated are unavailable.[31]

Using microchip gene expression arrays, the same group analyzed the endometrium of oocyte donors treated with the standard long protocols in comparison to natural cycles in the same patients. The authors created a control group by first comparing gene expression in the early luteal phase to mid luteal phase in the same patients to determine which genes changed as the endometrium became receptive. Then, they compared mid luteal endometrium

gene expression in natural cycles and stimulated cycles. The difference in gene expression between these two groups was then compared to the differences in the luteal states of the control group. Over 550 genes were noted to be different between the natural and stimulated endometrium; 351 genes that were regulated between early and mid luteal endometrium were also differentially regulated in stimulated endometrium compared to natural cycle endometrium but, for many of these genes, in the opposite direction. The stimulation of the endometrium with gonadotropins and then hCG in IVF cycles changes the quality of gene expression in comparison to natural cycles.[37]

Another group evaluated endometrial molecular characteristics in oocyte donors undergoing IVF and natural cycles. Pinopode maturation was advanced in stimulated endometrium, as was reported previously, with fewer pinopodes visible by electron microscopy in the mid luteal phase. Estrogen and progesterone receptor development was found to be accelerated. Gene expression profiling done in this group showed changes in the stimulated endometrium but only in a small number of genes. After further analysis, the authors questioned whether these changes in such a small number of genes was clinically relevant.[38] Differences in integrin expression and endometrial dating were evaluated in natural and stimulated cycles in oocyte donors. Using the Noyes' criteria, the endometrial glandular maturation was more often *delayed* in the stimulated cycles (60%) compared to the control cycles (25%). This delayed glandular development contributed to the additional finding of increased glandular/stromal dyssynchrony in COH cycles (80%) compared to controls (30%); $\alpha_v\beta_3$ integrin expression was detected significantly more often in the control cycles than in the COH cycles.[39] In-vitro studies of endometrial cell cultures obtained from hysterectomy specimens demonstrated a significant inhibition of cellular proliferation when treated with high doses of gonadotropins.[40]

Human chorionic gonadotropin and/or LH alone may contribute to maturation of the endometrium. In-vitro studies of human endometrial stromal and glandular cells stimulated with hCG showed an increase in cyclooxygenase 2 (COX-2) expression. This may increase prostaglandin synthesis in the endometrium and aid in development of decidualized endometrium, therefore playing a part in preparing the uterus for implantation.[41,42] It has also been proposed that hCG may be an angiogenic factor that acts during early implantation to adapt the uterus to a new pregnancy.[43]

In conclusion, molecular and histological changes in the endometrium of gonadotropin-stimulated patients have been noted by many investigators. Some have noted delayed maturation, while others have noted accelerated development. While not consistent, they suggest significant alterations in endometrial development in at least some gonadotropin cycles. This may have clinical relevance, as these changes may limit the success seen after gonadotropin therapy. Further work in this area is needed. Molecular marker analysis and gene expression profiles are also inconclusive to date, but represent very promising areas for future investigation.

CLINICAL MANAGEMENT OF THE ENDOMETRIUM AFTER GONADOTROPINS

Treatment of recurrent miscarriage

Li et al investigated the effect of gonadotropins on the endometrium when used in treatment of recurrent miscarriage. In patients with three or more miscarriages, endometrial biopsies were evaluated in both unstimulated and stimulated cycles in the same patients. A significant difference was seen in the delay in endometrial dating between the two groups. The control, unstimulated cycles had more delayed endometrium than endometrium treated with gonadotropins. It is possible that this mechanism accounts for the improvement in pregnancy rate in recurrent miscarriage patients treated with gonadotropins. In the same study, the outcome of pregnancies achieved with or without gonadotropins in patients with a history of recurrent pregnancy loss was evaluated. In patients achieving pregnancy after gonadotropin therapy, significantly fewer first trimester miscarriages were seen compared to pregnancies achieved without treatment (2/13 vs 7/12), although the actual numbers studied were quite small.[44]

There is no doubt that gonadotropin therapy increases pregnancy rates and usually results in a thicker endometrium as compared to the natural menstrual cycle. Unfortunately, endometrial dyssynchrony (delayed or accelerated development) may occur with gonadotropin use and can potentially lower the effectiveness of these agents.

Aromatase inhibitors

Aromatase inhibitors are a new option for ovarian stimulation. They competitively inhibit the final step in the conversion of androgens and testosterone into estrogen. Since they have a much shorter half-life in comparison to clomiphene citrate, it has been proposed that they may have less deleterious effects upon endometrial development. In patients with unexplained infertility, when used on days 3–7 of the menstrual cycle at a dose of 5 mg daily, the endometrial thickness achieved was not different from natural cycles (12.3 vs 12.1, respectively). Pinopode appearance was similar between the two groups. However, with this regimen, the difference in endometrial dating was apparent, with the control cycles more delayed than the study cycles.[45] Al-Fadhli and colleagues investigated the effects of either 2.5 mg or 5 mg of letrozole on the endometrium in a small pilot study of eight patients. With a higher dose of aromatase inhibitor, no difference was seen in the thickness of the endometrium, but an increase was seen in the pregnancy rate. This increase was from 5.9% to 26.3%.[46] Bayar et al found thicker endometria after letrozole as compared to CC, but equal pregnancy rates.[47] In polycystic ovary syndrome patients, Mitwally and Casper investigated the effects of ovulation induction with aromatase inhibitor after poor responses to CC. Normal ovulatory women with a history of thin endometrium measurements on CC were used as controls. Comparison of the two groups showed a thicker endometrium in the letrozole cycles compared to the CC cycles in both groups.[48]

More work is needed in this area, in particular to determine whether the presumed advantages of aromatase inhibitors upon endometrial development will translate into more successful livebirth pregnancies.

REFERENCES

1. Homburg R. Clomiphene citrate – end of an era? A mini-review. Hum Reprod 2005; 20(8): 2043–51.
2. Imani B, Eijkemans MJC, te Velde ER et al. A nomogram to predict the probability of live birth after clomiphene citrate induction of ovulation in normogonadotropic oligoamenorrheic infertility. Fertil Steril 2002; 77(1): 91–7.
3. Messinis IE. Ovulation induction: a mini review. Hum Reprod 2005; 20(10): 2688–97.
4. Lacin S, Vatansever S, Kuscu NK et al. Clomiphene citrate does not affect the secretion of alpha3, alphav and beta1 integrin molecules during the implantation window in patients with unexplained infertility. Hum Reprod 2001; 16(11): 2305–9.
5. Dickey RP, Holtkamp DE. Development, pharmacology and clinical experience with clomiphene citrate. Hum Reprod Update 1996; 2(6): 483–506.
6. Kolibianakis EM, Zikopoulos KA, Fatemi HM et al. Endometrial thickness cannot predict ongoing pregnancy achievement in cycles stimulated with clomiphene citrate for intrauterine insemination. Reprod Biomed Online 2004; 8(1): 115–18.
7. Nakamura Y, Ono M, Yoshida Y et al. Effects of clomiphene citrate on the endometrial thickness and echogenic pattern of the endometrium. Fertil Steril 1997; 67(2): 256–60.
8. Tsai HD, Chang CC, Hsieh YY et al. Artificial insemination. Role of endometrial thickness and pattern, of vascular impedance of the spiral and uterine arteries, and of the dominant follicle. J Reprod Med 2000; 45(3): 195–200.
9. Hock DL, Bohrer MK, Ananth CV et al. Sonographic assessment of endometrial pattern and thickness in patients treated with clomiphene citrate, human menopausal gonadotropins, and intrauterine insemination. Fertil Steril 1997; 68(2): 242–5.
10. Speroff L, Fritz MA. Clinical Gynecologic Endocrinology and Infertility, 7th edn. Philadelphia: Lippincott Williams & Wilkins, 2005.

11. Noyes RW, Hertig AT, Rock J. Dating the endometrial biopsy. Am J Obstet Gynecol 1975; 122(2): 262–3.

12. Sereepapong W, Suwajanakorn S, Triratanachat S et al. Effects of clomiphene citrate on the endometrium of regularly cycling women. Fertil Steril 2000; 73(2): 287–91.

13. Palomino WA, Fuentes A, Gonzalez RR et al. Differential expression of endometrial integrins and progesterone receptor during the window of implantation in normo-ovulatory women treated with clomiphene citrate. Fertil Steril 2005; 83(3): 587–93.

14. Bonhoff AJ, Naether OG, Johannisson E. Effects of clomiphene citrate stimulation on endometrial structure in infertile women. Hum Reprod 1996; 11(4): 844–9.

15. Kuscu NK, Koyuncu FM, Var A et al. Clomiphene citrate does not adversely affect endometrial leukemia inhibitory factor levels. Gynecol Endocrinol 2002; 6(2): 151–4.

16. Dawood MY, Lau M, Khan-Dawood FS. E-cadherin and its messenger ribonucleic acid in periimplantation phase human endometrium in normal and clomiphene-treated cycles. Am J Obstet Gynecol 1998; 178(5): 996–1001.

17. Dawood MY, Lau M, Khan-Dawood FS. Localization and expression of oxytocin receptor and its messenger ribonucleic acid in peri-implantation phase human endometrium during control and clomiphene-treated cycles. Am J Obstet Gynecol 1999; 181(1): 50–6.

18. Triwitayakorn A, Suwajanakorn S, Triratanachat S et al. Effects of initiation day of clomiphene citrate on the endometrium of women with regular menstrual cycles. Fertil Steril 2002; 78(1): 102–7.

19. Cheung W, Ng EH, Ho PC. A randomized double-blind comparison of perifollicular vascularity and endometrial receptivity in ovulatory women taking clomiphene citrate at two different times. Hum Reprod 2002; 17(11): 2881–4.

20. Dickey RP, Taylor SN, Curole DN et al. Relationship of clomiphene dose and patient weight to successful treatment. Hum Reprod 1997; 12(3): 449–53.

21. Shimoya K, Tomiyama T, Hashimoto K et al. Endometrial development was improved by transdermal estradiol in patients treated with clomiphene citrate. Gynecol Obstet Invest 1999; 47(4): 251–4.

22. Unfer V, Costabile L, Gerli S et al. Low dose of ethinyl estradiol can reverse the antiestrogenic effects of clomiphene citrate on endometrium. Gynecol Obstet Invest 2001; 51(2): 120–3.

23. Gerli S, Gholami H, Manna C et al. Use of ethinyl estradiol to reverse the antiestrogenic effects of clomiphene citrate in patients undergoing intrauterine insemination: a comparative, randomized study. Fertil Steril 2000; 73(1): 85–9.

24. Casper RF. Phytoestrogens, clomiphene, and the uterus. J Soc Gynecol Investig 2004; 11(5): 261–2.

25. Unfer V, Casini ML, Costabile L et al. High dose of phytoestrogens can reverse the antiestrogenic effects of clomiphene citrate on the endometrium in patients undergoing intrauterine insemination: A randomized trial. J Soc Gynecol Investig 2004; 11(5): 323–8.

26. ACOG Practice Bulletin. Clinical Management Guidelines for Obstetrician-Gynecologists. Use of botanicals for management of menopausal symptoms. Obstet Gynecol 2001; 97(6): Suppl 1–11.

27. Leibovitz Z, Grinin V, Rabia R et al. Assessment of endometrial receptivity for gestation in patients undergoing in vitro fertilization, using endometrial thickness and the endometrium–myometrium relative echogenicity coefficient. Ultrasound Obstet Gynecol 1999; 14(3): 194–9.

28. Oliveira JB, Baruffi RL, Mauri AL et al. Endometrial ultrasonography as a predictor of pregnancy in an in-vitro fertilization programme after ovarian stimulation and gonadotrophin-releasing hormone and gonadotrophins. Hum Reprod 1997; 12(11): 2515–18.

29. Bohrer MK, Hock DL, Rhoads GG et al. Sonographic assessment of endometrial pattern and thickness in patients treated with human menopausal gonadotropins. Fertil Steril 1996; 66(2): 244–7.

30. Isaacs JD Jr, Wells CS, Williams DB et al. Endometrial thickness is a valid monitoring parameter in cycles of ovulation induction with menotropins alone. Fertil Steril 1996; 65(2): 262–6.

31. Simon C, Oberye J, Bellver J et al. Similar endometrial development in oocyte donors treated with either high- or standard-dose Gnrh antagonist compared to treatment with a Gnrh agonist or in natural cycles. Hum Reprod 2005; 20(12): 3318–27.

32. Nikas G, Develioglu OH, Toner JP, Jones HW Jr. Endometrial pinopodes indicate a shift in the window of receptivity in IVF cycles. Hum Reprod 1999; 14(3): 787–92.

33. Develioglu OH, Hsiu J-G, Nikas G et al. Endometrial estrogen and progesterone receptor and pinopode expression in stimulated cycles of oocyte donors. Fertil Steril 1999; 71(6): 1040–7.

34. Develioglu OH, Nikas G, Hsiu J-G et al. Detection of endometrial pinopodes by light microscopy. Fertil Steril 2000; 74(4): 767–70.

35. Acosta AA, Elberger L, Borghi M et al. Endometrial dating and determination of the window of implantation in healthy fertile women. Fertil Steril 2000; 73(4): 788–98.

36. Ohno Y, Fujimoto Y. Endometrial oestrogen and progesterone receptors and their relationship to sonographic appearance of the endometrium. Hum Reprod Update 1998; 4(5): 560–4.

37. Horcajadas JA, Riesewijk A, Polman J et al. Effect of controlled ovarian hyperstimulation in IVF on endometrial gene expression profiles. Mol Hum Reprod 2005; 11(3): 195–205.

38. Mirkin S, Nikas G, Hsiu JG. Gene expression profiles and structural/functional features of the peri-implantation endometrium in natural and gonadotropin-stimulated cycles. J Clin Endocrinol Metab 2004; 89(11): 5742–52.

39. Meyer WR, Novotny DB, Fritz MA et al. Effect of exogenous gonadotropins on endometrial maturation in oocyte donors. Fertil Steril 1999; 71(1): 109–14.

40. Ku SY, Choi YM, Suh CS et al. Effect of gonadotropins on human endometrial stromal cell proliferation in vitro. Arch Gynecol Obstet 2002; 266(4): 223–8.

41. Han SW, Lei ZM, Rao CV. Up-regulation of cyclooxygenase-2 gene expression by chorionic gonadotropin during the differentiation of human endometrial stromal cells into decidua. Endocrinology 1996; 137(5): 1791–7.

42. Zhou XL, Lei ZM, Rao CV. Treatment of human endometrial gland epithelial cells with chorionic gonadotropin/luteinizing hormone increases the expression of the cyclooxygenase-2 gene. J Clin Endocrinol Metab 1999; 84(9): 3364–77.

43. Zygmunt M, Herr F, Keller-Schoenwetter S et al. Characterization of human chorionic gonadotropin as a novel angiogenic factor. J Clin Endocrinol Metab 2002; 87(11): 5290–6.

44. Li TC, Ding SH, Anstie B et al. Use of human menopausal gonadotropins in the treatment of endometrial defects associated with recurrent miscarriage: preliminary report. Fertil Steril 2001; 75(2): 434–7.

45. Cortinez A, De Carvalho I, Vantman D et al. Hormonal profile and endometrial morphology in letrozole-controlled ovarian hyperstimulation in ovulatory infertile patients. Fertil Steril 2005; 83(1): 110–15.

46. Al-Fadhli R, Sylvestre C, Buckett W et al. A randomized trial of superovulation with two different doses of letrozole. Fertil Steril 2006; 85(1): 161–4.

47. Bayar U, Basaran M, Kiran S et al. Use of an aromatase inhibitor in patients with polycystic ovary syndrome: a prospective randomized trial. Fertil Steril 2006; 86(5): 1447–51.

48. Mitwally MF, Casper RF. Use of an aromatase inhibitor for induction of ovulation in patients with an inadequate response to clomiphene citrate. Fertil Steril 2001; 75(2): 305–9.

44 Reproductive freedom and access to assisted reproductive technologies

Vardit Ravitsky and Art Caplan

INTRODUCTION

The desire to procreate is one of the most essential aspects of being human. It is a basic biological and psychological drive. Reproductive freedom is therefore a fundamental human interest. The right to establish a family has been recognized by the Universal. Declaration of Human Rights[1] and the right to protection from state intervention in matters related to reproduction has been legally acknowledged in the USA[2] and many other nations.

As assisted reproductive technologies (ART) become more common and effective, and as the problem of infertility affects a larger number of individuals, an increasing number of them turn to these technologies in their attempts to conceive a child. Through the end of 2002, almost 300 000 babies had been born in the USA as a result of reported ART procedures. In 2002, approximately 1 in every 100 babies born in the USA was conceived using ART.[3]

Whereas the process of natural coital conception is occurring in the most private of circumstances, the need for ART involves a dramatic change. The act of conception is carried from the privacy of the home into the more public domain of the clinic, and necessarily entails the participation of a group of professionals. Moreover, even when privately funded, it entails the use of resources that society helps create and maintain, such as the research leading to the development of newer technologies and clinical approaches. Society must also bear the cost for some of the unintended consequences of ART, such as the cost of caring for premature infants or children born with disabilities that might be linked to some ART practices.

As a result, questions arise regarding the limits of reproductive freedom. Does society – as represented by legislators, regulators, public opinion, or those who run fertility clinics – have the right to deny access to ART in certain cases? In the case of natural conception, regulating parenthood entails a level of intrusion into the private lives of individuals and families that can hardly be justified in a liberal society. In contrast, denying access to ART does not require such levels of intrusion. It simply requires refusing to help individuals who approach a fertility clinic. It is important to acknowledge, however, that denial of access can have devastating effects on people's lives.

It is therefore necessary and urgent to offer a comprehensive ethical analysis of possible justifications for denial. This is particularly true in the current US context, in which access to ART is not regulated[4] and where no national or professional guidelines for screening candidates are available.

A recent study that presented ethically complex case scenarios to directors of ART clinics in the USA[5] showed that there is little agreement on whether or not patients in the scenarios should or would be treated. Another recent study[6] that surveyed 210 ART programs in the USA showed that the majority believe they have the right and responsibility to screen candidates, mostly based on the prospective child's safety and welfare and the risk that pregnancy poses to the mother. The vast majority of programs collect information about physical and psychological attributes that could place a prospective child at risk, such as drug use or HIV (human immunodeficiency virus) status. Most programs also collect information that could have relevance to the child's future welfare, such as marital status, sexual orientation, income, mental health, physical and mental health of existing children, and stability of the relationship with a partner.

However, considering the substantial variation in the answers to hypothetical questions about turning away candidates based on such characteristics, this information is likely to be used differently by different programs. For example, a couple receiving welfare, or a gay couple, is likely to be granted access to ART in some programs but denied in others, depending on the values of the program they approach. Considering this social reality, it is vital to ethically evaluate different approaches to screening, in order to provide guidelines to ART programs, as well as recommendations for possible regulation or legislation.

The ethical framework offered in this chapter can be applied not only to current practices of in-vitro fertilization (IVF) and gamete donations but also to newer and emerging technologies such as prenatal genetic diagnosis (PGD), cryopreservation of ovaries, or procurement of sperm from deceased men. Such emerging possibilities are likely to result in a growing number of requests to use them as a part of ART practices. When analyzing the ethical implications of denying access to such emerging technologies, the same ethical principles offered here can be applied.

THREE CONCEPTUAL FRAMEWORKS

Three conceptual frameworks suggest themselves when considering the ethical aspects of access to ART. The first framework views ART to be comparable to natural conception and argues that denying access is never justified, having a child is seen as a basic human right. The second framework considers ART to be comparable to adoption. ART is seen as a mode of creating children and families that is not akin to sexual reproduction. Taking this view of ART leads to the normative position that society has the right and responsibility to screen candidates and deny access based on an assessment of the prospective child's welfare and best interest. The third framework offers a middle-ground approach that places ART somewhere between natural conception and adoption and therefore requires a distinctive set of criteria for screening but is more lenient toward granting and entitling access to ART services.

ART as comparable to natural conception

The first framework presumes that the right to have children is a fundamental and universal human right. It points out that ART modifies the method of conception, but not the fundamental interest in becoming a parent. It therefore argues that because liberal societies do not regulate natural conception, they should not regulate access to ART either. A few have even argued that access to ART should be constitutionally protected to the same extent as natural conception:

> Consider the analogous effect of blindness on the First Amendment right to read books. Surely a blind person has the same right to acquire information from books that a sighted person has. The inability to read visually would not bar the person from using Braille, recordings or a sighted reader to acquire the information contained in the book. ... Similarly, if bearing, begetting, or parenting children is protected as part of personal privacy or liberty, those experiences should be protected whether they are achieved coitally or noncoitally.[7]

If this argument is accepted, then denial of access is never ethically justified and all who wish to should be allowed to benefit from ART. However, this approach is problematic for a number of reasons.

First, the social investment in the creation and the maintenance of ART has no parallel in the case of natural conception. This investment justifies a degree of social input into the way ART is used. Whereas the right to conceive a child by sexual intercourse is a right to non-interference (i.e. a 'negative right'), the right to access ART in order to conceive a child, even when treatment is privately funded, is in some respects a right to services that are supported by social resources (i.e. a 'positive right'). In this respect, the right to access ART is more analogous to the right to medical care or to welfare benefits, which are typically regulated in liberal states.

The involvement of a professional team means that other parties' views and values come into play. Professionals have the autonomy not to participate in actions that conflict with their own set of moral values, as already established in cases of euthanasia, the provision of contraceptives, or abortion. Professionals may find themselves in a situation in which the services provided lead to the birth of a child under circumstances that are perceived as morally wrong. In such a case, the healthcare professional has the autonomy to refuse participation. In this respect as well, access to ART is not purely a matter of non-interference, but also a matter of being helped by others. It therefore raises the issue of whether these individuals share the view that the birth of a specific child is morally appropriate.

Some forms of ART require the involvement of third parties, such as gamete donors or surrogate mothers. It is very reasonable to argue that society carries a responsibility to protect the interests of these third parties. This is particularly important in cases where the well-off can afford to pay for the services that the less-well-off are likely to provide. Possible concerns regarding exploitation must therefore be addressed through a regulatory mechanism. There also need to be assurances given about such matters as privacy and responsibility for child support.

ART as comparable to adoption

The second approach to framing ART gives the welfare of the child paramount importance. It emphasizes the social responsibility to protect children from harm. It therefore argues that the screening of candidates for ART should be similar to the screening of candidates for adoption.

Admittedly, the same argument can be made for putting child welfare first in the case of natural conception. Indeed, some philosophers have argued that 'licensing parents' is the responsibility of the state in all cases.[8]

Yet, achieving parenthood through natural conception requires, after all, nothing but freedom from intrusion. Conception by ART is more analogous to adoption in the sense that in both cases potential parents are seeking *help*. In both cases they will be unable to become parents without a social structure that facilitates the process. This second framework therefore argues that in the case of ART, third parties (e.g. the state and its designated agencies) should have the right to screen candidates, based on criteria that focus on the welfare and best interest of the prospective child.

However, this approach is problematic as well because of the crucial difference between ART and adoption. In the case of adoption, society evaluates the adoptive parents in order to protect the interests of an *existing* child. The liberal state operates in this case under its traditional role of *parens patriae* ('father of the nation') and provides necessary protection to vulnerable individuals who already exist – in this case, the adopted child. In the case of ART, however, the child does *not* exist, and it is precisely its creation that is at the heart of the question.[9]

Creating another child that would be better-off, means creating a *different* child than the one in question, which is the reason this issue is often referred to as 'the non-identity problem' in the bioethical literature.[10] In order to argue that the birth of *this* child is not in her or his best interest, one must assume that the future circumstances of the child's life are so bleak, that non-existence is a preferable option. This argument may be convincing in very extreme cases such as knowingly creating a child with Tay–Sachs or Canavan's disease. However, it is implausible to assume that non-existence is preferable to the life of a child who will admittedly have to deal with some challenging circumstances, such as parents with disabling cognitive or emotional disorders or growing up amidst severe poverty.

A middle-ground approach

The third possibility is a 'middle-ground approach'. This framework maintains that society ought to have some say in screening candidates for ART, but that the criteria for evaluation should not be as restrictive as the ones employed in the case of an existing child, i.e. in adoption or foster care. This approach requires a careful assessment of different criteria for denying access to ART, under the assumption that in the case of a non-existing child, only the strongest justifications for denial should be accepted. The next section discusses and evaluates criteria that have been offered in the literature as potentially justifying the denial of access to ART.

POSSIBLE ETHICAL JUSTIFICATIONS FOR DENYING ACCESS TO ART

Welfare of the prospective child

Many attempts to ethically justify the denial of access to ART focus on the welfare of the prospective child. Such concerns can be divided into two broad categories: health or safety concerns and psychosocial concerns.

Health or safety concerns

One possible health concern involves passing on an undesirable inheritable condition, such as cystic fibrosis, to the future child. In such cases, it is important to refer the prospective parents to the available genetic counseling services in order to evaluate correctly the level of risk and to educate them about their possible options. Some genetic risks can justify the use of PGD, a technique in which one cell is removed from the pre-embryo and its DNA tested when it is still in vitro, so that a healthy embryo can be chosen and implanted.

More esoteric, but widely discussed in the bioethics literature, is the concern which arises in cases sometimes referred to as 'elective disability'. In these cases parents want to select for a baby that has a specific trait that is considered by many to be a disability, as in the case of choosing a deaf sperm donor in order to increase the chances for a deaf baby.[11] Whereas some of these cases may justify denying access to ART, when discussing choices with prospective parents, it is important to acknowledge and be sensitive to diverse perspectives about the value and meaning of certain biological traits to different people and communities.[12]

A second health concern arises when the prospective mother may pass on a disease, such as HIV, to the fetus. In such cases, it is important to assess her willingness to adhere to certain protocols during the pregnancy, in order to minimize the risk to the fetus. A similar concern arises when the prospective mother shows evidence of drug or alcohol abuse, which will have severe effects on the health of the developing fetus. In such cases, it is important to explore options for treating the dependency as a preliminary condition for ART. When such attempts fail, there is strong justification for denying access to ART, since the harm to the fetus is almost certain and the detrimental effect on its health and prospective life is severe. Since these effects are *avoidable* and are the outcome of the mother's *choice* to engage in unhealthy behaviors during pregnancy, it is justified to deny access to ART as long as these behaviors persist and no effort is made to manage them.

Possible safety concerns arise when there is proof of abuse or neglect of existing children, or when prospective parents may be unable to responsibly care for a child because of chronic drug or alcohol abuse, or because of a physical or mental disability, such as terminal cancer, retardation, or schizophrenia. When such concerns arise, it is important to assess on a case-by-case basis the existence of social support networks or extended family involvement, which can enhance parental capabilities and mitigate risk to the child of being without anyone willing to act as a parent.

In cases of this nature the level of risk depends on many contingencies and therefore varies greatly. General guidelines regarding such cases should point to possible safety concerns and recommend individual assessments of unique circumstances. When potential risks are assessed as probable and severe, they may justify denial. However, it is important to make sincere attempts to identify preventive strategies and to involve support networks before denying access to ART.

Psychosocial concerns

Concerns about the psychological or social conditions in which the prospective child will be raised can arise in various circumstances. Prospective parents may be living on welfare, so that concerns arise regarding their ability to provide suitable living conditions, health care, or educational opportunities. They may be a homosexual couple, so that concerns arise regarding the psychological effects on a child that is raised in a non-traditional family structure. They may be older, so that concerns arise regarding their ability to care for a child throughout the adolescent years. Or, a prospective mother may be single, so that concerns arise regarding her ability to raise a child on her own and the absence of a father figure for the optimal development of the child.

Overall, we argue that such circumstances do not provide justifications for denying access to ART. First, unlike unsafe behavior or non-adherence to a preventive protocol during pregnancy, such circumstances are not preventable but are rather an inherent component of the prospective parent's identity. One cannot become

miraculously rich or younger. Denial of access in such cases is not conditional upon some change in behavior. It is rather grounded in the belief that certain individuals do not deserve to become parents because of who they are.

The risks to the prospective child are unclear and speculative in nature. Unlike concerns about health and physical safety, it is very uncertain that any harm is likely to occur. To some degree, all children are at risk by the mere fact of being born to human parents who cannot provide an ideal environment. It is unjustified to deny certain individuals access to ART based on speculative risks that are common in the circumstances of natural conception.

In some cases, the concern arises because of a value judgment regarding what constitutes a good life. Such judgments should remain in the hands of individuals and not be made for them by institutions, professionals, or the state. A liberal society is supposed to protect liberty and respect diversity, not enforce certain ideals or a vision of what is best upon individuals.

In the context of speculative risks, it is important to highlight again the difference between assessing parental capabilities for adoption and making a decision regarding access to ART. When choosing adoptive parents, the state or its agencies are responsible for the welfare of an existing child. In the case of ART, denying access means that this child is better off not existing in the first place. This necessitates a different scale for evaluating risks than the one used for adoption.

When psychosocial concerns arise, a case-based approach is preferable to a regulatory framework that sets rigid limits on access, such as a predetermined age limit or a limitation based on family structure. In some cases, it is appropriate to assess the prospective parents' future needs and resources in order to recommend the necessary support in advance. For example, a single woman could benefit from an evaluation by a social worker that would help her assess her capability to cope with the demands of single motherhood and to identify the support networks that are available to her. In some extreme cases, such an evaluation could lead to the conclusion that the prospective parents are clearly incapable of caring for a child, in which case efforts should be made to confer resources upon them that will allow them to parent, or if such efforts fail, to dissuade them from proceeding.

Welfare of the prospective mother

In some cases, pregnancy poses significant risk to the prospective mother, as in the case of diabetes or multiple sclerosis. In such cases it is important to explain in detail the implication of the decision to become pregnant. However, if a woman chooses to proceed after she has been fully informed, denying her access to ART purely because it puts her at risk means deciding for her what is in her best interest against her explicit wishes. Such denial is based on paternalistic assumptions and is therefore unjustified.

However, two other related considerations must be mentioned. First, concerns for the safety and the health of the mother are intermingled with concerns for the welfare of the prospective child. Even if there is no risk to the developing fetus and the woman survives the pregnancy, she may suffer long-term adverse implications. She may die at an earlier age or become severely disabled, which reintroduces concerns about the quality of care the child will receive. Such concerns should be assertively discussed with the prospective mother as a part of the screening process.

Secondly, when pregnancy constitutes a serious health risk, a professional may feel that providing ART services conflicts with the basic principle of medical ethics which says 'do no harm'. The autonomy of professionals to refuse participation should be respected. In such cases, a woman should be presented with her options to seek care from another professional or at another clinic, as in the case of other controversial procedures, such as abortion, in which different professionals may hold different views regarding the service that they are asked to provide or have greater resources to bring to bear to support potential parents.

CONCLUSION

Reproductive freedom is a fundamental value. The presumption of those practicing ART should be that the interest of individuals in reproduction ought be recognized and respected. Regulations governing access to ART, and the actual practices of clinics, should be carefully scrutinized to ensure that any denial of access is ethically justified. Healthcare professionals and the organizations they work for bear the duty of justifying denials of ART services.

Serious predictable or probable risks to the health or the safety of the prospective child can justify denial of access, particularly when the risk occurs due to certain maternal behaviors during pregnancy or due to refusal to adhere to preventive protocols. Speculative concerns, especially those that are based on diverging values such as differences in culture, lifestyle, family structure, or socioeconomic status, do not provide sufficient justification for denial. The same conditions that seem to one person or community to be objectionable or even unacceptable, can be perceived by another as providing an adequate environment for raising a child. Furthermore, what some regard as the collapse of family values and the breakdown of the social fabric, others regard as a welcome emancipation that allows diverse individuals to be acknowledged as equal. Denying access to ART based on such differences is ethically unjustified and unacceptable.

REFERENCES

1. Universal Declaration of Human Rights, Adopted and proclaimed by General Assembly resolution 217 A (III) of 10 December 1948, Article 16. At: www.un.org/Overview/rights.html
2. Eisenstadt v. Baird, 405 U.S. 438 (1972); Griswold v. Connecticut, 381 US 479 (1965).
3. American Society for Reproductive Medicine (ASRM) Frequently asked questions about infertility. At: http://www.asrm.org/Patients/faqs.html
4. Cohen C. Unmanaged care: the need to regulate new reproductive technologies in the United States. Bioethics 1997; 1: 348–65.
5. Stern JE, Cramer CP, Green RM et al. Determining access to assisted reproductive technology: reactions of clinic directors to ethically complex case scenarios. Hum Reprod 2003; 18 (6): 1343–52.
6. Gurmankin AD, Caplan AL, Braverman AM. Screening practices and beliefs of assisted reproductive technology programs. Fertil Steril 2005; 83(1): 61–70.
7. Robertson J. Children of choice: freedom and the New Reproductive Technologies. Princeton, NJ: Princeton University Press, 1994.
8. LaFollette H. Licensing parents. Philosophy and Public Affairs 1980; 2: 182–97.
9. Davis DS. Genetic Dilemmas: Reproductive Technology, Parental Choices, and Children's Futures. New York: Routledge, 2001.
10. Heyd D. Genetics: Moral Issues in the Creation of People. Berkeley, CA: University of California Press 1992.
11. Dennis C. Genetics: deaf by design. Nature 2004; 431(7011): 894–6.
12. Davis DS. 'Choosing for disability.' In: Genetic Dilemmas: Reproductive Technology, Parental Choices, and Children's Futures. New York: Routledge, 2001.

45 The endometrium of polycystic ovary syndrome

Linda C Giudice and Bruce A Lessey

Synopsis

Background

- Polycystic ovary syndrome (PCOS) is the most common endocrine disorder in reproductive-aged women.
- Features of PCOS include hyperandrogenism, and ovulatory dysfunction, and many women have hyperinsulinemia and insulin resistance.
- Infertility and pregnancy loss are common features of PCOS and may reflect abnormal response of the endometrium to an altered hormonal milieu.
- Evidence suggests that the endometrium of women with PCOS may be prone to the development of hyperplasia or even cancer.

Basic Science

- Repair of the endometrium begins with the exposed ends of the endometrial glands, reconstituting an intact luminal surface.
- Ovarian estrogen stimulates the production of estrogen receptors providing the signal for proliferation, while at the same time increasing expression of progesterone and androgen receptors in the endometrium.
- Hypertrophy and thickening of the cycling endometrium is normally limited because progesterone from the corpus luteum arrests growth and promotes differentiation.
- The balance between cyclic estrogen and progesterone provides the endocrine signals that prepare the endometrium for implantation.
- Under the direction of progesterone and growth factors such as insulin-like growth factors (IGFs), the stroma of the endometrium normally undergoes a process of decidualization.
- Women with PCOS have endometrium that exhibits a loss of menstrual cyclicity due to oligo- or anovulation. As a result, many of the hormonal events that restrain cell proliferation are lacking.
- The loss of menstrual cyclicity and the altered hormonal milieu in PCOS women result in a host of molecular changes in the PCOS endometrium, many of which persist into the secretory phase, when these women undergo ovulation induction.
- Altered estrogen and progesterone receptors, defects in enzymatic activity, overexpression of androgen receptors and steroid receptor coactivators, and increased proliferation are all seen in PCOS endometrium, compared to normal endometrium.

Clinical

- Persistent anovulation in PCOS is frequently associated with hyperinsulinemia and clinical evidence of elevated serum androgen concentrations.
- Endometrial growth and differentiation in women with PCOS is influenced by the combined effects of androgens, insulin, and unopposed estrogens.
- Women with PCOS experience a higher than expected incidence of miscarriage and a lower overall cycle fecundability, compared to normal cycling women.
- Increased risk of endometrial hyperplasia and endometrial adenocarcinoma are seen in women with PCOS, especially those who do not seek treatment for anovulation or amenorrhea.

- Biomarkers of uterine receptivity are found to be altered in the endometrium or serum of women with PCOS, suggesting methods to evaluate the reproductive potential in women suspected of having this disorder.
- The goals for treatment of women with PCOS include reducing the impact of hyperandrogenism or hyper-insulinemia, restoring menstrual regularity, and preventing the development of endometrial hyperplasia or cancer.

ABSTRACT

Polycystic ovary syndrome (PCOS) is a common endocrinopathy, characterized by oligo/anovulation and elevated circulating androgens or evidence of hyperandrogenism, after all known potential causes have been excluded. In addition, insulin resistance and accompanying hyperinsulinemia commonly occur in women with PCOS. There is increasing evidence that the endocrinological and metabolic abnormalities in PCOS may have complex effects on the endometrium, contributing to infertility and endometrial disorders observed in women with this syndrome. Androgen receptors and steroid receptor coactivators are overexpressed in the endometrium of women with PCOS. Also, biomarkers of endometrial receptivity to embryonic implantation, such as $\alpha_v\beta_3$ integrin and glycodelin, are decreased, and epithelial expression of ERα abnormally persists in the window of implantation in endometrium in women with PCOS. In addition to being responsive to the steroid hormones estradiol, progesterone, and androgens, the endometrium is also a target for insulin, whose receptor is cyclically regulated in normo-ovulatory women. In vitro, insulin inhibits the normal process of endometrial stromal differentiation (decidualization). In addition, insulin-like growth factors (IGFs) and their binding proteins (IGFBPs) are regulated in and act on endometrial cellular constituents, and hyperinsulinemia down-regulates hepatic IGFBP-1, resulting in elevated free IGF-I in the circulation. Thus, elevated estrogen (without the opposing effects of progesterone in the absence of ovulation), hyperinsulinemia, elevated free IGF-I and androgens, and obesity probably contribute to endometrial dysfunction, infertility, increased miscarriage rate, endometrial hyperplasia, and endometrial cancer common in women with PCOS. The potential mechanisms underlying these disorders, specifically in women with PCOS, are complex and await additional transdisciplinary research for their complete elucidation.

INTRODUCTION

The endometrium, like breast and prostate, is regulated primarily by steroid hormones and growth factors. As a major target tissue for steroid hormones, the altered hormonal milieu in women with hyperandrogenism or hyperinsulinism associated with PCOS is reflected in the endometrium of affected women. Polycystic ovary syndrome is a common endocrine disorder, affecting approximately 6–8% of reproductive-age women.[1,2] Common symptoms include menstrual irregularity and ovulatory dysfunction. By definition, PCOS patients exhibit hyperandrogenism and approximately 75% of women with PCOS have insulin resistance and hyperinsulinemia and about 50% have elevated levels of circulation luteinizing hormone (LH).[3-5] A balanced and sequential exposure to both estrogen and progesterone yields an orchestrated pattern of gene expression, resulting in a synchronized period of uterine receptivity towards embryonic implantation.[6] Conversely, altered endocrine changes may render the endometrium aberrant in women with PCOS.

Infertility associated with PCOS derives from chronic anovulation, and there are emerging data that suggest higher implantation failure and rates of miscarriage in women with this disorder.[7-10] In addition, women with PCOS experience higher risks of endometrial hyperplasia and endometrial cancer.[11-14] Even once ovulatory status is restored, there now appear to be intrinsic differences between normal and PCOS endometrium that may predispose these women to poor reproductive outcome. In this chapter, we review the studies that support the clinical manifestations of implantation failure, miscarriage, endometrial hyperplasia, and cancer and the role of chronic, unopposed estrogens, hyperinsulinemia, and hyperandrogenism, and effects of members of the epidermal growth factor (EGF) and IGF family on endometrial structure and function.

THE MENSTRUAL CYCLE AND ITS DISTURBANCES IN PCOS

The cyclic changes observed as part of the normal menstrual cycle begin with the remnants of the shed endometrium following menstruation. Cells of the basalis layer rapidly regenerate and undergo hypertrophy and proliferation in response to estradiol from the developing ovarian follicle. From a thickness of approximately 2 mm, the endometrium thickens to 10–12 mm during the proliferative phase. Reconstitution of the luminal surface epithelium appears to be an early event. Members of the Wnt family, including Wnt7a from the luminal epithelium, provide a soluble signal to the underlying stroma to stimulate paracrine mechanisms of cell proliferation.[15] The rising concentration of ovarian estradiol regulates its own receptors (ERα) and those of progesterone (PR), priming the endometrium to full responsiveness by the time of ovulation.[16] This interval of proliferation is normally self-limited, followed by transformation of the thickened endometrium in response to progesterone during the secretory phase of the menstrual cycle. Progesterone, derived from the corpus luteum, arrests the proliferating endometrium and transforms it into a secretory structure that is capable of supporting embryonic growth and subsequent embryo implantation. Progesterone down-regulates both ERα and PR, and induces enzymes that reduce the impact of estradiol on the endometrium.[17] Besides its role in establishing uterine receptivity, progesterone also sets the stage for menstruation, should pregnancy not occur, and promotes apoptosis and cell death when progesterone is withdrawn.[18,19]

A recent global gene expression profiling study has demonstrated patterns of gene expression that recapitulate the functional characteristics of these phases of the cycle.[6] (For a complete review, see Chapter 14.) These studies reveal interesting and sharply defined segments of functional activity. The proteins expressed during the proliferative phase are primarily dedicated to DNA replication, cell proliferation, and tissue remodeling. After ovulation and the production of progesterone, the endometrium undergoes a striking series of changes, including inhibition of cellular proliferation, DNA synthesis, and cellular mitotic activity, and the onset of cellular differentiation, in preparation for an implanting conceptus. With the onset of uterine receptivity in the mid secretory phase, the endometrium shifts the emphasis of its cellular activity from the epithelium to the stromal compartment.

As outlined in Chapter 20, it is during this period of differentiation that the endometrium becomes receptive to embryonic implantation for a brief period, now commonly called the 'window of implantation'. Endometrial stromal cells undergo the process of decidualization, in response to progesterone, a process that is characterized by changes in the cytoskeleton (down-regulation of smooth muscle actin) and induction or up-regulation of prolactin, IGFs, IGFBPs, the insulin receptor, relaxin, and others.[9,13] Progesterone receptors continue to be strongly expressed in the decidua, while nearly absent in the epithelial compartment.[16,20] The stroma also adopts other epithelial phenotypes, including acquisition of certain integrins and cell adhesion molecules.[21] The decidualization of the stroma is important to the regulation of trophoblast invasion and to establish a cytokine milieu and immunomodulatory network in the stroma, should implantation occur. In the absence of embryonic implantation, withdrawal of progesterone initiates changes in gene expression that initiate inflammation, tissue digestion involving increased production of metalloproteinases and prostaglandins,[6] along with cellular apoptosis, resulting in endometrial tissue desquamation and menstruation. The menstrual phase also marks the initiation of the next wave of regeneration, with specific biochemical changes that support angiogenesis and increased steroid responsiveness.[22–24]

In women with PCOS, a loss of menstrual cyclicity due to oligo- or anovulation is a common finding.[5] With the loss of menstrual cyclicity, the regulatory roles of progesterone and progesterone withdrawal in the endometrium are suboptimal or absent. Moreover, an incessant stimulation by low-to-moderate levels of estrogen stimulates cell proliferation and hypertrophy. Thus, endometrial tissue in women with PCOS is in a state of a relatively enhanced response to estrogen and does not undergo the sequential changes in gene expression and associated biochemical processes that result in normal endometrial cellular growth, differentiation, and eventual tissue desquamation. The patterns of endometrial bleeding in women with PCOS vary from irregular menses to amenorrhea, reflecting the oligo-ovulatory and anovulatory states. Excessive endometrial hypertrophy may also lead to irregular endometrial breakdown, resulting in sporadic and sometimes prolonged episodes of menstrual-like bleeding.

Persistent anovulation in women with PCOS is frequently associated with hyperinsulinemia and hyperandrogenemia. Insulin resistance also leads to elevated levels of circulating fasting and postprandial insulin levels.[3] The mean total testosterone, free testosterone, androstenedione, dehydroepiandrosterone sulfate (DHEAS), and body mass index (BMI) are also higher in women with PCOS compared to control women.[4] The moderately elevated levels of estrogen encountered in PCOS are due in part to increased peripheral conversion of androstenedione to estrone in adipose tissue, and free estradiol and testosterone are elevated in the circulation in the setting of hyperinsulinemia, due, in part, to insulin down-regulation of sex hormone binding globulin (SHBG).[25,26] Furthermore, diminished progesterone

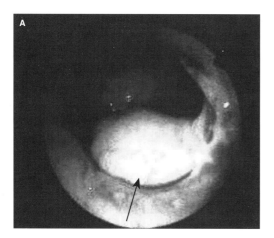
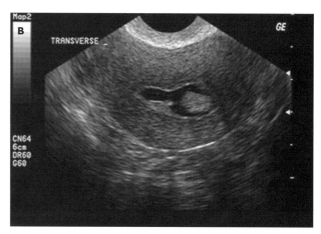

Figure 45.1   Sonohystogram of the endometrial cavity in a women with polycystic ovary syndrome, showing an endometrial polyp (**B**). The polyp was visualized and removed through operative hysteroscopy (**A**).

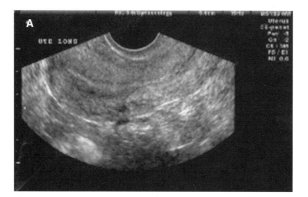
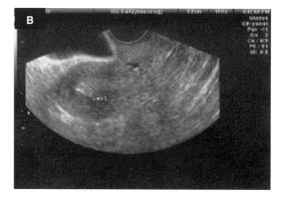

Figure 45.2   Ultrasound appearance of two patients with PCOS and 6 months of amenorrhea. (**A**) In this case, the endometrium was thin, despite prolonged amenorrhea. (**B**) In this patient with PCOS, the endometrium is thickened. Such differences may depend on the level of circulating estrogen, androgens, or intrinsic differences in the endometrium.

action reduces the enzymatic conversion of estradiol to its less active estrone.

Thus, endometrial growth and differentiation in women with PCOS are influenced by the combined effects of androgens, insulin, and unopposed estrogens. In the absence of ovulatory progesterone, the endometrium fails to undergo normal secretory transformation and is continuously exposed to a stimulatory and mitogenic effect of estrogen that can lead to endometrial overgrowth, unpredictable bleeding patterns, hyperplasia, and cancer.[12,13,27,28] Such a propensity for proliferation is also reflected in an increased risk for endometrial polyp formation[29] (Figure 45.1).

Lunenfeld and colleagues described the poor reproductive potential of women with PCOS compared to normal women and those with hypothalamic amenorrhea, once ovulatory function was restored.[30]

On ultrasound, the endometrial appearance in PCOS women is sometimes excessively thin and hyperechoic. Androgens, like progesterone, are antiproliferative in the endometrium.[31] While unopposed stimulatory effects of estrogen might lead to hyperplasia, another concern about the endometrium in PCOS is a thin and poorly responsive uterine lining. Unlike the typical trilaminar-appearing endometrium seen by ultrasound in normal cycling women, the lining in PCOS women is often hyperechoic in appearance. Response to prolonged amenorrhea may vary between PCOS women and depend on overall hormone levels as well as individual differences (Figure 45.2). As outlined below, the androgen receptors of PCOS endometrium are overexpressed in the PCOS endometrium compared to normal women, making this even more likely due to the hyperandrogenic state of PCOS.[32]

ALTERED STEROID HORMONE RECEPTORS AND COACTIVATORS IN PCOS ENDOMETRIUM

Steroid hormone receptor expression in human endometrium is cycle-dependent.[16,33] The main ER in cycling endometrium is ERα and it is up-regulated by estrogen, peaking in the late proliferative phase in epithelium and stroma. ERα expression in both epithelium and stroma is markedly inhibited in the mid secretory phase by progesterone.[20,34,35] ERβ is mainly expressed in the endometrial vascular endothelium.[35] Progesterone receptors peak at ovulation, similar to ERα, and decrease in the secretory phase under the regulation of progesterone.[16,20] Androgen receptors (ARs) are expressed in endometrial stroma and epithelium in normo-ovulatory women and decrease steadily from the early proliferative phase to the midsecretory phase with little, if any, immunostaining for the AR in the late luteal phase.[33] In-vitro studies of endometrial stroma and epithelial cells demonstrate that AR is up-regulated by estrogens and androgens and is inhibited by progestins and EGF.[32] In addition, administration of the antiprogestin mifepristone results in elevated AR expression in human and non-human primate endometrium,[36] although the mechanism of this effect remains poorly understood. Women with PCOS exhibit elevated endometrial AR expression compared to normal fertile controls,[32,37] probably due to elevated estrogen and androgens and diminished progesterone, supported by both in-vivo and in-vitro models.[38,39]

Like AR, elevations in ERα has been observed in PCOS endometrium, especially during the secretory phase.[37,40] As described in endometriosis, there appears to be a progesterone insensitivity in PCOS endometrium, even once ovulatory status has been achieved. Reduced progesterone action perhaps due to hyperandrogenemia, might explain the higher levels of secretory ERα observed in PCOS. There is increasing evidence of dysregulated expression of other progesterone-regulated endometrial biomarkers, including secretory products and some of the markers of uterine receptivity, in endometrial epithelium of women with PCOS. For example, in-vitro studies demonstrate that androstendione inhibits secretion of glycodelin, an important secretory product of endometrial epithelium during the receptive phase of implantation, and this effect is reversed by cyproterone acetate, an androgen antagonist.[41] While it is tempting to speculate that such dysregulation may be present in women with PCOS, leading to lower implantation rates, currently there are no data to support this.

Steroid receptor co-activators (SRCs) are accessory nuclear proteins that stabilize steroid receptor transcription complexes and greatly enhance the actions of steroid hormones.[42] While the studies of the p160 steroid receptor co-activators are limited, it appears that SRC1 is the predominant isoform present in normal endometrium.[40,43,44] It was shown that SRCs are overexpressed in the endometrium of PCOS.[40,45] In-vitro studies clearly show that overexpression of AIB1 and TIF2, two of these coactivators, renders the cells more responsive to estrogen.[40] That this heightened estrogen sensitivity could lead to hyperplasia or cancer is supported by the finding of increased coactivator expression in neoplastic endometrium.[43] Lessey and colleagues recently described the overexpression of estrogen responsive proteins in PCOS endometrium, including Cyr61, cFos, and markers of cell proliferation in PCOS endometrium, compared to normal controls.[46] These same markers of estrogen actions are increased in endometrial hyperplasia and cancer, as well.

BIOMARKERS OF UTERINE RECEPTIVITY IN PCOS ENDOMETRIUM

Glycodelin (also known as PP14) and insulin-like growth factor binding protein-1 (IGFBP-1; PP12) are two of the most highly expressed proteins in the secretory endometrium.[47–50] IGFBP-1 appears to have a role during embryo attachment and invasion[51–53] and is reduced in abnormal placentation.[54] IGFBP-1 has also been shown to be reduced in the endometrium of women with PCOS.[55] Glycodelin has been shown to be reduced in the endometrium of women with luteal phase defect and early pregnancy loss.[56–58] Both IGFBP-1 and glycodelin are reduced in women with PCOS compared to controls.[59] Interestingly, treatment of hyperinsulinemia with metformin resulted in an increase in both markers compared to the untreated controls.[59]

Another marker of uterine receptivity is integrin $\alpha_v\beta_3$.[60–62] This luminal surface marker appears during the mid secretory phase and is delayed or absent in many types of infertility.[63–65] This biomarker is delayed in its presentation on the endometrial surface in luteal phase defect;[60,66] it is either delayed in its expression or is not expressed at all in many cases of PCOS.[32] A critical regulator of this integrin is estrogen, functioning as an inhibitor of the $\alpha_v\beta_3$ integrin in endometrial epithelium.[67] As the down-regulation of ERα in epithelium heralds the opening of the window of implantation,[16,20] the expression of ERα in endometrium from women with PCOS in the mid secretory phase[40] might explain the reduced expression of this biomarker in PCOS endometrium. Taylor and colleagues have also shown that a key developmental gene, HOXA10 (an endometrial biomarker), stimulates integrin $\alpha_v\beta_3$ expression.[68] Since HOXA10 has been shown to be reduced by androgens, this could also account for the absence of integrin $\alpha_v\beta_3$ in the endometrium of PCOS women.[69] Collectively, these data on glycodelin, IGFBP-1, integrin $\alpha_v\beta_3$, HOXA10, and ERα suggest poor endometrial development in women with PCOS with occasional spontaneous ovulatory cycles, presumably due to inadequate progesterone action, although dysregulation by androgens or insulin cannot be excluded.

The endometrium is also a target for insulin, which probably acts through its own receptor and perhaps through the structurally similar IGF type I receptor.[70] The insulin receptor is up-regulated in the secretory phase of the cycle, a result of progesterone action in this tissue.[6] In vitro, insulin inhibits production of the endometrial stromal product, IGFBP-1, a biomarker of decidualization.[71] A recent study by Lathi et al[70] demonstrated that inhibition of IGFBP-1 in human endometrial stromal cells by low doses of insulin is mediated via the PIK3 (phosphatidylinositol 3-kinase) pathway, whereas at higher doses the MAPK (mitogen-activated protein kinase) pathway is also activated. Insulin may play a homeostatic role for energy metabolism in the endometrium at physiological levels, and in hyperinsulinemic states may activate cellular mitosis via the MAPK pathway, predisposing the endometrium to hyperplasia and/or cancer. In-vivo actions of insulin on the endometrium are difficult to distinguish from the actions of androgens, since hyperandrogenism and hyperinsulinemia are both frequently found in women with anovulation and PCOS.[72]

Like EGF, the IGF system is an important participant in endometrial proliferation, development, and implantation.[73] IGF-I is expressed primarily in the epithelium more than stroma, during the proliferative phase and, along with EGF, is one of two major growth factors that are 'estromedins' in this phase of the cycle.[73,74] IGF-II is expressed primarily in epithelium more than stroma in the secretory phase, is regulated by progesterone, and has been considered to be a 'progestomedin'.[74,75] IGF-I and IGF-II are mitogenic to endometrial cells in culture and can regulate secretory functions of stromal cells.[75,76] The decidualized endometrial stromal cells also inhibit IGF actions through the elaboration of the IGF binding proteins (primarily IGFBP-1), with binding affinities that are two orders of magnitude greater than the type I IGF receptor.[77] Conversely, IGFs (in addition to insulin) inhibit IGFBP-1 production and steady-state mRNA levels in human endometrial stromal cells in-vitro.[76] Thus, in PCOS endometrium, with hyperinsulinemia and prolonged unopposed estrogen, IGF-I may further augment the mitogenic activity of endometrial cells, leading to acceleration of hyperplasia and perhaps transformation to cancer.

CONCLUSIONS

PCOS is a complex disorder with metabolic and endocrine manifestations. Women with this disorder have both infertility and a heightened risk for endometrial neoplasia that appears to reflect an altered endocrine and paracrine milieu. Despite these emerging data to suggest the endometrium is abnormal, few studies have focused on the medical management of such defects. Increased cell proliferation and decreased expression of secretory endometrial biomarkers may be related to low progesterone, elevated insulin, free IGF-I, androgens, or altered steroid receptors or coactivators. Some of the data for these associations are firm; however, some of the data are conflicting, and further research is necessary to understand the poor reproductive performance in women with this disorder. Insulin and androgens have direct effects on endometrial function in vitro, including impairment of normal decidualization. Alternations in epithelial/stromal interactions may also be causative, although studies on paracrine interactions in PCOS are few. Chronic lack of progesterone and IGFBP production, accompanying anovulation, hyperinsulinemia, and hyperandrogenemia, may translate into a net stimulatory effect on endometrial proliferation, poor endometrial development, and endometrial hyperplasia and cancer. While preliminary studies using insulin sensitizers have shown improvement of circulating insulin and androgen levels, as well as improved reproductive performance,[59,78] further investigation is needed to determine the mechanism(s) of insulin action and the role of the IGF system in endometrial function and implantation. Development of optimal therapies for women with PCOS in the treatment of infertility and prevention of endometrial hyperplasia and cancer will require an integrated, concerted, and multidisciplinary research effort.

REFERENCES

1. Goodarzi MO, Azziz R. Diagnosis, epidemiology, and genetics of the polycystic ovary syndrome. Best Pract Res Clin Endocrinol Metab 2006; 20: 193–205.
2. Homburg R, Giudice LC, Chang RJ. Polycystic ovary syndrome. Hum Reprod 1996; 11: 465.

3. DeUgarte CM, Bartolucci AA, Azziz R. Prevalence of insulin resistance in the polycystic ovary syndrome using the homeostasis model assessment. Fertil Steril 2005; 83: 1454–60.

4. Kumar A, Woods KS, Bartolucci AA, Azziz R. Prevalence of adrenal androgen excess in patients with the polycystic ovary syndrome (PCOS). Clin Endocrinol (Oxf) 2005; 62: 644–9.

5. Azziz R, Carmina E, Dewailly D et al. Positions statement: criteria for defining polycystic ovary syndrome as a predominantly hyperandrogenic syndrome: an Androgen Excess Society guideline. J Clin Endocrinol Metab 2006; 91: 4237–45.

6. Talbi S, Hamilton AE, VO KC et al. Molecular phenotyping of human endometrium distinguishes menstrual cycle phases and underlying biological processes in normo-ovulatory women. Endocrinology 2006; 147: 1097–121.

7. Balen AH, Tan SL, Jacobs HS. Hypersecretion of luteinising hormone: a significant cause of infertility and miscarriage. Br J Obstet Gynaecol 1993; 100: 1082–9.

8. Balen AH, Tan SL, MacDougall J, Jacobs HS. Miscarriage rates following in-vitro fertilization are increased in women with polycystic ovaries and reduced by pituitary desensitization with buserelin. Hum Reprod 1993; 8: 959–64.

9. Okon MA, Laird SM, Tuckerman EM, Li TC. Serum androgen levels in women who have recurrent miscarriages and their correlation with markers of endometrial function. Fertil Steril 1998; 69: 682–90.

10. Fedorcsak P, Storeng R, Dale PO et al. Obesity is a risk factor for early pregnancy loss after IVF or ICSI. Acta Obstet Gynecol Scand 2000; 79: 43–8.

11. Speert H. Carcinoma of the endometrium in young women. Surg Gynecol Obstet 1949; 88: 332–6.

12. Pillay OC, Te Fong LF, Crow JC et al. The association between polycystic ovaries and endometrial cancer. Hum Reprod 2006; 21: 924–9.

13. Hardiman P, Pillay OC, Atiomo W. Polycystic ovary syndrome and endometrial carcinoma. Lancet 2003; 361: 1810–12.

14. Niwa K, Imai A, Hashimoto M et al. A case-control study of uterine endometrial cancer of pre- and post-menopausal women. Oncol Rep 2000; 7: 89–93.

15. Tulac S, Nayak LC, Kao LC et al. Identification, characterization, and regulation of the canonical Wnt signaling pathway in human endometrium. J Clin Endocrinol Metab 2003; 88: 3860–6.

16. Lessey BA, Killam AP, Metzger DA et al. Immunohistochemical analysis of human uterine estrogen and progesterone receptors throughout the menstrual cycle. J Clin Endocrinol Metab 1988; 67: 334–40.

17. Vihko R, Maentausta O, Isomaa V et al. Human 17 beta-hydroxy steroid dehydrogenase in normal and malignant endometrium. Ann NY Acad Sci 1991; 622: 392–401.

18. Dahmoun M, Boman K, Cajander S et al. Apoptosis, proliferation, and sex hormone receptors in superficial parts of human endometrium at the end of the secretory phase. J Clin Endocrinol Metab 1999; 84: 1737–43.

19. Lovely LP, Fazleabas AT, Fritz MA, McAdams DG, Lessey BA. Prevention of endometrail apoptosis: randomized prospective comparison of human chorionic gonadotropin versus progesterone treatment in the luteal phase. J Clin Endocrinol Metab 2005; 90: 235–6.

20. Garcia E, Bouchard P, De Brux J et al. Use of immunocyto chemistry of progesterone and estrogen receptors for endometrial dating. J Clin Endocrinol Metab 1988; 67: 80–7.

21. Ruck P, Marzusch K, Kaiserling E et al. Distribution of cell adhesion molecules in decidua of early human pregnancy. An immunohistochemical study. Lab Invest 1994; 71: 94–101.

22. Nayak NR, Critchley HOD, Slayden OD et al. Progesterone withdrawal up-regulates vascular endothelial growth factor receptor type 2 in the superficial zone stroma of the human and macaque endometrium: potential relevance to menstruation. J Clin Endocrinol Metab 2000; 85: 3442–52.

23. Wieser F, Schneeberger C, Hudelist G et al. Endometrial nuclear receptor co-factors SRC-1 and N-CoR are increased in human endometrium during menstruation. Mol Hum Reprod 2002; 8: 644–50.

24. Salamonsen LA, Kovacs GT, Findlay JK. Current concepts of the mechanisms of menstruation. Baillieres Best Pract Res Clin Obstet Gynaecol 1999; 13: 161–79.

25. Nestler JE, Powers LP, Matt DW et al. A direct effect of hyperinsulinemia on serum sex hormone-binding globulin levels in obese women with the polycystic ovary syndrome. J Clin Endocrinol Metab 1991; 72: 83–9.

26. Robinson S, Kiddy D, Gelding SV et al. The relationship of insulin insensitivity to menstrual pattern in women with hyperandrogenism and polycystic ovaries. Clin Endocrinol (Oxf) 1993; 39: 351–5.

27. Elliott JL, Hosford SL, Demopoulos RI et al. Endometrial adenocarcinoma and polycystic ovarian syndrome: risk factors, management, and prognosis. South Med J 2001; 94: 529–31.

28. Aksel S, Wentz AC, Jones GS. Anovulatory infertility associated with adenocarcinoma and adenomatous hyperplasia of the endometrium. Obstet Gynecol 1974; 43: 386–91.

29. Dallenbach-Hellweg G. The endometrium of infertility. A review. Pathol Res Pract 1984; 178: 527–37.

30. Dor J, Itzkowic DJ, Mashiach S,et al. Cumulative conception rates following gonadotropin therapy. Am J Obstet Gynecol 1980; 136: 102–5.

31. Brenner RM, Slayden OD, Nayak NR et al. A role for the androgen receptor in the endometrial antiproliferative effects of progesterone antagonists. Steroids 2003; 68: 1033–9.

32. Apparao KB, Lovely LP, Gui Y, et al. Elevated endometrial androgen receptor expression in women with polycystic ovarian syndrome. Biol Reprod 2002; 66: 297–304.

33. Mertens HJ, Heineman MJ, Theunissen PH et al. Androgen, estrogen and progesterone receptor expression in the human uterus during the menstrual cycle. Eur J Obstet Gynecol Reprod Biol 2001; 98: 58–65.

34. Lessey BA, Palomino WA, Apparao KB et al. Estrogen receptor-alpha (ER-alpha) and defects in uterine receptivity in women. Reprod Biol Endocrinol 2006; 4(Suppl 1): S9.

35. Hess A, Nayak NR, Giudice LC. Cyclic changes in primate oviduct and endometrium. In: Knobil E, Neill JD, eds. The Physiology of Reproduction. San Diego: Academic Press, 2005.

36. Slayden OD, Nayak NR, Burton KA et al. Progesterone antagonists increase androgen receptor expression in the rhesus macaque and human endometrium. J Clin Endocrinol Metab 2001; 86: 2668–79.

37. Villavicencio A, Bacallao K, Avellaira C et al. Androgen and estrogen receptors and co-regulators levels in endometria from patients with polycystic ovarian syndrome with and without endometrial hyperplasia. Gynecol Oncol 2006; 103: 307–14.

38. Fujimoto J, Nishigaki M, Hori M et al. The effect of estrogen and androgen on androgen receptors and mRNA levels in uterine leiomyoma, myometrium and endometrium of human subjects. J Steroid Biochem Mol Biol 1994; 50: 137–43.

39. Lovely LP, AppaRao KBC, Gui Y, Lessey BA. Characterization of the androgen receptor in a well-differentiated endometrial adenocarcinoma cell line (Ishikawa). J Steroid Biochem Mol Biol 2000; 74: 235–41.

40. Gregory CW, Wilson EM, Apparao KB et al. Steroid receptor coactivator expression throughout the menstrual cycle in normal and abnormal endometrium. J Clin Endocrinol Metab 2002; 87: 2960–6.

41. Tuckerman EM, Okon MA, LiTC, Laird SM. Do androgens have a direct effect on endometrial function? An in vitro study. Fertil Steril 2000; 74: 771–9.

42. McDonnell DP. The molecular determinants of estrogen receptor pharmacology. Maturitas 2004; 48(Suppl1): S7–12.

43. Uchikawa J, Shiozawa T, Shih HC et al. Expression of steroid receptor coactivators and corepressors in human endometrial hyperplasia and carcinoma with relevance to steroid receptors and Ki-67 expression. Cancer 2003; 98: 2207–13.

44. Shiozawa T, Shih HC, Miyamoto T et al. Cyclic changes in the expression of steroid receptor coactivators and corepressors in the normal human endometrium. J Clin Endocrinol Metab 2003; 88: 871–8.

45. Quezada S, Avellaira C, Johnson MC et al. Evaluation of steroid receptors, coregulators, and molecules associated with uterine receptivity in secretory endometria from untreated women with polycystic ovary syndrome. Fertil Steril 2006; 85: 1017–26.

46. MacLaughlin SD, Palomino WA, Mo B, Lessey BA. Cyr61 expression in normal and abnormal endometrium. ACOG National Meeting, 2006.

47. Joshi SG. Progestin-regulated proteins of the human endometrium. Semin Reprod Endocrinol 1983; 1: 221.

48. Julkunen M, Koistinen R, Sjoberg J et al. Secretory endometrium synthesizes placental protein 14. Endocrinology 1986; 118: 1782–6.

49. Bischof P. Three pregnancy proteins (PP12, PP14, and PAPP-A): their biological and clinical relevance. Am J Perinatol 1989; 6: 110–16.

50. Rutanen EM, Koistinen R, Seppala M et al. Progesterone-associated proteins PP12 and PP14 in the human endometrium. J Steroid Biochem 1987; 27: 25–31.

51. Giudice LC, Irwin JC, Dsupin BA et al. Insulin-like growth factor (IGF), IGF binding protein (IGFBP), and IGF receptor gene expression and IGFBP synthesis in human uterine leiomyomata. Hum Reprod 1993; 8: 1796–806.

52. Giudice LC, Mark SP, Irwin JC. Paracrine actions of insulin-like growth factors and IGF binding protein-1 in non-pregnant human endometrium and at the decidual–trophoblast interface. J Reprod Immunol 1998; 39: 133–48.

53. Irwin JC, Giudice LC. Insulin-like growth factor binding protein-1 binds to cytotrophoblast $\alpha_5\beta_1$ integrin and inhibits cytotrophoblast invasion into decidual multilayers. Soc Gynecol Invest Ann Mtg 1996; 3: 93A.

54. Irwin JC, Suen LF, Martina NA et al. Role of the IGF system in trophoblast invasion and pre-eclampsia. Hum Reprod 1999; 14(Suppl 2): 90.

55. Suikkari AM, Ruutiainen K, Erkkola R, Seppala M. Low levels of low molecular weight insulin-like growth factor-binding protein in patients with polycystic ovarian disease. Hum Reprod 1989; 4: 136–9.

56. Dalton CF, Laird SM, Serle E et al. The measurement of CA 125 and placental protein 14 in uterine flushings in women with recurrent miscarriage; relation to endometrial morphology. Hum Reprod 1995; 10: 2680–4.

57. Klentzeris LD, Bulmer JN, Seppälä M et al. Placental protein 14 in cycles with normal and retarded endometrial differentiation. Hum Reprod 1994; 9: 394–8.

58. Tulppala M, Julkunen M, Tiitinen A et al. Habitual abortion is accompanied by low serum levels of placental protein 14 in the luteal phase of the fertile cycle. Fertil Steril 1995; 63: 792–5.

59. Jakubowicz DJ, Seppälä M, Jakubowicz S et al. Insulin reduction with metformin increases luteal phase serum glycodelin and insulin-like growth factor-binding protein 1 concentrations and enhances uterine vascularity and blood flow in the polycystic ovary syndrome. J Clin Endocrinol Metab 2001; 86: 1126–33.

60. Lessey BA, Damjanovich L, Coutifaris C et al. Integrin adhesion molecules in the human endometrium. Correlation with the normal and abnormal menstrual cycle. J Clin Invest 1992; 90: 188–95.

61. Lessey BA, Castelbaum AJ, Buck CA et al. Further characterization of endometrial integrins during the menstrual cycle and in pregnancy. Fertil and Steril 1994; 62: 497–506.

62. Lessey BA, Castelbaum AJ. Integrins and implantation in the human. Rev Endocr Metab Disord 2002; 3: 107–17.

63. Lessey BA, Castelbaum AJ, Sawin SJ, Sun J. Integrins as markers of uterine receptivity in women with primary unexplained infertility. Fertil Steril 1995; 63: 535–42.

64. Meyer WR, Castelbaum AJ, Somkuti S et al. Hydrosalpinges adversely affect markers of endometrial receptivity. Hum Reprod 1997; 12: 1393–8.

65. Lessey BA, Castelbaum AJ, Sawin SW et al. Aberrant integrin expression in the endometrium of women with endometriosis. J Clin Endocrinol Metab 1994; 79: 643–9.

66. Creus M, Balasch J, Ordi J et al. Integrin expression in normal and out-of-phase endometria. Hum Reprod 1998; 13: 3460–8.

67. Somkuti SG, Yuan L, Fritz MA, Lessey BA. Epidermal growth factor and sex steroids dynamically regulate a marker of endometrial receptivity in Ishikawa cells. J Clin Endocrinol Metab 1997; 82: 2192–7.

68. Daftary GS, Troy PJ, Bagot CN et al. Direct regulation of beta3-integrin subunit gene expression by HOXA10 in endometrial cells. Mol Endocrinol 2002; 16: 571–9.

69. Cermik D, Selam B, Taylor HS. Regulation of HOXA-10 expression by testosterone in vitro and in the endometrium of patients with polycystic ovary syndrome. J Clin Endocrinol Metab 2003; 88: 238–43.

70. Lathi RB, Hess AP, Tulac S et al. Dose-dependent insulin regulation of insulin-like growth factor binding protein-1 in human endometrial stromal cells is mediated by distinct signaling pathways. J Clin Endocrinol Metab 2005; 90: 1599–606.

71. Giudice LC, Dsupin BA, Irwin JC. Steroid and peptide regulation of insulin-like growth factor-binding proteins secreted by human endometrial stromal cells is dependent on stromal differentiation. J Clin Endocrinol Metab 1992; 75: 1235–41.

72. Dunaif A. Insulin resistance and the polycystic ovarian syndrome: mechanisms and implications for pathogenesis. Endocr Rev 1997; 18: 774–800.

73. Nayak NR, Giudice LC. Comparative biology of the IGF system in endometrium, decidua, and placenta, and clinical implications for foetal growth and implantation disorders. Placenta 2003; 24: 281–96.

74. Zhou J, Dsupin BA, Giudice LC, Bondy CA. Insulin-like growth factor system gene expression in human endometrium during the menstrual cycle. J Clin Endocrinol Metab 1994; 79: 1723–34.

75. Frost RA, Mazella J, Tseng L. Insulin-like growth factor binding protein-1 inhibits the mitogenic effect of insulin-like growth factors and progestins in human endometrial stromal cells. Biol Reprod 1993; 49: 104–11.

76. Irwin JC, de las Fuentes L, Dsupin BA, Giudice LC. Insulin-like growth factor regulation of human endometrial stromal cell function: coordinate effects on insulin-like growth factor binding protein-1, cell proliferation and prolactin secretion. Regul Pept 1993; 48: 165–77.

77. Ballard FJ, Walton PE, Bastian S et al. Effects of interactions between IGFBPs and IGFs on the plasma clearance and in vivo biological activities of IGFs and IGF analogs. Growth Regul 1993; 3: 40–4.

78. Taylor AE. Insulin-lowering medications in polycystic ovary syndrome. Obstet Gynecol Clin North Am 2000; 27: 583–95.

46 Endometriosis

Erkut Attar and Serdar Bulun

INTRODUCTION

Endometriosis is a systemic disorder that is characterized by the presence of endometrium-like tissue in ectopic sites outside the uterus, primarily on pelvic peritoneum and ovaries.[1] Endometriosis affects nearly 1 in 7 women of reproductive age and often results in a vast array of gynecological problems, including dyspareunia, dysmenorrhea, pelvic pain, and infertility.[2-6] In the USA, endometriosis is the third most common gynecological disorder that requires hospitalization, and a leading cause of hysterectomy.

Endometriosis has been known for almost 300 years. In the late 17th century it was recognized as peritoneal ulcers in the abdomen. The association between pelvic pain, tissue damage, and scarring was recognized in the 18th century by Rokitansky. With the improvements in microscopy, Sampson first described the disease formally in 1921.[7] In the last century, various theories were proposed to explain the pathogenesis of endometriosis. Despite the extensive investigation of disease, the pathogenesis of this enigmatic disease is still poorly understood and remains controversial.

Classical theories for the pathogenesis of endometriosis can be divided into three main concepts: (1) coelomic metaplasia (in-situ development); (2) the induction theory; and (3) the transplantation or implantation theory. The theory of coelomic metaplasia proposes that endometriosis may develop from metaplasia of mesothelial cells lining the pelvic peritoneum and ovary. The induction theory is based on the assumption that specific substances, which are released by degenerating endometrium, induce the development of endometriosis from omnipotent stem cells present in connective tissue. These theories have been met with considerable opposition over the years and largely abandoned. Sampson proposed the hypothesis that the origin of peritoneal endometrial implants was tissue delivered by retrograde menstruation.[2] Retrograde menstruation is a nearly universal phenomenon among cycling women, but it is not clear why endometrial tissue will implant and grow in the peritoneal cavity of only a subgroup of women.[3,4] However, the transportation and implantation theory is still important at some point for the development of peritoneal endometriosis.

Current clinical observations and research on endometriosis revealed a new concept on the pathogenesis of the disease. In endometriosis, at least three different forms must be defined. It seems that peritoneal, ovarian, and rectovaginal endometriosis are different forms of the disease. *Therefore, with the current knowledge and understanding of the disease, pathogenesis of endometriosis can be explained by a combination of possible causes rather than a certain theory.* Furthermore, findings of an increased risk of ovarian cancer and the suggestion of increased risks of autoimmune diseases and breast and skin cancers support a need for multidisciplinary care for women with this disorder and long-term follow-up for surveillance of associated disorders that may develop in susceptible individuals.

PATHOGENESIS OF ENDOMETRIOSIS

Research on the pathogenesis of endometriosis currently interfaces with five areas of basic research:

- hormonal factors and steroidogenesis
- genetics
- environmental science
- immunology
- cancer biology.

Investigations about the role of genetics, the environment, the immune system, and estradiol in the pathogenesis of this disorder, as well as postgenomic study of intrinsic abnormalities in eutopic (i.e. within the uterus) and ectopic (i.e. endometriotic lesions) endometrium in women with the disease, are providing insights into the pathophysiology of the associated pain and infertility.

Hormonal factors and steroidogenesis

The clinical significance of estrogen biosynthesis in endometriosis is exemplified by the clinical observations that estrogen is essential for growth of endometriosis. The biologically active estrogen estradiol is produced from cholesterol through six serial enzymatic conversions in two ovarian cell types that cooperate in a paracrine fashion. The rate-limiting two steps include the entry of cholesterol into the mitochondrion facilitated by the steroidogenic acute regulatory protein (StAR) and the conversion of androstenedione to estrone by aromatase (Figure 46.1). StAR, aromatase, and all other steroidogenic enzymes are expressed in vivo in endometriosis, enabling this tissue to synthesize estradiol from cholesterol de novo.[8,9] Small but significant levels of aromatase enzyme activity and mRNA were also detected in eutopic endometrial tissue and stromal cells of women with endometriosis.[10,11] In contrast, StAR or aromatase expression or steroid hormone production is virtually undetectable in eutopic endometrial stromal cells from disease-free women and normal endometrium does not biosynthesize estradiol.[9–13] The recent demonstration of StAR and a complete set of steroidogenic enzymes including aromatase within the endometriotic stromal cell imply that estrogen is synthesized de novo from cholesterol and that endometriotic aromatase is not solely dependent for substrate on adrenal or ovarian secretion. These new findings revised our view of the pathogenesis of estrogen biosynthesis in endometriosis.

The eutopic endometrium of women with endometriosis contains low but significant levels of aromatase mRNA and enzyme activity and represents an intermediate state of this disease. It appears that upon retrograde menstruation and implantation of this inherently abnormal tissue on pelvic peritoneal surfaces, aromatase expression and enzyme activity are amplified by up to 400 times.[10,11]

Cyclooxygenase 2 (COX-2) expression that is important for prostaglandin E_2 (PGE_2) synthesis is increased markedly in both eutopic endometrium and endometriotic tissue of women with endometriosis.[14,15] PGE_2 plays a key role in the estrogen biosynthetic pathway in endometriotic tissue because it is a potent stimulator of key steroidogenic genes.[9,10,13,16] The most significantly induced steroidogenic genes are StAR and aromatase.[9,10,13,16] Thus, PGE_2 production in endometriosis is extremely important. The enzyme cyclooxygenase catalyzes the conversion of arachidonic acid to PGG_2, which is then converted to PGE_2 by the enzyme PGE_2 synthase. Two distinct genes, referred to as COX-1 and COX-2, encode the cyclooxygenase enzyme. Most importantly, COX-2 is strikingly up-regulated in stromal cells of endometriosis, whereas its expression is also significantly higher in endometrium of patients with endometriosis in comparison with the endometrium of disease-free patients.[14,15] Interleukin-1β (IL-1β) and PGE_2 itself induce COX-2 in endometriotic and endometrial stromal

cells, whereas vascular endothelial growth factor (VEGF) and estradiol (E_2) rapidly induce COX-2 in uterine endothelial cells.[17–19] Thus, a large number of pathways in endometriosis induce COX-2 to increase PGE_2 formation in this tissue. The regulation of PGE_2 synthase in endometriosis is not known.

Two basic pathological processes, namely growth and inflammation, are responsible for chronic pelvic pain and infertility, which are the primary devastating symptoms of endometriosis. Estrogen, growth factors, and metalloproteinases enhance the growth and invasion of endometriotic tissue, whereas prostaglandins and cytokines mediate pain, inflammation, and infertility.[20,21] Research work over the past 10 years has uncovered a molecular link between inflammation and estrogen production in endometriosis.[8] This is mediated by a positive feedback cycle that favors expression of key steroidogenic genes, most notably StAR and aromatase, expression of COX-2, and continuous local production of estradiol and PGE_2 in endometriotic tissue[9,10,13] (Figure 46.2).

Transcription of the aromatase gene in human tissues is regulated by at least 10 distinct promoters, each giving rise to aromatase mRNA species with variable 5 prime UTRs (untranslated regions) but an identical coding region.[22,23] Extraovarian endometriotic tissue and ovarian endometrioma-derived cells use almost exclusively promoter II, which is the PGE2/cAMP-responsive proximal promoter, for aromatase expression in vivo.[10,11,16] Thus, aberrant aromatase expression in endometriosis is primarily mediated by activation of promoter II.

A number of molecular abnormalities are responsible for PGE_2/cAMP-dependent aromatase expression in endometriosis. One critical mechanism is mediated by aberrantly expressed key transcriptional enhancers (e.g. steroidogenic factor 1, SF-1) in biopsied endometriotic tissues (in vivo) and cultured endometriotic stromal cells (in vitro). A flipside of this enhancer-mediated mechanism serves as a second mechanism to suppress steroidogenic gene expression in normal eutopic endometrial stromal cells exposed to PGE_2 or cAMP analogues. This involves the redundant presence and steroidogenic promoter-binding activity of multiple transcriptional inhibitors (chicken ovalbumin upstream transcription factor, COUP-TF) and co-repressors of SF-1 (e.g. Wilms' tumor 1, WT-1) serving as fail-safe mechanisms. COUP-TF is expressed in both eutopic endometrial and endometriotic cells, whereas SF-1 is expressed in endometriotic but not normal eutopic endometrial cells. COUP-TF is part of the transcriptional system that inhibits aromatase in eutopic endometrial

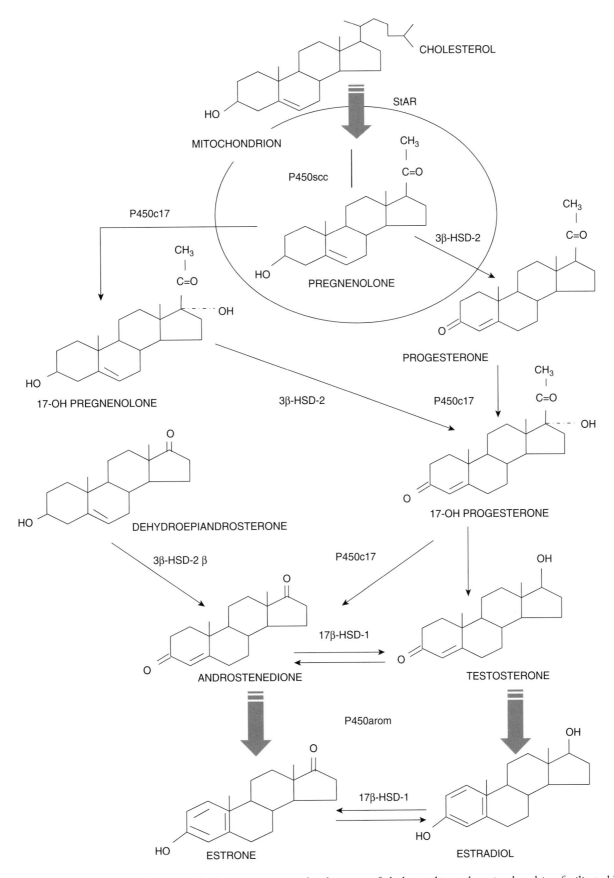

Figure 46.1 Ovarian steroidogenesis. The key steps seem to be the entry of cholesterol into the mitochondrion facilitated by the steroidogenic acute regulatory protein (StAR) for progesterone production and the conversion of androstenedione to estrone catalyzed by aromatase (P450arom) for estrogen production at the final step.

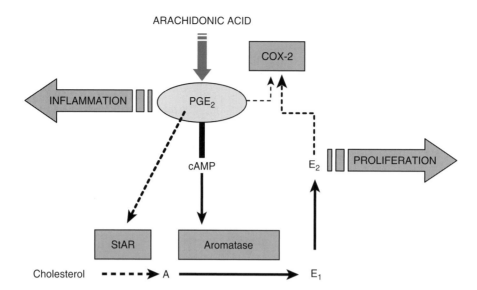

Figure 46.2   A positive feedback cycle for estrogen and prostaglandin fromation in endometriosis. Two basic pathological processes, namely growth and inflammation, are responsible for chronic pelvic pain and infertility, which are the primary devastating symptoms of endometriosis. Estrogen enhances the growth and invasion of endometriotic tissue, whereas prostanglandins and cytokines mediate pain, inflammation, and infertility. Estradiol is produced locally in endometriotic tissue. The precursor, androstenedione (A) of ovarian, adrenal, or local origin becomes converted to estrone (E1), which is in turn reduced to estradiol (E_2) in endometriotic implants. Endometriotic tissue is capable of synthesizing androsterione from cholesterol via the activity of steroidogenic acute regulatory protein (StAR). Estradiol directly induces cyclooxygenase 2 (COX-2), which gives rise to elevated concentrations of prostaglandin E_2 (PGE_2) in endometriosis. PGE_2 in trun, is the most potent known stimulator of StAR and aromatase in endometriotic stromal cells. This establishes a positive feedback loop in favor of continuous estrogen and prostaglandin formation in endometriosis.

stromal cells; in contrast, aberrantly expressed SF-1 in endometriotic stromal cells overrides this inhibition by competing for the same regulatory element. Thus, the mechanism here is differential expression of an enhancer in endometriosis but not in eutopic endometrium favoring aromatase expression[16] (Figure 46.3).

There are additional redundant mechanisms that serve to inhibit aromatase in normal endometrium and stimulate it in endometriosis.[24] For example, over-expression of C/EPBα stimulated, while C/EBPβ inhibited, P450arom promoter in endometriotic and eutopic endometrial cells.[24] Moreover, C/EBPβ was selectively down-regulated in vivo in endometriosis but not in eutopic endometrium, indicating that differential down-regulation of a transcriptional inhibitor in endometriosis is an additional mechanism for aromatase expression in this pathological tissue. Dosage-sensitive sex reversal, adrenal hypoplasia critical region, on chromosome X, gene 1 (DAX-1), a co-repressor of SF-1, inhibits SF-1-dependent expression of aromatase in endometriotic and endometrial cells.[25] Moreover, WT-1, another co-regulator of SF-1, also acts as a co-repressor and inhibits SF-1-dependent activity of the aromatase promoter II in endometriotic/endometrial stromal cells.[12,25] Intriguingly, WT-1 but

not DAX-1 is selectively down-regulated in vivo in endometriotic stromal cells.[12] Thus, WT-1 seems to be a physiologically significant co-repressor for the inhibition of steroidogenesis in eutopic endometrium. On the other hand, p300/CBP (CREB-binding protein), which is a co-activator of SF-1, enhances promoter II activity in endometriotic and endometrial stromal cells. These findings together are suggestive that SF-1 acts as a masterswitch to activate the promoters of aromatase and other key steroidogenic genes. Co-repressors or co-activators of SF-1 in endometrial vs endometriotic cells may further modify SF-1-dependent transcriptional activity.

Genetics

Endometriosis has long been recognized as having familial tendencies.[26] There is increasing evidence that endometriosis has a genetic basis.[27–30] The evidence was confined initially to small, case-control studies. Subsequently, compelling evidence of the genetic basis of endometriosis has emerged from the analysis of large clinical databases. Endometriosis probably shows a complex trait, like diabetes mellitus, hypertension, and

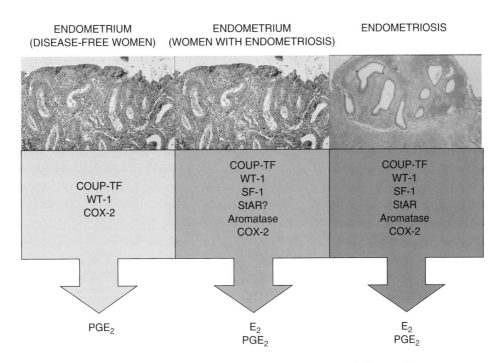

ENDOMETRIUM
(DISEASE-FREE WOMEN)

ENDOMETRIUM
(WOMEN WITH ENDOMETRIOSIS)

ENDOMETRIOSIS

COUP-TF
WT-1
COX-2

COUP-TF
WT-1
SF-1
StAR?
Aromatase
COX-2

COUP-TF
WT-1
SF-1
StAR
Aromatase
COX-2

PGE$_2$

E$_2$
PGE$_2$

E$_2$
PGE$_2$

Figure 46.3 Molecular abnormalities in endometriosis. In the endometrium of disease-free woman, steroidogenic acute regulatory protein (StAR) and aromatase are not expressed because the stimulatory transcription factor SF-1 is absent, and inhibitory factors COUP-TF (chicken ovalbumin upstream transcription factor) and WT-1 (Wilms' tumor 1) are present. In the endometrium of patients with endometriosis, very small quantities of SF-1 (steroidogenic factor 1) and aromatase are detectable and give rise to low levels of estrogen production, whereas COX-2 (cyclooxygenase 2) expression and PGE$_2$ (prostaglandin E$_2$) formation are markedly elevated. In the ectopic lesions (endometriotic tissue), elevated levels of SF-1, StAR, and aromatase are the basis of significant estradiol (E$_2$) formation. High COX-2 expression enhances formation of large amounts of PGE$_2$.

asthma. This implies that the disease is caused by an interaction between multiple genes and the environment. Such conditions do not have a clear Mendelian pattern of inheritance, and multiple gene loci conferring susceptibility to the condition interact with each other and the environment to produce the phenotype. Surgically confirmed disease in general occurs 6–9 times more commonly in the first-degree relatives of affected women than in controls.[31–33] This effect may be more pronounced in the relatives of women with severe disease.[34] Nevertheless, defining the familial tendency more thoroughly in the whole population is difficult because surgery is required to establish the diagnosis. The best available data indicate that the risk of the sister of an affected woman having endometriosis compared with the risk in the general population probably lies between 2 and 9 for all disease severities, although this risk may be as high as 15 in women with severe endometriosis.

The heritability of endometriosis is also apparent in non-human primates, which develop the disease spontaneously.[30] The appearance of clinical features at surgery and histological characteristics of the disease in the rhesus monkey mimic those in humans.[28,35]

Therefore, a clearer understanding of the epidemiology and inheritability of the disease may emerge from studying spontaneous endometriosis in rhesus monkey colonies (*Macaca mulatta*).[28] The Oxford Group identified 121 (8.3%) affected rhesus monkeys among the autopsy records of the 1459 female animals aged ≥4 years old, that died in the colony in the period 1982–1996 at California Regional Primate Research Center (CRPRC).[36] Hadfield et al studied the autopsy records of 399 rhesus monkeys that died in the colony between 1980 and 1995 and reported a prevalence rate of 20% in animals aged ≥4 years old and 29% in animals aged ≥10 years old.[37] Over a 20-year period, at the Wisconsin Regional Primate Research Center (WRPRC), 142 rhesus macaques with endometriosis have been identified principally from necropsy records, giving a prevalence of 31.4%.[38] These cases have been used to construct an extended multigenerational pedigree and 9 nuclear families consisting of 1602 females in total. A high degree of heritability is suggested, as in the human data among affected compared with unaffected animals, and a higher recurrence risk for full sibs compared with paternal and maternal half-sibs.

Quantitative genetic analysis is based on the principle that any region in the genome could encode a gene of importance. The most commonly used method of quantitative genetic analysis is sibling-pair analysis. The general principle is that affected relatives inherit identical copies of any given causative allele more often than expected by chance alone. Sibling-pair analysis begins by searching not for causative genes per se, but rather for polymorphic loci closely linked to causative genes. However, this approach is limited by the need for multigenerational families of affected and unaffected individuals. In addition, misclassification is a special problem, with difficulty in verifying absence of the disease in ostensibly affected or unaffected individuals.[26,39] The OXEGENE (Oxford Endometriosis Gene) Study and the Genes Behind Endometriosis Study started independently in 1995 based on previous research.[27,31,40] Both groups have mainly collected affected sister pairs using recruitment methods similar to those described elsewhere.[27] The International Endogene Study originated from the combined data set of these studies and consists of >2500 families.[27,41] This study showed a suggestive linkage for one chromosomal locus based on the analysis of marker data (400 markers at 10 cM) generated for a total of 289 families from the complete data set, containing 374 sister pairs plus other affected relatives.[41,42] However, the results of the full genome-wide scan of all the collected families have not yet been published. A web site has been developed to collect these reports.[43]

The use of linkage analysis alone is often insufficient to localize susceptibility genes in complex traits because of the limited resolution of the method for fine mapping. As a complementary approach, candidate genes need to be investigated in association studies by comparing the frequency of marker alleles in affected cases and normal controls. Increasing numbers of reports are exploring whether endometriosis is associated with perturbation of a hypothesized candidate gene involving point mutations or polymorphisms.[44–46] One of these candidate genes is the GALT gene. The disease has been proposed to be associated with inborn errors of galactose metabolism, in particular with a specific mutation, N314D, in the GALT gene.[47] The polymorphism causes reduced activity of the enzyme galactose-1-phosphate uridyl transferase, which is involved in galactose metabolism. Association was initially reported between the N314D polymorphism and endometriosis by Cramer et al in a US population: i.e. 30% in cases and 14% in controls.[47] Three studies involving more patients, however, failed to replicate

the association.[48,49] Subsequently, phase II detoxification genes that encode enzymes involved in detoxification, such as the glutathione S-transferase (GST) family, have been investigated. Enzymes belonging to the glutathione S-transferase family are involved in the two-stage detoxification of 2,3,7,8-tetrachlorodibenzo-P-dioxin (dioxin) which is a potential pollutant for endometriosis development.[50] In previous studies, homozygotes for a null mutation in one of the GST family genes, GSTM1 (glutathione S-transferase M1), were more common in endometriosis cases. However, subsequent studies have failed to replicate this association, and no association has been found for a mutation in a similar gene, GSTT1.[51–53]

Phase I detoxification genes (Ah receptor, CYP1A1, NAT2), the estrogen receptor, and aromatase genes (CYP19) were also studied as candidate genes. However, no consistent relationship has been shown in different studies. Sample size, standardization in phenotype definition, and the choice of control populations are the likely features to influence results, and could partly explain the lack of consistency in the findings. A recent review of general applications using polymorphisms and pharmacogenomics in endometriosis is now available.[54]

Genetic alterations in endometriotic tissue have been described in loss of heterozygosity studies and in studies using comparative genomic hybridization and fluorescence in-situ hybridization.[55–59] These alterations involve chromosomal regions that contain known tumor suppressor genes and oncogenes previously implicated in ovarian cancer. Evidence suggests involvement of oncogenes and tumor suppressor genes such as PTEN, K-ras, and p53 in the pathogenesis of endometriosis.

DNA microarray is an effective tool for the identification of differentially expressed genes between uterine and ectopic endometrium. Studies using microarray to assess gene expression levels in endometriosis are now under way. It has been shown that several gene products are differentially expressed in endometriotic tissue and in the endometrium of the patients with endometriosis compared to the normal controls. In these studies, results from the arrays were verified using real-time polymerase chain reaction (PCR). Alternatively, tissue microarray (TMA) analysis can be performed to complement cDNA microarrays.[60,61]

Kao et al analyzed more than 12 000 genes.[62] Giudice and colleagues and Taylor and colleagues compared expression profiles in eutopic endometrium from women with and without endometriosis.[63,64] Eyster and colleagues analyzed 4133 genes to detect differential gene expression between eutopic endometrium and endometriotic implants.[65] In these studies, microarray expression profiling revealed that several known cell adhesion molecules, endometrial epithelial secreted proteins, cytokine and immune system-related genes, and genes in signaling pathways are differently expressed in patients with endometriosis. Further analysis of the up-regulated or down-regulated genes identified will expand our understanding of the nature of endometriosis and assist in the eventual development of new treatments for endometriosis.

Environmental science

Dioxin is a potent chemical toxicant that serves as the reference compound for a large class of halogenated aromatic hydrocarbons. The dioxin connection to endometriosis was discovered almost by accident. The aim of the original study was to investigate the long-term reproductive effects of exposure to dioxin in the rhesus monkey. Twelve years after the initiation of this work, in 1989 endometriosis was discovered at the autopsy of a dioxin-exposed animal.

Scientists who have been studying the disease for two decades or more, unsuccessfully seeking a cause, consider the recognition of dioxin as a contributor to the disease in rhesus monkeys as an exciting breakthrough. Now, new thinking about endometriosis has been stimulated by research linking dioxin exposure to the disease in rhesus monkeys.[66] In rhesus monkeys, the disease develops spontaneously and resembles the human disease both anatomically and clinically.[28] It seems that there is a dose–response relationship between the dioxin and severity of endometriosis.[50] Reproductivity of these monkeys was also affected when they were exposed to high levels of dioxin. Fetotoxicity was also reported in rhesus monkeys exposed to dioxin.[67]

The major source of dioxin in the environment (95%) is from incinerators burning chlorinated wastes. Dioxin pollution is also connected with paper mills, which use chlorine bleaching in their process, and with the production of polyvinyl chloride (PVC) plastics. The major sources of dioxin are in the diet. Since dioxin is fat-soluble, it bioaccumulates up the food chain and it is mainly (97.5%) found in meat and dairy products. Men have no way of getting rid of dioxin other than letting it break down according to its chemical half-lives. Women, on the other hand, have two ways in which it can exit their bodies: it crosses the placenta into the growing infant, causing recurrent pregnancy loss, and it is present in the fatty breast milk, which is also a route of exposure that doses the infant.

Dioxin also modulates various hormone receptor systems that play a role in uterine function, including estrogen receptor, progesterone receptor, epidermal growth factor receptor, and prolactin receptor.[68,69] Moreover, this toxin alters the action of estrogen in reproductive organs in a manner which is both age-dependent and target organ specific.[69,70] It modulates steroid receptor expression, resulting in altered tissue-specific responses to hormones.[69] In addition to effects on the reproductive system, dioxin also adversely affects immunocompetence.[71–74] Dioxin shows immunosuppressive activities and is a potent inhibitor of T-lymphocyte function.[72–74]

Target genes for the action of dioxin include cytochrome p450 and growth regulatory genes involved in both inflammation and differentiation, including plasminogen activator inhibitor-2 and IL-1β.[75,76] As previously stated in this chapter, GSTM1 is responsible for detoxification of dioxin and was proposed as a candidate gene for endometriosis development.[51] The discovery of genes that predispose some women to develop endometriosis and the identification of the interacting environmental factors that cause expression of the endometriosis phenotype may improve the clinical management of endometriosis.

Immunology

There are many immune and inflammatory changes relevant to endometriosis that can be considered as a cause and/or result of the disease development. Genetic characteristics and environmental factors could be responsible for the altered immune functions and disease development in patients with endometriosis. Because the ectopic implants of endometrial tissue are destroyed by a variety of immune and inflammatory reactions, research on cancer biology is a part of the full understanding of the disease development. Nonetheless, altered macrophage function itself and the role of peritoneal fluid have a special impact on the current endometriosis research.

Unlike the situation seen in women without endometriosis, macrophages do not appear to be as active in phagocytosis. They do, however, secrete high concentrations of substances as growth factors that restrict natural killer activity, increase angiogenesis and fibrosis, and induce endometrial cell proliferation in vitro (Figure 46.4). Macrophage-derived substances such as prostanoids, cytokines, growth factors, and

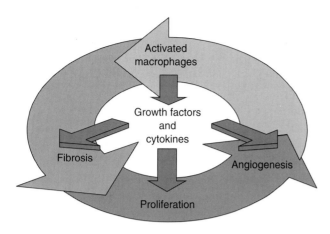

Figure 46.4 Macrophage- and endometriotic cell-derived cytokines and growth factors induce macrophage activitation, angiogenesis, and cell proliferation.

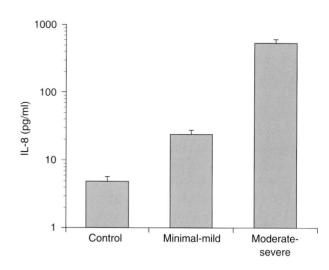

Figure 46.5 Interleukin-8 (IL-8) concentration in peritoneal fluid of patients with endometriosis.

angiogenic factors have been detected in the peritoneal fluid of women with endometriosis. These changes in the peritoneal milieu could also be responsible for the failure of fertilization, embryo development, and implantation.[77] In paricular, growth-promoting and angiogenic factors are considered to be substantially involved in the pathogenesis of endometriosis.[78] Interleukin 8 (IL-8) is a chemoattractant and activating factor for human neutrophils and a potent angiogenic agent. IL-8 concentrations in peritoneal fluid show higher levels in patients with endometriosis according to the stage of the disease compared to the control (Figure 46.5). However, potential sources of IL-8 in peritoneal fluid are not only the macrophages but also mesothelial cells of the peritoneum and the endometrium itself. It has been found that cultured mesothelial cells constitutively express IL-8 mRNA and secrete IL-8 protein, and the expression of IL-8 from mesothelial cells is modulated by other cytokines such as IL-1 and tumor neurosis factor α (TNF α).[79] These latter cytokines appear to play some role in the constitutive secretion of IL-8 as well as being capable of greatly stimulating further production and secretion.[80] Peritoneal macrophages, therefore, may play an important role in the initiation of the pathogenic cascade as a source of IL-1 and TNFα.

Monocyte chemotactic protein-1 (MCP-1) is also an active participant in the pathogenesis of endometriosis. The level of the MCP-1 was found to be significantly higher in patients with severe disease.[81] Elevated MCP-1 levels in peritoneal fluid of patients with endometriosis may play a role in growth and maintenance of ectopic endometrial tissue by directly stimulating endometrial cell proliferation.[82]

Activated macrophages in the peritoneal cavity produce a large amount of VEGF,[83] a growth factor related to angiogenesis. After the attachment phase, the high VEGF levels could provoke an increase in the subperitoneal vascular network and facilitate implantation and viability of the endometrial cells.[84]

Cancer biology

Endometriosis has many features in common with neoplasia, such as clonal proliferation and a tendency to metastasis and tissue invasion.[85–87] Although it is not a malignant disorder, endometriosis exhibits cellular proliferation and invasion. The invasive phenotype in endometriosis shares aspects with tumor metastasis.[88] T-cell-mediated invasion may be similar to that which occurs with metastatic neoplasia, wherein immune surveillance systems are inadequate or unable to respond to the seeding tissue.[89,90] Accumulation of various growth factors and the occurrence of angiogenesis to produce a self-contained blood supply are the features that implicate the relationship of cancer biology and ectopic endometriotic tissue development.

Women with endometriosis are at increased risk of malignant tumors of the pelvis. There have been several reports suggesting that women with endometriosis also have an increased risk of other types of cancers. A study of 876 women admitted to hospital with the diagnosis of endometriosis during a 25-year period found increased risks of ovarian cancer, non-Hodgkin's lymphoma, and breast cancer. Endometriosis is found in significantly higher frequency in women undergoing surgery for endometroid, clear cell, and mixed subtypes of ovarian cancers than in women with serous, mucinous, and other subtypes of cancers.[87] The synchronous occurrence of endometriosis with ovarian cancer and clear cell carcinoma and endometroid subtypes suggests transformation of endometriosis constituents into tumor cells. Endometrioid ovarian carcinomas are frequently associated with endometriosis. It is likely that most low-grade, relatively indolent ovarian carcinomas of endometrioid type arise from pre-existing endometriosis via mutations in CTNNB1 (the gene encoding β-catenin) and PTEN. Dinulescu et al recently presented a genetic model of peritoneal endometriosis and endometrioid ovarian adenocarcinoma in mice, both based on the activation of an oncogenic K-ras allele.[91] They found that expression of oncogenic K-ras or conditional PTEN deletion within the ovarian surface epithelium gives rise to preoplastic ovarian lesions with an endometrioid glandular morphology. The combination of the two mutations in the ovary leads to the induction of invasive and widely metastatic endometrioid ovarian adenocarcinomas. A high frequency of p53 mutations in atypical endometriosis and ovarian cancer associated with endometriosis has been shown. Endometriotic cysts similarly have been found to have loss of heterozygosity and partial deletions of chromosomes 9p, 11q, and 22q. There have been suggestions that the clonality and the high rate of aneuploidy predispose to malignant transformation of endometriotic lesions, especially into ovarian cancer of the endometroid and clear cell subtypes.

The process of new blood vessel development is called angiogenesis. There is considerable interest in the field of cancer for attacking these blood vessels as a means of preventing the growth of tumors. Endometriosis is a disease in the family of angiogenic diseases and excessive endometrial angiogenesis is proposed as an important mechanism in the pathogenesis of endometriosis.[92] Endometrial tissue develops its own vascular supply and becomes an independent growing mass.[93] In ways similar to the spread of a neoplasm, a piece of implanted tissue may subsequently break off from the primary site and travel elsewhere in the peritoneal cavity, setting up a peritoneal location or may enter a blood or lymph vessel and disseminate to distant body sites. As the free floating pieces of endometrial tissue themselves implant, grow, and develop their own blood supply, the process repeats itself. Endometrium is a rich source of growth factors which promote angiogenesis, including the fibroblast growth factors FGF1 and FGF2 and the VEGF.[94–96] It has been shown that the cell adhesion molecule

integrin $\alpha_v\beta_3$ is expressed in more blood vessels in the endometrium of women with endometriosis than in normal women.[97]

Dysmenorrhea is associated with increased plasma levels of vasopressin.[98,99] Vasopressin induces uterine contractions, but also increases contractility of the uterine artery and resistance.[100] Peptides such as oxytocin, endothelin, and norepinephrine contribute to the effect of vasopressin. The consequence is a large reduction in blood flow in the uterus, particularly to the endometrium during uterine contractions. Hypoxia is a critical activator of genes, especially for VEGF, and results in increased translation for VEGF protein in glandular and stromal cells of endometrium.[101] Thus, the greater hypoxia in the uteri of women with severe dysmenorrhea results in increased production of VEGF, facilitating angiogenesis at the implantation site of desquamated endometrium (Figure 46.6).

In peritoneal endometriosis, a delicate equilibrium seems to exist between the attacking forces and the defense mechanisms. If this active milieu is impaired, or if the number of regurgitated cells is too large, the surviving cells can adhere to exposed extracellular matrix (ECM) of a damaged peritoneal lining. In the pathogenesis of endometriosis, interactions of endometriotic cells with ECM can be postulated. Therefore, specific cell adhesion receptors and their ECM ligands are being investigated to understand the invasive features of endometriosis. Indeed, it has been shown that ECM turnover in patients with endometriosis is altered.[102]

A group of enzymes, matrix metallproteinases (MMPs), are responsible for ECM and endometrium remodeling. Considerable evidence indicates that MMPs play an active role in the establishment and progression of endometriosis.[103,104] It has been shown that MMP-1 expression is correlated with the activity of endometriotic tissue, suggesting its involvement in tissue remodeling and invasion of endometriotic cells.[105,106] MMPs mediate angiogenesis by degrading ECM in preparation for migration and tube formation of endothelial cells. Suppression of MMP inhibits establishment of ectopic lesions by human endometrium.[107] Tumor promotors, growth factors, cytokines, steroids, and oncogenes play a role in regulation of MMPs.

Cell adhesion molecules (CAMs) have been the focus of numerous studies addressing the genesis of the metastatic lesions in cancer. CAMs fall into four major groups: cadherins, selectins, members of the immunoglobulin superfamily, and integrins. Different molecules in each group may potentially play a role in the development and progression of disease.[108,109] Members of the integrin and cadherin family,

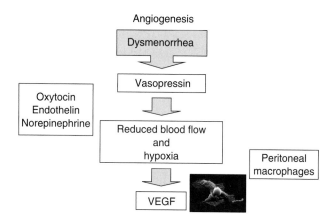

Figure 46.6 Hormonal and immune-mediated vascular endothelial growth factor (VEGF) production in endometriosis.

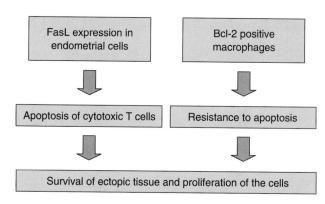

Figure 46.7 Expression of Fas ligand (FasL) in endometrial cells and increased number of Bcl-2 positive macrophages lead to survival of ectopic endometrial tissue.

important cell adhesion molecules, have been reported to be expressed in endometriotic lesions and in cells and tissues that are involved in the development of endometriosis.[110,111]

Programmed cell death (apoptosis) has been implicated in the pathogenesis of endometriosis.[112] Several investigations have revealed that uterine endometrium in mammals can be regulated by apoptosis. It has been suggested that decreased susceptibility of endometrial tissue to apoptosis contributes to the etiology or pathogenesis of endometriosis.[113] The increased proportion of Bcl-2 positive macrophages found in women with endometriosis may predispose these cells to resist apoptosis.[114] The continued survival of these active cells could have important consequences for the survival and proliferation of the ectopic tissue. Moreover, up-regulated Fas ligand (FasL) expression in endometrial cells may be relevant for the development of a relative local immunotolerance in endometriosis by inducing apoptosis of cytotoxic T lymphocytes.[115,116] Decreased apoptosis in endometrial cells of patients with endometriosis may lead to acquiring the capacity to utilize the products of an activated immune system to establish ectopic foci of disease (Figure 46.7).

SUMMARY FOR ETIOPATHOGENESIS OF PERITONEAL ENDOMETRIOSIS

Endometriosis is a multifactorial disease possibly caused by an interaction between multiple gene loci and the environment. Immune or inflammatory deficiency seen in endometriosis may be the result of the stress on immune functioning, or may be genetically determined. Environmental factors such as dioxin can

be responsible for immunosuppressive activities in patients with endometriosis. In addition, this toxin modulates steroid receptor expression, resulting in altered tissue-specific responses to hormones. Chronic immunosuppression in combination with hormonal regulation may facilitate the aberrant growth of ectopic endometrial tissue. It seems that genetic, environmental, immunological, and hormonal (autocrine and paracrine) factors are overlapping and affecting each other during the disease progression. However, the mechanism appears to require endometrium and retrograde menstruation in most cases with peritoneal disease. In conclusion, we have just started to bring together the more obvious clinical observations such as retrograde menstruation and/or dysmenorrhea and the results of the basic research on genetics, cancer biology, and immunology to explain the pathogenesis of disease (Figure 46.8). We believe that disseminated peritoneal endometriosis and the deep endometriosis are distinct forms of the disease. It is possible that oncogenes and tumor suppressor genes play an important role in the disseminated form of the peritoneal endometriosis.

TREATMENT OF ENDOMETRIOSIS

Endometriosis presents with a group of symptoms, including pain, dysmenorrhea, dyspareunia, dysfunctional uterine bleeding, and infertility. None of these symptoms is specific for endometriosis. The most consistent symptom is the chronic pelvic pain, with a prevalence of 30–70% in adults and 45–58% in adolescents. Dysmenorrhea is associated with endometriosis in more than 50% of adults and in up to 75% of

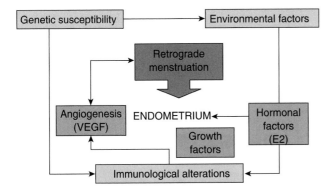

Figure 46.8 Pathogenesis and peritoneal endometriosis. VEGF, vascular endothelial growth factor; E$_2$, estradiol.

adolescents. Infertility is also a common symptom in endometriosis. It is estimated that 30% of women with endometriosis are infertile. A definitive diagnosis of most forms of endometriosis requires visual inspection of the pelvis at laparoscopy as the gold standard investigation. However, pain symptoms suggestive of the disease can be treated without a definitive diagnosis using a therapeutic trial of a hormonal drug to reduce menstrual flow. Traditionally, both surgical and medical therapies have focused on alleviation of pain, prevention of disease progression, and promotion of fertility. Therapeutic strategies must be tailored to the individual's symptoms, age, and desire for fertility.

TREATMENT OF INFERTILITY

In spite of significant developments in medical and surgical approaches, the optimal therapy for treating endometriosis-associated infertility has yet to be established. Most of the medical therapies used to treat endometriosis-associated pain have also been instituted in an attempt to treat the subfertility seen in women with endometriosis. Four randomized trials with five treatment arms have compared a medical treatment directed at endometriosis to placebo or no treatment, with fertility as the outcome measure.[117–120] Another eight randomized controlled trials compared danazol to a second medication.[121–128] The entire randomized controlled studies have been summarized by a meta-analysis (Figure 46.9). In none of these studies, has medical therapy been shown to be of any value.[129] Clearly, no increase in fertility can be demonstrated with these medications when compared to expectant management, nor has any medication proven superior to danazol in this regard. Thus, there appears to be no role for medical therapy in the treatment of

endometriosis-associated infertility. Medical therapy is even worse than no treatment in that the patient is unable to conceive while being medicated for several months.

It is widely accepted that severe endometriosis of sufficient severity to cause distortion of the pelvis impairs fertility by interfering with oocyte pickup and transport. Surgical treatment does improve fertility for all stages of disease. For severe disease, no randomized trials or meta-analyses exist to answer the question whether surgical excision of moderate–severe endometriosis enhances pregnancy rates. However, observational studies and numerous uncontrolled trials proving that pregnancies do occur after reparative surgery suggest the value of this approach.[130] Based upon three studies, there seems to be a negative correlation between the stage of endometriosis and the spontaneous cumulative pregnancy rate after surgical removal of endometriosis, but statistical significance was only reached in one study.[131–133] Treatment with danazol or a gonadotropin-releasing hormone (GnRH) agonist after surgery does not improve fertility compared with expectant management.[134–137]

More controversial is the situation with mimimal–mild endometriosis. The issue of efficacy of surgery in the enhancement of early-stage endometriosis-associated infertility remains unsettled. A meta-analysis of nonrandomized trials suggested that surgical treatment of early-stage endometriosis-associated infertility might be of value; however, there was sufficient heterogeneity among the studies to diminish confidence in such a conclusion.[138] A large-scale randomized controlled trial, termed ENDOCAN, was recently accomplished.[139] This study randomized 341 infertile women with stage I or II endometriosis to either diagnostic laparoscopy or surgical treatment of the disease. The women were followed for 36 weeks postoperatively and for up to 20 weeks if they conceived. The rate of pregnancy > 20 weeks was significantly higher in the surgically treated women (30.7% vs 17.7%). A similar but comparably small multicenter study with 101 patients demonstrated a live birthrate of 19.6% in the treatment group and 22.2% in the controls within 1 year of surgery. This study differed from the Canadian trial in that patients had a longer median duration of infertility and slightly more extensive disease. Combining the results of these two trials into a meta-analysis still favors surgical treatment.

Although the assisted reproductive techniques – controlled ovarian hyperstimulation/intrauterine inseminator (COH/IUI) or in-vitro fertilization (IVF) are clearly efficacious in endometriosis-related infertility,

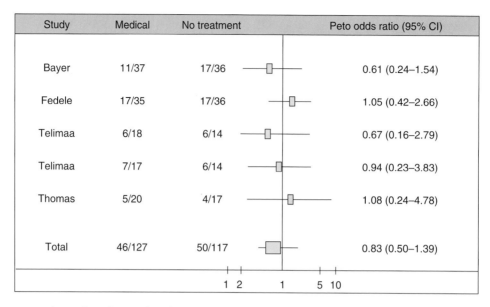

Study	Medical	No treatment	Peto odds ratio (95% CI)
Bayer	11/37	17/36	0.61 (0.24–1.54)
Fedele	17/35	17/36	1.05 (0.42–2.66)
Telimaa	6/18	6/14	0.67 (0.16–2.79)
Telimaa	7/17	6/14	0.94 (0.23–3.83)
Thomas	5/20	4/17	1.08 (0.24–4.78)
Total	46/127	50/117	0.83 (0.50–1.39)

Figure 46.9   Meta-analysis of randomized trials comparing medical therapy of endometriosis-associated infertility vs placebo or expectant management. (Reproduced from Olive and Pritts,[149] with permission.)

its degree of value, cost-effectiveness, and optimal method of employment have not yet been satisfactorily addressed. Three randomized trials have addressed the value of ovulation induction, and two have combined it with IUI.[140–142] From these results, it is apparent that fertility can be accelerated in women with endometriosis by using these approaches. IVF is an appropriate treatment, especially if there are coexisting causes of infertility and/or other treatments have failed, but IVF pregnancy rates are lower in women with endometriosis than in those with tubal infertility.

Combination of IVF and either medical or surgical therapy may be beneficial with advanced endometriosis. The idea that surgery increases IVF pregnancy rates is not supported by the available evidence.[143] It has been shown that down-regulation with GnRH agonist for 6 months increases the IVF success in patients with endometriosis. However, it is a fact that down-regulation with GnRH agonist in any patient produces a higher pregnancy rate. The issue of whether 2 weeks of down-regulation is sufficient in these patients or if 6 months of treatment is required remains unresolved and further study is required.

The laparoscopic excision of ovarian endometriomas appears to increase the chances of spontaneous conception, but the value of this treatment in women selected for IVF-ICSI (intracytoplasmic sperm injection) cycles is debatable. There are no randomized trials comparing laparoscopic excision to expectant management before IVF-ICSI cycles. Studies recruiting women with unilateral disease and comparing

ovarian responsiveness in the affected and contralateral intact gonads indicate that excision of endometriomas is associated with a quantitative damage to ovarian reserve.

TREATMENT OF PAIN

Established treatments

Current treatment regimens used to manage the disease are primarily designed to induce a hypoestrogenic state which leads to a reduction in disease and associated symptoms. Although these regimens have been used with great success, there are still drawbacks and limitations to these types of therapies. Established regimens for the treatment of endometriosis include estrogen–progesterone combinations, progestogens, danazol, and GnRH agonists. These drugs are equally effective in reducing pelvic pain associated with endometriosis.[136,144,145]

Oral contraceptives and progestins

Typically, oral contraceptives and non-steroidal anti-inflammatory drugs (NSAIDs) are first-line therapy because of their low cost and mild side effects. Oral contraceptives have been widely used in the treatment of minimal and mild endometriosis or even after surgical treatment, in order to minimize the relapses of endometriosis. Combined oral contraceptives with medium-dose estrogen and progestogens were shown

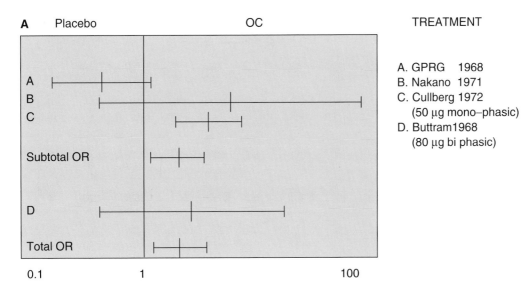

A Placebo   OC   TREATMENT

A. GPRG   1968
B. Nakano 1971
C. Cullberg 1972
     (50 μg mono–phasic)
D. Buttram1968
     (80 μg bi phasic)

A
B
C

Subtotal OR

D

Total OR

0.1   1   100

Figure 46.10   Meta-analysis of randomized trials comparing oral contraceptives to placebo for endometriosis-related pain. (Reproduced from Procter et al,[146] with permisson.)

to be more effective than placebo for pain relief[146] (Figure 46.10). Patients can be administered both uninterrupted and cyclical courses. Combined oral contraceptives that contain 20–35 μg of ethinyl estradiol are used daily and continuously for 6–12 months or until the patient decides to become pregnant. Symptomatic relief may be achieved in 75–100% of women. Cyclic use of oral contraceptives has proved significantly inferior to GnRH agonists for relief of dysmenorrhea, nearly as effective for relief of dyspareunia, and equally efficacious in the treatment of non-specific pelvic pain.[147]

Progestins have been used successfully to treat symptomatic endometriosis. They are characterized by side effects of relatively limited clinical importance, good overall tolerability, and low costs.[148] Either alone or combined with estrogens as in birth control pills, progestins might constitute an optimal choice for long-term treatment of symptomatic endometriosis. The available data suggest that the efficacy of progestins for temporary relief of endometriosis-associated pelvic pain is good and comparable to that of other, less-safe treatments.[145]

GnRH agonists

GnRH agonists have been shown to provide virtually identical pain relief to danazol.[149] Treatment of endometriosis with GnRH agonists is limited to 6 months because of possible adverse effects on bone metabolism. Treatment for 3 months with a GnRH agonist may be as effective as 6 months in terms of pain relief (Figure 46.11). In addition, the use of GnRH

agonists is associated with physical side effects such as vasomotor instability, headache, hot flashes, and depressive mood symptoms.[150–153] This adverse effect on bone density can be overcome by hormone add-back therapy. GnRHa therapy coupled with steroid add-back provides effective suppression of endometriosis and endometriosis-associated symptoms.

Experimental treatments

Experimental treatments of endometriosis include aromatase inhibitors (AIs), mifepristone, selective progesterone receptor modulators (SPRMs), modulators of the immune system (TNFα inhibitors), angiogenesis inhibitors, and levonorgestrel-releasing IUD (intrauterine device). Selective estrogen-receptor modulators (SERMs) are thought to act like estrogen in some tissues but behave like estrogen blockers (antiestrogens) in others. It has recently been reported that SERMs worsen endometriosis.

Progesterone antagonists and selective progesterone receptor modulators

Many progesterone antagonists and SPRMs display antiproliferative effects on the endometrium and thus have application in the treatment of endometriosis without being associated with hypoestrogenism and bone loss. A type II progesterone receptor modulator, RU486 (mifepristone) has been used to treat endometriosis.[154,155] RU486 is a complete antagonist that can disrupt endometrial integrity. It causes periarteriolar

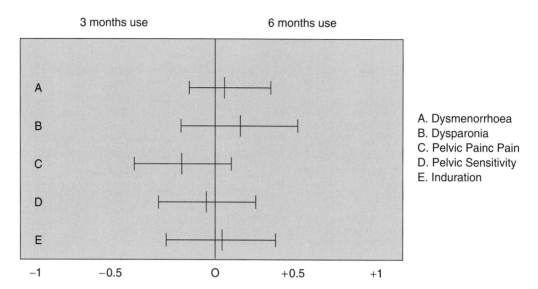

Figure 46.11   Effectiveness of gonadotropin releasing hormone analogues in the treatment of the painful symptoms of endometriosis. (Reproduced from Prentice et al,[189] with permission.)

degeneration of spiral arteries in endometrium. Mifepristone has some mild side effects, such as hot flashes, nausea, fatigue, and transient liver transaminase changes. No effects on bone density and lipid profile have been reported. SPRMs are partial antagonists of progesterone receptor. They have a mixed agonist–antagonists effect and can inhibit endometrial growth while not producing other systemic effects of progesterone.[156] Early clinical trials suggested that mifespristone and SPRMs are effective on endometriosis-associated pain with minimal side effects.[157]

Immunomodulators and antiangiogenesis treatment

Based upon the knowledge that MMPs are relevant to the development of endometriosis, anti-MMP therapies may be viable candidates for use in the treatment of endometriosis. Abnormal production of TNFα is also required for the establishment and maintenance of endometrial implants. Infliximab, which blocks TNFα function, could be used in the treatment of endometriosis.[158] There is now little doubt that the VEGF family has an essential role in the regulation of angiogenic processes in endometriosis.[159] VEGF inhibits pathological angiogenesis in a wide variety of tumor models, a phenomenon that has led to the clinical development of a variety of VEGF inhibitors.[160] It has been postulated that blocking the activity of VEGF could also be a possible treatment for endometriosis.[161,162] Preliminary results from experimental studies support this hypothesis.[163] Further studies are now needed to demonstrate the efficacy of this approach in clinical practice.

Intrauterine administration of levonorgestrel

Levonorgestrel down-regulates endometrial cell proliferation, increases apoptotic activity, induces endometrial glandular atrophy and extensive decidual transformation of the stroma, and has anti-inflammatory and immunomodulatory effects. Intrauterine administration of levonorgestrel with direct distribution to pelvic tissues would imply a local concentration greater than plasma levels. An intrauterine device (IUD) releasing levonorgestrel has proven effective in relieving dysmenorrhea associated with endometriosis, as well as pain associated with rectovaginal endometriosis.[164] It is also effective for the treatment of adenomyosis-associated menorrhagia.[165] In a randomized controlled trial, a levonorgestrel-bearing IUD was shown to be effective in the treatment of pelvic pain comparable to a GnRH analogue.[166] Although leakage of levonorgestrel in IUD into the circulation may potentially cause side effects associated with systemically adminstered progestins this approach appears to be promising in the long-term management of endometiosis.[167]

Aromatase inhibitors

The observation that local estrogen biosynthesis takes place in endometriotic implants prompted investigators to target aromatase in endometriosis using its third-generation inhibitors. The AIs are classified into two types: competitive inhibitors and inactivators of the aromatase enzyme.[168,169] Currently, three highly specific AIs are available in the USA. The competitive aromatase inhibitors are anastrozole and letrozole, and

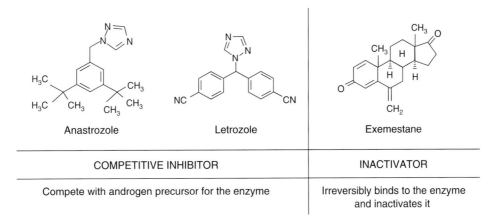

COMPETITIVE INHIBITOR	INACTIVATOR
Compete with androgen precursor for the enzyme	Irreversibly binds to the enzyme and inactivates it

Figure 46.12   FDA-approved aromatase inhibitors.

the inactivator compound is exemestane (Figure 46.12). Among these inhibitors, anastrozole and letrozole were used successfully to treat endometriosis in both postmenopausal and premenopausal women.[170–175]

The first article reporting the treatment of postmenopausal endometriosis with an aromatase inhibitor was published in 1998.[170] This postmenopausal woman had her uterus and both ovaries surgically removed and was therefore postmenopausal but continued to have a large persistent pelvic mass and severe pain.[170] An aromatase inhibitor effectively eradicated the mass and eliminated her pain.[170] This was followed by another case report confirming that an aromatase inhibitor is the medical treatment of choice in postmenopausal endometriosis, which is a relatively rare condition.[174]

In the treatment of premenopausal endometriosis, some form of ovarian suppression needs to be added to the currently available doses of aromatase inhibitors. If the ovary is not suppressed concomitantly, estrogen depletion in the hypothalamus may cause follicle-stimulating hormone (FSH) secretion and ovarian stimulation. Thus, an aromatase inhibitor was administered together with a GnRH agonist, a progestin, progesterone, or a combination oral contraceptive in four phase II trials.[171–173,175] All four studies showed a significant benefit of an aromatase inhibitor in reducing pelvic pain. One study showed laparoscopic evidence of eradicating visible pelvic endometriotic implants and significantly decreasing pain.[172] Another study that was randomized combined an aromatase inhibitor with a GnRH agonist and showed that 54.7% of the patients in the GnRH agonist + aromatase inhibitor arm vs only 10% of the patients in the GnRH agonist-only arm were symptom - free within 24 months from the completion of the treatment.[171] The combination of an aromatase inhibitor with an oral progestin or an oral contraceptive gave rise to similar results, and we

predict that many patients and physicians will prefer these simpler oral regimens.[172,173]

The side-effect profile for AIs is reasonably benign. Mild headache, nausea, and diarrhea have been encountered in some patients. Compared to GnRH analogues, hot flashes are milder and infrequent. The regimens that combine AIs with add-back progestins or oral contraceptives do not appear to be associated with significant bone loss after 6 months of treatment.[176, 177] In a randomized prospective study, goserelin + anastrozole treatment caused significantly higher bone loss at the spine compared with goserelin-only treatment at the completion of the 6-month treatment. However, no significant difference between these groups was observed at 24-month follow-up.[171]

These preliminary data indicate that aromatase inhibitors effectively treat pelvic pain associated with endometriosis that is resistant to existing therapeutic modalities. The use of the currently available doses of aromatase inhibitors in premenopausal women with endometriosis requires ovarian suppression via the addition of a GnRH analogue, progestin, or combination oral contraceptive. The side-effect profiles were quite favorable and did not include bone loss in the majority of these regimens. Therefore, aromatase inhibitors (in combination with an ovarian suppressive treatment) may soon become one of the most commonly used treatments of endometriosis.[178]

Surgical therapy for endometriosis-related pain

Depending upon the severity of disease found, ideal practice is to diagnose and remove endometriosis surgically at the same time. This approach is becoming standard practice in the management of endometriosis.

Surgical treatment of endometriosis can be classified as conservative or radical. The aim of conservative surgery is to return the appearance of the pelvis to as normal as possible. Laparoscopic management has the advantage of needing a minimal hospital stay; it is usually possible to go home the same or the following day. Improvement in pain symptoms following this type of surgery can be expected in 70% of cases. Recurrence risk for endometriosis has been estimated to be 10% per year after conservative surgery.

Auxiliary surgical procedures for pain associated with endometriosis may involve interruption of pathways of pain conduction via uterosacral nerve ablation or presacral nerve resection. Two nerve-interrupting adjunctive procedures can be used in the treatment of endometriosis-associated pain, but their value has not yet been clearly demonstrated.[179,180] Regardless of the cause, there is also insufficient evidence to recommend the use of nerve interruption in the management of dysmenorrhea.[181] Both procedures are reserved for patients with midline pelvic pain and may be performed by either laparoscopy or laparotomy.

Radical surgery means performing a hysterectomy with removal of both ovaries, it is reserved for women with very severe symptoms, who have not responded to medical treatment or conservative operations. Hysterectomy is an end-stage treatment for women who have completed their family. It is usual to suggest removal of the ovaries.[182] Thus, all visible endometriotic tissue can be removed at the same time.[183] There is a six times higher risk of recurrence after hysterectomy if the ovaries are not removed. However, radical surgery is not a definitive approach because recurrence may occur even after the radical surgery.

There are no data to justify hormonal treatment prior to surgery to improve the success of surgery.[184] A treatment with danazol or a GnRH agonist for 6 months after surgery reduces endometriosis-associated pain and delays recurrence at 12 and 24 months compared with placebo and expectant management. However, postoperative treatment with a combined oral contraceptive is not effective.[134–137,185–188]

REFERENCES

1. Giudice L, Kao L. Endometriosis. Lancet 2004; 364: 1789–99.
2. Houston DE, Noller K, Melton LJ, Selwyn BJ. The epidemiology of pelvic endometriosis. Clin Obstet Gynecol 1988; 31: 787–800.
3. Cramer DW, Missmer SA. The epidemiology of endometriosis. Ann NY Acad Sci 2002; 955: 11–22; discussion 34–6, 396–406.
4. Missmer SA, Cramer DW. The epidemiology of endometriosis. Obstet Gynecol Clin North Am 2003; 30: 1–19, vii.
5. Eskenazi, B, Warner ML. Epidemiology of endometriosis. Obstet Gynecol Clin North Am 1997; 24: 235–58.
6. Sensky TE, Liu DT. Endometriosis: associations with menorrhagia, infertility and oral contraceptives. Int J Gynaecol Obstet 1980; 17: 573–6.
7. Sampson JA. Peritoneal endometriosis due to the menstrual dissemination of endometrial tissue into the peritoneal cavity. Am J Obste Gynecol 1927; 14: 422–45.
8. Bulun SE, Yang S, Fang Z et al. Role of aromatase in endometrial disease. J Steroid Biochem Mol Biol 2001; 79: 19–25.
9. Tsai SJ, Wu MH, Lin CC et al. Regulation of steroidogenic acute regulatory protein expression and progesterone production in endometriotic stromal cells. J Clin Endocrinol Metab 2001; 86: 5765–73.
10. Noble LS, Takayama K, Putman JM et al. Prostaglandin E_2 stimulates aromatase expression in endometriosis-derived stromal cells. J Clin Endocrinol Metab 1997; 82: 600–6.
11. Noble LS, Simpson ER, Johns A, Bulun SE. Aromatase expression in endometriosis. J Clin Endocrinol Metab 1996; 81: 174–9.
12. Gurates B, Sebastian S, Yang S et al. WT1 and DAX-1 inhibit aromatase P450 expression in human endometrial and endometriotic stromal cells. J Clin Endocrinol Metab 2002; 87: 4369–77.
13. Sun HS, Hsiao KY, Hsu CC et al. Transactivation of steroidogenic acute regulatory protein in human endometriotic stromal cells is mediated by the prostaglandin EP2 receptor. Endocrinology 2003; 144: 3934–42.
14. Wu M, Wang C, Lin C et al. Distinct regulation of cyclooxygenase-2 by interleukin-1β in normal and endometriotic stromal cells. J Clin Endocrinol Metab 2005; 90: 286–95.
15. Ota H, Igarashi S, Sasaki M, Tanaka T. Distribution of cyclooxygenase-2 in eutopic and ectopic endometrium in endometriosis and adenomyosis. Hum Reprod 2001; 16: 561–66.
16. Zeitoun K, Takayama K, Michael MD, Bulun SE. Stimulation of aromatase P450 promoter (II) activity in endometriosis and its inhibition in endometrium are regulated by competitive binding of SF-1 and COUP-TF to the same cis-acting element. Mol Endocrinol 1999; 13: 239–53.
17. Tamura M, Sebastian S, Yang S et al. Vascular endothelial growth factor upregulates cyclooxygenase-2 expression in human endothelial cells. J Clin Endocrinol Metab 2002; 87: 3504–7.
18. Tamura M, Sebastian S, Yang S et al. Interleukin-1beta elevates cyclooxygenase-2 protein level and enzyme activity via increasing its mRNA stability in human endometrial stromal cells: an effect mediated by extracellularly regulated kinase 1 and 2. J Clin Endocrinol Metab 2002; 87: 3263–73.
19. Tamura M, Sebastian S, Tang S et al. Up-regulation of cyclooxygenase-2 expression and prostaglandin synthesis in endometrial stromal cells by malignant endometrial epithelial cells: a paracrine mechanism mediated by PGE_2 and nuclear factor-κ B. J Biol Chem 2002; 277: 26208–16.
20. Ryan IP, Taylor RN. Endometriosis and infertility: new concepts. Obstet Gynecol Surv 1997; 52: 365–71.
21. Bruner KL, Matrisian LM, Rodgers WH et al. Suppression of matrix metalloproteinases inhibits establishment of ectopic lesions by human endometrium in nude mice. J Clin Invest 1997; 99: 2851–7.
22. Sebastian S, Bulun SE. A highly complex organization of the regulatory region of the human CYP19 (aromatase) gene revealed by the human genome project. J Clin Endocrinol Metab 2001; 86: 4600–2.
23. Sebastian S, Takayama K, Shozu M, Bulun S. Cloning and characterization of a novel endothelial promoter of the human CYP19 (aromatase P450) gene that is up-regulated in breast cancer tissue. Mol Endocrinol 2002; 16: 2243–54.
24. Yang S, Fang Z, Takashi S et al. Regulation of aromatase P450 expression in endometriotic and endometrial stromal cells by

CCAT/enhancer binding proteins: decreased C/EBPβ in endometriosis is associated with overexpression of aromatase. J Clin Endocrinol Metab 2002; 87: 2336–45.

25. Gurates B, Amsterdam A, Tamura M et al. WT1 and DAX-1 regulate SF-1-mediated human P450arom gene expression in gonadal cells. Mol Cell Endocrinol 2003; 208: 61–75.

26. Simpson JL, Bischoff FZ. Heritability and molecular genetic studies of endometriosis. Ann NY Acad Sci 2002; 955: 239–51; discussion 293–5, 396–406.

27. Kennedy S, Bennett S, Weeks DE. Affected sib-pair analysis in endometriosis. Hum Reprod Update 2001; 7: 411–18.

28. MacKenzie WF, Casey HW. Animal model of human disease. Endometriosis. Animal model: endometriosis in rhesus monkeys. Am J Pathol 1975; 80: 341–4.

29. Zondervan KT, Cardon LR, Kennedy SH. The genetic basis of endometriosis. Curr Opin Obstet Gynecol 2001; 13: 309–14.

30. Zondervan K, Cardon L, Desrosiers R et al. The genetic epidemiology of spontaneous endometriosis in the rhesus monkey. Ann NY Acad Sci 2002; 955: 233–8; discussion 293–5, 396–406.

31. Kennedy S, Mardon H, Barlow D. Familial endometriosis. J Assist Reprod Genet 1995; 12: 32–4.

32. Kennedy S, Hadfield R, Mardon H et al. Age of onset of pain symptoms in non-twin sisters concordant for endometriosis. Hum Reprod 1996; 11: 403–5.

33. Moen MH. Endometriosis in monozygotic twins. Acta Obstet Gynecol Scand 1994; 73: 59–62.

34. Hadfield RM, Mardon HJ, Barlo DH et al. Endometriosis in monozygotic twins. Fertil Steril 1997; 68: 941–2.

35. Fazleabas AT, Brudney A, Gurates B et al. A modified baboon model for endometriosis. Ann NY Acad Sci 2002; 955: 308–17; discussion 340–2, 396–406.

36. Smith SK. Genetic factors in endometriosis pathogenesis and work-up. In: Female Infertiliy. London: Martin Dunitz, 1997: 363–71.

37. Hadfield RM, Yudkin PL, Coe CL et al. Risk factors for endometriosis in the rhesus monkey (*Macaca mulatta*): a case-control study. Hum Reprod Update 1997; 3: 109–15.

38. Zondervan KT, Weeks DE, Colman R et al. Familial aggregation of endometriosis in a large pedigree of rhesus macaques. Hum Reprod 2004; 19: 448–55.

39. Bischoff FZ, Simpson JL. Heritability and molecular genetic studies of endometriosis. Hum Reprod Update 2000; 6: 37–44.

40. Treloar SA, O'Connor DT, O'Connor VM, Martin NG, Genetic influences on endometriosis in an Australian twin sample. sueT@qimr.edu.au. Fertil Steril 1999; 71: 701–10.

41. Treloar S, Hadfield R, Montgomery G et al. The International Endogene Study: a collection of families for genetic research in endometriosis. Fertil Steril 2002; 78: 679–85.

42. Kennedy S. Genetics of endometriosis: a review of the positional cloning approaches. Semin Reprod Med 2003; 21: 111–18.

43. Zondervan K, Cardon L, Kennedy S. Development of a web site for the genetic epidemiology of endometriosis. Fertil Steril 2002; 78: 777–81.

44. Baranova H, Bothorishvilli R, Canis M et al. Glutathione S-transferase M1 gene polymorphism and susceptibility to endometriosis in a French population. Mol Hum Reprod 1997; 3: 775–80.

45. Baranov VS, Ivaschenko T, Bakay B et al. Proportion of the GSTM1 0/0 genotype in some Slavic populations and its correlation with cystic fibrosis and some multifactorial diseases. Hum Genet 1996; 97: 516–20.

46. Nakago,S, Hadfield RM, Zondervan KT et al. Association between endometriosis and N-acetyl transferase 2 polymorphisms in a UK population. Mol Hum Reprod 2001; 7: 1079–83.

47. Cramer DW, Hornstein MD, Ng WG, Barbieri RL. Endometriosis associated with the N314D mutation of galactose-1-phosphate uridyl transferase (GALT). Mol Hum Reprod 1996; 2: 149–52.

48. Hadfield RM, Manek S, Nakago S et al. Absence of a relationship between endometriosis and the N314D polymorphism of galactose-1-phosphate uridyl transferase in a UK population. Mol Hum Reprod 1999; 5: 990–3.

49. Morland SJ, Jiang X, Hitchcock A et al. Mutation of galactose-1-phosphate uridyl transferase and its association with ovarian cancer and endometriosis. Int J Cancer 1998; 77: 825–7.

50. Rier SE, Martin DC, Bowman RE et al. Endometriosis in rhesus monkeys (*Macaca mulatta*) following chronic exposure to 2,3,7,8-tetrachlorodibenzo-p-dioxin. Fundam Appl Toxicol 1993; 21: 433–41.

51. Hadfield RM, Manek S, Weeks DE et al. Linkage and association studies of the relationship between endometriosis and genes encoding the detoxification enzymes GSTM1, GSTT1 and CYP1A1. Mol Hum Reprod 2001; 7: 1073–8.

52. Morizane M, Yoshida S, Nakago S et al. No association of endometriosis with glutathione S-transferase M1 and T1 null mutations in a Japanese population. J Soc Gynecol Investig 2004; 11: 118–21.

53. Guo SW, The association of endometriosis risk and genetic polymorphisms involving dioxin detoxification enzymes: a systematic review. Eur J Obstet Gynecol Reprod Biol 2006; 124: 134–43.

54. Tempfer CB, Schneeberger C, Huber JC. Applications of polymorphisms and pharmacogenomics in obstetrics and gynecology. Pharmacogenomics 2004; 5: 57–65.

55. Thomas EJ, Campbell IG. Molecular genetic defects in endometriosis. Gynecol Obstet Invest 2000; 50(Suppl 1): 44–50.

56. Goumenou AG, Arvanitis DA, Matalliotakis IM et al. Loss of heterozygosity in adenomyosis on hMSH2, hMLH1, p16Ink4 and GALT loci. Int J Mol Med 2000; 6: 667–71.

57. Gogusev J, Bouquet de Joliniere J, Telvi L et al. Detection of DNA copy number changes in human endometriosis by comparative genomic hybridization. Hum Genet 1999; 105: 444–51.

58. Shin JC, Ross HL, Elias S et al. Detection of chromosomal aneuploidy in endometriosis by multi-color fluorescence in situ hybridization (FISH). Hum Genet 1997; 100: 401–6.

59. Bischoff FZ, Heard M, Simpson JL. Somatic DNA alterations in endometriosis: high frequency of chromosome 17 and p53 loss in late-stage endometriosis. J Reprod Immunol 2002; 55: 49–64.

60. Bubendorf L, Nocito A, Moch H, Sauter G. Tissue microarray (TMA) technology: miniaturized pathology archives for high-throughput in situ studies. J Pathol 2001; 195: 72–9.

61. Taylor RN, Lebovic DI, Mueller MD. Angiogenic factors in endometriosis. Ann NY Acad Sci 2002; 955: 89–100; discussion 118, 396–406.

62. Kao LC, Germeyer A, Tulac S et al. Expression profiling of endometrium from women with endometriosis reveals candidate genes for disease-based implantation failure and infertility. Endocrinology 2003; 144: 2870–81.

63. Giudice LC, Telles TL, Lobo S, Kao L. The molecular basis for implantation failure in endometriosis: on the road to discovery. Ann NY Acad Sci 2002; 955: 252–64; discussion 293–5, 396–406.

64. Taylor RN, Lundeen SG, Giudice LC. Emerging role of genomics in endometriosis research. Fertil Steril 2002; 78: 694–8.

65. Eyster KM, Boles AL, Brannian JD, Hansen KA. DNA microarray analysis of gene expression markers of endometriosis. Fertil Steril 2002; 77: 38–42.

66. Rier S, Foster WG. Environmental dioxins and endometriosis. Semin Reprod Med 2003; 21: 145–54.

67. McNulty WP. Toxicity and fetotoxicity of TCDD, TCDF and PCB isomers in rhesus macaques (*Macaca mulatta*). Environ Health Perspect 1985; 60: 77–88.

68. Jones MK, Weisenburger WP, Sipes IG, Russell DH. Circadian alterations in prolactin, corticosterone, and thyroid hormone

levels and down-regulation of prolactin receptor activity by 2,3,7,8-tetrachlorodibenzo-p-dioxin. Toxicol Appl Pharmacol 1987; 87: 337–50.

69. Safe S, Astroff B, Harris M et al. 2,3,7,8-Tetrachlorodibenzo-p-dioxin (TCDD) and related compounds as antioestrogens: characterization and mechanism of action. Pharmacol Toxicol 1991; 69: 400–9.

70. DeVito MJ, Thomas T, Martin E et al. Antiestrogenic action of 2,3,7,8-tetrachlorodibenzo-p-dioxin: tissue-specific regulation of estrogen receptor in CD1 mice. Toxicol Appl Pharmacol 1992; 113: 284–92.

71. Allen JR, Barsotti DA, Lambrecht LK, Van Miller J. Reproductive effects of halogenated aromatic hydrocarbons on nonhuman primates. Ann NY Acad Sci 1979; 320: 419–25.

72. Holsapple MP, Snyder NK, Wood SC, Morris DL. A review of 2,3,7,8-tetrachlorodibenzo-p-dioxin-induced changes in immunocompetence: 1991 update. Toxicology 1991; 69: 219–55.

73. Neubert R, Jacob-Muller U, Helge H et al. Polyhalogenated dibenzo-p-dioxins and dibenzofurans and the immune system. 2. In vitro effects of 2,3,7,8-tetrachlorodibenzo-p-dioxin (TCDD) on lymphocytes of venous blood from man and a non-human primate (*Callithrix jacchus*). Arch Toxicol 1991; 65: 213–19.

74. Tomar RS, Kerkvliet NI. Reduced T-helper cell function in mice exposed to 2,3,7,8-tetrachlorodibenzo-p-dioxin (TCDD). Toxicol Lett 1991; 57: 55–64.

75. Whitlock JP Jr. Genetic and molecular aspects of 2,3,7,8-tetrachlorodibenzo-p-dioxin action. Annu Rev Pharmacol Toxicol 1990; 30: 251–77.

76. Sutter TR, Guzman K, Dold KM, Greenlee WF. Targets for dioxin: genes for plasminogen activator inhibitor-2 and interleukin-1 beta. Science 1991; 254: 415–18.

77. Attar E, Genc S, Bulgurcuoglu S et al.Increased concentration of vascular endothelial growth factor in the follicular fluid of patients with endometriosis does not affect the outcome of in vitro fertilization-embryo transfer. Fertil Steril 2003; 80: 1518–20.

78. Wu MY, Ho HN. The role of cytokines in endometriosis. Am J Reprod Immunol 2003; 49: 285–96.

79. Arici A. Local cytokines in endometrial tissue: the role of interleukin-8 in the pathogenesis of endometriosis. Ann NY Acad Sci 2002; 955: 101–9; discussion 118, 396–406.

80. Arici A, Tazuke SI, Attar E et al. Interleukin-8 concentration in peritoneal fluid of patients with endometriosis and modulation of interleukin-8 expression in human mesothelial cells. Mol Hum Reprod 1996; 2: 40–5.

81. Kayisli UA, Mahutte NG, Arici A. Uterine chemokines in reproductive physiology and pathology. Am J Reprod Immunol 2002; 47: 213–21.

82. Arici A, Oral E, Attar E et al. Monocyte chemotactic protein-1 concentration in peritoneal fluid of women with endometriosis and its modulation of expression in mesothelial cells. Fertil Steril 1997; 67: 1065–72.

83. Liu Y, Lv L. Mechanism of elevated vascular endothelial growth factor levels in peritoneal fluids from patients with endometriosis. J Huazhong Univ Sci Technolog Med Sci 2004; 24: 470–2.

84. Donnez J, Smoes P, Gillerot S et al. Vascular endothelial growth factor (VEGF) in endometriosis. Hum Reprod 1998; 13: 1686–90.

85. Jimbo H, Hitomi Y, Yoshikawa H et al. Evidence for monoclonal expansion of epithelial cells in ovarian endometrial cysts. Am J Pathol 1997; 150: 1173–8.

86. Mayr D, Amann G, Siefert C et al. Does endometriosis really have premalignant potential? A clonal analysis of laser-microdissected tissue. FASCH J 2003; 17: 693–5.

87. Swiersz LM. Role of endometriosis in cancer and tumor development. Ann NY Acad Sci 2002; 955: 281–92; discussion 293–5, 396–406.

88. Starzinski-Powitz A, Gaetje R, Zeitvogel A et al. Tracing cellular and molecular mechanisms involved in endometriosis. Hum Reprod Update 1998; 4: 724–9.

89. Gaetje R, Kotzian S, Herrmann G et al. Invasiveness of endometriotic cells in vitro. Lancet 1995; 346: 1463–4.

90. Dmowski WP, Gebel HM, Braun DP. The role of cell-mediated immunity in pathogenesis of endometriosis. Acta Obstet Gynecol Scand Suppl 1994; 159: 7–14.

91. Dinulescu DM, Ince TA, Quade BJ et al. Role of K-ras and pten in the development of mouse models of endometriosis and endometrioid ovarian cancer. Nat Med 2005; 11: 63–70.

92. Girling JE, Rogers PA. Recent advances in endometrial angiogenesis research. Angiogenesis 2005; 8: 89–99.

93. Healy DL, Rogers PA, Hii L,Wingfield M. Angiogenesis: a new theory for endometriosis. Hum Reprod Update 1998; 4: 736–40.

94. Ferriani RA, Charnock-Jones DS, Prentice A et al. Immunohistochemical localization of acidic and basic fibroblast growth factors in normal human endometrium and endometriosis and the detection of their mRNA by polymerase chain reaction. Hum Reprod 1993; 8: 11–16.

95. Charnock-Jones DS, Sharkey AM, Rajput-Williams J et al. Identification and localization of alternately spliced mRNAs for vascular endothelial growth factor in human uterus and estrogen regulation in endometrial carcinoma cell lines. Biol Reprod 1993; 48: 1120–8.

96. Sangha RK, Li XF, Shams M, Ahmed A. Fibroblast growth factor receptor-1 is a critical component for endometrial remodeling: localization and expression of basic fibroblast growth factor and FGF-R1 in human endometrium during the menstrual cycle and decreased FGF-R1 expression in menorrhagia. Lab Invest 1997; 77: 389–402.

97. Hii LL, Rogers PA. Endometrial vascular and glandular expression of integrin alpha(v)beta3 in women with and without endometriosis. Hum Reprod 1998; 13: 1030–5.

98. Akerlund M, Stromberg P, Forsling ML. Primary dysmenorrhoea and vasopressin. Br J Obstet Gynaecol 1979; 86: 484–7.

99. Ekstrom P, Akerlund M, Forsling M et al. Stimulation of vasopressin release in women with primary dysmenorrhoea and after oral contraceptive treatment–effect on uterine contractility. Br J Obstet Gynaecol 1992; 99: 680–4.

100. Ekstrom P, Alm P, Akerlund M. Differences in vasomotor responses between main stem and smaller branches of the human uterine artery. Acta Obstet Gynecol Scand 1991; 70: 429–33.

101. Dmowski WP, Gebel HM, Rawlins RG. Immunologic aspects of endometriosis. Obstet Gynecol Clin North Am 1989; 16: 93–103.

102. Sillem M, Prifti S, Neher M, Runnebaum B. Extracellular matrix remodelling in the endometrium and its possible relevance to the pathogenesis of endometriosis. Hum Reprod Update 1998; 4: 730–5.

103. Osteen KG, Yeaman GR, Bruner-Tran KL. Matrix metalloproteinases and endometriosis. Semin Reprod Med 2003; 21: 155–64.

104. Seli E, Berkkanoglu M, Arici A. Pathogenesis of endometriosis. Obstet Gynecol Clin North Am 2003; 30: 41–61.

105. Kokorine I, Marbaix E, Henriet P et al. Focal cellular origin and regulation of interstitial collagenase (matrix metalloproteinase-1) are related to menstrual breakdown in the human endometrium. J Cell Sci 1996; 109 (Pt 8): 2151–60.

106. Wenzl RJ, Heinzl H. Localization of matrix metalloproteinase-2 in uterine endometrium and ectopic implants. Gynecol Obstet Invest 1998; 45: 253–7.

107. Bruner KL, Matrisian LM, Rodgers WH et al. Suppression of matrix metalloproteinases inhibits establishment of ectopic lesions by human endometrium in nude mice. J Clin Invest 1997; 99: 2851–7.

108. Lessey BA, Young SL. Integrins and other cell adhesion molecules in endometrium and endometriosis. Semin Reprod Endocrinol 1997; 15: 291–9.

109. Regidor PA, Vogel C, Regidor M et al. Expression pattern of integrin adhesion molecules in endometriosis and human endometrium. Hum Reprod Update 1998; 4: 710–18.

110. van der Linden PJ, de Goeij AF, Dunselman GA et al. Expression of integrins and E-cadherin in cells from menstrual effluent, endometrium, peritoneal fluid, peritoneum, and endometriosis. Fertil Steril 1994; 61: 85–90.

111. van der Linden PJ, de Goeij AF, Dunselman GA et al. P-cadherin expression in human endometrium and endometriosis. Gynecol Obstet Invest 1994; 38: 183–5.

112. Harada T, Kaponis A, Iwabe T et al. Apoptosis in human endometrium and endometriosis. Hum Reprod Update 2004; 10: 29–38.

113. Gebel HM, Braun DP, Tambur A et al. Spontaneous apoptosis of endometrial tissue is impaired in women with endometriosis. Fertil Steril 1998; 69: 1042–7.

114. McLaren J, Prentice A, Charnock-Jones DS et al. Immunolocalization of the apoptosis regulating proteins Bcl-2 and Bax in human endometrium and isolated peritoneal fluid macrophages in endometriosis. Hum Reprod 1997; 12: 146–52.

115. Garcia-Velasco JA, Arici A. Apoptosis and the pathogenesis of endometriosis. Semin Reprod Med 2003; 21: 165–72.

116. GarciaVelasco JA, Mulayim N, Kayisli UA, Arici A. Elevated soluble Fas ligand levels may suggest a role for apoptosis in women with endometriosis. Fertil Steril 2002; 78: 855–9.

117. Bayer SR, Seibel MM, Saffan DS et al. Efficacy of danazol treatment for minimal endometriosis in infertile women. A prospective, randomized study. J Reprod Med 1988; 33: 179–83.

118. Fedele L, Bianchi S, Arcaini L et al. Buserelin versus danazol in the treatment of endometriosis-associated infertility. Am J Obstet Gynecol 1989; 161: 871–6.

119. Telimaa S. Danazol and medroxyprogesterone acetate inefficacious in the treatment of infertility in endometriosis. Fertil Steril 1988; 50: 872–5.

120. Thomas EJ, Cooke ID. Successful treatment of asymptomatic endometriosis: does it benefit infertile women? Br Med J (Clin Res Ed) 1987; 294: 1117–19.

121. Henzl MR, Corson SL, Moghissi K et al. Administration of nasal nafarelin as compared with oral danazol for endometriosis. A multicenter double-blind comparative clinical trial. N Engl J Med 1988; 318: 485–9.

122. Fedele L, Bianchi S, Arcaini L et al. Buserelin versus danazol in the treatment of endometriosis-associated infertility. Am J Obstet and Gynecol 1989; 161: 871–76.

123. Fedele L, Bianchi S, Viezzoli T et al. Gestrinone versus danazol in the treatment of endometriosis. Fertil Steril 1989; 51: 781–5.

124. Noble AD, Letchworth AT. Medical treatment of endometriosis: a comparative trial. Postgrad Med J 1979; 55(Suppl 5): 37–9.

125. Fraser IS, Shearman RP, Jansen RP, Sutherland PD. A comparative treatment trial of endometriosis using the gonadotrophin-releasing hormone agonist, nafarelin, and the synthetic steroid, danazol. Aust N Z J Obstet Gynaecol 1991; 31: 158–63.

126. Rolland R, van der Heijden PF. Nafarelin versus danazol in the treatment of endometriosis. Am J Obstet Gynecol 1990; 162: 586–8.

127. Shaw RW. An open randomized comparative study of the effect of goserelin depot and danazol in the treatment of endometriosis. Zoladex Endometriosis Study Team. Fertil Steril 1992; 58: 265–72.

128. Dmowski WP, Radwanska E, Binor Z et al. Ovarian suppression induced with Buserelin or danazol in the management of endometriosis: a randomized, comparative study. Fertil Steril 1989; 51: 395–400.

129. Hughes E, Fedorkow D, Collins J, Vandekerckhove P. Ovulation suppression for endometriosis. Cochrane Database Syst Rev 2003: CD000155.

130. Olive DL, Lee KL. Analysis of sequential treatment protocols for endometriosis-associated infertility. Am J Obstet Gynecol 1986; 154: 613–19.

131. Guzick DS, Silliman NP, Adamson GD et al. Prediction of pregnancy in infertile women based on the American Society for Reproductive Medicine's revised classification of endometriosis. Fertil Steril 1997; 67: 822–9.

132. Osuga Y, Koga K, Tsutsumi O et al. Role of laparoscopy in the treatment of endometriosis-associated infertility. Gynecol Obstet Invest 2002; 53(Suppl 1): 33–9.

133. Adamson GD, Hurd SJ, Pasta DJ, Rodriguez BD. Laparoscopic endometriosis treatment: is it better? Fertil Steril 1993; 59: 35–44.

134. Parazzini F, Fedele L, Busacca M et al. Postsurgical medical treatment of advanced endometriosis: results of a randomized clinical trial. Am J Obstet Gynecol 1994; 171: 1205–7.

135. Bianchi S, Busacca M, Agnoli B et al. Effects of 3 month therapy with danazol after laparoscopic surgery for stage III/IV endometriosis: a randomized study. Hum Reprod 1999; 14: 1335–7.

136. Vercellini P, Crosignani PG, Fadini R et al. A gonadotropin-releasing hormone agonist compared with expectant management after conservative surgery for symptomatic endometriosis. Br J Obstet Gynaecol 1999; 106: 672–7.

137. Busacca M, Somigliana E, Bianchi S et al. Post-operative GnRH analogue treatment after conservative surgery for symptomatic endometriosis stage III–IV: a randomized controlled trial. Hum Reprod 2001; 16: 2399–402.

138. Hughes EG, Fedorkow DM, Collins JA. A quantitative overview of controlled trials in endometriosis-associated infertility. Fertil Steril 1993; 59: 963–70.

139. Marcoux S, Maheux R, Berube S. Laparoscopic surgery in infertile women with minimal or mild endometriosis. Canadian Collaborative Group on Endometriosis. N Engl J Med 1997; 337: 217–22.

140. Fedele L, Bianchi S, Marchini M et al. Superovulation with human menopausal gonadotropins in the treatment of infertility associated with minimal or mild endometriosis: a controlled randomized study. Fertil Steril 1992; 58: 28–31.

141. Deaton JL, Gibson M, Blackmer KM et al. A randomized, controlled trial of clomiphene citrate and intrauterine insemination in couples with unexplained infertility or surgically corrected endometriosis. Fertil Steril 1990; 54: 1083–8.

142. Tummon IS, Asher LJ, Martin JS, Tulandi T. Randomized controlled trial of superovulation and insemination for infertility associated with minimal or mild endometriosis. Fertil Steril 1997; 68: 8–12.

143. Somigliana E, Vercellini P, Vigano P et al. Should endometriomas be treated before IVF-ICSI cycles? Hum Reprod Update 2006; 12: 57–64.

144. Vercellini P, De Giorgi O, Mosconi P et al. Cyproterone acetate versus a continuous monophasic oral contraceptive in the treatment of recurrent pelvic pain after conservative surgery for symptomatic endometriosis. Fertil Steril 2002; 77: 52–61.

145. Vercellini P, Cortesi I, Crosignani PG. Progestins for symptomatic endometriosis: a critical analysis of the evidence. Fertil Steril 1997; 68: 393–401.

146. Proctor ML, Roberts H, Farquhar CM. Combined oral contraceptive pill (OCP) as treatment for primary dysmenorrhoea. Cochrane Database Syst Rev 2001: CD002120.

147. Vercellini P, Trespidi L, Colombo A et al. A gonadotropin-releasing hormone agonist versus a low-dose oral contraceptive for pelvic pain associated with endometriosis. Fertil Steril 1993; 60: 75–9.

148. Moghissi KS. Treatment of endometriosis with estrogen-progestin combination and progestogens alone. Clin Obstet Gynecol 1988; 31: 823–8.

149. Olive DL, Pritts EA. The treatment of endometriosis: a review of the evidence. Ann NY Acad Sci 2002; 955: 360–72; discussion 389–93, 396–406.

150. Watanabe Y, Nakamura G, Matsuguchi H et al. Efficacy of a low-dose leuprolide acetate depot in the treatment of uterine leiomyomata in Japanese women. Fertil Steril 1992; 58: 66–71.

151. Wheeler JM, Knittle JD, Miller JD. Depot leuprolide acetate versus danazol in the treatment of women with symptomatic endometriosis: a multicenter, double-blind randomized clinical trial. II. Assessment of safety. The Lupron Endometriosis Study Group. Am J Obstet Gynecol 1993; 169: 26–33.

152. Warnock JK, Bundren JC, Morris DW. Depressive symptoms associated with gonadotropin-releasing hormone agonists. Depress Anxiety 1998; 7: 171–7.

153. Rachman M, Garfield DA, Rachman I, Cohen R. Lupron-induced mania. Biol Psychiatry 1999; 45: 243–4.

154. Jiang J, Lu J, Wu R. [Mifepristone following conservative surgery in the treatment of endometriosis]. Zhonghua Fu Chan Ke Za Zhi 2001; 36: 717–20.

155. Kettel LM, Murphy AA, Morales AJ et al. Treatment of endometriosis with the antiprogesterone mifepristone (RU486). Fertil Steril 1996; 65: 23–8.

156. Chabbert-Buffet N, Meduri G, Bouchard P, Spitz IM. Selective progesterone receptor modulators and progesterone antagonists: mechanisms of action and clinical applications. Hum Reprod Update 2005; 11: 293–307.

157. Chwalisz K, Perez MC, Demanno D et al. Selective progesterone receptor modulator development and use in the treatment of leiomyomata and endometriosis. Endocr Rev 2005; 26: 423–38.

158. Bullimore DW. Endometriosis is sustained by tumour necrosis factor-alpha. Med Hypotheses 2003; 60: 84–8.

159. McLaren J. Vascular endothelial growth factor and endometriotic angiogenesis. Hum Reprod Update 2000; 6: 45–55.

160. Augustin HG. [Angiogenesis research – quo vadis?]. Ophthalmologe 2003; 100: 104–10.

161. Fraser HM, Lunn SF. Angiogenesis and its control in the female reproductive system. Br Med Bull 2000; 56: 787–97.

162. Taylor RN, Mueller MD. Anti-angiogenic treatment of endometriosis: biochemical aspects. Gynecol Obstet Invest 2004; 57: 54–6.

163. Nap AW, Dunselman GA, Griffioen AW et al. Angiostatic agents prevent the development of endometriosis-like lesions in the chicken chorioallantoic membrane. Fertil Steril 2005; 83: 793–5.

164. Vercellini P, Vigano P, Somigliana E. The role of the levonorgestrel-releasing intrauterine device in the management of symptomatic endometriosis. Curr Opin Obstet Gynecol 2005; 17: 359–65.

165. Fedele L, Bianchi S, Raffaelli R et al. Treatment of adenomyosis-associated menorrhagia with a levonorgestrel-releasing intrauterine device. Fertil Steril 1997; 68: 426–9.

166. Petta CA, Ferriani RA, Abrao MS et al. Randomized clinical trial of a levonorgestrel-releasing intrauterine system and a depot GnRH analogue for the treatment of chronic pelvic pain in women with endometriosis. Hum Reprod 2005; 20: 1993–8.

167. Lockhat FB, Emembolu JO, Konje JC. The efficacy, side-effects and continuation rates in women with symptomatic endometriosis undergoing treatment with an intra-uterine administered progestogen (levonorgestrel): a 3 year follow-up. Hum Reprod 2005; 20: 789–93.

168. Goss PE, Strasser K. Aromatase inhibitors in the treatment and prevention of breast cancer. J Clin Oncol 2001; 19: 881–94.

169. Buzdar A, Howell A. Advances in aromatase inhibition: clinical efficacy and tolerability in the treatment of breast cancer. Clin Cancer Res 2001; 7: 2620–35.

170. Takayama K, Zeitoun K, Gunby RT et al. Treatment of severe postmenopausal endometriosis with an aromatase inhibitor. Fertil Steril 1998; 69: 709–713.

171. Soysal S, Soysal M, Ozer S et al. The effects of post-surgical administration of goserelin plus anastrozole compared to goserelin alone in patients with severe endometriosis: a prospective randomized trial. Hum Reprod 2004; 19: 160–7.

172. Ailawadi R, Jobanputra S, Kataria M et al. Treatment of endometriosis and chronic pelvic pain with letrozole and norethindrone acetate: a pilot study. Fertil Steril 2004; 81: 290–6.

173. Amsterdam L, Gentry W, Rubin S et al. Treatment of endometriosis-related pelvic pain with a combination of an aromatase inhibitor (anastrozle) plus a combination oral contraceptive: a novel approach. Proceedings of the 85th Annual Endocrine Society Meeting 2003; 1: 360.

174. Razzi S, Fava A, Sartini A et al. Treatment of severe recurrent endometriosis with an aromatase inhibitor in a young ovariectomised woman. BJOG 2004; 111: 182–4.

175. Shippen E, West WJ. Successful treatment of severe endometriosis in two premenopausal women with an aromatase inhibitor. Fertil Steril 2004; 81: 1395–8.

176. Ailawadi RK, Jobanputra S, Kataria M et al. Treatment of endometriosis and chronic pelvic pain with letrozole and norethindrone acetate: a pilot study. Fertil Steril 2004; 81: 290–6.

177. Amsterdam LL, Gentry W, Jobanputra S et al. Anastrazole and oral contraceptives: a novel treatment for endometriosis. Fertil Steril 2005; 84: 300–4.

178. Attar E, Bulun SE. Aromatase and other steroidogenic genes in endometriosis: translational aspects. Hum Reprod Update 2006; 12: 49–56.

179. Wilson ML, Farquhar CM, Sinclair OJ, Johnson NP. Surgical interruption of pelvic nerve pathways for primary and secondary dysmenorrhoea. Cochrane Database Syst Rev 2000: CD001896.

180. Vercellini P, Aimi G, Busacca M et al. Laproscopic uterosacral ligament resection for dysmenorrhea associated with endometriosis: results of a randomized, controlled trial. Fertil Steril 2003; 80: 310–19.

181. Proctor M, Latthe P, Farquhar C et al. Surgical interruption of pelvic nerve pathways for primary and secondary dysmenorrhoea. Cochrane Database Syst Rev 2005: CD001896.

182. Namnoum AB, Hickman TN, Goodman SB et al. Incidence of symptom recurrence after hysterectomy for endometriosis. Fertil Steril 1995; 64: 898–902.

183. Lefebvre G, Allaire C, Jeffrey J et al. SOGC clinical guidelines. Hysterectomy. J Obstet Gynaecol Can 2002; 24: 37–61; quiz 74–6.

184. Muzii L, Marana R, Caruana P, Mancuso S. The impact of pre-operative gonadotropin-releasing hormone agonist treatment on laparoscopic excision of ovarian endometriotic cysts. Fertil Steril 1996; 65: 1235–7.

185. Telimaa S, Puolakka J, Rönnberg L, Kauppila A. Placebo-controlled comparison of danazol and high-dose medroxyprogesterone acetate in the treatment of endometriosis after conservative surgery. Gynecol Endocrinol 1987; 1: 363–71.

186. Hornstein MD, Hemmings R, Yuzpe AA, Heinrichs WL. Use of nafarelin versus placebo after reductive laparoscopic surgery for endometriosis. Fertil Steril 1997; 68: 860–4.

187. Morgante G, Ditto A, La Marca A, De Leo V. Low-dose danazol after combined surgical and medical therapy reduces the incidence of pelvic pain in women with moderate and severe endometriosis. Hum Reprod 1999; 14: 2371–4.

188. Muzii L, Marana R, Caruana P et al. Postoperative administration of monophasic combined oral contraceptives after laparoscopic treatment of ovarian endometriomas: a prospective, randomized trial. Am J Obstet Gynecol 2000; 183: 588–92.

47 The pathophysiology of dysfunctional uterine bleeding

Romana A Nowak

INTRODUCTION

Dysfunctional or abnormal uterine bleeding is a common but significant problem in women's health. Women may be affected at various times throughout their reproductive years due to the different types of abnormal uterine bleeding that can occur. Some of the causes include bleeding disorders such as Von Willebrand's disease and thrombocytopenia or anatomical problems such as the presence of uterine leiomyomas, polyps, adenomyosis, or cancer. Hormonal disturbances due to anovulation can cause abnormal uterine bleeding in perimenarcheal girls or women entering the perimenopause. The use of more effective, long-acting progestin contraceptives has also led to an increased incidence of abnormal uterine bleeding in women. This chapter focuses on the cellular and molecular mechanisms that are thought to contribute to the etiology of abnormal uterine bleeding. An overview of the normal menstrual cycle is first presented. A review of current hypotheses for two main causes of abnormal uterine bleeding, first in response to hormonal disturbances due to anovulation or progestin-only contraceptives and, secondly, due to anatomical factors, will follow. This overview will highlight the importance of matrix metalloproteinases (MMPs) and local changes in the immune environment within the endometrium in regulating the structural integrity of the cell and vascular structures. Loss of this structural integrity appears to be the underlying causative factor in the onset of abnormal uterine bleeding, regardless of the initial abnormality. An increased understanding of the mechanisms involved in blood vessel destabilization and bleeding in the endometrium will lead clinicians to explore new types of therapies for treatment of this condition.

THE MENSTRUAL CYCLE

Menstruation is a process that is unique to women and some primates. The cyclic breakdown and subsequent regrowth of the endometrial layer of the uterus throughout each menstrual cycle are critical for maintenance of a functional endometrium. These cyclical changes in the endometrium result from the production of the ovarian steroids estradiol and progesterone. Both stromal and glandular components of the endometrium show specific morphological changes that occur in response to the rise and fall of estrogen and progesterone during the normal menstrual cycle. The basic histological pattern, first described in 1950 by Noyes et al, is still used today.[1]

The progression of changes in the morphology of glands and stroma is paralleled by changes in the vascular structures. These changes start in the myometrium underlying the endometrium. Arcuate arteries arising in the myometrium give off radial branches (also known as basal arteries) that become coiled and form the so-called spiral arteries as they penetrate the endometrium. The spiral arteries, unlike the basal arteries, are sensitive to estrogen and progesterone.[2] These vessels form the rich network of interdigitating capillaries that supply the functional layer of endometrium that is later shed during menstruation. Menstruation is preceded by an ischemic phase characterized by vasoconstriction of these spiral arteries and arterioles, and bleeding ensues after these vessels relax.[2] Blood components, including clotting factors and platelets, appear to form clots that limit blood loss until regeneration is complete. For many years menstruation was thought to be a process that occurred in response to this localized ischemia. However, in recent years it has become clear that menstruation is actually a process that involves an active tissue breakdown which leads to a destabilization of the vascular structures in the endometrium, and this subsequently results in menstrual bleeding.

Factors regulating endometrial tissue breakdown at menstruation

The fall in the steroid hormones estradiol and progesterone preceding menstruation results in disruption of the endometrial cells and the extracellular matrix (ECM).[3] Disruption in the expression of molecules including desmoplakin I/II, E-cadherin and α- and β-catenins, and the loss of F-actin occur in the functionalis layer to allow for menstrual bleeding.[4] Apoptosis increases late in the secretory phase in the endometrial glands and thus prepares this tissue for disruption.[3] This breakdown of the ECM is regulated primarily by MMPs.[5] Matrix metalloproteinases are a group of zinc-containing proteolytic enzymes that are involved in several biological events involving extensive matrix remodeling.[6] These events include embryonic development, angiogenesis, wound healing, tumor invasion, and reproduction. The activity of this family of enzymes is controlled by growth factors, steroid hormones, cytokines, and tissue inhibitors of metalloproteinases (TIMPs).[7,8]

The MMPs can be classified into four broad classes based upon the substrate that they act upon. These classes are collagenases, gelatinases, stromelysins, and membrane-type enzymes (MT-MMPs). Collagenases include MMPs -1, -8, and -13, which degrade fibrillar and non-fibrillar collagen to form gelatin. Gelatinases include MMPs -2 and -9. They can act not only on gelatin but also on type IV collagen, laminin, and fibronectin. This group can also use interleukins and tumor necrosis factor α (TNFα) as substrates to activate the function of these cytokines.[9] Stromelysins include MMPs -3, -7, -10, and -11. These act on the substrates collagen, laminin, and fibronectin. A unique feature of the stromelysin family of enzymes is that they can activate other MMPs by cleaving the proenzymatic portion of the protein. They use this same feature to activate several different growth factors and cytokines.[9] The final group of MMPs is the membrane-associated MMPs. These proteins contain a transmembrane domain at their carboxy terminus, localizing them to the plasma membrane. The extracellular region of these MMPs can bind to proteins to either activate them (MMP-2) or inactivate them (TIMPs). Several of the MMPs are expressed by the stromal cells of the uterine endometrium, including MMPs -1, -2, -3, -9, -10, and -11.[5] MMP-7 is expressed by the endometrial epithelial cells. Expression of these various MMPs is restricted to specific phases of the menstrual cycle[11,12] and is regulated by ovarian steroid hormones. Progesterone decreases MMP expression by endometrial stromal cells and that is why levels of most of the MMPs are quite low during the secretory phase of the menstrual cycle. Once progesterone levels fall prior to menstruation, the expression of most of these MMPs in the endometrial stroma increases. Expression of MMPs in the endometrium is also regulated by local factors such as growth factors and cytokines. These factors are produced by the stromal cells themselves as well as by vascular cells and infiltrating leukocytes.[5,13]

Menstruation is preceded by an influx of inflammatory leukocytes into the endometrium. These leukocytes include macrophages, eosinophils, neutrophils, and mast cells.[14] How the recruitment of these immune cells to the endometrium is regulated is not clear, but it appears to occur in response to changing steroid hormone levels. Uterine glandular and stromal cells express steroid receptors in a cyclical fashion during the menstrual cycle. Estrogen receptor α (ERα) is expressed by both the epithelial and stromal cells during the proliferative phase, but expression drops precipitously by the end of the secretory phase.[15] Progesterone receptors A and B (PR-A and PR-B) are both expressed in glandular epithelial and stromal cells during the proliferative phase but during the secretory phase only the PR-A is present in endometrial stromal cells, while the glandular epithelial cells no longer express any progesterone receptor. Leukocytes do not express progesterone receptors,[13,16] suggesting that influx of these cells into the endometrium must occur in response to other local factors expressed by cells residing in the endometrium.

Recent studies support the hypothesis that the infiltration of the uterine endometrium by leukocytes from the circulation is regulated by cytokines and chemokines produced by uterine stromal or glandular epithelial cells.[17] Studies have shown that cyotokines such as interleukin-1 (IL-1) and TNFα are produced by endometrial stromal and epithelial cells and their expression peaks during the mid–late secretory phase of the menstrual cycle.[18] These increases in cytokines are coincident with the increases in leukocytes that occur late in the secretory phase. Chemokines of the CC and CXC groups have also been identified in the human uterine endometrium. The CXC chemokines are known to act primarily on neutrophils, while the CC chemokines act on monocytes, lymphocytes, and eosinophils.[17] Some of the specific chemokines that have been identified as products of uterine stromal or epithelial cells, or of perivascular cells, include RANTES (regulated on activation, normal T cell expressed and secreted), IL-8, monocyte chemotactic protein MCP-1 and -2, and eotaxin.[17] These cytokines and chemokines are known not only to attract leukocytes to the endometrium but also to increase their proliferation and activation. Figure 47.1 summarizes the interactions between uterine stromal cells and infiltrating leukocytes that lead to activation of MMP production and subsequent breakdown of the endometrium functionalis during menstruation.

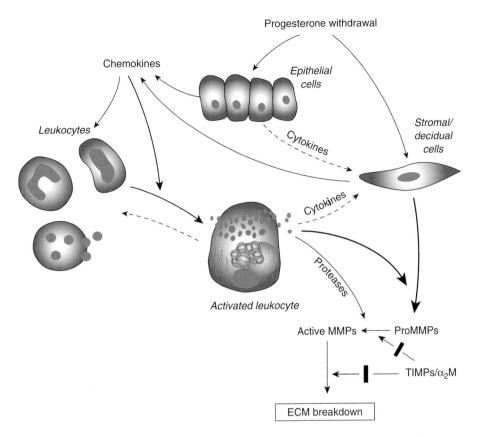

Figure 47.1 Hypothetical scheme for the molecular and cellular events within the endometrium that govern the initiation of menstruation. These events follow the withdrawal of progesterone in the secretory phase of the human menstrual cycle. This results in the production of chemokines, cytokines, and other factors from endometrial epithelial, stromal, and decidualized stromal cells. Leukocytes enter the tissue and become activated in response to chemokine signaling. Cytokines and other regulatory molecules from leukocytes, epithelial, and other resident cells stimulate the production of matrix metalloproteinases (MMPs) from stromal cells. Leukocytes also produce MMPs and other proteases that activate latent MMPs. The result is a cascade of MMP production and activation and an alteration in the balance between MMPs and tissue inhibitors of metalloproteinases (TIMPs) in favor of MMP action, resulting in degradation of tissue. (Reprinted with permission from Salamonsen.[14])

Local factors involved in endometrial remodeling

Extracellular matrix metalloproteinase inducer (EMM-PRIN) is a member of the immunoglobulin superfamily, which includes T-cell receptors, neural cell adhesion molecules, and major histocompatibility antigens. EMM-PRIN has been identified as tumor cell collagenase stimulatory factor (TCSF), a tumor cell surface molecule that stimulates nearby fibroblasts to produce MMPs.[18–20] EMMPRIN has been shown to play a role in monocarboxylic acid transport and reproduction. Null mutant embryos of EMMPRIN knockout mice have a high rate of implantation failure and the few null mutant male and female embryos that do successfully implant and survive to adulthood are infertile.[21] Female infertility appears to be due to a defect in the uterus, since wild-type embryos transferred into the uterus of a null mutant female fail to implant successfully.

One of the best characterized functions of EMM-PRIN is that it regulates MMP production in fibroblasts and also tumor cells.[19,20,22] EMMPRIN is expressed primarily by epithelial cells and promotes the production of MMPs -1, -2, -3, and -9 by nearby fibroblast cells. Glycosylation of EMMPRIN appears to be important for its MMP-stimulating functions.[23] The majority of this transmembrane protein is expressed on the cell surface but some EMMPRIN protein is released as a soluble form through microvesicle shedding.[24] EMMPRIN is expressed in the endometrium of both mice and humans. Recent studies by Noguchi et al[25] and Braundmeier et al[26] have reported that EMMPRIN protein is expressed in a cyclical manner in the human endometrium throughout the menstrual cycle. EMM-PRIN is expressed predominantly by uterine epithelial cells during the proliferative phase of the menstrual cycle, while increased expression occurs in the stroma during the mid–late secretory and menstrual phases.

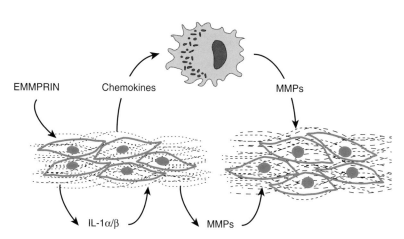

Figure 47.2 The effects of extracellular matrix metalloproteinase inducer (EMMPRIN) on matrix metaltoproteinase (MMP) production by uterine stromal cells. EMMPRIN can directly stimulate the production of several MMPs, including MMPs-1, -2, and -3 by uterine stromal cells. In addition, EMMPRIN is a potent inducer of interleukin-1α/β and several chemokines. IL-1 can act on uterine stromal cells to increase MMP production, while the chemokines help to recruit and activate leukocytes. These leukocytes produce a number of MMPs that can act on the surrounding tissues. EMMPRIN is thus able to stimulate local MMP production and contribute to tissue remodeling in the uterus by several mechanisms. (Drawing courtesy of Dr Robert Belton Jr.)

The pattern of EMMPRIN protein expression in the epithelial cells correlates with maximal expression of estrogen and progesterone receptors by these cells. EMMPRIN has also been shown to stimulate production of MMPs -1, -2, and -3 by uterine stromal cells.[26] Since the uterine stroma shows widespread expression of EMMPRIN protein during the late secretory and menstrual phases of the cycle, this supports a role for EMMPRIN as a regulator of ECM remodeling at the time of menstruation.

Recent findings point to an additional role for EMMPRIN in the tissue breakdown and remodeling that occur at the end of each menstrual cycle. Microarray data analyzing differences in gene expression between mouse uterine stromal cells treated with recombinant EMMPRIN and compared with uterine stromal cells that were not treated with EMMPRIN showed that EMMPRIN up-regulated expression of a number of cytokines and chemokines in these stromal cells (unpublished results). These include interleukin-1α and -1β and chemokines such as chemokine (C-C motif) ligand 3, ligand 7, and ligand 20. These findings suggest that EMMPRIN may also play an important role in helping to recruit various leukocytes such as macrophages into the uterine endometrium prior to the onset of menstruation. EMMPRIN may therefore be able to increase the production of MMPs locally through both a direct as well as an indirect mechanism (Figure 47.2).

Other factors that are produced by endometrial stromal cells and that may affect MMP production locally have recently been described. These include LEFTY-A/endometrial bleeding-associated factor and activin-A.[27,28] LEFTY-A mRNA levels increase in the endometrium prior to menstruation and precede the increase in MMP-9 expression.[27] Treatment of endometrial explants in vitro with recombinant LEFTY-A protein resulted in an increase in MMP-9 secretion into

culture medium. Activin expression by endometrial stromal cells is up-regulated during decidualization in parallel with increases in MMPs-2, -3, and -9.[28] Endometrial stromal cells cultured in vitro and treated with recombinant activin-A showed increases in the production of proMMPs -2, -3, -7, and -9 as well as active MMP-2. Treatment of endometrial stromal cells with activin-A can hasten decidualization, suggesting that activin plays an important role during this process. Decidualization involves dramatic morphological changes in stromal cells and occurs on a background of extensive tissue remodeling. Activin-A appears to regulate MMP production during this time and it is likely that alterations in the normal pattern of activin-A expression could lead to aberrant MMP expression in the endometrium, which could contribute to increased tissue breakdown and fragility.

ABNORMAL UTERINE BLEEDING ASSOCIATED WITH THE PERIMENOPAUSE OR USE OF PROGESTIN-ONLY CONTRACEPTIVES

Perimenopausal women

Women approaching menopause often experience changes in their normal menstrual bleeding patterns. The most common change is that the bleeding pattern becomes much more irregular, although some women may also experience menorrhagia. The causes of abnormal uterine bleeding in perimenopausal women may be anatomical (leiomyomas, adenomyosis, uterine polyps) or hormonal. This section addresses the hormonal changes that may contribute to the increased incidence of abnormal uterine bleeding in these women.

Perimenopausal women experience periods of ovulation and anovulation interspersed with periods of hypergonadotropism and hyperestrogenism.[29] Several different mechanisms have been suggested to explain the abnormal patterns of bleeding observed in these women. The first is that early in perimenopause ovulation does occur, but with a longer follicular phase that leads to a longer period of exposure to rising estrogen. This slower increase in estrogen levels causes the endometrium to proliferate excessively and can lead to menorrhagia.[30] Once women progress further into perimenopause, there is an increase in the incidence of anovulatory cycles and the proliferative phase of the cycle begins to shorten. These anovulatory cycles result in a preovulatory follicle that is capable of producing significant quantities of estrogen but is unable to ovulate because the luteinizing hormone (LH) surge is inhibited. The prolonged period of estrogenic stimulation of the endometrium again results in increased proliferation, which is followed by bleeding once the estrogen levels do decline. Such cycles, in which there is a relatively long period of estrogenic stimulation followed by little if any progesterone support, can also lead to a weakening of endometrial tissue structure, increased disorganization and fragility of the vascular elements, and irregular periods of bleeding.[31] Finally, as women reach the end of their perimenopausal period, their cycles become more infrequent and, due to a lack of any developing follicles, the uterine environment becomes hypoestrogenic.

The most commonly used medical treatments for perimenopausal women with abnormal uterine bleeding are non-steroidal anti-inflammatory drugs (NSAIDs). The NSAIDs can reduce blood loss at menstruation by inhibiting production of prostaglandins E_2 and $F_{2\alpha}$. These drugs are usually used as a first-line treatment, but have limited effectiveness in treating anovulatory bleeding. More commonly, women with anovulatory bleeding are treated with combined oral contraceptives or with progestin-only regimens that are administered for 10–14 days every month followed by a withdrawal bleed.[29,32] The use of combined oral contraceptives is particularly useful since not only can they provide cyclic control during anovulatory bleeding but also they can improve problems with abnormal uterine bleeding that are due to the presence of leiomyomas.[32] Progestin-only contraceptives such as medroxyprogesterone acetate (MPA) have also been shown to reduce uterine bleeding in anovulatory women. The MPA is usually given for 10–14 days each month in order to provide progesterone support for the normal transition to a secretory endometrium and thus overcome the hyperestrogenic environment that occurs in anovulatory cycles. These types of treatments can provide relief from irregular bleeding until the woman becomes menopausal.

Effects of using progestin-only contraceptives

Abnormal uterine bleeding is the primary reason that women decide to discontinue use of long-acting progestin contraceptives. These include such progestins as the levonorgestrel implant (Norplant), the injectable progestin Depo-Provera, and the intrauterine-administered progestin Mirena. The irregular or breakthrough bleeding that occurs in these patients is not caused by a loss in progesterone receptor expression in the endometrium.[33] Results from recent studies suggest that this breakthrough bleeding occurs in response to changes in the structural integrity of the endometrium that are accompanied by a loss in support for the vessel structures within it. Consequently, there is a marked increase in vessel fragility due to a loss of basement membrane support for the endothelial cells and the development of gaps between these cells that leads to leakiness of the vessels.[34,35]

The microvasculature of the endometrium in women using long-term progestin contraceptives has been analyzed and a number of changes associated with increased vessel fragility have been observed. These include an increase in the diameter of microcapillaries and venules on the endometrial surface, gaps in the basement membranes of vessels and between the endothelial cells lining these vessels, contact bleeding from dilated vessels, and a number of subepithelial hemorrhages.[34,36,37] Some studies have reported an increase in endometrial microvascular density in women using the levonorgestrel contraceptive implant system for 3–12 months.[36,37] However, other studies analyzing tissues from women who had been on medium- or high-dose progestins found that there was a decrease in endometrial microvessel density.[38] Thus, a change in the numbers of small vessels may also contribute to the problems with breakthrough bleeding that are often seen during the first several months of use of these long-acting progestins. It should be noted that the problems with breakthrough bleeding tend to be resolved after the first year of use of these types of contraceptives because the endometrium becomes atrophic and the women then develop amenorrhea.

The endometrium of women on long-acting progestin contraceptives shows other characteristic changes that occur fairly rapidly in response to the elevated levels of progesterone. There is extensive decidualization of the stromal cells, which is accompanied by a marked increase in leukocyte infiltration.[14,35] There is also a reduction in proliferation of the glandular components, which leads to general thinning of the endometrium and atrophy of the glands. The extensive decidualization is accompanied by an influx of leukocytes similar to that seen late in the secretory phase of the normal menstrual cycle.[14,39] The influx of leukocytes leads to increased expression of various MMPs in the endometrial stroma as well as increased production of prostaglandins, vascular endothelial growth factor (VEGF), thrombin, and IL-8.[14,40,41]

Lockwood et al[41] examined the effects of progesterone, hypoxia, and thrombin production on IL-8 production by uterine stromal cells. They hypothesized that in women treated with progestin-only contraceptives for extended periods the stromal cells would experience some hypoxia due to impaired endometrial perfusion. This local hypoxia would lead to increased thrombin production, which in turn could lead to elevated production of IL-8, a potent chemoattractant for neutrophils. In-vitro studies confirmed that uterine stromal cells treated with progesterone and cultured under hypoxic conditions showed a substantial increase in thrombin and IL-8 production. A study by Jones et al[42] showed that a number of chemokines, including macrophage-derived chemokine, hemofiltrate CC chemokine-1, MCP-3, eotaxin, and IL-8 were strongly expressed in the epithelial glands and in decidualized stromal cells of endometrium from women using levonorgestrel. The greatest immunoactivity for these chemokines was observed in the decidualized tissues. Expression of other chemokines such as macrophage inflammatory protein-1β and hemofiltrate CC chemokine-4 were greatly reduced in the endometrium of the women on levonorgestrel. Thus, the normal pattern of chemokine expression is altered in women using long-term progestin contraceptives, and this alters the leukocyte populations within the endometrium. This alteration in the normal balance of leukocytes within the endometrium can lead to increases in the levels of enzymes such as tryptase, chymase, and neutrophil elastase, which can further activate MMPs (Figure 47.3).[14]

Vascular endothelial cells may also be direct targets of steroid hormone action. Studies have shown that vascular endothelial cells from the endometrium do express progesterone receptors.[43,44] The progesterone receptors in these cells are functional and activation leads to cell cycle arrest, and inhibition of proliferation and migration.[43] Treatment of vascular endothelial cells isolated from endometrial tissues with progesterone for 3–6 days showed that progesterone could increase the secretion of MMP-9 by vascular endothelial cells. Thus, the direct effects of progesterone on endothelial cells to inhibit proliferation and increase MMP production could lead to a breakdown of the basement membrane components of endometrial microvessels, an increase in vessel fragility, and result in breakthrough bleeding.

LEIOMYOMA-RELATED ABNORMAL UTERINE BLEEDING

Changes in vascular structures

Leiomyomas are benign smooth muscle cell (SMC) tumors of the uterus that develop during a woman's reproductive years. These tumors are characterized by increased proliferation of uterine SMCs and an abundant ECM of interstitial collagens. Leiomyomas are monoclonal and originate in the myometrium, but they can protrude through the endometrium (Figure 47.4). Leiomyoma-related menorrhagia is a significant medical and social problem for many women. Effective treatment strategies are limited by a narrow understanding of the pathogenesis of this disease. Classic studies suggest that there is a fundamental alteration in the vascular structures of the myomatous uterus (see Figure 47.4). Recent progress in defining the molecular mechanisms of angiogenesis in the uterus lends support to this theory by demonstrating local dysregulation of vasoactive growth factors or growth factor receptors in leiomyomas or leiomyomatous myometrium. Thus, the molecular mechanisms underlying the process of leiomyoma-related menorrhagia are being delineated.

Although ectasia of the venules is the best characterized vascular abnormality in the myomatous uterus, multiple defects of arterioles, veins and the ECM surrounding them are probably responsible for this heterogeneous disorder. Understanding this dysregulation will not only define the pathophysiology of this important clinical problem, but it may also lead to innovative treatments.

Approximately 30% of women with leiomyomas experience menstrual abnormalities, with menorrhagia being most common.[45,46] There is no evidence that this abnormal bleeding is related to either an increased surface area of the uterine cavity or to an increased incidence of ovulatory dysfunction.[45,47] The theory that best explains leiomyoma-related abnormal bleeding states that the primary event is a change in venous structures in the endometrium and myometrium,

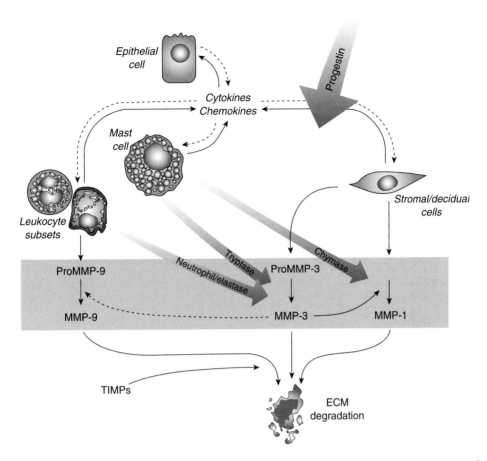

Figure 47.3   Postulated interactions between different endometrial constituents in women using progestin-only contraceptives leading to an alteration in the matrix metalloproteinase/tissue inhibitors of metalloproteinase (MMP/TIMP) balance and subsequent extracellular matrix (ECM) breakdown contributing to abnormal uterine bleeding. Different progestins may exert differing effects on endometrial epithelial and stromal cells, changing the chemokine/cytokine environment and thereby contributing to the different endometrial morphological and functional differences observed between different contraceptive agents. The changes in the chemokine/cytokine milieu are likely to result in infiltration and activation of leukocytes, production and activation of MMPs by both leukocytes and stromal/epithelial cells, and resultant degradation of the ECM, contributing to endometrial tissue loss and vascular fragility. (Reprinted with permission from Vincent and Salamonsen.[42])

resulting in venule ectasia.[47,48] Among the evidence to support this theory of vascular dysregulation in leiomyoma-related bleeding is the classic descriptive study by Sampson.[49] Sampson injected the vasculature of over 100 uteri and was able to show that the myometrium in leiomyomatous uteri had a great increase in the venous plexus, particularly at the periphery of leiomyomas. These findings were later confirmed by Faulkner.[50] Subsequent studies utilizing light microscopy demonstrated ectasia of the venules in both the myometrium and the endometrium of uteri containing leiomyomas.[48]

The classic premise of this theory suggests that leiomyomas in a variety of sites within the uterus can cause venule ectasia by compressing veins.[47,48] Current evidence suggests that it is not only physical compression but also the local action of vasoactive growth factors, which have altered synthesis, expression, or sequestration in leiomyomas, that accounts for these vascular abnormalities.[51] With ectasic venules, the hemostatic actions of the platelet and fibrin plug may be overwhelmed by the increased diameter of the vessels, which causes the 'flooding' clinically seen in women with menorrhagia.

These early studies also suggested abnormalities in arterial structures in leiomyomatous uteri, with leiomyomas having an increased arterial supply.[49,50] Several mechanisms of vascular dysregulation are consistent with both the heterogeneous clinical presentation of women with leiomyomas and the diversity of chromosomal abnormalities found in this neoplasm.[52] Thus, multiple somatic mutations can result in the same phenotypic changes. This paradigm of dysregulation of growth factor function that results in the

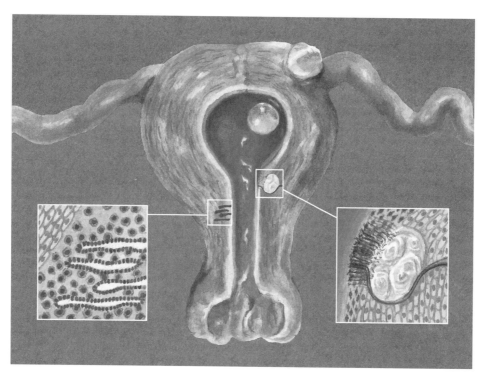

Figure 47.4 The presence of leiomyomas and/or adenomyosis within the uterus often leads to abnormal uterine bleeding. Leiomyomas (shown on the right side of the uterus) cause marked venule ectasia and may also increase microvessel density in the surrounding endometrium. These changes probably occur in response to a combination of physical factors as well as increased secretion of angiogenic growth factors by leiomyomas. Adenomyosis (shown on the left side of the uterus) leads to an influx of macrophages and other immune cells into affected areas of the myometrium. This alteration in the normal balance of leukocytes may lead to increased matrix metalloproteinase (MMP) production and tissue instability, leading to the breakdown of blood vessels and increased bleeding. (Drawing courtesy of Melissa Lynch.)

disruption of normal vascular function appears also to be relevant for non-uterine bleeding disorders. Hereditary hemorrhagic telangiectasia is characterized by profuse bleeding from mucosal surfaces, including the gastrointestinal tract and nasal epithelium, and by mucosal venule ectasia.[53] The molecular defect causing this disease is a mutation in endoglin, a binding protein that regulates the function of transforming growth factor β_1 (TGFβ_1).[54]

Differential growth factor expression: myometrium vs leiomyomas

The myometrium is a huge potential reservoir for paracrine or endocrine factors that regulate endometrial function. The apposition of these two tissues and the directional blood flow from the myometrium to the endometrium facilitate this interaction. After the functionalis layer is shed, regeneration proceeds from the endometrial basalis. With the basalis in direct contact with the myometrium, a mechanism is established whereby myometrial growth factors influence

endometrial regeneration in a paracrine fashion. This includes regeneration of both the supporting tissue components as well as the microvasculature. Growth factors that stimulate angiogenesis or relax vascular tone and that show overexpression of either ligand or receptor in leiomyomatous uteri are candidates to cause abnormal uterine bleeding in these women and thus become targets for potential therapies. Alternatively, underexpression of angiogenic inhibitory factors or vasoconstricting factors or their receptors in leiomyomas may also result in abnormal bleeding.

It is clear that numerous genes are differentially regulated in neoplastic leiomyomas and in normal myometrium. Both the estrogen receptor and progesterone receptor, as well as the enzyme aromatase, are constitutively up-regulated in leiomyomas compared with myometrium.[55–52] Leiomyomas also express higher levels of receptors for insulin-like growth factor I (IGF-I) and mRNA for IGF-II.[58,59] Leiomyomas also show an approximately five-fold increase in expression of TGFβ_3 compared to autologous myometrium.[60,61] Data from this laboratory also demonstrated the overexpression in leiomyomas of both mRNA and protein for parathyroid hormone-related protein (PTHrP) and basic fibroblast growth factor (bFGF).[62,63]

Growth factors or their receptors that are differentially regulated in leiomyomas or the endometrium of leiomyomatous uteri are potential mediators of leiomyoma-related complications. These differentially regulated factors, which are known to act on vascular tissue by increasing proliferation or changing vessel caliber, are potential causes of leiomyoma-related menorrhagia. This would include factors such as bFGF, VEGF, heparin-binding epidermal growth factor (HB-EGF), platelet-derived growth factor (PDGF), TGFβ, and PTHrP. Several of these factors (bFGF, VEGF, PDGF) belong to the heparin-binding group of growth factors. Because these factors all bind to heparin sulfate proteoglycans found in ECM, leiomyomas with their large ECM content may prove to be a reservoir for these factors. Both bFGF and VEGF primarily regulate endothelial cell migration vital to the angiogenic process. PDGF primarily regulates fibroblast and SMC function and thus may influence vascular SMCs, leiomyoma, or myometrial cells themselves, or the endometrial stromal cells.

Angiogenesis is an important process that must occur with each menstrual cycle in order to regenerate the vascular system within the endometrium. The sequence of events involved in angiogenesis is (i) basement membrane degradation, (ii) endothelial cell migration, (iii) endothelial cell proliferation, and (iv) capillary tube formation and stabilization.[64] Basement membrane degradation involves stromelysins, collagenases, and other MMPs to degrade specific elements of the ECM[64] so that endothelial cells can proliferate and migrate to the end of a vessel. This migratory process is believed to be favored by an environment rich in collagen types I and III and to be stimulated by bFGF, VEGF, PDGF, and TGFβ.[64,65] Several of these growth factors, along with cytokines such as TNFα, are potent stimulators of MMP production by endothelial and SMC cells. Recent studies have confirmed the importance of MMPs during the process of angiogenesis in tumor development, wound repair, and in the reproductive tract.[64,66] In fact the use of MMP inhibitor to inhibit angiogenesis in tumors is becoming a new area of therapeutic treatment for cancer.[66] Such findings are also helping investigators to understand how dysregulated expression of angiogenic growth factors in the uterus of women with leiomyomas contributes to the development of abnormal uterine bleeding through destabilization of the endometrium and changes in the vascular structures.

Basic fibroblast growth factor

Basic fibroblast growth factor promotes angiogenesis through a number of mechanisms, including the induction of endothelial cell proliferation, chemotaxis, and the production of matrix remodeling enzymes such as collagenase and plasminogen activator.[67] In human endometrial transformed cell lines, estradiol treatment stimulates bFGF-like activity, which is lost when cells are treated by progesterone. This model mimics hormonal influences regulating angiogenesis in vivo.[67] bFGF has also been shown to be the major mitogen causing the proliferation of vascular SMCs after injury.[68] Basic FGF has been detected by polymerase chain reaction (PCR) in human endometrium throughout the menstrual cycle and shown by immunohistochemistry to localize primarily to the glandular epithelial cells.[69]

It is known, however, that bFGF is stored in ECM bound to heparin sulfate proteoglycans, which may increase its local bioavailability.[78] Leiomyomas, which have large quantities of ECM, may serve as stores of heparin-binding growth factors, which, in turn, may affect surrounding endometrial tissue function. Studies by Mangrulkar et al[63] have shown that leiomyomas do indeed contain significant stores of bFGF. Immunohistochemistry for bFGF revealed only light staining within the myometrial, leiomyoma, or vascular SMCs. However, the large areas of ECM that distinguish leiomyomas from normal myometrium showed strong immunoreactivity for bFGF. Leiomyomas also displayed higher amounts of bFGF mRNA than autologous myometrium. Thus, leiomyomas synthesize and store significantly more bFGF than normal myometrium. A recent study[70] reported that pituitary tumor-transforming gene-1 (PTTG-1), a novel protooncogene overexpressed in numerous cancer cell lines, is up-regulated in leiomyomas. Interestingly, this study also reported that bFGF stimulated PTTG-1 expression in leiomyoma SMCs and that PTTG-1, in turn, increased both bFGF and VEGF expression in leiomyoma SMCs, resulting in a positive feedback loop between these factors.

Basic FGF can act through several different receptors, but acts most commonly through the type I receptor (FGFR-1) or the type II receptor (FGFR-2).[71] The two alternatively spliced isotypes of FGFR-1 have been localized to the human fetal uterus, as well as adult uterine endometrium, myometrium, and leiomyomas throughout the menstrual cycle.[72] However, immunohistochemical staining suggests that there is differential expression of these receptors within the uterine tissues as the menstrual cycle progresses. Immunoreactivity for the receptor was consistently stronger in myometrium than in leiomyomas during the proliferative phase. In addition, there was menstrual cycle-specific regulation of FGFR-1 protein in the endometrial stroma of normal women but not in women with leiomyomas and abnormal uterine bleeding.[72] Stromal FGFR-1 expression was suppressed in the early luteal phase in normal women but not in women with leiomyoma-related abnormal uterine bleeding. Thus, it appears that the presence of leiomyomas can alter FGFR expression in the surrounding endometrium. These findings support a role for bFGF in the pathogenesis of abnormal uterine bleeding caused by leiomyomas.

Vascular endothelial growth factor

VEGF is an angiogenic growth factor that is a potent mitogen for endothelial cells.[73] There appears to be menstrual cycle-specific expression of VEGF in the uterus. During the proliferative phase, VEGF mRNA was detected in distinct cells in the stroma by in-situ hybridization, with weak expression in the glands.[73] In contrast, during the secretory phase there was increasing expression in the glands, peaking in menstrual endometrium with the disappearance of stromal expression. Evidence from the human fetal model suggests that VEGF is secreted by epithelial cells and myocytes to modulate the function of endothelial cells in a paracrine fashion.[74] In the human uterus, VEGF concentrations were found to be similar in both myometrium and leiomyoma and to have no significant menstrual cycle variability in one study,[75] while another study reported that the levels of VEGF-A were significantly higher in leiomyomas than in corresponding myometrium.[76] The latter investigators also reported that treatment of women with gonadotropin-releasing hormone agonists (GnRHa) caused a significant reduction in VEGF-A expression in leiomyomas. Similar studies by Di Lieto et al[77,78] reported that treatment with GnRHa reduced not only VEGF expression in leiomyomas but also the expression of PDGF and bFGF. This decrease in growth factor expression was accompanied by a decrease in leiomyoma blood vessel density and uterine volume. These data also support a role for angiogenic growth factors in the growth and development of uterine leiomyomas.

Transforming growth factor β

The TGFβ family comprises five dimeric polypeptides encoded by distinct but closely related genes.[79]

TGFβ$_1$, -β$_2$, and -β$_3$ have been identified in a variety of normal and transformed mammalian cells and tissues.[79,80] TGFβ are multifunctional growth factors that regulate many aspects of cellular function, including proliferation, differentiation, ECM production, and chemotaxis. Three distinct proteins have been identified as TGFβ receptors and have been designated receptor types I–III.[79] mRNAs for TGFβ$_1$, -β$_2$, and -β$_3$, as well as for all three receptors, have been detected in both leiomyomas and myometrium.[60,61] TGFβ$_3$ has been shown to cause increased proliferation of both leiomyoma and myometrial cells, and a neutralizing antibody to this peptide causes a decrease in proliferation.[60,61] TGFβ has also been shown to play an important role in the accumulation of ECM in leiomyomas. Studies have shown that both fibronectin and collagen type I and type III production are regulated by TGFβ. Leiomyomas express up to five-fold higher amounts of mRNA for TGFβ$_3$ than do normal myometrial cells at all stages of the menstrual cycle.[60,61,81] Thus, the numbers of the TGFβ family probably play an important role in the overall growth of leiomyomas and may also have a significant impact on the surrounding myometrium and endometrium, including the vasculature.

Other factors involved in angiogenesis

A recent focus in the study of Mendelian tumor syndromes such as hereditary leiomyomatosis and renal cell cancer (HLRCC) and hereditary paragangliomatosis with pheochromocytomas (HPGL) has been on the role of Krebs cycle enzymes as tumor suppressors. Germline mutations in two Krebs cycle enzymes, fumarate hydratase (FH) and succinate dehydrogenase (SDHB, -C, -D), have been shown to predispose affected individuals to either HLRCC or HPGL. While it was not clear initially how a down-regulation of these Krebs cycle enzymes might lead to the development of these tumor syndromes, it has now become apparent that inactivation of these enzymes leads to the accumulation of specific Krebs cycle intermediates which activate the hypoxia/angiogenesis pathway. Studies have shown that the leiomyomas of HLRCC patients show an up-regulation in expression of hypoxia-inducible factor 1α and VEGF and also have an increased microvessel density.[82,83] These results suggest that the growth of leiomyomas may occur in response to inappropriate signaling to the SMCs that they are in a hypoxic state, and this may lead to subsequent growth of an SMC tumor. The increased expression of angiogenic growth factors such as bFGF and

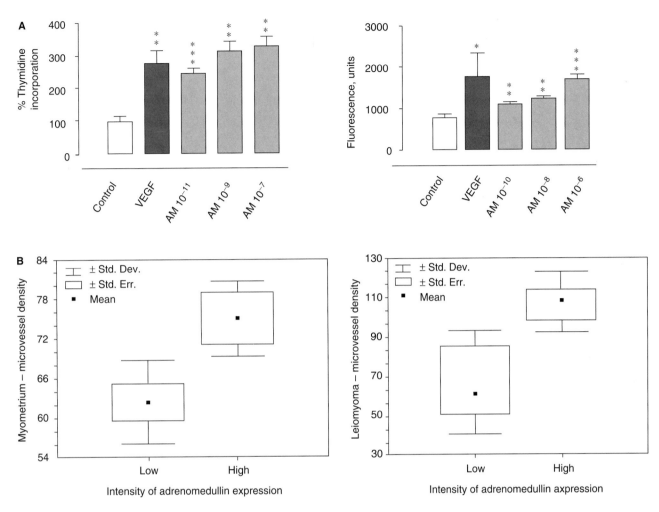

Figure 47.5 (A) Angiogenic effects of adrenomedullin (AM) in vitro. Adrenomedullin promotes proliferation of human endometrial microvascular endothelial cells. The effect is comparable to that seen with 10^{-9}mol/L VEGF. (Reprinted with permission from Nikitenko et al.[106]) (B) Expression of adrenomedullin correlates with vascular density in the myometrium and leiomyomas of patients with leiomyomas. (Reprinted with permission from Hague S et al.[99])

VEGF by leiomyomas may lead to increased vessel formation in the surrounding endometrium and may also contribute to enhanced fragility and destabilization of the blood vessels.

Another angiogenic factor that has been shown to be up-regulated in leiomyomas is adrenomedullin (ADM).[84] ADM has been shown to stimulate proliferation of endometrial microvascular endothelial cells using both a thymidine incorporation assay to assess changes in DNA synthesis and a fluorescence-based assay to measure relative changes in cell number (Figure 47.5A).[85] Expression of this angiogenic factor regulated by hypoxia in leiomyomas is positively correlated with microvessel density in leiomyomas (see Figure 47.5B).[84] In addition, these investigators reported that expression of ADM and VEGF was higher in the endometrium of patients with leiomyomas as compared to women who did not have leiomyomas.

Expression of MMPs in leiomyomas has also been studied. One would expect intuitively that MMP levels would be lower in leiomyomas since these tumors show such an abundant accumulation of fibronectin, interstitial collagens, and glycosaminoglycans. In addition, the levels of TGFβ are much higher in leiomyomas and this growth factor has been shown to down-regulate the expression of most MMPs while up-regulating TIMPs. Several studies have compared expression of MMPs in leiomyomas with autologous myometrium.[86,87] These groups found that while MMP-1, -2, and -3 levels are decreased in leiomyomas, the levels of MMP-11 are actually increased in these tumors. A study by Inagaki et al[88] reported that levels of MMP-2, MMP-9, and the cytokines IL-1β and TNFα were elevated in the uterine cavity fluid of women with leiomyomas as compared to women who did not have leiomyomas. These findings suggest that the presence of leiomyomas, and the secretion of various growth factors by leiomyomas into the surrounding myometrium and endometrium, may alter cytokine and MMP production within these tissues and contribute to a destabilization of the vascular structures in the endometrium that could lead to abnormal uterine bleeding.

Clinical therapies for treatment of leiomyomas

The most common treatments for leiomyomas are surgery-based and include hysterectomy, myomectomy, and endometrial ablation. These will not be discussed in detail here. In addition, uterine artery embolization and high-energy focused ultrasound are more recent approaches that are showing signs of success as less-invasive methods for treating leiomyomas.[51,89] Much interest exists in finding new drug-based therapies for the treatment of these tumors and their symptoms. Currently, the only drugs used for leiomyomas are the GnRHa, and these cause serious side effects when used for longer than 6 months.[45] The recurrence rate after use of these drugs is also fairly high.[45] Newer drugs that are being considered are drugs that block the actions of one or more of the growth factors that have been shown to be produced by leiomyoma SMCs and that stimulate SMC proliferation and/or matrix production. These drugs include pirfenidone, which inhibits cell proliferation and collagen production by leiomyoma SMCs and has been shown to block the actions of TGFβ, bFGF, and PDGF in other cell types.[90] Other drugs that show promise include interferons and halofuginone, which both have antiproliferative as well as antifibrotic effects in leiomyomas as well as other fibrotic diseases.[91,92]

ADENOMYOSIS

Adenomyosis is a common gynecological disorder found in approximately 20–30% of hysterectomy specimens.[93,94] Adenomyosis is characterized by the benign growth of endometrial glands and stroma within the myometrium. The degree of invasion is variable and can involve the entire uterine wall up to the serosa. A definitive diagnosis of adenomyosis is usually made if glandular extension into the uterine myometrium is >2.5 cm.[95,96] Adenomyosis is often associated with abnormal uterine bleeding, with the incidence of menorrhagia ranging from 40 to 50%. Despite the high frequency of adenomyosis found in the general population, neither the pathological nor the molecular causes of the abnormal uterine bleeding seen in women with adenomyosis have been elucidated.

Early theories about the origins of adenomyosis hypothesized that this disease occurs because of the abnormal in-growth of the endometrium basalis into the underlying myometrium.[97] However, more recent pathological studies have suggested that adenomyosis may actually arise as a result of disruption of the continuity between the endometrial basalis and the underlying myometrium. This could occur in response to mechanical injury or pregnancy and could cause displacement of the endometrial basalis into the myometrial layer. Thus, adenomyosis appears to be similar to endometriosis in that both diseases involve abnormal displacement of endometrium into either the underlying myometrium or into the pelvic cavity. Both adenomyosis and endometriosis involve a local dysregulation in immune function and appear as inflammatory processes[96,98] (see Figure 47.4). The endometrial glands of adenomyosis are characterized by increased expression of cell-surface antigens, heat shock proteins, adhesion molecules, and increased numbers of macrophages and other immune cells.[94,98] In addition, these glands also display increased levels of superoxide dismutase, cyclooxygenase, and xanthine oxidase.[99–101] Glandular epithelial cells from adenomyosis also show increased expression of bFGF, bFGF receptor, and granulocyte–macrophage colony-stimulating factor (GM-CSF).[94,102] GM-CSF is a hematopoietic cytokine that stimulates the proliferation and maturation of macrophages, eosinophils, and neutrophils. Elevated levels of GM-CSF in adenomyosis might be involved in the recruitment or activation of macrophages, leading to increased numbers of activated macrophages in the surrounding environment. Activated macrophages can synthesize and release an array of cytokines, prostaglandins, and MMPs.[13] Stromal cells of adenomyosis also show altered responses to the presence of macrophages. A recent study[103] reported that stromal cells from women with endometriosis showed increased levels of IL-6 production when co-cultured with macrophages in comparison with endometrial stromal cells obtained from women without adenomyosis. Increases in cytokine production by the stromal cells can also lead to further recruitment of immune cells and increases in local MMP production. Thus, adenomyosis may also cause abnormal uterine bleeding through a destabilization of the ECM due to increased production of MMPs by macrophages and endometrial stromal cells.

Treatment options for patients with adenomyosis remain quite limited. The most common treatment is to perform endoscopic endometrial ablation or hysterectomy. However, neither one of these treatments allows for preservation of subsequent fertility. Currently, the non-surgical treatment options can be divided into three categories. The first category consists of the use of hormonal therapies that have been used to treat other gynecological diseases such as uterine leiomyomas and endometriosis. The GnRH agonists such as leuprolide have been used to treat patients with adenomyosis for relatively short periods of up to 6 months. This type of treatment has led to an improvement in menorrhagia and even to subsequent pregnancies in some of the patients who were infertile due to the adenomyosis.[96] However, just as in patients treated for leiomyoma-related abnormal uterine bleeding, the length of treatment with GnRHa must be carefully controlled and be for a limited time due to the menopausal side effects that occur as a consequence of such treatment. There are also some reports on the use of long-acting progesterone release systems, namely the levonorgestrel-releasing intrauterine system, for treatment of adenomyosis.[104] Treatment with this drug for 12 months resulted in a significant reduction in uterine size and in menorrhagia.

Uterine arterial embolization, which is now considered a proven treatment option for leiomyomas, is now being tested for use in adenomyosis. A small number of pilot studies have reported that embolization of arteries near the areas of adenomyosis has led to an improvement in symptoms for most of the patients and have even resulted in some successful pregnancies.[105,106] A third treatment option that is now being considered is the use of high-intensity focused ultrasound. This technique has been recently approved for the treatment of uterine leiomyomas and involves the use of ultrasound guided by magnetic resonance imaging (MRI). The ultrasound can be focused quite specifically to destroy tissue in a non-invasive way.

SUMMARY

The normal menstrual cycle is a unique process that occurs in the endometrium of women and some primates. During this process there is a building and organizing of the endometrial structures, including the luminal and glandular epithelial cells, stromal cells, and vascular structures in the proliferative phase of the cycle. The endometrium is thus prepared for a potential implantation and further differentiation occurs during the secretory phase. However, if no successful implantation occurs, circulating progesterone levels drop and the endometrial functionalis is shed at menstruation. This process is tightly controlled by the changes in circulating steroid hormones and is dependent on a very specific pattern of changes in these hormones. Increasing evidence supports the hypothesis that menstruation is a process that involves local tissue destruction and vascular structure destabilization in response to increasing production of MMPs within the endometrium. These MMPs are secreted by uterine stromal cells as well as by various populations of leukocytes that infiltrate the endometrium in response to the fall in circulating progesterone levels near the end of the cycle.

Dysfunctional or abnormal uterine bleeding occurs in a number of women in response to anatomical problems such as leiomyomas or adenomyosis, or it can be caused by disturbances in the normal pattern of circulating steroid hormone levels which occur during the perimenopause or with the use of progestin-only contraceptives. While these causes may seem to be rather unrelated, they share some common features. In each case there is a change in the underlying integrity and organization of the endometrium, which leads to a destabilization of the tissue structures and blood vessels. This destabilization and breakdown of matrix involves MMPs produced by endometrial stromal cells or by infiltrating leukocytes in response to angiogenic growth factors, cytokines, or chemokines. Clinical therapies to provide relief from abnormal uterine bleeding are beginning to focus on identification of compounds that can regulate this influx of immune cells or the production of MMPs in order to prevent the destabilization of the vascular system from occurring. It is anticipated that within the next few years such new therapies will begin to undergo testing in a clinical setting and that successful treatment options will be identified.

REFERENCES

1. Noyes RW, Hertig AT, Rock J. Dating the endometrial biopsy. Fertil Steril 1950; 1: 3–25.
2. Kaiserman-Abramof LR, Padykula HA. Angiogenesis in the postovulatory primate endometrium: the coiled arteriolar system. Anat Rec 1989; 224: 479–89.
3. Tabibzadeh S. The signals and molecular pathways involved in human menstruation, a unique process of tissue destruction and remodeling. Mol Hum Reprod 1996; 2: 77–92.
4. Tabibzadeh S, Babknia A, Korg QF et al. Menstruation is associated with disordered expression of desmoplakin I/II and cadherin/catenins and conversion of F- to G-actin in endometrial epithelium. Hum Reprod 1995; 10: 776–84.
5. Curry TE Jr, Oster KG. Cyclic changes in the matrix metalloproteinase system in the ovary and uterus. Biol Reprod 2001; 64: 1285–96.

6. Mott JD, Werb Z. Regulation of matrix biology by matrix metalloproteinases. Curr Opin Cell Biol 2004; 16: 558–64.

7. Matrisian LM. The matrix-degrading metalloproteinases. Bioessays 1992; 14: 455–63.

8. Brew K, Dinakarpandian D, Nagase H. Tissue inhibitors of metalloproteinases: evolution, structure and function. Biochem Biophys Acta 2000; 1477: 267–83.

9. Mohan R, Chintala SK, Jung JC et al. Matrix metalloproteinase gelatinase B (MMP-9) coordinates and effects epithelial regeneration. J Biol Chem 2002; 277: 2065–72.

10. Rodgers WH, Matrisian LM, Giudice LC et al. Patterns of matrix metalloproteinase expression in cycling endometrium imply differential functions and regulation by steroid hormones. J Clin Invest 1994; 94: 946–53.

11. Rawdanowicz TJ, Hampton AL, Nagase H et al. Matrix metalloproteinase production by cultured human endometrial stromal cells: identification of interstitial collagenase, gelatinase-A, gelatinase-B and stromelysin-1 and their differential regulation by interleukin-1 alpha and tumor necrosis factor-alpha. J Clin Endocrinol Metab 1994; 79: 530–6.

12. Lockwood CJ, Krikun G, Hausknecht VA et al. Matrix metalloproteinases and matrix metalloproteinase inhibitor expression in endometrial stromal cells during progestin-initiated decidualization and menstruation-related progestin withdrawal. Endocrinology 1998; 139: 4607–13.

13. Salamonsen LA. Tissue injury and repair in the female human reproductive tract. Reproduction 2003; 125: 301–11.

14. Vincent AJ, Salamonsen LA. The role of matrix metalloproteinases and leukocytes in abnormal uterine bleeding associated with progestin-only contraceptives. Hum Reprod 2000; 15(Suppl 3): 135–43.

15. Wang H, Critchley HOD, Kelley RW et al. Progesterone receptor subtype B is differentially regulated in human endometrial stroma. Mol Hum Reprod 1998; 4: 407–12.

16. Salamonsen LA, Zhang J, Brasted M. Leukocyte networks and human endometrial remodeling. J Reprod Immunol 2002; 57: 95–108.

17. Salamonsen LA, Lathbury LJ. Endometrial leukocytes and menstruation. Hum Reprod Update 2000; 6: 16–27.

18. Salamonsen LA, Zhang J, Hampton A et al. Regulation of matrix metalloproteinases in human endometrium. Hum Reprod 2000; 15(Suppl 3): 112–19.

19. Biswas C, Zhang Y, DeCastro R et al. The human tumor cell-derived collagenase stimulating factor (renamed EMMPRIN) is a member of the immunoglobulin superfamily. Cancer Res 1995; 55: 434–9.

20. Guo H, Zucker S, Gordon MK et al. Stimulation of matrix metalloproteinase production by recombinant extracellular matrix metalloproteinase inducer from transfected Chinese hamster ovary cells. J Biol Chem 1997; 272: 24–7.

21. Igakura T, Kadomatsu K, Kaname T et al. A null mutation in basigin, an immunoglobulin superfamily member, indicates its important roles in peri-implantation development and spermatogenesis. Dev Biol 1998; 194: 152–65.

22. Kataoka H, DeCastro R, Zucker S et al. Tumor cell-derived collagenase-stimulatory factor increases expression of interstitial collagenase, stromelysin and 72–kDa gelatinase. Cancer Res 1993; 53: 3154–8.

23. Sun J, Hemler M. Regulation of MMP-1 and MMP-2 production through CD147/extracellular matrix metalloproteinase inducer interactions. Cancer Res 2001; 61: 2276–81.

24. Sidhu SS, Mengistab AT, Tauscher AN et al. The microvesicle as a vehicle for EMMPRIN in tumor–stromal interactions. Oncogene 2004; 23: 956–63.

25. Noguchi Y, Sato T, Hirata M et al. Identification and characterization of extracellular matrix metalloproteinase inducer in human endometrium during the menstrual cycle in vivo and in vitro. J Clin Endocrinol Metab 2003; 88: 6063–72.

26. Braundmeier A, Fazleabas A, Lessey BA et al. Extracellular matrix metalloproteinase inducer regulates metalloproteinases in human uterine endometrium. J Clin Endocrinol Metab 2006; 91: 2358–65.

27. Cornet PB, Galant C, Eeckhout Y et al. Regulation of matrix metalloproteinase-9/gelatinase B expression and activation by ovarian steroids and LEFTY-A/endometrial bleeding-associated factor in the human endometrium. J Clin Endocrinol Metab 2005; 90: 1001–11.

28. Jones RL, Findlay JK, Farnworth PG et al. Activin A and inhibin A differentially regulate human uterine matrix metalloproteinases: potential interactions during decidualization and trophoblast invasion. Endocrinology 2006; 147: 724–32.

29. Jain A, Santoro N. Endocrine mechanisms and management for abnormal uterine bleeding due to perimenopausal changes. Clin Obstet Gynecol 2005; 48: 295–311.

30. Sowers MR, La Pietra MT. Menopause: its epidemiology and potential association with chronic diseases. Epidemiol Rev 1995; 17: 287–302.

31. Brill AI. What is the role of hysteroscopy in the management of abnormal uterine bleeding? Clin Obstet Gynecol 1995; 38: 319–45.

32. Lumbiganon P, Rugpao S, Phandhu-fung S et al. Protective effects of depot-medroxyprogesterone acetate on surgically treated uterine leiomyomas: a multicenter case-control study. Br J Obstet Gynecol 1996; 103: 909–14.

33. Lockwood CJ, Runic R, Wan L et al. The role of tissue factor in regulating endometrial hemostasis: implications for progestin-only contraceptives. Hum Reprod 2000; 15: 144–51.

34. Hickey M, Fraser LS. A functional model for progestogen-induced breakthrough bleeding. Hum Reprod 2000; 15(Suppl 3): 1–6.

35. Jones RL, Critchley HOD. Morphological and functional changes in human endometrium following intrauterine levonorgestrel delivery. Hum Reprod 2000; 15(Suppl 3): 162–72.

36. Hickey M, Dwarte D, Fraser IS. Precise measurements of intrauterine vascular structures at hysteroscopy in menorrhagia and during Norplant use. Hum Reprod 1998; 13: 3190–6.

37. Hickey M, Simbar M, Markham R et al. Changes in endometrial vascular density in Norplant users. Contraception 1999; 59: 123–9.

38. Song JY, Markham R, Russell P et al. The effect of high dose medium and long-term progestogen exposure on endometrial vessels. Hum Reprod 1995; 10: 797–800.

39. Critchley HOD, Wang H, Jones RL et al. Morphological and functional features of endometrial decidualization following long-term intrauterine levonorgestrel delivery. Hum Reprod 1998; 13: 1218–24.

40. Schatz F, Krikun G, Caze R et al. Progestin-regulated expression of tissue factor in decidual cells: implications in endometrial hemostasis, menstruation and angiogenesis. Steroids 2003; 68: 849–60.

41. Lockwood CJ, Kumar P, Krikun G et al. Effects of thrombin, hypoxia, and steroids on interleukin-8 expression in decidualized human endometrial stromal cells: implications for long-term progestin-only contraceptive-induced bleeding. J Clin Endocrinol Metab 2004; 89: 1467–75.

42. Jones RL, Morison NB, Hannan NJ et al. Chemokine expression is dysregulated in the endometrium of women using progestin-only contraceptives and correlates to elevated recruitment of distinct leukocyte populations. Hum Reprod 2005; 20: 2724–35.

43. Vasquez F, Rodriguez-Manzaneque JC, Lydon JP et al. Progesterone regulates proliferation of endothelial cells. J Biol Chem 1999; 274: 2185–92.

44. Rodriguez-Manzaneque JC, Graubert M, Iruela-Arispe ML. Endothelial cell dysfunction following prolonged activation of progesterone receptor. Hum Reprod 2000; 15(Suppl 3): 39–47.

45. Stewart EA. Uterine fibroids. Lancet 2001; 357: 293–8.

46. Walker CL, Stewart EA. Uterine fibroids: the elephant in the room. Science 2005; 308: 1589–92.

47. Buttram VC Jr, Reiter RC. Uterine leiomyomas: etiology, symptomology and management. Fertil Steril 1981; 36: 433–45.

48. Farrer-Brown G, Beilby JOW, Tarbit MH. Venous changes in the endometrium of myomatous uteri. Obstet Gynecol 1971; 38: 743–51.

49. Sampson JA. The blood supply of uterine myomata. Surg Gynecol Obstet 1912; 14: 215–30.

50. Faulkner RI. The blood vessels of the myomatous uteri. Am J Obstet Gynecol 1945; 47: 185–97.

51. Stewart EA, Nowak RA. Leiomyoma-related bleeding: a classic hypothesis updated for the molecular era. Hum Reprod Update 1996; 2: 295–306.

52. Rein MS, Friedman AJ, Barbieri RI et al. Cytogenetic abnormalities in uterine leiomyomata. Obstet Gynecol 1991; 77: 923–6.

53. Guttmacher AE, Marchuk DA, White RI. Hereditary hemorrhagic telangiectasia. N Engl J Med 1995; 333: 918–24.

54. McAllister KA, Grogg KM, Johnson DW et al. Endoglin, a TGF-β binding protein of endothelial cells, is the gene for hereditary hemorrhagic telangiectasia type 1. Nat Genet 1994; 8: 345–51.

55. Rein MS, Friedman AJ, Stuart JM et al. Fibroid and myometrial steroid receptors in women treated with the gonadotropin-releasing hormone agonist luprolide acetate. Fertil Steril 1990; 53: 1018–23.

56. Brandon DD, Bethea CL, Strawn EY et al. Progesterone receptor messenger ribonucleic acid and protein are overexpressed in human leiomyomas. Am J Obstet Gynecol 1993; 169: 78–85.

57. Bulun SE, Simpson ER, Word RA. Expression of the CYP19 gene and its product aromatase cytochrome P450 in human uterine leiomyoma tissues and cells in culture. J Clin Endocrinol Metab 1994; 78: 736–43.

58. Gloudemans T, Prinsen L, Van Unnik JA et al. Insulin-like growth factor gene expression in human smooth muscle cell tumors. Cancer Res 1990; 50: 6689–95.

59. Vollenhoven BJ, Herrington AC, Healy DL. Messenger ribonucleic acid expression of the insulin-like growth factors and their binding proteins in uterine fibroids and myometrium. J Clin Endocrinol Metab 1993; 76: 1106–10.

60. Lee BS, Nowak RA. Human leiomyoma smooth muscle cells show increased expression of transforming growth factor-beta 3 (TGF beta 3) and altered responses to the antiproliferative effects of TGF beta 3. J Clin Endocrinol Metab 2001; 86: 913–20.

61. Sozen I, Arici A. Interactions of cytokines, growth factors, and the extracellular matrix in the cellular biology of uterine leiomyomata. Fertil Steril 2002; 78: 1–12.

62. Weir EC, Goad DI, Daifotis AG et al. Relative overexpression of the parathyroid hormone-related peptide gene in human leiomyomas. J Clin Endocrinol Metab 1994; 78: 784–9.

63. Mangrulkar RS, Ono M, Ishikawa M et al. Isolation and characterization of heparin-binding growth factors in human leiomyomas and normal myometrium. Biol Reprod 1995; 53: 636–46.

64. Rundhaug JE. Matrix metalloproteinases and angiogenesis. J Cell Mol Med 2005; 9: 267–85.

65. Playford RJ, Ghosh S. Cytokines and growth factor modulators in intestinal inflammation and repair. J Pathol 2005; 205: 417–25.

66. Handsley MM, Edwards DR. Metalloproteinases and their inhibitors in tumor angiogenesis. Int J Cancer 2005; 115: 849–60.

67. Klagsbrun M, Dluz S. Smooth muscle cell and endothelial cell growth factors. Trends Cardiovasc Med 1993; 3: 213–7.

68. Lindner V, Reidy MA. Proliferation of smooth muscle cells after vascular injury is inhibited by an antibody against basic fibroblast growth factor. Proc Natl Acad Sci USA 1991; 88: 3739–43.

69. Ferriani RA, Charnock-Jones DS, Prentis A et al. Immunohistochemical localization of acidic and basic fibroblast growth factors in normal human endometrium and endometriois and the detection of their mRNA by polymerase chain reaction. Hum Reprod 1993; 8: 11–16.

70. Tsai SJ, Lin SJ, Cheng HM et al. Expression and functional analysis of pituitary tumor transforming gene-1 in uterine leiomyomas. J Clin Endocrinol Metab 2005; 90: 3715–23.

71. Fernig DG, Gallagher JT. Fibroblast growth factors and their receptors: an information network controlling tissue growth, morphogenesis and repair. Prog Growth Factor Res 1994; 5: 353–77.

72. Anania CA, Stewart EA, Quade B et al. Expression of the fibroblast growth factor receptor in women with leiomyomas and abnormal uterine bleeding. Mol Hum Reprod 1997; 3: 685–91.

73. Charnock-Jones DS, Sharkey AM, Rajput-Williams J et al. Identification and localization of alternatively spliced mRNAs for vascular endothelial growth factor in human uterus and estrogen regulation in endometrial carcinoma cell lines. Biol Reprod 1993; 48: 1120–8.

74. Shifren JL, Doldi N, Ferrara N et al. In the human fetus, vascular endothelial growth factor is expressed in epithelial cells and myocytes, but not vascular endothelium: implications for mode of action. J Clin Endocrinol Metab 1994; 79: 316–22.

75. Harrison-Woolrych ML, Sharkey AM, Charnock-Jones DS et al. Locallization and quantification of vascular endothelial growth factor messenger ribonucleic acid in human myometrium and leiomyomata. J Clin Endocrinol Metab 1995; 80: 1853–8.

76. Gentry CC, Okolo SO, Gong LF et al. Quantification of vascular endothelial growth factor-A in leiomyomas and adjacent myometrium. Clin Sci (Lond) 2001; 101: 691–5.

77. Di Lieto A, DeFalco M, Mansueto G et al. Preoperative administration of GnRH-a plus tibolone to premenopausal women with uterine fibroids: evaluation of the clinical response, the immunohistochemical expression of PDGF, bFGF and VEGF and the vascular pattern. Steroids 2005; 70: 95–102.

78. DiLieto A, DeFalco M, Pollio F et al. Clinical response, vascular change and angiogenesis in gonadotropin-releasing hormone analogue-treated women with uterine myomas. J Soc Gynecol Investig 2005; 12: 123–8.

79. Massague J. The transforming growth factor-β family. Annu Rev Cell Biol 1990; 6: 597–641.

80. Massague J. Receptors for the TGF-β family. Cell 1992; 69: 1067–70.

81. Chegini N, Verala J, Luo X et al. Gene expression profile of leiomyoma and myometrium and the effect of gonadotropin releasing hormone analogue therapy. J Soc Gynecol Investig 2003; 10: 161–71.

82. Pollard P, Wortham N, Barclay E et al. Evidence of increased microvessel density and activation of the hypoxia pathway in tumours from the hereditary leiomyomatosis and renal cell cancer syndrome. J Pathol 2005; 205: 41–9.

83. Pollard PJ, Briere JJ, Alam NA et al. Accumulation of Krebs cycle intermediates and overexpression of H1F1-alpha in tumours which result from germline FH and SDH mutations. Hum Mol Genet 2005; 14: 2231–9.

84. Hague S, Zhang L, Oehler MK et al. Expression of the hypoxically regulated angiogenic factor adrenomedullin correlates with uterine leiomyoma vascular density. Clin Cancer Res 2000; 6: 2808–14.

85. Nikitenko LL, Fox SB, Kehoe S et al. Adrenomedullin and tumor angiogenesis. Br J Cancer 2006; 94: 1–7.

86. Palmer SS, Haynes-Johnson D, Diehl T et al. Increased expression of stromelysin 3 mRNA in leiomyomas (uterine fibroids) compared with myometrium. J Soc Gynecol Investig 1998; 5: 203–9.

87. Dou Q, Tarnuzzer RW, Williams RS et al. Differential expression of matrix metalloproteinases and their tissue inhibitors in leiomyomata: a mechanism for gonadotropin releasing hormone agonist-induced tumor regression. Mol Hum Reprod 1997; 3: 1005–14.

88. Inagaki N, Ung L, Otani T et al. Uterine cavity matrix metalloproteinases and cytokines in patients with leiomyoma adenomyosis or endometrial polyp. Eur J Obstet Gynecol Reprod Biol 2003; 111: 197–203.

89. Stewart EA, Rabinovici J, Tempany CM et al. Clinical outcomes of focused ultrasound surgery for the treatment of uterine fibroids. Fertil Steril 2006; 85: 22–9.

90. Lee B, Margolin SB, Nowak RA. Pirfenidone: a novel pharmacological agent that inhibits leiomyoma cell proliferation and collagen production. J Clin Endocrinol Metab 1998; 132: 491–6.

91. Nowak RA. Novel therapeutic strategies for leiomyomas: targeting growth factors and their receptors. Environ Health Perspect 2000; 108: 849–53.

92. Nowak RA. Drug therapies for uterine fibroids: a new approach to an old problem. Drug Discov Today: Therap Strateg 2004; 1: 237–42.

93. Parazzini F, Vercellini P, Pannazas et al. Risk factors for adenomyosis. Hum Reprod 1997; 12: 1275–9.

94. Propst AM, Quade BJ, Nowak RA et al. Granulocyte macrophage colony-stimulating factor in adenomyosis and autologous endometrium. J Soc Gynecol Investig 2002; 9: 93–7.

95. Uduwela AS, Perrera MD, Aiging L et al. Endometrial–myometrial interface: relationship to adenomyosis and changes in pregnancy. Obstet Gynecol Surv 2000; 55: 390–400.

96. Devlieger R, D'Hooghe T, Timmerman D. Uterine adenomyosis in the infertility clinic. Hum Reprod Update 2003; 9: 139–42.

97. Leyendecker G, Herbertz M, Kung G et al. Endometriosis results from the dislocation of basal endometrium. Hum Reprod 2002; 10: 2725–36.

98. Ota H, Igarashi S, Hatazawa J et al. Is adenomyosis an immune disease? Hum Reprod Update 1998; 4: 360–7.

99. Ota H, Igarashi S, Hatazawa J et al. Immunohistochemical assessment of superoxide dismutase expression in endometriosis and adenomyosis. Fertil Steril 1999; 72: 129–34.

100. Ota H, Igarashi S, Sasaki M et al. Distribution of cyclooxygenase-2 in eutopic and ectopic endometrium in adenomyosis and endometriosis. Hum Reprod 2001; 16: 561–6.

101. Ota H, Igarashi S, Tanaka T. Xanthine oxidase in eutopic and ectopic endometrium in endometriosis and adenomyosis. Fertil Steril 2001; 75: 785–90.

102. Propst AJ, Quade BJ, Gargiulio AR et al Adenomyosis demonstrates increased expression of the basic fibroblast growth factor receptor/ligand system compared with autologous endometrium. Menopause 2001; 8: 368–71.

103. Yang JH, Wu MY, Cheng DY et al. Increased interleukin-6 messenger RNA expression in macrophage-cocultured endometrial stromal cells in adenomyosis. Am J Reprod Immunol 2006; 55: 181–7.

104. Fong YF, Singh K. Medical treatment of a grossly enlarged adenomyotic uterus with the levongestrel-releasing intrauterine system. Contraception 1999; 60: 173–5.

105. Siskin GP, Tublin ME, Stainken BF et al. Uterine artery embolization for the treatment of adenomyosis: clinical response and evaluation with MR imaging. AJR Am J Roengenol 2001; 177: 297–302.

106. Timmerman D, Van den Bosch T, Peeraer K et al. Vascular malformation in the uterus: ultrasonographic diagnosis and conservative management. Eur J Obstet Gynecol Reprod Biol 2000; 92: 171–8.

48 Colonization and infection of the endometrium

David A Eschenbach

Synopsis

The diagnosis of endometritis depends on the clinical presentation and histologic criteria. Microbial assessment of cervical fluids is not reliable in diagnosis due to large numbers of vaginal microflora contaminating ervical fluid.

Plasma cells in endometrium are pathognomonic of endometritis

DEFINITION

Microorganisms ascend from the cervical–vaginal flora by a canalicular spread through the cervix into the endometrium and into the Fallopian tubes to cause salpingitis.[1] Endometritis results when the ascending vaginal cervical flora reaches the endometrium; thus, endometritis represents an intermediate stage of infection between the well-defined infections of cervicitis and salpingitis. In developed countries, pelvic tuberculosis is rare; so in these countries, endometritis results from non-tuberculosis cervical–vaginal microbes. The diagnosis of cervicitis is made by finding an increase in polymorphonuclear leukocytes (PMNs), or frank pus in the cervical canal, or identifying pathological bacteria such as *Neisseria gonorrhoeae*, *Chlamydia trachomatis*, or *Mycoplasma genitalium*.[2,3] The diagnosis of salpingitis can be made at laparoscopy by the detection of swollen, inflamed, or pus-filled Fallopian tubes or with less accuracy by clinical findings. However, endometritis, as an intermediate state of infection, is not easily accessible to visualization and a visual diagnosis through hysteroscopy is not well established.[4] Furthermore, microbial samples taken through the cervix contain so much cervical flora contamination as to be totally unreliable.[1,5] Thus, the diagnosis of endometritis does not rely upon visual or microbial but, instead, upon histological criteria. However, since PMNs are present in the endometrium during menses, PMNs alone can not be used for the histological diagnosis. Plasma cells are present in tissue, including endometrium, presumably in response to the presence of microbes. Thus, endometritis is defined by the presence of both plasma cells in the stroma together with PMNs in the superficial endometrial epithelium.[6] While histological endometritis is most closely associated with pelvic infection, other potential causes include stromal breakdown causing bleeding from hormonal effect on the endometrium.[7,8]

MICROBIAL ETIOLOGY

Sexually transmitted microbes that cause cervicitis, such as *N. gonorrhoeae*, *C. trachomatis*, and *M. genitalium*, are strongly linked with histological endometritis.[3,9–12] These same microbes were isolated from the endometrium of women with histological endometritis, albeit using transcervical catheters.[12,14] From 25 to 50% of young women with endometritis have one or more of these microbes in the cervix.[12] However, most of these reports are from women at high risk for sexually transmitted disease (STD), and other causes may become evident in populations at low risk for STD. Another condition examined in relation to endometritis is bacterial vaginosis. In bacterial vaginosis, the vaginal flora contains 10–1000 times more bacteria than the normal vaginal flora. Two studies found that histological endometritis was associated with the recovery of microbes associated with bacterial vaginosis from the endometrium.[14,15] However, bacterial vaginosis itself has a less consistent link to endometritis.[5,9,10] This discrepancy may be explained by the fact that catheters threaded through the cervix were used to recover microbes from the endometrium. As noted previously, contamination of this sample from vaginal cervical flora makes the microbial findings difficult to interpret. For example, the presence of 10–1000 times more bacteria in the vagina is expected to markedly increase contamination of the transcervically obtained endometrial sample by vaginal cervical flora. Furthermore, many women with bacterial vaginosis in these studies were at high risk for pelvic infection and they also had present the sexually transmitted microbes mentioned above; adjustment for these microbes among women with bacterial vaginosis has generally not occurred. Thus, it is possible that the STD microbes and not those microbes present in bacterial vaginosis caused the endometritis. The role of bacterial vaginosis per se as a cause for endometritis remains unclear, particularly among women without suspected salpingitis.

Two caveats are in order:

- new DNA technology to identify difficult to culture genital microbes[16,17] has not been used in the setting of endometritis
- *Mycoplasma tuberculosis* causes a distinct caseating histology in the endometrium; this chapter discusses only non-tuberculosis endometritis.

PATHOGENESIS

The relatively long, 3–4 cm cervix has a small 1–2 mm canal. The cervical canal is filled with cervical mucus that contains immunoglobulins and other antimicrobial molecules that provide a relative barrier to the transit of vaginal cervical microbes into the endometrium. Thus, at present, the normal endometrial cavity is considered to be a relatively sterile anatomical site. However, during menses, the cervical mucus barrier is lost. Furthermore, some vaginal infections, most notably bacterial vaginosis, produce sialidase and mucinase that potentially allow bacteria to more readily penetrate the cervical mucus barrier and enter the endometrial cavity. In fact, carbon particles (and fluid) readily pass from the vagina through the endometrium into Fallopian tubes and out into the pelvic cavity.[18] The cervix then probably represents a relative and not an absolute barrier to the entry of bacteria into the endometrium. It is even possible that a small number of cervical vaginal microbes constantly enter the endometrial cavity and either die spontaneously or are killed by the innate or acquired immune system.

The complexity of the immune system operative in the endometrium is just now under investigation.[19] Two cytokines associated with inflammation and cell trafficking were associated with abnormal bleeding among levonorgestrel users.[20] Abnormal bleeding is common in women with endometritis. In a population of women with endometritis, some women could have inflammation as a result of acute infection as described above, but with other women the inflammation might result from a combination of acute infection and immune signaling from a prior infection. For example, in women with a history of prior pelvic inflammatory disease (PID), endometritis was present in 43% of those with and in 28% of those without a current *C. trachomatis* or *N. gonorrhoeae* infection. In women without prior PID, endometritis was present in 23% of those with and 12% of those without current *C. trachomatis* or *N. gonor-*

rhoeae infection.[12] Thus, a prior infection appears to increase the rate or even perhaps the severity of inflammation in those with acute infection. An increased number of B cells, but not of macrophages or T cells in endometritis, further suggests a role of the adaptive immune system.[21] Furthermore, certain human leukocyte antigen (HLA) alleles were associated with endometritis, which suggests a genetic influence on the development of endometritis.[22] Finally, pre-existing endometrial inflammation would be expected to impact the carefully ordered immune environment necessary in the endometium for successful implantation.[23]

EPIDEMIOLOGY AND RISK FACTORS

Histological endometritis has a wildly divergent prevalence dependent upon the population. Endometritis is found in 5–10% of asymptomatic women undergoing infertility investigation,[4,9] in 25–40% of women with cervical infection,[9,10,12,24] and in a surprisingly high number (40%) of women with a recent delivery.[5] Women with human immunodeficiency virus (HIV) infection also had a high (40%) prevalence of endometritis.[25] The postpartum population might have been exposed to bacteria during delivery. HIV-infected women might lack an optimal mucosal defense system to handle normal bacterial traffic through the cervix into the endometrium.

However, in most young women, the epidemiology supports the idea of ascending infection as one cause of endometritis. Young women with endometritis tend to have selected risk factors associated with STD, including a young age,[12] a new sexual partner in the past 30 days,[14] a history of prior STD,[26] and non-white ethnicity.[10,14] In one report, women with endometritis had an elevated rate of prior PID;[12] in another report, they had an elevated rate of perceived infertility, but not of prior PID.[14]

CLINICAL MANIFESTATIONS

Endometritis was first suspected of causing abnormal uterine bleeding based upon finding an unexpected level of endometritis in the biopsies taken of reproductive-age women.[9] Subsequent prospective studies also demonstrated that endometritis was associated with intermenstrual bleeding[9] and heavy menses.[10]

In a mixed population of women with cervicitis only and symptoms of PID, the finding of histological endometritis was associated with a seven-fold increase in pelvic pain.[26] Abnormal vaginal bleeding and pelvic pain certainly are not specific for endometritis. The question of whether endometritis leads to distinct signs continues to be debated. Women with endometritis tend to have evidence of pelvic inflammation, but these signs are also common in women without endometritis. Furthermore, many women with endometritis are asymptomatic. Among consecutive women without clinical PID but either with cervicitis or at high risk for STD, histological endometritis was associated with cervical motion tenderness[12] and in a weak association with uterine tenderness.[9,10] However, even these associations are not consistently reported.[27]

Still, histological endometritis was associated with clinical manifestations consistent with pelvic infection, with the presence of *C. trachomatis* and *N. gonorrhoeae*, and with risk factors associated with infection. These clinical manifestations and the prevalence of cervical infection with *C. trachomatis* and *N. gonorrhoeae* in endometritis indicate a severity of disease that is intermediate between women with diagnosed salpingitis and signs of neither endometritis nor salpingitis.[28,29] A further indication that endometritis is infectious is the finding that antibiotic treatment of endometritis resulted in a significant reduction of vaginal bleeding, mucopurulent cervicitis, and uterine tenderness.[12] In conclusion, endometritis appears to cause distinct but very non-specific clinical symptoms and signs, and many women with endometritis have neither symptoms nor signs, leading of the difficulty of clinically diagnosing endometritis.

DIAGNOSIS

The diagnosis of endometritis is a pathological diagnosis based on histology at this time. Among young women who undergo endometrial biopsy, histological endometritis is found more often in those biopsied during the proliferative rather than the lateral phase of the menstrual cycle,[10,14] suggesting a uterine response to an increased exposure of microbes or other molecules at menses. A less likely but possible explanation is an effect of the proliferative phase milieu to reduce the endometrial inflammation response. The histological definition of endometritis includes the presence of both plasma cells in the endometrial stroma and of PMN in the superficial layers of endometrial tissue.[2] Findings used for the clinical diagnosis of endometritis are non-specific and subtle, as mentioned. Clinical findings present in women with endometritis include mild abdominal pain and mild cervical and uterine tenderness. Other non-specific tests include an increased number of vaginal inflammatory cells.[30,31] These findings are also present in women with cervicitis only without endometritis and in women with salpingitis (where endometritis is usually present).[14] More specific molecular testing of cervical fluid for endometrial inflammation has not yet been developed. This leads

to a situation where many, if not most, women with endometritis are simply not diagnosed.

Of special interest is the infertility work-up where the presence of endometritis could identify a patient at high risk for tubal infertility. It was further suggested that histological endometritis could even reduce the ability to become pregnant in such patients.[32] Microbial products and inflammatory molecules such as cytokines and chemokines could cause damage to implantation events and/or trophoblasts and the embryo itself, leading to reproductive failure. Such inflammation could affect this orderly inflammatory process necessary for normal implantation.[23] A reduced rate of pregnancy with in-vitro fertilization (IVF) occurs among women with a hydrosalpinx compared to those without a hydrosalpinx. Women with a hydrosalpinx have an increased number of endometrial inflammatory cells and a marked increase in interleukin-2 within endometrial tissue.[33] A reduced rate of conception also occurs when the IVF transfer catheter is contaminated with bacteria or vaginal infection is present.[34] In keeping with the possibility that vaginal cervical flora affects conception following IVF, pregnancy rates were highest in women with high concentration of lactobacilli.[34,35] However, an antibiotic treatment trial to reduce pregnancy loss is needed to further explore these possibilities.

TREATMENT

To date, few treatment trials of endometritis have been reported. Treatment using oral cefixime and azithromycin in a one-time dose and metronidazole for 7 days reduced the prevalence of endometritis in 48 women biopsied before and after antibiotics from 38% to 4%.[12] Antibiotic treatment was also associated with a reduction of abnormal bleeding from 60% to 30%, mucopurulent cervicitis from 20% to 6%, and uterine tenderness from 20% to 6% in this study. These treatment results need confirmation. Furthermore, no study has used a non-antibiotic comparison group to determine how often endometritis clears after endometrial sloughing at menses.

PROGNOSIS

Infection limited to the uterus is expected to have little effect on subsequent infertility and chronic pelvic pain, unlike salpingitis, which potentially causes Fallopian tube damage and peritoneal inflammation. To date, limited data reinforce the concept that endometritis represents an intermediate stage of infection between cervicitis and salpingitis. In a prospective follow-up of 613 antibiotic-treated women with and without endometritis, neither subsequent infertility nor chronic pelvic pain were elevated in those with endometritis.[36] The effect of endometritis on women not treated with antibiotics awaits further study.

REFERENCES

1. Westrom L, Eschenbach D. Pelvic inflammatory disease. In: Holmes KK, Sparling PF, Mardh PA et al, eds. Sexually Transmitted Disease, 4th edn. New york: McGraw Hill, 1999.
2. Centers for Disease Control and Prevention. Sexually transmitted diseases treatment guidelines, 2006. Centers for Disease Control and Prevention. MMWR 2006; 55: 1–93.
3. Manhart LE, Critchlow CW, Holmes KK, et al. Mucopurulent cervicitis and *Mycoplasma genitalium*. J Infect Dis 2003; 187: 650–7.
4. Polisseni F, Bambirra EA, Camargos AF. Detection of chronic endometritis by diagnostic hysteroscopy in asymptomatic infertile patients. Gynecol Obstet Invest 2003; 55(4): 205–10.
5. Andrews WW, Hauth JC, Cliver SP et al. Association of asymptomatic bacterial vaginosis with endometrial microbial colonization and plasma cell endometritis in nonpregnant women. Am J Obstet Gynecol 2006; 195(6): 1611–16.
6. Kiviat NB, Wolner-Hanssen P, Eschenbach DA et al. Endometrial histopathology in patients with culture-proven upper genital tract infection and laparoscopically diagnosed acute salpingitis. Am J Surg Pathol 1990; 14: 167–75.
7. Gilmore H, Fleischhacker D, Hecht JL. Diagnosis of chronic endometritis in biopsies with stromal breakdown. Hum Pathol 2007; 38: 581–4.
8. Thurman AR, Soper DE. Endometrial histology of depomedroxyprogesterone acetate users: a pilot study. Infect Dis Obstet Gynecol 2006; 14(2): 69402.
9. Paavonen J, Kiviat N, Brunham RC et al. Prevalence and manifestation of endometritis among women with cervicitis. Am J Obstet Gynecol 1985; 152: 280–6.
10. Korn AP, Hessol NA, Padian HS et al. Risk factors for plasma cell endometritis among women with cervical *Neisseria gonorrhoeae*, cervical *Chlamydia trachomatis*, or bacterial vaginosis. Am J Obstet Gynecol 1998; 187: 987–90.
11. Peipert JF, Ness RB, Blume J et al. Pelvic Inflammatory Disease Evaluation and Clinical Health Study Investigators. Clinical predictors of endometritis in women with symptoms and signs of pelvic inflammatory disease. Am J Obstet Gynecol 2001; 184(5): 856–63; discussion 863–4.
12. Eckert LO, Thwin SS, Hillier SL et al. The antimicrobial treatment of subacute endometritis: a proof of concept study. Am J Obstet Gynecol 2004; 190: 305–13.
13. Cohen CR, Manhart LE, Bukusi EA et al. Association between *Mycoplasma genitalium* and acute endometritis. Lancet 2002; 359(9308): 765–6.
14. Hillier SL, Kiviat NB, Hawes SE et al. Role of bacterial vaginosis-associated microorganisms in endometritis. Am J Obstet Gynecol 1996; 175: 435–41.
15. Haggerty CL, Hillier SL, Bass DC, Ness RB. PID Evaluation and Clinical Health Study Investigators. Bacterial vaginosis and anaerobic bacteria are associated with endometritis. Clin Infect Dis 2004; 39(7): 990–5.
16. Fredricks DN, Fiedler TL, Marrazzo JM. Molecular identification of bacteria associated with bacterial vaginosis. N Engl J Med 2005; 353: 1899–911.
17. Hyman RW, Fukushima M, Diamond L et al. Microbes on the human vaginal epithelium. Proc Natl Acad Sci USA 2005; 102: 7952–7.
18. Egli G, Newton M. The transported carbon particles in the human female reproductive tract. Fertil Steril 1961; 12: 151–6.
19. Talbi S, Hamilton AE, Vo KC et al. Molecular phenotyping of human endometium distinguishes menstrual cycle phases and underlying biological processes in normo-ovulatory women. Endocrinology 2006; 147(3): 1097–121.
20. Rhoton-Vlasak A, Chegini N, Hardt N, Williams RS. Histological characteristics and altered expression of interleukins (IL) IL-13 and IL-15 in endometria of levonorgestrel users with different uterine bleeding patterns. Fertil Steril 2005; 83(3): 659–65.
21. Disep B, Innes BA, Cochrane HR et al. Immunohistochemical characterization of endometrial leucocytes in endometritis. Histopathology 2004; 45(6): 625–32.
22. Ness RB, Brunham RC, Shen C, Bass DC; PID Evaluation Clinical Health (PEACH) Study Investigators. Associations among human leukocyte antigen (HLA) class II DQ variants, bacterial sexually transmitted diseases, endometritis, and fertility among women with clinical pelvic inflammatory disease. Sex Transm Dis 2004; 31(5): 301–4.
23. Lobo SC, Huang ST, Germeyer A et al. The immune environment in human endometrium during the window of implantation. Am J Reprod Immunol 2004; 52(4): 244–51.
24. Korn AP, Bolan G, Padian N et al. Plasma cell endometritis in women with symptomatic bacterial vaginosis. Obstet Gynecol 1995; 85: 387–90.
25. Eckert LO, Watts DH, Thwin SS et al. Histologic endometritis in asymptomatic human immunodeficiency virus-infected women: characterization and effect of antimicrobial therapy. Obstet Gynecol 2003; 102(5 Pt 1): 962–9.
26. Nelson DB, Ness RB, Peipert JF et al. Factors predicting upper genital tract inflammation among women with lower genital tract infection. J Womens Health 1998; 7(8): 1033–40.
27. Heatley MK. The association between clinical and pathological features in histologically identified chronic endometritis. J Obstet Gynaecol 2004; 24(7): 801–3.
28. Eckert LO, Hawes SE, Wolner-Hanssen PK et al. Endometritis: the clinical-pathologic syndrome. Am J Obstet Gynecol 2002; 186(4): 690–5.
29. Wiesenfeld HC, Sweet RL, Ness RB et al. Comparison of acute and subclinical pelvic inflammatory disease. Sex Transm Dis 2005; 32(7): 400–5.
30. Peipert JF, Ness RB, Soper DE, Bass D. Association of lower genital tract inflammation with objective evidence of endometritis. Infect Dis Obstet Gynecol 2000; 8(2): 83–7.
31. Yudin MH, Hillier SL, Wiesenfeld HC et al. Vaginal polymorphonuclear leukocytes and bacterial vaginosis as markers for histologic endometritis among women without symptoms of pelvic inflammatory disease. Am J Obstet Gynecol 2003; 188(2): 318–23.
32. Romero R, Espinoza J, Mazor M. Can endometrial infection/inflammation explain implantation failure, spontaneous abortion, and preterm birth after in vitro fertilization? Fertil Steril 2004; 82(4): 799–804.
33. Copperman AB, Wells V, Luna M et al. Presence of hydrosalpinx correlated to endometrial inflammatory response in vivo. Fertil Steril 2006; 86(4): 972–6.
34. Eckert LO, Moore DE, Patton DL et al. Relationship of vaginal bacteria and inflammation with conception and early pregnancy loss following in-vitro fertilization. Infect Dis Obstet Gynecol 2003; 11(1): 11–17.
35. Moore DE, Soules MR, Klein NA et al. Bacteria in the transfer catheter tip influences the live-birth rate after in vitro fertilization. Fertil Steril 2000; 74: 1118–24.
36. Haggerty CL, Ness RB, Amortegui A et al. Endometritis does not predict reproductive morbidity after pelvic inflammatory disease. Am J Obstet Gynecol 2003; 188(1): 141–8.

49 Ectopic pregnancy

John E Buster

INTRODUCTION

Unruptured ectopic pregnancy is evolving into a medical disease. With timely diagnosis, this condition can now be identified and treated without surgery in its early stages – even before symptoms. In many cases, systemic methotrexate, a strategy targeted directly at proliferating trophoblasts, is now preferred to surgery as the first-line intervention. Surgery is always first choice for cases where there is hemorrhage and hemodynamic instability. It is the default strategy for medical failures, neglected cases, and circumstances where methotrexate is contraindicated.

Ectopic pregnancy remains a serious, even fatal disease. Although in the United States, there has been a considerable decrease in maternal mortality, deaths still occur because of patient self-neglect and caregiver failures that include delays in diagnosis, poor treatment choices, and failure to follow established treatment guidelines. Early diagnosis and timely intervention are keys to preventing complications, preserving fertility, controlling costs, and the elimination of maternal mortality.

PREVALENCE

In the United States, ectopic pregnancy prevails at more than 100 000 cases per year.[1] This figure is probably an underestimate because only surgically managed cases obtained from hospital registries have been tabulated in the past by the Centers for Disease Control.[2] In more recent experience, patients are treated medically in outpatient facilities where they are not recorded in hospital registrations. Although there are some statistics suggesting that ectopic pregnancy prevalence is leveling, it will still continue to be a major epidemiological problem.[2,3] There appear to be three reasons for this:

1. There is a very high presence of risk factors (Table 49.1) in a society with unprecedented sexual liberties.
2. There is continued ascertainment bias from diagnostic methods that are more sensitive and specific than those used in the past. Ectopic pregnancies are thus reported in very early stages, where in the past they might have resolved without being diagnosed.
3. With the increasing use of in-vitro fertilization (IVF) and related fertility treatments, ectopic pregnancy is a common complication.

Ectopic pregnancy still accounts for approximately 5% of the maternal mortality in the United States.[4]

PATHOGENESIS

Factors impairing tubal transport of gametes and embryos increase risk of ectopic implantation.[5-7] Many ectopic pregnancies, however, implant in tubes or other pelvic structures that are grossly normal, so it is not always clear whether the etiology is disturbed pelvic anatomy or problems intrinsic to gametes and embryos themselves. The site of implantation influences clinical presentation.[7] Thus, in surgical series, approximately 98% of all ectopic pregnancies implant in fallopian tubes, with 80% being ampullary, 12% isthmic, 6% fimbrial, and the remaining 2% implanting in the cornua (Figure 49.1).[7] Implantation sites following assisted reproductive technology (ART) treatments show a higher percentage of cornual, cervical, and ovarian gestations (see Figure 49.1). Distal (ampullary and fimbrial) are more likely to resolve spontaneously, whereas proximal (isthmic and cornual) implantations are more likely to rupture.[7,8] In contrast, from a series of surgeries performed for ectopic ruptures during methotrexate therapy, the incidence of isthmic implantations appears much higher.[9] It is possible that the isthmic implantation may have been a selective factor in these methotrexate-related ruptures.[9]

With tubal implantations, proliferating trophoblasts invade all layers of surrounding oviduct wall.[5] The degree of trophoblastic invasion, the viability of the pregnancy, and the site of implantation determine the clinical course.[7-9] As trophoblasts proliferate, the growth may extend from the luminal mucosa, into the muscularis and lamina propria, into the serosa and, ultimately, the full thickness to disrupt large blood vessels in the broad ligament.[5] With vascular invasion,

Table 49.1   Risk factors[a] associated with ectopic pregnancy

Risk factor	Odds ratio[b]
High risk	
Tubal surgery	21.0
Tubal ligation	9.3
Previous ectopic pregnancy	8.3
In-utero exposure to DES	5.6
Use of IUD	4.2–45.0
Tubal pathology	3.8–21.0
Assisted reproduction	4.0
Morning-after pill	High
Moderate risk	
Infertility	2.5–21.0
Previous genital infections	2.5–3.7
Multiple sexual partners	2.1
Salpingitis isthmica nodosa	1.5
Low risk	
Previous pelvic infection	0.9–3.8
Cigarette smoking	2.3–2.5
Vaginal douching	1.1–3.1
First intercourse <18 years old	1.6

[a]Factors identifying patients at increased risk for ectopic pregnancy. Patients at increased risk need aggressive monitoring of their pregnancies immediately after fires missed menses.
[b]Single values, common odds ratio from homogenous studies; point estimates, range of values from heterogenous studies.
DES, diethylstilbestrol; IUD, intrauterine device.
Adapted from Heard and Buster.[34]

bleeding distorts the tube, stretches the serosa, and causes pain. If the embryo is abnormal (aneuploid in many cases), it may degenerate and abort as it does in about 80% of cases.[7–10] If the embryo is normal (euploid in many cases), it may continue to grow and differentiate with fetal elements, be resistant to methotrexate, and then rupture.[9,10] Spontaneous tubal abortion occurs in about 50% of tubal ectopic pregnancies and is often clinically silent. Spontaneous tubal abortion with hemorrhage can occur with bleeding that is self-limited.[8] Tubal rupture is usually associated with significant hemorrhage. As mentioned above, this complication is most likely when the implantation is located in the isthmus, which has limited distensibility. Chronic tubal rupture with extension into the broad ligament can produce a pelvic hematoma. Such implantations can produce a chronic course, with persistently elevated β-human chorionic gonadotropin (β-hCG) levels that may last for weeks.[7,8]

RISK FACTORS

Ectopic pregnancy is often associated with risk factors, leading to tubal epithelial damage. Meta-analyses have identified risk factors listed in Table 49.1 as the most influential.[11–25]

Tubal damage and infection

Pre-existing tubal pathology carries a 3.5-fold common adjusted odds ratio for ectopic pregnancy. Patients with a previous ectopic pregnancy are 6–8 times more likely to experience another ectopic pregnancy. Furthermore, some 8–14% of patients experience more than one ectopic pregnancy. Patients with a history of tubal surgery have a 21-fold common adjusted odds ratio of ectopic pregnancy.[14,23]

Endosalpingitis commonly results from pelvic infections. Thus, patients with histories of gonorrhea, serologically confirmed *Chlamydia*, and non-specific pelvic inflammatory disease, have a two-fold to four-fold higher risk of developing an ectopic pregnancy. The ectopic pregnancy rate is 4% in women with laparoscopically demonstrated salpingitis, compared with 0.7% in women with normal tubes.[13,21]

Salpingitis isthmica nodosa

This diagnosis increases the incidence of ectopic pregnancy by 52% over age- and race-matched controls.[17]

Diethylstilbestrol

Prenatal exposure to diethylstilbestrol (DES) alters fallopian tubal morphology, resulting in absent or minimal fimbrial tissue, a small tubal os, and decreased length and caliber of the tube. DES-related anomalies are associated with a five-fold increase in risk of ectopic pregnancy.[13]

Cigarette smoking

Cigarette smoking is associated with a slightly increased ectopic pregnancy risk. It is difficult to understand this association. Theories include impaired immunity that predisposes pregnant smokers to pelvic infections, alterations in tubal motility, or overrepresentation of lifestyles at increased risk of tubal injection.[26]

Contraception

Intrauterine devices

Intrauterine devices (IUDs) have been associated with ectopic pregnancy. IUDs effectively prevent intrauterine

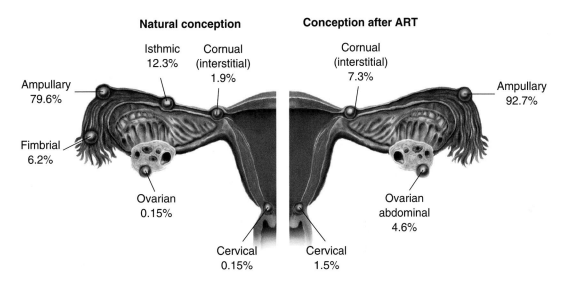

Figure 49.1 Implantation sites for ectopic pregnancy following natural cycles and assisted reproductive technologies (ART). Ectopic pregnancies are more likely to implant in the cornual and cervix than arise spontaneously. Heterotropic pregnancies are relatively common following ART and very rare in spontaneous conceptions. (Modified from Heard and Buster.[34])

implantation; however, if pregnancy occurs, there is increased likelihood that the pregnancy will be ectopic.[19,23]

Tubal ligation

Tubal ligation carries a similar risk for ectopic pregnancy to what is observed with current IUD use. As with the IUD, tubal ligations effectively prevent pregnancy, but if pregnancy does occur, suspicion for an ectopic pregnancy should be heightened.[13,23]

Electrocoagulation

Electrocoagulation is associated with higher ectopic pregnancy risk than other forms of tubal sterilization, possibly from tubal recanalization or uteroperitoneal fistula formation. Uteroperitoneal fistulas have been found in up to 75% of hysterectomy specimens from women with previous tubal ligations in which the tubes were cauterized in the corneal region of the uterus.[14,23]

Oral contraceptives

Oral contraceptives are associated with a substantially reduced risk of ectopic pregnancy when the comparison is with non-pregnant controls.[23] The risk is elevated, however, when the comparison is against pregnant controls. This protection is presumably due to the suppression of ovulation by oral contraceptives.[23] It is therefore not surprising that patients who take emergency contraception, such as oral contraceptives after fertilization, are at increased risk for an ectopic pregnancy. This has been attributed to altered tubal motility.[23,25]

Barrier contraceptives

Barrier contraceptives (condoms, spermicides, and diaphragms) reduce the odds ratio of ectopic pregnancy.[23]

CLINICAL PRESENTATION

Many ectopic pregnancies never express symptoms.[27–29] Some pass without notice except for delayed menses. Others are immediately diagnosed and treated because the patient is identified as high risk.[27–29] Table 49.1 summarizes and weighs risk factors that should be examined in every woman who has just been diagnosed as pregnant. Early diagnosis is not always achievable. In these cases, the triad of amenorrhea, irregular vaginal bleeding, and lower abdominal pain will be observed. Sudden, severe, lower abdominal pain is the most common complaint and occurs in 90–100% of women with symptomatic ectopic pregnancy. Pain radiating to the shoulder, syncope, and shock are associated with rupture and hemoperitoneum.

Abdominal tenderness with rebound is usually present. Pelvic examination usually reveals parametrial and cervical motion tenderness. A pelvic mass can be felt approximately 50% of the time.[27–29]

DIAGNOSIS

Diagnosis is possible as early as 4.5 weeks' gestation but is usually achievable at 5.5 to 6 weeks.[27–31] Unfortunately, visualizing an ectopic pregnancy at

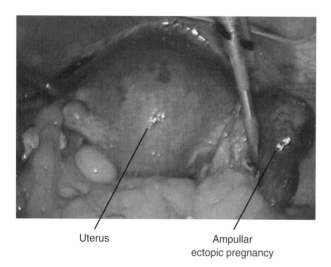

Uterus   Ampullar
                  ectopic pregnancy

Figure 49.2 Ampullary ectopic pregnancy. Many ampullary implantations abort spontaneously with few symptoms. (Courtesy of Dr David Zepeda. See also color plate section.)

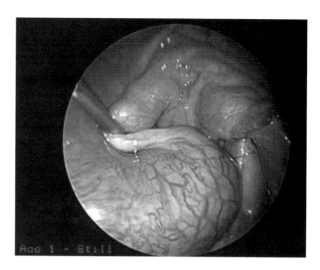

Figure 49.4 Cornual ectopic pregnancy. Cornual implantation may rupture catastrophically if diagnosis is delayed. (Courtesy of Dr David Zepeda. See also color plate section.)

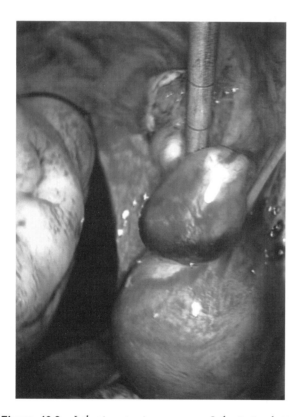

Figure 49.3 Isthmic ectopic pregnancy. Isthmic implantations have a higher likelihood of rupture than ampullary sites. A high percentage of isthmic implantations are associated with methotrexate failure. (Courtesy of Dr David Zepeda. See also color plate section.)

these early stages by ultrasound or laparoscopy is frequently not possible because they are under 2 cm, in size. More importantly, traditional laparoscopic visualization (Figures 49.2–49.4) is not really necessary for

diagnosis. Rather, combined use of diagnostic tests in algorithms that include serial measurements of β-hCG, ultrasonography, and uterine curettage will lead to timely diagnosis.[27-31]

A representative algorithm shown in Figure 49.5 has been efficacious in our hands.[27] Variations on this algorithm have been described.[27-29]

Serial β-human chorionic gonadotropin

β- hCG determinations in clinical use today are based on the enzyme-linked immunosorbent assay (ELISA), which detects β-hCG concentrations in urine and serum at 20 mIU/ml down to 1 mIU/ml, respectively. β-hCG produced by trophoblastic cells in normal pregnancy, even with first trimester bleeding, rises by at least 50% every 2 days.[30] This generally applies to β-hCG values below 10 000 mIU/mL. Eighty-five percent of abnormal pregnancies, whether intrauterine or ectopic, have impaired β-hCG production with a prolonged doubling time. This impairment is recently associated with transcriptional failure of the hCG β subunit gene in embryonic tissues undergoing miscarriage or in some ectopic pregnancies.[32] β-hCG levels that plateau or fail to rise normally concomitant with low serum progesterone should be considered nonviable. If a viable intrauterine gestation is not visible by transvaginal ultrasonography when the β-hCG is above 2000 mIU/ml (First International Reference Preparation [IRP]) and no fetal heartbeat can be visualized in the adnexa, uterine curettage can be performed.[27-32] In this situation, treatment of a nonviable intrauterine pregnancy is performed or ectopic

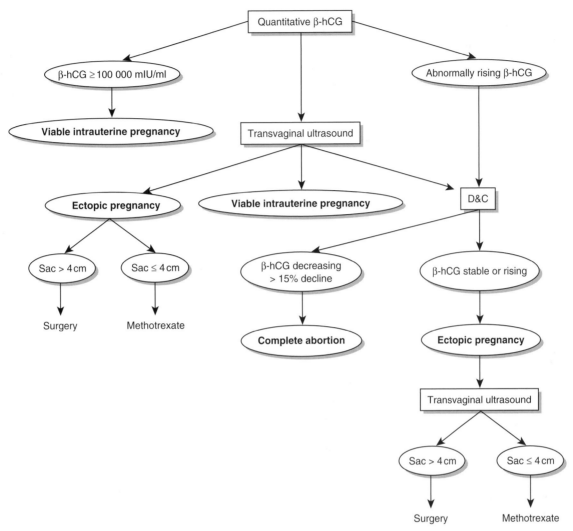

Figure 49.5   Representative algorithm for diagnosis of pregnancy. β-hCG, β-human chorionic gonadotropin; D&C, dilatation and curettage. (Adapted from Buster and Carson.[27])

pregnancy is diagnosed when the β-hCG levels do not fall.[29] This β-hCG threshold (2000 mIU/ml) is used in our clinic. This level is not universal, and each institution must identify its own values to avoid terminating normal intrauterine pregnancies.[27,33]

β-hCG determinations are further employed for diagnosis after uterine curettage. If the β-hCG fails to decline by 15% from a level drawn immediately before surgery, the pregnancy is presumed ectopic and treatment should be initiated.[29–35]

Ultrasound

Transvaginal ultrasound can first image intrauterine gestations when β-hCG is between 1000 and 2000 mIU/ml (First IRP), as early as 1 week after missed menses. In our clinic, an intrauterine gestation should

almost always be visualized when β-hCG is greater than 2000 mIU/ml (discrimination zone). In some circumstances, such as with twin gestations, this number is too low and an additional 1–2 days and a repeat ultrasound that identifies an intrauterine gestation are worth the wait in a stable patient.[27,34]

Diagnosis of an ectopic pregnancy can be made with 100% specificity but with low sensitivity (15–20%) if an extrauterine gestational sac is identified. A complex adnexal mass without an intrauterine pregnancy improves sensitivity to 21–84% at the expense of lower specificity (93.0–99.5%).[28] In reviewing the literature, the presence of any non-cystic, extraovarian adnexal mass in the absence of an intrauterine gestation was diagnostic of an ectopic pregnancy with 98.9% specificity, 96.3% positive predictive value, 84.4% sensitivity, and a 94.8% negative predictive value.[28] Despite the high resolution of transvaginal ultrasonography, an adnexal mass will not be found in 15–35% of patients with an ectopic pregnancy, particularly in early stages.[28] Some sonographic images, such as the pseudogestational sac, may mislead even an experienced examiner to diagnose a gestational sac incorrectly.[27–29]

Serial β-hCG and transvaginal ultrasound predict ectopic pregnancy with a positive predictive value of 95%.[28] Diagnosis is made routinely by the absence of an intrauterine pregnancy (i.e. gestational sac) at a designated β-hCG concentration. The vast majority of viable intrauterine pregnancies can be identified by ultrasonography when the β-hCG is >1500 mIU/ml (First IRP).[28] However, in those patients with an 'indeterminate' ultrasound, one-fourth have an ectopic pregnancy. Therefore, serial β-hCG and ultrasonography alone cannot diagnose all ectopic pregnancies.[27–31]

Uterine curettage

Uterine curettage is necessary when transvaginal ultrasound and a rising or plateauing β-hCG level below cut-off values are not sufficient for diagnosis.[29,35] A decrease in the β-hCG level of 15% or more 8–12 hours after curettage diagnoses complete abortion. If the β-hCG titer plateaus or rises after curettage, an ectopic pregnancy is likely.[29–34] It is essential that an intrauterine pregnancy be ruled out. One of the most significant complications of methotrexate is administration of the drug into a woman who is carrying a normal pregnancy.[36] Methotrexate embryopathy is a very serious, if not lethal, complication to the fetus.[36] Even when methotrexate is given to a patient experiencing a spontaneous abortion, the patient may blame the treatment for the miscarriage.[34,35]

TREATMENT OF ECTOPIC PREGNANCY

Medical management

Systemic methotrexate has been the mainstay of medical therapy since the mid 1980s.[37] A folic acid antagonist, methotrexate inhibits de-novo synthesis of purines and pyrimidines, interfering with DNA synthesis and cell multiplication.[38] Rapidly proliferating trophoblasts are hugely vulnerable to methotrexate.[38] Hemodynamically stable patients with unruptured ectopic pregnancy measuring ≤4.0 cm by ultrasound are eligible for methotrexate therapy. Patients with larger masses or evidence of acute intra-abdominal

Table 49.2   Methotrexate: single vs multiple dose

Single-dose methotrexate protocol

Day 1:	Baseline studies	
	Methotrexate	50 mg/m² i.m.
Day 4:	hCG titer	
Day 7:	hCG titer	
	CBC and platelet count	
	Liver and renal function tests	
Weekly:	hCG titer until negative	

Multiple-dose methotrexate protocol

Treatment is discontinued when a decline is observed in two consecutive daily hCG titers, or after four doses of methotrexate

Day 1:	Baseline studies	
	Methotrexate	1.0 mg/kg i.m.
Day 2:	Citrovorum	0.1 mg/kg i.m.
Day 3:	Methotrexate	1.0 mg/kg i.m.
Day 4:	Citrovorum	0.1 mg/kg i.m.
	hCG titer	
Day 5:	Methotrexate	1.0 mg/kg i.m.
	hCG titer	
Day 6:	Citrovorum	0.1 mg/kg i.m.
	hCG titer	
Day 7:	Methotrexate	1.0 mg/kg i.m.
	hCG titer	
Day 8:	Citrovorum	0.1 mg/kg i.m.
	CBC and platelet count	
	Renal and liver function tests	
Weekly:	hCG titer until negative	

hCG, human chorionic gonadotropin; CBC, complete blood count; i.m., intramuscular.

bleeding should undergo surgical treatment. Details of the two commonly employed methotrexate treatment regimens ('multiple-dose' and 'single-dose') are shown in Table 49.2.[27,34]

Multiple-dose methotrexate

Multiple-dose methotrexate therapy is tailored to the patient's weight and ectopic pregnancy responsiveness.[27,34] In 1996, a randomized clinical trial comparing laparoscopic salpingostomy with systemic multiple-dose methotrexate for treatment of unruptured ectopic pregnancies below 4 cm diameter was reported.[39] In this trial, 100 patients with laparoscopy-confirmed ectopic pregnancy were randomly treated with systemic methotrexate or laparoscopic salpingostomy. In the 51 patients treated with methotrexate, three (8%) required surgical intervention for active bleeding or tubal rupture. An additional course of methotrexate was required in two patients (5%) for persistent trophoblast, basal on β-hCG secretion. Of the 44 patients in the salpingostomy group, two patients (5%) failed and required salpingectomies, and eight patients

Table 49.3 Outcome of different treatments for ectopic pregnancy from case series publications

Method	Number of studies[a]	Number of patients	Number with successful resolution	Tubal patency rate	Subsequent fertility rate Intrauterine pregnancy	Subsequent fertility rate Ectopic pregnancy
Conservative laparoscopic surgery	32	1626	1516 (93%)	170/223 (76%)	366/647 (57%)	87/647 (13%)
Variable-dose methotrexate	12	338	314 (93%)	136/182 (75%)	55/95 (58%)	7/95 (7%)
Single-dose methotrexate	7	393	340 (87%)	61/75 (81%)	39/64 (61%)	5/64 (8%)
Direct-injection methotrexate	21	660	502 (76%)	130/162 (80%)	87/152 (57%)	9/152 (6%)
Expectant management	14	628	425 (68%)	60/79 (76%)	12/14 (86%)	1/14 (7%)

[a] References available on *The Lancet* website (http: www.thelancet.com) or from the journal's London office.
Adapted from Pisarska et al.[40]

(22%) required treatment with methotrexate for persistent trophoblast. Tubal patency was present in 67% of the patients in the methotrexate group and in 61% in the salpingostomy group.[39] This randomized study, combined with the case series comparisons reported through 1997, demonstrated convincingly that systemic methotrexate therapy produced outcomes comparable to laparoscopic salpingostomy.[40,41] A summary of case series reported through 1997 is given in Table 49.3.

Single-dose methotrexate

Single-dose methotrexate is much more convenient than the multiple dose (see Table 49.2).[42–44] It is, however, associated with a higher rupture rate.[45,46] The high success rates in the initial studies using single-dose methotrexate were most likely due to the inclusion of spontaneously aborting intrauterine pregnancies.[42] Subsequent studies of single-dose methotrexate therapy involving 304 patients were reported.[43] Although overall success of treatment, measured as no surgical intervention, is 87.2%, 11.5% of additional patients required more than one dose of methotrexate.[43] Of the patients considered successfully treated (with one or more doses), tubal patency was found in 81.3% of the women evaluated. The subsequent intrauterine pregnancy rate was 61%, and for ectopic pregnancies.[43]

Multiple vs single-dose methotrexate

Methotrexate as a single-dose intramuscular regimen is probably not as effective as multiple dosages. However, single-dose therapy is a standard according to a Practice Committee Report of the American College of Obstetricians and Gynecologists.[44] With this background, a recent meta-analysis of 26 studies (totaling 1372 cases) evaluating methotrexate dosing for ectopic pregnancy by Barnhart et al showed an odds ratio of 1.96 higher likelihood of rupture with use of single-dose

methotrexate over multidose therapy.[45] This odds ratio of rupture on single dose increased to 4.75 (95% confidence interval [CI] 1.77–12.62) when the authors controlled for baseline β-hCG values. In another study using a more indirect method of indirect comparison, the relative risk was 1.48 (95% CI 1.12–1.95). Very likely, the differences become smaller when methotrexate is being given to good prognosis patients.[45,46]

Special precautions during methotrexate

Patients being treated with methotrexate should be examined by a single examiner – only once. Transient pain ('separation' or 'tearing pain') is common.[47] Transient pelvic pain from resolution tubal bleeding of the ectopic pregnancy frequently occurs 3–7 days after the start of therapy, lasts 4–11 hours, and is presumably due to tubal abortion. Perhaps the most difficult aspect of methotrexate therapy is learning to distinguish the transient abdominal pain of successful therapy from that of a rupturing ectopic pregnancy.[47] Isthmic ectopic pregnancies are probably at high risk for rupture, and there is simply no way to identify these in advance.[9] A review of ectopic ruptures after methotrexate therapy revealed a higher prevalence of isthmic (47%) ectopic pregnancies than was unexpected from previous surgical series without methotrexate.[9] These ectopic pregnancies are frequently euploid and, because they are normal, may have an early normal doubling time and rise in β-hCG titers after methotrexate dosing.[9,10] Physicians must therefore carefully observe for clinical indications that an operation is necessary (Table 49.4). Thus, surgical intervention is required when pain is worsening and persistent beyond 12 hours. Orthostatic hypotension or a falling hematocrit should lead to immediate surgery. Sometimes it is necessary to hospitalize the patient with pain for observation (usually about 24 hours). In addition, colicky abdominal pain is common during the first 2 or 3 days of methotrexate therapy, and the

Table 49.4   When to operate

1. Rupture with hemodynamic instability
2. Anemia
3. Renal disease
4. Heptic dysfunction
5. Contraindications to methotrexate
6. Severe and unremitting pain
7. Unreliable patient

Table 49.5   Circumstances predicting failure of methotrexate treatment

1. Initial hCG >10 000 mIU/ml
2. Rapid hCG increments (>50% in 48 hours before and during methotrexate)
3. Persistent and severe pain, particularly following #1 and #2
4. Adnexal fetal heart activity
5. Gestational mass >4.0 cm

Table 49.6   Precautions for using methotrexate

1. No intercourse – gynecological examination or vaginal ultrasound – treat like placenta previa
2. Avoid sun exposure
3. Avoid folic acid in prenatal vitamins
4. Avoid gas-forming food, e.g. leeks, cabbages, and corn

woman should avoid gas-producing foods, such as leeks and cabbage. Patients should avoid exposure to the sun, because photosensitivity can be a complication of methotrexate.[34,48]

Methotrexate should not be administered into a woman pregnant with a viable gestation. Methotrexate embryopathy is a serious, if not lethal, complication to the fetus and newborn.[36] Every effort should be made to establish a correct diagnosis of ectopic pregnancy prior to methotrexate.

Methotrexate failure is predictable. In addition to falling hematocrit and hypotension, Table 49.5 lists several other predictors of treatment failure. High initial hCG diminishes prognosis for successful outcome, but there is no consensus in the literature as to what that threshold should be. Recommended thresholds have ranged from 1500 to 10 000 mIU/ml.[49,50] Other indices of treatment failure include adnexal heart activity, rapidly rising hCG both before and after starting methotrexate, and severe abdominal pain. In our experience, when hCG continues to rise rapidly during methotrexate and passes into the >10 000 mIU/ml range and is associated with severe and unremitting pain, surgery is indicated.[8]

Table 49.6 lists precautions for avoiding complications with methotrexate.

Direct injection of methotrexate and cytotoxins

Methotrexate by direct injection into the ectopic pregnancy is widely used in Europe. It is more cumbersome than systemic methotrexate.[51,52] Outcomes appear comparable to experience with systemic methotrexate, but comparisons are difficult because of differences in patient selection. Methotrexate side effects may be less because the agent is injected directly into the gestation sac but they do still occur. Prostaglandins, hyperosmolar glucose, potassium chloride, and saline by direct injection have been reported. The limited experience with prostaglandins and hypertonic glucose, poor success rates, and the need for laparoscopic or transvaginal aspiration makes these treatment alternatives unattractive.

Side effects of methotrexate therapy

High-dose methotrexate, as used in cancer chemotherapy, causes bone marrow suppression, hepatotoxicity, stomatitis, pulmonary fibrosis, alopecia, and photosensitivity.[38] These side effects are infrequent in the short treatment schedules used in ectopic pregnancy and can be attenuated by the administration of leucovorin (citrovorum factor). With ectopic pregnancy schedules, impaired liver function with transient transaminase elevations is common.[38] Other side effects include stomatitis, gastritis and enteritis, and bone marrow suppression. Cases of life-threatening neutropenia and febrile morbidity can occur after single or multidose intramuscular methotrexate, requiring hospitalization.[53] Cases of transient pneumonitis[41] from methotrexate therapy for ectopic pregnancy have been observed.[54] Reversible alopecia (a loss of 33–50% of the scalp hair) on two separate occasions following single-dose therapy for an ectopic pregnancy has also been reported. Mortalities have been reported, particularly when methotrexate is given to patients with compromised renal or liver function.[55] Rarely, hematosalpinx and pelvic hematoceles have been noted as late sequelae of methotrexate following the normalization of β-hCG levels. These patients may have pelvic pain, abnormal bleeding, or a pelvic mass, requiring surgery.

Surgery

Surgery is first choice for ectopic pregnancy where there is hemorrhage and hemodynamic instability. It is the default strategy for medical failures, neglected cases, and circumstances where methotrexate is contraindicated.

Ruptured ectopic pregnancy

Laparotomy or laparoscopy with salpingectomy is first choice for rupture. Laparoscopic salpingectomy is successful even in patients in hypovolemic shock. In the hands of a skilled laparoscopist, laparoscopic salpingectomy is an acceptable alternative to laparotomy.

Unruptured ectopic pregnancy

When methotrexate is contraindicated, laparoscopic salpingostomy is the first surgical choice. Salpingectomy can be performed either during laparotomy or laparoscopy using cautery or sutures (laparoscopic or endoloops).[56,57] Subsequent to salpingostomy, 53% of patients have intrauterine pregnancies, compared with 49.3% after salpingectomy. Recurrent ectopic pregnancy rates were slightly higher after conservative surgery, 14.8% compared with 9.9%.[40,56,57] Laparoscopic salpingectomy is preferred over salpingostomy in cases of uncontrollable bleeding not resolving with conservative measures when extensive tubal damage is present, if the ectopic pregnancy is in the same tube, and if sterilization is desired.

The recommended conservative surgical procedure for an ampullary ectopic pregnancy is linear salpingostomy, because the ectopic nidation typically is located between the endosalpinx and serosa rather than in the tubal lumen. A linear salpingostomy is created through a longitudinal incision by electrocautery, scissors, or laser over the bulging antimesenteric border of the Fallopian tube. The products of conception are removed with forceps or gentle flushing or suction. After maintaining hemostasis, the incision is closed primarily or left to heal by secondary intention. Some surgeons will administer a single dose of methotrexate after linear salpingostomy to avoid persistence of trophoblastic tissue and need for reoperation.[58,59]

Isthmic implantations are treated with segmental excision, followed by intraoperative or delayed microsurgical anastomosis. The tubal lumen is narrower and the muscularis is thicker in the isthmus than in the ampulla, predisposing the isthmus to greater damage after salpingostomy and greater rates of proximal tubal obstruction.

Manual fimbrial expression, also known as 'milking', can be used when trophoblastic tissue is aborting spontaneously through the fimbriae.

Laparoscopy has advantages over laparotomy, including less blood loss, decreased need for analgesia, and improved postoperative recovery.[60,61] Cost analysis has demonstrated significant savings in randomized trials.[60,61]

When evaluating subsequent fertility, intrauterine pregnancy rates are comparable for laparoscopy and laparotomy, as are rates of recurrent ectopic pregnancy.[60,61]

ECTOPIC PREGNANCY PERSISTING AFTER SALPINGOSTOMY

Persistent ectopic pregnancy is diagnosed by a plateauing or rising β-hCG concentration following conservative surgical therapy. Although the number of reported successful cases is small, women with persistent ectopic pregnancies are treated successfully using single-dose systemic methotrexate.[53,54]

ECTOPIC PREGNANCY ASSOCIATED WITH ASSISTED REPRODUCTIVE TECHNOLOGIES

Ectopic pregnancy after ART is increasingly common because of widespread use of IVF and allied procedures. Infertile patients are innately at increased risk for ectopic pregnancy compared to the normally fertile population.

Incidence

Information on ectopic pregnancies resulting from ART comes from data obtained from institutions in the United States and Canada reporting to the Society for Assisted Reproductive Technology and the United States Center for Disease Control. The rate of pregnancies per IVF cycle and 31 348 clinical pregnancies in 91 032 cycles that resulted in ectopic pregnancies after IVF in 2003 was only 0.7%.[62] This included outcome of ART cycles using fresh non-donor eggs or embryos in embryo.[63] This lower percentage probably reflected the trend toward performing salpingectomies when hydrosalpinges are present to improve the success of ART/IVF.

Location

As in naturally occurring ectopic pregnancies, the Fallopian tube is the most common site for ectopic pregnancies following IVF. The distribution does differ from spontaneously occurring ectopic pregnancies (see Figure 49.1). Data obtained from three studies reveal that 82.2% of ectopic pregnancies were tubal.[64,65] The risk of heterotopic pregnancy is significant at 11.7%.[64,65]

Tubal disease

The most important predisposing factor for ectopic pregnancy in patients undergoing IVF is tubal disease. Ectopic pregnancies are four times higher in patients with tubal factor infertility compared with patients with normal tubes.[65] Hydrosalpinges are associated more commonly with ectopic pregnancy than other types of tubal pathology. Prior tubal reconstructive surgery (salpingostomy) increases the risk of ectopic pregnancy by 10% above that in patients with tubal factor infertility without prior surgery.[65] Thus, it is not surprising that patients with previous pelvic inflammatory disease have a six-fold increase in ectopic pregnancy after IVF.[65] However, a history of prior ectopic pregnancy does not seem as important a risk factor in IVF cycles as in natural cycles.[63,65]

Salpingectomy, particularly with hydrosalpinx, decreases risks of ectopic pregnancy while increasing pregnancy rates after IVF. Meta-analysis has demonstrated that the presence of hydrosalpinges decreases the chance for viable pregnancy by approximately 50% when compared with patients with tubal disease but without hydrosalpinges.[64] The uterine implantation rate was also noted to be 50% lower, with a higher chance of miscarriage and ectopic gestation. It thus appears that when a hydrosalpinx is present there are decreased pregnancy rates following IVF. In addition, patients are at decreased risk for pelvic infection as well as future ectopic pregnancy.[64]

Ectopic pregnancy following ovulation induction

Hormone alterations during ovulation induction theoretically alter tubal function. In animal models, estrogen administration results in functional tubal blockage and embryo arrest in the fallopian tube. In humans, steroid hormones alter tubal function and contractility, thus affecting tubal peristalsis. There remains controversy as to whether ovulation-inducing agents, including clomiphene citrate, increase ectopic pregnancy rates.[66,67]

Heterotopic pregnancy following ART

Heterotopic pregnancies are rare, but occur in about 1% of pregnancies following an ART procedure, are usually diagnosed incidentally, and constitute 11.7% of ectopic pregnancies on routine follow-up ultrasonographic studies (see Figure 49.1). This increased prevalence of heterotopic pregnancies following ART may be related to ovarian hyperstimulation and multiple ovum development. Of 111 reported heterotopic pregnancies following ART, 88.3% were tubal, 6.3% cornual, 2.7% abdominal, 1.8% cervical, and 0.9% ovarian. Because of the significant risk of heterotopic pregnancy, ART pregnancies should have at least one ultrasound late in the first trimester after the hyperstimulated ovaries have resolved.[62,68]

EXPECTANT MANAGEMENT

Ectopic pregnancies may resolve spontaneously. In a cavalier experiment in 1955, Lund hospitalized 119 women with ectopic pregnancy for observation.[69] All were at least 6 weeks' gestation. Some required multiple blood transfusions, and many were hemodynamically unstable. However, 68 cases resolved without surgery. Additional studies reported in the literature since Lund's study found similar results.[70–73] Thus, both conservative medical and surgical therapy overtreats a substantial number of women with ectopic pregnancy. Falling β-hCG levels under 1000 mIU/ml have been followed with conservative expectant management. Although patients with an equivocal diagnosis of ectopic pregnancy may be treated in this fashion, there are very limited data to support expectant management in clinical practice.

COSTS OF CARING FOR ECTOPIC PREGNANCY

In 1990, total costs for ectopic pregnancies in the United States were estimated to be $1.1 billion. It is probably much higher today.[74] Laparoscopic surgery is less expensive than laparotomy for uncomplicated ectopic pregnancy.[75] Systemic methotrexate therapy is the most cost-efficient. Savings from methotrexate are highly dependent on patient selection. A study, undertaken to compare the costs of systemic methotrexate with surgery, concluded that there would be a reduction in overall costs when hCG levels were below 3000 mIU/ml; otherwise, there was not a substantial cost saving over surgery. Cost savings expected from methotrexate are lost when there are complications requiring emergency surgery or large number of clinic visits.[76–81]

UNUSUAL ECTOPIC PREGNANCIES

Abdominal pregnancy

The incidence of abdominal pregnancy is estimated at 1 in 8000 births and represents 1.4% of all ectopic pregnancies. The prognosis is poor, with an estimated maternal mortality rate of 5.1 per 1000 cases. The risk of dying from an abdominal pregnancy is 7.7 times higher than from other forms of ectopic pregnancy. The high rate of morbidity and mortality from abdominal pregnancy often results from a delay in diagnosis.[82,83]

Abdominal pregnancies can be categorized as primary or secondary. Abdominal pregnancies may become apparent throughout gestation, from the first trimester to fetal viability. Symptoms may vary from those considered normal for pregnancy to severe abdominal pain, intra-abdominal hemorrhage, and hemodynamic instability. Primary abdominal pregnancies are rare and are thought to occur as a result of primary peritoneal implantation. They usually abort early in the first trimester due to hemorrhagic disruption of the implantation site and hemoperitoneum. Secondary abdominal pregnancies occur with reimplantation after a partial tubal abortion or intraligamentary extension following tubal rupture. Historical criteria to distinguish between primary and secondary abdominal pregnancies are moot, because treatment is directed by the clinical picture.

Ultrasonography is the diagnostic tool of choice and usually can identify the empty uterus along with the extrauteral products of conception. If the fetus is near viability, hospitalization is recommended. If time permits, bowel preparation, administration of prophylactic antibiotics, and adequate blood replacement should be made available prior to an operative delivery. Unless the placenta is implanted on major vessels or vital structures, it should be removed. Although complications may occur, including sepsis, abscess formation, secondary hemorrhage, intestinal obstruction, wound dehiscence, amniotic fluid cyst formation, hypofibrinogenemia, and preeclampsia, the placenta can be left in place to prevent further hemorrhage at the time of surgery. In contrast to the typical tubal ectopic pregnancy, methotrexate is unlikely to accelerate retained placental absorption, because the trophoblastic cells are no longer actively dividing.

Ovarian pregnancy

Ovarian pregnancy, the most common form of abdominal pregnancy, is rare.[85,86] Clinical findings are similar to those of tubal ectopic gestations: abdominal pain, amenorrhea, and abnormal vaginal bleeding. In addition, hemodynamic instability as a result of rupture occurs in 30% of patients. Women with ovarian pregnancies are usually young and multiparous, but the factors leading to ovarian pregnancies are not clear.

Diagnosis is usually is made by the pathologist, because many ovarian pregnancies are mistaken for a ruptured corpus luteum or other ovarian tumors. Only 28% of cases were diagnosed correctly at the time of laparotomy.[85,86] The recommended treatment is cystectomy, wedge resection, or oophorectomy during laparotomy, although laparoscopic removal has been successful.

Cornual pregnancy

Cornual or interstitial pregnancy accounts for 1.9% of spontaneous but 7.3% of ART ectopic gestations. Historically, it has carried a 2.2% maternal mortality when almost all cases were diagnosed after the patient was symptomatic.[87] The most frequent symptoms are menstrual aberration, abdominal pain, abnormal vaginal bleeding, and shock, resulting from the brisk hemorrhage associated with uterine rupture. Due to myometrial distensibility, rupture is usually delayed, occurring at 9–12 weeks' gestation.[87] Today, the majority are diagnosed by ultrasound at 6–8 weeks and the course is far less morbid.

A unique risk factor for interstitial pregnancy is previous salpingectomy. Only a high index of suspicion and repeated ultrasonographic examination with Doppler flow studies allows early diagnosis. With timely early diagnosis, alternatives to the traditional cornual resection during laparotomy have been performed successfully. These include laparoscopic cornual resection, systemic methotrexate administration, local injection of methotrexate, potassium chloride injection, and removal by hysteroscopy.[88,89] Regardless of the initial treatment attempted, if uncontrolled hemorrhage occurs, hysterectomy may be the only choice.

Cervical pregnancy

The incidence of cervical pregnancy ranges from 1 in 2500 to 1 in 12 422 pregnancies. The most common predisposing factor is a prior dilatation and curettage, present in 68.6% of patients.[89,90] Interestingly, 31% of these were performed for termination of pregnancy. Other predisposing factors implicated in cervical pregnancies are previous cesarean delivery and IVF.

The most common initial symptom of cervical pregnancy is painless vaginal bleeding. These ectopics are usually diagnosed incidentally during routine ultrasonography or at the time of surgery for a suspected abortion in progress. In reported cases, most patients sought treatment for vaginal bleeding, and many had massive bleeding. The cervix is usually enlarged, globular, or distended. On occasion, it appears cyanotic, hyperemic, and soft in consistency. Sonography and magnetic resonance imaging have improved diagnosis of cervical pregnancy. Most patients are diagnosed correctly with ultrasonographic identification of the gestational sac in the cervix below a closed internal cervical os, with trophoblastic invasion into the endocervical tissue.[89,90]

When the patient is hemodynamically stable, conservative therapy commonly is employed. There are no large studies, only several case series. These have shown that use of methotrexate and uterine artery embolization are safe and effective for treatment in the stable patient with a cervical pregnancy. Unfortunately, massive hemorrhage may occur despite conservative measures, and hysterectomy is warranted.[89,90]

Heterotopic pregnancy

Heterotopic pregnancy is the coexistence of an intrauterine and ectopic gestation, and occurs in 1 in 3889 to 1 in 6778 pregnancies. In a review of 66 heterotopic pregnancies by Reece et al, 93.9% were tubal and 6.1% ovarian.[62]

Simultaneous existence of intra- and extrauterine pregnancies poses serious diagnostic pitfalls. Heterotopic pregnancies are diagnosed in most cases after clinical signs and symptoms develop, and most patients are admitted for emergency surgery following rupture. The delay in diagnosis is secondary to the finding of an intrauterine pregnancy, with the assumption that any symptoms will be self-limited.

Similar to tubal ectopic pregnancies, the most common complaint is lower abdominal pain. Routine ultrasonography detects only about half of tubal heterotopic pregnancies, and the remainder are diagnosed during laparoscopy or laparotomy when patients become symptomatic. Serial levels of the β subunit of hCG are not helpful, owing to the effect of the intrauterine pregnancy.[83]

Laparotomy is warranted if the diagnosis is suspected or the patient is symptomatic but hemodynamically stable. Expectant management is not recommended because β-hCG levels cannot be monitored adequately. Systemic methotrexate is contraindicated if a viable intrauterine pregnancy is present and desired. Local injection of methotrexate with potassium chloride has been described in small case series.[83]

SUMMARY

Ectopic pregnancy remains a serious and potentially fatal disease. In most circumstances, it can be diagnosed before symptoms develop and treated definitively with few complications. Quantitative β-hCG testing, ultrasonography, and curettage allow early diagnosis of ectopic pregnancy and use of medical therapy as the initial therapy option. Conservative surgical therapy and medical therapy for ectopic pregnancy are comparable in terms of success rates and subsequent fertility. Medical therapy is the preferred choice because of the freedom from surgical complications and lower cost. Surgery is the treatment of choice for hemorrhage, medical failures, neglected cases, and when medical therapy is contraindicated. Multiple-dose methotrexate is preferable to single-dose methotrexate, direct injection, or tubal cannulation and is the first choice for unruptured, uncomplicated ectopic pregnancy. Laparoscopic salpingostomy or salpingectomy is favored for cases of intra-abdominal hemorrhage, medical failure, neglected cases, and complex cases when medical therapy is contraindicated. Prophylactic postoperative systemic methotrexate (a single dose) can prevent virtually all cases of persistent ectopic pregnancy following salpingostomy. Salpingectomy prior to ART decreases ectopic pregnancy incidence while increasing pregnancy rates in select patients with pre-existing tubal disease.

REFERENCES

1. National Center for Health Statistics. Advance report of final mortality statistics, 1992. Hyattsville, MD: US Department of Health and Human Services, Public Health Service, CDC. Mon Vital Stat Rep 1994; 43(Suppl).
2. Zane SB, Kieke BA Jr, Kendrick JS et al. Surveillance in a time of changing health care practices: estimating ectopic pregnancy incidence in the United States. Matern Child Health J 2002; 6: 227–36.
3. Van den Eeden SK, Shan J, Bruce C et al. Ectopic pregnancy rate and treatment utilization in a large managed care organization. Obstet Gynecol 2005; 105: 1052–7.
4. Berg CJ, Chang J, Callaghan WM et al. Pregnancy-related mortality in the United States, 1991–1997. Obstet Gynecol 2003; 101: 289–96.
5. Budowick M, Johnson TRB, Genadry R et al. The histopathology of the developing tubal ectopic pregnancy. Fertil Steril 1980; 34: 169–71.
6. Westrom L. Effect of acute pelvic inflammatory disease on fertility. Am J Obstet Gynecol 1975; 121: 707–13.
7. Wong JA, Clark JF. Correlation of symptoms with age and location of gestation in tubal pregnancy. J Natl Med Assoc 1968; 60: 221–3.
8. Breen JL. A 21-year survey of 654 ectopic pregnancies. Am J Obstet Gynecol 1970; 106: 1004–19.
9. Dudley P, Heard MJ, Sangi-Haghpeykar H et al. Characterizing ectopic pregnancies that rupture despite treatment with methotrexate. Fertil Steril 2004; 82: 1374–8.

10. McKenzie LJ, El-Zimaity H, Krotz S et al. Comparative genomic hybridization of ectopic pregnancies that fail methotrexate therapy. Fertil Steril 2005; 84: 1517–19.

11. Bouyer J, Coste J, Shojaei T et al. Risk factors for ectopic pregnancy: a comprehensive analysis based on a large case-control, population-based study in France. Am J Epidemiol 2003; 157: 185–94.

12. Bouyer J, Rachou E, Germain E et al. Risk factors for extrauterine pregnancy in women using an intrauterine device. Fertil Steril 2000; 74: 899–908.

13. Ankum WM, Mol BWJ, Van der Veen F et al. Risk factors for ectopic pregnancy: a meta-analysis. JAMA 1996; 65: 1093–9.

14. Brenner PF, Benedetti T, Mishell DR. Ectopic pregnancy following tubal sterilization surgery. Obstet Gynecol 1977; 49: 323–4.

15. Dubuisson JB, Abriot FX, Mathieu L et al. Risk factors for ectopic pregnancy in 556 pregnancies after in vitro fertilization: implications for preventive management. Fertil Steril 1991; 56: 686–90.

16. Kranz SG, Gray RH, Damewood MD et al. Time trends in risk factors and clinical outcome of ectopic pregnancy. Fertil Steril 1990; 54: 42–6.

17. Majmudar B, Henderson PH, Semple E. Salpingitis isthmica nodosa: a high-risk factor for tubal pregnancy. Obstet Gynecol 1983; 62: 73–8.

18. Mol BWJ, Ankum WM, Bossuyt PMM et al. Contraception and the risk of ectopic pregnancy: a meta-analysis. Contraception 1995; 52: 337–41.

19. Xiong X, Buekens P, Wollast E. IUD use and the risk of ectopic pregnancy: a meta-analysis of case-control studies. Contraception 1995; 52: 23–34.

20. Fernandez H, Gerviase A. Ectopic pregnancies after infertility treatment: modern diagnosis and therapeutic strategy. Hum Reprod 2004; 10: 503–13.

21. Hillis SD, Owens LM, Marchbanks PA et al. Recurrent chlamydial infections increase the risks of hospitalisation for ectopic pregnancy and pelvic inflammatory disease. Am J Obstet Gynecol 1997; 176: 103–7.

22. Strandell A, Thorburn J, Hamberger L. Risk factors for ectopic pregnancy in assisted reproduction. Fertil Steril 1999; 71: 282–6.

23. Furlong LA. Ectopic pregnancy risk when contraception fails: a review. J Reprod Med 2002; 47: 881–5.

24. Peterson H, Xia Z, Hughes JM et al. The risk of ectopic pregnancy after tubal sterilization. N Engl J Med 1997; 336: 762–7.

25. Pereira PP, Cabar FR, Raiza LCP et al. Emergency contraception and ectopic pregnancy: report of 2 cases. Clinics 2005; 60: S1807.

26. Talbot P, Riveles K. Smoking and reproduction: the oviduct as a target of cigarette smoke. Reprod Biol Endocrinol 2005; 28; 3: 52.

27. Buster JE, Carson SA. Ectopic pregnancy: new advances in diagnosis and treatment. Curr Opin Obstet Gynecol 1995; 7: 168–76.

28. Garcia CR, Barnhart KT. Diagnosing ectopic pregnancy: decision analysis comparing six strategies. Obstet Gynecol 2001; 97: 464–70.

29. Seeber BE, Barnhart KT. Suspected ectopic pregnancy. Obstet Gynecol 2006; 107: 399–413.

30. Barnhart KT, Sammel MD, Rinaudo PF et al. Symptomatic patients with an early viable intrauterine pregnancy; hCG curves redefined. Obstet Gynecol 2004; 104: 50–5.

31. Barnhart KT, Katz I, Hummel A et al. Presumed diagnosis of ectopic pregnancy. Obstet Gynecol 2002; 100: 505–10.

32. Rull K, Laan M. Expression of beta-subunit of hCG genes during normal and failed pregnancy. Hum Reprod 2005; 20: 3360–8.

33. Barnhart KT, Sammel MD, Chung K et al. Decline of serum human chorionic gonadotropin and spontaneous complete abortion: defining the normal curve. Obstet Gynecol 2004; 104: 975–81.

34. Heard MJ, Buster JE. In: Scott JR, Gibbs RS, Karlan BY, Haney AF, eds. Danforth's Obstetrics and Gynecology. Philadelphia: Lippincott Williams & Wilkins, 2003: 89–104.

35. Ailawadi M, Lorch SA, Barnhart KT. Cost effectiveness of presumptively medically treating women at risk for ectopic pregnancy compared to first performing a D&C. Fertil Steril 2005; 83: 376–82.

36. Adam MP, Manning MA, Beck AE et al. Methotrexate/misoprostol embryopathy: report of four cases resulting from failed medical abortion. Am J Med Genet 2003; 123A: 72–8.

37. Rodi IA, Sauer MV, Gorrill MJ et al. The medical treatment of unruptured ectopic pregnancy with methotrexate and citrovorum rescue: preliminary experience. Fertil Steril 1986; 46: 811–13.

38. Barnhart K, Coutifaris C, Esposito M. The pharmacology of methotrexate. Expert Opin Pharmacother 2001; 2: 409–17.

39. Hajenius PH, Englesbel S, Mol BW et al. Randomised trial of systemic methotrexate versus laparoscopic salpingostomy in tubal pregnancy. Lancet 1997; 350: 1554–5.

40. Pisarska MD, Carson SA, Buster JE. Ectopic pregnancy. The Lancet 1998; 351: 1115–20.

41. Hajenius PH, Mol BW, Bossuyt PM et al. Interventions for tubal ectopic pregnancy. Cochrane Database Syst Rev 2000; CD000324.

42. Stovall TG, Ling FW. Single-dose methotrexate: an expanded clinical trial. Am J Obstet Gynecol 1993; 168: 759–72.

43. Lipscomb GH, Bran D, McCord ML et al. Analysis of three hundred fifteen ectopic pregnancies treated with single-dose methotrexate. Am J Obstet Gynecol 1998; 178: 1354–8.

44. Medical Management of Tubal Pregnancy. ACOG Practice Bulletin. Clinical Management Guidelines for Obstetrician-Gynecologists, December 1998; 3: 410–16.

45. Barnhart KT, Gosman G, Ashby R, Sammel M. The medical management of ectopic pregnancy: a meta-analysis comparing "single dose" and "multidose" regimens. Obstet Gynecol 2003; 101: 778–84.

46. Molinaro T, Gracia C, Sammel MD et al. Indirect analysis of single dose versus multiple dose methotrexate in the treatment of ectopic pregnancy. Fertil Steril 2006; in press.

47. Lipscomb GH, Puckett KJ, Bran D et al. Management of separation pain after single-dose methotrexate therapy for ectopic pregnancy. Obstet Gynecol 1999; 93: 590–3.

48. Buster JE, Heard MJ. Current issues in medical management of ectopic pregnancy. Curr Opin Obstet Gynecol 2000; 12: 525–7.

49. Lipscomb GH, Stovall TG, Ling FW. Nonsurgical treatment of ectopic pregnancy. N Engl J Med 2000; 343: 1325–9.

50. Lipscomb GH, McCord ML, Stovall TG et al. Predictors of success of methotrexate treament in women with tubal ectopic pregnancies. N Engl J Med 1999; 341: 1974–8.

51. Shalev E, Peleg D, Bustan M et al. Limited role for intratubal methotrexate treatment of ectopic pregnancy. Fertil Steril 1995; 63: 20–4.

52. Atri M, Bret PM, Tulandi T et al. Ectopic pregnancy: evolution after treatment with transvaginal methotrexate. Radiology 1992; 185: 749–53.

53. Isaacs JD, McGehee RP, Cowan BD. Life-threatening neutropenia following methotrexate treatment of ectopic pregnancy: a report of two cases. Obstet Gynecol 1996; 88: 694–6.

54. Schoenfeld A, Mashiach R, Vardy M et al. Methotrexate pneumonitis in nonsurgical treatment of ectopic pregnancy. Obstet Gynecol 1992; 80: 520–1.

55. Kelly H, Harvey D, Moll S. A cautionary tale: fatal outcome of methotrexate therapy given for management of ectopic pregnancy. Obstet Gynecol 2006; 107: 439–41.

56. Vermesh M, Silva PD, Rosen GF et al. Management of unruptured ectopic gestation by linear salpingostomy: a prospective, randomized clinical trial of laparoscopy versus laparotomy. Obstet Gynecol 1989; 73: 400–4.

57. Seifer DB, Guttmann JN, Grant WD et al. Comparison of persistent ectopic pregnancy after laparoscopic salpingostomy versus salpingostomy at laparotomy for ectopic pregnancy. Obstet Gynecol 1993; 81: 378–82.

58. Gracia C, Brown H, Barnhart K. Prophylactic methotrexate after linear salpingostomy: a decision analysis. Fertil Steril 2001; 76: 1191–5.

59. Gracia CR, Brown HA, Barnhart KT. Prophylactic methotrexate after linear salpingostomy: a decision analysis. Fertil Steril 2001; 76: 1191–5.

60. Lundorff P, Thorburn J, Hahlin M et al. Laparoscopic surgery in ectopic pregnancy: a randomized trial versus laparotomy. Acta Obstet Gynecol Scand 1991; 70: 343–8.

61. Murphy AA, Nager CW, Wujek JJ et al. Operative laparoscopy versus laparotomy for the management of ectopic pregnancy: a prospective trial. Fertil Steril 1992; 57: 1180–5.

62. Reece EA, Petrie RH, Sirmans MF et al. Combined intrauterine and extrauterine gestations: a review. Am J Obstet Gynecol 1983; 146: 323–30.

63. CDC Reproductive Health. 2003 Assisted reproductive technology success rates: NIH summary and fertility clinic reports. US Department of Health and Human Services 2003: 1–510.

64. Camus E, Poncelet C, Goffinet F et al. Pregnancy rates after in-vitro fertilization in cases of tubal infertility with and without hydrosalpinx: a meta-analysis of published comparative studies. Hum Reprod 1999; 14: 1243–9.

65. Abusheikha N, Salha O, Brinsden P. Extra-uterine pregnancy following assisted conception treatment. Hum Reprod Update 2000; 6: 80–92.

66. Dickey RP, Holtkamp DE. Development, pharmacology and clinical experience with clomiphene citrate. Hum Reprod Update 1996; 2: 483–506.

67. Fernandez H, Gervaise A. Ectopic pregnancies after infertility treatment: modern diagnosis and therapeutic strategy. Hum Reprod Update 2004; 10: 503–13.

68. Chin HY, Chen FP, Wang CJ et al. Heterotopic pregnancy after in vitro fertilization-embryo transfer. Int J Gynaecol Obstet 2004; 86: 411–16.

69. Lund J. Early ectopic pregnancy; comments on conservative treatment. J Obstet Gynaecol Br Emp 1955; 62: 70–6.

70. Fernandez H, Lelaidier C, Baton C et al. Return of reproductive performance after expectant management and local treatment for ectopic pregnancy. Hum Reprod 1991; 6: 1474–7.

71. Garcia AJ, Aubert JM, Sama J et al. Expectant management of presumed ectopic pregnancies. Fertil Steril 1987; 48: 395–400.

72. Shalev E, Peleg D, Tsabari A et al. Spontaneous resolution of ectopic tubal pregnancy: natural history. Fertil Steril 1995; 63: 15–19.

73. Ylöstalo P, Cacciatore B, Korhonen J et al. Expectant management of ectopic pregnancy. Eur J Obstet Gynecol Reprod Biol 1993; 49: 83–4.

74. Washington AE, Katz P. Ectopic pregnancy in the United States: economic consequences and payment source trends. Obstet Gynecol 1993; 81: 287–92.

75. Mol BWJ, Hajenius PH, Engelsbel S et al. An economic evaluation of laparoscopy and open surgery in the treatment of tubal pregnancy. Acta Obstet Gynecol Scand 1997; 76: 596–600.

76. Yao M, Tulandi T, Kaplow M et al. A comparison of methotrexate versus laparoscopic surgery for treatment of ectopic pregnancy: a cost analysis. Hum Reprod 1996; 11: 2762–6.

77. Stovall TG, Bradham DD, Ling FW et al. Cost of treatment of ectopic pregnancy: single-dose methotrexate versus surgical treatment. J Womens Health 1994; 3: 445–50.

78. Alexander JM, Rouse DJ, Varner E et al. Treatment of the small unruptured ectopic pregnancy: a cost analysis of methotrexate versus laparoscopy. Obstet Gynecol 1996; 88: 123–7.

79. Vaissade L, Gerbaud L, Pouly JL et al. Cost-effectiveness analysis of laparoscopic surgery versus methotrexate: comparison of data recorded in an ectopic pregnancy registry. J Gynecol Obstet Biol Reprod (Paris) 2003; 32: 447–58.

80. Morlock RJ, Lafata JE, Eisenstein D. Cost-effectiveness of single-dose methotrexate compared with laparoscopic treatment of ectopic pregnancy. Obstet Gynecol 2000; 95: 407–12.

81. Sowter MC, Farquhar CM, Gudex G. An economic evaluation of single dose systemic methotrexate and laparoscopic surgery for the treatment of unruptured ectopic pregnancy. BJOG 2001; 108: 204–12.

82. Atrash HK, Friede A, Hogue CJR. Abdominal pregnancy in the United States: frequency and maternal mortality. Obstet Gynecol 1987; 69: 333–7.

83. Fernandez H, Gervaise A. Ectopic pregnancies after infertility treatment: modern diagnosis and therapeutic strategy. Hum Reprod Update 2004; 10: 503–13.

84. Wicherek L, Galazka K, Popiela TJ et al. Metallothionein expression and infiltration of cytotoxic lymphocytes in uterine and tubal implantation sites. J Reprod Immunol 2006; 70: 119–31.

85. Grimes HG, Nosal RA, Gallagher JC. Ovarian pregnancy: a series of 24 cases. Obstet Gynecol 1983; 61: 174–80.

86. Hallatt JG. Primary ovarian pregnancy: a report of twenty-five cases. Am J Obstet Gynecol 1982; 143: 55–60.

87. Budnick SG, Jacobs SL, Nulsen JC et al. Conservative management of interstitial pregnancy. Obstet Gynecol Surv 1993; 48: 694–8.

88. Goldenberg M, Bider D, Oelsner G et al. Treatment of interstitial pregnancy with methotrexate via hysteroscopy. Fertil Steril 1992; 58: 1234–6.

89. Ushakov FB, Elchalal U, Aceman PH et al. Cervical pregnancy: past and future. Obstet Gynecol 1996; 52: 45–59.

90. Cepni I, Ocal P, Erkan S et al. Conservative treatment of cervical ectopic pregnancy with transvaginal ultrasound-guided aspiration and single-dose methotrexate. Fertil Steril 2004; 81: 1130–2.

50 Preeclampsia and intrauterine growth restriction

*Alexander EP Heazell, Justine Nugent, Rebecca L Jones,
Lynda K Harris, and Philip N Baker*

Synopsis

General

- Preeclampsia is a disorder of pregnancy in which the placenta causes maternal hypertension, systemic vascular endothelial dysfunction, and proteinuria.
- Intrauterine growth restriction (IUGR) results from insufficient transfer of nutrients and oxygen to the developing fetus. It can occur even in well-fed mothers.
- While these conditions normally present in the latter half of pregnancy, it is thought that events in early pregnancy lead to their development.

Basic Science

- Preeclampsia and IUGR are characterized by high resistance flow in the maternal arteries perfusing the placenta, due to defective trophoblast-mediated remodeling of the myometrial and decidual arteries.
- The placenta in preeclampsia is thought to be hypoxic.
- Preeclampsia is associated with exaggerated maternal vasoconstriction.
- Trophoblast invasion of the uterus is shallower in preeclampsia than in normal pregnancy.
- Villous trophoblast proliferation is reduced in IUGR.
- Villous vascular architecture is altered in some types of IUGR with reduced branching.
- Villous trophoblast proliferation is increased in preeclampsia but turnover is also faster, with an increased rate of trophoblastic particle shedding from the surface of the placenta into maternal circulation.
- Microparticles shed from the placenta interact with the maternal immune system, cause inflammatory changes, and impair maternal endothelial function.

Clinical

- Preeclampsia and IUGR are associated with increased perinatal morbidity and mortality.
- They present a significant global health problem.
- At the present time there are no effective interventions for either preeclampsia or IUGR, except delivery of the infant.
- Preeclampsia and IUGR have the potential to leave both infants and mothers with lifelong health problems, especially in the cardiovascular system.

INTRODUCTION

Preeclampsia and intrauterine growth restriction (IUGR) represent the most commonly encountered placental disorders in clinical practice; they may occur in isolation or coexist. Preeclampsia is a multisystem disorder, in which hypertension and endothelial dysfunction lead to end-organ malfunction. IUGR results from insufficient transfer of nutrients and oxygen to the developing fetus. Both preeclampsia and IUGR originate from dysfunction of the uteroplacental interface. While these conditions normally present in the latter half of pregnancy, current understanding of these complex conditions proposes that changes occurring early in pregnancy, from implantation onwards, are important in the development of both preeclampsia and IUGR.

Preeclampsia and IUGR are associated with an increased perinatal morbidity and mortality rate; 43% of stillbirths have evidence of IUGR,[1] while preeclampsia is also associated with an increase in maternal mortality, accounting for 13% of maternal deaths in the UK.[2] At the present time there are no effective interventions for either preeclampsia or IUGR, except for delivery of the infant. This leads to an increase in iatrogenic prematurity, which is associated with lifelong disability. In addition, IUGR is associated with an increased risk of cardiovascular disease in later life, leading to the 'developmental origins of adult health and disease' hypothesis.[3] Increased understanding of the uteroplacental interface in these pregnancy pathologies may provide potential therapeutic options that ideally prolong pregnancy and so reduce the associated perinatal morbidity and mortality.

DEFINITION OF PREECLAMPSIA AND IUGR

Preeclampsia is characterized by maternal hypertension and proteinuria. Although several definitions have been used, the most widely accepted definition of preeclampsia is newly diagnosed hypertension >140/90 mmHg on two separate occasions, and proteinuria >300 mg/24 hours developing after 20 weeks' gestation.[4] This definition excludes women with preexisting hypertension, in whom the presence of de-novo proteinuria is termed 'superimposed pre-eclampsia'.

IUGR is defined as the failure of a fetus to reach its optimal growth in utero. It should not be confused with small for gestational age, a statistical derivation that an infant lies under the 5th or 10th centile for birthweight. At least half of the infants with a birthweight under the 10th centile for their gender and gestation will have been normally nourished in utero. Conversely, infants who have a birthweight greater than the 10th centile may have failed to reach their growth potential. Until the advent of high-definition ultrasound scanning, the antenatal detection of IUGR was difficult. However, a variety of measurements used to estimate fetal weight in utero may be used to demonstrate suboptimal growth. In addition, a reduction in amniotic fluid volume and/or a loss of umbilical artery end-diastolic flow have been related to a diagnosis of IUGR. The individualized birthweight ratio, which takes account of maternal height, weight, and ethnicity, should be used when assessing whether an infant has IUGR.[5]

Table 50.1 Risk factors for the development of preeclampsia and IUGR

Variable	Risk ratio for developing preeclampsia	Risk ratio for developing IUGR
Chronic renal disease	20:1	3:1
Chronic hypertension	10:1	2-3:1
Family history of hypertensive disease of pregnancy	5:1	–
Twin pregnancy	4:1	3.5:1
Nulliparity	3:1	–
Previous pregnancy affected	7:1	6:1
Maternal age <18 years old	2:1	2:1
Maternal age >40 years old	3:1	–
Cigarette smoking	0.6:1	2.4:1
Diabetes mellitus	2:1	–

– = no data available.

EPIDEMIOLOGY OF PREECLAMPSIA AND IUGR

Preeclampsia and IUGR represent a significant global health problem; the World Health Organization estimates over 60 000 women die worldwide from preeclampsia each year. The majority of these cases occur within the developing world. However, preeclampsia has been an important cause of maternal death in the UK over recent decades, causing 13% of maternal deaths from pregnancy-related complications.[2] It has been estimated that at least 1 in 6 stillbirths and neonatal deaths occur in pregnancies complicated by maternal hypertension. Furthermore, preeclampsia and IUGR are responsible for the occupancy of approximately 20% of special care baby unit facilities, due to the necessity to expedite delivery to prevent a deterioration in maternal and fetal health.

The reported incidence of preeclampsia varies between 0.5% and 9.7%. This wide range may be explained by variations in the definition of preeclampsia and the population studied.[6] It is accepted that, in the developed world, the incidence of preeclampsia lies between 3% and 5%.[6] A summary of important risk factors which predispose women to develop preeclampsia and IUGR is shown in Table 50.1.[6–8] They demonstrate that maternal genotype and phenotype play an important part in the development of preeclampsia. The incidence of preeclampsia is increased in women who already have endothelial dysfunction, such as those with chronic hypertension and renal disease. There is also a significant genetic component to preeclampsia, although the genes involved have yet to be identified. An increased volume of placental tissue increases the incidence of preeclampsia, as seen in molar and multiple pregnancies.

IUGR is defined as the failure of a fetus to attain its growth potential. It occurs in approximately 8% of all pregnancies, and may coexist with preeclampsia.[9] It is associated with increased perinatal mortality and morbidity. Infants are at an increased risk of perinatal complications such as fetal distress, asphyxia, neonatal encephalopathy, hypothermia, hypoglycemia, and poor feeding, as well as risks of long-term neurological and developmental disorders. IUGR has been demonstrated to increase the risk of hypertension, coronary artery disease, type 2 diabetes, and stroke in later life,[3] and this gives rise to the developmental origins of adult disease hypothesis, which claims that the fetus is programmed in utero in response to undernutrition, leading to permanent changes in physiological function in later life.

PATHOPHYSIOLOGICAL MODELS OF PREECLAMPSIA AND IUGR

Many pathophysiological hypotheses have been developed to describe changes observed at the utero–placental interface in pregnancies complicated by preeclampsia and IUGR, including aberrant implantation, reduced invasion of the decidua by trophoblast, inadequate transformation of uteroplacental arteries, changes in villous trophoblast, altered maternal vascular responses, and the presence of circulating factors within maternal plasma in preeclampsia. Indeed, preeclampsia has been termed the 'disease of theories'. Research into these conditions has increased understanding of their development.

The endometrium and decidua

Preeclampsia and IUGR are characterized by high resistance flow in the maternal arteries perfusing the placenta, due to defective trophoblast-mediated remodeling of the myometrial and decidual arteries.[10] This suggests that these disorders have early origins, caused by insufficient trophoblast colonization of the maternal tissues during the establishment of pregnancy.

Blastocyst implantation and trophoblast invasion of the decidua are complex and highly orchestrated events, involving intimate physical and biochemical contact between maternal and fetal tissues. These processes are regulated by active two-way communication between the uterine and embryonic cells, mediated by a wealth of locally produced growth factors, cytokines, adhesion molecules, and proteases. Human implantation

and trophoblast invasion are challenging to study; this is increased with respect to preeclampsia and IUGR, as these conditions manifest much later in pregnancy, and patients who will go on to develop preeclampsia or IUGR cannot be reliably identified at present. Thus, knowledge in this area is mainly derived from studies on term placenta, in-vitro models, and extrapolation from animal studies. However, from delineation of the regulatory steps and factors involved during the establishment of normal pregnancy, it is possible to speculate about abnormalities and dysregulation that cause abnormal implantation, and thus may be potentially involved in the development of preeclampsia and IUGR.

The embryo is influenced by the maternal environment from the moment of conception. Cleavage, embryonic genome activation, and the first differentiation events during blastocyst development occur within a specialized environment created primarily by the epithelial cells lining the oviduct and uterus. Maternally derived nutrients and growth factors facilitate embryo development and growth, and the lack thereof in an in-vitro culture environment impacts upon embryo development.[11] Cultured mouse blastocysts contain fewer cells and their development is retarded compared to the in-vivo condition. Microarray experiments demonstrate global alterations in gene expression in cultured vs in-vivo matured mouse blastocysts.[12] This effect may play a role in human development, as the incidence of IUGR is increased in human pregnancies following assisted reproductive technologies involving in-vitro embryo culture.[13] Trophectoderm cells surrounding the embryo appear to be exceptionally sensitive to alterations in the environment, for example, in the loss of imprinting of the H19 gene in the placenta, but not embryonic cells, following embryo culture.[14] It is therefore hypothesized that through alterations in gene methylation and expression patterns, the placenta can be 'programmed' for abnormal development during early gestation.

Invasion of trophoblast into the uterine wall occurs at points of contact between anchoring placental villi and the decidua.[15] Cytotrophoblast cells in the anchoring villi proliferate rapidly, generating a cell column. At the distal portion of the column, cytotrophoblast cells differentiate into invasive extravillous cytotrophoblasts (EVTs), which detach from the column and migrate into the decidua. Decidual invasion and colonization of maternal arteries are critical processes in the establishment of the pregnancy, to enable sufficient placental perfusion later in pregnancy. EVT migration is tightly regulated by the environment at the maternal–fetal interface. Decidual-derived growth factors, autocrine

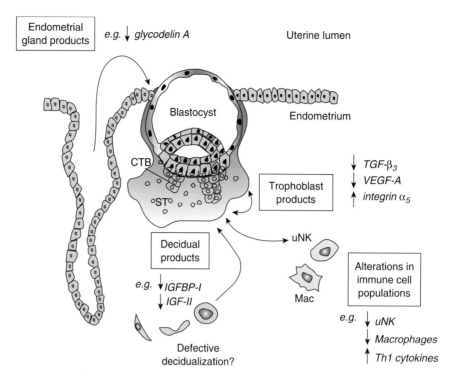

Figure 50.1 Summary of early embryo implantation events, illustrating potential defects in bidirectional communication between maternal and fetal cells in preeclampsia/IUGR. Endometrial products secreted by epithelial glands promote peri-implantation embryo development. Trophoblast differentiation: syncytial (ST) fusion and cytotrophoblast (CTB) outgrowth is regulated by autocrine trophoblast-derived factors and by paracrine signals from decidual cells. In addition, immune cells, particularly uterine natural killer cells (uNK) and macrophages (Mac), contribute to the unique immunological environment of the implantation site. There is evidence for aberrant expression of a number of maternal and trophoblast factors in the implantation site of pregnancies complicated by preeclampsia or IUGR, potentially contributing to the defective implantation and placentation evident in these disorders.

trophoblast factors, and oxygen tension all participate in modulating these processes. There is some evidence for altered expression of several regulatory factors in the implantation site in pregnancies complicated by preeclampsia and IUGR that may contribute to the abnormal/insufficient trophoblast invasion observed.

Decidualization is initiated spontaneously every menstrual cycle in anticipation of pregnancy. Decidual cells are a critical component of the implantation site; they produce an extracellular matrix conducive to trophoblast invasion, and secrete a wide array of paracrine factors that modulate cytotrophoblast proliferation and differentiation. Disruption or inhibition of decidualization in mouse models results in implantation failure, for example in the cyclooxygenase 2 (COX-2)[16] or interleukin-11 (IL-11) knockout mouse,[17] suggesting that insufficient decidualization in humans could contribute to pregnancy pathologies.[18] Indeed, a reduction in prolactin secretion (an established marker of decidualization) by decidua from preeclamptic pregnancies has already been demonstrated.[19]

A number of factors involved in creating the decidual environment have been studied in women with preeclampsia and IUGR, to examine their potential role in the decidualization process and on trophoblast development and function. Insulin-like growth factor binding protein 1 (IGFBP-1) is a major product of human decidua, indicating that the tight regulation of insulin-like growth factor (IGF) bioactivity is important during placentation. Overexpression of IGFBP-1 in mice results in abnormal trophoblast differentiation and invasion.[20] In women with preeclampsia, raised levels of circulating IGFBP-1 have been detected, and an elevation in placental and decidual production of IGFBP-1 and IGF-2 has been demonstrated.[21] Alterations in decidual angiogenesis have also been reported in women with preeclampsia, with increased microvascular density in the decidua basalis.[22] This is coincident with an up-regulation of angiogenic promoting factors such as tenascin, and elevated production of COX-1,[22] the biosynthetic enzyme for vasoactive prostaglandins.[23]

The decidua contains a highly specialized immunological environment, mediated primarily by the presence of a large population of uterine natural killer (uNK) cells (Figure 50.1). These constitute up to 40% of decidual cells in the first trimester of pregnancy, and can interact with cytotrophoblast cells via their expression of the human leukocyte antigen HLA-G.[24] This unique combination of low polymorphic MHC (major histocompatibility complex) class I antigen expression by trophoblasts and a population of NK cells with a decreased cytotoxic capacity is believed to be instrumental in allowing implantation of the semi-allogeneic embryo. Alterations in immune cell populations have been reported in the decidua of women with abnormal trophoblast invasion associated with IUGR and preeclampsia, including a reduction in uNK cells and elevated infiltration of cytotoxic NK cells.[25] This, coupled with a decrease in trophoblast HLA-G expression in preeclampsia placentas,[26] could impact upon normal immunomodulatory mechanisms and contribute to abnormal placentation.[27] Other abnormalities in immune cells have been reported in the decidual bed in preeclampsia, including reduced presence of lymphocyte subpopulations, and a shift in their cytokine production to a proinflammatory Th1 profile,[28] thought to be incompatible with pregnancy.[29] In addition, macrophages, which fulfill a major phagocytotic role, appear to be depleted in the decidual basal plate in preeclampsia,[30] suggesting a possible impairment of the clearance of apoptotic cells. This may contribute to inflammation and maternal immune system activation, caused by accumulation of cellular debris bearing paternal antigens.[31] Furthermore, there is some evidence for altered expression of immunomodulatory factors by the decidua; glycodelin A is secreted from the time of implantation and is presumed to confer a degree of protective effect to the placenta through promoting maternal tolerance. In decidual tissue from pregnancies complicated by IUGR, glycodelin A expression was significantly reduced, although this was not the case in preeclampsia.[32]

Trophoblast invasion is regulated by the balanced production of cytokines/growth factors such as activin A and IL-15 promoting invasion, or those which inhibit trophoblast invasion, e.g. transforming growth factor (TGF) βs and IL-10. TGFβ3 in particular, is a potent inhibitor of cytotrophoblast outgrowth from villous tips in vitro, and its expression pattern in early pregnancy confirms a physiological role, with low expression during early invasion, and up-regulated expression between 9 and 12 weeks, coincident with a reduction in invasive potential.[33] In pregnancies complicated by preeclampsia, TGFβ3 production by trophoblast cells is elevated, corresponding to reduced invasion. Moreover, inhibition of TGFβ3 using antisense technology or neutralizing antibodies restores invasive potential.[33] Aberrant expression

of TGFβ3 in decidua of pregnancies complicated by preeclampsia could be related to hypoxia, as hypoxia-inducible factor 1α (HIF-1α) is a potent stimulator of TGFβ3 expression.[34] Therefore, inadequate perfusion of the implantation site, and resultant hypoxia, could disrupt normal regulation of trophoblast invasion by oxygen, exacerbating the reduced invasion phenotype. Vascular endothelial growth factor (VEGF) is also potently stimulated by HIF-1α, and has been implicated in the pathogenesis of preeclampsia via effects on regulating trophoblast differentiation and survival. VEGF isoforms (especially VEGF-A) are up-regulated in EVTs, as they invade the decidua and vasculature, and in-vitro studies demonstrate a functional role in promoting their invasion and preventing apoptosis.[35] Cytotrophoblasts isolated from placentas of pregnancies complicated by preeclampsia exhibit a marked reduction in VEGF production, and while there is some controversy about the expression levels of the receptor Flt (Fms-like tyrosine kinase), the soluble receptor sFlt, which acts as a negative regulator of VEGF activity, is significantly increased in preeclampsia.[35]

Remodeling of the uterine spiral arteries during pregnancy

Following the initial colonization of the decidua by trophoblast derived from anchoring placental villi, these cells target and remodel uterine spiral arteries. This process, termed physiological change, leads to an increase in arterial diameter and enhanced uteroplacental perfusion.[36] It has been shown that early alterations in spiral artery structure occur as a maternal response to pregnancy.[37] However, in the absence of trophoblast, remodeling of the spiral arteries is significantly reduced, implicating these cells as an essential component in the process.[38,39] Early in normal pregnancy, interstitial EVTs detach from anchoring placental villi and invade the decidual stroma, preferentially homing towards the uterine spiral arteries (Figure 50.2). In addition, endovascular EVTs probably enter the distal openings of the spiral arteries and migrate through the lumen in a retrograde manner. These cells also form plugs within the spiral arteries, preventing maternal blood flow into the implantation site until between 9 and 12 weeks of gestation. The combined actions of interstitial and endovascular EVTs result in profound changes to the structure of the arterial wall as far as the first third of the myometrium.[38,40,41] Endothelial cells and smooth muscle cells are lost from the spiral arteries and are replaced by trophoblasts embedded in an amorphous

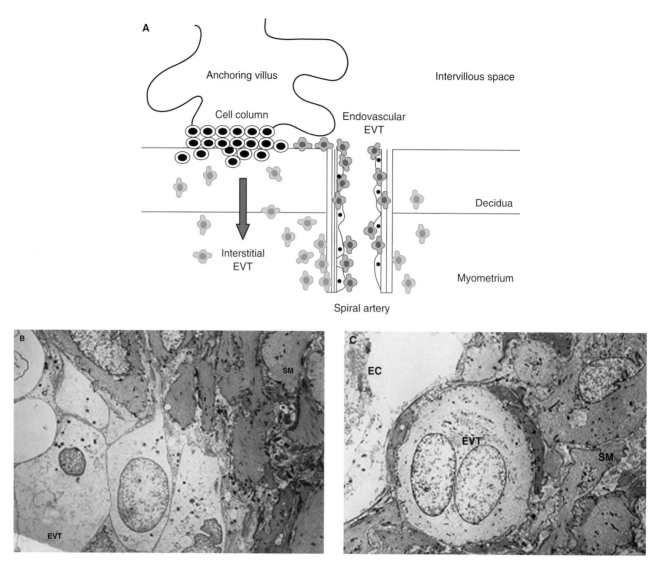

Figure 50.2 (A) Invasion of extravillous trophoblasts (EVT) from the cell column of an anchoring villus, differentiating into interstitial EVT and endovascular EVT. The endovascular EVT are shown invading through the endothelium of the decidual artery. (B,C) Electron micrographs of endovascular EVT adjacent to smooth muscle following in-vitro culture of EVT in the lumen of a spiral artery.

fibrinoid matrix.[36,38] Invading cytotrophoblasts directly target the endothelium and underlying smooth muscle, inducing these cells to undergo apoptosis. This process is partly mediated by cell–cell contact and partly via the release of soluble proapoptotic factors from the cytotrophoblasts.[42,43] Cytotrophoblasts also produce a variety of proteases that facilitate the breakdown of extracellular matrix components in the vessel wall and aid invasion through the internal elastic lamina. These include matrix metalloproteinases,[44] caspases,[45,46] cathepsins,[47,48] and urokinase plasminogen activator.[49,50] Degradation of the extracellular matrix, in particular elastin fibers, is necessary to attain the required increase in vessel diameter and to create high-flow, low-resistance conduits needed to meet the increasing demands of

the fetus for nutrients and oxygen. Transformation of the spiral arteries leads to loss of maternal vasomotor control, thus guaranteeing a constant supply of blood to the placenta despite maternal attempts to alter blood distribution.[51] Interestingly, uterine veins are rarely targeted or transformed by invading cytotrophoblasts, suggesting that vascular remodeling is only required in the uteroplacental arterial system, to enhance the delivery of nutrients to the fetoplacental unit.

Incomplete remodeling of the spiral arteries is commonly observed in pregnancies complicated by pre-eclampsia and/or IUGR. Indeed, shallow trophoblast invasion, a decreased population of invasive trophoblast, and narrow bore arteries retaining muscular walls have all been reported in the placental bed of women with preeclampsia and/or IUGR.[52-55] Areas of acute atherosis and medial smooth muscle cell hyperplasia are also observed with a higher frequency in spiral arteries from women with hypertensive disorders of pregnancy.[53,56] Furthermore, placental bed biopsies from women with preeclampsia contain a greater percentage of apoptotic trophoblasts than biopsies from healthy pregnant women,[57] although intravascular EVTs show reduced apoptosis in uterine vessels taken from pregnancies complicated by preeclampsia.[54]

Maternal macrophages may also play an important role in regulating the invasion process. In normal pregnancy, maternal macrophages are observed in the stroma in association with transformed spiral arteries. However, in preeclampsia, larger numbers of activated macrophages appear between invading cytotrophoblasts and the spiral arteries, and may play a role in preventing trophoblast from accessing vessel media, leading to poorly transformed vessels that contain little or no trophoblast.[58,59]

At present, the molecular mechanisms controlling trophoblast invasion and vascular remodeling are poorly understood. In normal pregnancy, endovascular cytotrophoblasts detaching from anchoring placental villi alter their adhesion molecule repertoire to promote invasion. This transformation is characterized by down-regulation of E-cadherin and integrin $\alpha_6\beta_4$, and up-regulation of VE-cadherin, $\alpha_1\beta_1$, and $\alpha_V\beta_3$.[60] In pregnancies complicated by preeclampsia, invasive cytotrophoblasts fail to express some of the molecules thought to mimic a vascular adhesion phenotype. These cells continue to express markers associated with cytotrophoblast progenitor cells and fail to up-regulate receptors associated with invasion, such as VE-cadherin, $\alpha_1\beta_1$, $\alpha_V\beta_3$, vascular cell adhesion molecule 1 (VCAM-1), and platelet–endothelial cell adhesion molecule 1 (PECAM-1).[61] The failure of cytotrophoblasts to attain a pseudovascular phenotype may, in part, explain why preeclampsia is characterized by shallow or inadequate invasion. It has also been shown that placental explants from pregnancies complicated by preeclampsia fail to exhibit spontaneous invasion in vitro,[33] and cytotrophoblasts isolated from preeclamptic placentas secrete a lower level of invasive proteases than cytotrophoblasts isolated from healthy placentas.[62] The molecular mechanisms underlying these phenomena are currently unknown. Oxidative stress in the implantation site may affect cytotrophoblast invasion through the modulation of adhesion molecules and their ligands. Interestingly, placental integrin α_5 is elevated in hypoxic conditions,[63] and the marker of oxidative stress 8-isoprostane is also increased in the decidua of pregnancies complicated by preeclampsia.[64]

The reduction of cytotrophoblast invasion, and subsequent failure of the spiral arteries to be remodeled in preeclampsia/IUGR is thought to lead to alterations in maternal uterine arterial blood flow. In normal pregnancy, Doppler ultrasound of the uterine artery demonstrates high flow in diastole, with a reduction in pulsatility, indicating a high-flow, low-resistance vascular bed. However, where spiral arteries have not been remodeled, the uterine artery Doppler shows low flow in diastole, a high pulsatility, and the notch seen in large arteries in early diastole remains, indicating a high-resistance uteroplacental circulation. When these changes are present between 24 and 30 weeks' gestation, the risk of developing preeclampsia or IUGR is increased seven-fold and three-fold, respectively.[65] Furthermore, there is an increase in apoptosis of villous trophoblast in pregnancies with abnormal uterine artery Doppler waveforms at 10–14 weeks' gestation, compared to those with normal waveforms.[66] This suggests that the failure of conversion of spiral arteries may lead to direct damage to the villous trophoblast. Although the nature of this damage is not clear at present, the changes in blood flow have been hypothesized to lead to a reduction in the delivery of oxygen and nutrients, or create local areas of ischemia–reperfusion within the placenta.

Uteroplacental arterial dysfunction in preeclampsia and IUGR

In addition to the morphological changes described in uterine arteries, important differences in vascular function have been demonstrated. As well as widespread endothelial dysfunction, markers of which are raised in both preeclampsia and IUGR, there is evidence that uteroplacental arterial function is altered in preeclampsia and IUGR. Wire myography studies performed on myometrial arteries from pregnancies complicated by IUGR show increased vasoconstriction and reduced endothelial-dependent relaxation compared with vessels obtained from normal pregnancies (Figure 50.3A).[67] In contrast, similar vessels taken from pregnancies complicated by preeclampsia show no increase in vasoconstriction, but demonstrate a greater decrease in endothelial-dependent relaxation than those taken from women with IUGR (Figure 50.3B).[68] In addition, there is evidence that maternal vessels taken from women with preeclampsia have exaggerated vasomotion – oscillations in vascular smooth muscle tone – compared with those from normal pregnancies.[69]

The increased vasoconstriction observed in vessels from preeclampsia/IUGR pregnancies can be attenuated

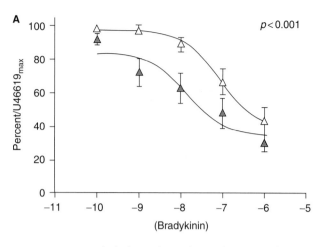
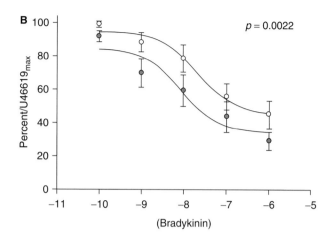

Figure 50.3 Endothelium-dependent relaxation of U46619-constricted myometrial small arteries. Data are expressed as percent maximal response to U46619. All data are mean ± SEM. The x-axis concentration of [Bradykinin] × 10^{-x}. (A) Normal pregnant (▲, $N = 14$), IUGR (△, $n = 16$ vessels from $N = 12$). This graph demonstrates the impaired endothelium-dependent relaxation of vessels taken from pregnancies complicated by IUGR compared with normal pregnancy. (B) Normal pregnant (○, $N = 13$), Preeclampsia (●, $N = 19$). This graph demonstrates impaired endothelial-dependent relaxation of vessels taken from pregnancies complicated by preeclampsia, which is greater than that of those complicated by IUGR.

by a phosphodiesterase-5 (PDE5) inhibitor, which potentiates the actions of intracellular guanosine monophosphate (GMP) by reducing GMP breakdown.[67,68] Interestingly, PDE5 inhibition does not modify bradykinin-induced endothelial-dependent relaxation in myometrial small arteries taken from normal pregnancies, but does improve in relaxation of small arteries from growth-restricted pregnancies, suggesting that there may be distinct changes to vascular physiology in IUGR.[67] Therefore, changes in the uteroplacental vascular structure and function may have important consequences for the delivery of oxygen and nutrients to the placenta.

Villous trophoblast

Following implantation and vascular remodeling, fetal growth and maintenance of a successful pregnancy is dependent on normal structure and function of the placental villus. Both macroscopic and microscopic changes have been described in placentas from pregnancies complicated by preeclampsia and IUGR. The principal macroscopic features of the placenta in preeclampsia and IUGR are areas of infarction resulting from occlusion of decidual arteries. These infarcts represent necrotic placental tissue, and may involve the full thickness of the placenta.[51] In addition, there are a number of microscopic changes described in villous trophoblast in pregnancies complicated by preeclampsia and IUGR. The majority of these changes reflect 'aging' and cell death of both cytotrophoblast and syncytiotrophoblast, and changes in the proliferation and differentiation of cytotrophoblast.

Syncytiotrophoblast is maintained by proliferation and fusion of underlying cytotrophoblast cells, which become progressively less densely packed as pregnancy progresses (Figure 50.4A). Following fusion, the nuclei degenerate, condense, and are sequestered into syncytial knots, which are then shed into the maternal circulation.[70]

In preeclampsia, the number of villi is not decreased, although there is a reduction in the volume of syncytiotrophoblast compared to villous area.[71] This is accompanied by an increase in the number of pyknotic syncytial nuclei, and an increase in the number of syncytial knots (Figure 50.4B).[72] This is associated with an increase in syncytiotrophoblast particles and fetal DNA within the maternal circulation.[73] In contrast, there is an increase in the number of cytotrophoblasts in pregnancies complicated by preeclampsia. It is hypothesized that this is due to increased proliferation of the cytotrophoblasts to repair the damaged syncytiotrophoblast.

In IUGR, the tertiary chorionic villi show decreased branching and a reduction in surface area, although there is no reduction in the volume of syncytiotrophoblast compared to villous area.[71] There are also reduced numbers of proliferating cytotrophoblast (Figure 50.4C),[74] and a reduction in the activity of nutrient transport across the syncytiotrophoblast membrane in vivo and in vitro. This affects the kinetics of amino acid and glucose delivery to the fetus.[75]

Preeclampsia and IUGR are both associated with an increase in the rate of apoptosis within villous trophoblast. In placentas taken from normal pregnancies, approximately 0.15% of all nuclei showed appearances of apoptosis;[76] this was increased to 0.25% and 0.5% in villous trophoblasts of pregnancies complicated by

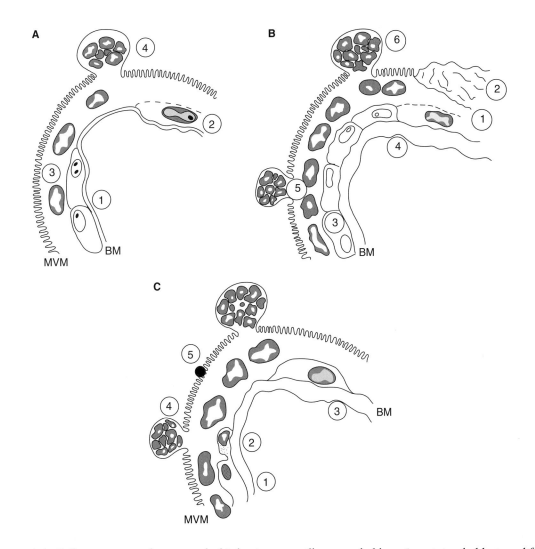

Figure 50.4 (A) Cell turnover within normal third trimester villous trophoblast: 1, cytotrophoblast proliferation; 2, cytotrophoblast fusion with overlying syncytiotrophoblast; 3, syncytiotrophoblast nuclei aging, showing signs of peripheral chromatin condensation of nuclei; 4, degenerate syncytiotrophoblast nuclei are gathered together in syncytial knots, prior to being lost into the maternal circulation. (B) Changes observed in villous trophoblast in preeclampsia: 1, loss of syncytiotrophoblast; 2, fibrin deposition; 3, cytotrophoblast proliferation; 4, thickened basement membrane; 5, increased number of apoptotic syncytiotrophoblast nuclei; 6, increased number of syncytial knots. (C) Changes observed in villous trophoblast in IUGR: 1, decreased cytotrophoblast proliferation; 2, cytotrophoblast apoptosis; 3, thickened basement membrane; 4, increased number of syncytial knots; 5, altered transport across syncytiotrophoblast membrane. BM, basement membrane; MVM, microvillous membrane.

IUGR and preeclampsia, respectively.[77,78] Apoptosis is also increased in villous trophoblasts adjacent to syncytiotrophoblast damage and fibrin deposition.[79] In tissue taken from normal pregnancy, the majority of nuclei exhibiting features of apoptosis are situated in the syncytiotrophoblast. Preeclampsia and IUGR show increased features of apoptosis in syncytiotrophoblast, but there is an increase in the formation of syncytial knots, in which apoptotic syncytial nuclei are gathered.[72] The evidence for apoptosis of cytotrophoblasts is more complicated; in preeclampsia there is an increase in the number of cytotrophoblasts, suggesting that there is increased proliferation, rather than cell

death.[72] An increase in cytotrophoblast apoptosis may be responsible for the decrease in proliferation described in villous trophoblast in IUGR.[80]

Apoptotic changes within syncytial nuclei in preeclampsia are associated with an imbalance of proteins controlling cell death. These changes are mostly found within the syncytiotrophoblast, including an increase in the expression of proapoptotic proteins p53, p21, Bak, and Bax, and a decrease in expression of antiapoptotic protein Mdm2.[81,82] Several other antiapoptotic proteins have been described within the syncytiotrophoblast, including Bcl-2, which antagonizes the effects of Bak and Bax, and the inhibitors of apoptosis (IAPs), which inhibit the action of caspases.[83–85] It is hypothesized that under normal circumstances the syncytiotrophoblast is protected from apoptotic cell death, although in preeclampsia the balance of pro- and antiapoptotic proteins is altered, leading to syncytiotrophoblast apoptosis.

In IUGR, the expression of p53 is up-regulated within cytotrophoblast nuclei, although there is no corresponding increase in Bax, Bak, or Bcl-2 expression.[86] The increased expression of p53 is associated with an increase in fibrin deposition. A further study demonstrated increased expression of activated caspase-3, an essential enzyme in the apoptotic pathway in cytotrophoblasts taken from pregnancies complicated by IUGR; this may occur in response to activation of p53.[80]

The cause of these changes in protein expression remains unclear, although the elevation of p53 suggests that, in preeclampsia and IUGR, villous trophoblast is exposed to noxious stimuli. In vitro, p53 is elevated in response to a variety of agents, especially those which damage DNA, such as radiation, hypoxia, hypoxia–reoxygenation, and reactive oxygen species;[87] p53 is stabilized and activated by a number of intracellular signaling proteins, including oxygen-sensing proteins such as HIF-1α and -2α. Both HIF1α and HIF2α have been localized to the syncytiotrophoblast in term placental tissue.[88,89] The expression of HIF1α is increased in villous trophoblast taken from pregnancies complicated by preeclampsia, and is degraded at a slower rate in preeclamptic tissue compared to that taken from normal pregnancy.[88]

These findings indicate that trophoblast expresses mediators of the apoptotic pathway necessary to detect hypoxia or reactive oxygen species and initiate a coordinated apoptotic response. Syncytiotrophoblast of normal placental villous explants does not incorporate radiolabeled uracil, suggesting that the syncytiotrophoblast does not synthesize RNA but instead relies on the constant fusion of cytotrophoblasts to maintain sufficient mRNA for transcription of essential protein.[90] Further research is required to determine how the signaling pathways such as the transcription-dependent effects of p53 are activated in syncytiotrophoblast.

It is likely that the increased rate of apoptosis observed in villous trophoblast in pregnancies complicated by preeclampsia not only impairs trophoblast function but also produces a maternal systemic response. In preeclampsia, an increase in deported syncytiotrophoblast fragments is detected within the maternal uterine vein.[91] Such fragments have an apoptotic appearance. Increased fetal DNA has also been reported in maternal plasma prior to the onset of preeclampsia.[73] It is hypothesized that an elevated rate of apoptotic degeneration of syncytiotrophoblast in preeclampsia leads to the release of substances that promote endothelial activation. Several factors have been suggested and the strongest candidates, syncytiotrophoblast debris and sFlt-1 (soluble fms-like tyrosine kinase 1), are described below.[92]

ENDOTHELIAL DYSFUNCTION IN PREECLAMPSIA AND IUGR

The vascular endothelium is a highly specialized, metabolically active interface between the blood and underlying tissues. Its functions are diverse: mediating vascular tone, maintaining thromboresistance, and participating in the inflammatory response. Under normal circumstances, the endothelium prevents inappropriate coagulation by the production of antithrombotic compounds such as thrombomodulin. In addition, endothelium-derived prostaglandin and nitric oxide have also been shown to inhibit platelet aggregation and adhesion. The endothelium is also able to respond to damage by producing substances that promote coagulation, e.g. tissue factor. Dysfunction of vascular endothelial cells can explain the wide range of maternal symptoms and signs – e.g. hypertension, proteinuria, edema, and coagulopathy – that characterize the preeclampsia syndrome.[93] The pathophysiological changes associated with preeclampsia are indicative of a profoundly vasoconstricted maternal circulation with a reduced plasma volume leading to decreased systemic organ perfusion.

There is plentiful evidence for endothelial dysfunction in preeclampsia: plasma concentrations of von Willebrand factor, thrombomodulin, cellular fibronectin, tissue plasminogen activator (t-PA), and plasminogen activator inhibitor 1 are all raised,[94] leading to the widespread deposition of fibrin. Furthermore, levels of endothelin 1 are increased in the maternal circulation, reflecting an increase in its synthesis by activated endothelial cells. In addition, there is also an increase in factors known to modify endothelial cell behavior, including cell adhesion molecules such as VCAM-1 and growth factors, e.g. VEGF.

The most consistent pathophysiological abnormality in preeclampsia is increased sensitivity to vasopressor agents such as angiotensin II. A widespread altered endothelial response has been demonstrated; thus, while subcutaneous arteries of non-pregnant and pregnant subjects respond comparably to endothelium-dependent

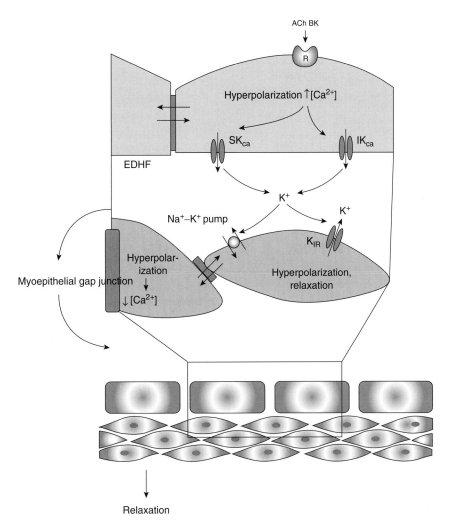

Figure 50.5 The role of K$^+$ ions and EDHF. Endothelial cell stimulation by receptor-dependent (e.g. acetylcholine [ACh]; bradykinin [BK]) initiates endothelial cell hyperpolarization by activating small- and intermediate-conductance K_{Ca} channels (SK_{Ca} and IK_{Ca} channels). Endothelial cell hyperpolarization leads to the accumulation of K$^+$ ions in the subendothelial space in concentrations sufficient to activate inwardly rectifying K$^+$ (K_{IR}) channels and/or the Na$^+$–K$^+$ pump. The hyperpolarization of the endothelial cells, following K_{Ca} channel activation, can be transmitted along the monolayer of endothelial cells or towards the smooth muscle cells through gap junctions. It is hypothesized that there is a reduction in EDHF activity in preeclampsia, leading to a reduction of endothelial-dependent relaxation.

(acetylcholine) and endothelium-independent (sodium nitroprusside) vasodilators, vessels taken from women with preeclampsia had an impaired response to acetylcholine. A similar impairment of relaxation to bradykinin was also seen in systemic vessels from women with preeclampsia. Both acetylcholine and bradykinin are endothelium-dependent vasodilators; i.e. when the endothelium is completely removed, relaxation does not occur.

Endothelial release of nitric oxide (NO) was thought to be the mediator for endothelium-dependent relaxation. However, resistance arteries from different vascular beds remain susceptible to endothelium-dependent vasodilators when COX and NO synthase enzymes are inhibited. This suggests the presence of another

mediator, termed endothelium-derived hyperpolarizing factor (EDHF).[94] EDHF-mediated relaxation is initiated by an increase in intracellular Ca^{2+} in endothelial cells (Figure 50.5). This leads to activation of both small conductance (SK_{Ca}) and intermediate conductance (IK_{Ca}) potassium (K$^+$) channels in endothelial cells. Although EDHF does not have any direct effect on K$^+$ channels on smooth muscle cells, opening of SK_{Ca} and IK_{Ca} channels results in an accumulation of K$^+$ in the myoendothelial space and endothelial cell hyperpolarization. This could then spread to adjacent smooth muscle cells through myoendothelial gap junctions or via activation of inwardly rectifying K$^+$(K_{IR}) channels and/or Na$^+$–K$^+$-ATPase. Therefore, smooth muscle cell hyperpolarization brings about relaxation and vasodilation.[95] It has been hypothesized that EDHF mediates endothelium-dependent responses in pregnancy, via the pathway described above, and that the release of EDHF is diminished in preeclampsia, leading to a net increase in vascular tone.[96]

ENDOTHELIAL RESPONSE TO CIRCULATING FACTORS IN PREECLAMPSIA

Normal pregnancy is associated with a mild systemic inflammatory response, which is thought to be exaggerated in preeclampsia. Proinflammatory factor(s) are hypothesized to originate from the placenta, as delivery of the placenta leads to a resolution of symptoms.[92] The evidence for circulating factor(s) is strong, as plasma taken from women with preeclampsia impairs endothelial-dependent relaxation of vessels taken from women with normal pregnancies.

Thus, putative proinflammatory factors and vasoconstrictors may be released into the maternal circulation in small amounts from a normal placenta, and in increased amounts in preeclampsia. Debris from the syncytiotrophoblast layer is constantly lost into the maternal circulation, as trophoblast fragments are detectable in the uterine vein blood in both normal and preeclamptic pregnancies. Peripheral blood taken from the same women contains few trophoblast fragments, as relatively large fragments become trapped in pulmonary capillaries.[91] It is unlikely that large fragments are responsible for a systemic reaction. Instead, subcellular particles of syncytiotrophoblast, which can be detected throughout the maternal circulation, may be the stimulus. Subcellular particles of syncytiotrophoblast have been found in plasma from normal pregnancies, with increased levels noted in preeclampsia. Levels of cytokeratin, a cytoskeletal protein of trophoblast, and fetal cell-free DNA are also significantly higher in plasma from pregnancies complicated by preeclampsia than in normal pregnancies.[73,97]

Syncytiotrophoblast microparticles appear to activate an inflammatory response, causing endothelial cell damage. Specifically, they can inhibit endothelial cell function and even cause endothelial cell death in vitro.[98,99] Monocytes, an important component in the cellular immune response, interact with syncytiotrophoblast microparticles both in vivo and in vitro. In vitro, monocytes bound to syncytiotrophoblast microparticles are stimulated to produce the proinflammatory cytokines tumor necrosis factor-α (TNFα) and IL-12. In normal pregnancy, it has been shown that monocyte production of IL-12 is enhanced, possibly as a result of stimulation by syncytiotrophoblast microparticles.[100] Cell-mediated immunity is also suppressed in normal pregnancy, possibly because of inhibition of lymphocyte proliferation by syncytiotrophoblast microparticles. In preeclampsia, it is hypothesized that excess stimulation of monocytes and production of proinflammatory cytokines activate T lymphocytes.[100] Variations in the sensitivity of the maternal immune system in preeclampsia may also contribute to the magnitude of the systemic response.

Another potential factor produced by and released from trophoblast is sFlt-1, a variant of the VEGF receptor Flt-1, which lacks the transmembrane and cytoplasmic domains and therefore binds and sequesters VEGF and placenta-derived growth factor (PlGF). The factor sFlt-1 is released into the maternal circulation throughout normal pregnancy, and is increased in both maternal plasma and at the mRNA and protein level in placental tissue in preeclampsia, although not in IUGR.[101] This increase in sFlt-1 reduces the free VEGF and PlGF in the maternal circulation, causing a loss of microvascular relaxation and endothelial dysfunction, which can be reversed in vitro by adding excess exogenous VEGF and PlGF. Interestingly, unlike syncytiotrophoblast debris, sFlt-1 has been shown to induce the maternal syndrome in vivo.[102] Adenoviral gene transfer of sFlt-1 into rats results in a preeclampsia-like illness (in the absence of pregnancy), including hypertension, proteinuria, and glomerular endotheliosis.[103]

Excess sFlt-1 production may occur as a result of placental hypoxia, caused by impaired oxygen delivery following inadequate transformation of the uterine spiral arteries. However, both sFlt-1 and VEGF are hypoxia-inducible genes and the net effect of these anti- and proangiogenic factors differs between trophoblast and endothelial cells. A reduction from 20% O_2 to 8% O_2 and further to 2% O_2 in primary cytotrophoblast cell culture increases trophoblast proliferation and the expression of sFlt-1 mRNA.[104] As a consequence, production of total VEGF is increased, although free active VEGF is undetectable. These changes are unique to cytotrophoblasts and are not seen in umbilical vein endothelial cells or villous fibroblasts. In addition, levels of sFlt in vivo are greater in the umbilical vein than in the umbilical artery. These two findings strongly suggest that the placenta is the source of increased sFlt-1 production during preeclampsia.[104] Furthermore, altered placental production of sFlt-1 in preeclampsia may lead to further placental dysfunction, creating a positive feedback loop of sFlt-1 production that eventually causes the clinical syndrome.

Despite the in-vitro effects of both syncytiotrophoblast debris and sFlt-1, preeclampsia is unlikely to be caused by a single circulating factor. This is supported by the demonstration that fractionation of plasma taken from patients with preeclampsia reduces the inhibitory effect on endothelial-dependent relaxation of myometrial arteries, while this inhibitory effect is recovered when the plasma fractions are recombined.[105] This suggests that the vasoactive effects of preeclamptic plasma result from the synergistic action of two or more factors. At the present time, new high-throughput multiparametric technologies such as high-definition mass spectroscopy and infrared spectroscopy are being employed to detect molecular differences between plasma from normal and preeclamptic pregnancies.

SUMMARY

Preeclampsia and IUGR remain important multisystem medical disorders of pregnancy which have the potential to leave infants and mothers with lifelong sequelae, including neurological disability and increased risk of cardiovascular disease. These disorders have a complex etiology, with the current pathophysiological models described in this chapter highlighting abnormalities of implantation, invasion of the cytotrophoblast cells, transformation of decidual and myometrial spiral arteries, placental damage, and endothelial dysfunction. The multifactorial nature of the development of preeclampsia and IUGR may account for the wide variation in clinical presentation of these conditions, including the gestation and speed of onset and the severity of symptoms.

Recent evidence highlighting potential pathophysiological events may allow targeted therapy in the future. However, further investigation is required to develop a better understanding of the links between defective implantation, failure of the spiral arteries to be transformed, placental dysfunction, and endothelial activation, with particular attention paid to the mechanism by which placental damage produces circulating factors with such potent vasoactive properties. Underlying these pathologies may be a generalized disorder of trophoblast function, affecting both villous and extravillous lineages. Therefore, an understanding of the nature of the noxious insult to villous trophoblast may allow therapeutic interventions to reduce the onset or magnitude of damage.

Ultimately, the goals of research within this field are to identify trophoblast dysfunction, enabling accurate detection of patients at risk of preeclampsia or IUGR, and to develop effective interventions to prevent the abnormal events early in pregnancy, leading to better maternal and fetal health in late pregnancy. Current pathophysiological models provide a framework on which to test current theories, and to improve understanding of these disorders, which present with problems in late pregnancy, despite having their origins in early gestation.

REFERENCES

1. Gardosi J, Kady SM et al. Classification of stillbirth by relevant condition at death (ReCoDe): population based cohort study. BMJ 2005; 331(7525): 1113–17.
2. Confidential Enquiry into Maternal and Child Health. Why Mothers Die 2000–2002. London, RCOG Press, 2004.
3. Godfrey KM, Barker DJ. Fetal nutrition and adult disease. Am J Clin Nutr 2000; 71(Suppl 5): 1344S–52S.
4. Davey DA, MacGillivray I. The classification and definition of the hypertensive disorders of pregnancy. Am J Obstet Gynecol 1988; 158(4): 892–8.
5. Sanderson DA, Wilcox MA et al. The individualised birthweight ratio: a new method of identifying intrauterine growth retardation. Br J Obstet Gynaecol 1994; 101(4): 310–14.
6. Myers JE, Brockelsby J. The epidemiology of pre-eclampsia. In: Barker PN, Kingdom JCP, eds. Pre-eclampsia: Current Perspectives on Management. London: Parthenon, 2004.
7. Bernstein PS, Divon MY. Etiologies of fetal growth restriction. Clin Obstet Gynaecol 1997; 40(4): 723–9.
8. Duckitt K, Harrington D. Risk factors for pre-eclampsia at antenatal booking: systematic review of controlled studies. BMJ 2005; 330(7491): 565.
9. Brar HS, Rutherford SE. Classification of intrauterine growth retardation. Semin Perinatol 1988; 12(1): 2–10.
10. Redline RW, Patterson P. Pre-eclampsia is associated with an excess of proliferative immature intermediate trophoblast. Hum Pathol 1995; 26(6): 594–600.
11. Kwong WY, Wild AE et al. Maternal undernutrition during the preimplantation period of rat development causes blastocyst abnormalities and programming of postnatal hypertension. Development 2000; 127(19): 4195–202.
12. Rinaudo P, Schultz RM. Effects of embryo culture on global pattern of gene expression in preimplantation mouse embryos. Reproduction 2004; 128(3): 301–11.
13. Schieve LA, Meikle SF et al. Low and very low birth weight in infants conceived with use of assisted reproductive technology. N Engl J Med 2002; 346(10): 731–7.
14. Doherty AS, Mann MR et al. Differential effects of culture on imprinted H19 expression in the preimplantation mouse embryo. Biol Reprod 2000; 62(6): 1526–35.
15. Cross JC, Werb Z et al. Implantation and the placenta: key pieces of the development puzzle. Science 1994; 266(5190): 1508–18.
16. Lim H, Paria BC et al. Multiple female reproductive failures in cyclooxygenase 2-deficient mice. Cell 1997; 91(2): 197–208.
17. Robb L, Li R et al. Infertility in female mice lacking the receptor for interleukin 11 is due to a defective uterine response to implantation. Nat Med 1998; 4(3): 303–8.
18. Brosens JJ, Pijnenborg R et al. The myometrial junctional zone spiral arteries in normal and abnormal pregnancies: a review of the literature. Am J Obstet Gynecol 2002; 187(5): 1416–23.
19. Golander A, Kopel R et al. Decreased prolactin secretion by decidual tissue of pre-eclampsia in vitro. Acta Endocrinol (Copenh) 1985; 108(1): 111–13.
20. Crossey PA, Pillai CC et al. Altered placental development and intrauterine growth restriction in IGF binding protein-1 transgenic mice. J Clin Invest 2002; 110(3): 411–18.

21. Giudice LC, Martina NA et al. Insulin-like growth factor binding protein-1 at the maternal–fetal interface and insulin-like growth factor-I, insulin-like growth factor-II, and insulin-like growth factor binding protein-1 in the circulation of women with severe preeclampsia. Am J Obstet Gynecol 1997; 176(4): 751–7; discussion 757–8.

22. Ribatti D, Loverro G et al. Expression of tenascin is related to angiogenesis in pre-eclampsia. Eur J Clin Invest 1998; 28(5): 373–8.

23. Wetzka B, Nusing R et al. Cyclooxygenase-1 and -2 in human placenta and placental bed after normal and pre-eclamptic pregnancies. Hum Reprod 1997; 12(10): 2313–20.

24. King A, Hiby SE et al. Recognition of trophoblast HLA class I molecules by decidual NK cell receptors – a review. Placenta 2000; 21 (Suppl A): S81–5.

25. Eide IP, Rolfseng T et al. Serious foetal growth restriction is associated with reduced proportions of natural killer cells in decidua basalis. Virchows Arch 2006; 448: 269–76.

26. Colbern GT, Chiang MH et al. Expression of the nonclassic histocompatibility antigen HLA-G by preeclamptic placenta. Am J Obstet Gynecol 1994; 170(5 Pt 1): 1244–50.

27. Le Bouteiller P, Pizzato N et al. HLA-G, pre-eclampsia, immunity and vascular events. J Reprod Immunol 2003; 59(2): 219–34.

28. Wilczynski JR, Tchorzewski H et al. Lymphocyte subset distribution and cytokine secretion in third trimester decidua in normal pregnancy and preeclampsia. Eur J Obstet Gynecol Reprod Biol 2003; 109(1): 8–15.

29. Wegmann TG, Lin H et al. Bidirectional cytokine interactions in the maternal–fetal relationship: is successful pregnancy a TH2 phenomenon? Immunol Today 1993; 14(7): 353–6.

30. Burk MR, Troeger C et al. Severely reduced presence of tissue macrophages in the basal plate of pre-eclamptic placentae. Placenta 2001; 22(4): 309–16.

31. Abrahams VM, Kim YM et al. Macrophages and apoptotic cell clearance during pregnancy. Am J Reprod Immunol 2004; 51(4): 275–82.

32. Jeschke U, Mylonas I et al. Expression of glycodelin protein and mRNA in human ductal breast cancer carcinoma in situ, invasive ductal carcinomas, their lymph node and distant metastases, and ductal carcinomas with recurrence. Oncol Rep 2005; 13(3): 413–19.

33. Caniggia I, Grisaru-Gravnosky S et al. Inhibition of TGF-beta 3 restores the invasive capability of extravillous trophoblasts in preeclamptic pregnancies. J Clin Invest 1999; 103(12): 1641–50.

34. Caniggia I, Mostachfi H et al. Hypoxia-inducible factor-1 mediates the biological effects of oxygen on human trophoblast differentiation through TGFbeta(3). J Clin Invest 2000; 105(5): 577–87.

35. Zhou Y, McMaster M et al. Vascular endothelial growth factor ligands and receptors that regulate human cytotrophoblast survival are dysregulated in severe preeclampsia and hemolysis, elevated liver enzymes, and low platelets syndrome. Am J Pathol 2002; 160(4): 1405–23.

36. Brosens I, Robertson WB et al. The physiological response of the vessels of the placental bed to normal pregnancy. J Pathol Bacteriol 1967; 93(2): 569–79.

37. Craven CM, Morgan T et al. Decidual spiral artery remodelling begins before cellular interaction with cytotrophoblasts. Placenta 1998; 19(4): 241–52.

38. Pijnenborg R, Bland JM et al. Uteroplacental arterial changes related to interstitial trophoblast migration in early human pregnancy. Placenta 1983; 4(4): 397–413.

39. Kam EP, Gardner L et al. The role of trophoblast in the physiological change in decidual spiral arteries. Hum Reprod 1999; 14(8): 2131–8.

40. Pijnenborg R, Dixon G et al. Trophoblastic invasion of human decidua from 8 to 18 weeks of pregnancy. Placenta 1980; 1(1): 3–19.

41. Kaufmann P, Black S et al. Endovascular trophoblast invasion: implications for the pathogenesis of intrauterine growth retardation and preeclampsia. Biol Reprod 2003; 69(1): 1–7.

42. Ashton SV, Whitley GS et al. Uterine spiral artery remodeling involves endothelial apoptosis induced by extravillous trophoblasts through Fas/FasL interactions. Arterioscler Thromb Vasc Biol 2005; 25(1): 102–8.

43. Harris LK, Keogh R, Wareing M et al. Invasive trophoblasts stimulate vascular smooth muscle cell apoptosis by a fas ligand-dependent mechanism. Am J Pathol 2006; 169: 1863–74.

44. Xu P, Wang Y et al. Effects of matrix proteins on the expression of matrix metalloproteinase-2, -9, and -14 and tissue inhibitors of metalloproteinases in human cytotrophoblast cells during the first trimester. Biol Reprod 2001; 65(1): 240–6.

45. De Falco M, Fedele V et al. Immunohistochemical distribution of proteins belonging to the receptor-mediated and the mitochondrial apoptotic pathways in human placenta during gestation. Cell Tissue Res 2004; 318(3): 599–608.

46. Kam DW, Charles AK et al. Caspase-14 expression in the human placenta. Reprod Biomed Online 2005; 11(2): 236–43.

47. Divya P, Chhikara P et al. Differential activity of cathepsin L in human placenta at two different stages of gestation. Placenta 2002; 23(1): 59–64.

48. Nakanishi T, Ozaki Y et al. Role of cathepsins and cystatins in patients with recurrent miscarriage. Mol Hum Reprod 2005; 11(5): 351–5.

49. Floridon C, Nielsen O et al. Localization and significance of urokinase plasminogen activator and its receptor in placental tissue from intrauterine, ectopic and molar pregnancies. Placenta 1999; 20(8): 711–21.

50. Bauer S, Pollheimer J et al. Tumor necrosis factor-alpha inhibits trophoblast migration through elevation of plasminogen activator inhibitor-1 in first-trimester villous explant cultures. J Clin Endocrinol Metab 2004; 89(2): 812–22.

51. Benirschke K, Kaufmann P. Pathology of the Human Placenta. New York, Springer, 2000.

52. Khong TY, De Wolf F et al. Inadequate maternal vascular response to placentation in pregnancies complicated by pre-eclampsia and by small-for-gestational age infants. Br J Obstet Gynaecol 1986; 93(10): 1049–59.

53. Pijnenborg R, Anthony J et al. Placental bed spiral arteries in the hypertensive disorders of pregnancy. Br J Obstet Gynaecol 1991; 98(7): 648–55.

54. Kadyrov M, Schmitz C et al. Pre-eclampsia and maternal anaemia display reduced apoptosis and opposite invasive phenotypes of extravillous trophoblast. Placenta 2003; 24(5): 540–8.

55. Naicker T, Khedun SM et al. Quantitative analysis of trophoblast invasion in preeclampsia. Acta Obstet Gynecol Scand 2003; 82(8): 722–9.

56. Meekins JW, Pijnenborg R et al. A study of placental bed spiral arteries and trophoblast invasion in normal and severe pre-eclamptic pregnancies. Br J Obstet Gynaecol 1994; 101(8): 669–74.

57. DiFederico E, Genbacev O et al. Preeclampsia is associated with widespread apoptosis of placental cytotrophoblasts within the uterine wall. Am J Pathol 1999; 155(1): 293–301.

58. Reister F, Frank HG et al. The distribution of macrophages in spiral arteries of the placental bed in pre-eclampsia differs from that in healthy patients. Placenta 1999; 20(2–3): 229–33.

59. Reister F, Frank HG et al. Macrophage-induced apoptosis limits endovascular trophoblast invasion in the uterine wall of preeclamptic women. Lab Invest 2001; 81(8): 1143–52.

60. Zhou Y, Fisher SJ et al. Human cytotrophoblasts adopt a vascular phenotype as they differentiate. A strategy for successful endovascular invasion? J Clin Invest 1997; 99(9): 2139–51.

61. Zhou Y, Damsky CH et al. Preeclampsia is associated with failure of human cytotrophoblasts to mimic a vascular adhesion phenotype. One cause of defective endovascular invasion in this syndrome? J Clin Invest 1997; 99(9): 2152–64.

62. Graham CH, McCrae KR. Altered expression of gelatinase and surface-associated plasminogen activator activity by trophoblast cells isolated from placentas of preeclamptic patients. Am J Obstet Gynecol 1996; 175(3 Pt 1): 555–62.

63. Iwaki T, Yamamoto K et al. Alteration of integrins under hypoxic stress in early placenta and choriocarcinoma cell line BeWo. Gynecol Obstet Invest 2004; 57(4): 196–203.

64. Staff AC, Ranheim T et al. Augmented PLA2 activity in preeclamptic decidual tissue – a key player in the pathophysiology of 'acute atherosis' in pre-eclampsia? Placenta 2003; 24(10): 965–73.

65. El-Hamedi A, Shillito J et al. A prospective analysis of the role of uterine artery Doppler waveform notching in the assessment of at-risk pregnancies. Hypertens Pregnancy 2005; 24(2): 137–45.

66. Prefumo F, Ayling LJ et al. Uterine artery resistance at 10–14 weeks of gestation is correlated with trophoblast apoptosis. Ultrasound Obstet Gynaecol 2004; 24: 234.

67. Wareing M, Myers JE et al. Sildenafil citrate (Viagra) enhances vasodilatation in fetal growth restriction. J Clin Endocrinol Metab 2005; 90(5): 2550–5.

68. Wareing M, Myers JE et al. Effects of a phosphodiesterase-5 (PDE5) inhibitor on endothelium-dependent relaxation of myometrial small arteries. Am J Obstet Gynecol 2004; 190(5): 1283–90.

69. Nilsson H, Aalkjaer C. Vasomotion: mechanisms and physiological importance. Mol Interv 2003; 3(2): 79–89, 51.

70. Mayhew TM, Leach L et al. Proliferation, differentiation and apoptosis in villous trophoblast at 13–41 weeks of gestation (including observations on annulate lamellae and nuclear pore complexes). Placenta 1999; 20(5–6): 407–22.

71. Crocker IP, Daayana SL et al. An image analysis technique for the investigation of human placental morphology in preeclampsia and intrauterine growth restriction. J Soc Gynecol Invest 12004; 1(2(Suppl)): 347A.

72. Soma H, Yoshida K et al. Morphologic changes in the hypertensive placenta. Contrib Gynecol Obstet 1982; 9: 58–75.

73. Zhong XY, Holzgreve W et al. The levels of circulatory cell free fetal DNA in maternal plasma are elevated prior to the onset of preeclampsia. Hypertens Pregnancy 2002; 21(1): 77–83.

74. Macara L, Kingdom JC et al. Structural analysis of placental terminal villi from growth-restricted pregnancies with abnormal umbilical artery Doppler waveforms. Placenta 1996; 17(1): 37–48.

75. Pardi G, Marconi AM et al. Placental–fetal interrelationship in IUGR fetuses – a review. Placenta 2002; 23(Suppl A): S136–41.

76. Smith SC, Baker PN et al. Placental apoptosis in normal human pregnancy. Am J Obstet Gynecol 1997; 177(1): 57–65.

77. Smith SC, Baker PN et al. Increased placental apoptosis in intrauterine growth restriction. Am J Obstet Gynecol 1997; 177(6): 1395–401.

78. Leung DN, Smith SC et al. Increased placental apoptosis in pregnancies complicated by preeclampsia. Am J Obstet Gynecol 2001; 184(6): 1249–50.

79. Nelson DM. Apoptotic changes occur in syncytiotrophoblast of human placental villi where fibrin type fibrinoid is deposited at discontinuities in the villous trophoblast. Placenta 1996; 17(7): 387–91.

80. Endo H, Okamoto A et al. Frequent apoptosis in placental villi from pregnancies complicated with intrauterine growth restriction and without maternal symptoms. Int J Mol Med 2005; 16(1): 79–84.

81. Heazell AE, Brown LM et al. Expression of oncoproteins p53 and Mdm2 within trophoblast of normal and pre-eclamptic pregnancies. J Soc Gynecol Investig 2005; 12(2 Suppl): 362A.

82. Heazell AE, Brown LM et al. Expression of Oncoproteins p53, BAK and p21 in normal pregnancies and those complicated by pre-eclampsia. Placenta 2005; 26: A59.

83. Qiao S, Nagasaka T et al. p53, Bax and Bcl-2 expression, and apoptosis in gestational trophoblast of complete hydatidiform mole. Placenta 1998; 19(5–6): 361–9.

84. Gruslin A, Qiu Q et al. X-linked inhibitor of apoptosis protein expression and the regulation of apoptosis during human placental development. Biol Reprod 2001; 64(4): 1264–72.

85. Ka H, Hunt JS. Temporal and spatial patterns of expression of inhibitors of apoptosis in human placentas. Am J Pathol 2003; 163(2): 413–22.

86. Levy R, Smith SD et al. Trophoblast apoptosis from pregnancies complicated by fetal growth restriction is associated with enhanced p53 expression. Am J Obstet Gynecol 2002; 186(5): 1056–61.

87. Prives C, Hall PA. The p53 pathway. J Pathol 1999; 187(1): 112–26.

88. Rajakumar A, Doty K et al. Impaired oxygen-dependent reduction of HIF-1alpha and -2alpha proteins in pre-eclamptic placentae. Placenta 2003; 24(2–3): 199–208.

89. Rajakumar A, Brandon HM et al. Evidence for the functional activity of hypoxia-inducible transcription factors overexpressed in preeclamptic placentae. Placenta 2004; 25(10): 763–9.

90. Huppertz B, Kingdom J et al. Hypoxia favours necrotic versus apoptotic shedding of placental syncytiotrophoblast into the maternal circulation. Placenta 2003; 24(2–3): 181–90.

91. Johansen M, Redman CW et al. Trophoblast deportation in human pregnancy – its relevance for pre-eclampsia. Placenta 1999; 20(7): 531–9.

92. Redman CW, Sargent IL. Latest advances in understanding preeclampsia. Science 2005; 308(5728): 1592–4.

93. Roberts JM, Taylor RN et al. Preeclampsia: an endothelial cell disorder. Am J Obstet Gynecol 1989; 161(5): 1200–4.

94. Hayman R, Brockelsby J et al. Preeclampsia: the endothelium, circulating factor(s) and vascular endothelial growth factor. J Soc Gynecol Investig 1999; 6(1): 3–10.

95. Busse R, Edwards G et al. EDHF: bringing the concepts together. Trends Pharmacol Sci 2002; 23(8): 374–80.

96. Kenny LC, Baker PN et al. Differential mechanisms of endothelium-dependent vasodilator responses in human myometrial small arteries in normal pregnancy and preeclampsia. Clin Sci (Lond) 2002; 103(1): 67–73.

97. Hefler LA, Tempfer CB et al. Placental expression and serum levels of cytokeratin-18 are increased in women with preeclampsia. J Soc Gynecol Investig 2001; 8(3): 169–73.

98. Cockell AP, Learmont JG et al. Human placental syncytiotrophoblast microvillous membranes impair maternal vascular endothelial function. Br J Obstet Gynaecol 1997; 104(2): 235–40.

99. Gupta AK, Rusterholz C et al. A comparative study of the effect of three different syncytiotrophoblast microparticles preparations on endothelial cells. Placenta 2005; 26(1): 59–66.

100. Sargent IL, Germain SJ et al. Trophoblast deportation and the maternal inflammatory response in pre-eclampsia. J Reprod Immunol 2003; 59(2): 153–60.

101. Shibata E, Rajakumar A et al. Soluble fms-like tyrosine kinase 1 is increased in preeclampsia but not in normotensive pregnancies with small-for-gestational-age neonates: relationship to circulating placental growth factor. J Clin Endocrinol Metab 2005; 90(8): 4895–903.

102. Maynard SE, Min JY et al. Excess placental soluble fms-like tyrosine kinase 1 (sFlt1) may contribute to endothelial dysfunction, hypertension, and proteinuria in preeclampsia. J Clin Invest 2003; 111(5): 649–58.

103. Karumanchi SA, Bdolah Y. Hypoxia and sFlt-1 in preeclampsia: the "chicken-and-egg" question. Endocrinology 2004; 145(11): 4835–7.

104. Nagamatsu T, Fujii T et al. Cytotrophoblasts up-regulate soluble fms-like tyrosine kinase-1 expression under reduced oxygen: an implication for the placental vascular development and the pathophysiology of preeclampsia. Endocrinology 2004; 145(11): 4838–45.

105. Myers JE, Hart S et al. There is no single circulating factor in pre-eclampsia (toxaemia). B J Obstet Gynaecol 2005; 112: 1450.

51 Aging of the endometrium

David F Archer

CHRONOLOGICAL AGE AND THE ENDOMETRIUM

The uterus has only one significant but extremely important function: the continuation of the species. The implantation of an embryo, the provision of a blood supply to the developing fetus, the formation of a mechanism for transmission of nutrients from the mother to the fetus, and resultant parturition all take place in the uterus. The uterus is composed of two distinctly different tissues – the endometrium and the myometrium. The endometrium consists of two discrete layers – the basalis and the functionalis. The functionalis is shed regularly through the necrosis and sloughing associated with menstruation.[1] The basalis portion remains intact and is the site of the normal endometrial reparative process.[2]

The endometrium has a diversity of cell types and secretes or metabolizes numerous proteins, cytokines, growth factors, and receptors for protein and steroid hormones.[3] The cells that make up the endometrial glands and stroma are specifically and exclusively responsive to estrogen or estrogen-like molecules. Estrogens initiate a variety of actions, most prominent of which is the growth of the endometrium, and ultimately the induction of progesterone receptors. Withdrawal of estrogen results in a thin endometrium with morphological characteristics described as inactive or atrophic, reflecting the lack of estrogen stimulation. The application of a progestin without preceding estrogen stimulation does not result in any endometrial growth or evidence of a functional response.[4]

As women age, there is a reduction in fecundity and an increase in early pregnancy loss.[5] These findings are attributed to aging of the oocyte and resultant dysfunction in the embryo. Use of donor oocytes in older women undergoing assisted reproductive technology (ART) find that implantation and successful pregnancy outcome is an oocyte factor rather than an alteration in endometrial function.[6–8] Women with premature ovarian failure who wish to become pregnant require donor oocytes for fertilization, and subsequent embryo development and pregnancy. Women with premature loss of ovarian function following administration of exogenous estrogen and progestogens to synchronize the endometrium have normal embryo implantation and resultant pregnancy.[7,9] Postmenopausal women treated with exogenous estrogen and progestogen have had successful pregnancies following transfer of an embryo into their uterus.[10,11] These data indicate that normal endometrial physiology and function exist in response to appropriate endogenous or exogenous hormonal stimulation, irrespective of the woman's age.

There is accelerated ovarian follicular atresia associated with declining ovarian function as women age.[12–14] This phenomenon is linked to an altered responsiveness of the hypothalamic–pituitary–ovarian axis to circulating estrogen, specifically reflected in a loss of pituitary luteinizing hormone (LH) release secondary to rising levels of estrogen, along with other identifiable changes in serum levels of pituitary and ovarian hormones.[15–19] These changes are clinically manifest as a prolonged follicular phase and/or anovulatory cycles.[19] During this perimenopausal transition, the endometrial morphology (histology) reflects the hormonal status of the individual woman. Proliferative endometrium is found associated with anovulation and secretory endometrium when ovulation and corpus luteal function are normal.

The postmenopausal woman is characterized by the cessation of reproductive function due to the loss of ovarian follicles and the resultant reduction in peripheral serum estrogen levels. Postmenopausal women who are not on exogenous hormonal medication have a thin endometrial lining. The atrophic postmenopausal endometrium is composed of a surface epithelium, stroma, and small straight tubular glands.[20]

The endometrium of a postmenopausal woman is described as atrophic or inactive based on histology. This reflects the lack of mitotic activity in the glands and the resultant involutional changes in the stroma. There is a thin endometrial stripe with transvaginal ultrasound and an inability to obtain any tissue on biopsy due to the lack of significant amounts of endometrial tissue. The atrophic endometrium is related to the hormonal status, since the use of exogenous hormones will re-establish endometrial growth and differentiation. Although the woman ages, the endometrium continues to be able to respond to estrogen stimulation and its functionality is not lost or reduced with aging. An endometrial response to exogenous estrogen can occur in women over 70 years old.

All estrogenic substances have a common mechanism of action. They must bind to the estrogen receptor (ER), dimerize the receptor after binding, and enter the nucleus where the estrogen receptor complexes with the estrogen response element (ERE) on the DNA.[21] Each estrogenic molecule has different binding affinity for the ER. The interaction between the individual estrogen molecule and the ER results in unique conformational changes in the estrogen receptor complex.[22] The estrogen/estrogen receptor complex after interacting with the ERE initiates a variety of nuclear events, involving activator and repressor molecules that appear to be specific to the unique estrogen/ER complex.[22,23] Despite these individual molecular biological events, the morphological response of the endometrium appears to be similar despite the structural differences of the exogenous estrogenic substance. The extent of the histological endometrial response is related to the dose, duration, and 'potency' of the estrogen.

ESTROGEN ALONE IN POSTMENOPAUSAL WOMEN

Estrogens administered to postmenopausal women who have an intact uterus elicit a rapid growth response of the endometrium.[24] Clinical studies have found that the dose of the estrogen and its clinical strength (activity) is important in determining the ultimate endometrium outcome. The proliferative response using histology can be variable between women and there is no quantitative method for comparing the endometrial response to the dose or serum estrogen concentration. Endometrial hyperplasia is a histological endpoint that has been used in prospective clinical trials of estrogen (ET) and estrogen + progestin therapy (EPT).[25,26] The initial response to estrogen exposure is that of proliferation of the glands and stroma with accompanying vascular growth. With continued estrogen exposure there is an increasing incidence of endometrial hyperplasia.[25–30] The variation in the incidence of hyperplasia is reflective of the population under investigation and the dose and duration of the treatment and ranges from 8.0% to 53%.[31]

Conjugated equine estrogens (CE) have been associated with a variable incidence of hyperplasia based on the study population, dose, and duration of treatment. The use of CE 0.625 mg alone in prospective

studies of ≥1 years' duration has resulted in an 8–20% incidence of endometrial hyperplasia at 1 year.[26,27,32] The continued use of CE 0.625 mg is associated with a further increase in endometrial hyperplasia during the second year, to an incidence of 27.3%.[27,32] The Postmenopausal Estrogen and Progestin Interventions study found that the women in the CE 0.625 mg group were more likely to develop simple (cystic) 27.7% vs 0.8%, complex (adenomatous) 22.7% vs 0.8%, or atypical hyperplasia 11.8% vs 0% compared to placebo ($p < 0.001$) during the 3 years of the trial.

Lower doses of CE (0.45 mg and 0.3 mg) were found to have a decrease in endometrial hyperplasia rates (3.23% and 0.37%, respectively), compared with 8.03% for CE 0.625 mg over 1 year of treatment.[33] The incidence of hyperplasia in the second year with continued use was CE 0.625 mg 27.27%; CE 0.45 mg 14.93% ; and CE 0.3 mg 3.17%.[32] These data support the effect of estrogen dose and duration on endometrial hyperplasia.

The use of oral estradiol (E_2) 1.0 mg for 1 year resulted in an overall incidence of endometrial hyperplasia of 14.6%, with simple hyperplasia 12.2%, complex without atypia 1.6%, and complex with atypia 0.8%.[25] The endometrial response to oral E_2 is rapid, with proliferation of the endometrium being present within 3 months along with an increased thickness of the endometrial stripe by transvaginal ultrasound (TVUS).[24] Discontinuing the exogenous E_2 withdraws the stimulus and the endometrium reverts to its atrophic (unstimulated) condition.

Ethinyl estradiol (EE_2) in doses of 0.5, 1.0, 2.5, 5.0, and 10.0 μg had a statistically increased incidence of hyperplasia only at the 10 μg dose. This study in 1278 women was carried out over 1 year.[34]

Esterified estrogens only in doses of 0.625 or 1.25 mg were associated with an increased incidence of endometrial hyperplasia.[35] There was no significant increase in endometrial hyperplasia with the 0.3 mg/ day dose during the study, which lasted 2 years.[35,36]

Estrone sulfate 1.25 mg alone was not associated with an increase in endometrial hyperplasia after 2 years.[37]

ENDOMETRIAL HYPERPLASIA AND ENDOMETRIAL CANCER

Unopposed estrogen used in postmenopausal women with a uterus results in an increased incidence of endometrial cancer.[28] There are limited data that implicate both low doses of estrogen (0.3 mg) and estriol, a 'weak' estrogen, as increasing the incidence of endometrial cancer.[38,39] The increased risk of endometrial cancer with unopposed estrogen has resulted in the addition of a progestin to the estrogen regimen in postmenopausal women.[28] EPT has been shown to reduce the risk of endometrial cancer to that found in women with no prior hormone use.[28,40,41] The Women's Health Initiative prospective randomized blinded clinical trial of CE/MPA (medroxyprogesterone acetate (0.625/2.5 mg)) found no evidence of increased endometrial cancer over the 6.2 years of the study compared to placebo.[41]

The incidence of endometrial cancer, like all cancers, increases with age.[42] There appears to be an ethnic disparity in the incidence of endometrial cancer.[43–46] This may be partly due to the increased incidence of hysterectomy in African-American women.[47] Other risk factors are obesity and diabetes mellitus.[48–53] The risk of obesity on the incidence of endometrial cancers appears to transcend ethnic background.[52,54–56] Endometrial cancer presents with vaginal bleeding as an early sign. Appropriate diagnostic studies are endometrial sampling and the use of TVUS evaluation of the endometrium in symptomatic (bleeding) post-menopausal women.[57–62]

Endometrial cancer occurs at an incidence of approximately 1–2 cases per 1000 women per year. Because of this low incidence, most prospective clinical trials of EPT have used the occurrence of endometrial hyperplasia as the outcome measure of risk. Endometrial hyperplasia per se is not a risk factor for endometrial cancer.[63,64] Atypical endometrial hyperplasia is a risk factor for endometrial cancer. Although we have used endometrial morphology to identify women at risk for malignancy (premalignant disease), the interpretation of the endometrial histology is variable between pathologists.[32,65] Recently, the use of a more sophisticated system called endometrial intraepithelial neoplasia (EIN) has been found to have a high predictive ability for progression of endometrial abnormalities to endometrial cancer.[66–73] This method uses biomarkers in the endometrium, most notably the absence of PTEN, a tumor suppressor gene, to identify endometrial cancer.[66,67,69,71]

ESTROGEN + PROGESTIN

The increased incidence of endometrial hyperplasia with unopposed estrogens is well established.[29,30,74] Current clinical trials of hormonal products have often used an approved estrogen and progestin as the comparator for the occurrence of endometrial hyperplasia and bleeding.[75–78]

There are several methods for adding the progestin to concurrent ET in women with an intact uterus. The estrogen is usually given continuously and the progestin can be added for 14 days for each 28-day cycle or month (this results in 13 cycles/year): this is called cyclic estrogen + progestin therapy (csEPT). Continuous estrogen plus progestin therapy (ccEPT) is the use of daily delivery of the estrogen + progestin by the oral route. There is a long cycle of estrogen, with the progestin added for 14 days every 3 months, or at 6-month intervals. A novel intermittent use of a progestin every 3 days has been called pulsed progestin.[31] All of the approved therapies have resulted in the interdiction of endometrial hyperplasia.[29–31] A prospective clinical trial of long-cycle progestin with E_2 was stopped because of an unacceptable incidence of endometrial hyperplasia.[30,79]

Conjugated estrogens and medroxyprogesterone acetate in various doses have been the most extensive preparation studied. Prospective clinical trials of both cyclic use of MPA (14 days per cycle) and continuous use of MPA with CE do not increase the incidence of endometrial hyperplasia.[26,33] Lower doses of CE and MPA have been shown not to increase the incidence of endometrial hyperplasia after 1 or 2 years of treatment.[32,33]

EE_2 5 μg with norethindrone acetate (NETA) 1.0 mg had no cases of endometrial hyperplasia over the 2 years of this study.[34,80] The lower dose, containing EE_2 2.5 μg and NETA 0.5 mg, did not find any evidence of endometrial hyperplasia.[80]

Estradiol combined with NETA 0.5, 0.25, and 0.1 mg reported a low incidence of endometrial hyperplasia compared with E_2 1.0 mg alone over a 1-year period.[25] The incidence of endometrial hyperplasia with the different doses was NETA 0.1 mg, 0.8%; NETA 0.25 mg, 0.4%; and NETA 0.5 mg, 0.4%.[25]

The intermittent use of norethindrone every 3 days (pulsed progestin) in conjunction with piperazine estrone sulfate 0.625 mg was not associated with an increase in endometrial hyperplasia.[81] The pulsed progestin regimen with E_2 + norgestimate (NGM) found a dose–response for the progestin in interdicting endometrial hyperplasia.[82] The use of E_2 1.0 mg + NGM 90 μg or E_2 1.0 mg + NGM 180 μg was not associated with endometrial hyperplasia, but there were 16 (6%) cases of endometrial hyperplasia in subjects who received E_2 1.0 mg + NGM 30 μg and 74 cases (28%) in the E_2 1.0 mg unopposed group.[82]

Drospirenone, a novel progestogen derived from spironolactone, in doses of 0.5, 1.0, 2.0, and 3.0 mg, inhibited the effect of E_2 1.0 mg and prevented endometrial hyperplasia.[83] Other progestins that have been reported in the literature, e.g. nomogestrel, levonorgestrel, and dydrogesterone, as well as all approved combinations of estrogen and progestin products, inhibit the development of endometrial hyperplasia.[29,30,84]

Trimegestone a 19-norprogesterone has also been studied with E_2 and CE in both cyclic and continuous regimens.[85–88] There was good endometrial protection, with endometrial hyperplasia < 1.0% in these studies.

The use of the long-cycle regimen of estrogen continuously with progestin administered every 3 or 6 months is not an approved regimen. Several reports have indicated that there is no increased risk of hyperplasia with this method.[89,90] Conversely, in a large prospective clinical trial of long-cycle progestin use, there was an increased incidence of endometrial hyperplasia with the use of E_2 2.0 mg and NETA.[79] The difference in endometrial hyperplasia rates between a 3-month interval group 5.6% was statistically significant compared to 1.0% in the monthly group.[79] It is of note that the progestin NETA 1.0 mg was only given for 10 days of each cycle. This duration of progestin use may be insufficient to protect the endometrium.[28]

TRANSDERMAL ESTRADIOL AND PROGESTINS

Transdermal estradiol alone was initially used to treat menopausal symptoms. The addition of transdermal progestin came later because of the need to add a progestin to the transdermal system. Progestins are not well absorbed across the epidermis. The transport of estradiol and norethindrone appears to be along the lipid layers of the interface between adjacent epithelial cells.[91] Several advantages of transdermal administration have been noted, principally the stable serum concentration of the estradiol and progestin. There is an improved compliance with a once or twice a week administration of a transdermal system compared to the daily requirement with oral medication. Two recent publications have indicated that transdermal estrogen compared to oral estrogen does not appear to increase the risk of deep vein thrombosis. These two studies are observational in character and should be considered as hypothesis-generating rather than as conclusive evidence for a diminished incidence of venous thrombosis in postmenopausal women using transdermal estrogen.[92,93]

Estradiol and norethindrone have been studied in several clinical trials. The norethindrone dose ranges from 125 to 400 mg/day with several doses of estrogen. The majority of the clinical trials have not found any evidence of hyperplasia.[94,95] Several of the clinical trials have had a low (<1.0%) incidence of endometrial hyperplasia in the participants. The significance of these findings is not known at the present time.[96–98]

Estradiol and levonorgestrel have been studied in two clinical trials, where efficacy for menopausal symptom relief was found. No cases of endometrial hyperplasia were identified in either trial of continuous EPT.[99] One of the trials was a comparison to estradiol only administered transdermally. The combination of E_2 and levonorgestrel was not associated with endometrial hyperplasia, whereas E_2 0.045 mg alone had a 12.8% incidence.[99] A study of transdermal estradiol and sequential levonorgestrel at three doses for 14 days identified two cases of endometrial hyperplasia, one in each of the two higher-dose levonorgestrel arms.[100]

TIBOLONE: A SELECTIVE TISSUE ESTROGEN ACTIVITY REGULATOR

Tibolone should not be considered as an estrogen–progestin combination. Tibolone is a prodrug that is metabolized into three active compounds in the body:[101] two of these are estrogenic and one, the Δ_4-tibolone, has been shown to have progestational properties.[102] Clinical studies have not found any evidence of endometrial stimulation in women using tibolone.[103–106] There were three cases of endometrial cancer in one clinical trial of osteoporosis prevention in older women.[107] There was a significant increase in the incidence of endometrial cancer in one observational study.[40] This may have been due to prescribing bias by physicians.[108,109] A prospective randomized trial of tibolone compared to conjugated estrogen with MPA has been studied in a multinational, multicentered trial. There was no evidence of endometrial hyperplasia in this study after 2 years' exposure to tibolone.[76]

ENDOMETRIAL RESPONSE TO SELECTIVE ESTROGEN RECEPTOR MODULATORS

Selective estrogen receptor modulators (SERMs) have unique activities based on their interaction with the ER. SERMs do not appear to stimulate the endometrium or breast while having a positive effect on bone.[110,111] This selectivity of response in ER-rich target tissues (breast and endometrium) has led to their utilization in postmenopausal women. The SERMs bind to the ER but, owing to their altered configuration, they have tissue-selective responses.[22] They can behave as estrogens in some tissues, but should not have estrogenic activity in the endometrium.

Tamoxifen has been used for many years to reduce the recurrence rate of breast cancer in women with ER-positive tumors. The recent publication of the Study of Tamoxifen and Raloxifene (STAR) trial has indicated that both of these SERMs reduce the recurrence rate of ER-positive breast cancers in high-risk women.[112]

Tamoxifen (TAM) is an antiestrogen when used in premenopausal women. Alone in postmenopausal women, TAM has a weak estrogen effect.[110] The endometrial response to continuous use of TAM is variable. There are many observational and anecdotal reports that implicate TAM with an increased risk of endometrial abnormalities,[113–118] ranging from polyps through hyperplasia and neoplasia. A current prospective trial, the STAR trial, compared TAM to raloxifene for prevention of breast cancer in 19 747 women: endometrial cancer occurred in 36 cases with tamoxifen and 23 with raloxifene (relative risk [RR] = 0.62; 95% confidence interval [CI] 0.35–1.08).[112] Tamoxifen has a weak estrogenic effect in postmenopausal woman that necessitates regular surveillance for endometrial abnormalities using a variety of methods.[119–128] The best means of monitoring these women should involve regular evaluation of the endometrium using ultrasound and histology.

The effects of raloxifene on the endometrium were analyzed from the database of 1157 postmenopausal women participating in four clinical trials.[129] There were no cases of endometrial hyperplasia in this group of women. The principal means of monitoring the endometrium was the use of TVUS, which did not show a statistically significant increase in thickness of the endometrial lining over placebo in the clinical trials.[129–132] The incidence of endometrial bleeding, as another indirect assessment of lack of endometrial stimulation, was similar between the raloxifene and placebo groups.[129,132–134]

Bazedoxifene is a SERM under development for prevention of bone loss.[135] At doses of 2.5, 5.0, 10, 20, and 40 mg/day, bazedoxifene was not associated with any evidence of endometrial stimulation in a 6-month trial using TVUS and endometrial biopsy results.[136] These data are consonant with preclinical studies, where there was no evidence of uterine growth.[135]

There are no published clinical data on lasofoxifene. It has undergone phase 3 trials for prevention of bone loss. Preclinical data indicate no effect on uterine weight compared with controls, but evidence for prevention of bone loss.[137–139]

Levormeloxifene was in a phase 3 clinical trial that was halted when it was found to have an increased incidence of reproductive tract problems. Two of the side effects were increased endometrial thickness on ultrasound scan (19% vs 1%) and enlarged uterus (17% vs 3%) compared with placebo.[140]

Ospemifene was found to have a weak estrogen effect on the vaginal epithelium, but no significant change in endometrial thickness based on ultrasound evaluation and endometrial biopsy.[141,142] The two clinical studies used either raloxifene or placebo as a comparator but only lasted for 3 months.[141,142]

ENDOMETRIAL BLEEDING

Each clinical trial of estrogen with or without a progestin, and all of the SERMs, have addressed the occurrence and duration of endometrial bleeding. This symptom is one that is best correlated with continuation of hormone therapy for the individual woman. The actual number of days of bleeding or spotting varies between studies, and is predicated on the study design and criteria of bleeding and spotting. It would be helpful to have an overall acceptable definition and method of describing this side effect of the therapy.[143] The occurrence of bleeding during EPT does not predict the endometrial histology.[144] The sensitivity of ultrasound endometrial measurements is low in women on hormone therapy in predicting the endometrial histological pattern.[145]

The incidence of bleeding appears to be related to the estrogen dose in most instances, with reduced bleeding associated with lower estrogen doses.[34,146] Increasing the progestin dose may reduce the incidence of bleeding during use of hormone therapy.[85,147] The exact mechanism(s) involved in the bleeding in postmenopausal women using hormone therapy is unknown. There is evidence that bleeding from an atrophic endometrium induced by progestins may be similar to that which occurs in the hypoestrogenic postmenopausal woman.[148] The same group more recently has found changes in levels of metalloproteinases, and the ratio of metalloproteinases to tissue inhibitors of metalloproteinases to be a better indicator of the occurrence of bleeding in hormone therapy users.[149,150] It is possible that multiple factors contribute to the onset of irregular endometrial bleeding in the postmenopausal woman on continuous EPT.[151–153]

SUMMARY

The endometrium is capable of responding to the hormone milieu at any age. This response using estradiol and progestins can result in a 'normal' endometrium in terms of physiology and function. The number of women who are exposed and the extent of the endometrial response to each estrogen is highly variable. The use of unopposed estrogen in a woman with an intact uterus is not appropriate. The use of estrogen + a progestin in marketed products has been found to interdict the development of endometrial hyperplasia, a surrogate marker for endometrial cancer in prospective clinical trials. SERMs have a role in the management of postmenopausal women, but in some instances regular surveillance of the endometrium is indicated. The use of exogenous hormones in postmenopausal women can result in endometrial bleeding. Appropriate evaluation by the healthcare provider is required in each instance.

REFERENCES

1. Ferenczy A. Pathophysiology of endometrial bleeding. Maturitas 2003; 45(1): 1–14.
2. Ludwig H, Spornitz UM. Microarchitecture of the human endometrium by scanning electron microscopy: menstrual desquamation and remodeling. Ann NY Acad Sci 1991; 622: 28–46.
3. Jabbour HN, Kelly RW, Fraser HM, Critchley HO. Endocrine regulation of menstruation. Endocr Rev 2006; 27(1): 17–46.
4. Wallach EE. Physiology of menstruation. Clin Obstet Gynecol 1970; 13(2): 366–85.
5. Heffner LJ. Advanced maternal age – how old is too old? N Engl J Med 2004; 351(19): 1927–9.
6. Pal L, Santoro N. Age-related decline in fertility. Endocrinol Metab Clin North Am 2003; 32(3): 669–88.
7. Toner JP, Flood JT. Fertility after the age of 40. Obstet Gynecol Clin North Am 1993; 20(2): 261–72.
8. Abdalla HI, Wren ME, Thomas A, Korea L. Age of the uterus does not affect pregnancy or implantation rates; a study of egg donation in women of different ages sharing oocytes from the same donor. Hum Reprod 1997; 12(4): 827–9.
9. Society for Assisted Reproduction Technology: American Society for Reproductive Medicine. Assisted reproductive technology in the United States: 2001 results generated from the American Society for Reproductive Medicine/Society for Assisted Reproductive Technology registry. Fertil Steril 2007; 87: 1253–66.
10. Paulson RJ, Boostanfar R, Saadat P et al. Pregnancy in the sixth decade of life: obstetric outcomes in women of advanced reproductive age. JAMA 2002; 288(18): 2320–3.
11. Sauer MV, Paulson RJ, Lobo RA. Pregnancy in women 50 or more years of age: outcomes of 22 consecutively established pregnancies from oocyte donation. Fertil Steril 1995; 64(1): 111–15.
12. Gosden RG. Follicular status at the menopause. Hum Reprod 1987; 2(7): 617–21.
13. Faddy MJ, Gosden RG, Gougeon A, Richardson SJ et al. Accelerated disappearance of ovarian follicles in mid-life: implications for forecasting menopause. Hum Reprod 1992; 7(10): 1342–6.
14. Gosden RG, Faddy MJ. Ovarian aging, follicular depletion, and steroidogenesis. Exp Gerontol 1994; 29(3–4): 265–74.
15. Santoro N. The menopausal transition. Am J Med 2005; 118 (Suppl 12B): 8–13.
16. Jain A, Santoro N. Endocrine mechanisms and management for abnormal bleeding due to perimenopausal changes. Clin Obstet Gynecol 2005; 48(2): 295–311.
17. Santoro N, Brown JR, Adel T, Skurnick JH. Characterization of reproductive hormonal dynamics in the perimenopause. J Clin Endocrinol Metab 1996; 81(4): 1495–501.
18. Burger HG, Dudley EC, Robertson DM, Dennerstein L. Hormonal changes in the menopause transition. Recent Prog Horm Res 2002; 57: 257–75.
19. Dudley EC, Hopper JL, Taffe J et al. Using longitudinal data to define the perimenopause by menstrual cycle characteristics. Climacteric 1998; 1(1): 18–25.
20. Sherman M, Mazur M, Kurman R. Benign diseases of the endometrium. In: Kurman R, ed. Blaustein's Pathology of the Female Genital Tract, 5th edn. New York: Springer, 2002: 421–67.
21. Turgeon JL, McDonnell DP, Martin KA, Wise PM. Hormone therapy: physiological complexity belies therapeutic simplicity. Science 2004; 304(5675): 1269–73.
22. McDonnell DP. The molecular determinants of estrogen receptor pharmacology. Maturitas 2004; 48(Suppl 1): S7–12.
23. McDonnell DP, Norris JD. Connections and regulation of the human estrogen receptor. Science 2002; 296(5573): 1642–4.
24. Ettinger B, Bainton L, Upmalis DH et al. Comparison of endometrial growth produced by unopposed conjugated estrogens or by micronized estradiol in postmenopausal women. Am J Obstet Gynecol 1997; 176(1 Pt 1): 112–17.
25. Kurman RJ, Felix JC, Archer DF et al. Norethindrone acetate and estradiol-induced endometrial hyperplasia. Obstet Gynecol 2000; 96(3): 373–9.
26. Woodruff JD, Pickar JH. Incidence of endometrial hyperplasia in postmenopausal women taking conjugated estrogens (Premarin) with medroxyprogesterone acetate or conjugated estrogens alone. The Menopause Study Group. Am J Obstet Gynecol 1994; 170(5 Pt 1): 1213–23.
27. Effects of hormone replacement therapy on endometrial histology in postmenopausal women. The Postmenopausal Estrogen/Progestin Interventions (PEPI) Trial. The Writing Group for the PEPI Trial. JAMA 1996; 275(5): 370–5.
28. Archer DF. The effect of the duration of progestin use on the occurrence of endometrial cancer in postmenopausal women. Menopause 2001; 8(4): 245–51.
29. Lethaby A, Farquhar C, Sarkis A et al. Hormone replacement therapy in postmenopausal women: endometrial hyperplasia and irregular bleeding. Cochrane Database Syst Rev 2000(2): CD000402.
30. Lethaby A, Suckling J, Barlow D et al. Hormone replacement therapy in postmenopausal women: endometrial hyperplasia and irregular bleeding. Cochrane Database Syst Rev 2004(3): CD000402.
31. Role of progestogen in hormone therapy for postmenopausal women: position statement of The North American Menopause Society. Menopause 2003; 10(2): 113–32.
32. Pickar JH, Yeh IT, Wheeler JE et al. Endometrial effects of lower doses of conjugated equine estrogens and medroxyprogesterone acetate: two-year substudy results. Fertil Steril 2003; 80(5): 1234–40.

33. Pickar JH, Yeh I, Wheeler JE et al. Endometrial effects of lower doses of conjugated equine estrogens and medroxy-progesterone acetate. Fertil Steril 2001; 76(1): 25–31.

34. Speroff L, Rowan J, Symons J et al. The comparative effect on bone density, endometrium, and lipids of continuous hormones as replacement therapy (CHART study). A randomized controlled trial. JAMA 1996; 276(17): 1397–403.

35. Genant HK, Lucas J, Weiss S et al. Low-dose esterified estrogen therapy: effects on bone, plasma estradiol concentrations, endometrium, and lipid levels. Estratab/Osteoporosis Study Group. Arch Intern Med 1997; 157(22): 2609–15.

36. Crandall C. Low-dose estrogen therapy for menopausal women: a review of efficacy and safety. J Womens Health (Larchmt) 2003; 12(8): 723–47.

37. Nand SL, Webster MA, Baber R, O'Connor V. Bleeding pattern and endometrial changes during continuous combined hormone replacement therapy. The Ogen/Provera Study Group. Obstet Gynecol 1998; 91(5 Pt 1): 678–84.

38. Weiderpass E, Baron JA, Adami HO et al. Low-potency estrogen and risk of endometrial cancer: a case-control study. Lancet 1999; 353(9167): 1824–8.

39. Van Gorp T, Neven P. Endometrial safety of hormone replacement therapy: review of literature. Maturitas 2002; 42(2): 93–104.

40. Beral V, Bull D, Reeves G. Endometrial cancer and hormone-replacement therapy in the Million Women Study. Lancet 2005; 365(9470): 1543–51.

41. Anderson GL, Judd HL, Kaunitz AM et al. Effects of estrogen plus progestin on gynecologic cancers and associated diagnostic procedures: the Women's Health Initiative randomized trial. JAMA 2003; 290(13): 1739–48.

42. Amant F, Moerman P, Neven P et al. Endometrial cancer. Lancet 2005; 366(9484): 491–505.

43. Bray F, Dos Santos Silva I, Moller H, Weiderpass E. Endometrial cancer incidence trends in Europe: underlying determinants and prospects for prevention. Cancer Epidemiol Biomarkers Prev 2005; 14(5): 1132–42.

44. Somoye G, Olaitan A, Mocroft A, Jacobs I. Age related trends in the incidence of endometrial cancer in South East England 1962–1997. J Obstet Gynaecol 2005; 25(1): 35–8.

45. Beard CM, Hartmann LC, Keeney GL et al. Endometrial cancer in Olmsted County, MN: trends in incidence, risk factors and survival. Ann Epidemiol 2000; 10(2): 97–105.

46. Sherman ME, Devesa SS. Analysis of racial differences in incidence, survival, and mortality for malignant tumors of the uterine corpus. Cancer 2003; 98(1): 176–86.

47. Sherman ME, Carreon JD, Lacey JV Jr, Devesa SS. Impact of hysterectomy on endometrial carcinoma rates in the United States. J Natl Cancer Inst 2005; 97(22): 1700–2.

48. Anderson KE, Anderson E, Mink PJ et al. Diabetes and endometrial cancer in the Iowa Women's Health Study. Cancer Epidemiol Biomarkers Prev 2001; 10(6): 611–16.

49. Vuento MH, Pirhonen JP, Makinen JI et al. Screening for endometrial cancer in asymptomatic postmenopausal women with conventional and colour Doppler sonography. Br J Obstet Gynaecol 1999; 106(1): 14–20.

50. Weiderpass E, Persson I, Adami HO et al. Body size in different periods of life, diabetes mellitus, hypertension, and risk of postmenopausal endometrial cancer (Sweden). Cancer Causes Control 2000; 11(2): 185–92.

51. Jain MG, Rohan TE, Howe GR, Miller AB. A cohort study of nutritional factors and endometrial cancer. Eur J Epidemiol 2000; 16(10): 899–905.

52. Salazar-Martinez E, Lazcano-Ponce EC, Lira-Lira GG et al. Case-control study of diabetes, obesity, physical activity and risk of endometrial cancer among Mexican women. Cancer Causes Control 2000; 11(8): 707–11.

53. Friberg E, Mantzoros CS, Wolk A. Diabetes and risk of endometrial cancer: a population-based prospective cohort study. Cancer Epidemiol Biomarkers Prev 2007; 16(2): 276–80.

54. Schouten LJ, Goldbohm RA, van den Brandt PA. Anthropometry, physical activity, and endometrial cancer risk: results from the Netherlands Cohort Study. J Natl Cancer Inst 2004; 96(21): 1635–8.

55. Xu WH, Matthews CE, Xiang YB et al. Effect of adiposity and fat distribution on endometrial cancer risk in Shanghai women. Am J Epidemiol 2005; 161(10): 939–47.

56. Bjorge T, Engeland A, Tretli S, Weiderpass E. Body size in relation to cancer of the uterine corpus in 1 million Norwegian women. Int J Cancer 2007; 120(2): 378–83.

57. Briley M, Lindsell DR. The role of transvaginal ultrasound in the investigation of women with post-menopausal bleeding. Clin Radiol 1998; 53(7): 502–5.

58. Goldstein SR. The endometrial echo revisited: have we created a monster? Am J Obstet Gynecol 2004; 191(4): 1092–6.

59. Bakos O, Smith P, Heimer G. Transvaginal ultrasonography for identifying endometrial pathology in postmenopausal women. Maturitas 1994; 20(2-3): 181–9.

60. Elsandabesee D, Greenwood P. The performance of Pipelle endometrial sampling in a dedicated postmenopausal bleeding clinic. J Obstet Gynaecol 2005; 25(1): 32–4.

61. Robertson G. Screening for endometrial cancer. Med J Aust 2003; 178(12): 657–9.

62. Markovitch O, Tepper R, Fishman A et al. The value of transvaginal ultrasonography in the prediction of endometrial pathologies in asymptomatic postmenopausal breast cancer tamoxifen-treated patients. Gynecol Oncol 2004; 95(3): 456–62.

63. Burke TW, Tortolero-Luna G, Malpica A et al. Endometrial hyperplasia and endometrial cancer. Obstet Gynecol Clin North Am 1996; 23(2): 411–56.

64. Montgomery BE, Daum GS, Dunton CJ. Endometrial hyperplasia: a review. Obstet Gynecol Surv 2004; 59(5): 368–78.

65. Nucci MR, Castrillon DH, Bai H et al. Biomarkers in diagnostic obstetric and gynecologic pathology: a review. Adv Anat Pathol 2003; 10(2): 55–68.

66. Baak JP, Van Diermen B, Steinbakk A et al. Lack of PTEN expression in endometrial intraepithelial neoplasia is correlated with cancer progression. Hum Pathol 2005; 36(5): 555–61.

67. Baak JP, Mutter GL, Robboy S et al. The molecular genetics and morphometry-based endometrial intraepithelial neoplasia classification system predicts disease progression in endometrial hyperplasia more accurately than the 1994 World Health Organization classification system. Cancer 2005; 103(11): 2304–12.

68. Hecht JL, Ince TA, Baak JP et al. Prediction of endometrial carcinoma by subjective endometrial intraepithelial neoplasia diagnosis. Mod Pathol 2005; 18(3): 324–30.

69. Mutter GL, Ince TA, Baak JP et al. Molecular identification of latent precancers in histologically normal endometrium. Cancer Res 2001; 61(11): 4311–14.

70. Mutter GL. Histopathology of genetically defined endometrial precancers. Int J Gynecol Pathol 2000; 19(4): 301–9.

71. Mutter GL, Lin MC, Fitzgerald JT et al. Altered PTEN expression as a diagnostic marker for the earliest endometrial precancers. J Natl Cancer Inst 2000; 92(11): 924–30.

72. Mutter GL, Baak JP, Crum CP et al. Endometrial precancer diagnosis by histopathology, clonal analysis, and computerized morphometry. J Pathol 2000; 190(4): 462–9.

73. Mutter GL. Endometrial intraepithelial neoplasia (EIN): will it bring order to chaos? The Endometrial Collaborative Group. Gynecol Oncol 2000; 76(3): 287–90.

74. Sturdee DW. Endometrial morphology and bleeding patterns as a function of progestogen supplementation. Int J Fertil Menopausal Stud 1996; 41(1): 22–8.

75. Simon JA, Symons JP. Unscheduled bleeding during initiation of continuous combined hormone replacement therapy: a direct comparison of two combinations of norethindrone acetate and ethinyl estradiol to medroxyprogesterone acetate and conjugated equine estrogens. Menopause 2001; 8(5): 321–7.

76. Archer DF, Hendrix S, Gallagher C et al. Endometrial effects of tibolone. J Clin Endocrinol Metab 2007; 92: 911–18.

77. Johnson JV, Davidson M, Archer D, Bachmann G. Postmenopausal uterine bleeding profiles with two forms of continuous combined hormone replacement therapy. Menopause 2002; 9(1): 16–22.

78. Yildirim G, Tugrul S, Uslu H et al. Effects of two different regimens of continuous hormone replacement therapy on endometrial histopathology and postmenopausal uterine bleeding. Arch Gynecol Obstet 2006; 273(5): 268–73.

79. Bjarnason K, Cerin A, Lindgren R, Weber T. Adverse endometrial effects during long cycle hormone replacement therapy. Scandinavian Long Cycle Study Group. Maturitas 1999; 32(3): 161–70.

80. Rowan JP, Simon JA, Speroff L, Ellman H. Effects of low-dose norethindrone acetate plus ethinyl estradiol (0.5 mg/2.5 µg) in women with postmenopausal symptoms: updated analysis of three randomized, controlled trials. Clin Ther 2006; 28(6): 921–32.

81. Casper RF, Chapdelaine A. Estrogen and interrupted progestin: a new concept for menopausal hormone replacement therapy. Am J Obstet Gynecol 1993; 168(4): 1188–94; discussion 1194–6.

82. Corson SL, Richart RM, Caubel P, Lim P. Effect of a unique constant-estrogen, pulsed-progestin hormone replacement therapy containing 17β-estradiol and norgestimate on endometrial histology. Int J Fertil Womens Med 1999; 44(6): 279–85.

83. Archer DF, Thorneycroft IH, Foegh M et al. Long-term safety of drospirenone-estradiol for hormone therapy: a randomized, double-blind, multicenter trial. Menopause 2005; 12(6): 716–27.

84. Sitruk-Ware R. Progestogens in hormonal replacement therapy: new molecules, risks, and benefits. Menopause 2002; 9(1): 6–15.

85. Al-Azzawi F, Wahab M, Thompson J, Whitehead M, Thompson W. Acceptability and patterns of uterine bleeding in sequential trimegestone-based hormone replacement therapy: a dose-ranging study. Hum Reprod 1999; 14(3): 636–41.

86. Bouchard P, De Cicco-Nardone F, Spielmann D, Garcea N. Bleeding profile and endometrial safety of continuous combined regimens 1 mg 17β-estradiol/trimegestone versus 1 or 2 mg 17β-estradiol/norethisterone acetate in postmenopausal women. Gynecol Endocrinol 2005; 21(3): 142–8.

87. Grubb G, Spielmann D, Pickar J, Constantine G. Clinical experience with trimegestone as a new progestin in HRT. Steroids 2003; 68(10–13): 921–6.

88. Koninckx PR, Spielmann D. A comparative 2-year study of the effects of sequential regimens of 1 mg 17β-estradiol and trimegestone with a regimen containing estradiol valerate and norethisterone on the bleeding profile and endometrial safety in postmenopausal women. Gynecol Endocrinol 2005; 21(2): 82–9.

89. Ettinger B, Selby J, Citron JT et al. Cyclic hormone replacement therapy using quarterly progestin. Obstet Gynecol 1994; 83(5 Pt 1): 693–700.

90. Ettinger B, Pressman A, Van Gessel A. Low-dosage esterified estrogens opposed by progestin at 6-month intervals. Obstet Gynecol 2001; 98(2): 205–11.

91. Neelissen JA, Arth C, Wolff M et al. Visualization of percutaneous ³H-estradiol and ³H-norethindrone acetate transport across human epidermis as a function of time. Acta Derm Venereol Suppl (Stockh) 2000; 208: 36–43.

92. Canonico M, Oger E, Plu-Bureau G et al. Hormone therapy and venous thromboembolism among postmenopausal women: impact of the route of estrogen administration and progestogens: the ESTHER study. Circulation 2007; 115(7): 840–5.

93. Scarabin PY, Oger E, Plu-Bureau G. Differential association of oral and transdermal estrogen-replacement therapy with venous thromboembolism risk. Lancet 2003; 362(9382): 428–32.

94. Johannisson E, Holinka CF, Arrenbrecht S. Transdermal sequential and continuous hormone replacement regimens with estradiol and norethisterone acetate in postmenopausal women: effects on the endometrium. Int J Fertil Womens Med 1997; 42 (Suppl 2): 388–98.

95. Samsioe G, Boschitsch E, Concin H et al. Endometrial safety, overall safety and tolerability of transdermal continuous combined hormone replacement therapy over 96 weeks: a randomized open-label study. Climacteric 2006; 9(5): 368–79.

96. Brynhildsen J, Hammar M. Low dose transdermal estradiol/norethisterone acetate treatment over 2 years does not cause endometrial proliferation in postmenopausal women. Menopause 2002; 9(2): 137–44.

97. Archer DF, Furst K, Tipping D et al. A randomized comparison of continuous combined transdermal delivery of estradiol–norethindrone acetate and estradiol alone for menopause. CombiPatch Study Group. Obstet Gynecol 1999; 94(4): 498–503.

98. Mattsson LA, Bohnet HG, Gredmark T et al. Continuous, combined hormone replacement: randomized comparison of transdermal and oral preparations. Obstet Gynecol 1999; 94(1): 61–5.

99. Shulman LP, Yankov V, Uhl K. Safety and efficacy of a continuous once-a-week 17β-estradiol/levonorgestrel transdermal system and its effects on vasomotor symptoms and endometrial safety in postmenopausal women: the results of two multicenter, double-blind, randomized, controlled trials. Menopause 2002; 9(3): 195–207.

100. Sturdee DW, van de Weijer P, von Holst T. Endometrial safety of a transdermal sequential estradiol–levonorgestrel combination. Climacteric 2002; 5(2): 170–7.

101. Kloosterboer HJ. Tissue-selectivity: the mechanism of action of tibolone. Maturitas 2004; 48(Suppl 1): S30–40.

102. Kloosterboer HJ. Tibolone: a steroid with a tissue-specific mode of action. J Steroid Biochem Mol Biol 2001; 76(1–5): 231–8.

103. Christodoulakos GE, Botsis DS, Lambrinoudaki IV et al. A 5-year study on the effect of hormone therapy, tibolone and raloxifene on vaginal bleeding and endometrial thickness. Maturitas 2006; 53(4): 413–23.

104. Volker W, Coelingh Bennink HJ, Helmond FA. Effects of tibolone on the endometrium. Climacteric 2001; 4(3): 203–8.

105. Morris EP, Wilson PO, Robinson J, Rymer JM. Long term effects of tibolone on the genital tract in postmenopausal women. Br J Obstet Gynaecol 1999; 106(9): 954–9.

106. Langer RD, Landgren BM, Rymer J, Helmond FA. Effects of tibolone and continuous combined conjugated equine estrogen/medroxyprogesterone acetate on the endometrium and vaginal bleeding: results of the OPAL study. Am J Obstet Gynecol 2006; 195(5): 1320–7.

107. Gallagher JC, Baylink DJ, Freeman R, McClung M. Prevention of bone loss with tibolone in postmenopausal women: results of two randomized, double-blind, placebo-controlled, dose-finding studies. J Clin Endocrinol Metab 2001; 86(10): 4717–26.

108. de Vries CS, Bromley SE, Thomas H, Farmer RD. Tibolone and endometrial cancer: a cohort and nested case-control study in the UK. Drug Saf 2005; 28(3): 241–9.

109. Velthuis-Te Wierik EJ, Hendricks PT, Martinez C. Preferential prescribing of tibolone and combined estrogen plus progestogen therapy in postmenopausal women. Menopause 2007; 14: 518–27.

110. Arun B, Anthony M, Dunn B. The search for the ideal SERM. Expert Opin Pharmacother 2002; 3(6): 681–91.

111. Mitlak BH, Cohen FJ. Selective estrogen receptor modulators: a look ahead. Drugs 1999; 57(5): 653–63.

112. Vogel VG, Costantino JP, Wickerham DL et al. Effects of tamoxifen vs raloxifene on the risk of developing invasive breast cancer and other disease outcomes: the NSABP Study of Tamoxifen and Raloxifene (STAR) P-2 trial. JAMA 2006; 295(23): 2727–41.

113. Al-Azemi M, Labib NS, Motawy MM et al. Prevalence of endometrial proliferation in pipelle biopsies in tamoxifen-treated postmenopausal women with breast cancer in Kuwait. Med Princ Pract 2004; 13(1): 30–4.

114. Gerber B, Krause A, Muller H et al. Effects of adjuvant tamoxifen on the endometrium in postmenopausal women with breast cancer: a prospective long-term study using transvaginal ultrasound. J Clin Oncol 2000; 18(20): 3464–70.

115. Maugeri G, Nardo LG, Campione C, Nardo F. Endometrial lesions after tamoxifen therapy in breast cancer women. Breast J 2001; 7(4): 240–4.

116. Schlesinger C, Kamoi S, Ascher SM et al. Endometrial polyps: a comparison study of patients receiving tamoxifen with two control groups. Int J Gynecol Pathol 1998; 17(4): 302–11.

117. Tregon ML, Blumel JE, Tarin JJ, Cano A. The early response of the postmenopausal endometrium to tamoxifen: expression of estrogen receptors, progesterone receptors, and Ki-67 antigen. Menopause 2003; 10(2): 154–9.

118. Goldstein SR. The effect of SERMs on the endometrium. Ann NY Acad Sci 2001; 949: 237–42.

119. Blumenfeld ML, Turner LP. Role of transvaginal sonography in the evaluation of endometrial hyperplasia and cancer. Clin Obstet Gynecol 1996; 39(3): 641–55.

120. Fong K, Causer P, Atri M et al. Transvaginal US and hysterosonography in postmenopausal women with breast cancer receiving tamoxifen: correlation with hysteroscopy and pathologic study. Radiographics 2003; 23(1): 137–50; discussion 151–5.

121. Hann LE, Gretz EM, Bach AM, Francis SM. Sonohysterography for evaluation of the endometrium in women treated with tamoxifen. AJR Am J Roentgenol 2001; 177(2): 337–42.

122. Achiron R, Lipitz S, Sivan E et al. Changes mimicking endometrial neoplasia in postmenopausal, tamoxifen-treated women with breast cancer: a transvaginal Doppler study. Ultrasound Obstet Gynecol 1995; 6(2): 116–20.

123. Cohen I, Rosen DJ, Shapira J et al. Endometrial changes with tamoxifen: comparison between tamoxifen-treated and non-treated asymptomatic, postmenopausal breast cancer patients. Gynecol Oncol 1994; 52(2): 185–90.

124. Anteby EY, Yagel S, Weissman A et al. Sonographic evaluation of the uterus in postmenopausal women receiving tamoxifen: characterization of mid-uterine abnormalities. Eur J Obstet Gynecol Reprod Biol 1996; 69(2): 115–19.

125. Ascher SM, Johnson JC, Barnes WA et al. MR imaging appearance of the uterus in postmenopausal women receiving tamoxifen therapy for breast cancer: histopathologic correlation. Radiology 1996; 200(1): 105–10.

126. Bese T, Kosebay D, Demirkiran F et al. Ultrasonographic appearance of endometrium in postmenopausal breast cancer patients receiving tamoxifen. Eur J Obstet Gynecol Reprod Biol 1996; 67(2): 157–62.

127. Jaeger BM, Grumbach K. Tamoxifen induced endometrial abnormalities: evaluation by saline infusion sonohysterography. Md Med J 1997; 46(8): 433–5.

128. Ismail SM. Endometrial changes during tamoxifen treatment. Lancet 1998; 351(9105): 838.

129. Davies GC, Huster WJ, Shen W et al. Endometrial response to raloxifene compared with placebo, cyclical hormone

130. Cohen FJ, Watts S, Shah A et al. Uterine effects of 3-year raloxifene therapy in postmenopausal women younger than age 60. Obstet Gynecol 2000; 95(1): 104–10.

131. Delmas PD, Bjarnason NH, Mitlak BH et al. Effects of raloxifene on bone mineral density, serum cholesterol concentrations, and uterine endometrium in postmenopausal women. N Engl J Med 1997; 337(23): 1641–7.

132. Jolly EE, Bjarnason NH, Neven P et al. Prevention of osteoporosis and uterine effects in postmenopausal women taking raloxifene for 5 years. Menopause 2003; 10(4): 337–44.

133. Boss SM, Huster WJ, Neild JA et al. Effects of raloxifene hydrochloride on the endometrium of postmenopausal women. Am J Obstet Gynecol 1997; 177(6): 1458–64.

134. Goldstein SR, Scheele WH, Rajagopalan SK et al. A 12-month comparative study of raloxifene, estrogen, and placebo on the postmenopausal endometrium. Obstet Gynecol 2000; 95(1): 95–103.

135. Komm BS, Kharode YP, Bodine PV et al. Bazedoxifene acetate: a selective estrogen receptor modulator with improved selectivity. Endocrinology 2005; 146(9): 3999–4008.

136. Ronkin S, Northington R, Baracat E et al. Endometrial effects of bazedoxifene acetate, a novel selective estrogen receptor modulator, in postmenopausal women. Obstet Gynecol 2005; 105(6): 1397–404.

137. Ke HZ, Foley GL, Simmons HA et al. Long-term treatment of lasofoxifene preserves bone mass and bone strength and does not adversely affect the uterus in ovariectomized rats. Endocrinology 2004; 145(4): 1996–2005.

138. Ke HZ, Qi H, Chidsey-Frink KL et al. Lasofoxifene (CP-336,156) protects against the age-related changes in bone mass, bone strength, and total serum cholesterol in intact aged male rats. J Bone Miner Res 2001; 16(4): 765–73.

139. Ke HZ, Qi H, Crawford DT et al. Lasofoxifene (CP-336,156), a selective estrogen receptor modulator, prevents bone loss induced by aging and orchidectomy in the adult rat. Endocrinology 2000; 141(4): 1338–44.

140. Goldstein SR, Nanavati N. Adverse events that are associated with the selective estrogen receptor modulator levormeloxifene in an aborted phase III osteoporosis treatment study. Am J Obstet Gynecol 2002; 187(3): 521–7.

141. Komi J, Lankinen KS, Harkonen P et al. Effects of ospemifene and raloxifene on hormonal status, lipids, genital tract, and tolerability in postmenopausal women. Menopause 2005; 12(2): 202–9.

142. Rutanen EM, Heikkinen J, Halonen K et al. Effects of ospemifene, a novel SERM, on hormones, genital tract, climacteric symptoms, and quality of life in postmenopausal women: a double-blind, randomized trial. Menopause 2003; 10(5): 433–9.

143. Archer DF, Pickar JH. The assessment of bleeding patterns in postmenopausal women during continuous combined hormone replacement therapy: a review of methodology and recommendations for reporting of the data. Climacteric 2002; 5(1): 45–59.

144. Pickar JH, Archer DF. Is bleeding a predictor of endometrial hyperplasia in postmenopausal women receiving hormone replacement therapy? Menopause Study Group (United States, Italy, Netherlands, Switzerland, Belgium, Germany, and Finland). Am J Obstet Gynecol 1997; 177(5): 1178–83.

145. Archer DF, Lobo RA, Land HF, Pickar JH. A comparative study of transvaginal uterine ultrasound and endometrial biopsy for evaluating the endometrium of postmenopausal women taking hormone replacement therapy. Menopause 1999; 6(3): 201–8.

146. Archer DF, Dorin M, Lewis V et al. Effects of lower doses of conjugated equine estrogens and medroxyprogesterone

acetate on endometrial bleeding. Fertil Steril 2001; 75(6): 1080–7.

147. Archer DF, Pickar JH. Hormone replacement therapy: effect of progestin dose and time since menopause on endometrial bleeding. Obstet Gynecol 2000; 96(6): 899–905.

148. Hickey M, Lau TM, Russell P et al. Microvascular density in conditions of endometrial atrophy. Hum Reprod 1996; 11(9): 2009–13.

149. Hickey M, Crewe J, Mahoney LA et al. Mechanisms of irregular bleeding with hormone therapy: the role of matrix metalloproteinases and their tissue inhibitors. J Clin Endocrinol Metab 2006; 91(8): 3189–98.

150. Hickey M, Higham J, Sullivan M et al. Endometrial bleeding in hormone replacement therapy users: preliminary findings regarding the role of matrix metalloproteinase 9 (MMP-9) and tissue inhibitors of MMPs. Fertil Steril 2001; 75(2): 288–96.

151. Hickey M, Crewe J, Goodridge JP et al. Menopausal hormone therapy and irregular endometrial bleeding: a potential role for uterine natural killer cells? J Clin Endocrinol Metab 2005; 90(10): 5528–35.

152. Hickey M, Fraser I. Human uterine vascular structures in normal and diseased states. Microsc Res Tech 2003; 60(4): 377–89.

153. Mirkin S, Navarro F, Archer DF. Hormone therapy and endometrial angiogenesis. Climacteric 2003; 6(4): 273–7.

52 The effects of hormone therapy and botanicals and dietary supplements on the endometrium

Stacie E Geller and Laura Studee

INTRODUCTION

Every year, millions of women begin the menopausal transition. By the year 2030, the World Health Organization estimates 1.2 billion women will be age 50 or over, which is nearly triple the number of women in that age bracket in 1990.[1] The vast majority of women will experience some symptoms during the menopausal transition. This is also a time when many women begin to experience the signs and symptoms of midlife and aging.[2,3] During this phase, many women turn to some form of therapy, either hormonal or non-hormonal, to treat menopausal symptoms and prevent or treat chronic disease.

Hormone therapy (HT)[*] has been prescribed for a number of years for both menopausal symptoms as well as some conditions associated with aging. Hormone therapy is still considered the first line of treatment for vasomotor symptoms and is a treatment option for osteoporosis. However, given the results of the Women's Health Initiative (WHI), HT may not be considered by providers or desired by patients as the first line of treatment for menopausal symptoms and chronic conditions related to aging.[4] Many women are turning to alternative therapies such as botanical and dietary supplements (BDS) for relief.[4,5] Although the efficacy of both hormonal and non-hormonal therapies is important to understand, evidence regarding long-term safety of these treatments is also crucial. This chapter reviews the safety of HT as well as the commonly used botanicals and dietary supplements on the endometrium.

HORMONE THERAPY AND THE ENDOMETRIUM

Endometrial cancer and hyperplasia

The relationship of endometrial hyperplasia to endometrial cancer has long been recognized.[6,7] Subsequently, the relationship of HT, either estrogen plus progestin (E+P) or estrogen alone (E), to endometrial hyperplasia was investigated. It is now widely accepted that estrogen alone, when used for women with an intact uterus, increases the risk of endometrial hyperplasia and, if untreated, subsequently of endometrial cancer.[8,9]

The annual incidence of endometrial hyperplasia for women using E alone is thought to be about 20%.[10–13] In the Postmenopausal Estrogen/Progestin Interventions (PEPI) trial, 67% of the women with an intact uterus treated with ET developed endometrial hyperplasia by the end of 3 years.[14] In the Women's Health, Osteoporosis, Progestin, Estrogen (HOPE) study, 8% of women on a standard dose of ET (0.625 mg) developed hyperplasia as compared to <0.4% of women using E+P for over 1 year.[15] In a study of 218 women on unopposed estrogen (1 mg of 17β-estradiol) for 3 years, 9.4% of women developed hyperplasia.[15a] The risk of hyperplasia increases with increasing dose and increasing duration of use. Figure 52.1 illustrates the relationship of the risk of endometrial hyperplasia to hormone use.

The estimated cumulative incidence of endometrial cancer in developed countries for women aged 50–64 who do not use HT is about 5 in every 1000 women. Use of E alone is estimated to result in an additional 4 endometrial cancers per 1000 women for 5 years' use and an additional 10 per 1000 women for 10 years' use.[16] Based on a meta-analysis of 30 studies, Grady et al found a 2.3 relative risk (RR) of endometrial cancer in women using E alone compared with non-users. A much higher relative risk was reported for longer duration of estrogen use (RR =9.5 for ≥10 years of use).[17] Most of these studies have been conducted using oral conjugated equine estrogen (CEE), although other formulations and modes of transmission of estrogen have not been proven to be any safer on the endometrium. Figure 52.2 illustrates the risk of endometrial cancer to hormone use.

---

[*]The phrase hormone therapy (HT) refers to the combination of estrogen plus progestin (E+P). Reference to estrogen alone (E) will always be noted as such.

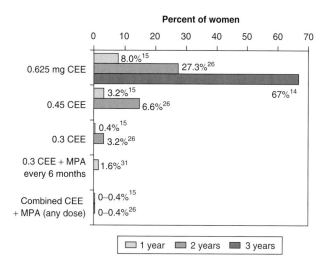

Figure 52.1 Percent of women with endometrial hyperplasia with hormone therapy use. CEE, conjugated equine estrogen; MPA, medroxyprogesterone acetate. As elsewhere in this chapter, superscript numbers refer to references.

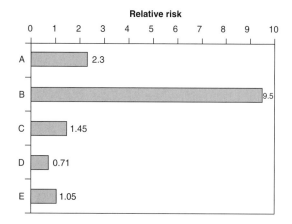

Figure 52.2 Relative risk of endometrial cancer with hormone therapy use. A=Estrogen only use (dose range 0.3–1.5 mg), all durations, from Grady meta-analysis.[17] B=Estrogen only use (dose range 0.3–1.5 mg), for >10 years, from Grady meta-analysis.[16] C=Estrogen only use, dose not specified, from Million Women Study. D=Continuous estrogen + progestin use, dose not specified, from Million Women Study.[16] E=Cyclic estrogen + progestin use, does not specified, from Million Women Study.[16] As elsewhere in this chapter, superscript numbers refer to references.

Combined hormone therapy (E+P)

Since use of unopposed estrogen alone is linked with a high risk of endometrial cancer, current hormonal treatment regimens combine continuous estrogen with continuous or sequential progestin in order to achieve the beneficial effects of estrogen while avoiding the potential for increased risk of endometrial cancer.

Progestin counteracts the proliferative effects of unopposed estrogens on endometrial tissue, thereby reducing the risks of both hyperplasia and, subsequently, endometrial cancer.[13,18,19] Several studies have documented this and most have been conducted using medroxyprogesterone acetate (MPA), although other doses and types of progestin are also highly effective.[14,20–22b]

In the WHI trial of estrogen (CEE) plus progestin (MPA), the endometrial cancer rates were low and were not increased by 5 years of E+P exposure. The Writing Group for the WHI Investigators suggest that is possible that close monitoring for bleeding and treatment of hyperplasia may contribute to the absence of increased risk of endometrial cancer.[4] In the estrogen-only (CEE) arm of the WHI, the issue of endometrial hyperplasia and endometrial cancer were not examined since all women were hysterectomized.[23]

For some women, progestins are associated with side effects such as bloating, weight gain, and breast tenderness, and many clinicians are prescribing cyclical or sequential use of progestin as opposed to continuous use to decrease these symptoms. A few studies have examined the safety issue of continuous vs cyclical use of progestin. One such study, the Million Women Study (MWS), was conducted in the UK in the period 1996–2001 to examine the effect of all hormone therapy (E+P or E alone) on the risk of incident and fatal breast cancer. The MWS also examined the effect of hormone use on endometrial cancer. They found that by comparison with never-users of hormones, continuous combined HT was associated with a reduced risk (RR=0.71), cyclical combined therapy with no alteration in risk (RR=1.05), and estrogen alone with increased risk of endometrial cancer (RR=1.45).[16] The risk of estrogen use alone was also significantly affected by a woman's body mass index (BMI), with the adverse effects of estrogen only in non-obese women. For women who reported use of tibolone, a synthetic steroid with estrogenic, progestagenic, and androgenic properties (not FDA [Food and Drug Administration] approved but used in UK and Europe), there was an even greater increased risk of endometrial cancer (RR =1.79).[16]

Other studies have shown that the more days every month that a progestin is used in a cyclic HT regimen, the lower the incidence of endometrial cancer.[10] Many of these studies found that women who received continuous combined HT had a lower risk of endometrial cancer than women who added a progestin for less than 10 days per month.[10,13,24,25] These data suggest that not only is the risk of endometrial cancer significantly reduced by adding progestin to estrogen therapy but also that increasing days per month may further reduce risk.[24]

Low-dose estrogen

In the wake of the results of the WHI, many providers are turning to lower doses of estrogen and progestin. The endometrial safety of lower doses of E+P was documented in the HOPE study. Healthy, postmenopausal women ($n = 2673$) with an intact uterus received one of the following treatments for 1 year: (a) CEE 0.625 mg/day, (b) CEE 0.625/MPA 2.5 mg/day, (c) CEE 0.45 mg/day, (d) CEE 0.45/MPA 2.5 mg/day, (e) CEE 0.45/MPA 1.5 mg/day, (f) CEE 0.3 mg/day, (g) CEE 0.3/MPA 1.5 mg/day, or (h) placebo.

At 1 year, endometrial hyperplasia rates ranged from 0 to 0.37% for all CEE/MPA doses. Ninety-one percent of the endometrial hyperplasia developed in women who were administered CEE 0.625 mg or CEE 0.45 mg without progestin. The incidence of endometrial hyperplasia increased with age for women administered CEE alone.[15] A subset of 822 women were followed for an additional year and at the end of 2 years there were no cases of endometrial hyperplasia in the four CEE/MPA groups. The results of this study suggest that 2 years of treatment with lower doses of CEE/MPA provided endometrial protection comparable to that seen with commonly prescribed higher doses.[26]

The endometrial safety of unopposed low-dose estrogen for women with an intact uterus (with no progestin) has rarely been studied. The limited available data do suggest that low-dose estrogen induces less hyperplasia than higher doses of estrogen.[27-29] In the HOPE study, for the CEE-alone groups, a dose-related increase in incidence rates of endometrial hyperplasia ranged from 3.17% with CEE 0.3 mg to 27.27% with CEE 0.625 mg (see Figure 52.1). More hyperplasia occurred with 0.45 mg or 0.625 mg/day than with 0.3 mg/day of CEE over 1 year.[15] A short-term (12-week) study comparing three doses of unopposed estrogen (0.25, 0.5, or 1.0 mg/day) showed less frequent endometrial thickening with 0.25 mg vs the higher doses.[30] One randomized controlled trial (RCT) using transdermal estrogen compared 25 vs 50 vs 150 μg/day for 12 weeks and found that metrorrhagia (bleeding between menstrual cycles) and endometrial hyperplasia were less frequent with the 25 μg than the higher doses (1 in 14 women). Given the limited data, despite a lower incidence of hyperplasia with low-dose estrogen, it should not be assumed to be safe on the endometrium, especially over the long term.

The other new trend in hormone use, along with low-dose estrogen, is use of progestin every 3–6 months for withdrawal bleeding to protect the uterus. The long-term safety of these regimens on the endometrium has received little study. One study, which used 0.3 mg/day of estrogen combined with a 14-day course of MPA (10 mg/day) every 6 months, found endometrial hyperplasia in only two women (1.6%, 95% confidence interval [CI] 0.3%, 6.2%).[31]

Some researchers suggest that for women using low-dose estrogen opposed by progestin at 6-month intervals, a 1–2% annual incidence of non-atypical hyperplasia is acceptable since histological progression occurs in only 20% of such cases.[31,32] Of course, this course of hormonal treatment demands more rigorous follow-up by the clinician, such as transvaginal ultrasounds and endometrial biopsies, to diagnose endometrial hyperplasia and treat these women before progression to endometrial cancer.

Conclusions

Use of an unopposed, standard dosage of estrogen conveys about a 15–20% annual risk of endometrial hyperplasia. Therefore, good medical practice dictates that for women who have an intact uterus, HT regimens should combine continuous estrogen with continuous or sequential progestin.[33] Women who receive any of several HT regimens of standard or low-dosage estrogen with progestin (daily, monthly cycle, or 3–6-month cycles) develop endometrial hyperplasia at a rate of about 1–2%.[14,34] The appropriate dosing and timing of progestin needed to adequately oppose the proliferative effect of estrogen on the endometrium is largely thought to be influenced by the dose of estrogen used.[25,35] Lower doses of estrogen suggest less hyperplasia than higher doses. However, most studies have insufficient sample size and duration of follow-up for conclusive information about long-term endometrial cancer risk with low-dose unopposed estrogen.

Lastly, it should be noted that lower doses of estrogen have not been proven any safer than higher doses of estrogen related to deep vein thrombosis, heart disease, stroke, and breast cancer and in fact providers are advised to assume equal risks until proven otherwise.[33] Notwithstanding, clinicians are increasingly prescribing lower doses of estrogen to treat menopausal symptoms. Consequently, the dose and duration of use for progestin with low-dose estrogenic treatment is undergoing a transformation. Since prevention of endometrial hyperplasia appears to depend on adequate dose and duration of progestin use, additional long-term safety studies (5 years or more) of these various regimens must be undertaken.

Treatment with lower doses of CEE/MPA have been shown to provide endometrial protection comparable to that seen with commonly prescribed higher doses. Other formulations and modes of transmission should also be studied. These regimens should be considered for postmenopausal women who are candidates for hormone therapy.

ENDOMETRIUM AND BOTANICAL AND DIETARY SUPPLEMENTS

Since the results of the Women's Health Initiative, many women are turning to botanical and dietary supplement products for relief of menopausal symptoms as well as prevention and treatment of chronic health conditions associated with aging. Women throughout the world have been using plant extracts for hundreds of years to treat uterine disorders, menstrual complaints, pregnancy, and childbirth, all apparently without toxic effects, although rigorous long-term safety trials are rare.[36,37] The use of BDS among menopausal women has increased exponentially in recent years.[38–40] In the USA and Britain, surveys show that 80% of peri- and postmenopausal women are current or former users of dietary supplements, and 60–70% of users cited the belief that these supplements are good for one's health. Most women report using alternative therapies because they find these options more congruent with their values, beliefs, and lifestyles. Women also believe that use of these herbal products is natural and safe and cannot hurt them.[38,41,42] Table 52.1 summarizes the studies which have reported on the effects of botanicals on the endometrium.

In the USA, botanicals are classified by the Dietary Supplement Health Education Act (DSHEA) as dietary supplements, not drugs, and are not intended for diagnosis, prevention, or treatment and therefore are not regulated by the FDA. This fact results in considerable variability of content, standardization, dosage, purity, and possible contamination of available products. In addition, careful long-term safety data, as seen with many of the hormone studies, are very limited.

Endometrium and phytoestrogens

Botanicals and dietary supplements can be divided into two broad categories – plants that exhibit estrogen-like properties (phytoestrogens which are weak estrogens) and plants that do not exhibit these characteristics. The major phytoestrogens with known estrogenic properties used by menopausal women are soy, red clover, and hops. Given that the development of endometrial cancer is largely related to prolonged exposure to unopposed estrogens, much investigation has been conducted to assess if phytoestrogens, which are thought to be weak estrogens found in plant foods, have estrogenic or antiestrogenic effects, especially on breast and endometrial tissue.

Soy and red clover have been the subject of much interest for the reduction of menopausal symptoms and conditions related to aging because of their high concentrations of phytoestrogens, specifically isoflavones, which are thought to be especially healthful. The studies of soy and red clover as a plant/food for alleviation of menopausal symptoms have not provided a clear answer to their role in reducing menopausal symptoms. A review of the literature from the more rigorous trials shows, at best, only a mild to modest effect on vasomotor symptoms.[43–45] However, many women continue to use isoflavones as they age because of their purported positive effect on cognition, bone, and lipid profiles. Careful examination of the endometrial safety of these products must be considered.

Soy isoflavones

Soy isoflavones have been consumed in large quantities across the world for centuries and are commonly used by midlife women, either in food, protein supplement, or isoflavone tablet form. Epidemiological studies over the past decade have suggested a protective effect for chronic diseases, including heart disease, as well as a number of cancers (breast, endometrial, and prostate). The FDA has approved a health claim for isoflavone-rich soy protein, stating that consumption of 25 g of soy protein daily can reduce cholesterol levels.[46] The German Commission E, a health regulatory body that regulates dietary supplements, has also approved soy (as soy lecithin or soy phospholipid) for hypercholesterolemia.[47]

Isoflavones belong to a class of compounds known as phytoestrogens which occur naturally in many plants and have structural and functional similarities to human estrogen, 17β-estradiol.[48,49] Soy, in particular, contains very high amounts of isoflavones, particularly genistein, daidzein, and glycitein. These are readily absorbed and metabolized in the gut and are well tolerated without reported adverse effects.[50]

Phytoestrogens, such as those found in soy, have been shown to lower endogenous estrogen levels.[51,52] Another effect of phytoestrogen is the stimulation of sex hormone-binding globulin (SHBG) production

Table 52.1 Clinical trials of botanicals and their effect on the endometrium

Reference	Description of groups, botanical type, and dosage	Study design[a]	Number of participants	Duration	Effect on the endometrium
Balk et al[64]	Soy cereal with 92 mg of isoflavones per serving Placebo	RCT	27 postmenopausal women	6 months	Phytoestrogens did not cause stimulation of the endometrium, as assessed by endometrial biopsy, compared to placebo
Nikander et al[65]	Soy isoflavone tablet with 114 mg of isoflavones Placebo	R, CO study	64 postmenopausal women with history of breast cancer	3 months	No changes in proliferation markers in the endometrium with isoflavone compared to placebo
Kaari et al[66]	Soy isoflavone tablet with 120 mg of isoflavones Conjugated estrogen: 0.625 mg Placebo	RCT	79 postmenopausal women	6 months	No significant differences in endometrial proliferation for isoflavone group after 6 months treatment compared to placebo. Significant increase in endometrial proliferation for estrogen group
Unfer et al[67]	Soy isoflavone tablet with 150 mg of isoflavones Placebo	RCT	376 postmenopausal women	5 years	After 5 years of treatment, incidence of endometrial hyperplasia was significantly higher in the isoflavone group compared to placebo (3.4% vs 0%)
Hale et al[81]	Red clover tablet with 50 mg of purified isoflavones Placebo	RCT	30 perimenopausal women	3 months	No proliferative effect of red clover isoflavones on the endometrium compared to placebo
Baber et al[80]	Red clover tablet with 40 mg of purified isoflavones Placebo	R, CO study	51 postmenopausal women	12 weeks	No changes in endometrial tissue after 3 months of treatment compared to placebo
Nappi et al[101]	Black cohosh: 40 mg/day Low-dose transdermal estradiol: 25 mg every 7 days	RCT	64 postmenopausal women	3 months	No changes in endometrial thickness after treatment compared to placebo
Wuttke et al[102]	Black cohosh: 40 mg Conjugated estrogen (CE): 0.6 mg Placebo	RCT	62 postmenopausal women	3 months	No changes in endometrial thickness after treatment with black cohosh compared to placebo. Estrogen significantly increased endometrial thickness
Liske et al[104]	Standard (S): 39 mg High (H): 127.9 mg dose of black cohosh	RCT	152 peri- and postmenopausal women	24 weeks	No changes in vaginal cell proliferation or vaginal ultrasound for both groups compared to baseline
Hirata et al[108]	Dong quai root: 4.5 g/day Placebo	RCT	71 postmenopausal women	24 weeks	Dong quai did not promote endometrial proliferation or increase maturation of vaginal epithelial cells compared to placebo

[a]RCT = randomized controlled trial; R = randomized; CO = cross-over.

in the liver. Higher SHBG levels result in less free estradiol, reducing the amount of estrogen available to bind to estrogen receptors (ERs).[53] Finally, phytoestrogens bind competitively to ER, thereby blocking binding by other estrogens.[54,55] Because the estrogenic potential of phytoestrogens is weak ($\leq 0.1\%$ of estradiol), and they do not elicit a strong estrogenic response, they are thought to have antiestrogenic effects that may inhibit growth and proliferation of estrogen-dependent cancer cells.[56]

Other investigators have also found a non-estrogenic mechanism of action. In a study by Teede et al, 50 women were randomized to consume either soy protein isolates (40 g of soy protein and 118 mg of isoflavone) or placebo, and then measures of hepatic proteins and gonadotropin concentrations were assessed. At the end of 3 months, there were no differences between the treatment and control group, suggesting that soy/isoflavones do not affect in-vivo biological indicators of estrogenicity and most likely act more like selective estrogen receptor modulators (SERMs) and, as such, may be safe for endometrial tissue and possibly protective.[57]

The data from animal, epidemiological, and clinical studies present a somewhat varied picture of soy safety. A series of animal studies on both mice and rats found significant increases in uterine weight after subcutaneous injections of isoflavones (genistein) with 2–4 weeks of treatment.[58,59] When newborn mice (1–5 days old) were given genistein subcutaneously, not only did uterine weight increase but also they exhibited atypical hyperplasia, squamous metaplasia, and uterine adenocarcinoma.[60] Since soy isoflavones were given subcutaneously to the animals, not in food, it is not possible to extrapolate these findings to humans.

In humans, soy is metabolized in the digestive system, and the adsorption, distribution, and metabolism of soy isoflavones by the digestive system can vary widely by individual.[50] In women, most research examining the relationship between soy isoflavones and endometrial safety has focused on epidemiological studies of endometrial cancer rates. These studies have compared the incidence of endometrial cancer of high soy consumers generally found in Asian countries, where women consume up to 40 mg of soy daily, to low soy consumers, generally found in North America and Europe, where women consume less than 2 mg of soy. These studies have found a decreased risk of endometrial cancer in areas of high soy consumption.[61] Two case-control studies conducted in the USA (Hawaii and San Francisco) found an inverse relationship between soy consumption and risk of endometrial cancer: the higher the soy consumption, the lower the risk of endometrial cancer.[62,63] However, in the San Francisco study, the reduction in risk was stronger for postmenopausal women than for premenopausal women.[63] This epidemiological evidence seems to suggest that soy has a protective effect against endometrial cancer. However, the presumed protective effect of soy isoflavones may have been a combination of several factors, including the consumption of soy early in life, a low-fat and high-fiber diet, as well as a less sedentary lifestyle.

The data from RCTs present a fairly positive, although somewhat different, picture. Short-term placebo-controlled studies of 3–6 months have found no stimulation of the endometrium with isoflavone supplementation.[64,65] A 6-month estrogen controlled trial of soy isoflavones found that while estrogen increased endometrium proliferation, isoflavone tablets had no effect on the endometrium.[66] However, the only long-term, 5-year trial, of soy isoflavone tablets (150 mg of isoflavones per day) vs placebo found an increased occurrence of endometrial hyperplasia in postmenopausal women who consumed isoflavone (3.3.% vs 0%), a rate similar to that seen with low-dose estrogen use.[67]

It does appear from epidemiological studies that high soy intake may show a protective effect on the endometrium and short-term clinical studies of soy (3–6 months) show no adverse effect on the endometrium. However, longer-term use (5 years) may pose some risk and requires additional clinical studies to determine the long-term safety.

Red clover (Trifolium pratense)

Red clover is another commonly used phytoestrogen for treatment of menopausal symptoms and conditions related to aging. It is native to Europe and the Middle East, but is now found throughout the world. Traditionally, it has been used as an abortifacient, anticancer treatment, antispasmodic, menstrual regulator, and wound healer. In recent years, it has been touted as a natural alternative to hormone therapy for menopausal women.[68]

Similar to soy, red clover is a rich source of isoflavones; however, it has a distinct chemical profile from soy, with higher levels of O-methylated isoflavones, formononetin and biochanin A, and less daidzein and genistein than soy.[69,70] The commercially available red clover extracts are the hydrolyzed form of the isoflavones; they enhance bioavailability by gut bacteria and are easily absorbed into the intestine.[71]

Red clover has been shown to have some estrogenic properties in vitro. Receptor-binding experiments have shown that the isoflavones present in red clover bind to both ERα and ERβ, but all of the isoflavones bind preferentially to ERβ.[72–74] Experiments have found that a methanolic extract of red clover up-regulates the estrogen-induced genes in a breast cancer cell line and endometrial adenocarcinoma cell line (Ishikawa cells).[73] There is little dispute, therefore, that in vitro, red clover exhibits weak estrogenic activity, although the tendency of isoflavones to bind preferentially to ERβ over ERα suggests that, similar to soy, they may protect against cancers rather than promote growth, but the potential effects on the endometrium are unclear.[71]

Animal studies have also confirmed an estrogenic effect on the uterus. Subterranean clover (T. subterranean), similar to red clover, contains large amounts of phytoestrogens, and its consumption by sheep in Australia in the 1940s resulted in infertility, abnormal lactation, dystocia, and prolapsed uterus.[75] In ovariectomized sheep, red clover caused clear estrogenic effects, including enlargement of the uterus.[76] In immature rats, phytoestrogens in feed containing red clover were directly related to uterotropic effects.[77] Also, in an ovariectomized rat model, red clover extract exhibited uterotropic effects.[78] It is difficult to conclude if these animal studies are applicable to humans, because of differences in physiology, metabolism, and supplement type and dose.

Of the red clover clinical trials for menopausal symptoms, most have not reported on endometrial effects, but three studies did report no increase in endometrial thickness.[79,80] Additionally, a placebo-controlled pilot study that examined, as its primary outcome, the endometrial effects of red clover during perimenopause, found no evidence of a proliferative effect of red clover on the endometrium.[81] As these studies were all conducted for less than 6 months, it appears that red clover, similar to soy, may be safe for short-term use, but more clinical studies need to be conducted to determine if red clover extracts are safe on the endometrium over the long term.

Hops (Humulus lupulus)

Hops is native to Asia, Europe, and North America, and is mostly known for its use in beer production. The therapeutic uses of hops, as approved by the German Commission E, are for mood disturbances and anxiety and it is used by women undergoing the menopausal transition.[47]

The class of phytoestrogens present in hops is known as prenylflavonoids (a class of non-steroidal phytoestrogens), but they are thought to be more potent than other phytoestrogens. In molecular binding assays, hops extracts have been shown to bind to both ERα and ERβ and up-regulate estrogen-dependent genes in a similar manner to red clover extracts.[71,73,82] Experiments performed on breast cancer cell lines have demonstrated the ability of hops extracts to cause proliferation in the absence of estrogen and inhibit proliferation in the presence of estrogen.[74,83]

Hops appears to exert estrogenic effects on the uterus and vaginal epithelium at the animal level, although the studies are somewhat contradictory. Early studies of immature mice showed a uterotropic effect of hops extract.[84] Other research has found no uterotropic effects after 3 weeks of treatment with hops in ovariectomized rats, but did find that hops' treatment increased vaginal epithelium, increased vascular permeability, and elevated hepatic levels, indicating estrogenic effects on these different tissues.[85]

No human trials have been done to examine the effects of hops on the endometrium. Hops has only been studied in combination with other botanicals, such as valerian and lemon balm, for use as a sleeping aid, but no safety studies have been reported on the endometrium. Given the clear estrogenic effects in vitro and in animal models, and the fact that hops appears not to exert SERM-like selectivity as seen with other phytoestrogens, it may pose negative effects on the endometrium. It is important to conduct future studies on the long-term safety effects of hops in menopausal women.

Endometrium and other botanicals used for menopause

A number of other botanicals are thought not to have an estrogenic mechanism of action and it would be hypothesized that these herbs would therefore be safe on the endometrium, although most have not been studied for endometrial safety.

Black cohosh (Cimicifuga racemosa)

Black cohosh is a plant native to North America and is commonly used for menopausal symptoms, including hot flashes, irritability, sleep disturbances, and vertigo.[86] The German Commission E has approved the use of 40 mg/day of black cohosh for 6 months for relief of menopausal symptoms, although in Germany, many women use this herbal remedy for longer periods of time with physician oversight.[47] There have been several clinical trials conducted in Germany since the

1940s and most have shown positive results for reduction of hot flashes. However, the methodology in some of these studies was weak, many were sponsored by the manufacturers, and limited long-term safety data have been reported.[73,74,87] There are currently several ongoing RCTs in the USA to further assess efficacy and long-term safety of black cohosh on the endometrium.

Black cohosh contains triterpine glycosides, flavonoids, aromatic acids, and other constituents, although the exact mechanism of action and whether black cohosh has estrogenic activity has been debated for a number of years.[88] There have been data both supporting and refuting the estrogenic activity of black cohosh. Early studies of ovariectomized rats found that black cohosh causes a selective reduction of luteinizing hormone (LH) but no increase in uterine weight.[89,90] An open clinical study of menopausal women also found that black cohosh inhibited LH, but not follicle-stimulating hormone (FSH) secretions, which led the authors to hypothesize that black cohosh had an estrogen-like effect in menopausal women.[91] However, this effect on LH has not been duplicated in other animal or clinical studies.

In fact, more recent studies have refuted the likelihood of estrogenic activity. Numerous studies of ER-positive cell lines have shown than black cohosh extracts do not stimulate growth or stimulate estrogen-dependent gene expression.[73,83,87,92] Human studies have shown no effect on serum hormone levels of LH, FSH, prolactin, SHBG, and estradiol.[93] Recent data, in fact, have demonstrated that black cohosh may be a partial agonist of the serotonin receptor, which may be the mechanism for relief of hot flashes and improvement in mood.[94–96] In particular, the work of Burdette et al indicates that black cohosh acts on serotonin receptors but not on estrogen receptors.[94]

Several animal studies in both mice and rats have found no negative effects of black cohosh specifically on uterine tissue, no increases in uterine weight, or stimulation of vaginal epithelium, all suggesting that black cohosh does not exert estrogenic effects. Large doses of black cohosh (600 mg/kg) administered orally or subcutaneously did not exert vaginotropic effects on ovariectomized rats or uterotropic effects on immature mice.[94,97–99] Uteri removed from rats treated with three doses (4, 40, 400 mg/kg daily) showed no increase in weight compared to controls. Animals that received black cohosh in conjunction with estrogen had similar uterine weights compared with estrogen alone.[94] Furthermore, a black cohosh extract in the dose of 60 mg/kg did not exhibit uterotropic effects or affect estrogen-dependent gene expression in the uterus of ovariectomized rats.[100]

Although there have been a number of clinical trials of black cohosh for relief of vasomotor symptoms, few have reported on the safety effects of black cohosh on the endometrium. Four short-term clinical trials (3 months) of black cohosh for menopausal symptoms found no changes in endometrial thickness after treatment compared to placebo.[96,101–103] Two studies of black cohosh extract lasting 6 months each found either no vaginal cell proliferation or no changes in vaginal ultrasound.[104,105] A one year study of a black cohosh extract (CR BNO 1055) recently reported no increase in endometrial thickness for either placebo or treatment groups.[105a]

In summary, black cohosh has an overall positive safety profile for up to 6 months. In fact, because black cohosh is thought to be serotonergic, it is considered a safe alternative for women in whom estrogen therapy is contraindicated, and has been suggested for relief of vasomotor symptoms for women with breast cancer who are prescribed tamoxifen. It is also considered safe on the endometrium, although long-term safety trials are needed.

Dong quai (Angelica sinesis)

Dong quai is one of the most commonly prescribed Chinese herbs for problems unique to women and has been traditionally known as 'a female tonic.' Traditional systems of medicine and folk medicine have used dong quai for a variety of complaints, including abnormal menstruation and menopausal symptoms.[106] Taken alone, dong quai does not appear to be beneficial for menopausal symptoms; however, it is mostly used in multibotanical formulations and is still considered to be a valuable female tonic by herbalists around the world.

It is debatable as to whether dong quai has any estrogenic activity, as in-vitro and animal studies present conflicting evidence. Molecular and cell culture experiments have shown dong quai to weakly bind to ERα and ERβ.[73] Amato et al analyzed the effects of 17β-estradiol and herbal extracts on the growth of an estrogen-dependent breast cancer cell line, MCF-7. At high doses, dong quai and ginseng significantly induced the growth of MCF-7 cells in a dose-dependent manner, although black cohosh and licorice root did not.[107] Other investigators have not observed estrogenic activity. Zava et al reported that dong quai did not bind to ERs and had no effect on breast cancer cell growth.[74]

Animal studies have also shown mixed effects of dong quai on the uterus. Amato et al compared several botanicals to assess estrogenic activity in ovariectomized mice and utilized a group treated with 17β-estradiol as a positive control group. As expected, the mean uterine weight of the estrogen-treated group was approximately 1.7-fold higher than that of the control group. There were no significant differences in uterine weight among any of the herb-treated groups (black cohosh, licorice, ginseng, dong quai) relative to the untreated controls. However, a study using an ovariectomized rat model observed a uterotropic effect after supplementation with dong quai for 3 weeks.[85]

Only one human study has examined the effects of dong quai on menopausal symptoms and endometrial tissue. Postmenopausal women were randomized to receive either dong quai or placebo for 24 weeks. The study demonstrated that dong quai did not significantly reduce hot flashes and did not promote endometrial proliferation or increase maturation of vaginal epithelial cells as compared to placebo.[108]

There have also been several case reports of increased bleeding due to the interaction of dong quai with anticoagulant medications.[109] Given its unproven clinical efficacy, the potential for adverse effects secondary to herb–drug interactions, and lack of long-term safety trials, dong quai should be used with care.

Other botanicals and dietary supplements

Chaste tree (*Vitex agnus-castus*) has been used for centuries to treat various female complaints, including premenstrual syndrome, cyclical breast discomfort, and menstrual cycle irregularities, and has been approved by the German Commission E for these uses.[47] The progesterone-like effect of *Vitex* has been verified by endometrial biopsy, analysis of blood hormone levels, and examination of vaginal secretions.[110]

Two recent in-vitro studies have examined the estrogenicity of chaste tree. In a receptor-binding assay, chaste tree was found to bind only to ERβ and not ERα.[111] Liu et al found that linoleic acid from chaste tree fruit can bind to both ERα and ERβ and that estrogen-induced genes were up-regulated in endometrial cells.[112] There are several clinical studies of chaste tree but no endometrial effects have been reported.

Ginkgo (*Ginkgo biloba*) has been approved by the German Commission E for cerebral insufficiency, vertigo and tinnitus, and peripheral vascular disease.[47] It is often taken by menopausal women who are concerned about memory loss and decreased cognition. One in-vitro study has examined the estrogenic effects of ginkgo and found it to have weak estrogenic activity on both ERα and ERβ in competitive binding assays, although the binding affinity was higher for ERβ than for ERα. Gingko induced cell proliferation in ER-positive breast

cell lines (MCF-7) but not in ER negative cells.[113] This suggests potential estrogenic activity, but further in-vitro, animal, and human studies are needed to elucidate the effects of ginkgo on the endometrium.

Licorice (*Glycyrrhiza glabra*) is approved by the German Commission E for inflammation of the mucous membrane of the upper respiratory tract and ulcers.[47] In menopausal women, licorice is not taken alone, but as part of a multibotanical supplement. In-vitro experiments of licorice extracts have documented a weak estrogen agonist effect of licorice.[73,74,114] In rat models, two components of licorice, glabridin and glabrene, increased uterine weight and induced estrogen-dependent proteins in uterine tissue.[115,116] Amato et al observed no change in uterine weight in mice after being fed a licorice extract for 4 days.[107] No published human studies have examined endometrium outcomes with licorice use. There is no scientific information to support the estrogenic properties of licorice. Doses of more than 500 mg/day have been associated with congestive heart failure.[117] Furthermore, excessive licorice ingestion has been associated with side effects due to its mineralocorticoid activity.[118]

Ginseng (*Panax ginseng*) is known as a traditional 'tonic' herb that is reported to cope with stress and to boost immunity. The German Commission E lists its uses as 'a tonic for invigoration and fortification in times of fatigue and debility and for declining capacity for work and concentration'.[47] Controversy exists in the scientific literature regarding the estrogenic activity of ginseng. It is structurally similar to estrogen, which suggests a possible estrogenic effect; however, there is no evidence of efficacy in menopausal women.[119] Amato et al found that at high doses, ginseng significantly induced the growth of MCF-7 cells in a dose-dependent manner.[107] Several human studies have showed no estrogenic effects, no improvement in vasomotor symptoms, but improvement in somatic complaints (fatigue, insomnia, depression) and a very favorable effect on depression and well-being health subscales compared with placebo.[120] Because of increased breast cell proliferation in vitro, its use is not advisable in the presence of breast cancer, although more research on ginseng's effects on breast cells in vivo is needed to know its true safety.[107] No safety trials have been conducted to test the effects of ginseng on endometrial tissue.

The botanicals motherwort, evening primrose, kava, valerian, St John's wort, and wild yam are commonly used for menopausal symptoms, generally in the form of a multibotanical and are thought not to be estrogenic. There are no published data on the endometrial effects of these herbs.

Motherwort (*Leonurus cardiaca*) is another botanical historically revered as a calmative agent for the heart, especially palpitations.[121] The German Commission E has approved its use for nervous cardiac disorders and as an adjuvant for thyroid hyperfunction.[47] It is also found in many menopausal formulas for women experiencing this symptom and was typically combined with black cohosh as a 'superior antispasmodic and nervine;' however, contemporary research is lacking on efficacy and safety.

Evening primrose (*Oenothera biennis*) contains gamolinolenic acid as its main active compound. It is an essential fatty acid, not a hormone or phytoestrogen, and is thought not to be estrogenic.[122] The only RCT of evening primrose for menopausal symptoms found no differences in the reduction of hot flashes between the two groups.[123]

Kava (*Piper methysticum*) is a South Pacific herb used medicinally and socially and data suggest efficacy for treatment of anxiety.[124] Two trials evaluating kava's effect on menopausal symptoms showed significant improvement in irritability and insomnia compared with placebo.[125] Although there have been no negative reports on the endometrium, there are a number of safety issues related to kava. The sale of kava has been banned in Canada, Australia, and several European countries because of potential hepatotoxicity. The FDA, American Botanical Council, and various industry trade organizations have advised consumers of rare but potential risks of severe liver injury associated with the use of kava-containing preparations.[126]

Valerian (*Valeriana officinalis*) has been used for centuries and is currently approved by the German Commission E for 'states of unrest and nervous sleep disturbances.'[47] The key active components of valerian are sesquiterpenes of the volatile oil. These compounds, along with others present in valerian, have been shown to have direct sedative effects and interact with neurotransmitters such as GABA (γ-aminobutyric acid).[127] Three RCTs have been conducted that have shown improved subjective sleep quality, although none of the studies was conducted with menopausal women.[43] There have been no reported drug interactions; side effects, such as nausea, headache, dizziness, and upset stomach, have been reported in less than 10% of subjects in RCTs.[128]

St John's wort (*Hypericum perforatum*) is one of the most heavily studied botanicals for treatment of depression and has been shown to be superior to placebo or equivalent to antidepressant medications.[129] St John's wort works in a similar manner to selective serotonin reuptake inhibitors (SSRIs) and is therefore presumed to be non-estrogenic and safe for the endometrium, although there are no published reports.

Wild yam (*Dioscorea villosa*) was formerly referred to as 'colic root' and has been promoted as effective for gastrointestinal irritation and spasm. Historically, it was also used for menstrual cramps and postpartum pain. Despite promotional claims, wild yam does not convert to a progesterone when taken internally or applied topically and has no estrogenic properties. One RCT of topical wild yam extract cream vs placebo showed no difference in alleviation of menopausal symptoms or serum/salivary hormone levels.[130] Although popular for menopause, there is no contemporary or historical evidence of benefit.

Conclusions on BDS

A growing body of scientific literature suggests that incorporation of some form of alternative therapy could result in improved clinical outcomes for menopausal and aging women. Several commonly used botanicals appear to be safe on the endometrium for short-term use; however, controversy exists in the scientific literature regarding the estrogenic activity of many of these herbs. Of the botanicals reviewed, black cohosh, due to its serotonergic action, may present the strongest safety profile for protection of the endometrium. Red clover and soy also appear to be safe with short-term use. The risk of endometrial hyperplasia after 5 years of soy isoflavones use is about equal to use of low-dose unopposed estrogen (0.3 mg) after 2 years (see Figure 52.1 and Table 52.1).[15,67] However, a diet rich in soy protein has also been shown to be beneficial in protecting against conditions of aging and may protect against estrogen-dependent cancers.

Many of the other botanicals may be safe for use; however, limited study has been conducted to assess long-term safety. Although there have been a number of observational, epidemiological, and clinical studies conducted for relief of menopausal symptoms, there is a continued need for further research on the effectiveness and long-term safety of botanicals and dietary supplements, especially on the endometrium. Double-blind, randomized, placebo-controlled trials assessing the safety and efficacy of these treatments are needed. Trials of these compounds used alone or in combination for treatment of menopausal symptoms or prevention of age-related conditions such as heart disease and osteoporosis should include assays on the effects of these herbs on the human endometrium. In addition, regulation of content, standardization of dosage, and accurate labeling of safety and efficacy should be required and would serve to increase public and professional confidence in these products.

PROS AND CONS OF ALTERNATIVE THERAPIES COMPARED TO STANDARD HORMONE THERAPY

Vasomotor symptoms are a major clinical complaint among menopausal women. HT is a proven effective treatment for relief of hot flashes and has also been shown to reduce fracture rates as women age, although there are several other therapeutic options to treat osteoporosis. HT regimens prescribed appropriately, combined continuous estrogen with continuous or sequential progestin, for women with an intact uterus, protects the endometrium at a rate similar to that of the general population. However, HT has well-proven risks associated with its use, including increased risk for breast cancer, cardiovascular disease, and pulmonary embolism. Also, the side effects associated with HT, generally from the progestin, are quite bothersome for some women. Additionally, HT is not considered a viable treatment for women with hot flashes who have ER-positive cancers and may be prescribed tamoxifen.

Non-hormonal pharmacological alternatives provide an option for women who are either reluctant to use exogenous hormones or cannot use HT, with seemingly fewer side effects than those of hormones. The clinical trials to date suggest that black cohosh is an effective herb for relief of hot flashes and, due to its serotonergic mechanism of action, is safe for the endometrium. Phytoestrogens, in the form of soy and red clover, although not proven effective for hot flashes, can provide positive health effects on plasma lipid concentrations and may be protective for cognitive decline and bone loss. In addition, epidemiological studies even suggest protection against estrogen-dependent cancers such as endometrial cancer, although the mechanism of action is not understood.

Other botanicals discussed may improve other clinical complaints associated with menopause and aging such as mood disorders, depression, sleep, and anxiety, but there are limited efficacy data and even less safety evidence. Theoretically, those botanicals that have a weak estrogenic effect may exhibit SERM-like behavior but it is unclear whether they pose any threat to women in general and ER-positive cancer patients in particular, although it is probably a reduced risk compared to hormones, given the evidence to date. However, until long-term safety has been proven, caution should be taken with breast cancer patients in particular.

There are both positive and negative aspects to any choice. Whatever decision menopausal women make related to the use of hormone therapy or botanicals for relief of menopausal symptoms as well as to promote long-term health, it is critical to discuss these issues with their healthcare providers so they can assist them in managing these choices through an evidence-based approach.

REFERENCES

1. World Menopause Day [website]. Available at: http://www.imsociety.org/pages/wmday.html. Accessed on December 1, 2005.
2. Whiteman MK, Staropoli CA, Benedict JC et al. Risk factors for hot flashes in midlife women. J Womens Health (Larchmt) 2003; 12: 459–72.
3. Grisso JA, Freeman EW, Maurin E et al. Racial differences in menopause information and the experience of hot flashes. J Gen Intern Med 1999; 14: 98–103.
4. Rossouw JE, Anderson GL, Prentice RL et al. Risks and benefits of oestrogen plus progestin in healthy postmenopausal women: principal results from the Women's Health Initiative randomized controlled trial. JAMA 2002; 288: 321–33.
5. Kolata G. Race to fill the void in menopause drug market. The New York Times September 1, 2002, 2002; National Desk: 1.
6. Novak E, Yui E. Relation of endometrial hyperplasia to adenocarcinoma of uterus. Am J Obstet Gynecol 1936; 32: 674–98.
7. Taylor HJ. Endometrial hyperplasia and carcinoma of the body of uterus. Am J Obstet Gynecol 1932; 23: 309–32.
8. Gusberg S. Precursors of corpus carcinoma estrogens and adenomatous hyperplasia. Am J Obstet Gynecol 1947; 54: 905–27.
9. Hertig A, Sommers S. Genesis of endometrial carcinoma. Cancer 1949; 2: 946–56.
10. Pike MC, Peters RK, Cozen W et al. Estrogen–progestin replacement therapy and endometrial cancer. J Natl Cancer Inst 1997; 89: 1110–16.
11. Jick SS, Walker AM, Jick H. Estrogens, progesterone, and endometrial cancer. Epidemiology 1993; 4: 20–4.
12. Brinton LA, Hoover RN. Estrogen replacement therapy and endometrial cancer risk: unresolved issues. The Endometrial Cancer Collaborative Group. Obstet Gynecol 1993; 81: 265–71.
13. Beresford SA, Weiss NS, Voigt LF et al. Risk of endometrial cancer in relation to use of oestrogen combined with cyclic progestagen therapy in postmenopausal women. Lancet 1997; 349: 458–61.
14. Effects of hormone replacement therapy on endometrial histology in postmenopausal women. The Postmenopausal Estrogen/Progestin Interventions (PEPI) Trial. The Writing Group for the PEPI Trial. JAMA 1996; 275: 370–5.
15. Pickar JH, Yeh I, Wheeler JE et al. Endometrial effects of lower doses of conjugated equine oestrogens and medroxyprogesterone acetate. Fertil Steril 2001; 76: 25–31.
15a. Steiner AZ, Xiang M, Mack WJ et al. Unopposed estradiol therapy in postmenopausal women: results from two randomized trials. Obstet Gynecol 2007; 108: 578–80.
16. Beral V, Bull D, Reeves G. Endometrial cancer and hormone-replacement therapy in the Million Women Study. Lancet 2005; 365: 1543–51.
17. Grady D, Gebretsadik T, Kerlikowske K et al. Hormone replacement therapy and endometrial cancer risk: a meta-analysis. Obstet Gynecol 1995; 85: 304–13.

18. Weiderpass E, Adami HO, Baron JA et al. Risk of endometrial cancer following estrogen replacement with and without progestins. J Natl Cancer Inst 1999; 91: 1131–7.

19. Gambrell RD Jr. Strategies to reduce the incidence of endometrial cancer in postmenopausal women. Am J Obstet Gynecol 1997; 177: 1196–204.

20. Randall TC, Kurman RJ. Progestin treatment of atypical hyperplasia and well-differentiated carcinoma of the endometrium in women under age 40. Obstet Gynecol 1997; 90: 434–40.

21. Wentz WB. Treatment of persistent endometrial hyperplasia with progestins. Am J Obstet Gynecol 1966; 96: 999–1004.

22. Woodruff JD, Pickar JH. Incidence of endometrial hyperplasia in postmenopausal women taking conjugated estragens (Premarin) with medroxyprogesterone acetate or conjugated estrogens alone. The Menopause Study Group. Am J Obstet Gynecol 1994; 170: 1213–23.

22a. Samsioe G, Dvorak V, Genazzani AR et al. One-year endometrial safety evaluation of a continuous combined transdermal matrix patch delivery low-dose estradiol-norethisterone acetate in postmenopausal women. Maturitas 2007; 57: 171–81.

22b. Wildemeersch D, Pylyser K, DeWever N, Pavwels P, Tjalma W. Endometrial safety after 5 years of continuous combined transdermal estrogen and intrauterine levonorgestrel delivery for postmenopausal hormone subsitution. Maturitas 2007; 57: 205–9.

23. Anderson GL, Limacher M, Assaf AR et al. Effects of conjugated equine estrogen in postmenopausal women with hysterectomy: the Women's Health Initiative randomized controlled trial. JAMA 2004; 291: 1701–12.

24. Hill DA, Weiss NS, Beresford SA et al. Continuous combined hormone replacement therapy and risk of endometrial cancer. Am J Obstet Gynecol 2000; 183: 1456–61.

25. Voigt LF, Weiss NS, Chu J et al. Progestagen supplementation of exogenous oestrogens and risk of endometrial cancer. Lancet 1991; 338: 274–7.

26. Pickar JH, Yeh IT, Wheeler JE et al. Endometrial effects of lower doses of conjugated equine estrogens and medroxyprogesterone acetate: two-year substudy results. Fertil Steril 2003; 80: 1234–40.

27. Utian WH, Burry KA, Archer DF et al. Efficacy and safety of low, standard, and high dosages of an estradiol transdermal system (Esclim) compared with placebo on vasomotor symptoms in highly symptomatic menopausal patients. The Esclim Study Group. Am J Obstet Gynecol 1999; 181: 71–9.

28. Genant HK, Lucas J, Weiss S et al. Low-dose esterified estrogen therapy: effects on bone, plasma estradiol concentrations, endometrium, and lipid levels. Estratab/Osteoporosis Study Group. Arch Intern Med 1997; 157: 2609–15.

29. Speroff L, Rowan J, Symons J et al. The comparative effect on bone density, endometrium, and lipids of continuous hormones as replacement therapy (CHART study). A randomized controlled trial. JAMA 1996; 276: 1397–403.

30. Prestwood KM, Kenny AM, Unson C et al. The effect of low dose micronized 17ss-estradiol on bone turnover, sex hormone levels, and side effects in older women: a randomized, double blind, placebo-controlled study. J Clin Endocrinol Metab 2000; 85: 4462–9.

31. Ettinger B, Pressman A, Van Gessel A. Low-dosage esterified estrogens opposed by progestin at 6-month intervals. Obstet Gynecol 2001; 98: 205–11.

32. Speroff L, Whitcomb RW, Kempfert NJ et al. Efficacy and local tolerance of a low-dose, 7-day matrix estradiol transdermal system in the treatment of menopausal vasomotor symptoms. Obstet Gynecol 1996; 88: 587–92.

33. Executive summary. Hormone therapy. Obstet Gynecol 2004; 104: 1S–4S.

34. Ettinger B, Selby J, Citron JT et al. Cyclic hormone replacement therapy using quarterly progestin. Obstet Gynecol 1994; 83: 693–700.

35. Casanas-Roux F, Nisolle M, Marbaix E et al. Morphometric, immunohistological and three-dimensional evaluation of the endometrium of menopausal women treated by oestrogen and Crinone, a new slow-release vaginal progesterone. Hum Reprod 1996; 11: 357–63.

36. McKenna DJ, Jones K, Humphrey S et al. Black cohosh: efficacy, safety, and use in clinical and preclinical applications. Altern Ther Health Med 2001; 7: 93–100.

37. Roemheld-Hamm B. Chasteberry. Am Fam Physician 2005; 72: 821–4.

38. Albertazzi P, Steel SA, Clifford E et al. Attitudes towards and use of dietary supplementation in a sample of postmenopausal women. Climacteric 2002; 5: 374–82.

39. Drivdahl CE, Miser WF. The use of alternative health care by a family practice population. J Am Board Fam Pract 1998; 11: 193–9.

40. Eisenberg DM, Davis RB, Ettner SL et al. Trends in alternative medicine use in the United States, 1990–1997: results of a follow-up national survey. JAMA 1998; 280: 1569–75.

41. Kass-Annese B. Alternative therapies for menopause. Clin Obstet Gynecol 2000; 43: 162–83.

42. Mahady GB, Parrot J, Lee C et al. Botanical dietary supplement use in peri- and postmenopausal women. Menopause 2003; 10: 65–72.

43. Geller SE, Studee L. Botanical and dietary supplements for menopausal symptoms: what works, what does not. J Womens Health (Larchmt) 2005; 14: 634–49.

44. Krebs EE, Ensrud KE, MacDonald R et al. Phytoestrogens for treatment of menopausal symptoms: a systematic review. Obstet Gynecol 2004; 104: 824–36.

45. Wuttke W, Jarry H, Westphalen S et al. Phytoestrogens for hormone replacement therapy? J Steroid Biochem Mol Biol 2002; 83: 133–47.

46. Food labeling: health claims; soy protein and coronary heart disease. Federal Register 1999, 64; 57699–733.

47. Blumenthal M, ed. Herbal Medicine: Expanded Commision E Monographs. Newton, MA: Integrative Medicine Communications, 2003.

48. Knight DC, Eden JA. A review of the clinical effects of phytoestrogens. Obstet Gynecol 1996; 87: 897–904.

49. Cassidy A. Physiological effects of phyto-estrogens in relation to cancer and other human health risks. Proc Nutr Soc 1996; 55: 399–417.

50. Munro IC, Harwood M, Hlywka JJ et al. Soy isoflavones: a safety review. Nutr Rev 2003; 61: 1–33.

51. Lu LJ, Anderson KE, Grady JJ et al. Decreased ovarian hormones during a soya diet: implications for breast cancer prevention. Cancer Res 2000; (60): 4112–21.

52. Xu X, Duncan AM, Merz BE et al. Effects of soy isoflavones on estrogen and phytoestrogen metabolism in premenopausal women. Cancer Epidemiol Biomarkers Prev 1998; 7: 1101–8.

53. Messina MJ, Persky V, Setchell KD et al. Soy intake and cancer risk: a review of the in vitro and in vivo data. Nutr Cancer 1994; 21: 113–31.

54. Miksicek RJ. Estrogenic flavonoids: structural requirements for biological activity. Proc Soc Exp Biol Med 1995; 208: 44–50.

55. Adlercreutz CH, Goldin BR, Gorbach SL et al. Soybean phytoestrogen intake and cancer risk. J Nutr 1995; 125: 757S–70S.

56. Molteni A, Brizio-Molteni L, Persky V. In vitro hormonal effects of soybean isoflavones. J Nutr 1995; 125: 751S–6S.

57. Teede HJ, Dalais FS, McGrath BP. Dietary soy containing phytoestrogens does not have detectable estrogenic effects on hepatic protein synthesis in postmenopausal women. Am J Clin Nutr 2004; 79: 396–401.

58. Ishimi Y, Arai N, Wang X et al. Difference in effective dosage of genistein on bone and uterus in ovariectomized mice. Biochem Biophys Res Commun 2000; 274: 697–701.

59. Brown NM, Lamartiniere CA. Genistein regulation of transforming growth factor-alpha, epidermal growth factor (EGF), and EGF receptor expression in the rat uterus and vagina. Cell Growth Differ 2000; 11: 255–60.

60. Newbold RR, Banks EP, Bullock B et al. Uterine adenocarcinoma in mice treated neonatally with genistein. Cancer Res 2001; 61: 4325–8.

61. de Kleijn MJ, van der Schouw YT, Wilson PW et al. Intake of dietary phytoestrogens is low in postmenopausal women in the United States: the Framingham study (1–4). J Nutr 2001; 131: 1826–32.

62. Goodman MT, Wilkens LR, Hankin JH et al. Association of soy and fiber consumption with the risk of endometrial cancer. Am J Epidemiol 1997; 146: 294–306.

63. Horn-Ross PL, John EM, Canchola AJ et al. Phytoestrogen intake and endometrial cancer risk. J Natl Cancer Inst 2003; 95: 1158–64.

64. Balk JL, Whiteside DA, Naus G et al. A pilot study of the effects of phytoestrogen supplementation on postmenopausal endometrium. J Soc Gynecol Investig 2002; 9: 238–42.

65. Nikander E, Rutanen EM, Nieminen P et al. Lack of effect of isoflavonoids on the vagina and endometrium in postmenopausal women. Fertil Steril 2005; 83: 137–42.

66. Kaari C, Haidar MA, Junior JM et al. Randomized clinical trial comparing conjugated equine estrogens and isoflavones in postmenopausal women: a pilot study. Maturitas 2006; 53: 49–58.

67. Unfer V, Casini ML, Costabile L et al. Endometrial effects of long-term treatment with phytoestrogens: a randomized, double-blind, placebo-controlled study. Fertil Steril 2004; 82: 145–8.

68. Fugh-Berman A, Kronenberg F. Red clover (Trifolium pratense) for menopausal women: current state of knowledge. Menopause 2001; 8: 333–7.

69. Beck V, Rohr U, Jungbauer A. Phytoestrogens derived from red clover: an alternative to estrogen replacement therapy? J Steroid Biochem Mol Biol 2005; 94: 499–518.

70. Piersen CE, Booth NL, Sun Y et al. Chemical and biological characterization and clinical evaluation of botanical dietary supplements: a phase I red clover extract as a model. Curr Med Chem 2004; 11: 1361–74.

71. Piersen CE. Phytoestrogens in botanical dietary supplements: implications for cancer. Integr Cancer Ther 2003; 2: 120–38.

72. Kuiper GG, Lemmen JG, Carlsson B et al. Interaction of estrogenic chemicals and phytoestrogens with estrogen receptor beta. Endocrinology 1998; 139: 4252–63.

73. Liu J, Burdette JE, Xu H et al. Evaluation of estrogenic activity of plant extracts for the potential treatment of menopausal symptoms. J Agric Food Chem 2001; 49: 2472–9.

74. Zava DT, Dollbaum CM, Blen M. Estrogen and progestin bioactivity of foods, herbs, and spices. Proc Soc Exp Biol Med 1998; 217: 369–78.

75. Lewis RA. Lewis' Dictionary of Toxicology. Boca Raton, FL: CRC press, 1998.

76. Nwannenna AI, Lundh TJ, Madej A et al. Clinical changes in ovariectomized ewes exposed to phytoestrogens and 17 beta-estradiol implants. Proc Soc Exp Biol Med 1995; 208: 92–7.

77. Saloniemi H, Wahala K, Nykanen-Kurki P et al. Phytoestrogen content and estrogenic effect of legume fodder. Proc Soc Exp Biol Med 1995; 208: 13–17.

78. Burdette JE, Liu J, Lantvit D et al. Trifolium pratense (red clover) exhibits estrogenic effects in vivo in ovariectomized Sprague-Dawley rats. J Nutr 2002; 132: 27–30.

79. Nachtigall LE, Nachtigall LB. The effects of isoflavone derived from red clover on vasomotor symptoms and endometrial thickness. Paper presented at: the 9th World Congress on Menopause, 2000; Yokohama, Japan.

80. Baber RJ, Templeman C, Morton T et al. Randomized placebo-controlled trial of an isoflavone supplement and menopausal symptoms in women. Climacteric 1999; 2: 85–92.

81. Hale GE, Hughes CL, Robboy SJ et al. A double-blind randomized study on the effects of red clover isoflavones on the endometrium. Menopause 2001; 8: 338–46.

82. Milligan S, Kalita J, Pocock V et al. Oestrogenic activity of the hop phyto-oestrogen, 8-prenylnaringenin. Reproduction 2002; 123: 235–42.

83. Dixon-Shanies D, Shaikh N. Growth inhibition of human breast cancer cells by herbs and phytoestrogens. Oncol Rep 1999; 6: 1383–7.

84. Zenisek A, Bednar J. Contribution to the identification of the estrogen activity of hops. Am Perfumer Arom 1960; 75: 61.

85. Eagon CL, Elm MS, Teepe AG, Eagon PK. Medicinal botanicals: estrogenicity in rat uterus and liver. Paper presented at American Association for Cancer Research, 1997.

86. Black cohosh. In: Blumenthal M, ed. The ABC Clinical Guide to Herbs. Austin, TX: American Botanical Council, 2002: 13–22.

87. Zierau O, Bodinet C, Kolba S et al. Antiestrogenic activities of Cimicifuga racemosa extracts. J Steroid Biochem Mol Biol 2002; 80: 125–30.

88. Black Cohosh Rhizome. American Herbal Pharmacopeia. Santa Cruz, CA, 2002.

89. Jarry H, Harnischfeger G. [Endocrine effects of constituents of Cimicifuga racemosa. 1. The effect on serum levels of pituitary hormones in ovariectomized rats]. Planta Med 1985: 1: 46–9. [in German]

90. Jarry H, Harnischfeger G, Duker E. [The endocrine effects of constituents of Cimicifuga racemosa. 2. In vitro binding of constituents to estrogen receptors]. Planta Med 1985; 4: 316–19. [in German]

91. Duker EM, Kopanski L, Jarry H, Wuttke W. Effects of extracts from Cimicifuga racemosa on gonadotropin release in menopausal women and ovariectomized rats. Planta Med 1991; 57: 420–4.

92. Nesselhut T, Schellhase C, Dietrich R et al. [Studies of mamma carcinoma cells regarding the proliferative potential of herbal medication with estrogenic-like effects]. Arch Gynecol Obstet 1993; 254: 817–18. [in German]

93. Dog TL, Powell KL, Weisman SM. Critical evaluation of the safety of Cimicifuga racemosa in menopause symptom relief. Menopause 2003; 10: 299–313.

94. Burdette JE, Liu J, Chen SN et al. Black cohosh acts as a mixed competitive ligand and partial agonist of the serotonin receptor. J Agric Food Chem 2003; 51: 5661–70.

95. Mahady GB. Is black cohosh estrogenic? Nutr Rev 2003; 61: 183–6.

96. Nesselhut T, Liske E. Pharmacological measures in postmenopausal women with an isopropanolic extract of Cimicifuga racemosa rhizoma. Paper presented at 10th Annual Meeting, North American Menopause Society, New York, 1999.

97. Einer-Jensen N, Zhao J, Andersen KP et al. Cimicifuga and Melbrosia lack oestrogenic effects in mice and rats. Maturitas 1996; 25: 149–53.

98. Freudenstein J, Dasenbrock C, Nisslein T. Lack of promotion of estrogen-dependent mammary gland tumors in vivo by an isopropanolic Cimicifuga racemosa extract. Cancer Res 2002; 62: 3448–52.

99. Seidlova-Wuttke D, Jarry H, Becker T et al. Pharmacology of Cimicifuga racemosa extract BNO 1055 in rats: bone, fat and uterus. Maturitas 2003; 44: S39–50.

100. Kretzschmar G, Nisslein T, Zierau O et al. No estrogen-like effects of an isopropanolic extract of Rhizoma Cimicifugae racemosae on uterus and vena cava of rats after 17 day treatment. J Steroid Biochem Mol Biol 2005; 97: 271–7.

101. Nappi RE, Malavasi B, Brundu B et al. Efficacy of Cimicifuga racemosa on climacteric complaints: a randomized study versus low-dose transdermal estradiol Gynecol Endocrinol. 2005; 20: 30–5.

102. Wuttke W, Seidlova-Wuttke D, Gorkow C. The Cimicifuga preparation BNO 1055 vs. conjugated estrogens in a double-blind placebo-controlled study: effects on menopause symptoms and bone markers. Maturitas 2003; 44: S67–77.

103. Georgiev DB, Iordanova E. Phytoestrogens – the alternative approach. Maturitas 1996; 27: 213.

104. Liske E, Hanggi W, Henneicke-von Zepelin HH et al. Physiological investigation of a unique extract of black cohosh (Cimicifugae racemosae rhizoma): a 6-month clinical study demonstrates no systemic estrogenic effect. J Womens Health Gend Based Med 2002; 11: 163–74.

105. Maamari R, Schreiber A. Cimicifuga racemosa and quality of life. Paper presented at 12th annual meeting, North American Menopause Society, New Orleans, LA, 2001.

105a. Raus K, Brucker C, Gorkow C, Wuttke W. First-time proof of endometrial safety of the special black cohosh extract (Actaea or Cimifuga racemosa extract) CR BNO 155. Menopause 2006; 13: 678–91.

106. Radix Angelicae Sinensis. In: WHO Monographs on Selected Medicinal Plants. Geneva, Switzerland: WHO, 2001.

107. Amato P, Christophe S, Mellon PL. Estrogenic activity of herbs commonly used as remedies for menopausal symptoms. Menopause 2002; 9: 145–50.

108. Hirata JD, Swiersz LM, Zell B et al. Does dong quai have estrogenic effects in postmenopausal women? A double-blind, placebo-controlled trial. Fertil Steril 1997; 68: 981–6.

109. Lo AC, Chan K, Yeung JH et al. Danggui (Angelica sinensis) affects the pharmacodynamics but not the pharmacokinetics of warfarin in rabbits. Eur J Drug Metab Pharmacokinet 1995; 20: 55–60.

110. Brown D. The use of Vitex agnus castus for hyperprolactinemia. Q Rev Nat Med 1997: 19–21.

111. Jarry H, Spengler B, Porzel A et al. Evidence for estrogen receptor beta-selective activity of Vitex agnus-castus and isolated flavones. Planta Med 2003; 69: 945–7.

112. Liu J, Burdette JE, Sun Y et al. Isolation of linoleic acid as an estrogenic compound from the fruits of Vitex agnus-castus L. (chaste-berry). Phytomedicine 2004; 11: 18–23.

113. Oh SM, Chung KH. Estrogenic activities of Ginkgo biloba extracts. Life Sci 2004; 74: 1325–35.

114. Maggiolini M, Statti G, Vivacqua A et al. Estrogenic and antiproliferative activities of isoliquiritigenin in MCF7 breast cancer cells. J Steroid Biochem Mol Biol 2002; 82: 315–22.

115. Tamir S, Eizenberg M, Somjen D et al. Estrogen-like activity of glabrene and other constituents isolated from licorice root. J Steroid Biochem Mol Biol 2001; 78: 291–8.

116. Tamir S, Eizenberg M, Somjen D et al. Estrogenic and antiproliferative properties of glabridin from licorice in human breast cancer cells. Cancer Res 2000; 60: 5704–9.

117. de Klerk GJ, Nieuwenhuis MG, Beutler JJ. Hypokalaemia and hypertension associated with use of liquorice flavoured chewing gum. BMJ 1997; 314: 731–2.

118. Chandler RF. Licorice, more than just a flower. Can Pharm J 1985; 118: 421–4.

119. Chandler RF. Herbal medicine: ginseng – an aphrodisiac? Can Pharm J 1988; 121: 36–8.

120. Wiklund IK, Mattsson LA, Lindgren R et al. Effects of a standardized ginseng extract on quality of life and physiological parameters in symptomatic postmenopausal women: a double-blind, placebo-controlled trial. Swedish Alternative Medicine Group. Int J Clin Pharmacol Res 1999; 19: 89–99.

121. Motherwort [website]. Available at: http://scienceviews.com/plants/motherwort.html Accessed on November 20, 2005.

122. McMillan TL, Mark S. Complementary and alternative medicine and physical activity for menopausal symptoms. JAMWA 2004; 59: 270–7.

123. Chenoy R, Hussain S, Tayob Y et al. Effect of oral gamolenic acid from evening primrose oil on menopausal flushing. BMJ 1994; 308: 501–3.

124. Pittler MH, Ernst E. Efficacy of kava extract for treating anxiety: systematic review and meta-analysis. J Clin Psychopharmacol 2000; 20: 84–9.

125. Warnecke G. [Psychosomatic dysfunctions in the female climacteric. Clinical effectiveness and tolerance of Kava Extract WS 1490]. Fortschr Med 1991; 109: 119–22. [in German]

126. Blumenthal M, ed. The ABC Clinical Guide to Herbs. Austin, TX: American Botanical Council, 2003.

127. Hadley S, Petry JJ. Valerian. Am Fam Physician 2003; 67: 1755–8.

128. Valeriana officinalis. Altern Med Rev 2004; 9: 438–40.

129. Linde K, Ramirez G, Mulrow CD et al. St John's wort for depression – an overview and meta-analysis of randomised clinical trials. BMJ 1996; 313: 253–8.

130. Komesaroff PA, Black CV, Cable V et al. Effects of wild yam extract on menopausal symptoms, lipids and sex hormones in healthy menopausal women. Climacteric 2001; 4: 144–50.

53 Uterine disease in midlife and beyond: the menopausal transition and postmenopause

Alex J Polotsky and Nanette Santoro

ABSTRACT

The hypothalamic–pituitary–gonadal axis changes functionally and structurally throughout life. It is becoming increasingly clear that the uterus is not merely a passive recipient of this dynamically changing input, but rather an exocrine, endocrine, and paracrine organ in its own right. The menopausal transition is a time in the life cycle of women during which complaints of bleeding irregularity and menorrhagia are common. The underlying changes in the hypothalamic–pituitary–gonadal axis that contribute to this clinical problem are beginning to be understood. There is little evidence that aging per se alters essential uterine and endometrial function. During the postmenopause, women not receiving hormonal replacement therapy are believed to have a quiescent endometrium. However, in this setting, aging favors the development of neoplasia. A basic appreciation of the contribution of the hormonal milieu and a woman's life cycle to uterine function assists greatly in the differential diagnosis of abnormal bleeding in the older reproductive-aged and postmenopausal woman.

EPIDEMIOLOGICAL CONSIDERATIONS

In 2001, an NIH (National Institutes of Health)-sponsored workshop[1] defined the menopausal transition as a stage characterized by variation in menstrual cycle length and ending with the final menstrual period (Figure 53.1). Abnormal uterine bleeding accounts for up to 20% of gynecological office visits and frequently leads to operative procedures.[2] One study of 500 consecutive perimenopausal patients found a 70% prevalence of oligomenorrhea and/or hypomenorrhea, and an 18% prevalence of menorrhagia, metrorrhagia, and/or hypermenorrhea.[3] In the USA, out of 600 000 hysterectomies performed annually, women aged 40–54 years old account for almost 45% of all procedures.[4] Data from the UK suggest that the primary reason for hysterectomy of women in this age group is menorrhagia.[5] Minimally invasive or medical options in the treatment of menorrhagia, including progesterone-containing intrauterine

systems[6] and endometrial ablation,[7] may offer a wider choice and significantly decreased cost for the patient and society at large. Although hysterectomy may be thought of as a drastic solution to menorrhagia, prospective cohort studies suggest very high rates of satisfaction when surgical therapy has been undertaken.[8] Further support comes from five randomized clinical trials (total of 752 participants) that have confirmed a small advantage in terms of patient satisfaction with hysterectomy over medical management of heavy menstrual bleeding.[9] The bleeding problems that plague women in the postreproductive and premenopausal years have been incompletely characterized and appear to arise from anatomical, hormonal, and functional alterations in the endometrium's ability to perform organized, monthly shedding and/or support the growth of a conceptus. This chapter attempts to integrate the current state of knowledge regarding possible clues to the common problem of unwanted, irregular, and excessively heavy bleeding in midlife women.

Postmenopausal women are presumed to have inactive endometrium. Studies utilizing large-scale transvaginal ultrasound screening have largely confirmed this assumption and suggested a useful clinical cut-off of 4 mm for pursuing an endometrial histological diagnosis of postmenopausal bleeding.[10] However, patterns of endometrial growth and other predictors of predisposition to endometrial polyps or cancers have not been defined in the postmenopausal woman. Some of the correlates of postmenopausal bleeding are described herein. A brief overview of the current clinical standards on the age-appropriate approach to the evaluation of abnormal vaginal bleeding is provided.

WHAT IS NORMAL?

Ascribing a pathological origin for the many possible causes of unexpected menstrual bleeding in women is a habit for the medical practitioner. Most textbooks of obstetrics and gynecology routinely recommend a screening endometrial biopsy for any woman over 35 years old with abnormal bleeding to rule out

					Final Menstrual Period (FMP)		

Stages:	−5	−4	−3	−2	−1	0 ▼	+1	+2
Terminology:	Reproductive			Menopausal Transition			Postmenopause	
	Early	Peak	Late	Early	Late*		Early*	Late
				Perimenopause				
Duration of stage:	variable			variable		(a) 1 year	(b) 4 years	until demise
Menstrual cycles:	variable to regular	regular		variable cycle length (>7 days different from normal)	≥2 skipped cycles and an interval of amenorrhea (≥60 days)	Amen × 12 months	none	
Endocrine:	normal FSH		↑ FSH	↑ FSH		↑ FSH		

*Stages most likely to be characterized by vasomotor symptoms   ↑ = elevated

Figure 53.1   The stages of reproductive aging. The reproductive years are divided into three stages: early (postmenarcheal); peak (about 16–35 years old); and late (about 35–45 years old). The menopausal transition usually has its onset in the mid-40s and is characterized by increased cycle variability in its early stages, and prolonged (> 60 days) amenorrhea in its late stage. FSH, follicle-stimulating hormone. (Reprinted from Fertility and Sterility, Volume 76, Soules et al, Executive summary: Stages of Reproductive Aging Workshop, pages 874–878. ©2001, with permission from the American Society for Reproductive Medicine.)[1] http://www.fertstert.org/article/PIIS0015028201029090/fulltext – fig1

hyperplasia or carcinoma. The actual number of cases which will be detected is so small that a threshold of age 35 years old is probably unduly conservative. Assessment of risk factors, such as obesity, chronic anovulation, and family history of colon cancer, may yield better pre-test probability for detection of endometrial pathology.[11] Nonetheless, any such policy begs the question of what, exactly, is normal uterine bleeding in women whose menstrual cycles are necessarily becoming irregular due to anovulation[12] and other hormonal alterations associated with reproductive aging.[13–17]

Clues from large studies

Treloar et al analyzed over 20 000 menstrual cycles throughout the reproductive lives of many women.[18] The normal menstrual cycle length in women is tightly regulated between the ages of 20 and 40 years old, ranging from approximately 25 to 35 days. There is a general trend towards cycle shortening with reproductive aging, with mean cycle length deviating downward to about 24 days by age 40 years old. Thereafter, menstrual cycle length becomes extremely variable, but becomes shorter on the mean before it lengthens near the menopause. These data indicate that very

short cycles (less than 21 days) are not unusual occurrences in the fifth decade of life. Similar findings of menstrual cycle, and in particular, follicular phase shortening, have been reported in large-scale studies from the UK[19] and Australia.[20]

Discerning what constitutes abnormal bleeding against this variable and changing baseline is a clinical challenge. Extremes of bleeding appear to become more common as women move through the menopausal transition.[21] Many women may find solace in the knowledge that their final menstrual period is imminent. However, it is not currently possible for the clinician to provide this information with good reliability. As menopause can only be diagnosed retrospectively at the present time, predictions about the timing of the final menstrual period remain imprecise. A prospective cohort study of women in Melbourne, Australia showed that bouts of protracted amenorrhea (at least three but not more than 11 consecutive months) predicted the final menstrual period in 95% of women within the following 4 years.[22] In another analysis of the same cohort, an increase in the 'running range' of cycle lengths (difference between the shortest and the longest cycles) to 42 days served as an indicator of the last 20 pre-final periods.[23] While these estimates provide some measure of precision, they lack applicability to the majority of women, who do not routinely keep track of their intermenstrual interval. Simpler methods of prediction are desirable and are currently under development.

Clues from the endocrine literature

As women enter their 40s, the follicular phase of the menstrual cycle becomes condensed, and the period of selection of the dominant follicle appears to be shorter.[15,19,24,25] In contrast, the luteal phase remains relatively constant, with a mean length of 14 days in ovulatory cycles.[16]

Along with these changes, ovulatory cycles appear to have increased estrogen secretion associated with them[15,17] and anovulatory cycles can have very high concentrations of estrogen.[12,15,17] As women progress further through the menopausal transition, cycles become longer, and periods of little or no estrogen production alternate with anovulatory and ovulatory cycles. Recent data from the Study of Women's Health Across the Nation (SWAN), a longitudinal study that includes detailed hormonal assessments of menstrual cycles in almost 1000 women, demonstrate relatively frequent episodes of anovulation with estrogen peaks but no preovulatory luteinizing hormone (LH) surge.[26] These findings suggest that there is central nervous system insensitivity to estrogen in menopausal transition, implying that exposure to acyclic estrogen unopposed by progesterone may be a clinically silent event, but might have implications for endometrial health.

Since ovulation appears to occur up to the final menstrual period,[16,25] conception is theoretically possible, although uncommon, until then. Increased secretion of estrogen may facilitate the development of hyperplasia or polyps of the endometrium. Very short follicular/proliferative phases may not allow for adequate endometrial development, and thus inhibited implantation may also occur on hormonal grounds. Little direct investigation of endometrial function has been made in women in this age group.

By 1 year after a woman's final menstrual period (FMP), hormonal patterns appear to be stable, with tonically elevated gonadotropins and minimal evidence of estrogen secretion or excretion.[25] Endometrial maturation is therefore believed to be suspended in an inactive state, unless neoplastic processes intervene.

Anatomical changes in uterine function with age

Leiomyomata represent the most common anatomical abnormality of the uterus. Although fibroids are clinically manifested in about 25–30% of women,[27] targeted pathological examination suggests the prevalence of up to 80% in surgically excised uteri.[28] Symptoms and interventions tend to increase with age. In the USA, myomata constitute the chief cause for hysterectomy for women in their 40s, with total numbers varying from 30% of all cases in Caucasians to over 50% in African-Americans.[27] Black race appears to be a strong independent risk factor for fibroids, with an adjusted relative risk of 3.25 compared to the frequency in white women in a large prospective cohort.[29] How leiomyomata impact upon endometrial function is unclear. Intrauterine location tends to be a better correlate with abnormal bleeding than size (Figure 53.2).

Myomata are estrogen-responsive benign muscle tumors of monoclonal origin. In apparent contradiction to well-established dogma, use of oral contraceptives is associated with a decreased prevalence of symptomatic myomas.[31] This might be taken to mean that oral contraceptives are a protective factor for some women and help to inhibit myoma growth. However, it is also possible that women at high risk for the development of uterine myomata are infrequently prescribed oral contraceptives, thus accounting for the observed association. The finding from the Nurses' Health Study that early teenage exposure to the oral contraceptive pill (OCP) may increase the risk of myomata[32] supports the latter explanation for the association between oral contraceptive use and myomata.

Submucosal leiomyomata appear to impact directly on menses and will increase the duration and flow of menses. However, how subtle changes in blood flow and contour of the uterine cavity caused by intramural or subserosal leiomyomata may present problems with bleeding or alter the endometrial environment is not well understood. Local dysregulation of several growth factors (transforming growth factor-β [TGFβ], fibroblast growth factor [FGF], vascular endothelial growth factor [VEGF], among others) affecting angiogenesis have been studied as putative molecular mechanisms for leiomyoma-induced menorrhagia.[33] Growth regulation of leiomyomata appears to be unique among benign mesenchymal tumors.[34] EBAF (endometrial bleeding associated factor), is overexpressed in leiomyomata and is structurally similar to the TGFβ growth factor.[35] Further study of the mutated genes found in myomata but not in normal myometrium (e.g. growth-promoting gene [HMGI-C]), may eventually help to explicate the pathogenesis and inform the clinical management of uterine leiomyomata.[36]

Endometrial polyps, localized overgrowths of endometrial glands and stroma with a central blood

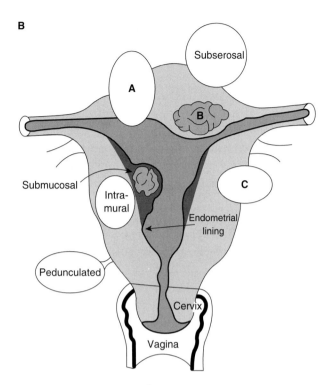

Figure 53.2 Location of uterine myomata. Most myomas are of mixed type, however, as illustrated by A, B, and C. (Reprinted from The Lancet, Volume 357, Stewart EA, Uterine fibroids, page 293. ©2001, with permission from Elsevier.[30])

vessel, peak in the fifth decade of life. A prevalence of up to 24% has been reported among symptomatic women undergoing histopathological examination.[37] Polyps are often asymptomatic and rarely neoplastic with a 0.8% incidence of carcinoma reported in one large Italian study.[38] In contrast, endometrial hyperplasia within polyps is not uncommon, with the rates ranging from 3% to 26% for atypical and non-atypical hyperplasia, respectively.[38] The pathogenesis of endometrial polyps is poorly understood. Their frequent association with endometrial hyperplasia implies that they are estrogen sensitive. Preliminary data indicate that mRNA for local endometrial aromatase is up-regulated in polyps and their adjacent endometrium.[39] Cytogenetic analysis reveals several heterogeneous clonal chromosomal rearrangements.[40] Of note, one specific chromosomal translocation, 6p21, correlates with abnormal expression of high-mobility group (HMG) proteins that are also identified in leiomyomata.[41]

Adenomyosis, defined as the presence of uterine glands and stroma within the myometrium, increases with age. The true prevalence of adenomyosis is unknown, in part due to the difficulty in clinical diagnosis. Definitive identification may only be made by histological examination. While its pathogenesis is not well understood, the higher risk in parous women is in contradistinction to endometriosis, which is more common in nulligravidae. Most etiological studies implicate endomyometrial invagination of the endometrium,[42] yet a de-novo formation theory was supported by a case of adenomyosis arising from a rudimentary uterine horn in a woman with Müllerian agenesis.[43]

Implantation efficiency decreases with age

Although the effect appears small compared to the vastly greater detriment that ovarian aging plays in female fertility, the uterus does indeed appear to perform less effectively in permitting implantation to occur with age. Studies of women receiving donated oocytes, in whom the ovarian factor has presumably been corrected, are conflicting, but most indicate a small but detectable detrimental effect of age.[44-47] In a large study of over 17 000 oocyte donation cycles, implantation rates declined as the age of the recipient increased to her late 40s and 50s.[48]

Biochemical assessment of the uterus using gly-codelin, also known as placental protein 14 (PP-14), as a marker of luteal adequacy failed to reveal any decline in this protein with aging in regularly cycling women up to 52 years.[49] However, PP-14 may be a relatively insensitive marker protein. Assessment of other known endometrial products such as $\alpha_v\beta_3$ integrin[50] or insulin-like growth factor binding protein 1 (IGFBP-1)[51] has not been carried out in the perimenopausal age group. Thus, although there does appear to be a small loss in uterine receptivity with aging, its genesis remains unknown. Clearly, the uterine effects of aging are minor in comparison with the ovarian effects, as reproductive capacity has been reported in women in their 60s.[52]

On the molecular level, no age-specific effects have been observed in expression patterns of markers of cellular proliferation and cell cycle progression. This finding implies that aging per se is not related to fundamental alterations in benign uterine proliferation processes.[53]

MECHANISMS OF MENSTRUATION

Normal menstruation is initiated by the withdrawal of estrogen and progesterone. Hormonal withdrawal results in rhythmic spasm of the steroid-sensitive spiral arterioles of the endometrium. These spasms result in progressive necrosis of the outer endometrial layers, the functionalis.[54] On the molecular level, withdrawal of progesterone increases levels of prostaglandins PGE_2 and $PGF_{2\alpha}$ via induction of cyclooxygenase 2 (COX-2) and inhibition of the inactivating enzyme prostaglandin dehydrogenase.[55] The importance of the elucidation of molecular mechanisms of menstruation is underscored by the effectiveness of non-steroidal anti-inflammatory drugs (NSAIDs) (drugs inhibiting COX-2) in the treatment of excessive menstrual bleeding. The prostaglandin-triggered vasoconstriction and cytokine changes are mediated by the PR (progesterone receptor)-positive perivascular stromal cells.[56] While these early processes are possibly rescued by progesterone, the subsequent stages of the menses appear to be irreversible.[57] The increased activity of the matrix metalloproteinases (MMPs), lytic enzymes that break down extracellular matrix and basement membranes, is thought to herald menstrual bleeding.[57] The end result of progesterone withdrawal leads to increased MMP output, with concomitant decreases in tissue inhibitors of metalloproteinases (TIMPs). The net effect is a rapid, well-organized autodigestion of the superficial endometrium with retention of the basalis layer.

Endometrial sloughing is typically organized, lasts for 3–7 days, and results in an average loss of about 30 ml of blood.[58,59] Platelet plugging and regeneration of the endometrial epithelium are the two mechanisms that are currently understood to control menstrual blood loss.[60] Processes that interfere with these mechanisms can be anatomical (i.e. myomata, polyps) or hormonal (failure to produce enough estrogen to regenerate the epithelium). Both of these possibilities are more likely to happen in perimenopausal women.

Seminal work by Noyes et al highlighted endometrial leukocytes as prominent morphological markers of menstrual cycle phase transition.[61] A subset of natural killer cells with an antigen profile distinct from their peripheral counterparts appear to have cyclical alterations in cell number.[55] It is postulated that these uterine natural killer (uNK) cells have a role in control of initiation of menstruation.[62] Of note, these uNK cells do not have appreciable expression of PR[63] that may support a special role of the stromal cells in mediating the decidualization-to-menstruation progression. Stromal cells retain PR through the late secretory phase and are most susceptible to progesterone withdrawal.[55] Detailed knowledge of specificity of progesterone responses and their link to molecular targets in menstrual endometrium is lacking and remains an active area of research. PR modulation is one of the promising investigational therapies that could potentially allow for differential activation of some of these specific progesterone-mediated actions.[64]

Causes of menorrhagia in the menopausal transition

Investigation of women with the complaint of excessive menstrual blood loss has not been revealing with regard to potential mechanisms underlying menorrhagia. Few studies of menorrhagia have included a systematic investigation of intrauterine pathology by hysteroscopy or sonographic enhancement with saline. Most have ruled out anatomical pathology by dilatation and curettage (D&C), which may not be satisfactory.[65] It remains a disappointing paradox that, in the 21st century, gynecologists cannot justify hysterectomy, one of the most common operations performed, with objective diagnostic criteria.

A classic study by Hallberg et al defined menorrhagia as a total menstrual loss of >80 ml, as this appeared to define a threshold for the development of anemia.[66] However, the quantification of the amount of blood lost at menstruation and its biological basis is not a straightforward clinical task. Substantiating the claim of menorrhagia is problematic to begin with. When uterine weight and surface area were examined in the proportion of women who ultimately had a hysterectomy (40 out of 92), no relationship could be established between measured menstrual blood loss and these variables.[67] Usage of pads and tampons did not correlate in these and many other studies with the actual measured menstrual blood loss. However, these data have been recently revisited. In a Scottish cohort of 952 women, subjective measures such as passage of clots and changing rates during flow were able to predict clinically important blood loss in 76% of women.[68] This same group of investigators contested the clinical relevance of the 80 ml cut-off for the definition of menorrhagia by showing that it was neither predictive of iron status nor representative of a biologically relevant threshold.[69] Clinical studies of women with proven blood loss >80 ml with menses have not revealed any characteristic hormonal deviation from a control group.[59] These latter data are particularly important in that they contradict the dictum of women as poor judges of menstrual flow and reinstate the importance of historical information as one of the best, yet imperfect, tools available in guiding therapy.

Women with excessive menstrual blood loss appear in some studies to produce excess prostaglandin,[70] justifying the therapeutic usefulness of prostaglandin inhibitors. Decreased luteal progesterone may also be a feature of perimenopausal cycles[15] which is amenable to treatment. Interestingly, exogenous progesterone generally works poorly for excessive bleeding, whereas

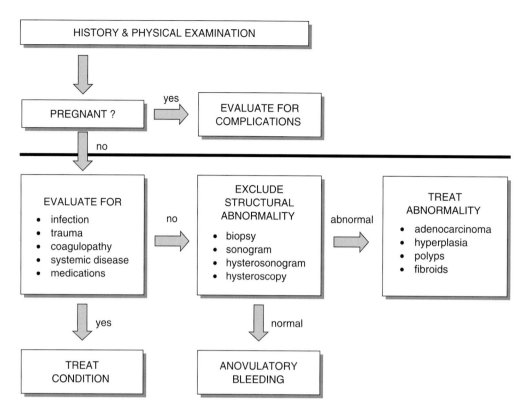

Figure 53.3   Evaluation of abnormal uterine bleeding in perimenopausal women. (Adapted from APGO educational series on women's health issues.[79])

intrauterine progestins perform quite well.[71,72] The hormonal milieu of the perimenopausal woman may well favor exuberant endometrial growth; however, the variability of menstrual cycle patterns may naturally protect women from widespread hyperplasia. Mifepristone, a progesterone antagonist, has also been used successfully in clinical studies to reduce menstrual bleeding.[70] While the use of antiprogestins may seem counterintuitive due to the antiestrogenic properties of progestins, they have been found to result in atrophy of the functionalis, probably due to atrophy of the endometrial spiral arteries in the non-human primate models.[73]

Molecular mechanisms of abnormal bleeding is an active area of research. One study detected increased luteal phase estrogen receptor-α (ERα) and PR in women with objectively confirmed menorrhagia who ranged in age from 19 to 52 years old.[74] Another recent investigation demonstrated elevated levels of proliferative phase ER and PR in ovulatory women with prolonged menses aged 18–45 years old.[75] These findings are consistent with excessive estrogen stimulation of the endometrium (leading to increases in both ER and PR) and inadequate progesterone down-regulation of ER and PR. Dysregulation of the mechanisms promoting extracellular matrix and vascular basement membrane degradation, vessel spasm and orderly shedding

of the functionalis, and regeneration may also occur in the absence of appropriate mediation of steroid hormone responsiveness. ER has been detected in arteriolar smooth muscle,[76] although one immunohistochemical study of vascular smooth muscle ER failed to confirm any abnormalities in women with menorrhagia.[77] Genetic variation may also provide insights, as the noncoding Pvu II ER polymorphism has been shown to be associated with earlier menopause and a two-fold greater risk for surgical menopause.[78] The molecular mechanisms underlying menorrhagia, break-through bleeding and endometrial bleeding associated with polyps, submucosal leiomyomata, or other abnormalities in the uterine cavity remain an important area of research in women's health.

DIAGNOSIS OF ABNORMAL BLEEDING

When confronting the clinical complaint of abnormal bleeding, the clinician needs to put the historical information into context. Bleeding sufficient to result in anemia clearly deserves further work-up regardless of the patient's age. In general, the older the patient, the higher the suspicion for endometrial pathology and the lower the threshold for endometrial evaluation, although a lower age limit of 35 may be too stringent.[11] Although standardized age-specific work-up algorithms are available[79] (Figure 53.3), it is advisable to tailor specific evaluation to the risk factors of an individual patient.

Diagnostic considerations in menopausal transition

Women who have not yet undergone their FMP may have several types of complaints. As women approach the menopausal transition, cycles become more irregular, as abnormal bleeding usually leads to a great deal of patient concern about possible cancer. Additional diagnostic techniques available in the office include transvaginal ultrasound (TVUS) and saline infusion sonography (SIS) or hysterosonography. SIS is probably most useful in the perimenopausal woman, as endometrial thickness 'norms' have been developed only for postmenopausal women (see below). SIS has proven to be another office-based, low-cost procedure that assists in screening women for anatomical lesions. It is exceptionally well suited to detecting small polyps or submucosal myomata that might otherwise be undetected. In one study of 106 women with menometrorrhagia, SIS had sensitivity and specificity of 93.1% and 93.9%, respectively, for detecting intracavitary lesions, significantly higher than those for ultrasonography.[80]

Cancers are rare in premenopausal women, and are not typical causes of menorrhagia. Recent data estimate that there are 24 cases of endometrial cancer per 100 000 woman-years among women aged 45–49 years old in the USA[81] or less than 2% of all biopsies in one study.[82] Cancers are more frequent in biopsies of postmenopausal women, with quoted incidences of 11% of women with postmenopausal bleeding[83] and up to 20% when heavy bleeding is the presenting symptom.[82]

Operative diagnostic procedures are on the wane in the USA. D&C procedures have been declining sharply since the 1980s, as they are notoriously inaccurate and may miss up to 30% of focal lesions.[84] Although diagnostic hysteroscopy has been largely replaced by operative hysteroscopy with pre-screening of patients using the above-referenced techniques, office or mini-hysteroscopy is inexpensive and allows for direct visualization of pathology and/or biopsy in an outpatient setting.[85] When specific anatomical abnormalities are suspected, the diagnostic modality should be tailored to the pathology sought: magnetic resonance imaging (MRI) is the best available test for adenomyosis, a rare cause of abnormal bleeding with pain being the most common symptom.

Measuring follicle-stimulating hormone (FSH) has long been used as a marker for the menopause transition, yet it has limited utility in evaluating abnormal vaginal bleeding. Granulosa cell products have been studied as possible markers of menopause. In one recent study, Müllerian-inhibiting substance was the hormone most closely associated with onset of the menopausal transition and was similar in magnitude to age and antral follicle counts as a predictor of menopause.[86] While there may be clinical value in forecasting the end of dysfunctional uterine bleeding for the perimenopausal patient, at present there is not a reliable and precise method that can be applied to this purpose. Menopause remains a retrospective clinical diagnosis that should guide the clinical decision-making for evaluation of abnormal clinical bleeding.

Postmenopausal bleeding

In the postmenopausal woman, there is a much greater need to rule out carcinoma on the initial presentation. Any bleeding occurring at least 1 year after the FMP should be investigated. TVUS is now becoming the standard of care first diagnostic test in evaluating the first episode of postmenopausal bleeding (PMB). In a study of 458 postmenopausal women, the negative predictive value of an endometrial stripe of <5 mm was found to be 99%.[87]

While the first prerogative of evaluating PMB is to rule out carcinoma, it should be noted that the most common etiology in this age group is atrophy. In one prospective study of 628 postmenopausal patients undergoing hysterectomy, the incidence of atrophic endometrium was 83% and endometrial carcinoma 11%.[83] It is noteworthy that recurrent bleeding was more common in carcinoma. Polyps are found less frequently in the postmenopause than in the perimenopause and have been reported in about 10% of women.[88]

One special consideration in evaluating postmenopausal women is a concern for disseminating cancer into the peritoneal cavity with SIS or hysteroscopy. The topic remains controversial, with one large Japanese study of 1040 hysteroscopies finding no effect on peritoneal washings,[89] whereas a smaller Austrian report showed a significant correlation between positive peritoneal cytology and history of hysteroscopy.[90] It remains to be seen if the association of positive peritoneal washings with hysteroscopy results in any detrimental effect on prognosis.

Table 53.1 Therapy of abnormal bleeding in the menopausal transition

Therapy	Modality	Advantages	Disadvantages
Medical management	Cyclic OCPs	Added benefit of contraception	Contraindicated in smokers, migraineurs
	Oral progesterone	Effective for endometrial hyperplasia	Ineffective, clinical data do not support use
	NSAIDs	Added benefit for dysmenorrhea	Possible GI side effects; less effective than hormonal therapy
	Depo-Provera	Added benefit of contraception; convenient injection schedule	Frequent break-through bleeding; may decrease bone density if long term
	Danazol	Effective in reducing menstrual loss	Androgen-related side effects; expensive
	Antifibrinolytics	To be taken only on the days of menses; effective for acute therapy	Potential risk of thromboembolic events. GI, leg cramps, dizziness, headaches
	GnRH analogues	Highly effective	Hot flushes; expensive; decreased bone density and need for add-back with long-term use
	Mifepristone	Effective in reducing menstrual loss	May be difficult to obtain due to local laws governing abortifacients
	SPRMs	Suppression of menses without interfering with ovulation	Investigational use only
Minimally invasive	Progestin-releasing IUD	Added benefit of contraception; highly effective	Requires normal or near-normal cavity
	Endometrial destruction or ablation	Office procedure (depending on technique)	Significant minority of patients ultimately require further surgery
	Uterine fibroid embolization	Effective for selected leiomyomata	Post-procedure pain, rare infectious side effects
Surgery	Hysterectomy	High rates of patient satisfaction	Major surgery with its inherent risks

OCPs, oral contraceptive pills; NSAIDs, non-steroidal anti-inflammatory drugs; GI, gastrointestinal; GnRH, gonadotropin-releasing hormone; SPRMs, selective progesterone receptor modulators; IUD, intrauterine device.

THERAPY OF ABNORMAL BLEEDING

Perimenopausal women

The perimenopausal woman experiencing abnormal bleeding should receive specific therapy if there is an anatomical lesion or hyperplasia/carcinoma. Certain therapeutic modalities are more effective for specific structural abnormalities, with operative hysteroscopy being a standard of care for endometrial polyps and hysterectomy for adenomyosis (Table 53.1). However, in the vast majority of cases the initial work-up will be negative. The next steps in therapy differ somewhat between the US and European medical practice.

A widespread practice in the USA is to attempt to administer a short course of a progestin in a cyclic fashion to perimenopausal women. There are limited clinical data to support this practice. On the contrary, several randomized studies have demonstrated that cyclic oral progestins are less efficacious than any other means of medical therapy.[91] Perimenopausal women have irregularly irregular patterns of cycling; therefore, progestin administration cannot be expected to be fortuitously timed to mature the endometrium in the face of adequate estrogen priming. More irregular and occasionally profuse bleeding may occur, leading to an unhappy patient and probably poor follow-up.

Perimenopausal women bleed irregularly because they cycle irregularly. In the face of a negative work-up, cycle control can usually be achieved with cyclic OCPs. Food and Drug Administration (FDA) labeling permits their usage up to the menopause in non-smokers. Clinicians tend to underutilize this very simple modality, which provides the added benefit of conception control. Patients whose chief complaint is cycle control can derive great benefit and predictable bleeding from oral contraceptives. Long-cycle (up to 3 months) oral contraception can reduce bleeding intervals dramatically and have high patient acceptance.[92] Drawbacks to oral contraceptive use in women in their 40s include increasing age-related risks of thromboembolism and myocardial infarction.[93]

Complaints centered around the time of menses may be more amenable to intermittent therapy. Prostaglandin inhibitors have been shown to be effective at reducing measured menstrual blood loss in many studies, primarily performed in the UK.[94] Uterine progestin administration has also been shown to be effective;[72] Mirena (levonorgestrel) is available for use in the USA. The unpopularity of the intrauterine device (IUD) in this country is a potential limitation on its use. However, it represents another method of providing both conception control and cycle control for the perimenopausal woman.

Antifibrinolytic agents, including tranexamic acid and aminocaproic acid, have been tested in several British and Scandinavian studies[95] as therapeutic agents; however, they have not gained popularity in the USA.[91] Danocrine (donazol), although expensive, has also been shown to be of benefit. A major drawback is androgen-related side effects occurring in approximately 40% of patients. The side-effect profile may be improved by lowering the dose.

Since the endocrine milieu of the perimenopausal woman is often progesterone deficient, Depo-Provera might be another useful adjunct that provides contraception. However, irregular, but light bleeding may occur while on Depo-Provera, which may be unacceptable to patients. Decreased bone density is of concern with long-term administration, but may be less of an issue with middle-aged women than it is with adolescents.[96]

An additional medical approach is to administer a long-acting gonadotropin-releasing hormone (GnRH) agonist with add-back supplemental estrogen or norethindrone if used for more than 6 months.[97] Although expensive, this regimen may be considered in refractory cases in which surgical management is not desired or advisable. GnRH antagonists may also be used; however their long-term use has the same disadvantages as GnRH agonists. Selective PR modulators have reached clinical trials and may present a unique option of suppressing menses without interfering with ovulation.[64]

Prior to consideration of hysterectomy, surgical intervention with endometrial ablation appears to be a reasonable alternative. Endometrial destructive techniques have been designed that include both hysteroscopy and the use of custom-made transcervical devices employing radiofrequency, microwave, or thermal balloons.[9] Uterine embolization is an effective minimally invasive technique for treatment of leiomyoma-caused bleeding. It should be stressed that both embolization and endometrial destructive technique should not be performed in women who contemplate future childbearing.

Systematic reviews of trials comparing hysterectomy with minimally invasive techniques demonstrate that up to 20% of endometrial destruction patients ultimately undergo hysterectomy.[9] While this finding

may be regarded as evidence for the definitive nature of hysterectomy, it also shows that the majority of minimally invasive patients are able to avoid major surgery. Women who undergo hysterectomy often report high degrees of satisfaction and many actively seek this surgical intervention to relieve their symptoms. This indicates the likelihood that symptoms other than bleeding per se cause the inconvenience that leads women to seek medical care. A recent randomized trial of hysterectomy vs medical therapy revealed significantly higher rates for improved sexual desire, quality of life, and symptom satisfaction in the hysterectomy group.[98] At the same time, refinements in surgical technique and increased utilization of laparoscopic hysterectomy could further reduce the morbidity of this major surgery.[99]

Postmenopausal bleeding

Since postmenopausal bleeding is by definition abnormal, the physician should perform a careful diagnostic work-up. A similar evaluation is warranted in the perimenopausal patient in which severe menorrhagia occurs. Granulosa cell tumors, epithelial ovarian cancers, and other non-uterine malignancies may precipitate bleeding by production of estrogen or excessive human chorionic gonadotropin (hCG), which, in turn, stimulates ovarian thecal production of androgens. Thus, even after uterine pathology has been ruled out, the physician should consider other potential sources of hormone excess.

SUMMARY

Perimenopausal women have altered endometrial behavior compared to their mid-reproductive age counterparts. Alterations in the cyclic pattern of endometrial growth, differentiation, and shedding and monthly regeneration occur, with frequent episodes of irregular and heavy menses. The perimenopausal hormonal milieu may be responsible for the tendency to develop hyperplasia and dysfunctional uterine bleeding. Implantation efficacy is reduced, although it is not clear if aging per se results in any fundamental alterations in uterine proliferation. Further clarification of the respective roles of hormones, anatomy, and biochemical mediators of endometrial function are critical to understanding the natural evolution of the menopausal process in the endometrium.

REFERENCES

1. Soules MR, Sherman S, Parrott E et al. Executive summary: Stages of Reproductive Aging Workshop (STRAW). Fertil Steril 2001; 76: 874–8.

2. Schwayder JM. Contemporary management of abnormal uterine bleeding. Obstet Gynecol Clin 2000; 27: 219–34.

3. Seltzer VL, Benjamin F, Deutsch S. Perimenopausal bleeding patterns and pathologic findings. J Am Med Womens Assoc 1990; 45: 132–4.

4. Lepine LA, Hillis SD, Marchbanks PA et al. Hysterectomy surveillance – United States, 1980–1993. MMWR CDC Surveillance Summaries 1997; 461: 1–16.

5. Bonnar J, Sheppard BL. Treatment of menorrhagia during menstruation: randomized controlled trial of ethamsylate, mefenamic acid, and tranexamic acid. BMJ 1996; 313: 579–82.

6. Hurskainen R, Teperi J, Rissanen P et al. Clinical outcomes and costs with the levonorgestrel-releasing intrauterine system or hysterectomy for treatment of menorrhagia: randomized trial 5-year follow-up. JAMA 2004; 291: 1456–63.

7. Lethaby A, Hickey M. Endometrial destruction techniques for heavy menstrual bleeding. Cochrane Database Syst Rev 2005; 4: CD00075320–00814.

8. Carlson KJ, Miller BA, Fowler FJ. The Maine Women's Health Study II: outcomes of surgical management of leiomyomas, abnormal bleeding and chronic pelvic pain. Obstet Gynecol 1994; 83: 566–72.

9. Lethaby A, Shepperd S, Cooke I et al. Endometrial resection and ablation versus hysterectomy for heavy menstrual bleeding. Cochrane Database Syst Rev 2005; 4: CD00075320–00813.

10. Gull B, Karlsson B, Milsom I et al. Can ultrasound replace dilation and curettage? A longitudinal evaluation of postmenopausal bleeding and transvaginal sonographic measurement of the endometrium as predictors of endometrial cancer. Am J Obstet Gynecol 2003; 188: 401–8.

11. Farquhar CM, Lethaby A, Sowter M et al. An evaluation of risk factors for endometrial hyperplasia in premenopausal women with abnormal menstrual bleeding. Am J Obstet Gynecol 1999; 181: 525–9.

12. van Look PFA, Lothian H, Hunter WM et al. Hypothalamic–pituitary–ovarian function in perimenopausal women. Clin Endocrinol 1997; 7: 13–31.

13. Burger HG, Dudley BC, Hopper JL et al. The endocrinology of the menopausal transition: a cross-sectional study of a population-based sample. Clin Endocrinol Metab 1995; 80: 3527–45.

14. Klein NA, Battaglia DE, Fujimoto VY et al. Reproductive aging: accelerated ovarian follicular development associated with a monotropic follicle-stimulating hormone rise in normal women. J Clin Endocrinol Metab 1996; 81: 1038–45.

15. Santoro N, Brown JR, Adel T et al. Characterization of perimenopausal reproductive hormonal dynamics. Clin Endocrinol Metab 1996; 81: 1495–501.

16. Sherman BM, West JH, Korenman SG. The menopausal transition: analysis of LH, FSH, estradiol and progesterone concentrations during menstrual cycles of older women. Clin Endocrinol Metab 1976; 42: 629–36.

17. Shideler SE, DeVane GW, Kaira PS et al. Ovarian–pituitary hormone interactions during the perimenopause. Maturitas 1989; 11: 331–9.

18. Treloar AE, Boynton RE, Behn BG et al. Variation of the human menstrual cycle through reproductive life. Int J Fertil 1967; 12: 77–127.

19. Ahmed-Ebbiary NA, Lenton EA, Cooke ID. Hypothalamic–pituitary ageing: progressive increase in FSH and LH concentrations throughout the reproductive life in regularly menstruation women. Clin Endocrinol 1994; 41: 199–206.

20. Burger HG, Dudley BC, Hopper JL et al. The endocrinology of the menopausal transition: a cross-sectional study of a population-based sample. Clin Endocrinol Metab 1995; 80: 3527–45.

21. Belsey EM, Pinol APY. Task force on long-acting systemic agents for fertility regulation: menstrual bleeding patterns in untreated women. Contraception 1997; 55: 57–65.

22. Garamszegi C, Dennerstein L, Dudley E et al. Menopausal status: subjectively and objectively defined. J Psychosom Obstet Gynaecol 1998; 19: 165–73.

23. Taffe JR, Dennerstein L. Menstrual patterns leading to the final menstrual period. Menopause 2002; 9: 32–40.

24. Klein NA, Battaglia D, Fujimoto V et al. Reproductive aging: accelerated ovarian follicular development associated with a monotropic follicle-stimulating hormone rise in normal older women. J Clin Endocrinol Metab 1996; 81: 1038–45.

25. Metcalf MG, Donald RA. Fluctuating ovarian function in a perimenopausal woman. NZ Med J 1979; 89: 45–7.

26. Weiss G, Skurnick JH, Goldsmith LT et al. Menopause and hypothalamic–pituitary sensitivity to estrogen. JAMA 2004; 292: 2991–6.

27. Management of Uterine Fibroids. Summary, Evidence Report/Technology Assessment: Number 34. AHRQ Publication No. 01–E051, January 2001. Agency for Healthcare Research and Quality, Rockville, MD. Accessed on December 2, 2005 at http://www.ahrq.gov/clinic/epcsums/utersumm.htm.

28. Cramer SF, Patel A. The frequency of uterine leiomyomas. Am J Clin Pathol 1990; 94: 435–8.

29. Marshall LM, Spiegelman D, Barbieri RL et al. Variation in the incidence of uterine leiomyoma among premenopausal women by age and race. Obstet Gynecol 1997; 90: 967–73.

30. Stewart EA. Uterine fibroids. Lancet 2001; 357: 293–8.

31. Ross RK, Pike MC, Vessey MP et al. Risk factors for uterine fibroids: reduced risk associated with oral contraceptives. BMJ (Clin Res Ed) 1986; 293: 359–62.

32. Marshall L, Spiegelman D, Goldman MB et al. A prospective study of reproductive factors and oral contraceptive use in relation to the risk of uterine leiomyomata. Fertil Steril 1998; 70: 432–9.

33. Stewart EA, Nowak RA. Leiomyoma-related bleeding: a classic hypothesis updated for the molecular era. Hum Reprod Update 1996; 2: 295–306.

34. Schoenberg C, Fejzo M, Ashar HR et al. Translocation breakpoints upstream of the HMGIC gene in uterine leiomyomata suggest dysregulation of this gene by a mechanism different from that in lipomas. Genes Chromosomes Cancer 1996; 17: 1–6.

35. Kothapalli R, Buyuksal I, Wu SQ et al. Detection of ebaf, a novel human gene of the transforming growth factor beta superfamily association of gene expression with endometrial bleeding. J Clin Invest 1997; 99: 2342–50.

36. Barbieri RL. Ambulatory management of uterine leiomyomata. Clin Obstet Gynecol 1999; 42: 196–205.

37. Van Bogaert L. Clinicopathologic findings in endometrial polyps. Obstet Gynecol 1988; 71: 771–3.

38. Savelli L, De Iaco, P Santini D et al. Histopathologic features and risk factors for benignity, hyperplasia, and cancer in endometrial polyps. Am J Obstet Gynecol 2003; 188: 927–31.

39. Pal L, Pollack S, Niklaus A et al. Focal over expression of endometrial aromatase may underlie pathogenesis of endometrial polyps. J Soc Gynecol Investig 2005; 12: 95A.

40. Dal Cin P, Vanni R, Marras S et al. Four cytogenetic subgroups can be identified in endometrial polyps. Cancer Res 1995; 55: 1565–8.

41. Tallini G, Vanni R, Manfioletti G et al. HMGI-C and HMGI(Y) immunoreactivity correlates with cytogenetic abnormalities in lipomas, pulmonary chondroid hamartomas, endometrial polyps, and uterine leiomyomas and is compatible with rearrangement

of the HMGI-C and HMGI(Y) genes. Lab Invest 2000; 80: 359–69.

42. Ferenczy A. Pathophysiology of adenomyosis. Hum Reprod Update 1998; 4: 312–22.

43. Enatsu A, Harada T, Yoshida S et al. Adenomyosis in a patient with the Rokitansky–Kuster–Hauser syndrome. Fertil Steril 2000; 73: 862–3.

44. Cano F, Simon C, Retnohi J et al. Effect of aging on the female reproductive system: evidence for a role of uterine senescence in the decline in female fecundity. Fertil Steril 1995; 64: 584–9.

45. Navot D, Drews MR, Bergh PA et al. Age-related decline in female fertility is not due to diminished capacity of the uterus to sustain embryo implantation. Fertil Steril 1994; 61: 97–101.

46. Sauer MV, Paulson RJ, Lobo RA. A preliminary report on oocyte donation extending reproductive potential to women over 40. N Engl J Med 1990; 323: 1157–60.

47. Yaron Y, Botchan A, Amit A et al. Endometrial receptivity: the age-related decline in pregnancy rates and the effect of ovarian function. Fertil Steril 1993; 60: 314–18.

48. Toner JP, Grainger DA, Frazier LM. Clinical outcomes among recipients of donated eggs: an analysis of the U.S. national experience, 1996–1998. Fertil Steril 2002; 78: 1038–45.

49. Batista MC, Cartledge TP, Zeilmer AW et al. Effects of aging on menstrual cycle hormones and endometrial maturation. Fertil Steril 1995; 64: 492–9.

50. Lessey BA, Young SL. Integrins and other cellular adhesion molecules in endometrium and endometriosis. Semin Reprod Endocrinol 1990; 15: 291–9.

51. Lee PD, Giudice LC, Conover CA, Powell DR. Insulin-like growth factor binding protein-1: recent findings and new directions. Proc Soc Exp Biol Med 1997; 216: 319–57.

52. Paulson RJ, Hatch IE, Lobo RA et al. Cumulative conception and live birth rates after oocyte donation: implications regarding endometrial receptivity. Hum Reprod 1997; 12: 835–9.

53. Aubuchon M, Niklaus AL, Zapantis G et al. Human endometrium from mid reproductive age to menopausal transition: mrna and protein expression of cell cycle markers and steroid hormone receptors in laser captured luminal and glandular epithelia. J Soc Gynecol Investig 2005; 12: 182A–3A.

54. Markee JE. Menstruation in intraocular endometrial transplants in the rhesus monkey. Contrib Embryol 1940; 28: 219–308.

55. Jabbour HN, Kelly RW, Fraser HM, Critchley HO. Endocrine regulation of menstruation. Endocr Rev 2006; 27: 17–46.

56. Kelly RW, King AE, Critchley HOD Cytokine control in human endometrium. Reproduction 2001; 121: 3–19.

57. Bruner KL, Rodgers WH, Gold L et al. Transforming growth factor beta mediates the progesterone suppression of an epithelial metalloproteinase by adjacent stroma in the human endometrium. Proc Natl Acad Sci USA 1995; 92: 7362–6.

58. Barer AP, Fowler WM. The blood loss during normal menstruation. Am J Obstet Gynecol 1936; 31: 979–86.

59. Haynes PJ, Anderson ABM, Turnbull AC. Patterns of menstrual blood loss in menorrhagia. Res Clin Forums 1979; 1: 73–8.

60. Christiaens GC, Sixma JJ, Haspeis AA. Hemostasis in menstrual endometrium: a review. Obstet Gynecol Surv 1982; 37: 281–303.

61. Noyes RW, Hertig AT, Rock J. Dating the endometrial biopsy. Fertil Steril 1950; 1: 3–25.

62. King A. Uterine leukocytes and decidualization. Hum Reprod Update 2000; 6: 28–36.

63. Henderson TA, Saunders PT, Moffett-King A et al. Steroid receptor expression in uterine natural killer cells. J Clin Endocrinol Metab 2003; 88: 440–9.

64. Chwalisz K, DeManno D, Garg R et al. Therapeutic potential for the selective progesterone receptor modulator asoprisnil in the treatment of leiomyomata. Semin Reprod Med 2004; 22: 113–19.

65. Grimes D. Diagnostic dilatation and curettage: a reappraisal. Am J Obstet Gynecol 1982; 142: 1–6.

66. Hallberg L, Hogdahl AM, Nilsson L et al. Menstrual loss – a population study. Variation at different ages and attempts to define normality. Acta Obstet Gynecol Scand 1966; 45: 320–51.

67. Chimbira TH, Anderson ABM, Turnbull AC. Relation between measured menstrual blood loss and patient's subjective assessment of loss, duration of bleeding, number of sanitary towels used, uterine weight and endometrial surface area. Br J Obstet Gynaecol 1980; 87: 603–9.

68. Warner PE, Critchley HO, Lumsden MA et al Menorrhagia I: measured blood loss, clinical features, and outcome in women with heavy periods: a survey with follow-up data. Am J Obstet Gynecol 2004; 190: 1216–23.

69. Warner PE, Critchley HO, Lumsden MA et al. Menorrhagia II: is the 80-ml blood loss criterion useful in management of complaint of menorrhagia? Am J Obstet Gynecol 2004; 190: 1224–9.

70. Cameron ST, Critchley HOD, Thong KJ et al. Effects of daily low dose mifepristone on endometrial maturation and proliferation. Hum Reprod 1996; 11: 2518–26.

71. Bergqvist A, Rybo G. Treatment of menorrhagia with intrauterine release of progesterone. Br J Obstet Gynaecol 1983; 90: 255–8.

72. Cameron IT. Dysfunctional uterine bleeding. Baillières Clin Obstet Gynecol 1989; 3: 315–27.

73. Okulicz WC, Balsamo M, Tast J. Progesterone regulation of endometrial estrogen receptor and cell proliferation during the late proliferative and secretory phase in artificial menstrual cycles in the rhesus monkey. Biol Reprod 1993; 49: 24–32.

74. Gleeson N, Jordan M, Sheppard B et al. Cyclical variation in endometrial oestrogen and progesterone receptors in women with normal menstruation and dysfunctional uterine bleeding. Eur J Obstet Gynecol Reprod Biol 1993; 48: 207–14.

75. Chakraborty S, Khurana N, Sharma JB et al. Endometrial hormone receptors in women with dysfunctional uterine bleeding. Arch Gynecol Obstet 2005; 272: 17–22.

76. Losordo DW, Kearney M, Kim EA et al. Variable expression of the estrogen receptor in normal and atherosclerotic coronary arteries of premenopausal women. Circulation 1994; 89: 1501–10.

77. Rogers PAW, Lederman F, Looy J et al. Endometrial vascular smooth muscle oestrogen and progesterone receptor distribution in women with and without menorrhagia. Hum Reprod 1996; 11: 2003–8.

78. Weel AE, Uitterlinden AG, Westendorp IC et al. Estrogen receptor polymorphism predicts the onset of natural and surgical menopause. J Clin Endocrinol Metab 1999; 84: 3146–50.

79. APGO Educational Series on Women's Health Issues. Clinical management of abnormal uterine bleeding. Association of Professors of Gynecology and Obstetrics, Crofton, MD, May 2002.

80. Kamel HS, Darwish AM, Mohamed SA. Comparison of transvaginal ultrasonography and vaginal sonohysterography in the detection of endometrial polyps. Acta Obstet Gynecol Scand 2000; 79: 60–4.

81. Ries LAG, Eisner MP, Kosary CL et al (eds). SEER Cancer Statistics Review, 1975–2000, National Cancer Institute. Bethesda, MD. Accessed December 1, 2005 at http://seer.cancer.gov/csr/1975_2000.

82. Allen DG, Correy JF, Marsden DE. Abnormal uterine bleeding and cancer of the genital tract. Aust NZ J Obstet Gynaecol 1990; 30: 81–3.

83. Iatrakis G, Diakakis I, Kourounis G et al. Postmenopausal uterine bleeding. Clin Exp Obstet Gynecol 1997; 24: 157.

84. Loffer FD. Hysteroscopy with selective endometrial sampling compared with D&C for abnormal uterine bleeding: the value of a negative hysteroscopic view. Obstet Gynecol 1989; 73: 16–20.

85. Cicinelli E, Parisi C, Galantino P et al. Reliability, feasibility, and safety of minihysteroscopy with a vaginoscopic approach: experience with 6,000 cases. Fertil Steril 2003; 80: 199–202.

86. van Rooij IAJ, den Tonkelaar I, Broekmans FJM et al. Anti-müllerian hormone is a promising predictor for the occurrence of the menopausal transition. Menopause 2004; 11: 601–6.

87. Langer RD, Pierce JJ, O'Hanlan KA et al. Transvaginal ultrasonography compared with endometrial biopsy for the detection of endometrial disease. Postmenopausal Estrogen/Progestin Interventions Trial. N Engl J Med 1997; 337: 1792–8.

88. Gredmark T, Kvint S, Havel G et al. Histopathological findings in women with postmenopausal bleeding. Br J Obstet Gynaecol 1995; 102: 133–6.

89. Tanizawa O, Miyake A, Sugimoto O. [Re-evaluation of hysteroscopy in the diagnosis of uterine endometrial cancer]. Nippon Sanka Fujinka Gakkai Zasshi 1991; 43: 622–6. [in Japanese]

90. Obermair A, Geramou M, Gucer F et al. Does hysteroscopy facilitate tumor cell dissemination? Incidence of peritoneal cytology from patients with early stage endometrial carcinoma following dilatation and curettage (D&C) versus hysteroscopy and D&C. Cancer 2000; 88: 139–43.

91. Lethaby A, Irvine G, Cameron I. Cyclical progestogens for heavy menstrual bleeding. Cochrane Database Syst Rev 2000; CD001016.

92. Miller L, Notter KM. Menstrual reduction with extended use of combination oral contraceptive pills: randomized controlled trial. Obstet Gynecol 2001; 98: 771–8.

93. Tanis BC, van den Bosch MA, Kemmeren JM et al. Oral contraceptives and the risk of myocardial infarction. N Engl J Med 2001; 345: 1787–93.

94. Lethaby A, Augood C, Duckitt K. Nonsteroidal anti-inflammatory drugs for heavy menstrual bleeding. Cochrane Database Syst Rev 2000; CD000400.

95. Irvine GA, Cameron IT. Medical management of dysfunctional uterine bleeding. Baillières Best Pract Res Clin Obstet Gynaecol 1999; 13: 189–202.

96. Beksinska MF, Smit JA, Kleinschmidt I et al. Bone mineral density in women aged 40–49 years using depot-medroxyprogesterone acetate, norethisterone enanthate or combined oral contraceptives for contraception. Contraception 2005; 71: 170–5.

97. Rogerson L, Hawe J, Duffy S. Modern approaches to management of menorrhagia. Hosp Med 2000; 61: 90–2.

98. Kuppermann M, Varner RE, Summitt RL Jr et al. Effect of hysterectomy vs medical treatment on health-related quality of life and sexual functioning: the medicine or surgery (Ms) randomized trial. JAMA 2004; 291: 1447–55.

99. Ribeiro SC, Ribeiro RM, Santos NC et al. A randomized study of total abdominal, vaginal and laparoscopic hysterectomy. Int J Gynaecol Obstet 2003; 83: 37–43.

54 Benign uterine disease: leiomyomata and benign polyps

Marcy Maguire and James H Segars

ABSTRACT

It is estimated that one-third of all gynecological visits are precipitated by uterine bleeding and an even greater proportion of women in the perimenopausal period seek care because of abnormal uterine bleeding. Benign diseases of the endometrium – endometrial polyps and uterine leiomyomata – are the most likely causes of such symptoms. The objective of this chapter is to review the current understanding of how these two benign conditions of the endometrium affect endometrial growth, leading to common gynecological problems such as abnormal uterine bleeding and infertility. Understanding of leiomyomata and endometrial polyps remains incomplete, although recent advances resulting from the application of genomic and proteomic methods to these diseases have provided insight. Additional basic, translational, and clinical research is needed to improve understanding and develop more effective preventive strategies for the disorders.

UTERINE LEIOMYOMATA AND ALTERED ENDOMETRIAL GROWTH

INTRODUCTION AND CLASSIFICATION OF UTERINE FIBROIDS

Uterine leiomyomata (commonly know as 'fibroids') are benign growths believed to arise from the expansion of single cells based on studies of clonality.[1] A role for sex steroids in the growth of fibroids is suggested by epidemiological, clinical, and experimental studies.[2,3] Pathologically, fibroids are composed of remarkably homogeneous cells surrounded by whorls of an abundant extracellular matrix (ECM). Clinical studies of fibroid growth confirm the importance of the ECM in fibroid growth, as growth >5 cm is largely due to increased deposition of extracellular proteins.[4] Although uterine fibroids commonly cause pelvic pressure and pain, since the effect of fibroids upon the endometrium is the focus of this chapter, the discussion here is

focused upon the altered endometrial development that is associated with uterine bleeding and infertility. Fibroids most likely to affect endometrial growth are those that are either intracavitary (IC), or those that are located in the myometrium just beneath the endometrium, often distorting the endometrial cavity, known as submucous myomas (SM). The description of a fibroid as 'submucous' is a misnomer, since there is no mucosal epithelium in the uterus, but the term is often used in the literature and will be used interchangeably with the more proper phrase 'subendometrial' fibroid.

Students of fibroid disease are confronted with a formidable obstacle, as there is not a current, universally accepted classification system for fibroid disease. As a result, investigators often improvise depending upon their needs, leading to difficulties when studies between investigators are compared. For the purposes of this review, the European Society of Human Reproduction and Embryology (ESHRE) hysteroscopic classification[5] will be used, as it is currently the most inclusive and clinically relevant (Figure 54.1). In addition, clinically there appears to be more than one type of fibroid disease.[6] This is obvious for the familial and genetic syndromes of fibroid disease,[7] but is also notable for common fibroids that may be solitary in some cases, but in other cases the uterus is largely replaced with fibroid change. Molecular characterization of fibroids suggests that the pathological entity of a fibroid may feature different genetic differences depending upon the race or genetic cause.[2,7]

INCIDENCE AND PREVALENCE OF UTERINE FIBROIDS

The incidence of uterine fibroids, and thus their ability to alter endometrial growth, varies according to age, race, population, and risk factors. It should be noted that fibroids are three-fold more common in African-American women than in Caucasian women based on population prevalence studies,[8] retrospective studies in infertility patients,[9] myomectomy, and hysterectomy

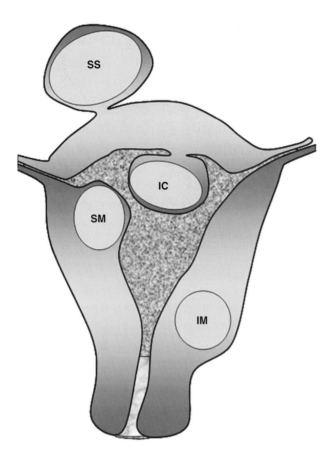

Figure 54.1   Subtypes of uterine leiomyomata. Uterine leiomyomata may be classified by location. Subserosal fibroids (SS) are fibroids that are located beneath the serosal surface of the uterus and do not extend into the corpus of the myometrium. Subserosal fibroids are unlikely to affect endometrial development. Intramural fibroids (IM) are localized primarily within the myometrium. Studies of intramural leiomyomata are conflicting, but if sufficiently large (4–6 cm), some reports indicate that endometrial development is affected. Submucosal leiomyomata (SM) are also located within the uterine muscle, but lead to distortion of the endometrial cavity. Submucosal leiomyomata are associated with altered endometrial development in many instances. Intracavitary fibroids (IC) are located primarily within the endometrial cavity and are most strongly associated with altered endometrial development.

rates.[10] Studies have also shown that the incidence of leiomyoma increases with age. In one study of hysterectomy specimens, 77% of specimens contained leiomyoma,[11] suggesting that by the perimenopause, the majority of hysterectomy specimens contained leiomyoma. Studies of fibroid growth suggested that the rate of growth was approximately 1 cm/year.[4] A review of leiomyomata growth supported this finding and supported the conclusion that in most cases, fibroids grew at a rate of 1.2 cm/2.5 year.[12] Cross-sectional studies and cohort studies of populations suggest that the prevalence and incidence of disease varies among different geographic populations.[6] It should be emphasized that the clinical prevalence of disease is affected by the diagnostic method used to detect disease (see below). Regardless of the differences in detection and variation in prevalence among different populations, it is clear that fibroids are one of the most commonly encountered gynecological diseases.

Relevant to consideration of the effect of fibroids on endometrial development is the question: given that fibroids are a very prevalent condition, how often do fibroids affect endometrial growth? It is not possible to fully address this question since most studies have focused on microscopic or ultrasound criteria, but fibroids may cause subtle alterations in endometrial differentiation that are not apparent by those criteria. Clinically, the effect of fibroids upon endometrial development in vivo may be grossly visualized by a thinning of the endometrium overlying the uterine fibroid that is observed on an ultrasound examination. Using this metric, it is clear that not all fibroids affect endometrial development. In a study from Michigan, the authors noted that only 40% of fibroids that distorted the endometrial cavity were associated with thinning of the endometrium.[13] Few studies have specifically addressed the prevalence of fibroids that alter endometrial growth, but it is clear that uterine location of fibroids influences their effect upon endometrial development.

EFFECTS OF UTERINE FIBROIDS ON ENDOMETRIAL GROWTH

Endometrial anomalies have been known to be associated with uterine fibroids for over 30 years. An interesting study by Deligdish and Loewenthal[14] examined 30 hysterectomy specimens by light microscopy and reported that endometrial change most commonly associated with leiomyoma was glandular atrophy overlying the leiomyoma. In addition, distorted or dilated endometrial glands were noted in 50% of cases. Furthermore, only 3/30 (10%) endometrial tissues overlying leiomyoma exhibited cyclic changes.[14] In general, subsequent reports have confirmed similar endometrial anomalies by light microscopy. For instance, in 1979 Sharma et al[15] reported a study of 40 uteri with submucous myoma and noted 'parallel oriented and elongated glands,' and in many cases endometrial atrophy. A remarkable finding noted by both studies[14,15] was the presence of muscle fibers in the endometrium overlying leiomyoma, a finding that may be considered strongly suggestive of the presence of uterine fibroids if noted on endometrial biopsy.

Patterson-Keels et al[13] examined 13 hysterectomy specimens with fibroids and compared these to 7 specimens without fibroids. The authors divided the samples into two groups based upon the distance of the fibroid to the endometrial cavity. In the group where the fibroid was closest to the endometrial cavity (average distance of 0.5 cm), the endometrial thickness was only 0.38 cm and no endometrial glands were seen. If the fibroid was 1.7 cm from the endometrial cavity, an average of 74.5 glands were noted, as compared to 82.6 in control specimens that lacked fibroids.[13] These observations are important, since they indicate that the proximity of the fibroid to the endometrium has a direct effect upon endometrial development overlying the fibroid. These data, supported by a number of studies, support the conclusion that leiomyomata closest to the endometrial cavity are those most likely to alter endometrial development.

A significant finding noted by Deligdish and Loewenthal[14] was that in 12/30 cases there were abnormal endometrial changes opposite the leiomyomata. The finding of 'subtotal atrophy' in the endometrial region opposite the leiomyoma was attributed to mechanical pressure exerted by the leiomyoma. Sharma et al[15] also noted endometrial anomalies opposite the fibroid and went further to correlate the glandular atrophy opposite the fibroid with the size of the leiomyoma in the uterus. In leiomyomata of 2–4 cm size, 0/10 specimens had endometrial changes opposite the leiomyoma. If the leiomyoma was 4–6 cm, 14/23 had changes in the endometrium opposite the leiomyoma. If the leiomyoma was 6–8 cm, 6/6 specimens had endometrial changes opposite the tumor.

The presence of endometrial changes opposite the leiomyoma is an important and significant observation because this means that a fibroid located in one portion of the uterus can exert a global effect upon endometrial development not limited to the region overlying the fibroid. Stated differently, a 4 cm leiomyoma may cause endometrial glandular atrophy not only overlying the tumor but also throughout the endometrial cavity (Figure 54.2). Alteration in endometrial development is of relevance to understanding the effect of fibroids regarding infertility, where a clear reduction in implantation rates is noted. In addition, the observation of endometrial effects opposite the leiomyoma is very provocative, since it would seem unlikely that locally secreted paracrine growth factors could contribute to the endometrial change because the vascular and cell contacts are remote from the endometrial changes on the opposite side of the uterus.

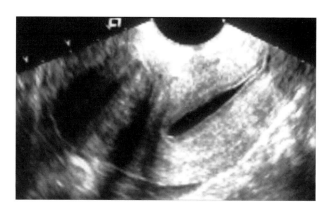

Figure 54.2 Subtle effects of a leiomyoma upon endometrial growth. Transvaginal saline sonography showing a 3.5×4.0 cm fundal fibroid that is located in the myometrium, but lies within 5 mm of the endometrial basalis. The endometrium is clearly visible as a band of tissue between the black uterine cavity and the myometrium. Endometrial thickness in this case may be subtly reduced (by 1–2 mm) adjacent to the leiomyoma, in comparison with endometrium overlying myometrium opposite the leiomyoma.

DO VASCULAR CHANGES ASSOCIATED WITH LEIOMYOMATA EXPLAIN THE ENDOMETRIAL EFFECTS?

The fact that uterine fibroids are associated with vascular congestion was recorded by Sampson in 1913 and, based on this observation, for many years menorrhagia associated with fibroids was assumed to be a direct result of vascular changes, especially venous congestion.

In their 1960 study, Sehgal and Haskins[16] reasoned that since estrogen treatment reduced menorrhagia in cases with leiomyoma, venous congestion could not be responsible for menorrhagia associated with fibroids because estrogen would not be expected to influence vascular congestion of the endometrium. The authors used direct plaster casts of the endometrial lining in 26 specimens. They noted that the average surface area was 14.5 cm² without leiomyomata, but increased to an average area of 87 cm² in the group with Hgb <11%.[16] The authors suggested that increased surface area, not venous congestion per se, accounted for the increased menorrhagia with leiomyoma.

The remarkable vascular effects associated with leiomyomata then raise the question: were the observed endometrial changes due to vascular effects? In their 1970 study of the vascular patterns of uterine leiomyomata, Farrer-Brown et al[17] used injection of radiographic contrast and X-ray studies to examine specimens. The authors noted it was difficult to inject the veins in many specimens, but in many cases there were large dilated veins very close to the endometrial cavity. In addition, the authors[17] observed similar endometrial changes to Deligdish and Loewenthal,[14] although that was not the purpose of the study. In a follow-up study of 28 specimens Farrer-Brown et al[18] specifically commented on endometrial changes and suggested that dilatation of the veins in the endometrium may contribute to the anomalies overlying the leiomyoma. In published micrographs, the specimens are noted to have leiomyomata immediately beneath the endometrium. The authors noted that there was no specific pattern to the vascular supply of the leiomyomata, but that larger fibroids tended to be associated with larger vessels.

Subsequent studies suggested that there was a direct relationship between blood flow and size[19] – the larger the fibroid, the greater the flow. Casey et al[20] examined 10 uteri with vascular markers and noted greater diameter ($p = 0.04$) in large fibroids vs myometrium, but no evidence of increased blood supply to fibroids. This observation was supported by Doppler measurement,[21] which revealed than fibroids tumors themselves had a lower flow than surrounding normal myometrium.

In summation, available evidence supports the conclusion that while venous congestion is certainly associated with leiomyomata, the tumors themselves do not have increased blood flow and the tumors appear to recruit vascular supply from adjacent myometrium. In rare cases there may be erosion of vascular channels located under the endometrium. Current evidence indicates that in most cases excessive menorrhagia associated with leiomyomata is related to endometrial changes (especially atrophy) caused by the leiomyomata, as well as the increased surface area of the endometrial cavity in the presence of a leiomyomata.

WHAT IS THE MECHANISM OF ENDOMETRIAL ATROPHY ASSOCIATED WITH LEIOMYOMATA?

Despite recent studies directed to define the molecular features of uterine fibroids, the mechanism(s) responsible for the endometrial atrophy overlying fibroids, and the endometrial changes opposite leiomyomata, remain unclear. Few studies have been specifically directed at the endometrium, possibly because the tissue is extremely thin and difficult to study.

Of note, Bulun et al[22,23] reported that leiomyomata were a source of estrogen and there were increased tissue concentrations of estrogen in leiomyomata and in surrounding tissues compared to myometrium without

leiomyomata. The mechanism was production of aromatase by leiomyomata. In contrast, normal myometrium does not produce aromatase.[22] Since locally produced estrogen may then diffuse around the leiomyoma, the increased estrogen might then influence endometrial development, provided the leiomyomata is adjacent to the endometrium. If locally produced estrogen is a mechanism that contributes to endometrial effects of fibroids, it is not clear why the effect is glandular atrophy, not endometrial proliferation and glandular mitoses – effects usually associated with estrogen. However, the possibility of a direct or local effect of leiomyomata has inherent appeal. If locally produced, possibly estrogen-responsive, growth factors act by a paracrine mechanism to alter endometrial development, it is somewhat difficult to account for effects upon endometrium opposite the fibroid, unless the factor(s) diffuses across the endometrial lumen.

Recently Rackow and Taylor[24] reported that presence of leiomyomata altered expression of *Hoxa-10*, a gene that regulates segmental development in tissues as well as other genes in adult tissues. This observation is noteworthy because *Hoxa-10*-deficient mice exhibit a block to endometrial implantation, suggesting that *Hoxa-10* expression in the endometrium is required for nidation.[25] The presence of fibroids that were submucosal led to a reduction in *Hoxa-10* expression not only in the endometrium overlying the fibroid but also in the endometrial tissue opposite the fibroid,[24] suggesting a global effect upon endometrial development. The effect was limited to fibroids that were submucosal and was not observed with intramural fibroids.[24] Reduction in *Hoxa-10* expression might correlate with a molecular deficiency in endometrial development and therefore be associated with a reduction in implantation, consistent with clinical observations (see below). As the observation was recently reported, it is not known how fibroids might cause such a reduction, or the specific endometrial defect that might correlate or result from this reduction in *Hoxa-10*.

One possible mechanism that might explain how leiomyomata exert effects across the endometrial lumen is that of mechanotransduction, a signaling pathway that has been elucidated in the cardiovascular[26] and breast cancer literature.[27] In addition to the soluble growth factor signaling cascades usually considered and well-elucidated, there is a solid-state cell signaling mechanism important for cell differentiation (for brief review, see Huang and Ingber[28]). Such mechanisms influence dilation of vessels,[26] and as noted above, endometrial and myometrial changes associated with leiomyomata often feature vascular dilatation. At present there are no studies that have directly analyzed solid-state mechanotransduction in endometrial tissues. A plausible mechanism is that mechanotransduction signaling in endometrial tissue is activated by pressure of the fibroid upon the endometrium, thus leading to endometrial atrophy. This explanation has appeal, since it might also explain:

- the effects of fibroid distention upon endometrium overlying the leiomyoma
- effect and size-relationship of leiomyomata on endometrium opposite the leiomyoma
- trans-differentiation of endometrial cells to form myofibers, as noted by several authors
- why vascular dilatation is often associated with endometrial atrophy.

Studies to evaluate the role of mechanotransduction in endometrial development are needed.

A related possibility is that the ECM of the tissue surrounding the leiomyoma may influence endometrial growth and differentiation. Altered ECM has been associated with fibroid growth,[29] and fibroids are known to secrete an ECM that is altered in amount, content,[30] and structure.[31] Alteration of ECM also influences the mechanical properties of the tissue.[27,28] Alteration of the ECM may alter the effects of estrogen at the level of the endometrium,[32] in keeping with clinical and pathological observations of impairment in estrogen effect in the endometrium. The relationship of the ECM to cell signaling has been most clearly elucidated in other tissues,[26,27] but might also play a role in endometrial development.

It is possible that endometrial effects of uterine fibroids may involve dysregulation in several signaling pathways that influence endometrial development. Additional research is needed to elucidate the precise mechanism of how the presence of uterine fibroids alters endometrial growth and differentiation not only of tissue overlying the fibroid but also of endometrial tissue lying opposite the fibroid.

CLINICAL CONSEQUENCES OF FIBROIDS

Several of the clinical problems associated with leiomyomata appear to be related to their effect upon endometrial growth. Fibroids are associated with several common gynecological symptoms: pelvic pain, pelvic pressure, excessive bleeding, infertility, and miscarriage. Of these symptoms, excessive bleeding, infertility, and miscarriage may be the indirect effects of leiomyomata

upon endometrial development. Obstetrical complications are significant and include an increased likelihood of preterm birth, cesarean section, placental abruption, abnormal fetal presentations, premature rupture of membranes, and dysfunctional labor.[33] It is possible, but not established, that altered endometrial development may predispose to the altered decidual relationships that may cause problems such as placental abruption. Gynecological symptoms such as pain, pressure, and bleeding often lead to hysterectomy or myomectomy. Fibroids are the leading indication for hysterectomy in the USA. For some women with fibroids, uterine artery embolization (UAE) and magnetic resonance imaging (MRI)-guided ultrasound are suitable interventions that may be beneficial, although the long-term durability and consequences of UAE and MRI-guided ultrasound have not been studied.[34]

MEDICAL STRATEGIES FOR TREATMENT OF BLEEDING ASSOCIATED WITH FIBROIDS

Medical therapy is presently almost solely limited to preoperative management, as there is no Food and Drug Administration (FDA)-approved effective, long-term treatment to reduce fibroid size or prevent fibroid development. Strategies such as gonadotropin-releasing hormone (GnRH) agonist treatment are limited by hypestrogenic symptoms and bone loss, unless 'add-back' hormone replacement is given. Contrary to expectations, the levonorgestrel-releasing intrauterine device (IUD) has been shown to be of considerable benefit in reducing bleeding, even in the presence of fibroids that grossly distort the endometrial cavity,[35] again emphasizing that the endometrial development overlying the fibroids is the proximate cause of bleeding associated with fibroids and not erosion of large vascular channels.

Bleeding symptoms, especially preoperatively to augment hemoglobin levels, are effectively managed by short-term GnRH agonist treatment, optimally as a depot injection, with or without 'add-back' hormonal replacement. Acute bleeding episodes often, but not always, respond to oral contraceptive pill therapy with stabilization or marked reduction in bleeding. Since fibroids are progestin-responsive, antiprogestins have been shown to reduce fibroid size.[36] While sizable reductions in fibroid size can be obtained with pure antiprogestins, this medical strategy is limited by the associated endometrial hyperplasia, which has been noted in 28% of women due to the inhibition of the progestin action at the level of the endometrium.[36]

The endometrial hyperplasia observed with pure antiprogestins fueled development of selective progesterone receptor modulators (SPRMs), compounds that act in a mixed agonist–antagonist manner. The selective progestin modulator asoprisnil (J867-TAP) has shown promise in clinical trials, with a significant reduction in bleeding and a reduction in fibroid size.[37] A significant clinical finding with asoprisnil was that bleeding stopped immediately, even before there was reduction in fibroid size, consistent with immediate stabilization of endometrial shedding associated with fibroids.[37] Again, this beneficial response underscores the fact that endometrial effects, not vascular erosion, is most often the mechanism of menorrhagia in bleeding caused by fibroids. Trials are currently underway to evaluate this promising compound which might be able to serve as a long-term medical option, since treatment with asoprisnil is not accompanied by a hypoestrogenic state.

Another medication currently under investigation is pirfenidone. This compound is an antifibrotic and antitumor agent that has been shown to interfere with transforming growth factor-β (TGFβ) action in vitro and inhibit leiomyoma cell growth.[38] Pirfenidone was shown by Stewart et al[39] to reduce fibroid volume in small clinical trials, presumably via inhibition of TGFβ action. Whether pirfenidone will show benefit upon endometrial development in women with fibroid disease remains to be determined, but the reduction in fibroid volume associated with treatment was significant.

CONSEQUENCES OF THE EFFECT OF FIBROIDS UPON THE ENDOMETRIUM: INFERTILITY AND MISCARRIAGE

Fibroids that distort the endometrial cavity and affect endometrial development have been clearly linked to a reduction in implantation and miscarriage (for review, see Pritts[40]). Because the time-to-pregnancy comparisons are simplest to control in women undergoing assisted reproductive technologies (ART) such as in-vitro fertilization/intracytoplasmic sperm injection (IVF-ICSI), the effect of fibroids upon infertility is most apparent and the contribution of fibroids to infertility is most readily defined. If the endometrial cavity was distorted in women pursuing ART, implantation rates were reduced (the likelihood of a conceptus establishing a healthy relationship with the endometrium), miscarriage rates were increased, and overall pregnancy rates were lower.[40] The effect was strongest and most apparent for those fibroids that were entirely located within the endometrial cavity (Figure 54.3), the

intracavitary leiomyomata.[40] As was observed for effects upon the endometrium,[13] the fibroids that distorted the cavity were associated with reductions in fertility, whereas fibroids located on the outer surface of the uterus (peritoneal), subserosal fibroids, had little impact upon fertility. The strong effect of location of fibroids upon fertility has been consistently observed in many studies by a number of investigators, not only in women pursuing ART but also in women interested in pregnancy who are not pursuing ART.

For women interested in pregnancy who have fibroids that distort the cavity, or those women who desire to preserve the option to pursue childbearing in the future, myomectomy is the preferred course of therapy. Myomectomy may be performed either hysteroscopically if the leiomyomata are accessible and of suitable size (≤ 2 cm), or via laparotomy. A recent Cochrane review[41] considered the question of whether evidence was sufficient to consider UAE for women interested in fertility and concluded that possible impairment of ovarian function in women following UAE made myomectomy a better choice for women interested in fertility.

Evidence is currently rather limited, but since there is collateral circulation between the uterus and ovary, embolization of the uterine artery (note: the uterus, not the fibroid, is embolized) may lead to ovarian insufficiency as documented by elevated follicle-stimulating hormone (FSH) levels or early menopause in some women.[41] Another concern for treatment of women with UAE who are interested in fertility is the associated abnormalities in placentation, such as placenta accreta, which is markedly increased.[42] In addition, there are anecdotal reports of complete endometrial atophy following UAE. For these reasons, current recommendations for women interested in fertility who have fibroids likely to impair establishment of pregnancy are not UAE, but rather operative normalization of the uterine cavity. The anecdotal reports of pregnancy following UAE are not sufficient evidence of the safety and efficacy of the method in women desirous of childbearing and most centers offering UAE consider desire for future pregnancy to be a relative contraindication.

An exciting option for women interested in future childbearing is MRI-guided ultrasound ablation of uterine fibroids.[43] Since this treatment does not impair ovarian function, it is reasonable to consider in women interested in future childbearing. Also, endometrial damage is unlikely to result from the treatment. At present the therapy is offered only in a few centers and is relatively costly. A very attractive feature of the

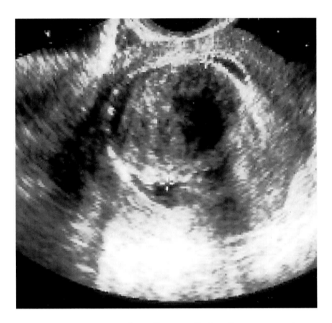

Figure 54.3 Impaired endometrial development with an intracavitary leiomyoma. Transvaginal saline sonography of an intracavitary leiomyoma. Note the thin endometrium surrounding the leiomyomata. While such a thin endometrium may be associated with menses, or be related to the timing of this examination, the finding of a thin endometrium with atrophic changes at biopsy is frequent.

method is that no incision is required and recovery has been reported to be rapid. Whether this method will prove of benefit for women with endometrial anomalies related to fibroid disease remains to be shown.

Since the fibroids most clearly associated with impairment of fertility are precisely those that are likely to adversely impact endometrial development, it is quite reasonable to suggest that the endometrial effects of fibroids are responsible for the observed reduction in implantation and pregnancy. Consistent with this notion, the endometrial lining overlying the fibroid that abuts or distorts the endometrial cavity is abnormally thinned and fails to develop normally. As present there is no satisfactory treatment to reverse the endometrial effects of uterine fibroids other than removal of the fibroid.

CLINICAL MANAGEMENT OF FIBROIDS WITH PAIN, BLEEDING, OR PRESSURE SYMPTOMS

As mentioned, if bleeding is the primary symptom and fertility is not desired, the levonorgestrel-releasing IUD may be used.[35] For women with no desire for future childbearing and symptoms of pelvic pressure or pain, UAE and MRI-guided ultrasound are non-surgical procedures that have shown benefit.[41,43]

Myomectomy is often the best option for women interested in preserving the uterus or childbearing. Hysterectomy remains a definitive surgical therapy for fibroid disease. Although not FDA-approved for the indication, a GnRH agonist is often used clinically to reduce fibroid size preoperatively in order to facilitate removal of a fibroid uterus vaginally instead of via an abdominal approach.

DIAGNOSIS OF FIBROID DISEASE

Ultrasound is the principal method used for the diagnosis of fibroid disease. Physical examination can be misleading, since other pelvic tumors may also present with a pelvic mass and similar symptoms. For proper assessment of fibroid disease, transvaginal saline hysterosonography is the preferred imaging method.[44] Occasionally, for assessment of the uterus with very large leiomyomata, or with multiple lesions, MRI is extremely useful.[45] Hysterosalpingography has been used in the past, but is inferior to saline sonography and transvaginal sonography.

The diagnostic accuracy for fibroid disease is often considered in terms of detection, but rarely are false positives addressed. False-positive diagnosis of fibroids can create clinical problems. There are several cases that the authors have encountered where a false-positive diagnosis was made (Figure 54.4). In every instance that the authors have encountered, a false diagnosis was made based on an intramural fibroid and later disproved at surgery, occasionally including a biopsy of the region in question. At least one study also supports the false-positive diagnosis: in the study by DeWaay et al,[46] fibroids were initially documented, but were not found again when ultrasound examinations were repeated months later. The disappearing fibroids were small, with a mean diameter of 1.1 cm.[46] Since true fibroids are composed of dense fibrous tissue and studies correlating pathology with imaging have not observed regression of fibroids,[4] these 'disappearing fibroids' most likely represent false-positive diagnoses of leiomyoma in up to 27% of small leiomyomata. It is reasonable to conclude that false-positive diagnosis of fibroids is caused by the confusion of a persistent uterine contraction with a fibroid, since in both cases there may be a difference in sonolucency, but other conditions may be present, such as adenomyosis. Because the diagnosis of fibroids may lead to surgery, it is prudent to confirm any suspected fibroids either on two serial studies, or by another modality, whether it be examination or another imaging technique, before proceeding to surgery.

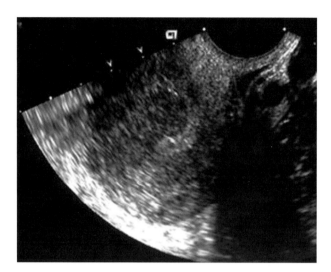

Figure 54.4 Incorrect diagnosis of leiomyoma by ultrasound. Transvaginal sonogram of a sagittal plane through the uterus. Note the 1.5–2.0 cm echolucent appearance of the myometrium that appears to distort the more echodense endometrium. A laparotomy was performed to remove the fibroid, but no fibroid was found at surgery.

BENIGN ENDOMETRIAL POLYPS

DEFINITION

Endometrial polyps are benign overgrowths of endometrial tissue containing endometrial glands in a fibrous stroma.[47,48] Structurally, endometrial polyps can be broad-based or pedunculated with a thin stalk and are typically 0.5–3 cm in diameter. Most investigators draw a distinction between polyps arising in premenopausal women and those in postmenopausal women.[49,50] Microscopic examination of polyps in premenopausal women revealed irregular proliferative glands in a fibrotic stroma with thick-walled blood vessels. Postmenopausal polyps usually contain cuboidal tissue in a dense, cellular stroma lacking mitotic activity. It is not clear whether the differences between pre- and postmenopausal polyps reflect true differences in polyp formation or a response to the different hormonal milieu of the patient. However, the risk of malignant change in an endometrial polyp is related to the menopausal status of the patient.[51]

INCIDENCE AND PREVALENCE OF ENDOMETRIAL POLYPS

Endometrial polyps are very common. It is difficult to accurately estimate the incidence of polyps in asymptomatic women, but studies have reported that endometrial polyps are found in approximately 24–25% of the general female population.[52] Polyps occur most commonly in women between the ages of 40 and 50 years old.[47,53] The prevalence of polyps in premenopausal women is about 15%. In one study, polyps were multiple in 26% of premenopausal women and 15% of postmenopausal women.[53] Endometrial polyps may arise at any location within the endometrial cavity.

SUBTYPES OF ENDOMETRIAL POLYPS

Endometrial polyps can be categorized by their appearance as well as by their cytogenetic traits. Based on histological appearance, there are two premenopausal and one postmenopausal histological subtypes of polyps. Premenopausal polyps can be functional or hyperplastic. Functional polyps resemble the surrounding endometrium and respond to the cyclic hormonal changes of the menstrual cycle. By contrast, hyperplastic polyps resemble the basalis layer of the endometrium and respond to estrogen but not progesterone.[50] The majority of postmenopausal endometrial polyps are atrophic and the stroma in the polyps has undergone fibrotic transformation.

Endometrial polyps may be divided into four cytogenetic subtypes.[54] Polyps in subgroup I contain a rearrangement of chromosome 6p21–22. Subgroup II polyps have a rearrangement of the chromosome 12q13–15 region.[54] Of note, leiomyomata also often harbor this rearrangement. In fact, the multiple aberration regions on chromosome 12q15 harbor recurrent breakpoints found in a variety of benign tumors. A gene encoding a high-mobility group (HMG) protein has been mapped to this region of chromosome 12.[55] Endometrial polyps in subgroup III have rearrangements of chromosome 7q22. Lastly, polyps in subgroup IV have a normal female karyotype.

ETIOLOGY OF BENIGN ENDOMETRIAL POLYPS

The etiology of endometrial polyps remains unclear. Three central causes of endometrial polyps have been suggested:

- polyps are local outgrowths of the basalis endometrium;
- polyps form in response to an imbalance of estrogen and progesterone receptors
- polyps are a product of genetic mutations that increase mitosis and decrease apoptosis.

Although they are not mutually exclusive, each of these possibilities entails fundamental assumptions that relate to the differential effects of steroid hormones on polyp origin and growth. One, or several, of these possible explanations may contribute to the disordered profile of growth factors found in benign endometrial polyps.

As discussed elsewhere in this book, the endometrium may be divided into two layers – a deeper basalis and a more superficial functionalis. While the basalis is relatively unresponsive to steroid hormones, the functionalis undergoes cyclic stages of growth and regression in accordance with the changing hormonal milieu of the menstrual cycle. It is possible that endometrial polyps are local outgrowths of the basalis endometrium and, as such, retain the basal cell characteristic of not responding to progesterone.[48] Because basalis cells respond to estrogen, but not progesterone, polyps are stimulated to undergo hyperplasia, but could be resistant to the antiproliferative effects of progesterone.

A second possible etiology of endometrial polyps is that polyp growth results from differential expression of estrogen and progesterone receptors. Due to imbalances in steroid receptor function, or response of the tissue to sex steroids, polyps develop and grow in response to estrogen but are relatively insensitive to the antiproliferative effects of progesterone.[50] Consistent with this hypothesis, polyps arise more commonly in hyperestrogenic environments. Similar to the normal endometrium, some endometrial polyps do exhibit changes in estrogen and progesterone receptor expression corresponding to different stages of the menstrual cycle.

However, several investigators have reported that polyps exhibited aberrant steroid receptor expression. Maia et al[48] found that endometrial polyps have an increased number of estrogen receptors relative to progesterone receptors. Subsequent studies examined endometrial polyps removed during specific phases of the menstrual cycle and found that, compared to the normal endometrium, glandular cells in polyps expressed fewer progesterone receptors during the proliferative phase and more estrogen receptors during the secretory phase.[56] Other studies have reported increased estrogen receptor expression in glandular epithelium of polyps than in surrounding endometrium and in the stromal cells of polyps than in surrounding endometrium.[57] Similarly, in postmenopausal women, elevated estrogen receptor expression has been found in endometrial polyps compared to the surrounding endometrium.[57] This was true regardless of whether a woman's steroid levels were artificially elevated through hormone replacement therapy (HRT) or tamoxifen.[56]

Another possible origin of endometrial polyps is that genetic mutations may cause an imbalance between growth and apoptosis. There is very little apoptosis in the basalis layer of the endometrium throughout the menstrual cycle.[58] In the normal cycling endometrium, there are low levels of apoptosis in the functionalis zone during the proliferative phase. The level of apoptosis rises toward the latter half of the secretory phase and peaks during the menstrual phase. In support of this possibility, there are several studies that indicate altered expression of apoptosis and growth regulatory factors in endometrial polyps.

For example, Ki-67, Bcl-2, inhibins, and cyclooxygenase 2 (COX-2) are four of the many cell cycle regulatory proteins that are differentially expressed in endometrial polyps. Ki-67 is a marker of cell mitosis, whereas Bcl-2 is an inhibitor of apoptosis. Of note, Ki-67 and Bcl-2 are hormonally responsive proteins. Bcl-2 expression increases in response to estrogen in the proliferative phase; this response is blunted by progesterone.[59] Supplemental estrogen has been shown to raise Ki-67 levels.[60] In the glandular cells of the functionalis layer of the normal endometrium, Ki-67 and Bcl-2 were elevated during the proliferative phase relative to the secretory phase of the menstrual cycle.[59]

Several studies have found aberrant expression of these proteins in endometrial polyps. One group found that Bcl-2 expression was markedly elevated in polyps relative to the endometrium during the proliferative phase.[56] This finding suggests that polyps might result from reduced apoptosis and perhaps a failure of tissue shedding during menstruation. Risberg et al[61] observed a pattern of low Ki-67 and high Bcl-2 in the stroma and glands of endometrial polyps, suggesting that polyps may develop from an imbalance between proliferation and apoptosis. However, another group found Ki67 and Bcl-2 expression varied in polyps in accordance with the menstrual cycle and that expression of both was sharply reduced in the luteal phase.[59] This same group noted that Ki-67-positive cells were significantly greater in polyps than cycling endometrium in the late proliferative phase, but there were no significant differences between Bcl-2 expression in polyps vs endometrium.[59] Of note, polyps staining positively for Ki-67 were also noted to stain positively for c-erbB2, suggesting a possible role for paracrine factors in polyp development.[62]

Other studies reported differences in inhibin expression in polyps vs the normal cycling endometrium. Inhibins are key inhibitory proteins that regulate many cell functions. A study by Mylonas et al[63] found that inhibins (INH-α and INH-βA) were reduced in polyps during the secretory phase of the menstrual cycle. The comparatively low level of inhibins in polyps during the secretory phase is consistent with the hyperplastic nature of polyps. While inhibins rise during the secretory phase in the normal endometrium, restricting cell division and encouraging differentiation, polyps appear to lack adequate amounts of these inhibitory proteins to normalize their growth.

Increased COX-2 expression may also be involved in endometrial polyp development. COX-2 enzymes play a critical role in the development of polyps in the colorectal and gastric mucosa. Indeed, although COX-2 is barely detectable in the normal intestinal mucosa, up to 50% of colorectal polyps and 80% of colorectal carcinomas overexpressed COX-2.[64] It is cyclically expressed in the endometrium of menstruating women and peaks during late proliferative/early luteal phase and again during menstruation.[60] These changes may be caused by changing levels of estrogen and progesterone during the menstrual cycle. In support of this possibility, HRT and oral contraceptive pills, medications that suppress normal variations in sex steroid concentrations, reduce COX-2 expression.[65]

Consistent with an important role for COX-2, its expression was increased in endometrial cancer,[66] and tumor grade and invasiveness correlated with COX-2 expression. Lesions with the deepest myometrial invasion had the highest COX-2 expression.[67] The importance of COX-2 in the development of intestinal polyps, and subsequently colorectal carcinoma, and the preponderance of COX-2 in endometrial carcinoma suggests that increased COX-2 expression may contribute, at least in part, to endometrial polyp development.

The different theories of endometrial polyp origin suggest that polyps may arise from a combination of alterations in steroid receptor expression and cell growth regulatory proteins. The unique features of basalis cells may contribute to these alterations. Collectively, the altered expression of these factors may contribute to the generation of a benign endometrial growth that is responsive to estrogen, but resistant, in part, to progesterone.

IS THERE A RELATIONSHIP BETWEEN BENIGN ENDOMETRIAL POLYPS AND ENDOMETRIAL CANCER?

One important question that has received much attention is whether endometrial polyps represent an early stage in the development of endometrial cancer.

The question is whether polyps result from early genetic mutations in the progression to endometrial hyperplasia, which can then evolve into endometrial carcinoma similar to colonic polyps. Opponents of this theory believe that polyps are benign tumors, which, although monoclonal and hyperplastic, lack the ability to transform into malignant tissue.

Studies report an incidence of malignancy from 0.42 to 3.2% within endometrial polyps, with most studies recording an incidence around 1%.[68,69] Interestingly, the rate of hyperplasia with and without atypia in polyps is a bit higher (3.1% and 25.7%, respectively).[51] Conversely, endometrial polyps were found in 12–34% of uteri containing endometrial carcinoma. A retrospective review found malignant polyps in 32% of 107 unselected cases of stage 1A endometrial cancer.[70] Nonetheless, the actual rate of malignancy in polyps is quite low. These data support the viewpoint that polyps are rarely an early event on the path to endometrial carcinoma, and that other genetic or molecular events are required for malignant transformation. A clinically important point is that the association between endometrial polyps and cancer is much greater in postmenopausal women than in premenopausal women. In a postmortem study of uteri, less than 1% of the polyps discovered in pre-menopausal women were associated with endometrial cancer, whereas 9.6% of postmenopausal polyps were associated with malignancy.[71]

Endometrial adenocarcinoma is the most common endometrial malignancy. Although there is strong evidence that endometrial hyperplasia gives rise to adenocarcinoma, there is less evidence suggesting that hyperplasia and/or malignancy evolves from polyps. However, serous carcinoma, a rare and aggressive endometrial cancer, frequently arises in endometrial polyps.[72,73] This observation is somewhat counterintuitive because while endometrial polyps have a strong association with estrogen, serous carcinoma is not an estrogen-responsive carcinoma.

Despite the apparent link between polyps and endometrial cancer, there is also evidence that polyps are not associated with endometrial malignancy. Whereas normal and anovulatory endometria are polyclonal, endometrial polyps, hyperplasias, and endometrial carcinomas are monoclonal.[74] However, using preferential X chromosome inactivation, Jovanovic et al[74] were able to determine that endometrial hyperplasias, but not polyps, were potentially precancerous. Additionally, whereas polyps display an increased expression of estrogen receptors, loss of sex steroid receptors is an early event in endometrial carcinogenesis.[75,76] On a cytogenetic level, polyps express more

Bcl-2 and less Ki-67 compared to the normal endometrium whereas endometrial cancer cells exhibit extremely high Bcl-2 expression.[61] Moreover, Bcl-2, the antiapoptotic protein, is increased in endometrial polyps but is seldom overexpressed in complex atypical hyperplasia or endometrial cancer.[77] In summary, the relationship of polyps to endometrial carcinogenesis suggests that polyps are not usually premalignant lesions on a continuum with a high likelihood of progression to cancer, but rather the same changes in the endometrium that predispose to cancer may also predispose to development of polyps.

RISK FACTORS FOR BENIGN ENDOMETRIAL POLYPS

Several risk factors predispose women to developing endometrial polyps. Age, obesity, hypertension, tamoxifen, HRT, anovulation, endometriosis, and age at menopause have all been associated with polyp occurrence. Consistent with the likely role of estrogen in polyp origin described above, many of these risk factors are associated with elevated estrogen levels.

As mentioned previously, endometrial polyps are found most commonly in women between 40 and 50 years old.[53] In a study of over 500 women who underwent polypectomy, increasing age was associated with an increased risk that polyps were premalignant or malignant.[51]

Obesity may also contribute to the development of endometrial polyps. Researchers have hypothesized that the hyperestrogenic environment generated by increased peripheral adipose stimulates hyperplasia in endometrial cells. Although obesity in combination with increased age and/or elevated blood pressure has been linked to endometrial polyps, no studies have been able to show that obesity alone causes polyp growth.[53] Interestingly, in patients with a high body mass index, estrogen receptor expression was not reduced in endometrial polyps, as was noted in normal endometrium, consistent with the notion that estrogen receptor regulation is altered in endometrial polyps.[78]

Hypertension is a risk factor for developing endometrial polyps. Moreover, endometrial polyps in hypertensive individuals are more likely to be premalignant or malignant.[53]

There is a strong association between tamoxifen and endometrial polyp growth.[79,80] Tamoxifen is a SERM (selective estrogen receptor modulator) that has estrogen agonist effects in uterine tissue; however, because of its antiestrogenic effect on breast tissue, it is frequently used as an adjunct treatment in estrogen receptor-positive breast cancer. It is likely that the estrogen agonist effect of tamoxifen initiates or promotes endometrial polyp growth. One study reported a 39% incidence of polyps in asymptomatic women receiving tamoxifen.[80] Another study found an elevated proliferation index (as measured through an antibody to Ki-67) in the endometrium of individuals taking tamoxifen as compared to untreated women.[81] Further supporting the role of tamoxifen's estrogen-receptor-mediated stimulatory role in polyp growth, raloxifene, a SERM with antiestrogenic effects in both the breast and the endometrium, causes a decrease in endometrial polyp formation.[82] Of note, a study showed that administering progesterone through a levonorgestrel-releasing IUD to women receiving tamoxifen decreased the occurrence of endometrial polyps.[83]

Hormone replacement therapy has also been associated with endometrial polyp development in some reports, yet in other studies appears to reduce polyp development. A rational explanation for the differences may be that, with certain regimens, the estrogenic component of HRT might contribute to the development of endometrial polyps. Several studies have reported an increased incidence of endometrial polyps in women taking HRT.[84,85] Other researchers have found that HRT is not a risk factor for polyps,[79] while still others have shown that HRT is protective against endometrial polyps.[86] Much of the controversy in these studies revolves around doses of estrogens administered in HRT. The higher the dose of estrogen relative to progesterone, the more likely the patients are to develop polyps.

Lastly, anovulation and age at menopause have been linked to development of endometrial polyps.[84] As in the prior risk factors associated with polyp development, these conditions are associated with increased estrogen exposure. Anovulatory patients frequently experience a persistently estrogen-dominant hormonal milieu. Women who go through menopause later in life are exposed to cyclically high levels of estrogen for a longer period. Interestingly, endometriosis is also associated with an increased frequency of endometrial polyps.[87]

CLINICAL CONSEQUENCES OF BENIGN ENDOMETRIAL POLYPS

The major symptoms associated with endometrial polyps are abnormal uterine bleeding, infertility, and miscarriage. Abnormal uterine bleeding (AUB) is unscheduled intramenstrual bleeding or any bleeding after menopause. A clinically important fact is that 13–50% of women with AUB have polyps.[88] Polyps account for approximately 30% of postmenopausal bleeding.[89] While premenopausal AUB can be managed somewhat conservatively, any uterine bleeding after menopause must be investigated expeditiously as the risk of endometrial cancer is higher in that age group.

Endometrial polyps appear to contribute to infertility. There is great variation in the reported incidence of endometrial polyps in infertile women. Fabres et al[90] reported a 34.9% incidence of polyps in infertile women. In contrast, in a case series of 642 infertile women, La Torre et al[91] reported only a 2.8% incidence of endometrial polyps. Several studies report an improvement in fertility following polypectomy. For instance, one prospective randomized controlled clinical trial[92] showed that polypectomy prior to intrauterine insemination (IUI) improved pregnancy rates by roughly two-fold. The mechanism of precisely how benign polyps reduce fertility is not entirely clear, but a number of studies have suggested the beneficial effect of polypectomy in the patient with infertility.

DIAGNOSIS OF BENIGN ENDOMETRIAL POLYPS

Although hysterosalpingography (HSG), transvaginal ultrasound, pipelle biopsy, and even MRI have been used to diagnose endometrial polyps, saline infusion sonohysterography (SIS) has emerged as the most accurate, non-invasive tool for identifying polyps. Hysteroscopy remains the 'gold standard' for identifying endometrial polyps. It enables direct visualization of the uterine cavity as well as possible excision of endometrial lesions. However, there are several less-invasive methods used for evaluation of the uterine cavity.

Saline infusion sonohysterography is currently the best minimally invasive technique for identifying endometrial polyps. Sterile saline is injected into the uterus under direct ultrasound observation and the saline distends the uterine cavity, facilitating evaluation of individual sides of the endometrial lining. Endometrial polyps typically appear as well-defined lesions that are isoechoic with the endometrium (Figure 54.5), with preservation of the endometrium–myometrium interface.[93] In premenopausal women, SIS is typically performed during the early proliferative phase (days 4–6) of the menstrual cycle when the endometrium is thin.[93] SIS should not be performed after day 10 of the menstrual cycle due to the risk of concurrent pregnancy. The ability of SIS to detect intrauterine pathology is similar to that of hysteroscopy.

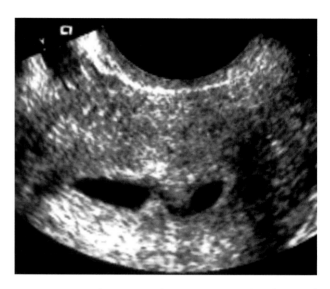

Figure 54.5 Ultrasonographic appearance of endometrial polyps in a premenopausal woman. Transvaginal saline sonogram of two endometrial polyps viewed on a transverse section through the uterine cavity. Two sessile lesions are noted to arise from the inferior and superior endometrium that extend into the endometrial cavity.

SIS has been shown to have both a sensitivity and specificity of 100%, a positive predictive value of 90%, and a diagnostic accuracy of 90.6% for the diagnosis of endometrial polyps.[44,94] Because SIS is quite accurate at identifying endometrial polyps, but lacks adequate power to differentiate benign from malignant pathology, many focal abnormalities identified on SIS must be biopsied.

Hysterosalpingography, injection of radioopaque dye through the cervix into the uterus and Fallopian tubes, can be used to diagnose endometrial polyps. Polyps appear as echogenic masses with smooth margins on HSG.[95] However, the sensitivity and specificity of HSG for polyps were only 50% and 82.5%, respectively.[94]

Transvaginal ultrasound was a slightly better diagnostic tool for endometrial polyps, with a sensitivity of 75% and a specificity of 96.5%.[94] By transvaginal ultrasound, endometrial polyps appear as diffusely thickened endometrium or hyperechoic masses surrounded by a hypoechoic endometrium.[96] In contrast to submucosal myomas, which are surrounded by myometrium on one side and endometrium on the other side, polyps are uterine cavity contour defects completely surrounded by endometrium.[96] There may be cystic spaces in polyps – these are fairly specific for benign disease. The presence of a single blood vessel on Doppler ultrasound is highly suggestive of a polyp.[96]

Infrequently, polyps are diagnosed by office biopsy of the endometrium. When a postmenopausal woman has an episode of bleeding, her endometrium should be biopsied and analyzed for evidence of hyperplasia or cancer. The pipelle is a convenient instrument to sample the endometrium. The pipelle catheter is placed through a patient's cervix into her uterine cavity, and endometrial tissue is removed by creating negative pressure within the catheter and moving the pipelle back and forth several times. This technique retrieves an adequate endometrial specimen in 91% of all patients, and 81% of postmenopausal women. However, pipelle biopsy of the endometrial cavity is a poor method for the identification of endometrial polyps. In a study of endometrial polyps in tamoxifen-treated women by Hann et al[97] endometrial biopsy had a sensitivity of only 4% for diagnosing endometrial polyps.

Occasionally, endometrial polyps are identified on MRI. Polyps are intermediate in signal intensity on T1-weighted images. On T2-weighted images, polyps are slightly hypointense relative to the normal endometrium.[98] Large polyps are usually more heterogeneous in signal intensity.[98] It can be difficult to differentiate endometrial polyps from submucosal fibroids, focal hyperplasia, and endometrial carcinoma on MRI. Gadolinium enhancement of the MRI images can be helpful in increasing polyp detection. T1-weighted images have 83% sensitivity, 92% specificity, and 89% accuracy for distinguishing malignant from benign central uterine masses. T2-weighted images have 50% sensitivity, 97% specificity, and 82% accuracy in identifying benign vs malignant intrauterine lesions.

TREATMENT OF BENIGN ENDOMETRIAL POLYPS

There are three basic approaches to the treatment of endometrial polyps: expectant management, medical treatment, and polypectomy. Small endometrial polyps have been reported to regress without treatment.[46] In one study of asymptomatic women surveyed for endometrial polyps, polyps that regressed were on average 0.7 cm in diameter, whereas polyps that persisted were an average of 1.3 cm on diagnosis.[46] Therefore, in some situations, it may be acceptable to follow a patient with serial saline infusion sonohysterograms and pay close attention to their symptoms. Whether the 'disappearing polyps' may represent a false-positive diagnosis is uncertain, since only one method was used for diagnosis. Expectant management of polyps risks delay in diagnosis of premalignant or malignant intrauterine lesions and therefore should only be considered in a patient whose risk of endometrial hyperplasia and/or cancer is very low. For example, it would not be advisable to follow an endometrial polyp discovered in a postmenopausal

woman following an episode of bleeding. In contrast, a young woman incidentally found to have a small asymptomatic polyp might be followed for three or four menstrual cycles and then rescanned for evidence of polyp regression.

Alternatively, some physicians have treated polyps with medications. Progestins have been given under the assumption that endometrial polyps regress in response to progesterone. As mentioned above, when given simultaneously with tamoxifen, progesterone has been shown to decrease polyp occurrence. Other clinicians have suggested that non-steroidal anti-inflammatory drugs (NSAIDs) might have efficacy. However, a study by Tjarks et al[88] showed that neither progestins nor NSAIDs are helpful in relief of symptoms caused by polyps.

In most cases the definitive and appropriate treatment of endometrial polyps is polypectomy, a surgical removal of the polyp. Patients who have undergone polypectomy have a subjective decline in their menorrhagia/metrorrhagia symptoms.[88] This improvement in symptomatology is the same for both pre- and postmenopausal patients.[88] One study reported an 88% success rate 3 years after hysteroscopic polypectomy in 51 postmenopausal women.[99] Moreover, this method enables histological examination of the polyp and, therefore, definitive assessment of the polyp's malignant potential.

In the past, polypectomy was performed blindly (with polyp forceps and/or dilatation and curettage [D&C]), but the preferred method is hysteroscopic resection. In one study, D&C alone completely removed endometrial polyps in only 8% of test subjects.[100] Dilatation and curettage in combination with the polyp forceps completely removed polyps in 41% of the cases.[100] Hysteroscopy confirms removal of the polyp by allowing the surgeon to directly inspect the endometrial cavity. Moreover, using an operative hysteroscope, a surgeon can resect an endometrial polyp under direct visualization. This technique has the advantage of ensuring excision of the entire polyp, including the base. Some investigators have suggested that removal of the polyp base is essential for cure, as the polyp originates in the basalis layer of the endometrium.[53] As it ensures polyp excision in virtually 100% of cases, hysteroscopy is the preferred method of polyp removal.

CONCLUSIONS

Many clinical consequences of fibroids, such as reduction in implantation, increased miscarriage, infertility, and menorrhagia, are probably related to altered growth and development of the endometrium. The most important feature that determines whether a fibroid will affect endometrial growth and differentiation is the location of the fibroid and its proximity to the endometrium. The second characteristic of relevance is the size of the fibroid: larger fibroids are more likely to influence endometrial development. Intramural leiomyomata of 4–6 cm may be associated with altered endometrial development not only adjacent to the fibroid but also to the endometrium opposite the fibroid by mechanisms that remain unclear.

Light microscopy frequently reveals endometrial atrophy, with a reduction in glandular development in endometrial tissue overlying a fibroid. In addition to light microscopic changes, there may be subtle changes associated with altered differentiation of the endometrium, such as a reduction in *HoxA-10*. Subtle alterations may be clinically important, but there are no clinically available tests to define such effects.

Endometrial polyps may also affect endometrial development and are associated with abnormal uterine bleeding, increased miscarriage, and possibly infertility. Conclusive proof of the clinical effects of endometrial polyps is limited by the paucity of randomized controlled trials.

Microscopic features observed with polyps depend upon the menopausal status of the woman. In premenopausal women, polyps exhibit irregular proliferation of glands associated with a fibrotic stroma and thick-walled vessels. In postmenopausal women, polyps usually contain cuboidal epithelium with a dense cellular stroma. Clinically, the effects of polyps resemble those of uterine fibroids, suggesting that altered endometrial differentiation may explain many of the clinical symptoms.

Medical treatment options for symptomatic uterine leiomyomata and endometrial polyps are limited, and surgical excision is usually pursued. Non-surgical options, such as selective antiprogestins, the levonorgestrel-releasing IUD, focused ultrasound, and UAE may provide symptomatic relief for some patients with fibroids.

ACKNOWLEDGMENTS

The authors wish to thank Dr Alicia Armstrong for helpful suggestions and critical reading of the manuscript. The authors thank Dr Frederick Larsen for assistance with clinical materials.

REFERENCES

1. Ligon AH, Morton CC. Genetics of uterine leiomyomas. Genes Chromosomes Cancer 2000; 28: 235–45.
2. Walker CL, Stewart EA. Uterine fibroids: the elephant in the room. Science 2005; 308: 1589–92.
3. Flake GP, Andersen J, Dixon D. Etiology and pathogenesis of uterine leiomyomas: a review. Environ Health Perspect 2003; 111: 1037–54.
4. Davis BJ. The NIEHS Uterine Fibroid Study: preliminary results. Presented at: Advances in Leiomyoma Research: 2nd NIH International Congress, Bethesda, MD, February 24–25, 2005.
5. Bajekal N, Li TC. Fibroids, infertility and pregnancy wastage. Hum Reprod Update 2000; 6: 614–20.
6. Payson M, Leppert P, Segars J. Epidemiology of myomas. Obstet Gynecol Clin North Am 2006; 33: 1–11.
7. Stewart EA, Morton CC. The genetics of leiomyomata: what clinicians need to know. Obstet Gynecol 2006; 107: 917–21.
8. Baird DD, Dunson DB, Hill MC et al. High cumulative incidence of uterine leiomyoma in black and white women. Am J Obstet Gynecol 2003; 188: 100–7.
9. Feinberg EC, Larsen FW, Catherino WH et al. Comparison of assisted reproductive technology utilization and outcomes between Caucasian and African American patients in an equal-access-to-care setting. Fertil Steril 2006; 85: 888–94.
10. Roth TM, Gustilo-Ashby T, Barber MD et al. Effects of race and clinical factors on short-term outcomes of abdominal myomectomy. Obstet Gynecol 2003; 101: 881–4.
11. Cramer SF, Patel A. The frequency of uterine leiomyomas. Am J Clin Pathol 1990; 94: 435–8.
12. Ryan GL, Syrop CH, Van Voorhis BJ. Role, epidemiology, and natural history of benign uterine mass lesions. Clin Obstet Gynecol 2005; 48: 312–24.
13. Patterson-Keels LM, Selvaggi SM, Haefner HK et al. Morphologic assessment of endometrium overlying submucosal leiomyomas. J Reprod Med 1994; 39: 579–84.
14. Deligdish L, Loewenthal M. Endometrial changes associated with myomata of the uterus. J Clin Pathol 1970; 23: 676–80.
15. Sharma SP, Misra SD, Mittal VP. Endometrial changes – a criterion for the diagnosis of submucous uterine leiomyoma. Indian J Pathol Microbiol 1979; 22: 33–6.
16. Sehgal N, Haskins AL. The mechanism of uterine bleeding in the presence of fibromyomas. Am Surg 1960; 26: 21–3.
17. Farrer-Brown G, Beilby JO, Tarbit MH. The vascular patterns in myomatous uteri. J Obstet Gynaecol Bronw Comm 1970; 77: 967–75.
18. Farrer-Brown G, Beilby JO, Tarbit MH. Venous changes in the endometrium of myomatous uteri. Obstet Gynecol 1971; 38: 743–51.
19. Huang SC, Yu CH, Huang RT et al. Intratumoral blood flow in uterine myoma correlated with a lower tumor size and volume, but not correlated with cell proliferation or angiogenesis. Obstet Gynecol 1996; 87: 1019–24.
20. Casey R, Rogers PAW, Vollenhoven BJ. An immunohistochemical analysis of fibroid vasculature. Hum Reprod 2000; 15: 1469–75.
21. Kurjak A, Kupesic-Urek S, Miric D. The assessment of benign uterine tumor vascularization by transvaginal color Doppler. Ultrasound Med Biol 1992; 18: 645–9.
22. Bulun SE, Simpson ER, Word RA. Expression of the CYP19 gene and its product aromatase cytochrome P450 in human leiomyoma tissues and cells in culture. J Clin Endocrinol Metab 1994; 78: 736–43.
23. Bulun SE, Imir G, Utsunomiya H et al. Aromatase in endometriosis and uterine leiomyomata. J Steroid Biochem Mol Biol 2005; 95: 57–62.
24. Rackow BW, Taylor HS. Uterine leiomyomas affect molecular determinants of endometrial receptivity. Fertil Steril 2006; 86: S10.
25. Benson GV, Lim H, Paria BC et al. Mechanisms of reduced fertility in Hoxa-10 mutant mice: uterine homeosis and loss

of maternal Hoxa-10 expression. Development 1996; 122: 2687–96.

26. Ingber DE. Mechanical signaling and the cellular response to extracellular matrix in angiogenesis and cardiovascular physiology. Circ Res 2002; 91: 877–87.

27. Paszek MJ, Weaver VM. The tension mounts: mechanics meets morphogenesis and malignancy. J Mammary Gland Biol Neoplasia 2004; 9: 325–42.

28. Huang S, Ingber DE. Cell tension, matrix mechanics, and cancer development. Cancer Cell 2005; 8: 175–6.

29. Sozen K, Arici A. Interactions of cytokines, growth factors, and the extracellular matrix in the biology of uterine leiomyomata. Fertil Steril 2002; 78: 1–12.

30. Catherino WH, Leppert PC, Stenmark MH et al. Reduced dermatopontin expression is a molecular link between uterine leiomyomas and keloids. Genes Chromosomes Cancer 2004; 40: 204–17.

31. Leppert PC, Baginski T, Prupas C et al. Comparative ultrastructure of collagen fibrils in uterine leiomyomas and normal myometrium. Fertil Steril 2004; 82: 1182–7.

32. Cox DA, Helvering LM. Extracellular matrix integrity: a possible mechanism for differential clinical effects among selective estrogen receptor modulators and estrogens? Mol Cell Endocrinol 2006; 247: 53–9.

33. Coronado GD, Marshall LM, Schwartz SM. Complications in pregnancy, labor, and delivery with uterine leiomyoma: a population-based study. Obstet Gynecol 2000; 95: 764–9.

34. Spies JB, Myers ER, Worthington-Kirsch R et al. The FIBROID registry: symptom and quality-of-life status 1 year after therapy. Obstet Gynecol 2005; 106: 1309–18.

35. Soysal S, Soysal ME. The efficacy of levonorgestrel-releasing intrauterine device in selected cases of myoma-related menorrhagia: a prospective controlled trial. Gynecol Obstet Invest 2005; 59: 29–35.

36. Steinauer J, Pritts EA, Jackson R et al. Systematic review of mifepristone for the treatment of uterine leiomyomata. Obstet Gynecol 2004; 103: 1331–6.

37. DeManno D, Elger W, Garg R et al. Asoprisnil (J867): a selective progesterone receptor modulator for gynecological therapy. Steroids 2003; 68: 1019–32.

38. Lee BS, Margolin SB, Nowak RA. Pirfenidone: a novel pharmacological agent that inhibits leiomyoma cell proliferation and collagen production. J Clin Endocrinol Metab 1998; 83: 219–23.

39. Stewart EA, Disalvo D, Sharif NA et al. Pirendione for the treatment of uterine leiomyomas: pilot study data. J Soc Gynecol Invest 1999; 6: 229A.

40. Pritts EA. Fibroids and infertility: a systematic review of the evidence. Obstet Gynecol Surv 2001; 56: 483–91.

41. Gupta JK, Sinha AS, Lumsden MA et al. Uterine artery embolization for symptomatic uterine fibroids. Cochrane Database Syst Rev 2006; CD005073.

42. Pron G, Mocarski E, Bennett J et al. Pregnancy after uterine artery embolization for leiomyomata: the Ontario multicenter trial. Obstet Gynecol 2005; 105: 67–76.

43. Stewart EA, Rabinovici J, Tempany CM et al. Clinical outcomes of focused ultrasound surgery for the treatment of uterine fibroids. Fertil Steril 2006; 85: 22–9.

44. Nass Duce M, Oz U, Ozer C et al. Diagnostic value of sonohysterography in the evaluation of submucosal fibroids and endometrial polyps. Aust NZ J Obstet Gynaecol 2003; 43: 448–52.

45. Imaoka I, Sugimura K, Masui T et al. Abnormal uterine cavity: differential diagnosis with MR imaging. Mag Reson Imaging 1999; 17: 1445–55.

46. DeWaay DJ, Syrop CH, Nygaard IE et al. Natural history of uterine polyps and leiomyomata. Obstet Gynecol 2002; 100: 3–7.

47. Van Bogaert L-J. Clinicopathologic findings in endometrial polyps. Obstet Gynecol 1988; 71: 771–3.

48. Maia H, Maltez A, Calmon LC et al. Histopathology and steroid receptors in endometrial polyps of postmenopausal patients under hormone replacement therapy. Gynaecol Endosc 1998; 7: 267–72.

49. McGurgan P, Taylor LJ, Duffy SR et al. Are endometrial polyps from premenopausal women similar to postmenopausal women? An immunohistochemical comparison of endometrial polyps from pre- and postmenopausal women. Maturitas 2006; 54: 277–84.

50. Mittal K, Schwartz L, Goswami S et al. Estrogen and progesterone receptor expression in endometrial polyps. Int J Gynecol Pathol 1996; 15: 345–8.

51. Savelli L, De Iaco P, Santini D et al. Histopathologic features and risks factors for benignity, hyperplasia, and cancer in endometrial polyps. Am J Obstet Gynecol 2003; 188: 927–31.

52. Sherman ME, Mazur MT, Kurman RJ. Benign diseases of the endometrium. In: Kurman RJ, ed. Blaustein's Pathology of the Female Genital Tract. New York: Springer, 2002: 421–66.

53. Reslova T, Tosner J, Resl M et al. Endometrial polyps. Arch Gynecol Obstet 1999; 262: 133–9.

54. Dal-Cin P, Vanni R, Marras S et al. Four cytogenetic subgroups can be identified in endometrial polyps. Cancer Res 1995; 55: 1565–8.

55. Hennig Y, Wanschura S, Diechert U et al. Rearrangements of the high mobility group protein family genes and the molecular genetic origin of uterine leiomyomas and endometrial polyps. Mol Hum Reprod 1996; 2: 277–83.

56. Taylor LJ, Jackson TL, Reid JG et al. The differential expression of oestrogen receptors, progesterone receptors, Bcl-2, and Ki67 in endometrial polyps. BJOG 2003; 100: 794–8.

57. Sant'Ana de Almeida EC, Nogueira AA, Candido dos Reis FJ et al. Immunohistochemical expression of estrogen and progesterone receptors in endometrial polyps and adjacent endometrium in postmenopausal women. Maturitas 2004; 49: 229–33.

58. Arends MJ. Apoptosis in the endometrium. Histopathology 1999; 35: 174–8.

59. Maia H, Maltez A, Studart E et al. Ki-67, Bcl-2 and p53 expression in endometrial polyps and in the normal endometrium during the menstrual cycle. BJOG 2004; 111: 1242–7.

60. Maia H, Corriea T, Freitas LA et al. Cyclooxygenase-2 expression in endometrial polyps during menopause. Gynecol Endocrinol 2005; 21: 336–9.

61. Risberg B, Karlsson K, Abeler V et al. Dissociated expression of Bcl-2 and Ki-67 in endometrial lesions: diagnostic and histogenetic implications. Int J Gynecol Pathol 2002; 21: 155–60.

62. Maia H, Maltez A, Athayde C et al. Proliferation profile of endometrial polyps in post-menopausal women. Maturitas 2001; 40: 273–81.

63. Mylonas I, Makovitzky J, Fernow A et al. Expression of the inhibin/activin subunits alpha (α) and beta-A(βA) and beta-B (βB) in benign human endometrial polyps and tamoxifen-associated polyps. Arch Gynecol Obstet 2005; 272: 59–66.

64. Smadar S, Arber N. Cyclooxygenase-2 inhibition prevents colorectal cancer: from the bench to the bed side. Oncology 2005; 69: 33–7.

65. Hsu SC, Long C-Y, Yang C-H et al. Cycolooxygenase-2 expression in the endometrium at the end of two years' continuous combined hormone replacement therapy. Maturitas 2003; 46: 295–9.

66. Fujiwaki R, Iida K, Kanasaki H et al. Cyclooxygenase-2 expression in endometrial cancer: correlation with microvessel count and expression of vascular endothelial growth

factor and thymidine phosphorylase. Hum Pathol 2002; 33: 213–9.

67. Ferrandina G, Legge F, Ranelletti FO et al. Cyclooxygenase-2 expression in endometrial carcinoma: correlation with clinicopathologic parameters and clinical outcome. Cancer 2002; 95: 801–7.

68. Anastasiadis PG, Koutlaki NG, Skaphida PG et al. Endometrial polyps: prevalence, detection, and malignant potential in women with abnormal uterine bleeding. Eur J Gynaecol Oncol 2000; 21: 180–3.

69. Shushan A, Revel A, Rojansky N. How often are endometrial polyps malignant? Gynecol Obstet Invest 2004; 58: 212–15.

70. Farrell R, Scurry J, Otton G et al. Clinicopathologic review of malignant polyps in stage 1A carcinoma of the endometrium. Gynecol Oncol 2005; 98: 254–62.

71. Peterson WF, Novak ER. Endometrial polyps. Obstet Gynecol 1956; 8: 40–9.

72. Silva EG, Jenkins R. Serous carcinoma in endometrial polyps. Mod Pathol 1990; 3: 120–8.

73. McCluggage WG, Sumathi VP, McManus DT. Uterine serous carcinoma and endometrial intraepithelial carcinoma arising from endometrial polyps: report of 5 cases, including 2 associated with tamoxifen therapy. Hum Pathol 2003; 34: 939–43.

74. Jovanovic AS, Boynton KA, Mutter GL. Uteri of women with endometrial carcinoma contain a histopathological spectrum of monoclonal putative precancers, some with microsatellite instability. Cancer Res 1996; 56: 1917–21.

75. Pickartz H, Beckmann R, Fleige B et al. Steroid receptors and proliferative activity in non-neoplastic and neoplastic endometria. Virchows Arch A Pathol Anat Histopathol 1990; 417: 163–71.

76. Li SF, Shiozawa T, Nakayama K et al. Stepwise abnormality of sex steroid hormone receptors, tumor suppressor gene products (p53 and Rb), and cyclin E in uterine endometrioid adenocarcinoma. Cancer 1996; 77: 321–9.

77. Niemann TH, Trgovac TL, McGaughty VR et al. Bcl-2 expression in endometrial hyperplasia and carcinoma. Gynecol Oncol 1996; 63: 318–22.

78. Belisario MS, Vassallo J, Andrade LA et al. The expression of hormone receptors in the endometrium and endometrial polyps in postmenopausal women and its relationship to body mass index. Maturitas 2006; 53: 114–18.

79. Bakour SH, Gupta JK, Khan KS. Risk factors associated with endometrial polyps in abnormal uterine bleeding. Int J Gynecol Obstet 2002; 76: 165–8.

80. Fong K, Kung R, Lytwyn A et al. Endometrial evaluation with transvaginal US and hysterosonography in asymptomatic postmenopausal women with breast cancer receiving tamoxifen. Radiology 2001; 220: 765–73.

81. Mourits MJ, Ten Hoor KA, van der Zee AGJ et al. The effects of tamoxifen on proliferation and steroid receptor expression in postmenopausal endometrium. J Clin Pathol 2002; 55: 514–19.

82. Neven P, Quail D, Lévrier M et al. Uterine effects of Estrogen Plus Progestin Therapy and Raloxifene: Adjudicated Results From the EURALOX Study. Obstet Gynecol 2004; 103: 881–91.

83. Gardner FJ, Konje JC, Abrams KR et al. Endometrial protection from tamoxifen-stimulated changes by a levonorgestrel-releasing intrauterine system: a randomised controlled trial. Lancet 2000; 356: 1711–17.

84. Oguz S, Sargin A, Kelekci S et al. The role of hormone replacement therapy in endometrial polyp formation. Maturitas 2005; 50: 231–6.

85. Van den Bosch T, Van Schoubroeck D, Ameye L et al. Ultrasound assessment of endometrial thickness and endometrial polyps in women on hormone replacement therapy. Am J Obstet Gynecol 2003; 188: 1249–53.

86. Perrone G, DeAngelis C, Critelli C et al. Hysteroscopic findings in postmenopausal abnormal uterine bleeding: a comparison between HRT users and non-users. Maturitas 2002; 43: 251–5.

87. Kim MR, Kim YA, Jo MY et al. High frequency of endometrial polyps in endometriosis. J Am Asso Gynecol Laparosc 2003; 10: 46–8.

88. Tjarks M, Van Voorhis BJ. Treatment of endometrial polyps. Obstet Gynecol 2000; 96: 886–9.

89. Cohen MA, Sauer MV, Ketz M. Utilizing routine sonohysterography to detect intrauterine pathology before initiating hormone replacement therapy. Menopause 1999; 6: 68–70.

90. Fabres C, Alam V, Balmaceda J et al. Comparison of ultrasonography and hysteroscopy in the diagnosis of intrauterine lesions in infertile women. J Am Assoc Gynecol Laparosc 1998; 5: 375–8.

91. La Torre R, De Felice C, De Angelis C et al. Transvaginal sonographic evaluation of endometrial polyps: a comparison of two-dimensional and three-dimensional contrast sonography. Clin Exp Obstet Gynecol 1999; 26: 171–3.

92. Pérez-Medina T, Bajo-Arenas J, Salazar F et al. Endometrial polyps and their implication in the pregnancy rates of patients undergoing intrauterine insemination: a prospective, randomized study. Hum Reprod 2005; 20: 1632–5.

93. Davis PC, O'Neill MJ, Yoder IC et al. Sonohysterographic findings of endometrial and subendometrial conditions. Radiographics 2002; 22: 803–16.

94. Soares SR, Barbosa dos Reis MB, Camargos AF. Diagnostic accuracy of sonohysterography, transvaginal sonography, and hysterosalpingography in patients with uterine cavity diseases. Fertil Steril 2000; 73: 406–11.

95. Fong K, Causer P, Atri M et al. Transvaginal US and hysterosonography in postmenopausal women with breast cancer receiving tamoxifen: correlation with hysteroscopy and pathologic study. Radiographics 2003; 23: 137–55.

96. Davidson KG, Dubinsky TJ. Ultrasonographic evaluation of the endometrium in postmenopausal vaginal bleeding. Radiol Clin North Am 2003; 41: 769–80.

97. Hann LE, Kim CM, Gonen M et al. Sonohysterography compared with endometrial biopsy for evaluation of the endometrium in tamoxifen-treated women. J Ultrasound Med 2003; 22: 1173–9.

98. Chaudhry S, Reinhold C, Guermazi A et al. Benign and malignant disorders of the endometrium. Top Magn Reson Imaging 2003; 14: 339–58.

99. Cravello L, de Montgolfier R, D'Ercole C et al. Hysteroscopic surgery in postmenopausal women. Acta Obstet Gynecol Scand 1996; 75: 536–6.

100. Gebauer G, Hafner A, Siebzehnrübl E et al. Role of hysteroscopy in detection and extraction of endometrial polyps: results of a prospective study. Am J Obstet Gynecol 2001; 184: 59–63.

55 Models of endometrial carcinogenesis

Mark E Sherman and James V Lacey Jr

Synopsis

Background

- Endometrial carcinoma is the 5th most common cancer in women, with a projected 39 000 new cases expected in the USA in 2007.
- It can be divided into type I or hormone-dependent, and type II or hormone-independent cancers. Alternatively, classification can be made on histopathological criteria. Sometimes a mixture of types is present in one lesion.

Basic Science

- A majority of endometrial carcinomas are type 1. Most of these are histologically classified as endometrioid adenocarcinoma.
- Type I carcinoma occurs partially as the result of cell growth stimulation by estrogen that is unopposed by progesterone.
- A reversible state of proliferation known as endometrial hyperplasia can persist and eventually give rise to carcinoma (type I).
- Tissue aging with accumulating mutations in conserved progenitor cells is important in the mechanism of carcinogenesis.
- Mutations associated with type I endometrial carcinoma occur in mismatch repair genes (*mlh1,msh2,msh6*), *PTEN, Ki-ras,*and *β-catenin*.
- Type II carcinoma appears to develop rapidly from atrophic rather than hyperplastic tissue. These tumors are poorly differentiated (often with serous, clear cell, or other non-endometrioid features), and generally, more deeply invasive and more often metastatic when diagnosed.
- Many type II carcinomas appear histologically to arise from uterine luminal (surface) epithelium, which is commonly referred to as endometrial intraepithelial carcinoma (EIC).
- Mutations in *p53* are associated with most type II carcinomas (especially serous carcinomas).

Clinical

- Currently, histopathological classifications of endometrial hyperplasia cannot accurately predict which carcinoma precursors will definitely progress to carcinoma if untreated and which will regress. However, data suggest that classifications stratify patients according to risk.
- Increased risk for type I carcinoma is associated with aging; obesity; diabetes; nulliparity; and use of unopposed estrogen. Use of birth control pills with high progesterone content and smoking are associated with lower risk.
- Type I carcinomas are frequently slow-growing and curable by hysterectomy.
- Hysterectomy for benign indications is extremely common, which leads to an underestimation of carcinoma rates among women with intact uteri. These procedures may also affect our ability to understand causes of endometrial cancer by altering the population at risk.
- Serous carcinomas are often associated with polyps. Early dissemination is common, often manifested as growth along peritoneal surfaces and ascites, leading to a presentation resembling that for ovarian carcinoma.

ABSTRACT

Models of carcinogenesis represent both a coherent synthesis of current knowledge and a tool for identifying gaps in our understanding that require further investigation. Accordingly, all models epitomize a certain planned obsolescence, and this chapter is presented with the expectation that time will modify and perhaps erase some of what is proposed.

For purposes of presentation, we will divide the current discussion into two main models, hormone-dependent, or type I, and hormone-independent, or type II, pathways, with all of their attendant simplifications and assumptions. Each discussion begins with a brief summary of relevant epidemiological, clinical, experimental/molecular, and pathological data followed by a presentation of the model, a critique of its limitations, and proposals for future investigation.

TWO TYPES OF ENDOMETRIAL CARCINOMAS: HISTORICAL PERSPECTIVE

Over two decades ago, Bokhman, a Russian gynecologist, offered a novel hypothesis about the process of carcinogenesis: the etiology of cancer represents an important determinant of its pathogenesis, biological characteristics, and clinical behavior.[1] Specifically, he proposed that endometrial carcinomas are divisible into two main types (designated, 'type I' and 'type II'), which contrast in etiology, clinical features, pathological appearance, and biological aggressiveness. Despite substantial advances in our understanding of endometrial carcinogenesis since Bokhman's concept was introduced, his original insights provide a useful starting point and a framework for developing contemporary models. In fact, the concept that tumors have defined 'molecular portraits' that are identifiable at inception, remain relatively invariant over time, and influence the biology and clinical course of disease in patients is gaining acceptance in breast cancer research and other tumor systems.[2]

As originally proposed, type I carcinomas were envisioned to constitute about two-thirds of endometrial carcinomas. Type I carcinomas were characterized as presenting with stereotypical clinical attributes: obesity, hypercholesterolemia, diabetes mellitus, anovulatory bleeding, ovarian stromal hyperplasia, and endometrial hyperplasia adjacent to the tumor.[1] These tumors seemed to develop through a slow multistage process, resulting in the growth of biologically indolent carcinomas that were

frequently curable by hysterectomy. The development of these tumors was understood as representing a process of hormonal carcinogenesis, in which the growth-promoting effects of estrogen exposure are inadequately opposed by intermittent progesterone stimulation.

The earliest events in the type I pathway were considered highly reversible endometrial proliferations, termed endometrial hyperplasia (EH), which had the potential to persist and progress to endometrial carcinoma after many years in the absence of treatment. More recently, it has been observed that most, though not all, type I tumors are histologically classified as endometrioid endometrial adenocarcinoma,[3,4] which constitute approximately 80% of all endometrial carcinomas. This high percentage exceeds the initial estimated proportion of type I tumors and raises questions about the extent to which the type I carcinoma (an etiological designation) and endometrioid carcinoma (a histopathological category) overlap.

In contrast, type II tumors were diagnosed at older ages and lacked the clinical features suggestive of hormonal imbalances.[1,3,4] The etiology of these tumors remains largely unknown; neither risk factors nor protective factors for these neoplasms have been well-characterized. Type II tumors seem to rapidly develop from atrophic rather than from hyperplastic endometrium. Generally, these tumors are poorly differentiated and deeply invasive, and frequently invade lymphatic channels and metastasize. Many type II carcinomas are histopathologically classified as serous or other non-endometrioid histopathological types, especially clear cell carcinoma. Mixed tumors containing areas of clear cell and serous carcinoma are relatively common. Recently, several investigators have suggested that serous carcinomas, and possibly other examples of type II tumors, develop from malignant change in endometrial surface epithelium, a lesion variously termed endometrial intraepithelial carcinoma (EIC), carcinoma in situ, or serous surface carcinoma.[5–8]

All histopathological types of endometrial carcinoma probably include some mixture of type I and type II endometrial cancers as described originally by Bokhman; the correspondence of etiological factors and histopathological type is imperfect. Many patients diagnosed with endometrioid carcinoma do not have classic risk factors associated with hyperestrinism and some women with classic risk factors for endometrioid carcinoma develop serous tumors. Furthermore, tumor classifications developed for clinical management may not prove equally informative for understanding etiology. Specifically, it is logical to classify tumors of mixed histology according to their most clinically aggressive component, because treatments should be directed towards combating the most lethal threat to the patient. Accordingly, for clinical purposes, mixed carcinomas containing serous components are usually reported as serous carcinomas rather than as mixed carcinomas.[8] However, some of these 'serous carcinomas' may develop initially as endometrioid carcinomas through a type I pathway, and only secondarily develop non-endometrioid areas typical of type II carcinomas. Accumulation of p53 protein as a result of stabilizing gene mutations or other factors may be implicated in the secondary development of these histopathological growth patterns.[9] Such mixed tumors demonstrate features that combine aspects of both type I and type II carcinomas: hormonal etiology, a mixture of endometrioid and non-endometrioid histology, and clinically aggressive behavior.

ETIOLOGY OF TYPE I ENDOMETRIAL CARCINOMAS

Life course

Even though most endometrial carcinomas are diagnosed after menopause, some established risk factors and protective factors exert effects before menopause. Therefore, these factors likely produce long-lasting, if not permanent, changes in the endometrium. Given that malignant transformation requires the accumulation of multiple molecular alterations within cells, one effect of risk factors might be to impede endometrial shedding, thereby increasing the chances that a clone of abnormal cells will persist within the endometrium. Therefore, for purposes of understanding endometrial carcinogenesis, it is fruitful to parse the reproductive life of women into three phases – premenopause, the menopausal transition (often referred to as peri-menopause), and postmenopause – that are each characterized by different patterns of endometrial shedding. During premenopause, risk is set, so to speak. During the menopausal transition, local events modify, magnify, or reduce risk. During postmenopause, promoting events can lead to the emergence of precursors and carcinomas.

The usual dichotomous categorization of a woman's adult life into pre- and postmenopausal phases neglects the potential importance of the perimenopausal transition in establishing the baseline status of the postmenopausal endometrium. In some women, the perimenopause is characterized by periods of prolonged anovulation and spiking estrogen levels that could in

theory promote persistence and growth of preneoplastic cells, although this proposal is difficult to study and has not been fully explored.[10,11] Unfortunately, most epidemiological studies collect exposure information by interviewing cancer patients, the majority of whom are postmenopausal when diagnosed and, therefore, cannot always provide accurate, precise, and complete information about critical early life events.

Conceptualizing the life course of mature women in three phases invites speculation about how each phase might affect cancer risk. In the premenopause, rapid regeneration of the endometrium following menses results predictably in uncorrected molecular alterations that might promote carcinogenesis; however, the clonal expansion of such cells is opposed by menstrual shedding, DNA repair mechanisms, apoptosis, and other factors. If cells that remain permanently within the endometrium (i.e. cells in the basalis, possibly stem cells) do not accumulate cancer-causing alterations, cancer risk is reduced. The characteristics of a woman's perimenopause, including overall duration, frequency and length of anovulatory intervals, and the occurrence of spiking serum estrogen levels unopposed by progesterone may influence whether abnormal cells that are present within the endometrium during the menopausal transition will regress, persist, or progress to clinical disease. After menopause, when menstrual shedding has ceased, abnormal cells that are present will likely persist. The hormonal milieu and other factors may represent determinants of whether these potentially neoplastic cells grow to produce a carcinoma precursor, undergo apoptosis or senescence, or persist as occult foci without producing clinical manifestations.

Hormonal imbalance

Type I carcinomas reflect the effects of excess exposure to estrogen unopposed by sufficient exposure to progesterone. Extensive support for this principle includes:

- the observation that endometrial proliferation is maximal during the follicular phase of the menstrual cycle, when serum estrogen levels peak[12]
- the marked dose- and duration-dependent increase in risk for EH and endometrial carcinoma associated with unopposed exogenous estrogen use after menopause[13]
- the observation that oral contraceptive regimens that contain high doses of estrogen and modest doses of progestins increase endometrial carcinoma risk, whereas regimens that contain weak estrogens and potent progestins are highly protective.[14]

Additional support for the importance of hormonal imbalances in the etiology of endometrial carcinoma comes from case-control and cohort studies that have found that endometrial carcinoma risk is elevated among postmenopausal women with high serum levels of estrogens (or androgens, as discussed below) and low levels of sex hormone-binding globulin (SHBG binds estrogens and reduces the bioavailable fraction).[15,16]

Although the etiological importance of estrogens in endometrial carcinoma has been emphasized, understanding the balance between different hormonal exposures, the interactions among hormones and other factors, and the intricacies of sequence and timing are critical for elucidating the complex process of endometrial carcinogenesis. Notably, among premenopausal women, relative progesterone deficiency and anovulation may represent more important factors than elevated estrogen levels per se. In addition, elevated androgen levels seem to increase endometrial carcinoma risk, but the responsible mechanisms may differ among pre- and postmenopausal women. Among premenopausal women, excess androgen exposure may provoke follicular atresia, anovulation, and progesterone deficiency, whereas among older women, androgens may serve as a substrate for aromatization to estrogens in peripheral adipose tissue (see Kaaks et al[17] for summary).

Although excess estrogen stimulation relative to progesterone has dominated etiological thinking about endometrial carcinogenesis, other mechanisms that are involved in malignant tumor formation at other sites are undoubtedly operative in the uterus. These processes include inflammation, angiogenesis, and disruption of normal tissue architecture leading to abnormal epithelial–stromal interactions.

Tissue aging

Most risk factors for type I endometrial carcinomas are related to menstrual and reproductive characteristics. To account mechanistically for the effects of these factors on endometrial cancer risk, Key and Pike proposed the 'tissue aging' hypothesis of hormonal carcinogenesis.[18]

Conceptually, tissue aging is viewed as the net effect of accumulated mutations in stem cells and factors that affect the fate of such cells, such as proliferation, differentiation, and apoptosis. This hypothesis was developed to account for the observed age-specific population-based incidence rates for endometrial cancer (and other hormonally related tumors), which are characterized by a linear increase until menopause,

followed by a slower rate of rise at older ages. Note that although incidence rates of endometrial carcinoma are higher after menopause, the rates of increase are slowed, pointing towards a central role of premenopausal hormones and possibly other early life factors in the etiology of these tumors.

A central tenet of this model is that physiological proliferation of normal glandular cells is maximal when serum estradiol levels reach 50 pg/ml; higher levels do not produce greater proliferation.[12] This finding is interpreted to indicate that among women with high estradiol levels (such as normally cycling premenopausal women) the main factor accounting for abnormal endometrial proliferation and neoplastic change is progesterone deficiency, not estrogen excess. In contrast, most postmenopausal women have low serum estrogen levels and lack progesterone; therefore, after menopause, excess estrogen exposure achieves primacy in the pathogenesis of type I endometrial carcinomas.

The tissue aging hypothesis accommodates many established reproductive and menstrual risk factors for type I endometrial carcinomas. For example, early menarche, late menopause, and nulliparity result in a greater number of lifetime menstrual cycles, which is hypothesized to raise the potential that endometrial progenitor cells will develop uncorrected molecular alterations and expand into neoplastic clones. Similarly, anovulation occurring in the setting of polycystic ovary syndrome (PCOS) or other conditions is characterized by failure to form corpora lutea and, therefore, results in progesterone deficiency.

Recent data suggesting that cumulative epigenetic changes in endometrial tissues represent surrogates for the total number of lifetime progenitor cell divisions provide support for the tissue aging hypothesis of endometrial carcinoma.[19] These experiments are predicated on two postulates: (1) epigenetic changes are preserved in the progeny of dividing somatic cells; (2) cumulative changes reflect the status of the endometrial (progenitor) cell compartment because other cells are cyclically shed and, therefore, cannot accumulate molecular changes. In this investigation, quantitative assessment of methylation of two genes, CSX and CSX6, is viewed as a cumulative measure of the epigenetic errors that have occurred in progenitor cells, which in turn reflect the lifetime number of progenitor cell divisions ('epigenetic molecular clock'). As predicted, the percentage methylation of these genes was progressively higher among women at older ages until menopause, and then remained relatively stable. In addition, women who were older than 52 years of age and had endometrial carcinoma risk factors (i.e.

nulliparity or obesity) had more frequent methylation events than women who did not have these factors. These findings are consistent with the view that aging, nulliparity, and obesity increase endometrial carcinoma risk because they are associated with a higher number of progenitor cell divisions, leading to a higher cumulative number of epigenetic errors. It is likely that similar conclusions would apply to somatic mutations and other measures of DNA damage.

Inflammation

The potential importance of inflammation in endometrial carcinogenesis has received recent attention.[20] This concept emphasizes that menstrual shedding is an inflammatory process that results in increased levels of cytokines and other factors that might augment the growth-promoting effects of estrogen-related proliferation or magnify other estrogen-related procarcinogenic effects. Menstrual events are associated with cellular injury and release of lysosomal enzymes, bleeding, formation of platelet thrombi, hypoxia, and ischemia. It is postulated that these processes lead to increased levels of inflammatory cytokines, formation of reactive oxygen species, and activation of the transcription factor nuclear factor-κB (NF-κB), which promotes cellular proliferation and inhibits apoptosis. It remains unknown whether the inflammatory processes associated with menses differ fundamentally among women who develop carcinoma as opposed to those who do not.

Arguably, increased lifetime number of menstrual cycles among women with early menarche or late menopause would lead to greater DNA damage secondary to increased exposure to free radicals and the growth-promoting effects of cytokines. It has also been postulated that obesity, which is a strong endometrial carcinoma risk factor, is an inherently proinflammatory state. In addition, it has been proposed that carcinoma risk factors promote the formation of proinflammatory estrogen metabolites, whereas protective factors such as smoking do not. Finally, it is hypothesized that parity could reduce endometrial carcinoma risk in two ways, by (1) decreasing the total lifetime exposure to inflammatory intermediates produced during menses and (2) creating a noninflammatory endometrial milieu during pregnancy.

If the development of a proinflammatory endometrial microenvironment and systemic milieu are important factors in endometrial carcinogenesis, anti-inflammatory interventions might be preventive. However, a major challenge to this perspective is that neither endometritis nor factors associated with endometritis such as sexually transmitted diseases (STDs) have been shown to increase endometrial carcinoma risk. Differences in the patterns of inflammation that are associated with STDs and endometrial carcinoma risk factors might reconcile this possible inconsistency. It is of interest that the development of endometrioid carcinoma is often accompanied by the accumulation of foamy macrophages, which could produce growth-promoting cytokines that contribute to carcinogenesis.[21]

Stromal aging

Increasingly, studies of carcinogenesis in many organ systems are exploring the role of the tissue microenvironment, including epithelial–stromal interactions. Endometrial stroma has a central role in embryological development and endometrial physiology. In particular, stroma seems to function as a critical intermediary of the effects of hormones on endometrial proliferation. Studies performed using co-cultures of endometrial glandular epithelium and stroma obtained from wild-type and estrogen receptor (ER) knockout mice have demonstrated that estrogen-stimulated glandular proliferation requires wild-type ER-expressing stroma, but not wild-type ER-expressing glandular epithelium (see Chapter 9). Therefore, mounting evidence suggests that estrogen may act by stimulating ER-expressing stroma to produce growth factors, possibly including insulin-like growth factors (IGFs) and others.[22] Although endometrial stroma appears to act in a paracrine fashion to physiologically regulate epithelial proliferation, stroma may also function to suppress carcinogenesis.

In experimental systems, stroma seems to have anti-carcinogenic effects that weaken with age. For example, data suggest that young stroma secretes soluble factors that can inhibit anchorage-independent growth of the endometrial carcinoma cell lines RL95-2 and HEC1-B, whereas this capacity is markedly reduced with stromal aging. In addition, data suggest that aged endometrial stroma secretes increased amounts of interleukin-1 (IL-1) and demonstrates increased expression of IL-1 responsive genes. IL-1 may produce endometrial stromal senescence, which could reduce the ability of stroma to produce effects that oppose malignant transformation of glandular epithelium.[23]

Specific factors

Most studies of endometrial carcinoma risk factors have not considered differences by histopathological type.

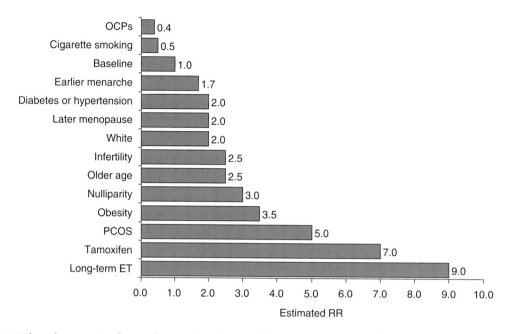

Figure 55.1   Risk and protective factors for type I endometrial carcinoma. OCPs, oral contraceptive pills; PCOS, polycystic ovary syndrome; ET, estrogen therapy; RR, relative risk.

Therefore, risk factor data for endometrial carcinoma implicitly relate mainly to endometrioid carcinomas, which account for approximately 80% or more of these cancers. For purposes of discussion, we will assume that these data are related to risk for type I tumors, although endometrioid histopathological type and etiological type I are not synonymous terms (Figure 55.1).

Endometrial carcinoma is a disease of aging and high socioeconomic status. Population-based incidence rates rise more slowly after menopause, but rates continue to rise with advancing age. In the USA, rates are higher among white than black women.[24] Although women living in Asia have low rates of endometrial carcinoma, rates increase substantially when they immigrate to the USA, implicating the potential importance of both mid-life or later-in-life factors and genetics in causality.[25]

Endometrial carcinoma risk is related to three reproductive factors that reflect a woman's lifetime number of menstrual cycles: parity, age at menarche, and age at menopause.[14] Nulliparous women are at increased risk for endometrial carcinoma, whereas childbearing is protective and the effect may increase in relation to the total number of live births. Some data suggest that parity is particularly protective against endometrial carcinoma diagnosed at young ages. Early menarche and late menopause have been found to also increase risk in several studies, with somewhat more consistent data for the latter.

Use of unopposed estrogens is perhaps the best characterized endometrial carcinoma risk factor. Risk seems to increase with both dose and duration of exposure, reaching approximately a 10-fold elevation after 10 years of use.[13] The impact of unopposed estrogen use produced a dramatic increase in endometrial carcinoma rates in the US population in the late 1970s, which subsequently fell once the link with endometrial carcinoma was recognized and its use among women with intact uteri was curtailed.[14] Administration of combined regimens including estrogen and progesterone in sufficient doses and for adequate periods markedly reduces or perhaps eliminates risk for EH and carcinoma. Most data suggest that risk associated with unopposed estrogen is not abolished by exposure to protective factors such as smoking, oral contraceptive use, or parity and that it persists for many years after use has stopped.

Exogenous estrogen is considered a carcinogen based largely on its association with endometrial carcinomas. Not only do menopausal estrogens increase risk but also the selective estrogen receptor modulator tamoxifen, which has agonist properties in the uterus, clearly increases endometrial cancer risk. Women given tamoxifen as adjuvant therapy for estrogen receptor-positive breast carcinomas have greater than a two-fold increased risk of endometrial carcinoma.[26] Risk persists for many years after administration. Clinical reports have also found that hormone-producing tumors such as ovarian granulosa cell tumors increase risk for endometrial carcinoma and its precursors.

Obesity, which is probably the strongest contemporary risk factor for sporadic endometrial carcinoma type I, may act through several mechanisms. Understanding the role of obesity in endometrial carcinogenesis is particularly important:

- obesity confers relative risks of three- to four-fold
- obesity may contribute causally to the development of ~40% of cancers ('attributable fraction')
- the prevalence of obesity has increased markedly in developed nations in recent decades.[17,27]

The current understanding of the metabolic derangements and functional consequences of obesity have been comprehensively reviewed,[17,27] although many fundamental issues remain uncertain. For example, it is unclear whether endometrial cancer risk rises linearly with increasing body mass or added risk only occurs among women who exceed a certain threshold, such as obesity defined by body mass index (BMI; kg/m^2) cut-offs. Although obesity seems to increase risk both among pre- and postmenopausal women, the mechanisms that have been hypothesized to account for risk among younger and older women differ.

Among premenopausal women, data suggest that obesity is not associated with increased bound or bioavailable estrogens, and in fact, may be associated with lower circulating hormone levels.[28] However, obesity has been linked to anovulation, providing the theoretical basis for such women having a progesterone deficiency, although this remains unproven. It is hypothesized that obese premenopausal women synthesize increased amounts of androgens in both the adrenals and the ovaries, and the latter may cause anovulation. Obesity is also linked to high serum insulin and IGF-1 levels, which could inhibit hepatic synthesis of SHBG, thereby increasing the unbound metabolically active circulating fraction of several hormones. Finally, distribution of adipose tissue may have an impact on its contribution to hormone imbalances; some data suggest that central obesity in particular produces greater risk than similar levels of excess weight distributed differently.[29]

Most studies have suggested that adult-onset diabetes is associated with twofold increased risk for endometrial carcinoma, presumably through increased insulin levels in the setting of insulin resistance.[17] However, many diabetics are obese, which makes it difficult to untangle the independent effect of these factors. For similar reasons, it is challenging to determine whether physical activity reduces endometrial carcinoma risk independent of its inverse correlation with obesity.

Endometrial cancers related to high-penetrance genes are uncommon but provide important insights into endometrial carcinogenesis. Women with hereditary non-polyposis colorectal cancer syndrome (HNPCC), a disorder characterized by mutations in mismatch repair genes, *mlh1* and *msh2*, have increased risk for endometrial cancer colon cancer, and other tumors.[30–34] Although mutations of these genes are not found among sporadic endometrial cancer cases, loss of expression of these genes in association with methylation of CpG islands in their promoter regions has been found in approximately 25% of sporadic tumors.[35,36] Similarly, patients with Cowden's disease have germline mutations in *PTEN* and increased risk for endometrial carcinoma[37] and perhaps 40–50% of sporadic type I carcinomas and their precursors demonstrate somatic *PTEN* point mutations.[38–40] Therefore, studies of women with germline mutations may provide mechanistic insights that are relevant to understanding the development of sporadic tumors.

Of equal interest in developing models of endometrial carcinogenesis is the recognition that certain factors produce long-lasting reduction in risk that persists for years after cessation of the specific exposures.[14] High-dose progesterone-containing oral contraceptives produce risk reduction of approximately 50% with long-term use. Similarly, smoking produces long-lasting protection against endometrial cancer. Although it is often presumed that the smoking effect is mediated through an antiestrogenic process, this may be explained by an increased metabolism of estrogens to comparatively inactive 2-hydroxylated metabolites (as opposed to more active 16-hydroxylated metabolites) rather than to a direct reduction in serum estrogens.[41]

Research challenges

Several factors complicate continued exploration of endometrial cancer etiology: hysterectomy for benign indications, exogenous hormone use, and lack of screening for precursors. Hysterectomy alters the at-risk pool in complex ways. Exogenous hormone use modifies the natural history of precursors. Finally, the lack of effective screening methods for endometrial carcinoma complicates attempts to understand the natural history of early potential precursor lesions. These topics are discussed briefly below.

In the USA and other developed nations, approximately one-third to one-half of women >50 years old have undergone hysterectomy for benign indications such as leiomyomata, adenomyosis, prolapse, and other disorders.[42] Many of these benign lesions share risk factors with endometrial carcinoma. Consequently, hysterectomy procedures both reduce the at-risk population numerically and preferentially remove higher-risk women, leaving behind a smaller group of

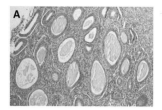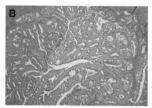

Figure 55.2   (A) Slightly crowded dilated glands compatible with non-atypical simple hyperplasia. (B) Substantially crowded glands with minimal intervening stroma (right) approaching glandular fusion (left) compatible with atypical complex hyperplasia with features of early endometrioid carcinoma, grade 1. (See also color plate section.)

women that has been partially depleted of those at greatest cancer risk. The higher prevalence of hysterectomy among black women, and the fact that many black women who undergo hysterectomy have strong risk factors for endometrial carcinoma, may partly explain the lower incidence of endometrial carcinoma in this racial group in the USA.[43]

A large percentage of women in developed nations use exogenous hormones for varying periods for contraception, irregular vaginal bleeding, menopausal symptoms, and other indications. Many women have used multiple products that differ in chemical content and biological effects and interaction with other exposures.[44] In addition to the uncertain risks associated with different combinations of exposures, these hormones often produce side effects that can influence the detection of endometrial carcinoma. Some estrogen + progestin regimens generate monthly bleeding, which may be predictable or irregular, and these symptoms can prompt diagnostic work-ups that heighten detection or lead to clinical interventions that probably alter natural history.

Our inability to effectively screen for endometrial carcinoma means that we know relatively little about how risk factors and protective factors affect normal endometrium and influence early events in carcinogenesis. Few etiological studies of endometrial carcinoma precursors have been performed and these studies have enrolled women who presented with endometrial bleeding, which represents a biased subset of women, limited to those with symptomatic disease.

TYPE I ENDOMETRIAL CARCINOMA PRECURSORS

EH constitutes a morphologically and biologically heterogeneous category of lesions that range in clinical behavior

from innocuous, highly reversible proliferations to incipient endometrial carcinoma. Although EH is the only frequently occurring precursor of type I endometrial carcinomas, it is typically detected in less than 50% of uteri removed for carcinoma, even if the endometrium is extensively examined histologically. In some cases, carcinomas may replace or obliterate the EH from which they developed, whereas in other cases, carcinomas may have arisen from uncharacterized precursors. Rarely, microscopic examination reveals the development of carcinoma directly from non-hyperplastic endometrium.

Multiple lines of evidence support the view that EH is a precursor lesion. Longitudinal studies suggest that women with EH are at increased risk for a subsequent diagnosis of carcinoma.[45] In addition, in uteri removed for carcinoma, EH is often topographically related to and merges with the tumor. Molecular studies have found clonal linkages between EH and carcinoma.[46]

EH is defined histopathologically as an abnormal proliferation of endometrial glands showing a spectrum of architectural and cytological abnormalities. The morphological features of the mildest forms of EH overlap with anovulatory endometrium, whereas the most severe lesions are essentially indistinguishable from well-differentiated endometrioid adenocarcinoma (Figure 55.2). The histopathological classification of EH is based on features such as glandular crowding (a reduced amount of endometrial stroma between glands), irregular glandular outlines, and nuclear atypia.

In the USA and other countries, clinical reporting of EH is based mainly on the World Health Organization (WHO) classification. In this classification, glands with dilated lumina displaying minor degrees of crowding are categorized as simple EH, whereas lesions composed of irregularly shaped severely crowded glands (nearly back-to-back) are designated as complex EH. Lesions are further classified as nonatypical or atypical based on whether the glandular cell nuclei appear markedly abnormal. Generally, the severity of glandular crowding and cytological atypia develop in parallel. Most simple EH is classified as non-atypical, whereas nearly all atypical EH is also designated as complex.

Other classification systems have also been proposed. In the endometrial intraepithelial neoplasia (EIN) classification, lesions are divided into EH (roughly reflecting a response to excessive estrogen exposure) and EIN, a clonal carcinoma precursor.[47,48] The EIN system is based on multivariate statistical analyses of data derived from quantitative image cytometry showing that lesions with an abnormal 'D score' predict which women with EH are most likely to progress to carcinoma. Approximately 75% of lesions classified as EIN, based upon abnormal D scores, are monoclonal. Morphometric data were used to develop criteria permitting the diagnosis of EIN with routine light microscopy. The EIN classification represents an attempt to translate computer-generated D scores into criteria applicable to routine light microscopic diagnosis. EIN is defined as cytologically distinctive lesions measuring 1–2 mm that demonstrate a volume percentage stroma of less than 55%. In the EIN classification, carcinoma precursors (i.e. EIN) are defined mainly on the basis of glandular crowding, whereas in the WHO system, nuclear atypia is paramount (i.e. atypical EH).

The WHO classification system is the most widely used classification in clinical practice. Clinical implementation of the classification was based largely on a retrospective review of 170 curettages collected in the period 1940–1970.[45] In this study, non-atypical simple EH accounted for approximately 55% of EH lesions; however, 80% of these lesions regressed and only 1% progressed to carcinoma. In fact, even atypical complex EH, the lesion with the highest neoplastic potential, progressed to carcinoma in only 29% of women while regressing in 57%. Although this study provided much of the evidence supporting the adoption of the WHO classification, this investigation was limited by several factors: (1) small numbers of EH lesions and carcinoma outcomes; (2) lack of a population-based sample; (3) absence of a masked histopathological review; (4) failure to control for treatment and other confounders; and (5) failure to use multivariate or time-dependent statistical models. In addition, some etiological exposures that were common during the calendar period of case accrual, such as administration of unopposed estrogen to women with intact uteri, are no longer relevant. In short, there is a pressing need for updated 'natural history' studies of EH. Identifying lesions with minimal risk for progression to carcinoma would provide substantial benefit to many women by allowing them to avoid hysterectomy and its related complications.

Clinical studies based on the WHO classification have revealed other concerns, including the lack of quantitative criteria for glandular crowding (to distinguish simple from complex EH) and nuclear atypia (to distinguish non-atypical from atypical EH), which contribute to suboptimal histopathological reproducibility.[49] Expert reviews of community diagnoses of endometrial biopsies and curettages have consistently demonstrated that variants of normal endometrium that display metaplastic changes (altered differentiation in benign epithelium) are frequently misclassified as EH.[50] However, usual endometrial sampling methods such as biopsy and curettage remove only a fraction of the total endometrial surface, which inevitably leads to sampling errors and underdiagnosis. Data suggest that carcinoma may be present in over 40% of uteri removed for treatment following a diagnosis of atypical EH on a biopsy or curettage.[51] In short, pathologists' tendencies to overdiagnose biopsies, gynecologists' concerns about underdiagnosis secondary to inadequate sampling, and women's historical acceptance of hysterectomy for benign indications has almost certainly led to substantial overtreatment of many reversible benign proliferating lesions.

Population-based incidence data for EH are not routinely collected; consequently, data related to rates of EH are sparse and inconsistent. For example, a tabulation of diagnoses of 2662 curettages performed at 11 hospitals in the Netherlands found that the ratio of EH:carcinoma was 4.5:1.0; however, markedly atypical EH diagnoses constituted a minor fraction of total EH lesions and were much less prevalent than carcinoma.[52] These data are consistent with evidence that most EH lesions do not progress to carcinoma. However, Koss et al,[53] using a cytological technique to assess asymptomatic mainly postmenopausal women, identified a rate of EH of 8.1 per 1000 as compared to 7.0 per 1000 for carcinoma. These data are more difficult to reconcile with the frequent reversion of EH to normal. Given the wide discrepancy in these data and changes in the prevalence of key risk factors that have occurred since these analyses were performed, contemporary population-based studies are needed. Unfortunately, accurate ascertainment of EH rates is difficult and, as mentioned above, the natural history of these lesions is frequently modified by medical treatment.

Risk factor data for EH are extremely limited. Exposures were compared among 109 women with hyperplasia and 111 with cancer identified in a population of 25 000 women aged 40–65 years old participating in a breast cancer screening study.[54] Although use of unopposed estrogen and obesity were risk factors for both EH and carcinoma, parity, age at first birth, number of children, age at menopause, and body mass were only related to carcinoma risk. An older population-based case-control study conducted between 1977 and 1978 found that unopposed estrogen use and elevated body mass were risk factors for adenomatous EH (i.e. complex EH) among postmenopausal women, but were protective among premenopausal women.[55] A retrospective clinical study of 46 cases of EH and 5 of carcinomas among premenopausal women found that age ≥45 years old, weight ≥90 kg, infertility, family history of colon cancer, and nulliparity were associated with increased risk.[56] Another recent clinical study suggested that patient characteristics differ for women with atypical and non-atypical EH.[57] In summary, data related to factors associated with EH are sparse, conflicting, and sometimes inconsistent with data for endometrial carcinoma. The inability to accurately and reproducibly identify true carcinoma precursors is central to this problem.

The goal of refining the classification of EH is to develop a method for reproducibly distinguishing true carcinoma precursors that have limited potential to regress and should prompt hysterectomy, from the much larger, morphologically heterogeneous set of lesions that would either regress spontaneously or could be effectively treated pharmacologically. The ability to accurately identify proximate endometrial precursors would also facilitate prevention research by permitting assessment of exposures among younger women in whom most precursors occur as opposed to studies of older women with carcinoma. Notably, endometrial precursors typically develop in the late premenopausal and perimenopausal periods, whereas carcinomas are typically diagnosed after menopause. Accordingly, carcinoma case-control studies typically enroll menopausal women to assess risk factors that were operative before menopause, leading to incomplete and possibly inaccurate evaluations. On these bases, the relative merits of the WHO and EIN systems have been debated.[58] Other clinicians have suggested that the classification of EH in biopsies would be improved by combining the categories of complex EH and atypical EH into a unified category of endometrial neoplasia, which would be distinguished from less severe lesions that would be reported as EH.[49]

TYPE I ENDOMETRIAL CARCINOMAS: MOLECULAR AND EXPERIMENTAL DATA

HNPCC is an autosomal dominant disorder caused by inheritance of a germline mutation in a mismatch repair gene.[30-34] The molecular hallmark of carcinomas associated with HNPCC is microsatellite instability (MSI), which is manifested by loss of fidelity in maintaining the lengths of DNA sequences consisting of simple highly repetitive motifs. Loss of function for a gene involved in DNA repair may result in a 'mutator phenotype',[59] characterized by a likelihood of developing multiple mutations within cells or single clones that predispose to the development of carcinoma.

Criteria for the recognition of HNPCC were expanded in 1999 to include endometrial carcinoma, which is now recognized as the second most frequent malignancy associated with the syndrome.[30-34] HNPCC probably accounts for only a few percent of unselected endometrial carcinomas and even among women with carcinoma <55 years old, probably a relatively low percentage have the syndrome.

In addition to HNPCC, there is some evidence for the existence of site-specific endometrial carcinoma syndromes. Ollikainen et al[60] identified 23 such potential families in an unselected group of cases in 519 women with endometrial carcinomas. Loss of immunohistochemical expression of at least one or more mismatch repair proteins (*mlh1*, *msh2*, or *msh6*) was identified in only 52% of tumors and multiple affected women within families did not always have tumors that demonstrated identical immunostaining results. Further exploration of the genetic factors that are operative in these families is warranted.

Although HNPCC is relatively rare, MSI has been reported to occur in about 10–40% of cases in series of unselected endometrial carcinomas.[33,61-65] Two large series reported MSI in 29%[33] and 45%[64] of patients. Variation in reported frequencies probably reflects differences in patient populations, molecular methods, and criteria for MSI. The majority of sporadic tumors with MSI do not demonstrate mutations in mismatch repair genes, but methylation of CpG islands in the promoter regions of these genes has been found frequently in association with loss of expression.

Limited data suggest that immunohistochemical staining for mismatch repair genes may indicate which EH lesions will progress to carcinoma. In one study that compared staining for *mhl1*, *msh2*, and *msh6* in 50 EH lesions (13 complex atypical) that did not progress and 18 EH lesions (16 complex atypical EH) that were associated with a subsequent diagnosis of carcinoma, negative stains were significantly more frequent in EH that was associated with a future diagnosis of carcinoma.[66] However, the lesions that progressed were more severe by histopathological criteria and only univariate analyses were performed.

PTEN is a tumor suppressor gene that is altered in many forms of carcinoma. The protein product is a phosphatase that interacts with important cell regulatory molecules leading to growth suppression or apoptosis.[67] In normal endometrial glands, PTEN protein can be detected immunohistochemically and the most intense staining is found during the secretory phase of the menstrual cycle, when progesterone up-regulates expression.[68]

In carcinoma and EH, immunostains can identify diffuse loss of PTEN expression, arising via mutation, methylation, or other mechanisms. In addition, germline mutations occur in Cowden's disease, which is characterized by the development of multiple harmartomas and tumors, including an increased risk of endometrial carcinoma[37] and PTEN knockout mice with mismatch repair deficiency that are chronically exposed to estrogen rapidly develop EH and endometrial carcinoma.[69] Reports have demonstrated PTEN mutations in about one-third to one-half of endometrial cancers, with a slightly lower percentage in EH.[38–40] Mutations have been identified in 83% of tumors and 55% of precursors using a denaturing gradient gel electrophoresis method.[70] PTEN mutations may be found more often in tumors associated with EH and those which demonstrate MSI; therefore, differences in study subjects may contribute to variable reporting of PTEN alterations.

Absence of immunohistochemical staining for PTEN has been associated with detection of PTEN point mutations in microdissected PTEN-null glands. Small foci of PTEN-null glands have been identified in 12 of 34 biopsies performed for clinical indications that were classified histopathologically as normal endometrium.[71] Repeat biopsies performed an average of 400 days later demonstrated PTEN-null glands again in 10 of 12 women. The risk of EH and carcinoma developing in women with histopathologically unremarkable PTEN-null glands is unknown.

Activating point mutations at codon 12 of the Ki-*ras* protooncogene have been identified in approximately 10–30% of type I carcinomas, with lower estimates obtained in US studies and higher estimates found in Japanese populations.[72–75] Several studies have also identified *ras* mutations in EH, although data are inconsistent concerning whether these alterations are found in all degrees of EH or only atypical EH. These mutations are hypothesized to result in constitutive growth signaling through the mitogen-activated protein kinase pathway. The true prevalence of *ras* mutations in different populations and among women with different risk factors for endometrial carcinoma is unknown because large population-based epidemiological investigations have not been performed. Data are inconsistent with respect to whether *ras* mutations affect prognosis.

β-catenin is another gene that is frequently mutated or abnormally expressed in type I endometrial carcinomas, especially in endometrioid carcinomas with squamous differentiation. Mutation and other mechanisms may lead to stabilization and accumulation of β-catenin protein within the nuclei of glandular cells. In one investigation, increased nuclear staining was found in 85% of endometrioid carcinomas with squamous 'morules' (nodular foci of squamous epithelium), 46% with squamous metaplasia, and only 13% of carcinomas without evidence of squamous differentiation.[76] Accumulation of β-catenin may be associated with upregulation of the p53-p21WAF1 pathways and suppression of proliferation.[77]

Studies have compared gene expression patterns in endometrial carcinoma vs benign endometrium and in type 1 vs type 2 tumors.[78–83] Differences in methods of sample preparation, RNA isolation, array platforms, and analytical approaches may account for some of the inconsistent results. In addition, defining the transcriptome of 'normal' endometrium has been challenging (see Chapter 14) and little is understood about variation in gene expression among women with different menstrual and reproductive characteristics, including those that represent risk factors for carcinoma.[84] Although several common somatic alterations have been identified in type I endometrial carcinomas, many endometrial carcinomas lack mutations in *PTEN*, *p53*, *CTNBBI*, and mismatch repair genes.[85] This observation highlights the importance of additional research to discover genes and pathways involved in endometrial carcinogenesis.

Other studies have demonstrated differences between type I and type II carcinomas in the expression of genes involved in many different cellular functions as well as alterations common to both carcinoma types that distinguish them from benign endometrium. For these ongoing discovery efforts to produce maximal information gain, parallel efforts are needed to incorporate information learned from gene expression studies into models that include epidemiological risk factors, clinical presentation, and outcomes.

TYPE II ENDOMETRIAL CARCINOMAS: OVERVIEW

Bokhman's seminal observation that some endometrial carcinoma patients lack the usual features suggestive of hormonal imbalances and have an unusually poor prognosis was followed by efforts in pathology to identify tumors with clinically aggressive features. Whereas Bokhman's research focused on clinical features, pathologists investigated the microscopic appearance of endometrial carcinomas as predictors of behavior. In particular, pathologists had recognized that some endometrial tumors formed papillary structures, consisting of tumor cells lining fibrovascular cores associated with spherical calcifications termed 'psammoma bodies,' features that were commonly found in ovarian carcinomas. However, papillary endometrial carcinomas varied greatly in behavior; some tumors were clinically aggressive, whereas others behaved in an indolent fashion more typical of endometrial carcinomas overall. In large part, the confusion regarding the diagnosis of papillary endometrial carcinomas was clarified when Hendrickson et al published their landmark paper providing a detailed clinicopathological description of uterine serous carcinoma, which represents the best characterized example of a type II carcinoma.[86]

EPIDEMIOLOGY OF TYPE II ENDOMETRIAL CARCINOMAS

The epidemiology of type II endometrial carcinomas has received limited attention. To date, attempts to define a subset of endometrioid carcinomas that might develop via a type II pathway have been unsuccessful. Data suggest that risk factors for endometrioid carcinoma are generally similar, irrespective of other histopathological features such as coexisting EH, squamous differentiation, grade, and stage.[87] Data comparing risk factors for endometrioid and serous carcinomas as a means of identifying risk factor differences for type I and type II carcinomas are also limited.

Although non-endometrioid types of carcinoma represent the best candidates for development via the type II pathway, these carcinomas account for less than 20% of endometrial tumors overall, which has limited the power of epidemiological studies to reach firm conclusions. Studies have employed several approaches, including comparisons of risk factors by histopathological type, age at diagnosis, and other pathological features. Some information about risk factors can be inferred from larger case series that have collected clinical information.

Clinical reports and population-based registry data have consistently found that serous carcinomas are virtually restricted to postmenopausal women who are ≥5 years older on average than women with endometrioid carcinomas.[24] The incidence rate of serous carcinomas among blacks is considerably higher than among whites in the USA, whereas data for endometrioid carcinomas show a strong predominance among whites.[24] The differences in age at diagnosis and the racial disparities in rates support the view that the etiology of serous carcinoma differs from that of endometrioid carcinomas, and provide coherent general support for the etiological type I vs type II dichotomy.

In an analysis of data from a case-control study that included 328 endometrioid carcinomas and 26 serous carcinomas confirmed by pathology review, elevated BMI and use of exogenous estrogen were associated with an expected increase in risk for endometrioid carcinomas but did not significantly increase risk for serous carcinomas. However, protective factors such as parity, smoking, and oral contraceptive use demonstrated similar risk associations with the two histopathological tumor types.[88] In addition, this study found that serum levels adjusted for age and BMI of all measured estrogens were lower among patients with serous carcinomas as compared to endometrioid carcinomas, although not all differences reached statistical significance. Serum SHBG levels were significantly higher among serous carcinoma patients. Another analysis of limited size failed to confirm these differences in risk factor associations and found that non-obese women with serous carcinoma were slightly heavier at 18 years old and had used exogenous estrogen more often.[89] In summary, older age and black race represent the most consistently identified risk factors for type II carcinomas; data for other factors are limited and inconsistent.

PATHOLOGY OF TYPE II CARCINOMA

The development of refined histopathological criteria for serous carcinoma has been linked to efforts to define clinically aggressive endometrial cancers. Serous carcinomas accounted for five times the expected number of recurrences among women with clinical stage I carcinomas. Important histopathological and clinical features of these tumors have been defined.[86]

Historically, histopathological grading of endometrial carcinoma was based on architectural differentiation; tumors consisting of well-formed glands or papillae were considered well differentiated and were assumed to portend a good prognosis. Given that approximately 80% of endometrial carcinomas are classified as endometrioid and, therefore, display concordant degrees of architectural and cytological differentiation, assessment of the latter was not considered essential for grading. However, serous carcinomas diverged from this paradigm by showing areas displaying excellent architectural differentiation combined with anaplastic cytology, typified by extreme nuclear pleomorphism, hyperchromasia, and macronucleoli. The tumor cells demonstrated frequent mitoses, including abnormal forms. Although the discordance between architectural and cytological differentiation initially posed a dilemma for histopathologists, it later proved useful in recognizing serous carcinomas.

The appearance and behavior of serous carcinomas clearly contrast with those of the more usual types of endometrial carcinomas; however, the pathological evidence that serous carcinomas reflect the type II pathway of endometrial carcinogenesis is best supported by the appearance of the non-invasive endometrium in uteri containing these tumors.[5] Uteri that contain minimal volume serous carcinomas are typically small and possess thin endometrial and myometrial layers. Unlike the thickened endometrium of type I carcinomas, which can be appreciated on ultrasound, gross inspection, and microscopic examination, the uninvolved endometrium in uteri containing serous carcinoma is atrophic, not hyperplastic, and demonstrates a small number of mitotically inactive glands. The endometrial surface epithelium adjacent to serous carcinomas typically shows atrophic cells replaced by anaplastic malignant tumor cells that cytologically resemble those of the tumor bulk invading the myometrium (Figure 55.3). These lesions may extend into glands and replace the cervical and tubal epithelium without invading through the basement membrane. This surface lesion, variously termed endometrial intraepithelial carcinoma (EIC), endometrial carcinoma in situ, and uterine surface carcinoma, is postulated to be an early non-invasive manifestation of serous carcinoma, which points to the origin of these tumors from malignant transformation of atrophic surface epithelium.[5–8]

Since its description, EIC has been identified with increasing frequency. EIC has been identified in up to 90% of uteri removed for serous carcinoma that have been extensively sampled for histopathological examination. EIC has also been identified in uteri that do not contain invasive carcinoma.[90–92] Retrospective reviews of biopsies preceding clinical diagnoses of EIC have demonstrated that in some cases EIC was present more than 1 year prior to hysterectomy without progressing to invasion. However, some women with EIC alone (which does not penetrate the endometrial basement membrane) may show dissemination of tumor outside the uterus. Analysis of a limited number of such cases has demonstrated that the extrauterine foci in such cases are clonally related to the lesions within the endometrium, suggesting metastatic spread rather than a multifocal tumor origin.[93] One possible mechanism that could account for invasive disease outside the uterus in the absence of invasion within the uterus is expulsion of EIC cells through the fallopian tube followed by implantation.

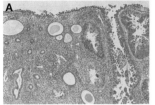
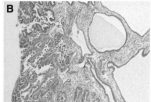

Figure 55.3 (A) Endometrial intraepithelial carcinoma (EIC) showing replacement of surface epithelium and superficial gland necks by malignant cells. Note: invasion through the basement membrane is not identified. (Adapted from Sherman et al.[8]) (B) Minimal uterine serous carcinoma (probably EIC) involving surface of endometrial polyp. (See also color plate section.)

Some investigators have proposed the term 'minimal uterine serous carcinoma' for EIC and small invasive serous carcinomas because assessing invasion may be difficult in these cases and both lesions may metastasize and therefore require surgical staging.[92] Minimal uterine serous carcinomas that have extrauterine disease have a guarded prognosis and generally require aggressive treatment.

A substantial proportion of serous carcinomas, especially small tumors, are associated with endometrial polyps.[92,94] EIC typically appears on the surface epithelium of the polyp and in such cases intrauterine tumor may be confined to the polyp. The relevance of this observation for the pathogenesis of serous carcinomas remains speculative. Limited data suggest that endometrial polyps consist of clonal proliferations of stroma associated with polyclonal glands. When involved by serous carcinoma, such polyps often demonstrate dilated atrophic glands, rather than hyperplastic ones. One interpretation of these descriptive data is that the relatively frequent discovery of serous carcinomas within polyps is merely coincidental, reflecting the tendency of polyps to bleed and prompt diagnostic biopsies. Alternatively, polyps might predispose to the development of serous carcinoma because of (1) the increased risk of hypoxia and ischemia secondary to compromise of polyp blood supply, (2) stromal alterations that create a microenvironment that predisposes to malignancy, or (3) abnormalities in the glandular component or surface epithelium. Serous carcinomas demonstrate a strong tendency to disseminate early, resembling ovarian carcinomas in their tendency to spread along peritoneal surfaces, produce malignant ascites, and recur in the upper abdomen. In contrast, endometrioid carcinomas tend to metastasize late in their development and to produce solid nodules rather than spreading diffusely on the peritoneal surface.

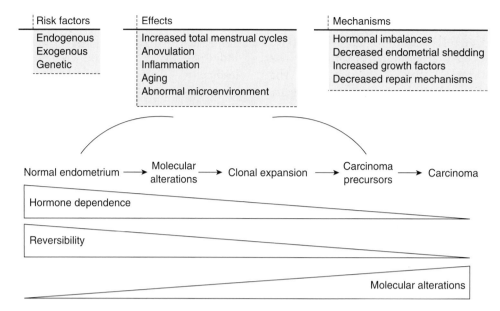

Figure 55.4   Pathogenesis of type I endometrial carcinoma.

MOLECULAR BIOLOGY OF TYPE II CARCINOMAS

Molecular changes found frequently in type I carcinomas such as mutations in *ras*, *PTEN*, or *β catenin* and methylation of mismatch repair genes are rare in type II carcinomas.[95] In contrast, up to 90% of invasive serous carcinomas and EIC demonstrate mutations in *p53*.[96] Detection of identical *p53* point mutations in EIC lesions and the serous carcinomas with which they were associated support the view that these lesions are related. Interestingly, women with Li–Fraumeni syndrome, who have germline *p53* protein mutations, are not known to develop endometrial carcinomas at an increased rate, although many may not survive into late adulthood.

Benign atrophic endometrium may remain mitotically active, even in the absence of exogenous hormone therapy. Limited data also suggest that abnormal *p53* expression may occur in surface endometrium of uteri removed for benign indications.[97] Assessing risk factors among women with abnormal p53 protein accumulation can provide clues to the genotoxic stresses that are associated with type II carcinomas. If *p53* mutation represents a critical event in the pathogenesis of type II carcinomas, then exploration of candidate exposures that have been linked to *p53* mutations in carcinomas, such as hypoxia, oxidative injury, or exposure to exogenous genotoxins, might provide insights into the development of these tumors.[98]

ENDOMETRIAL CARCINOMA TYPE I: MODEL OF PATHOGENESIS

Endometrial carcinogenesis requires the accumulation of multiple molecular changes in groups of cells that persist within the uterus over time and retain proliferative capacity (Figure 55.4). Molecular alterations may occur stochastically as a result of errors in DNA replication during normal menstrual cycling, but the rate at which these errors occur and the likelihood that cells with premalignant changes will persist, proliferate, and autonomously grow may represent the heretofore elusive biological correlates of epidemiological risk. Therefore, factors related to risk for type I endometrial carcinoma, including exposures, genetics, gene–environment interactions, medical interventions, competing risk of mortality, and other considerations, can be viewed in terms of their effects in causing molecular alterations. The mechanisms that mediate the procarcinogenic influence of risk factors are poorly understood, but may include hormonal imbalances that produce relative excess exposure to estrogen, increased exposure to growth factors, possibly including IGFs and others, exposure to proinflammatory cytokines, and reduced endometrial shedding. Protective factors favor relative excess exposure to progesterone, leading to endometrial differentiation, apoptosis, DNA repair, senescence, and others.

Several features of this process require emphasis. First, nuances related to particular characteristics of exposures, including combinations of exposures, sequence, and timing, may represent determinants of risk. For example, anovulation immediately after menarche is common, but its relationship to carcinoma risk may differ from anovulation during the perimenopause. Obesity increases risk, but weight gains, losses, and body fat distribution may also be important. Even with regard to risk related to well-defined exposures such as use of exogenous hormones, differences in dose, duration, and timing may be critical and effects may vary with other factors such as body mass, smoking, and other exposures.[44] Secondly, most EH lesions probably do not progress to carcinoma, and not all carcinomas seem to arise from EH. Similarly, the specific combinations of molecular events that result in tumor formation seem to vary greatly among cases. Whereas mutations of several genes have been implicated in the process, the importance of the sequence and combination of changes is poorly defined. Accordingly, the type I pathway seems to reflect a slow progressive accumulation of molecular changes that remains highly reversible, possibly even after histopathological criteria for carcinoma have been met. In fact, grade 1 endometrioid carcinomas may be curable with repeated curettage and progesterone treatment.[99]

The risk that particular grades of EH will progress to more severe stages remains ill-defined, as do the histopathological and molecular changes that indicate a transition from carcinoma precursor to carcinoma. Histopathologically, progression of EH is manifested as increasing glandular crowding and nuclear atypia, which usually develop in tandem. Fusion of glands that result in a cribriform or colander-like pattern have been interpreted as evidence of stromal invasion and have been considered the earliest pathological manifestation of endometrioid carcinoma. However, type I carcinomas rarely metastasize in the absence of myometrial invasion, which may indicate that some lesions that meet histopathological criteria for a diagnosis of carcinoma do not possess all of the biological attributes of clinical 'cancer,' such as the capacity to invade myometrium and lymphatics and metastasize.

From a morphological perspective, the development of carcinoma is characterized by disruption of the normal topographical relationships between glands, basement membrane, extracellular matrix, and stroma. Although the role of endometrial stroma in the development of carcinogenesis remains unclear, studies in animal models suggest that hormones influence glandular proliferation indirectly by inducing or inhibiting secretion of growth factors by stromal cells.[22] As EH progresses, glandular crowding is associated with a reduction in periglandular stroma, which may disrupt

normal paracrine regulatory mechanisms. Furthermore, whereas normal endometrium probably produces little estrogen, tumor stroma can possess aromatase, leading to estrogen synthesis and tumor growth at epithelial–stromal boundaries.[100] Desmoplastic stroma is usually associated with myometrial invasion, but not carcinoma confined to the endometrium.

Current models beg specific questions for which answers are needed to advance our understanding. From an etiological perspective, there are probably important risk factors that remain undiscovered, especially with regard to environmental exposures, diet, physical activity, alcohol, and other less-studied exposures. In addition, there are many gaps in the understanding of how established risk factors such as obesity, adipose distribution, diet, and physical activity interact. The incomplete understanding of how patient characteristics modify risks associated with exogenous hormone use continues to pose perplexing etiological concerns. In addition to the recognized importance of high-penetrance genes, it is likely that patients with specific profiles of low-penetrance genes may be at increased risk, and efforts to define associations are ongoing. Finally, refining our understanding of protective factors is a pressing need, as a fuller understanding of these associations may provide useful clues for prevention. Each of these issues would probably benefit from the development of novel ways to capitalize on the presumed lengthy natural history of type I endometrial carcinoma by attempting to isolate the critical events that occur early in life, during midlife, and at older ages.

ENDOMETRIAL CARCINOMA TYPE II: MODEL OF PATHOGENESIS

The main recognized risk factors for type II carcinomas are aging, somatic *p53* mutations, and possibly endometrial atrophy and endometrial polyps (Figure 55.5). If *p53* alterations occur in the absence of identifiable histopathological abnormalities, as has been suggested,[97] then *p53* mutations are not sufficient for the development of type II carcinomas, even if frequent.

A consistent characteristic of type II carcinomas is their association with advanced age. This may suggest cumulative processes which account for risk such as DNA damage, telomere crisis secondary to shortening following repeated cell divisions, or other mechanisms. Although DNA methylation increases with age, methylation represents a common event in the development of type I but not type II carcinomas. Presumably, the pathogenesis of type II endometrial carcinomas is related to

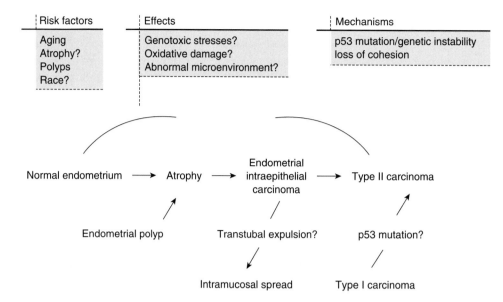

Figure 55.5   Pathogenesis of type II endometrial carcinoma.

an unrecognized late-life event that stimulates quiescent cells bearing molecular alterations to begin dividing, converting a molecular change into a neoplastic event. Interestingly, increasing recognition of EIC and minimal uterine serous carcinomas would suggest that there is some lag between the development of malignant transformation and the development of invasive carcinoma in the uterus. However, EIC cells may shed through the fallopian tube to produce extrauterine disease without infiltrating through the basement membrane.

Discovering more about the etiology of type II carcinomas will require collaborative efforts because these tumors are rare. These efforts may be justified because type II tumors are highly malignant and some of the information gleaned may improve our understanding of the pathogenesis of ovarian serous carcinoma, a tumor that is more common but shares some biological and clinical features with its endometrial counterpart. Defining whether use of estrogens is protective may also be helpful if it provides increased understanding of the biology of atrophy and genetic instability as it relates to tumors in the endometrium and in other organs. Although the investigation of serous carcinomas has provided an initial means for studying type II endometrial carcinoma, this etiological category probably includes tumors classified as endometrioid, clear cell, carcinosarcoma and other types. In fact these tumors, like serous carcinoma, may develop in a manner that is relatively independent of unopposed estrogen effects, yet differ sharply in etiology and pathogenesis from serous carcinoma. For example, there is some evidence that carcinosarcomas represent metaplastic carcinomas and that these tumors may contain epithelial components that resemble either endometrioid or serous carcinoma.

Perhaps such tumors are divisible into type I or type II based on the appearance and development of the carcinomatous portions, which seem to appear prior to the sarcomatous elements.[101] Clear cell carcinomas seem to represent a distinct category that may contain a mixture of type I and type II or perhaps constitute an entirely separate, but as yet undefined, type III.[102]

CONCLUSIONS

Our understanding of endometrial carcinogenesis has grown demonstrably since Bokhman introduced his original dualistic model. Undoubtedly, this knowledge will continue to grow, hopefully at an even faster pace by using molecular technology. In the future, enhanced understanding of the etiology and pathogenesis of these tumors will enable us to reduce overtreatment of innocuous lesions while improving prevention, detection, and treatment of lethal disease.

REFERENCES

1. Bokhman JV. Two pathogenetic types of endometrial carcinoma. Gynecol Oncol 1983; 15: 10–7.
2. Lacroix M, Toillon RA, Leclercq G. Stable 'portrait' of breast tumors during progression: data from biology, pathology and genetics. Endocr Relat Cancer 2004; 11: 497–522.
3. Deligdisch L, Holinka CF. Endometrial carcinoma: two diseases? Cancer Detect Prev 1987; 10: 237–46.
4. Sherman ME. Theories of endometrial carcinogenesis: a multidisciplinary approach. Mod Pathol 2000; 13: 295–308.
5. Ambros RA, Sherman ME, Zahn CM et al. Endometrial intraepithelial carcinoma: a distinctive lesion specifically associated with tumors displaying serous differentiation. Hum Pathol 1995; 26: 1260–7.

6. Spiegel GW. Endometrial carcinoma in situ in postmenopausal women. Am J Surg Pathol 1995; 19: 417–32.

7. Zheng W, Schwartz PE. Serous EIC as an early form of uterine papillary serous carcinoma: recent progress in understanding its pathogenesis and current opinions regarding pathologic and clinical management. Gynecol Oncol 2005; 96: 579–82.

8. Sherman ME, Bitterman P, Rosenshein NB et al. Uterine serous carcinoma: a morphologically diverse neoplasm with unifying clinicopathologic features. Am J Surg Pathol 1992; 16: 600–10.

9. Feng YZ, Shiozawa T. Horiuchi A et al. Intratumoral heterogeneous expression of p53 correlates with p53 mutation, Ki-67, and cyclin A expression in endometrioid-type endometrial adenocarcinomas. Virchows Arch 2005; 447: 816–22.

10. Hale GE, Hughes CL, Cline JM. Endometrial cancer: hormonal factors, the perimenopausal "window of risk," and isoflavones. J Clin Endocrinol Metab 2002; 87: 3–15.

11. Prior JC. Perimenopause: the complex endocrinology of the menopausal transition. Endocr Rev 1998; 19: 397–428.

12. Ferenczy A, Bertrand G, Gelfand MM. Proliferation kinetics of human endometrium during the normal menstrual cycle. Am J Obstet Gynecol 1979; 133: 859–67.

13. Lethaby A, Suckling J, Barlow D et al. Hormone replacement therapy in postmenopausal women: endometrial hyperplasia and irregular bleeding. Cochrane Database Syst Rev 2004; CD000402.

14. Cooke LS, Weiss NS. Endometrial cancer. In: Schottenfeld D, Fraumeni JF Jr, eds. Cancer Epidemiology and Prevention. New York: Oxford University Press, 2006.

15. Potischman N, Hoover RN, Brinton LA et al. Case-control study of endogenous steroid hormones and endometrial cancer. J Natl Cancer Inst 1996; 88: 1127–35.

16. Zeleniuch-Jacquotte A, Akhemedkhanov A, Kato I et al. Postmenopausal endogenous oestrogens and risk of endometrial cancer: results of a prospective study. Br J Cancer 2001; 84: 975–81.

17. Kaaks R, Lukanova A, Kurzer MS. Obesity, endogenous hormones, and endometrial cancer risk: a synthetic review. Cancer Epidemiol Biomarkers Prev 2002; 11: 153–43.

18. Key TJ, Pike MC. The dose–effect relationship between 'unopposed' oestrogens and endometrial mitotic rate: its central role in explaining and predicting endometrial cancer risk. Br J Cancer 1998; 57: 205–12.

19. Kim JY, Tavare S, Shibata D. Counting human somatic cell replications: methylation mirrors endometrial stem cell divisions. Proc Natl Acad Sci USA 2005; 102: 17739–44.

20. Modugno F, Ness RB, Chen C et al. Inflammation and endometrial cancer: a hypothesis. Cancer Epidemiol Biomarkers Prev 2005; 14: 2840–7.

21. Silver SA, Sherman ME. Morphologic and immunophenotypic characterization of foam cells in endometrial lesions. Int J Gynecol Pathol 1998; 17: 140–5.

22. Cooke PS, Buchanan DL, Young P et al. Stromal estrogen receptors mediate mitogenic effects of estradiol on uterine epithelium. Proc Natl Acad Sci USA 1997; 84: 6535–40.

23. Rinehart CA, Watson JM, Torti VR et al. The role of interleukin-1 in interactive senescence and age-related human endometrial cancer. Exp Cell Res 1999; 248: 599–607.

24. Sherman ME, Devesa SS. Analysis of racial differences in incidence, survival, and mortality for malignant tumors of the uterine corpus. Cancer 2003; 98: 176–86.

25. Parkin DM, Whelan SL, Ferlay J. Cancer Incidence in Five Continents. Lyon: IARC Scientific Publishers, 2006.

26. Curtis RE, Freedman DM, Sherman ME et al. Risk of malignant mixed müllerian tumors after tamoxifen therapy for breast cancer. J Natl Cancer Inst 2004; 96: 70–4.

27. Calle EE, Thun MJ. Obesity and cancer. Oncogene 2004; 23: 6365–78.

28. Potischman N, Swanson CA, Siiteri P et al. Reversal of relation between body mass and endogenous estrogen concentrations with menopausal status. J Natl Cancer Inst 1996; 88: 756–8.

29. Swanson CA, Potischman N, Wilbanks GD et al. Relation of endometrial cancer risk to past and contemporary body size and body fat distribution. Cancer Epidemiol Biomarkers Prev 1993; 2: 321–7.

30. Aarnio M, Sankila R, Pukkala E et al. Cancer risk in mutation carriers of DNA-mismatch-repair genes. Int J Cancer 1999; 81: 214–18.

31. Banno K, Susumu N, Yanokura M et al. Association of HNPCC and endometrial cancers. Int J Clin Oncol 2004; 9: 262–9.

32. Fornasarig M, Campagnutta E, Talamini R et al. Risk factors for endometrial cancer according to familial susceptibility. Int J Cancer 1998; 77: 29–32.

33. Goodfellow PJ, Buttin BM, Herzog TJ et al. Prevalence of defective DNA mismatch repair and MSH6 mutation an unselected series of endometrial cancers. Proc Natl Acad Sci USA 2003; 100: 5908–13.

34. Schmeler KM, Lynch HT, Chen LM et al. Prophylactic surgery to reduce the risk of gynecologic cancer in the Lynch syndrome. N Engl J Med 2006; 244: 261–9.

35. Esteller M, Catasus L, Matias-Guiu X et al. hMLH1 promoter hypermethylation is an early event in human endometrial tumorigenesis. Am J Pathol 1999; 155: 1767–72.

36. Esteller M, Levine R, Baylin SB et al. MLH1 promoter hypermethylation is associated with the microsatellite instability phenotype in sporadic endometrial carcinomas. Oncogene 1998; 17: 2413–17.

37. Pilarksi R, Eng C. Will the real Cowden syndrome please stand up (again)? Expanding mutational and clinical spectra of the PTEN hamartoma tumor syndrome. J Med Genet 2004; 41: 323–6.

38. Levine RL, Cargile CB, Blazes MS et al. PTEN mutations and microsatellite instability in complex atypical hyperplasia, a precursor lesion to uterine endometrioid carcinoma. Cancer Res 1998; 58: 3254–8.

39. Maxwell GL, Risinger JI, Gumbs C et al. Mutation of the PTEN tumor suppressor gene in endometrial hyperplasias. Cancer Res 1998; 58: 2500–3.

40. Risinger JI, Hayes K, Maxwell GL et al. PTEN mutation in endometrial cancers is associated with favorable clinical and pathologic characteristics. Clin Cancer Res 1998; 4: 3005–10.

41. Michnovicz JJ, Hershcopf RJ, Naganuma H et al. Increased 2-hydroxylation of estradiol as a possible mechanism for the anti-estrogenic effect of cigarette smoking. N Engl J Med 1986; 315: 1305–9.

42. Lepine LA, Hillis SC, Marchbanks PA et al. Hysterectomy surveillance – United States, 1980–1993. MMWR CDC Surveill Summ 1997; 46: 1–15.

43. Sherman ME, Carreon JD, Lacey JV et al. Impact of hysterectomy on endometrial carcinoma rates in the United States. J Natl Cancer Inst 2005; 97: 1700–2.

44. Beral V, Bull D, Reeves G. Endometrial cancer and hormone-replacement therapy in the Million Women Study. Lancet 2005; 365: 1543–51.

45. Kurman RJ, Kaminski PF, Norris HJ. The behavior of endometrial hyperplasia. A long-term study of "untreated" hyperplasia in 170 patients. Cancer 1985; 56: 403–12.

46. Mutter GL, Boynton KA, Faquin WC et al. Allelotype mapping of unstable microsatellites establishes direct lineage continuity between endometrial precancers and cancer. Cancer Res 1996; 56: 4483–6.

47. Baak JP, Mutter GL, Robboy S et al. The molecular genetics and morphometry-based endometrial intraepithelial neoplasia classification system predicts disease progression in endometrial hyperplasia more accurately than the 1994 World

Health Organization classification system. Cancer 2005; 103: 2304–12.

48. Mutter GL. Endometrial intraepithelial neoplasia (EIN): will it bring order to chaos? The Endometrial Collaborative Group. Gynecol Oncol 2000; 76: 287–90.

49. Bergeron C, Nogales FF, Masseroli M et al. A multicentric European study testing the reproducibility of the WHO classification of endometrial hyperplasia with a proposal of a simplified working classification for biopsy and curettage specimens. Am J Surg Pathol 1999; 23: 1102–8.

50. Winkler B, Alvarez S, Richart RM et al. Pitfalls in the diagnosis of endometrial neoplasia. Obstet Gynecol 1984; 64: 185–94.

51. Zaino RJ, Kauderer J, Trimble CL et al. Reproducibility of the diagnosis of atypical endometrial hyperplasia: Gynecologic Oncology Group study. Cancer 2006; 106: 804–11.

52. Ausems EW, van der Kamp JK, Baak JP. Nuclear morphometry in the determination of the prognosis of marked atypical endometrial hperplasia. Int J Gynecol Pathol 1985; 4: 180–5.

53. Koss LG, Schreiber K, Oberlander SG et al. Detection of endometrial carcinoma and hyperplasia in asymptomatic women. Obstet Gynecol 1984; 64: 1–11.

54. Baanders-van Halewyn EA, Blankenstein MA et al. A comparative study of risk factors for hyperplasia and cancer of the endometrium. Eur J Cancer Prev 1996; 5: 105–12.

55. Kreiger N, Marrett LD, Clarke EA et al. Risk factors for adenomatous endometrial hyperplasia: a case-control study. Am J Epidemiol 1986; 123: 291–301.

56. Farquhar CM, Lethaby A, Sowter M et al. An evaluation of risk factors for endometrial hyperplasia in premenopausal women with abnormal menstrual bleeding. Am J Obstet Gynecol 1999; 181: 525–9.

57. Abastasuadus PG, Skaphida PG, Koutlaki NG et al. Descriptive epidemiology of endometrial hyperplasia in patients with abnormal uterine bleeding. Eur J Gynaecol Oncol 2000; 21: 131–4.

58. Zaino RJ. Endometrial hyperplasia: is it time for a quantum leap to a new classification? Int J Gynecol Pathol 2000; 19: 314–21.

59. Loeb LA. Microsatellite instability: marker of a mutator phenotype in cancer. Cancer Res 1994; 54: 5059–63.

60. Ollikainen M, Abdel-Rahman WM, Moisio AL et al. Molecular analysis of familial endometrial carcinoma: a manifestation of hereditary nonpolyposis colorectal cancer or a separate syndrome? J Clin Oncol 2005; 23: 4609–16.

61. Burks RT. Kessis TD, Cho KR et al. Microsatellite instability in endometrial carcinoma. Oncogene 1994; 9: 1163–6.

62. Caduff RF, Johnston CM, Svoboda-Newman SM et al. Clinical and pathological significance of microsatellite instability in sporadic endometrial carcinoma. Am J Pathol 1996; 148: 1671–8.

63. Gurin CC, Federici MG, Kang L et al. Causes and consequences of microsatellite instability in endometrial carcinoma. Cancer Res 1999; 59: 462–6.

64. MacDonald ND, Salvesen HB, Ryan A et al. Frequency and prognostic impact of microsatellite instability in a large population-based study of endometrial carcinomas. Cancer Res 2000; 60: 1750–2.

65. Risinger JI, Berchuck A, Kohler MF et al. Genetic instability of microsatellites in endometrial carcinoma. Cancer Res 1993; 53: 5100–3.

66. Orbo A, Nilsen MN, Arnes MS et al. Loss of expression of MLH1, MSH2, MSH6, and PTEN related to endometrial cancer in 68 patients with endometrial hyperplasia. Int J Gynecol Pathol 2003; 22: 141–8.

67. Sansal I, Sellers WR. The biology and clinical relevance of the PTEN tumor suppressor pathway. J Clin Oncol 2004; 22: 2954–63.

68. Mutter GL, Lin MC, Fitzgerald JT et al. Changes in endometrial PTEN expression throughout the human menstrual cycle. J Clin Endocrinol Metab 2000; 85: 2334–8.

69. Wang H, Douglas W, Lia M et al. DNA mismatch repair deficiency accelerates endometrial tumorigenesis in Pten heterozygous mice. Am J Pathol 2002; 160: 1481–6.

70. Mutter GL, Lin MC, Fitzgerald JT et al. Altered PTEN expression as a diagnostic marker for the earliest endometrial precancers. J Natl Cancer Inst 2000; 92: 924–30.

71. Mutter GL, Ince TA, Baak JP et al. Molecular identification of latent precancers in histologically normal endometrium. Cancer Res 2001; 51: 5308–14.

72. Enomoto T, Inoue M Perantoni AO et al. K-ras activation in premalignant and malignant epithelial lesions of the human uterus. Cancer Res 2001; 61: 4311–14.

73. Ingar-Trowbridge D, Risinger JI et al. Mutations of the Ki-ras oncogene in endometrial carcinoma. Am J Obstet Gynecol 1992; 167: 227–32.

74. Ito K, Watanabe K, Nasim S et al. K-ras point mutation in endometrial carcinoma: effect on outcome is dependent on age of patient. Gynecol Oncol 1996; 63: 238–46.

75. Sasano H, Nishii H, Takahashi H et al. Mutation of the Ki-ras protooncogene in human endometrial hyperplasia and carcinoma. Cancer Res 1993; 53: 1906–10.

76. Saegusa M, Okayasi I. Frequent nuclear beta-catenin accumulation and associated mutations in endometrioid-type endometrial and ovarian carcinomas with squamous differentiation. J Pathol 2001; 194: 59–67.

77. Saegusa M, Hashimura M, Kuwata T et al. Beta-catenin simultaneously induces activation of the p53-p21WAF1 pathway and overexpression of cyclin D1 during squamous differentiation of endometrial carcinoma cells. Am J Pathol 2004; 164: 1739–49.

78. Maxwell GL, Chandramouli GV, Dainty L et al. Microarray analysis of endometrial carcinomas and mixed müllerian tumors reveals distinct gene expression profiles associated with different histologic types of uterine cancer. Clin Cancer Res 2005; 11: 4056–66.

79. Mutter GL, Baak JP, Fitzgerald JT et al. Global expression changes of constitutive and hormonally regulated genes during endometrial neoplastic transformation. Gynecol Oncol 2001; 83: 177–85.

80. Risinger JI, Maxwell GL, Chandramouli GV et al. Microarray analysis reveals distinct gene expression profiles among different histologic types of endometrial cancer. Cancer Res 2003; 63: 6–11.

81. Santin AD, Zhan F, Cane S et al. Gene expression fingerprint of uterine serous papillary carcinoma: identification of novel molecular markers for uterine serous cancer diagnosis and therapy. Br J Cancer 2005; 92: 1561–73.

82. Shedden KA, Kshirsagar MP, Schwartz DR et al. Histologic type, organ of origin, and Wnt pathway status: effect on gene expression in ovarian and uterine carcinomas. Clin Cancer Res 2005; 11: 2123–31.

83. Sugiyama Y, Dan S, Yoshida Y et al. A large-scale gene expression comparison of microdissected, small-sized endometrial cancers with or without hyperplasia matched to same-patient normal tissue. Clin Cancer Res 2003; 9: 5589–600.

84. Borthwick JM, Charnick-Jones DS, Tom BD et al. Determination of the transcript profile of human endometrium. Mol Hum Reprod 2003; 9: 19–33.

85. Risinger JI, Maxwell GL, Berchuck A et al. Promoter hypermethylation as an epigenetic component in Type I and Type II endometrial cancers. Ann NY Acad Sci 2003; 983: 208–12.

86. Hendrickson M, Ross J, Eifel P et al. Uterine papillary serous carcinoma: a highly malignant form of endometrial adenocarcinoma. Am J Surg Pathol 1982; 6: 93–108.

87. Sturgeon SR, Sherman ME, Kurman RJ et al. Analysis of histopathological features of endometrioid uterine carcinomas and epidemiologic risk factors. Cancer Epidemiol Biomarkers Prev 1998; 7: 231–5.

88. Sherman ME, Sturgeon S, Brinton LA et al. Risk factors and hormone levels in patients with serous and endometrioid uterine carcinomas. Mod Pathol 1997; 10: 963–8.

89. Elit L, Pal T, Goshen R et al. Familial and hormonal risk factors for papillary serous uterine cancer. Eur J Gynaecol Oncol 2002; 23: 187–90.

90. Carcangiu ML, Tan LK, Chambers JT. Stage IA uterine serous carcinoma: a study of 13 cases. Am J Surg Pathol 1997; 21: 1507–14.

91. Lee KR, Belinson JL. Recurrence in noninvasive endometrial carcinoma. Relationship to uterine papillary serous carcinoma. Am J Surg Pathol 2000; 24: 797–806.

92. Wheeler DT, Bell KA, Kurman RJ et al. Minimal uterine serous carcinoma: diagnosis and clinicopathologic correlation. Am J Surg Pathol 2000; 24: 797–806.

93. Baergen RN, Warren CD, Isacson C et al. Early uterine serous carcinoma: clonal origin of extrauterine disease. Int J Gynecol Pathol 2001; 20: 214–19.

94. Silva EG, Jenkins R. Serous carcinoma in endometrial polyps. Mod Pathol 1990; 3: 120–8.

95. Lax SF. Molecular genetic pathways in various types of endometrial carcinoma: from a phenotypical to a molecular-based classification. Virchows Arch 2004; 444: 213–23.

96. Tashiro H, Isacson C, Levine R et al. p53 gene mutations are common in uterine serous carcinoma and occur early in their pathogenesis. Am J Pathol 1997; 150: 177–85.

97. Maksem JA, Lee SS. Endometrial intraepithelial carcinoma diagnosed by brush cytology and p53 immunostaining, and confirmed by hysterectomy. Diagn Cytopathol 1998; 19: 284–7.

98. Oliver M, Hussain SP, de Fromentel CC et al. TP53 mutation spectra and load: a tool for generating hypotheses on the etiology of cancer. In: Buffer PRJ, Baan RBM, Boffetta P, eds. Mechanisms of Carcinogenesis: Contributions of Molecular Epidemiology. Lyon: International Agency for Research on Cancer (IARC), 2004.

99. Ramirez PT, Frumovitz M, Bodurka DC et al. Hormonal therapy for the management of grade 1 endometrial adenocarcinoma: a literature review. Gynecol Oncol 2004; 95: 133–8.

100. Watanabe K, Sasano H, Harada N et al. Aromatase in human endometrial carcinoma and hyperplasia. Immunohistochemical, in situ hybridization, and biochemical studies. Am J Pathol 1995; 146: 491–500.

101. Bitterman P, Chun B, Kurman RJ. The significance of epithelial differentiation in mixed mesodermal tumors of the uterus. A clinicopathologic and immunohistochemical study. Am J Surg Pathol 1990; 14: 317–28.

102. Lax SF, Pizer ES, Ronnett BM et al. Clear cell carcinoma of the endometrium is characterized by a distinctive profile of p53, Ki-67, estrogen, and progesterone receptor expression. Hum Pathol 1998; 29: 551–8.

56 Malignancy

Jean A Hurteau, BJ Rimel, Amy Hakim, and Yvonne Collins

INTRODUCTION

Endometrial cancer is the most common gynecological pelvic malignancy found in the Western world.[1] Each year, approximately 40 000 cases of endometrial cancer are diagnosed in the USA, making it the fourth most common cancer found in women after breast, lung, and colon cancer.[2]

Although endometrial cancer is a disease of the postmenopausal state, approximately 25% of cases are found in the premenopausal period. Even though 75% of endometrial cancers are confined to the uterus, mortality rates have continued to rise over the last decade, despite recent studies showing improved survival in patients with advanced endometrial cancers treated with adjuvant chemotherapy.[2,3]

ETIOLOGY AND RISK FACTORS

Most endometrial cancer is the result of unopposed estrogen states (Table 56.1). Administration of estrogen without progesterone is well known to induce endometrial hyperplasia, a condition that can progress to endometrial cancer.[4] In a prospective randomized trial, 20% of patients taking conjugated estrogen alone developed endometrial hyperplasia, while <1% of patients taking a combination of estrogen and progesterone developed hyperplasia.[4] Subsequent studies have confirmed increases in endometrial carcinoma with the use of exogenous estrogens alone.[5] These studies and others have confirmed that the proliferative and mitotic effects of estrogen lead to endometrial cancer when not abated by the antimitotic effects of progesterone.[6]

Although many conditions have been associated with unopposed estrogen states, obesity is the most common risk factor associated with an increased risk of endometrial cancer. This association is thought to arise from the excess estrogen derived from peripheral conversion of androgens to estrone through the aromatase enzymes situated in adipocytes.[7] Furthermore, obesity is associated with decreased levels of sex hormone-binding globulin (SHBG), thereby increasing levels of free estradiol.[8]

Table 56.1 Risk factors and protective factors for endometrial cancer

Risk factors	Protective factors
Unopposed estrogen	OCPs
Chronic anovulation	Exercise (?)
Obesity	Smoking
Nulliparity	
Tamoxifen	
Diabetes	
Hypertension	

OCPs, oral contraceptive pills.

Exogenous sources of estrogen in the form of pharmacological agents that include tamoxifen have also been associated with endometrial cancer. Tamoxifen is a competitive inhibitor of estrogen that has partial agonist activity on the endometrium. It is used in the treatment of breast cancer and to reduce breast cancer risk in specific high-risk patients. This partial agonist activity stimulates the endometrium with a variety of effects from benign polyps to endometrial cancer.[9] In a randomized, double-blind, controlled trial of tamoxifen for chemoprevention in women at high risk for breast cancer, the risk of endometrial cancer was noted to be twice the baseline.[10]

Nulliparity contributes a nearly three-fold risk for endometrial cancer.[11] In a case-controlled study of Danish women, completion of one-term pregnancy was associated with a 40% risk reduction compared to nulliparous women.[12] The risk reduction seems to be related to the pregnancy-related increase in progesterone and mechanical clearing of endometrium subsequent to the delivery process. Nulliparity related to infertility has also been associated with the development of endometrial cancer. This may be due to anovulatory cycles promoting unopposed estrogen states, the lack of complete sloughing of the endometrium, and/or elevated levels of androgens.

Chronic anovulation usually occurs with adequate estrogen but lacks the progesterone of the luteal phase. This has been associated with an increased risk of developing endometrial cancer.[13] Polycystic ovary syndrome (PCOS) is a frequent cause of anovulation, with a prevalence of 3–8% in the population.[6] These women also have high levels of androgens, which may increase peripheral conversion to estrone and subsequently increase their risk of endometrial cancer. Insulin resistance is also associated with PCOS. Hyperinsulinemia is associated with decreased SHBG, which may be another mechanism for increasing the risk of endometrial cancer.[6]

Other ovarian-related sources of estrogen include sex cord stromal tumors, of which granulosa cell tumors are well known to be estrogen-secreting. These tumors are known to stimulate the endometrium and are associated with endometrial hyperplasia and carcinoma in approximately 25–40% of cases.

Increasing age is also associated with increasing rates of endometrial cancer, possibly because of the cumulative effect of other risk factors over time or the lack of menses and thus progesterone. In some studies, increasing age at menopause was correlated with endometrial cancer risk. Decreasing age at menopause was similarly associated with a decreased risk of endometrial cancer.[14] It has been postulated that more anovulatory cycles in those women with late menopause may be the reason for the increased risk.

Diabetes has been associated with increased risk of endometrial cancer and with poorer prognosis. The Iowa Women's Health Study identified 415 women diagnosed with endometrial cancer and 39 deaths from the disease. Adjusted for age and stage at diagnosis, women with diabetes were noted to have a risk of death from endometrial cancer almost three times that of non-diabetic women.[15] The authors have hypothesized that a diabetes-related condition such as hyperglycemia or hyperinsulinemia may contribute to the poorer survival. In-vitro studies of endometrial cancer cells show high affinity for and proliferation in response to insulin.

Hypertension has been associated with increased risk of endometrial cancer; however, it is also found concurrently with diabetes and obesity, which have clear associations with increased risk. In a large retrospective study of hypertensive patients in Finland, obesity was noted to be a risk factor for endometrial cancer, but hypertension was not.[16] However, a recent study of both hypertensive and normotensive women demonstrated that the presence of angiotensin-converting enzyme polymorphism was associated with endometrial cancer in younger normotensive women.[17] The effect of the renin–angiotensin system on the endometrium is not well understood. The authors hypothesize that elevated levels of angiotensin receptor subtype II in the endometrium and decreased angiotensin II levels may have a role in proliferation, differentiation, and apoptosis.

Use of combination oral contraceptive pills has been associated with a 40–50% risk reduction in endometrial cancer compared to non-users.[18] This reduction appears to be cumulative, lasting 10–30 years after last use.[18] The copper and plastic intrauterine devices (IUDs) have been associated with decreased risk of endometrial cancer in several studies.[19] This may be due to a local inflammatory effect on the endometrium or to some mechanical process. The progesterone-releasing IUD Mirena has been used in a small series of patients for endometrial cancer treatment but has not been evaluated for risk reduction.[20] Given the known antimitotic effect of progesterone on the endometrium, it has been theorized to reduce risk.

The possible protective effects of exercise have not been well elucidated. Some studies have found this effect independent of body weight, but these results are not consistent.[21] A prospective study of US women evaluating exercise over 1 year showed little effect on risk, suggesting that longer-term studies on exercise may be necessary.[22]

Smoking is associated with a decreased risk of endometrial cancer. A large prospective study demonstrated an inverse relationship between both length of smoking and number of cigarettes and endometrial cancer risk.[23] Tobacco use increases circulating androgens and progesterone by decreasing their metabolism, while it does not appear to be associated with changes in estrogen levels.[23] This protective effect is probably related to increases in progesterone. However, smoking cannot be recommended due to its other deleterious health effects, including increased risk of ovarian cancer.

TYPE I OR TYPE II ENDOMETRIAL CANCERS

Endometrial cancers are divided into two categories based on clinical and molecular characteristics (Table 56.2). Type 1 cancers are estrogen-sensitive, arise in a background of endometrial hyperplasia, and occur in pre- and postmenopausal women. They tend to be low grade and lower stage and usually have an endometrioid histology. Type II cancers are not related to estrogen, usually arise in a background of endometrial atrophy, and usually occur in thinner and older women. These cancers tend to be more aggressive in nature with poorer histologies (papillary serous and clear cell) and grades.

Approximately 80% of endometrial cancer cases represent type I cancers.[24] On a molecular level, these tumors are associated with mutations in DNA mismatch

Table 56.2 Characteristics of type I and type II endometrial cancer

Characteristic	Type I	Type II
Age	< 50 years old	> 50 years old
Weight	Obese	Normal
Parity	Nulliparous	Parous
Sensitive to estrogen	Yes	No
Histology	Associated with endometrial hyperplasia, usually endometrioid carcinoma, low grade	Associated with endometrial atrophy, high grade, serous papillary or clear cell carcinoma
Tumor stage	Early	Late
Family history	Yes	No
Genes	DNA mismatch repair (hMSH-1, hMLH-2), k-Ras, PTEN, β-catenin	p53, Her-2/neu

repair genes (MLH, MSH), k-Ras, PTEN, and β-catenin. In sporadic type I endometrial cancer, inactivation and hypermethylation of MLH-1 and/or microsatellite instability (MSI) of other genes is more common than actual mutations.[25]

Type II endometrial cancers, representing only about 20% of spontaneous cancers, are associated with abnormalities of the p53 and Her-2/neu genes. These tumors tend to be more aggressive and are associated with a poorer prognosis despite adequate therapy.[24]

Approximately 10% of endometrial cancers are associated with a hereditary component. Most of these are attributed to the HNPCC (hereditary non-polyposis colorectal cancer) syndrome. HNPCC, also known as Lynch type II syndrome, is associated with founder mutations in DNA mismatch repair genes, most commonly hMSH2 or hMLH1. This autosomal dominant disorder increases a woman's lifetime risk of endometrial cancer to approximately 40–60%, which is even higher than her risk of colorectal (33%) or ovarian cancer (12%).[24] Endometrial cancers associated with this syndrome usually occur at a younger age and are associated with a lower stage and grade of disease, although these cancers do tend to be endometrioid.[24] HNPCC can also be associated with gastric, pancreatic, and upper urinary tract cancers.

PREMALIGNANT AND PATHOLOGICAL CHANGES IN THE HUMAN ENDOMETRIUM

Endometrial hyperplasia

Type I endometrial carcinomas are thought to arise in the setting of hyperestrogenism. Most women who develop type I endometrial adenocarcinomas have histories of anovulatory bleeding, infertility, obesity,

hyperlipidemia, diabetes, or hypertension.[26] These associated conditions in correlation with unopposed estrogen states are thought to cause changes in the normal endometrium. These changes were first evaluated by Kurman et al in their retrospective study of the natural history of endometrial hyperplasia and the potential for progression to carcinoma.[27] Their classification is currently endorsed by the International Society of Gynecologic Pathologists (ISGP) and the World Health Organization (WHO).[27,28] This classification includes simple and complex hyperplasia for changes that do not display cytologic atypia, and the subclassifications of simple and complex hyperplasia with atypia for lesions that display cytological atypia.[27,29]

Simple hyperplasia

Simple hyperplasia is a term used to describe a proliferative or thickened endometrium with an increase in the number of glands. These glands can be dilated and have outpouchings and invaginations.[28] There can be little crowding of the glands (mild or cystic hyperplasia) with stroma seen between the glands, or the glands can display irregular borders and have crowding (mild to moderate adenomatous hyperplasia or 'adenomatous hyperplasia') with reduced stroma between the glands.[27,30,31] Progression to carcinoma occurs in 1% of patients with simple hyperplasia.[27]

Complex hyperplasia

Complex hyperplasia is a term used to describe proliferative-appearing endometrium with glandular crowding (back-to-back) and irregular glandular borders. In addition, the glands are structurally complex.[27] Intraluminal bridges are seen, and the common appearance of two-to-four cell layers results from epithelial pseudostratification.[23] Progression to carcinoma occurs in 3% of patients with complex hyperplasia.[27]

Atypical hyperplasia

Atypical hyperplasia is a term used to describe a hyperplastic endometrium with glands that display cytological atypia. The hyperplasia can be simple or complex, while the cells of the glands are often increased in size, and have nuclear hyperchromatism and nuclear enlargement.[28] The nuclei tend to be enlarged, and pleomorphic, with prominent nucleoli, and clumped chromatin.[27] Cytological atypia without back-to-back crowding of the glands is termed simple atypical hyperplasia (SAH); cytological atypia with back-to-back crowding of the glands is termed complex atypical hyperplasia (CAH).[27] Progression to carcinoma occurs in 8% of patients with SAH and in 25% of patients with CAH.[27]

Treatment options and follow-up

There is no consensus on the optimal follow-up strategy for women with endometrial hyperplasia that does not display atypia. For these patients, progression to carcinoma is in the range of 1–3%.[26] In the past, many of these women were treated with traditional short courses of high-dose progestins or even hysterectomy.[30] High-dose progestins can result in profound side effects and, if the patient is premenopausal and desires fertility, hysterectomy is an extreme option in light of the low risk of disease progression.[30] Currently, other new and better-tolerated options are available and include the use of combined estrogen- and progestin-containing oral contraceptives or combined hormone replacement therapy, or localized progestogens in the form of the Mirena levonorgestrel-releasing intrauterine device.[30–33] Follow-up visits and repeat sampling of the endometrium should be the standard of care to check for disease progression in any woman treated with conservative management. In one study of 351 women diagnosed with all forms of endometrial hyperplasia, 35 of 108 (32%) who were treated conservatively had persistent or progressive disease noted during their follow-up.[30]

Patients with atypical hyperplasia should have a strict follow-up strategy tailored to their desire for fertility. In a recent Gynecologic Oncology Group (GOG) prospective study (GOG 167) of 289 women with a community diagnosis of atypical hyperplasia on diagnostic biopsy who underwent hysterectomy within 12 weeks of entry onto protocol without interval treatment, 123 of 289 specimens (42.6%) showed concurrent endometrial carcinoma, and of these 13 of 123 specimens (10.5%) were myoinvasive while 10 of 123

(10.6%) involved the outer 50% of the myometrium.[34] It is therefore recommended that patients with CAH undergo hysterectomy should fertility not be an issue. Should medical management be recommended, a patient can be offered megestrol acetate 20 mg twice per day, with titration of the dose secondary to endometrial sampling every 3–6 months. This was the strategy followed by Randall and Kurman in their study of premenopausal women with atypical hyperplasia and well-differentiated carcinoma.[35,36] They noted 16 of 17 women <40 years old with atypical hyperplasia who were treated with megestrol acetate or medroxyprogesterone acetate had regression of their lesions and one had persistence.[36] The median length of time for regression was 9 months.[36]

CLASSIFICATION OF EPITHELIAL ENDOMETRIAL CANCER (TABLE 56.3)

Endometrioid adenocarcinoma

Endometrioid adenocarcinomas are the most common subtype of endometrial cancer (60%).[37,38] Most often they arise in the setting of hyperestrogenism in women who have a history of obesity, anovulation, infertility, diabetes, and/or hypertension. These tumors tend to arise in the body of the uterus, but they can occur in the lower uterine segment.[37] They tend to have the appearance of proliferative endometrium with a glandular pattern. The glands can be complex, with cells containing round nuclei, prominent nucleoli, and clumped chromatin.[37] The tumors can be well-differentiated (G1), moderately differentiated (G2), or poorly differentiated (G3).

Villoglandular carcinoma

Villoglandular carcinoma is a variant of endometrioid adenocarcinoma. It is a low-grade tumor with a favorable prognosis.[38] It tends to have long slender papillae with bland cells and cigar-shaped nuclei.[38]

Secretory adenocarcinoma

Secretory adenocarcinoma is another but much less common variant of endometrioid adenocarcinoma with a good prognosis.[37] It has well-differentiated glands with columnar cells that contain subnuclear and/or supranuclear vacuoles.[28,37,39,40] These carcinomas tend

Table 56.3   Classification of endometrial tumors

Epithelial endometrial tumors	Sarcomatous endometrial tumors
Endometrioid adenocarcinoma	Leiomyosarcoma
Villoglandular carcinoma	Endometrial stromal nodule
Secretory adenocarcinoma	Endometrial stromal sarcoma
Ciliated carcinoma	Undifferentiated uterine sarcoma
Endometrioid carcinoma with squamous differentiation	Carcinosarcoma (homologous/heterologous)
Serous adenocarcinoma	Adenosarcoma
Mucinous carcinoma	
Clear cell adenocarcinoma	
Squamous cell carcinoma	
Mixed carcinoma	
Undifferentiated carcinoma	

to resemble secretory endometrium and are usually grade 1.[28,37]

Ciliated carcinoma

Another variant of endometrioid carcinoma is the rare ciliated carcinoma. At least 75% of a tumor's cells have to be ciliated for it to be designated as ciliated.[31,40] These tumors tend to be associated with prior estrogen use.[28,40]

Endometrioid carcinoma with squamous differentiation

Approximately 25% of endometrial adenocarcinomas present with areas of squamous differentiation.[37] Previously, these tumors were divided into benign and malignant types: adenoacanthoma, if the squamous component was benign; and adenosquamous carcinoma, if the squamous component was malignant.[38] Prognosis is better for adenoacanthoma and for endometrioid adenocarcinoma without squamous differentiation compared to adenosquamous carcinoma (90% survival for the former two categories vs 65% for the latter category).[38]

Serous carcinoma

Serous carcinoma of the endometrium is an aggressive form of endometrial carcinoma that is similar to serous carcinoma of the ovary and fallopian tube and accounts for 10% of endometrial cancers.[37,38] It tends to have nuclear atypia with mainly papillary architecture.[37] Twenty-five percent of cases contain psammoma

bodies.[37,41] These carcinomas tend to invade the myometrium and lymphatics. Depth of myometrial invasion do not appear to predict extrauterine disease.[37,42] Endometrial intraepithelial carcinoma (EIC) is a term coined to describe serous carcinoma precursor lesions which arise in the setting of atrophy or polyps.[37,43]

Mucinous carcinoma

Mucinous carcinoma of the endometrium represents about 1–9% of all endometrial cancers,[37,44,45] and is similar to mucinous carcinomas seen in the ovary and endocervix.[38] These cancers have columnar cells and cytoplasm that contains copious amounts of mucin.[37,38] Fifty percent of the cells in the tumor must contain mucin in order for the carcinoma to be labeled mucinous.[37,46] The nuclei are located in the basal layer. The cytoplasm of mucinous carcinoma of the endometrium is positive for carcinoembryonic antigen (CEA).[37,47] A primary mucinous carcinoma of the endocervix must be ruled out in any diagnosis of mucinous carcinoma of the endometrium. Most mucinous tumors of the endometrium are grade 1 and the prognosis is most often favorable.[37,44]

Clear cell carcinoma

Clear cell adenocarcinoma of the endometrium is seen in about 3–6% of endometrial cancers, and patients are usually menopausal and have a higher mean age at presentation (68 years) than in most other endometrial cancers.[37,48–50] These cancers tend to have cells with clear cytoplasm.[37,38] The cytoplasm contains glycogen, which is lost with fixation, giving the carcinoma its clear cell appearance with hematoxylin and eosin (H&E) staining.[37,38] These cancers tend to have a higher nuclear grade, with a 5-year survival rate of 20–65%.[38,48–52]

Squamous carcinoma

Pure squamous carcinoma of the endometrium is quite rare and extrauterine disease has a poor prognosis.[37,38,53] Grossly, it appears like endometrioid carcinoma, but microscopically it looks like squamous carcinomas found in the cervix.[37,38] Before 1967, it was thought to be associated with cervical stenosis, pyometria, and endometritis,[37,38] and since then it is known to be associated with squamous metaplasia of the endometrium.[37]

Mixed carcinoma

Mixed carcinomas are so named for tumors that contain at least 10% of a second histological cell type.[38]

Undifferentiated carcinoma

Undifferentiated carcinomas make up less than 2% of endometrial carcinomas,[56] have a poor prognosis, and refer to tumors that in general show no glandular, squamous, or sarcomatous differentiation when stained.[54] Some are of large cell type and appear to have some sort of gland formation, while others are of small cell type.[54]

Metastatic carcinoma

Cancers of the breast (in particular, lobular carcinoma), pelvis, ovary, cervix, pancreas, stomach, and less commonly kidney, bladder, gallbladder, thyroid, and cutaneous melanoma, can metastasize to the endometrium.[37,38]

THE MOLECULAR BIOLOGY OF ENDOMETRIAL CARCINOMA

In 1983, Bokhman first described endometrial cancer as an entity with two distinctly different types.[26] He studied 366 patients with endometrial carcinoma and found that one type of patient (type I) had medical histories that included one or more of the following: anovulatory bleeding, decreased fertility, obesity, hyperlipidemia, diabetes, hypertension, and coexistent precursor lesions such as complex hyperplasia with atypia that could also precede their cancer diagnosis.[26,55] These

cancers were arising more commonly in a setting of hyperestrogenism.

The second type of endometrial cancer (type II) appears to arise in patients with no signs of hyperestrogenism; in fact, their cancers develop in the setting of an atrophic endometrium.[56] In addition, type II patients generally do not have histories of anovulation, infertility, obesity, hyperlipemia, hypertension, or diabetes mellitus.

Bokhman showed that type I patients had tumors with more favorable prognoses, with mild to moderate differentiation (79.9%) and superficial invasion (69.6%) on histology. Type II tumors tended to be poorly differentiated with deep myometrial invasion (65.7%) and more likely to have metastases to the pelvic lymph nodes (27.8% vs 9.4% in type I patients).

Type I patients had a 5-year survival of 85.6% compared to 58.8% in type II patients.[56] Other clinicians have confirmed these findings in type I and type II cancers, and have identified different histological types.[59] Type I cancers tend to be endometrioid in origin, while type II cancers tend to include papillary, clear cell, and anaplastic cancers.[57]

Type I tumors tend to be associated with alterations in DNA mismatch repair genes, PTEN, k-Ras, and β-catenin, whereas type II tumors tend to be associated with alterations in p53 and HER-2/neu genes.[58]

Molecular alterations in type I endometrial cancers

Microsatellite instability (MSI)

Two of the major genetic alterations in endometrioid endometrial cancer (type I) are MSI and alterations in the tumor suppressor gene PTEN.[59] Microsatellite DNA sequences are short tandem repeats found throughout the genome. Genes involved in MSI are those that code for proteins associated with DNA mismatch repair such as hMLH-1, hMSH-2, MSH-6, hPMS1, or hPMS2.[59,60] Alterations in these genes affect the cell's ability to repair mutations that arise during DNA replication, allowing these mutations to be transcribed more often.[60–63] MSI was first noted in patients with HNPCC syndrome. Seventy-five percent of patients with endometrial cancer in the setting of HNPCC syndrome have MSI as compared to 25% of patients with sporadic endometrial cancers.[60] In addition, one study showed that MSI is present in 28% of sporadic endometrioid endometrial carcinomas compared to 0% in serous endometrial cancers.[64]

Patients with endometrial cancer in the setting of HNPCC syndrome tend to have an inherited mutation in one of the two genes: MLH-1 or MSH-2. These genes require two hits (deletions or mutations) in endometrial cells, which cause them to acquire MSI and to become deficient in their ability to repair mismatched pairs, insertions, or deletions during the replication of DNA.[59,60] Sporadic endometrial cancers associated with MSI are most commonly caused by inactivation of MLH-1 genes by the hypermethylation of normally unmethylated CpG islands in the promoter region of this gene, while loss of expression of MSH-2 and MSH-6 are the second most common causes of MSI in sporadic endometrial cancers.[59,65,66] Type II endometrial cancers do not tend to have hypermethylated gene loci.[25,59]

PTEN mutations

Mutations in PTEN, a tumor suppressor gene, are among the most common gene alterations (i.e. due to loss of expression or loss of heterozygosity [LOH]) in type I endometrial cancers (37–83%), especially when MSI is present.[67–71] PTEN encodes a 55 kDa protein that gets its name from its preserved tyrosine phosphatase domain, as well as its sequence homology with the matrix protein tensin.[59,67] It is found on chromosome 10 (10q23–24).[70] The PTEN protein has both lipid phosphatase and protein phosphatase activity, and therefore affects the PI3 kinase signal transduction pathway, leading to increased cell proliferation and survival,[58] and it affects the downstream AKT pathway.[59] PTEN also mediates agonist-induced apoptosis through up-regulation of caspases and BID, and down-regulates the antiapoptotic gene BCL-2.[59] Mutter et al showed that in endometrial cancers and precancers (endometrial intraepithelial neoplasia) the PTEN mutation rate was 83% (25 out of 30) in endometrial adenocarcinomas and 55% (16 out of 29) in precancerous lesion.[68] In addition, PTEN mutations have been shown to be associated with an early-stage non-metastatic disease, and a more favorable outcome,[71] as well as being linked to early events such as CAH, in the pathogenesis of endometrioid endometrial cancer.[70] PTEN mutations have been seen in just 1/21 (5%) of serous/clear cell tumors.[71]

Alterations in K-Ras oncogenes

Ras genes have GTPase activity and play a role in the control of cell growth and differentiation.[58] K-Ras codes for a small inner plasma cellular membrane GTPase that functions as a molecular switch during cell signaling.[59] GTPase activating proteins (GAPs) stop K-Ras signaling by stimulating intrinsic GTPase activity, while K-Ras variants with point mutations in codons 12, 13, or 61 become resistant to GTPase activity and are constantly activated.[58,72] Lax et al found K-Ras mutations at codon 12 in 26% of endometrioid endometrial cancers and in only 2% of serous endometrial cancers.[58,64] In addition, K-Ras mutations were noted to be quite high in grade 2 tumors (60%), while present in only 10% of grade 1 tumors and 21% of grade 3 tumors.[64] These results are consistent with those of Enemoto et al, who found that mutations in K-Ras were localized to a portion of endometrial cancer cells in an adenocarcinoma with a more aggressive histological pattern.[73] Esteller et al screened 55 endometrial cancer specimens for codon 12 K-Ras mutations and detected them in 8 of 55 (14.5%) patients with endometrial cancer.[71] K-Ras mutations were not significantly correlated with any clinicopathological features such as age at diagnosis, FIGO (International Federation of Gynecology and Obstetrics) stage, grade, histological subtype, or clinical status.[72]

Mutations in β-catenin

Initially identified as a submembranous protein of the cadherin-mediated cell–cell adhesion system encoded by the CTNNB1 gene at 3p21,[58,74] β-catenin has also been identified as a downstream transcriptional activator in the Wnt signal transduction pathway, where its activity is tightly controlled by the adenomatous polyposis coli (APC) tumor suppressor gene.[58,70,75,76] Some colon cancers and melanomas have been shown to be initiated by disruption of APC-mediated regulation of β-catenin up-regulation of cell proliferation, and by stabilization of β-catenin.[74,76,77] Fukuchi et al analyzed mutations in exon 3 of the β-catenin gene in endometrial cancers with LOH at the APC tumor suppressor gene locus to determine if β-catenin was stabilized (and therefore not degraded).[77] They found that 10 of 76 cases had β-catenin gene mutations, and all these mutations were identified as single-base missense mutations on serine/threonine residues (codons 33, 37, 41, and 45) which alter the glycogen synthase kinase-3β phosphorylation consensus motif, and provide for the degradation of β-catenin.[77] Thirty-eight percent of the endometrial cancer cases studied showed accumulation of β-catenin in the cytoplasm and/or nucleus, suggesting that stabilization of β-catenin secondary to mutations in exon 3 of the β-catenin gene may be important in endometrial cancer development:[77] 16–38% of unclassified endometrial cancers express nuclear β-catenin.[58,77,78] In addition, nuclear β-catenin expression is significantly more likely to be seen in endometrioid endometrial carcinomas (31–47%) than in non-endometrioid endometrial carcinomas (0–3%).[58,79,80]

Molecular alterations in type II endometrial cancers

Type II endometrial cancers are associated with an atrophic endometrium and do not appear to involve an estrogen-stimulated precursor lesion. These cancers are classified as non-endometrioid, tend to be serous papillary or clear cell carcinomas, and can have putative non-estrogen precursor lesions, namely endometrial intraepithelial carcinoma. The molecular alterations seen most frequently in type II endometrial cancers are p53 mutations and HER-2/neu overexpression.

Mutations in p53

The TP53 tumor suppressor gene is the most commonly altered gene in human cancers, and is located on the short arm of chromosome 17.[58,81–83] It encodes a nuclear protein that has as its primary role the prevention of propagation of DNA-damaged cells.[58] When DNA damage does occur, nuclear p53 accumulates and then, by way of p21, results in cell cycle arrest secondary to the inhibition of cyclin-D_1 phosphorylation of the Rb gene, and by the promotion of apoptosis, through BAX and Apaf-1 proteins.[58,81,84] Mutation of the p53 gene makes it non-functional but able to resist degradation, and therefore it accumulates (is overexpressed), resulting in it acting as a dominant negative inhibitor of wild-type p53.[58] Normal cells do not overexpress the p53 protein. Many cancer cells, however, have been shown to exhibit mutations and overexpression of p53, including 50–60% of lung and colon cancers and 25% of breast cancers.[81,85] Early in the study of p53 and gynecological malignancies, Kohler et al used immunohistochemistry to test for the overexpression of the p53 protein in 107 snap frozen endometrial adenocarcinomas and 15 benign uterine samples.[86] They found significant overexpression in 22 of 107 cancers (21%), with advanced stage cancers (stage III/IV) displaying more overexpression (41%) than early (stage I/II) cancers (9%).[86] They also showed a significant association between p53 overexpression and non-endometrioid endometrial cancers, positive peritoneal cytology, extrauterine metastasis, and negative progesterone receptor status.[86] Later, Kohler et al reported the results of immunohistochemical stained tissue from 179 endometrial cancers for p53 overexpression.[87] They demonstrated p53 overexpression in 35% of endometrial cancers. In addition, they showed that p53 overexpression was significantly associated

with race, lack of hormone replacement, and older age. Finally, after correcting for hormone use, they showed that p53 overexpression in advanced-stage endometrial cancers was an independent variable significantly associated with poor survival and was more likely to be seen in cancers from black women.[87] Pisani et al also studied p53 overexpression in endometrial cancers.[82,88] They found significant overexpression of p53 in 15% of tumors and a significant 12% probability of 5-year survival, compared to a 90% probability of 5-year survival in the p53 negative cohort.[88]

Mutations in p53 appear to be strongly associated with uterine papillary serous carcinomas (UPSCs) and with the putative type II endometrial precursor, EICs (90% in UPSCs and 78% in EICs).[80] These results are consistent with Lax et al, who showed that p53 mutations were found in 93% of uterine serous carcinoma and in only 17% of uterine endometrioid carcinomas, as well as with Sherman et al, who showed that p53 was significantly overexpressed in 86% of serous endometrial carcinomas as compared to 20% of endometrioid carcinomas.[90]

Finally, the fact that p53 mutations are found in a high percentage of serous carcinomas that are concurrent with EICs (79% of p53-overexpressing tumors contain both EICs and serous uterine carcinomas),[90] helps strengthen the hypothesis that p53 overexpression is an early event in serous uterine carcinomas, and that they develop from endometrial surface epithelium which has been transformed from an EIC.[90]

Mutations in HER-2/neu

The HER-2/neu oncogene encodes for a 185 kDa transmembrane receptor tyrosine kinase which is a cell-surface glycoprotein that has similarities with the epidermal growth factor receptor (EGFR).[58,91,92] It preferentially heterodimerizes with members of the EGFR family and is therefore important in ErbB signaling, which is responsible for cell growth and differentiation.[58,93] Early studies had shown that HER-2/neu occurred in one-third of breast and ovarian cancers, and that overexpression was associated with a poor outcome. Tumors that express high levels of HER-2/neu have been shown to be associated with decreased survival, resistance to hormone therapy, resistance to tumor necrosis factor-α (TNFα), as well as resistance to activated macrophages, and lymphocyte-activated killer cells.[94,95] In 1991, Berchuck et al, using immunohistochemistry, set out to determine the level of HER-2/neu expression in normal and malignant endometrium.[96] In 24 normal endometrial samples they found light to moderate staining (1 + to 2 +) in the glands and no variation in staining throughout the menstrual cycle.[96] Nine of 95 endometrial adenocarcinomas (9%) showed heavier staining for HER-2/neu than was seen in normal endometrium. High expression of HER-2/neu was found in 27% of patients with metastatic disease vs 4% of patients with cancer confined to the uterus.[96] At the time, the significance of these results was not clear.[96] Hetzel et al helped to elucidate the significance of HER-2/neu overexpression in endometrial cancer when they reported their findings in 247 patients.[91] They found overexpression of HER-2/neu to be strong in 37 patients (15%), mild in 144 (58%), and not present in 66 patients (27%).[91] The 5-year progression-free survival was 56% for the strong staining group, 83% for the mild staining group, and 95% for the non-staining group.[91] In addition, they showed that strong staining for HER-2/neu was associated with an overall 5-year survival of 51% vs 96% in patients with cancers with no staining.[84] Even in patients with stage I disease there was an inverse relationship with the degree of staining and prognosis. The 5-year progression-free survival was 62% when strong overexpression was noted vs 97% when there was no expression.[91]

Santin et al then examined HER-2/neu expression exclusively in UPSC.[97] They only studied a small number of specimens, but they found that 8 of 10 UPSCs (80%) strongly stained for HER-2/neu (2+ to 3+). They also studied primary UPSC cell lines, which they found expressed HER-2/neu even more strongly than HER-2/neu-positive breast or ovarian cell lines.[97] Similar results were shown by Diaz-Montes et al in their study of 25 patients with uterine serous carcinoma.[98] Using immunohistochemistry, they showed that 12 of 25 patients with UPSC (48%) overexpressed HER-2/neu, and that patients with overexpression tended to present with more advanced-stage disease than HER-2-negative patients.[98] In addition, they showed that ≥50% myometrial invasion was statistically significantly more likely in cases with HER-2/neu overexpression (7 of 12 cases [70%]) vs HER-2/neu-negative tumors (0 of 13 cases).[98] Finally, they showed that overexpression of HER-2/neu was present in 81.8% of patients with advanced-stage disease vs 28.6% of patients with early-stage disease.[98]

Other important factors in endometrial cancers: steroid receptors and angiogenesis

Steroid receptors

Estrogen receptors (ERs) and progesterone receptors (PRs) are members of the nuclear receptor superfamily, and they act as transcription factors when bound by their respective hormones.[58] Bound estrogen or progesterone receptors then bind to estrogen or progesterone response elements in the promoter regions of target genes in a cell. This binding causes the transcription of hundreds and perhaps thousands of these target genes, such as activating protein 1 (AP-1) and nuclear factor-κB (NF-κB).[58,99,100]

There are two subtypes of the estrogen receptor, ERα and ERβ, and the uterus has been shown to contain mainly ERα.[58] It is thought that estrogen-mediated tumorigenesis is critically affected by an imbalance in ERα and ERβ, and since ERα mRNA tends to decrease from normal or grade I lesions to grade III lesions, while ERβ expression is not changed, this leads to an increase in the ERα/ERβ ratio.[58,101,102]

The progesterone receptor has two isoforms (PR-A and PR-B). It is thought that PR-A down-regulates the action of estrogen in the endometrium by preventing the transactivation of ERα, while PR-B acts as an estrogen agonist in the endometrium.[58] PR-A is thought to partially inhibit estrogen-induced endometrial proliferation by PR-B.[58]

Finally, high levels of estrogen and progesterone receptors have been demonstrated to correspond to better tumor differentiation and a lower occurrence of nodal metastasis, and have been shown to be independent predictors of better survival.[103,105,107]

The role of angiogenesis

Angiogenesis is very important to the growth and spread of cancers.[58] Some tumors themselves produce angiogenic substances, while others recruit and stimulate local inflammatory cells such as macrophages, which then produce angiogenic substances.[92,106] Some angiogenic substances such as vascular endothelial growth factor (VEGF) and platelet-dependent endothelial cell growth factor (PD-EGF) have been isolated in gynecological malignancies.[92,107,108] Several studies have demonstrated that high intratumor microvessel density is associated with advanced stage, increased risk of recurrence, and a poor prognosis. Increasing progression of microvessel density has been observed from benign endometrium to atypical hyperplasia, and finally to invasive cancer.[58,109,110]

ENDOMETRIAL CANCER

Clinical symptoms

Symptoms related to endometrial cancer include abnormal vaginal bleeding, either intermenstrual, perimenopausal, or more commonly postmenopausal, abnormal vaginal discharge, and leukorrhea. Although endometrial cancer is not the most common cause of postmenopausal bleeding, it is the most serious. Other causes include atrophy, hyperplasia, or trauma. More advanced disease can present with pelvic pressure, back pain, or hemoptysis. In patients where the cervical os was found to be stenotic, they presented with foul purulent vaginal discharge secondary to a hematometra or pyometra and were associated with a poor prognosis.[111] Less than 5% of women diagnosed with endometrial cancer are asymptomatic.

Diagnosis

Endometrial carcinoma occurs most commonly in postmenopausal women in the sixth and seventh decades of life, with 75% in women > 50 years old. The standard method for evaluating women with postmenopausal or irregular uterine bleeding is with fractional dilatation and curettage (D&C). This entails curettage of the endocervical canal, sounding of the uterus, dilatation of the cervix, and then curettage of the uterus circumferentially. These specimens are then sent for pathological evaluation. An office endometrial biopsy positive for malignancy can also be used for diagnosis.[112] Grimes showed that the accuracy of diagnosing an endometrial cancer with office biopsy is 90–98% when compared with the results of D&C.[113] There are subsets of women who are diagnosed with endometrial cancer when being evaluated for malignant cells on Papanicolaou (Pap) smears. They tend to have more advanced disease according to DuBeshter.[114] In patients with an atypical hyperplasia, as many as 40% of patients can also have a carcinoma of the uterus.[115]

Hysteroscopy and D&C are used in situations where additional information is needed for the diagnosis. Stelmachow reports that this procedure is more accurate in diagnosing polyps and myomas when compared to biopsy or D&C alone.[116] Hysteroscopy is more commonly used in cases of persistent bleeding, inadequate biopsies, or cervical stenosis. Ultrasound with or without sonohysterography may be used in addition to biopsy. It can help distinguish the etiology behind the bleeding.

Primary treatment

Surgical staging

The staging for endometrial cancer was changed by FIGO in 1988 from a clinical staging to a surgical staging (Figure 56.1). The most minimal procedure is

intraperitoneal washings for cytopathological evaluation, examination of the abdominopelvic cavity for evidence of metastatic disease, total hysterectomy (extrafascial), bilateral salpingo-oophorectomy. Also, lymph nodes should be examined and removed if they appear suspicious. All specimens removed should be sent for pathological evaluation. This includes evaluation of the uterus immediately to determine the depth of tumor invasion, which may lead to further staging. Generally, for tumors confined to the endometrium, a lymph node sampling isn't warranted because <1% of patients will have nodal disease.[117] The indications for lymphatic sampling include greater than half myometrial involvement, grade III disease, cervical involvement, adnexal involvement, extrauterine spread, high-grade histologies (serous/clear cell/squamous/undifferentiated), suspicious adenopathy, or tumor size > 2 cm. However, most recently, some clinicians have advocated a lymph node dissection for all patients with endometrial cancer as a therapeutic maneuver and a measure to tailor adjuvant treatments.

A vaginal approach may be used in selected populations of patients. This procedure is limited, as is doesn't allow for exploration of the abdomen and lymph node assessment cannot be done. Therefore, it should be used in patients who are less likely to have extrauterine spread.

Laparoscopic procedures are also used in the surgical staging of endometrial cancers. It allows for a smaller incision along with abdominal assessment and lymph node sampling. Homesley et al reviewed 50 patients who underwent laparoscopic surgery for preoperative grade I endometrial cancers:[118] 10% of patients failed laparoscopy, most commonly secondary to dense adhesions; the median number of pelvic and aortic nodes, respectively, was 16 and 8; and the median operative time was 180 minutes. The authors concluded that this was a feasible procedure and is limited by the technical experience needed over a period of time.

The prognosis for endometrial cancer is based on pathological factors, including the histological cell type, grade of tumor, depth of myometrial invasion, lymphatic space invasion, and involvement of cervix, adnexa, or lymph nodes.

The more aggressive cell types are serous, clear cell, undifferentiated, and squamous. These types were relatively rare and the overall survival for patients with these histologies is approximately 30–40%.[119] Overall, the risk of extrauterine spread is as high as 62%.[119]

Creasman with the GOG demonstrated that the grade correlated directly with depth of myometrial

```
┌─────────────────────────────────────────────────────────┐
│ Corpus cancer surgical staging (FIGO 1988)              │
│                                                         │
│ IA G123    Tumor limited to endometrium                 │
│ IB G123    Invasion to < 1/2 myometrium                 │
│ IC G123    Invasion to > 1/2 myometrium                 │
│                                                         │
│ IIA G123   Endocervical glandular involvement           │
│ IIB G123   Cervical stromal invasion                    │
│                                                         │
│ IIIA G123  Tumor invades serosa or adnexa and/or positive│
│            peritoneal cytology                          │
│ IIIB G123  Vaginal metastases                           │
│ IIIC G123  Metastases to pelvic or para-aortic lymph nodes│
│                                                         │
│ IVA G123   Tumor invades bladder and/or bowel mucosa    │
│ IVB        Distant metastases, including intra-abdominal │
│            and/or inguinal lymph nodes                   │
│                                                         │
│ Histopathology – Degree of differentiation              │
│                                                         │
│ Cases should be grouped by the degree of differentiation of│
│ the adenocarcinoma:                                     │
│                                                         │
│ G1    5% ≤ of a non-squamous or non-morular solid growth│
│       pattern                                           │
│ G2    6–50% of a non-squamous or non-morular solid growth│
│       pattern                                           │
│ G3    > 50% of a non-squamous or non-morular solid growth│
│       pattern                                           │
└─────────────────────────────────────────────────────────┘
```

Figure 56.1 Corpus cancer surgical staging, (FIGO 1988)

invasion and lymphatic space invasion (both pelvic and para-aortic lymph nodes).[120] In a study of 621 patients, 42% with grade III disease had deep myometrial involvement. The current surgical staging of endometrial cancer by FIGO categorizes myometrial invasion as less than or greater than 50%. Myometrial involvement is the single most important factor which is associated with treatment failure and recurrent disease. Boronow et al and Piver et al have shown that invasion into the myometrium > 50% is related to greater extrauterine spread and recurrence.[121,122]

Grade directly correlates not only with myometrial involvement but also with nodal metastasis. Creasman et al showed that for patients with clinical stage I/II disease there were 11% (70 of 621 patients) with nodal metastasis:[120] 22/70 had metastasis to both the pelvic and para-aortic nodes and 12/70 had metastasis to the para-aortic nodes only. Cervical involvement, lymphatic space involvement, extrauterine disease, and positive peritoneal cytology were also correlated with nodal metastasis.

Observation

Patients with disease limited to the endometrium (stage IA), with either grade I or II, require no adjuvant postoperative therapy. Morrow et al analyzed 91 patients in this subset of patients, of which 72 received no additional therapy after hysterectomy.[117] There were no recurrences, with a 100% 5-year survival.

Adjuvant radiation therapy

Once the surgery and pathological evaluation has been completed, the treatment of endometrial carcinoma is variable. The treatment includes surgery, with the addition of radiotherapy and/or chemotherapy. The treatment planning is determined by the prognostic factors found on histological evaluation. Patients are determined to be low risk, intermediate risk, or high risk, based on the surgical/pathological staging and the risk of potential recurrence. The health of the patients and the co-morbidities are also a factor in treatment planning.

Low- and intermediate-risk patients

LOW RISK (< 5% risk)
Stage IA, GI and GII
No adjuvant therapy

INTERMEDIATE RISK (5–15% risk)
Stage IA, GIII
Stage IB, IC (all grades)
Stage IIA, IIB (any grade)
Adjuvant therapy (vaginal brachytherapy, whole pelvic radiotherapy)

This group of patients, although not high risk, may potentially benefit from adjuvant radiotherapy. Keys et al and the GOG performed a phase III clinical trial to study this question in surgically staged patients.[123] They randomized patients with intermediate-risk factors to surgery vs surgery + adjuvant pelvic radiotherapy to determine if there was any benefit to additional therapy. They found that the local regional recurrence rate was decreased in the radiation group but the overall survival was not affected. However, the study lacked power to conclude on survival and two-thirds of the recurrences in the non-radiated group were vaginal. This led some to conclude that vaginal cuff radiation would be as effective with less toxicity in this group of patients.

Creutzberg in the PORTEC trial also compared patients who underwent surgery alone vs surgery + adjuvant whole pelvic radiotherapy for patients with stage I disease.[124] Unlike the GOG trial where patients underwent surgical staging, the PORTEC trial did not require full staging as an entry criteria. There were 714 patients in the study and 339 received radiotherapy after surgery and 355 underwent surgery alone. It was concluded that adjuvant pelvic radiotherapy improved locoregional control but that there was not an overall survival benefit.[124]

High-risk patients

HIGH RISK (>15% risk)
  Stage IIIA, IIIB, IIIC (all grades)
  Stage IVA and IVB (all grades)
  Adjuvant therapies (whole pelvic radiotherapy + vaginal brachytherapy with or without para-aortic radiation, whole abdominal radiation, intraperitoneal P32 or chemotherapy)

Several groups have shown that their patients benefit from postoperative adjuvant therapy.[125–128] The GOG also showed that the risk of nodal metastasis increased with deep myometrial invasion, adnexal involvement, and extrauterine disease from 25%, 32%, and 51%, respectively.[117] The 5-year survival after treatment was 72% for the GOG study and 67% according to Potish et al.[128]

Therapy for the high-risk histological types is unclear; however, Kelly et al retrospectively reviewed 74 patients with papillary serous carcinoma of the uterus with stage I disease.[129] Patients were subdivided based upon residual disease in the uterus: those patients with no residual disease (stage IA) had no recurrences over 17 years, regardless of adjuvant therapy; those patients (stage 1A) treated with platinum therapy had no recurrences, whereas 43% of those with no adjuvant chemotherapy recurred. According to the authors, platinum-based chemotherapy was associated with an improved disease-free survival. Additionally, 43 patients who received vaginal cuff radiation did not recur locally, but the 31 who received no vaginal cuff radiation recurred in the vagina. It was concluded that vaginal cuff radiation improved local control.[129]

Adjuvant chemotherapy

Morrow and the GOG investigated the use of doxorubicin as adjuvant therapy in patients who have been previously surgically staged.[130] There were 181 patients with poor prognostic factors who were randomized to receive adjuvant pelvic and para-aortic radiotherapy followed by doxorubicin (92 patients) vs radiotherapy alone (89 patients). Upon review, there was no difference in the survival or recurrence rates between the two arms.

In 2000, the GOG completed a phase III trial comparing doxorubicin and cisplatin with or without paclitaxel + filgrastim in advanced endometrial carcinoma to determine if the addition of paclitaxel improved overall survival.[131] There were 129 patients randomized to doxorubicin/cisplatin and 134 randomized to the paclitaxel

arm, for a total of 263 patients. The response rate for the three-drug regimen was 57% (22% being complete responders) compared to the two-drug regimen, which was 34% (7% being complete responders). The toxicity with the three-arm regimen was higher than the two-arm regimen. Fleming et al concluded that doxorubicin/cisplatin/paclitaxel was well tolerated and had an improved response rate and survival when compared to the arm without paclitaxel.[132]

In 1993, the GOG reported a 45% response rate for patients with advanced or recurrent disease with the combination of doxorubicin and cisplatin, which was better than the 27% reported with doxorubicin alone.[133] The GOG subsequently investigated a 24-hour infusion of paclitaxel in patients with advanced endometrial carcinoma. There was a 36% response rate, with 14% complete responders. The GOG explored the addition of paclitaxel and evaluated patients with advanced and recurrent endometrial carcinoma. The addition of paclitaxel to doxorubicin and cisplatin improved response rates to 57%. The three-drug combination also improved progression-free survival and overall survival.[131] In 2004, the GOG completed a trial randomizing patients with advanced endometrial carcinoma to pelvic radiotherapy followed by cisplatin and doxorubicin vs cisplatin, doxorubicin, and paclitaxel; the results are pending.

Randall et al evaluated adjuvant chemotherapy with doxorubicin and cisplatin vs whole-abdomen radiotherapy in patients with stage III or IV disease.[134] There were 396 patients randomized: 202 patients to radiotherapy and 194 to chemotherapy. There was a statistically significant survival advantage in patients treated with chemotherapy. The 5-year overall survival was 42% for those who received chemotherapy and 38% for those randomized to radiotherapy. Additionally, there were 13% pelvic recurrences for those who received radiotherapy and 18% for those who received chemotherapy. The GOG recently completed a phase III trial that randomized patients to paclitaxel, doxorubicin, cisplatin vs paclitaxel and carboplatin; the results are still pending.

Hormonal therapy

Hormonal therapies have proven effective in the treatment of recurrent and metastatic endometrial cancer. Success has been seen with progestational agents and antiestrogens since the early 1960s when described by Kelley et al.[135] The overall response rates for progestins are approximately 25%, with a progression-free interval of approximately 4 months on average. In trials investigating tamoxifen, the response rates ranged from 0 to 53% with the higher responses being seen with higher doses.[136]

Ehrlich et al studied steroid receptors and the association with the patient's response to hormonal treatment in endometrial cancer.[137] They showed that receptor-positive tumors tended to be better differentiated with a better prognosis that correlated with improved overall survival and disease-free survival. Ayoub et al randomized patients to combination therapy with cyclophosphamide, doxorubicin, 5-fluorouracil (5-FU) along with medroxyprogesterone acetate alternating with tamoxifen.[136] This study showed a significant improvement in response rates with the addition of hormonal therapy, but that did not translate into a survival advantage.

There is currently an industry-sponsored phase II trial evaluating letrozole in the treatment of advanced and recurrent estrogen and/or progesterone receptor-positive endometrial cancer. In addition, the GOG is evaluating fulvestrant in a phase II trial in the treatment of recurrent, persistent, and metastatic endometrial cancers.

Estrogen therapy

In patients with endometrial cancers, the trials evaluating estrogen therapy were all retrospective until the completion of the GOG randomized clinical trial that evaluated estrogen replacement therapy vs placebo in patients with stage I and II endometrial cancers after surgery.[138] In this trial, there were 1236 eligible subjects for evaluation. The median follow-up time was 35.7 months. There were only 41.1% of patients who were compliant with the estrogen replacement therapy arm for the entire period of the study. For this population, the recurrence rate was 2.3%, deaths related to endometrial cancer were 0.8%, and 1.3% of patients developed a new malignancy. For the placebo arm, the recurrence rate was 1.9%, deaths related to endometrial cancer were 0.6%, and 1.6% of patients developed new malignancies.[138] It was concluded that this study could not support or refute the safety of estrogen replacement therapy in patients with endometrial cancer. The American College of Obstetrics and Gynecology states that:

> for women with a history of endometrial cancer, estrogen could be used for the same indications as for any other women, except that the selection of appropriate candidates should be based on prognostic indicators and the risk the patient is willing to accept.[139]

Non-surgical candidates

In patients with endometrial cancer who are not surgical candidates, whole pelvic radiotherapy along with intracavitary brachytherapy is an alternative treatment approach. Multiple studies have demonstrated respectable survivals with radiation treatment, especially for patients with early disease.[140] The survival rates vary from 43% to 85% with clinical stage I–II disease and from 10% to 50% with clinical stage III–IV disease.[140] However it is important to note that surgery remains the standard of care, with an improved survival rate of approximately 15–25% compared to radiotherapy alone.[140]

Biological therapy

Given the low response rates and decreased survival for advanced and recurrent endometrial cancers, biological therapies are now being investigated. The GOG is currently evaluating Trastuzumab in a phase II trial for the treatment of stage III, IV, or recurrent endometrial cancers. Other agents that are under evaluation include EGFR inhibitors, imatinib, and *Clostridium perfingens* enterotoxin.

Follow-up

Podczaski has shown that history and physical examination are the most effective tools for follow-up.[141] Generally, patients are followed every 3–4 months for the first 2 years and then every 6 months until the 5-year mark is reached. Approximately 80% of recurrences will be diagnosed on physical examination and within the first 2 years after treatment.[141] Chest X-ray helps in the detection of asymptomatic pulmonary metastases.

With the current obesity epidemic in the USA, it is likely that the incidence of endometrial cancer will continue to rise, thereby making this disease of continued importance in women's health issues in North America.

REFERENCES

1. Barakat RR. Contemporary issues in the management of endometrial cancer. Review. CA Cancer J Clin 1998; 48(5): 299–314.
2. Partridge EE, Shingleton HM, Menck HR. The National Cancer Data Base report on endometrial cancer. J Surg Oncol 1996; 61(2): 111–23.

3. Randall ME, Filiaci VL, Muss H et al. Gynecologic Oncology Group Study. Randomized phase III trial of whole-abdominal irradiation versus doxorubicin and cisplatin chemotherapy in advanced endometrial carcinoma: a Gynecologic Oncology Group Study. J Clin Oncol 2006; 24(1): 36–44.

4. Woodruff JD, Pickar JH. Incidence of endometrial hyperplasia in postmenopausal women taking conjugated estrogens (Premarin) with medroxyprogesterone acetate or conjugated estrogens alone. The Menopause Study Group. Am J Obstet Gynecol 1994; 170(5 Pt 1): 1213–23.

5. Henderson BE. The cancer question: an overview of recent epidemiologic and retrospective data. Am J Obstet Gynecol 1989; 161(6 Pt 2): 1859–64.

6. Kaaks R, Lukanova A, Kurzer MS. Obesity, endogenous hormones, and endometrial cancer risk: a synthetic review. Cancer Epidemiol Biomarkers Prev 2002; 11: 1531–43.

7. Folsom AR, Kaye SA, Potter JD, Prineas RJ. Association of incident carcinoma of the endometrium with body weight and fat distribution in older women: early findings of the Iowa Women's Health Study. Cancer Res 1989; 49(23): 6828–31.

8. Potischman N, Hoover RN, Brinton LA et al. Case-control study of endogenous steroid hormones and endometrial cancer. J Natl Cancer Inst 1996; 88(16): 1127–35.

9. Cohen I. Endometrial pathologies associated with postmenopausal tamoxifen treatment. Gynecol Oncol 2004; 94(2): 256–66.

10. Fisher B, Costantino JP, Wickerham L et al. Tamoxifen for prevention of breast cancer: report of the National Surgical Adjuvant Breast and Bowel Project P-1 Study. J Natl Cancer Inst 1998; 90: 1371–88.

11. Brinton A, Berman ML, Mortel R et al. Reproductive, menstrual, and medical risk factors for endometrial cancer: results from a case–control study. Am J Obstet Gynecol 1992; 167(5): 1317–25.

12. Parslov M, Lindegaard O, Klintorp S et al. Risk factors among young women with endometrial cancer: a Danish case-control study. Am J Obstet Gynecol 2000; 182(1): 23–9.

13. Coulam CB, Annegers JF, Kranz JS. Chronic anovulation syndrome and associated neoplasia. Obstet Gynecol 1983; 61(4): 403–7.

14. Kalandidi A, Tzonou A, Lipworth L et al. A case-control study of endometrial cancer in relation to reproductive, somatometric, and life-style variables. Oncology 1996; 53(5): 354–9.

15. Folsom AR, Anderson KE, Sweeney C, Jacobs DR. Diabetes as a risk factor for death following endometrial cancer. Gynecol Oncol 2004; 94: 740–5.

16. Lindgren AM, Nissinen AM, Tuomilehto JO, Pukkala E. Cancer pattern among hypertensive patients in North Karelia, Finland. J Hum Hypertens 2005; 19(5): 373–9.

17. Freitas-Silva M, Pereira D, Coelho C et al. Angiotensin I-converting enzyme gene insertion/deletion polymorphism and endometrial human cancer in normotensive and hypertensive women. Cancer Genet Cytogenet 2004; 155(1): 42–6.

18. Burkman RT, Collins JA, Shulman LP, Williams JK. Current perspectives on oral contraceptive use. Am J Obstet Gynecol 2001; 185(2 Suppl): S4–12.

19. Hubacher D, Grimes D, Lara-Ricalde R et al. The limited clinical usefulness of taking a history in the evaluation of women with tubal factor infertility. Fertil Steril 2004; 81(1): 6–10.

20. Dhar KK, NeedhiRajan T, Koslowski M, Woolas RP. Is levonorgestrel intrauterine system effective for treatment of early endometrial cancer? Report of four cases and review of the literature. Gynecol Oncol 2005; 97(3): 924–7.

21. Matthews CE, Xu WH, Zheng W et al. Physical activity and risk of endometrial cancer: a report from the Shanghai endometrial cancer study. Cancer Epidemiol Biomarkers Prev 2005; 14(4): 779–85.

22. Colbert LH, Lacey JV Jr, Schairer C et al. Physical activity and risk of endometrial cancer in a prospective cohort study (United States). Cancer Causes Control 2003; 14(6): 559–67.

23. Viswanathan AN, Feskanich D, De Vivo I et al. Smoking and the risk of endometrial cancer: results from the Nurses' Health Study. Int J Cancer 2005; 114(6): 996–1001.

24. Ryan AJ, Susil B, Jobling TW, Oehler MK. Endometrial cancer. Cell Tissue Res 2005; 322(1): 53–61.

25. Risinger JI, Maxwell GL, Berchuck A, Barrett JC. Promoter hypermethylation as an epigenetic component in Type I and Type II endometrial cancers. Ann NY Acad Sci 2003; 983: 208–12.

26. Bokhman JV. Two pathologic types of endometrial carcinoma. Gynecol Oncol 1983; 15(1): 7–10.

27. Kurman RJ, Kaminski PF, Norris HJ. The behavior of endometrial hyperplasia: a long-term study of "untreated" hyperplasia in 170 patients. Cancer 1985; 56: 403–12.

28. Tropé CG, Alektiar KM, Sabbatini PJ, Zaino R. Corpus: epithelial tumors. In: Hoskins WJ, Perez CA, Young RC et al, eds. Priniciples and Practice of Gynecologic Oncology. Philadelphia: Lippincott Williams & Wilkins, 2005: 825–7.

29. Montegomery BE, Daum GS, Dunton CJ. Endometrial hyperplasia: a review. Obstet Gynecol Surv 2004; 59(5): 368–78.

30. Clark TJ, Neelakantan D, Gupta JK. The management of endometrial hyperplasia: an evaluation of current practice. Eur J Obstet Gynecol 2006; 125: 259–64.

31. Wells M, Sturdee DW, Barlow DH et al. Effect on endometrium of long-term treatment with continuous combined oestrogen–progestogen replacement therapy: follow up study. BMJ 2002; 325: 239.

32. Perino A, Quartararo P, Catinella E et al. Treatment of endometrial hyperplasia with levonorgestrel releasing intrauterine devices. Acta Eur Fertil 1987; 18: 137–40.

33. Wildemeersch D, Dhont M. Treatment of non-atypical and atypical endometrial hyperplasia with a levonorgestrel-releasing intrauterine system. Am J Obstet Gynecol 2003; 188: 1297–8.

34. Trimble CL, Kauderer J, Zaino R et al. Concurrent endometrial cancer in women with a biopsy diagnosis of atypical endometrial hyperplasia. A Gynecologic Oncology Group study. Cancer 2006; 106: 812–19.

35. Kurman RJ, Norris HJ. Evaluation of criteria for distinguishing atypical endometrial hyperplasia from well-differentiated carcinoma. Cancer 1982; 49: 2547–59.

36. Randall TC, Kurman RJ. Progestin treatment of atypical hyperplasia and well-differentiated carcinoma of the endometrium in women under age 40. Obstet Gynecol 1997; 90: 434–40.

37. Anderson MC, Robboy SJ, Russell P, Morse A. Endometrial carcinoma. In: Robboy SJ, Anderson MC, Russell P, eds. Pathology of the Female Reproductive Tract. Philadelphia: Elsevier Science, 2002: 331–59.

38. Brosens JJ, Barker FG. Uterine junctional zone: function and disease. Lancet 1995; 346: 558–60.

39. Ioffe OB, Simsir A, Silverberg SG. Pathology. In: Berek JS, Hacker NF, eds. Practical Gynecologic Oncology, 4th edn. Philadelphia: Lippincott Williams & Wilkins, 2005: 196–212.

40. Hendrickson MR, Kempson RL. Ciliated carcinoma – a variant of endometrial carcinoma: a report of 10 cases. Int J Gynecol Pathol 1983; 2: 1–12.

41. Demopoulos RI, Genega E, Vamvakas E et al. Papillary carcinoma of the endometrium: morphometric predictors of survival. Int J Gynecol Pathol 1996; 15: 110–18.

42. Goff BA, Kato D, Schmidt RA et al. Uterine papillary serous carcinoma: patterns of metastatic spread. Gynecol Oncol 1994; 54: 264–8.

43. Ambros RA, Sherman ME, Zahn CM et al. Endometrial intraepithelial carcinoma: a distinctive lesion specifically

associated with tumors displaying serous differentiation. Hum Pathol 1995; 26: 1260–7.

44. Melhem MF, Tobon H. Mucinous adenocarcinoma of the endometrium: a clinicopathological review of 18 cases. Int J Gynecol Pathol 1998; 6: 347–55.

45. Ross JC, Eifel PJ, Cox RS et al. Primary mucinous adenocarcinoma of the endometrium. A clinicopathological and histochemical study. Am J Surg Pathol 1983; 7: 715–29.

46. Sherman ME, Silverberg SG. Advances in endometrial pathology. Clin Lab Med 1995; 15: 517–43.

47. Tiltman A. Mucinous carcinoma of the endometrium. Obstet Gynecol 1980; 55: 244–7.

48. Abler VM, Kjorstad KE. Clear cell carcinoma of the endometrium: a histopathological study of 97 cases. Gynecol Oncol 1991; 40: 207–17.

49. Christopherson W, Alberhasky R, Connelly P. Carcinoma of the endometrium II. Papillary adenocarcinoma: a clinicopathological study of 46 cases. Am J Clin Pathol 1982; 77: 534–40.

50. Webb GA, Lagios MD. Clear cell carcinoma of the endometrium. Am J Obstet Gynecol 1987; 156: 1486–91.

51. Lax SF, Pizer ES, Ronnett BM, Kurman RJ. Clear cell carcinoma of the endometrium is characterized by p53, Ki-67, estrogen, and progesterone receptor expression. Hum Pathol 1998; 29: 551–8.

52. Lackman FD, Craighead PS. Therapeutic dilemmas in the management of uterine papillary serous carcinoma. Curr Treat Options Oncol 2003; 4: 99–104.

53. Silverberg SG, Kurman RJ. In: Tumors of the uterine corpus and gestational trophoblastic disease. In: Atlas of Tumor Pathology, 3rd series, fascicle 3. Washington, DC: Armed Forces Institute of Pathology, 1992: 47–9.

54. Altrabulsi B, Malpica A, Deavers MT et al. Undifferentiated carcinoma of the endometrium. Am J Surg Pathol 2005; 29: 1316–21.

55. Deligdisch L, Holinka CF. Endometrial carcinoma: two distinct diseases? Cancer Detect Prev 1987; 10(3–4): 237–46.

56. Potischman N, Hoover RN, Briton LA et al. Case-control study of endogenous steroid hormones and endometrial cancer. J Natl Cancer Inst 1996; 88(16): 1127–35.

57. Kurman RJ, Kaminski PF, Norris. The behavior of endometrial hyperplasia: a long-term study or "untreated" hyperplasia in 170 patients. Cancer 1985; 56: 403–12.

58. Ryan Aj, Susil B, Jobling TW, Oehler M. Endometrial cancer. Cell Tissue Res 2005; 322: 53–61.

59. Abal M, Planaguma J, Gil-Moreno A et al. Molecular pathology of endometrial carcinoma: transcriptional signature in endometrial tumors. Histol Histopathol 2006; 21: 197–204.

60. Matias-Guiu X, Catasus L, Bussaglia E et al. Molecular pathology of endometrial hyperplasia and carcinoma. Hum Pathol 2001; 32: 569–77.

61. Aaltonen LA, Peltomaki P, Leach FS et al. Clues to the pathogenesis of familial colorectal cancer. Science 1993; 260: 812–16.

62. Ionov YM, Peinado A, Malkhosyan S et al. Ubiquitous somatic mutation in simple repeated sequences reveals a new mechanism of colonic carcinogenesis. Nature 1993; 363: 558–61.

63. Tribodeau SN, Bren G, Schaid V. Microsatellite instability in cancer of the proximal colon. Science 1993; 260: 816–19.

64. Lax SF, Kendall B, SLebos RJC, Ellenson LH. The frequency of p53, K-ras mutations, and microsatellite instability differs in uterine endometrioid and serous carcinoma: evidence of distinct molecular genetic pathways. Cancer 2000; 88: 814–24.

65. Esteller M, Levine R, Baylin SB et al. MLH1 promoter hypermethylation is associated with the microsatellite instability in sporadic endometrial carcinomas. Oncogene 1998; 17: 2413–17.

66. MacDonald ND, Salvesen HB, Ryan A et al. Molecular differences between RER+ and RER− sporadic endometrial carcinomas in a large population-based series. Int J Gynecol Cancer 2004; 14: 957–65.

67. MacWhinnie N, Monaghan H. The use of p53, PTEN, and Cerb-2 to differentiate uterine serous papillary carcinoma from endometrioid endometrial carcinoma. Int J Gynecol Cancer 2004; 14: 938–46.

68. Mutter GL, Lin M, Fitzgerald JT et al. Altered PTEN expression as a diagnostic marker for the earliest endometrial precancers. J Natl Cancer Inst 2000; 92: 924–31.

69. Steck PA, Pershouse MA, Jasser SA et al. Identification of a candidate tumor suppressor gene, MMAC1, at chromosome 10q23.3 that is mutated in multiple advanced cancers. Nat Genet 1997; 15: 356–62.

70. Levine RL, Cargile CB, Blazes MS et al. PTEN mutations and microsatellite instability in complex atypical hyperplasia, a precursor lesion to uterine endometrioid carcinoma. Cancer Res 1998; 58(15): 3254–8.

71. Risinger JI, Hayes K, Maxwell GL et al. PTEN mutation in endometrial cancers is associated with favorable clinical and pathologic characteristics. Clin Cancer Res 1998; 4(12): 3005–10.

72. Esteller M, Garcia A, Martinez-Palones JM et al. Clinicopathological significance of K-RAS point mutation and gene amplification in endometrial cancer. Eur J Cancer 1997; 33(10): 1572–7.

73. Enomoto T, Inoue M, Perantoni AO et al. K-ras activation in pre-malignant and malignant epithelial lesions of the human uterus. Cancer Res 1991; 51(19): 5308–14.

74. Inoue M. Current aspects of the carcinogenesis of the uterine endometrium. Int J Gynecol Cancer 2001; 11: 339–48.

75. Bullions LC, Levine AJ. The role of beta-catenin in cell adhesion, signal transduction, and cancer. Curr Opin Oncol 1998; 10: 81–7.

76. Tucker EL, Pignatelli M. Catenins and their associated proteins in colorectal cancer. Histol Histopathol 2000; 15: 251–30.

77. Fuckuchi T, Sakamoto M, Tsuda H et al. Beta-catenin mutation in carcinoma of the uterine endometrium. Cancer Res 1998; 58(16): 3526–8.

78. Scholten AN, Creutzberg CL, van den Broek LJ et al. Nuclear beta-catenin is a molecular feature of type I endometrial carcinoma. J Pathol 2003; 201: 460–5.

79. Moreno-Bueno G, Hardisson D, Sanchez C et al. Abnormalities of the APC/beta catenin pathway in endometrial cancer. Oncogene 2002; 21: 7981–90.

80. Schlosshauer PW, Ellenson LH, Soslow RA. Beta-catenin and E-cadherin expression patterns in high-grade endometrial carcinoma are associated with histological subtype. Mod Pathol 2002; 15: 1032–7.

81. Berchuck A, Kohler F, Marks JR et al. The p53 tumor suppressor gene is frequently altered in gynecologic cancers. Am J Obstet Gynecol 1994; 170(1): 246–52.

82. Miller C, Mohandas T, Wolf D et al. Human p53 gene localized to short arm of chromosome 17. Nature 1986; 319: 783–4.

83. Mazurek A, Pierzynski P, Kuc P et al. Evaluation of angiogenesis, p53 tissue protein expression and serum VEGF in patients with endometrial cancer. Neoplasm 2004; 51(3): 193–7.

84. Yin Y, Solomon G, Deng C, Barrett JC. Differential regulation of p21 by p53 and Rb in cellular response to oxidative stress. Mol Carcinog 1999; 24: 15–24.

85. Hollstein M, Sidransky D, Vogelstein B, Harris CC. p53 mutations in human cancers. Science 1991; 253: 49–53.

86. Kohler MF, Berchuck A, Davidoff AM et al. Overexpression and mutation of p53 in endometrial carcinoma. 1992; 52(6): 1622–7.

87. Kohler MF, Carney P, Dodge R et al. p53 overexpression in advanced-stage endometrial adenocarcinoma. Am J Obstet Gynecol 1996; 175: 1256–52.

88. Pisani AL, Barbuto DA, Chen D et al. HER-2/neu, p53, and DNA analysis as prognosticators for survival in endometrial carcinoma. Obstet Gynecol 1995; 85: 729–34.

89. Tashiro H, Isacson C, Levine R et al. p53 mutations are common in uterine serous carcinoma and occur early in their pathogenesis. Am J Pathol 1997; 150: 177–85.

90. Sherman ME, Bur ME, Kurman RJ. P53 in endometrial cancer and its putative precursors: evidence for diverse pathways of tumorigenesis. Hum Pathol 1995; 26(11): 1268–74.

91. Hetzel DJ, Wilson TO, Keeney GL et al. HER-2/neu expression: a major prognostic factor in endometrial cancer. Gynecol Oncol 1992; 47: 179–85.

92. Yamamoto T, Ikawa S, Akiyama T et al. Similarity of protein encoded by human c-erb-B-2 gene to epidermal growth factor receptor. Nature 1986; 319: 230–4.

93. Dougall WC, Qian X, Peterson NC et al. The neu-oncogene: signal transduction pathways, transformation mechanisms and evolving therapies. Oncogene 1994; 9: 2109–23.

94. Santin A. HER2/neu overexpression: has the Achilles' heel of uterine serous papillary carcinoma been exposed? Gynecol Oncol 2003; 88: 263–5.

95. Busse D, Doughty RS, Arteaga CL. HER-2/neu (erbB-2) and the cell cycle. Semin Oncol 2000; 27: 3–8.

96. Berchuck A, Rodriguez G, Kinney RB et al. Overexpression of HER-2/neu in endometrial cancer is associated with advanced stage disease. Am J Obstet Gynecol 1991; 164 (1 Pt 1); 15–21.

97. Santin A, Bellone S, Gokden M et al. Overexpression of HER-2/Neu in uterine serous papillary cancer. Clin Cancer Res 2002; 8: 1271–9.

98. Diaz-Montes TP, Ji H, Sehdev AES et al. Clinical significance of HER-2/neu overexpression in uterine serous carcinoma. Gynecol Oncol 2006; 100: 139–44.

99. Oehler MK, Rees MC, Bicknell R. Steroids and the endometrium. Curr Med Chem 2002; 7: 543–60.

100. Gielen S, Hanekamp EE, Hanifi-Moghaddam P et al. Growth and transcriptional activities of estrogen and progesterone in human endometrial cells. Int J Gynecol Cancer 2006; 16: 110–20.

101. Jazaeri AA, Nunes KJ, Dalton MS et al. Well-differentiated endometrial adenocarcinomas and poorly differentiated mixed Müllerian tumors have altered ER and PR isoform expression. Oncogene 2001; 20: 6965–9.

102. Saegusa M, Okayasu I. Changes in expression of estrogen receptors alpha and beta in relation to progesterone receptor and pS2 status in normal and malignant endometrium. Jpn J Cancer Res 2000; 915: 10–18.

103. Rose PG. Endometrial carcinoma. N Engl J Med 1996; 335(9): 640–9.

104. Zaino RJ, Satyaswaroop PG, Mortel R. The relationship of histologic and histochemical parameters to progesterone receptor status in endometrial adenocarcinoma. Gynecol Oncol 1983; 16: 196–208.

105. Creasman WT. Prognostic significance of hormone receptors in endometrial cancer. Cancer 1973; 71(Suppl): 1467–70.

106. Abukafia O, Sherer DM. Angiogenesis of the endometrium. Obstet Gynecol 1999; 94: 148–53.

107. Obermair A, Tempfer C, Wasicky R et al. Prognostic significance of tumor angiogenesis in endometrial cancer. Obstet Gynecol 1999; 93: 367–71.

108. Salvesen HB, Akslen LA. Significance of tumor-associated macrophages, endothelial growth factor and thrombospondin-1 expression for tumor angiogenesis and prognosis in endometrial carcinomas. Int J Cancer 1999; 84: 538–43.

109. Kirschner CV, Alani-Amezcua JM, Martin VG et al. Angiogenesis factor in endometrial carcinoma: a new prognostic

110. bulafia O, Triest WE, Sherer DM et al. Angiogenesis in endometrial hyperplasia and stage I endometrial carcinoma. Obstet Gynecol 1995; 86: 479–85.

111. Smith M, McCartney AJ. Occult, high-risk endometrial cancer. Gynecol Oncol 1985; 22: 154–61.

112. Walters D, Robinson D, Park RC, Patow WE. Diagnostic outpatient aspiration curettage. Obstet Gynecol 1975; 46: 160–4.

113. Grimes DA. Diagnostic office curettage; heresy no longer. Contemp Obstet Gynecol 1986; 27: 96.

114. DuBeshter B, Warshal DP, Angel C et al. Endometrial carcinoma: the relevance of cervical cytology. Obstet Gynecol 1991; 77: 458–62.

115. Trimble CL, Kauderer J, Zaino R et al. Concurrent endometrial carcinoma in women with a biopsy diagnosis of atypical endometrial hyperplasia: a Gynecologic Oncology Group study. Cancer 2006; 106(4): 812–19.

116. Stelmachow J. The role of hysteroscopy in gynecologic oncology. Gynecol Oncol 1982; 14: 392–5.

117. Morrow CP, Bundy BN, Kurman RJ, Creasman WT. Relationship between surgical–pathological risk factors and outcome in clinical stage I and II carcinoma of the endometrium: a Gynecologic Oncology Group study. Gynecol Oncol 1991; 40: 55–65.

118. Homesley HD, Boike G, Spiegel GW. Feasibility of laparoscopic management of presumed stage I endometrial carcinoma and assessment of accuracy of myoinvasion estimates by frozen section: a Gynecologic Oncology Group study. Int J Gynecol Cancer 2004; 14: 341–7.

119. Wilson TO, Podratz KC, Gaffey TA et al. Evaluation of unfavorable histologic subtypes in endometrial adenocarcinoma. Am J Obstet Gynecol 1990; 162: 418–23.

120. Creasman WT, Morrow CP, Bundy BN et al. Surgical pathologic spread patterns of endometrial cancer: a Gynecologic Oncology Group study. Cancer 1987: 60: 2035–41.

121. Boronow RC, Morrow CP, Creasman WT et al. Surgical staging in endometrial cancer: clinical pathologic findings of a prospective study. Obstet Gynecol 1984; 63: 825–32.

122. Piver MS, Hempling RE. A prospective trial of postoperative vaginal radium/cesium for grade 1–2 less than 50% myometrial invasion and pelvic radiation therapy for grade 3 or deep myometrial invasion in surgical stage I endometrial adenocarcinoma. Cancer 1990; 66: 1133–8.

123. Keys HM, Roberts JA, Brunetto VL et al. A Phase III trial of surgery with or without adjunctive external pelvic radiation therapy in intermediate risk endometrial adenocarcinoma: a Gynecologic Oncology Group Study. Gynecol Oncol 2004; 92(3): 744–51.

124. Creutzberg CL, van Putten WL, Koper PC et al. Surgery and postoperative radiotherapy versus surgery alone for patients with stage-I endometrial carcinoma: a multicentre randomized trial. PORTEC Study Group. Post Operative Radiation Therapy in Endometrial Carcinoma. Lancet 2000; 355: 1404–11.

125. Greer BE, Hamberger A. Treatment of intraperitoneal metastatic adenocarcinoma of the endometrium by whole-abdominal moving-strip technique and pelvic boost irradiation. Gynecol Oncol 1983; 16: 365–73.

126. Loeffler J, Rosen E, Niloff J et al. Whole abdominal irradiation for tumors of the uterine corpus. Cancer 1988; 61: 1332–5.

127. Martinez A, Schray M, Podratz K et al. Postoperative whole abdomino-pelvic irradiation for patients with high risk endometrial cancer. Int J Radiat Oncol Biol Phys 1989; 17: 371–7.

128. Potish RA, Twiggs LA, Adcock LL, Prem KA. Role of whole abdominal radiation therapy in the management of endometrial cancer; prognostic importance of factors indicating peritoneal metastases. Gynecol Oncol 1985; 21: 80–6.

129. Kelly MG, O'Malley DM, Hui P et al. Improved survival in surgical stage I patients with uterine papillary serous carcinoma

(UPSC) treated with adjuvant platinum-based chemotherapy. Gynecol Oncol 2005; 98: 353–9.

130. Morrow C, Bundy B, Homesley H et al. Doxorubin as an adjuvant following surgery and radiation therapy in patients with high-risk endometrial carcinoma, stage I and occult Stage II: a Gynecologic Oncology Group study. Gynecol Oncol 1990; 36: 166–71.

131. Fleming GF, Brunetto VL, Cella D et al. Phase III trial of doxorubicin plus cisplatin with or without paclitaxel plus fil-grastim in advanced endometrial carcinoma: a Gynecologic Oncology Group study. J Clin Oncol 2004; 22: 2159–66.

132. Fleming GF, Filiaci VL, Bentley RC et al. Phase III randomized trial of doxorubicin + cisplatin versus doxorubicin + 24-h pacli-taxel + filgrastim in endometrial carcinoma: a Gynecologic Oncology Group study. Ann Oncol 2004; 15: 1173–8.

133. Thigpen T, Blessing J, Homesley H et al. Phase III trial of dox-orubicin +/− cisplatin in advanced or recurrent endometrial carcinoma: a Gynecologic Oncology Group study. Proc Am Soc Clin Oncol 1993; 12: 261(Abstract 830).

134. Randall ME, Filiaci VL, Muss H et al. Randomized phase III trial of whole-abdominal irradiation versus doxorubicin and cisplatin chemotherapy in advanced endometrial carcinoma: a Gynecologic Oncology Group study. J Clin Oncol 2006; 24: 36–44.

135. Kelley RM, Baker WH. Progestational agents in the treatment of carcinoma of the endometrium. N Engl J Med 1961; 264: 216–22.

136. Ayoub J, Audet-Lapointe P, Methot Y et al. Efficacy of sequential cyclical hormonal therapy in endometrial cancer and its correlation with steroid hormone receptor status. Gynecol Oncol 1988; 31: 327–37.

137. Ehrlich CE, Young PCM, Stehman FB. Steroid receptors and clinical outcome in patients with adenocarcinoma of the endometrium. Am J Obstet Gynecol 1988; 158: 796–807.

138. Barakat RR, Bundy BN, Spirtos NM et al. Randomized dou-ble-blind trial of estrogen replacement therapy versus placebo in stage I or II endometrial cancer: a Gynecologic Oncology Group study. J Clin Oncol 2006; 24: 587–92.

139. American College of Obstetricians and Gynecologists: Estrogen Replacement Therapy Technical Bulletin. Washington, DC: American College of Obstetricians and Gynecologists, 1986.

140. Varia M, Rosenman J, Halle J et al. Primary radiation therapy for medically inoperable patients with endometrial carcinoma – stages I–II. Int J Radiat Oncol Biol Phys 1987; 13: 11–15.

141. Podczaski E, Kaminski P, Gurski K et al. Detection and pat-terns of treatment failure in 300 consecutive cases of "early" endometrial cancer after primary surgery. Gynecol Oncol 1992; 47: 323–7.

Index

N.B. Page numbers in *italic* denote figures or tables.

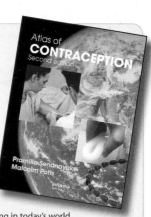